AF248909

PROGRESSIVE TYPOGRAPHERS, INC.
YORK COUNTY INDUSTRIAL PARK
P.O. BOX 1003
EMIGSVILLE, PA   17318

Immune Complexes in Clinical and Experimental Medicine

This volume is published as part of a long-standing cooperative program between Harvard University Press and the Commonwealth Fund, a philanthropic foundation, to encourage the publication of significant scholarly books in medicine and health.

Immune Complexes in Clinical and Experimental Medicine

Ralph C. Williams, Jr.

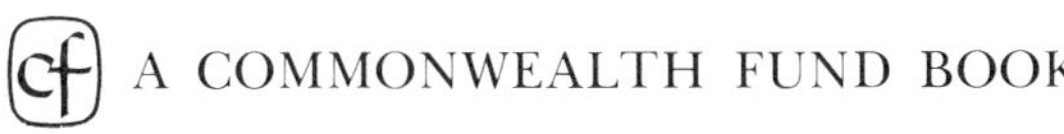 A COMMONWEALTH FUND BOOK

Harvard University Press   Cambridge, Massachusetts, and London, England   1980

Copyright © 1980 by the President and Fellows of Harvard College
All rights reserved
Printed in the United States of America

Library of Congress Cataloging in Publication Data

Williams, Ralph C   1928–
    Immune complexes in clinical and experimental medicine.

    "A Commonwealth Fund book."
    Bibliography: p.
    Includes index.
    1. Immune complexes.   2. Immune complex diseases.
I. Title. [DNLM: 1. Antigen-antibody complex.
QW570.3 W726li]
QR185.8.I45W54   616.07'9   79-21448
ISBN 0-674-44438-8

To Frank J. Dixon and Henry G. Kunkel

*who were among the first to recognize the importance of
immune complexes and who have clarified much of their
mystery*

Preface

There is today a rapidly growing mass of information relative to the physiological consequences of immune complexes. Interactions between cells, the evolution of important clinical syndromes, possibly the ultimate spread of metastatic cancer may be governed by mechanisms triggered by various types of immune complexes. Many physical and facultative effects of circulating as well as tissue-fixed immune complexes are not yet fully understood and await new approaches aimed at clarifying their behavior.

Within this volume I have attempted to assemble an overview of the subject, with the focus on areas where sufficient clinical or experimental information has accumulated to expand on what began as an explanation for some types of renal disease and is now recognized as an extremely significant aspect of the biologic response to many forms of tissue injury, infection, or neoplasia. The final importance of immune complexes in clinical medicine must still be determined; but it is now abundantly clear that immune regulation and many mechanisms of tissue destruction demand the precise understanding of this subject that will eventually be ours.

It is my hope that this book will provide a logical approach to a subject which during the past ten years has assumed more and more of a central role in the comprehension of many disease events as well as the more complex distant ripples that these disease states produce. A precise understanding of the physical, anatomic, theoretical, and practical effects of immune complexes will soon be fundamental to clear interpretation of the pathophysiology of a wide variety of diseases. I have not tried to set down a complete catalogue or encyclopedia of all diseases in which immune complexes have been implicated, but instead to present a broad view of the subject that I hope will be useful not only to the medical student or physician in training but to the practicing clinician, experimental pathologist, or basic research worker.

The first three chapters illustrate the importance of immune complexes in human bacterial, parasitic, and viral infections. Chapters 4 and 5 focus on physical and immunochemical factors, as well as host determinants, in the formation of immune complexes and their disposal in normal body homeostasis. Chapter 6 evaluates current methods used to detect immune complexes. Chapters 7 through 12 cover what is known of the role of immune complexes in a variety of specific organ sites or general disease states. Chapter 13 discusses the experimental models developed in animals for the study of immune complexes, and a brief Epilogue concludes the book.

I should like to express my deep gratitude to those who assisted in compiling this volume. I am particularly indebted to Carol Arnold, Jody Butterfield, Sophia Collaros, John Lingenfelter, Peggy Maddox, Carol Montman, Sophia Olona, Debbie Rindels, and Julie Weaks for their help with the manuscript. Sheila Foley, David McMullen, Donna Maurer, Mike Norviel, and David Tafoya assisted enormously with the illustrations and drawings, and the library staff at the Imperial Cancer Research Fund in London under Helen Flinders gave invaluable aid. I take pleasure in acknowledging the support of the Josiah Macy Foundation during a sabbatical leave in which the book was written, and the aid of the Commonwealth Fund in bringing the volume to fruition.

Contents

CHAPTER 1

Bacterial Infections

Most bacterial infections in both man and animals are associated with generation of an immune response in the host. In recent times—particularly in the immunosuppressed or immunologically compromised host—the immune response may be muted or low-key, but in general, infection by natural pathogens, potential pathogens, or relatively ubiquitous nosocomial agents engenders some kind of immunologic reaction in the host. Part of the immune response to foreign or infecting bacteria involves generation of humoral antibody. Early work on antibody response in experimental animals established that the primary or initial antibody formed may be largely IgM, whereas after the first week IgG antibody production is called forth, and as the immune response gains in momentum, IgG antibody gains ascendancy and IgM antibody declines (1–3).

Some modification of these basic principles may occur, depending largely on the types of antigen involved—protein, sugar, or protein-lipid-carbohydrate complex. Another important modulating factor is the actual antigenic load: very small doses of powerful immunogens may produce rapid but ephemeral 19 S IgM antibody responses and virtually no detectable 7 S IgG antibody. In all immune responses, whether principally 19 S IgM or 7 S IgG, memory cells are induced, which are then primed for a secondary, more prolonged IgG antibody response. As time of immunization or exposure to potential antigens increases, there is usually a marked increment in antibody-combining-site tightness of fit or avidity of IgG

antibody formed. This principle has been documented in the elegant studies of Siskind and colleagues (4–6). In addition, the level of 7 S IgG may actually regulate or monitor ongoing synthesis of antibody by the host (7, 8), through a process similar to feedback inhibition.

Some routes of immunization such as mucosal, oral, or even intrabronchial appear to be much more likely to produce an IgA or IgM antibody response than IgG. Although predominance of IgA antibody as the humoral product of mucosal immunization has been amply illustrated in studies by many groups (9–13), the totality of factors involved in determining immunoglobulin class of antibody molecules manufactured during the host response to any particular infecting bacterium is not yet clearly understood.

In bacterial infections several extenuating influences may substantially affect the humoral antibody response. First, the chemical characteristics of certain classes of antigens may predetermine a characteristic profile of humoral antibody. There is some evidence that many of the lipopolysaccharides found in a wide range of Gram-negative bacteria are particularly potent stimulators of IgM antibody. These same substances also appear to have powerful ancillary effects on the immune system—for instance in general activation of the reticuloendothelial system, direct activation of the complement pathways (14), or even in some circumstances as polyclonal B-cell activators (15).

Considerable adjuvant or antibody-enhancing activity of the lipopolysaccharides of Gram-negative bacteria has been documented in many laboratories. Digestion or partitioning off of some of the intrinsic immunologic properties of these materials was achieved by Parish and Ada (16), who showed that the immunogenic portion of *Salmonella adelaide* endotoxin could be separated from the mediating adjuvant effect by cyanogen bromide cleavage. The immunogenic fragment in this instance had a relatively low molecular weight (18,000 Daltons) compared to the whole endotoxin molecule. Another aspect that has been shown to be important in the humoral antibody response to bacterial antigens is the actual physical state of the antigen. There is now some evidence that particulate antigens, as in the case of *S. adelaide* studied by Ada and co-workers (17), preferentially stimulate an IgM response. In the same way it has been shown by others (18) that protein antigens such as thyroglobulin coated onto acrylic particles may result in a prolonged IgM antibody response, instead of inducing initial IgM antibody followed by gradually increasing IgG antibody of higher and higher avidity.

Other bacterial antigens, like the pneumococcal polysaccharides present in type III or type VIII pneumococci, are potent antigenic stimuli for the production of 7 S IgG antibody. Studies by Jaton and colleagues (19, 20) have shown that hyperimmunization of rabbits with such pneumococcal serotypes can produce monoclonal IgG antibodies with specificities against precisely defined chemical determinants on the repeating sugar linkages that make up the structure of the various pneumococcal capsular polysaccharide antigens. In addition, other selected bacterial polysaccharides (for instance, those obtained from some variant strains of group C or G streptococci) are capable of inducing formation of homogeneous monoclonal antibodies of IgG type in rabbits (21). These models for the production of monoclonal M-components in experimental animals have also been utilized to extend knowledge of the genetic control, as well as the precise combining specificities, of such responses.

Of great practical importance in studying the humoral immune response produced in infected patients is precisely how the complete immunologic apparatus of the host reacts when it encounters lipopolysaccharide released from an invading *Escherichia coli,* or when it sees the pneumococcus surrounded by its fluffy capsule of repeating sugar units. The immune response broken down into its simplest parts can be defined as essentially B-cell or humoral-antibody related, and T-cell or mediated by immunologically competent cells. Some antigens appear to require interaction between various specialized types of immunocompetent cells to promote an adequate immune reaction. Present evidence indicates that B cells are involved directly in humoral antibody formation and T cells in mediating cell-directed immune reactions. Certain bacterial antigens appear to require T-cell–B-cell interaction or intercommunication in order to produce a protective immune response, whereas others do not. Current knowledge of these processes as applied to a number of important human bacterial pathogens lags far behind understanding of host reactions to simple chemically defined haptens or to protein antigens such as bovine serum albumin, which have been studied extensively in various experimental animal models.

There are several possible pathways by which an immune reaction in an infected host may proceed. Bacterial antigen may interact with the producer of humoral antibody—the B cell—directly, or after being processed and refined by an intermediary cell such as the macrophage. The subsequent B-cell activation is then sufficient for a successful, progressive synthesis and release of humoral antibody and presumably neutralization, complement activation and opsonization, and phagocytosis with eventual elimination of the invading bacteria. Other pathogenic bacteria or bacterial antigens may require considerable B-cell–T-cell interaction for an effective immune response. Such antigens have been termed T-dependent, since they seem to require help by various soluble helping intermediary T-cell factors that act on B cells for maximal effective humoral immunity.

Clear understanding of these basic principles is important when we consider the immune response to specific infecting bacteria. It is not yet known, for instance, what complete repertoire of antigens exists in many of the important pathogens of man. Work in experimental animals has established that various pneumococcal polysaccharides are T-independent (22, 23). It is not known, however, whether other extracellular or intracellular pneumococcal antigens are T-dependent or independent. By the same token, we do not know whether the great variety of extracellular or cell-related bacterial antigens found in other common pathogens such as *Staphylococcus aureus*, β-hemolytic group A streptococci, *Klebsiella*, or even *Pseudomonas aeruginosa* are T-dependent or T-independent in evoking an immune response. In addition, it is clear that interactions between T cells and B cells in the immune response may be profoundly influenced by suppressor effects on B-cell function caused by T cells, macrophages, or other intermediary cells (24–27). Eventual complete understanding of the host response to individual bacterial pathogens must be based on a careful analysis of all of these factors, including antigenic repertoire, T-cell–B-cell interaction, knowledge of adjuvant properties of certain bacterial antigens, and the actual physical state of the key bacterial antigens involved.

Another extremely important aspect of the local tissue immune response to bacteria has recently been studied by Miller and associates (28), who showed that isolated renal cells were capable of in vitro suppression of T-cell proliferation. Such a phenomenon could obviate fundamental immunoregulatory cell processes, including T-cell support of the cell-mediated immune response. It seems likely that many local tissue factors may play an important role in the precise immune response associated with a variety of bacterial infections.

Of all sources of extrinsic antigens to which man is continually exposed, bacteria known to be associated with specific diseases have been the most elaborately characterized. Specific examples of the importance of immune complexes in determining the course or sequelae in a variety of bacterial reactions serve to illustrate the practical necessity for a clear understanding of the immune response in common clinical situations.

Subacute Bacterial Endocarditis (Infective Endocarditis)

Subacute bacterial endocarditis, recently termed infective endocarditis (IE), is a disorder associated with a low-grade, often indolent

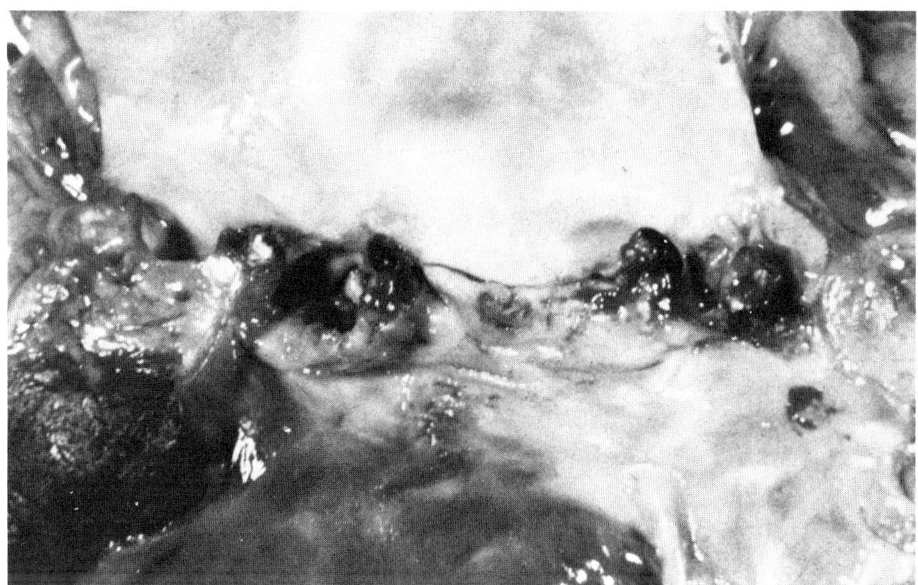

Figure 1-1 The typical gross appearance of aortic valvular vegetations seen in infective endocarditis. (Photograph courtesy of A. G. Stansfeld, St. Bartholomew's Hospital, London.)

infection in a nidus of fibrin, coagulum, and platelets within the arterial or venous circulation of the afflicted individual. Vegetations typical of this disease are shown in Figure 1-1. The most common organisms involved in this infection are represented by the α-hemolytic viridans streptococci, *Staphylococcus aureus, S. albus,* candida, or a wide variety of bacteria of low virulence or natural pathogenicity, but when entrenched as vegetations on heart valves fully capable of inducing severe disease and abundant distant sequelae.

Before the advent of antibiotics virtually all patients with IE died of cardiovascular complications as a consequence of progressive valvular dysfunction, embolic phenomena, heart

failure, or occasionally progressive renal failure (29–35). Infective endocarditis may be associated with several forms of renal injury, including segmental infarction, focal abscess formation, diffuse glomerulonephritis, or a more localized form of glomerular injury originally termed focal embolic nephritis. For many years the glomerular lesions in the kidney associated with IE were felt by most pathologists to represent microemboli from the infected heart valves; the term *focal embolic nephritis* was often used to describe these findings. Examples of these microscopic renal lesions from patients studied postmortem are shown in Figure 1-2.

Various aspects of the renal involvement recorded in some patients with IE did not fit the pathological concept of minute bacterial or fibrin emboli producing segmental glomerular lesions. First, a certain proportion of patients were shown at autopsy or by renal biopsy to have lesions more typical of an acute diffuse glomerulonephritis. Second, patients with IE

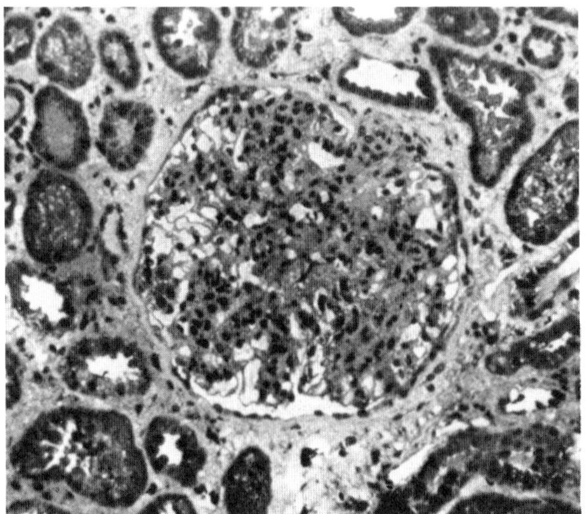

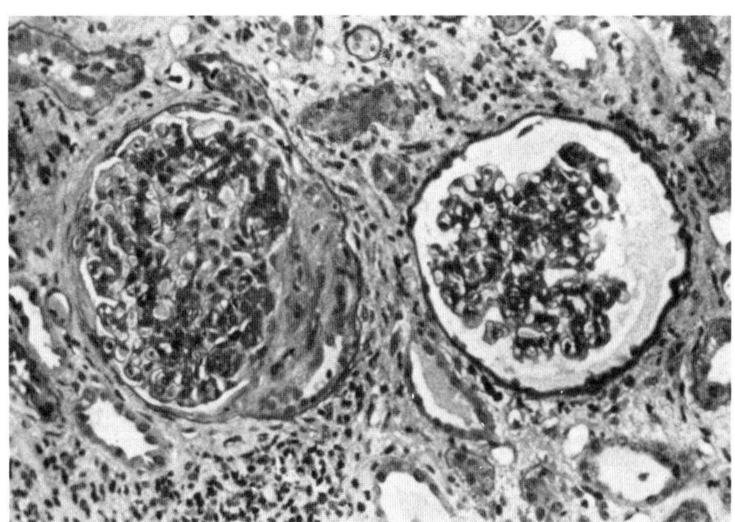

Figure 1-2 *Above,* light microscopy of renal tissue from a patient with culture-negative endocarditis showing diffuse glomerulonephritis with focal epithelial proliferation and crescent formation. *Below,* light microscopic picture of the same patient, again with culture-negative endocarditis showing diffuse glomerulonephritis with focal areas of fibrin deposition and necrosis. Magnification × 150. (Reproduced with permission, R. A. Gutman, G. E. Striker, B. C. Gilliland et al., *Medicine* 51:1, 1972.)

and the clinical or pathological picture of an acute glomerulonephritis sometimes showed vegetations only on the right side of the heart. In such instances direct embolization to the kidney through the efficient macrophage filter of the lungs seemed unlikely; however, in a series of 23 autopsied cases of right-sided IE studied by Bain and colleagues (36), renal lesions were noted in 14, and suppurative nephritis with either focal abscesses or involvement of the whole renal parenchyma was recorded in 8 patients. In this carefully studied group 3 patients were recorded with the lesion of so-called focal embolic nephritis.

Subsequently, a series of interrelated observations has provided a convincing body of evidence that the renal lesion in IE is often probably the result of glomerular deposition of circulating immune complexes. About half of a group of 51 patients with IE caused by a broad variety of organisms showed the presence of marked elevations of rheumatoid factors during the active phase of the disease (37). These anti-gamma-globulins or self-directed auto-reacting antibodies showed broad reactivity for human as well as rabbit gamma-globulin preparations. Of great interest was the finding that upon initiation of appropriate antimicrobial therapy, a striking fall and ultimate complete disappearance of rheumatoid factors were recorded in most of these subjects. An example is shown in Figure 1-3. By contrast such rapid disappearance in rheumatoid factor elevations is not generally seen in patients with positive latex fixation reactions in connective-tissue diseases such as rheumatoid arthritis. These findings suggested that the rheumatoid factors may be generated in IE as antibodies against altered autologous gamma globulins. Thus disappearance of anti-γ-globulins after the course of successful antibiotic therapy might be interpreted as evidence that removal of autologous bacterial-antigen-antibody complexes by treatment was capable of turning off the stimulus toward rheumatoid factor production. Furthermore, these observations, viewed now in perspective, indicate that an ongoing self-immunization with autologous complexes may be involved in continued rheumatoid factor production even in rheumatoid arthritis itself.

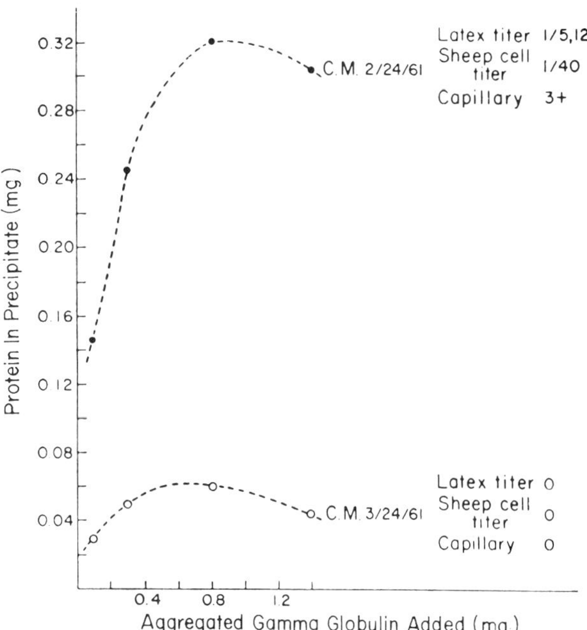

Figure 1-3 Serial changes in anti-γ-globulin activity before and after successful treatment for bacterial endocarditis. (Reproduced with permission, R. C. Williams, Jr., and H. G. Kunkel, *J. Clin. Invest.* 41: 666, 1962.)

Striking hypocomplementemia, as measured by total hemolytic complement or assay of individual complement components, has been documented in a substantial proportion of patients with acute diffuse nephritis and IE (37–39). Subsequent careful biopsy or postmortem studies of several groups of individual patients have also now provided strong evidence that glomerular immune complex deposition is fundamental to the pathogenesis of the lesion in such individuals (37–42). Pathological studies have demonstrated gamma globulin, complement components, and occasionally bacterial antigen by immunofluorescence in glomerular lesions. Moreover, a rabbit model that simulated the human disease using *Streptococcus viridans* showed that diffuse glomerulonephritis developed only in animals that had been immunized to the infecting agent prior to the experimental production of endocarditis (43). These results were of considerable interest, since they appeared to indicate that, for a diffuse proliferative glomerulonephritis to occur, immunity to infecting organisms might be necessary prior to development of IE. To our knowledge this particular point has not been reinvestigated recently in patients with IE and acute diffuse nephritis; it would of course require studies of such individuals before and after onset of the clinical disorder.

Electron microscopic studies of biopsy and autopsy material have provided additional abundant support for the concept that many of the renal lesions in IE are produced by immune complex deposition (38–40). Examples of immunofluorescence studies as well as the ultrastructural appearance of subendothelial dense glomerular deposits recorded in subjects with IE are shown in Figures 1-4 and 1-5.

Several features of the clinical situation in IE have an important bearing on other less chronic or perhaps less dramatic infections. First, in IE renal disease, renal immune-complex disposition has not been restricted or especially limited to any particular organism but has been recorded in association with a wide variety of infecting organisms, including the pneumococcus, gonococcus, *Haemophilus influenzae, Staphylococcus aureus,* and *S. albus* and microaerophilic species (37–39, 44–46). Lesions in the renal glomeruli, while tending in many instances to be localized in the mesangium as well as in a lobular distribution, are often diffuse or granular in type and often closely resemble an acute diffuse nephritis seen after group A β-hemolytic streptococcus infections. Thus, in valvular or endocardial infections by a wide variety of both Gram-positive and Gram-negative organisms, there is a common feature capable of inducing progressive renal deposition of complexes in a certain proportion of patients at risk. This is an important aspect of bacterial endocarditis, which emphasizes the fact that intravascular and particularly intraarterial infection with organisms as diverse as proteus or *S. albus* may afford an opportunity for the formation of immune complexes potentially very dangerous for the host.

An impressive parallel is presented by patients with infected intraventricular shunts. In this circumstance the causative organism is often an *S. albus* or *S. aureus* of relatively low virulence (47). Numerous examples of acute diffuse nephritis associated with such infections have now been documented (47–53). An example of the striking immune deposits associated with nephritis or nephrotic syndrome in such patients is shown in Figure 1-6. It is obvious that an infected nidus directly contiguous to the circulation provides a ready avenue for the infected patient to receive a small steady antigenic load over a prolonged period of time. Studies by several groups have indicated that the degree of bacteremia occurring in IE is remarkably constant, seldom varying over 100 organisms/ml, and more often falling in the range of 10 to 20 bacteria/ml (54, 55). Such prolonged low-dose antigenic stimulation provides an ideal opportunity for the infected individual to manufacture a steadily increasing and maximum humoral antibody response. In such a circumstance, from a theoretical standpoint, the humoral IgG antibody response would show progressive increments in antibody avidity over time. An increase in immu-

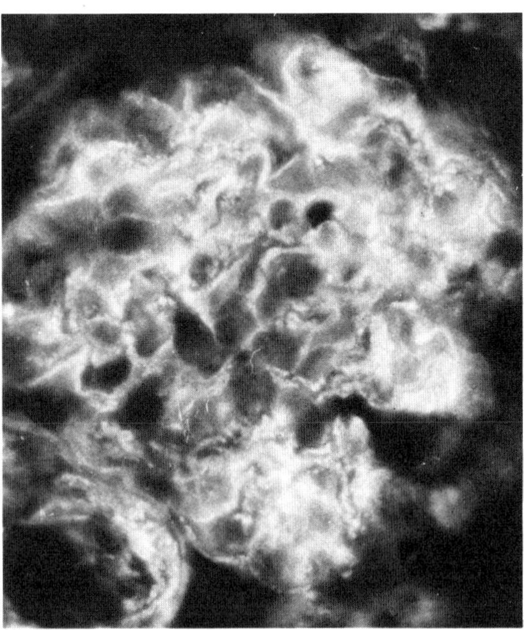

Figure 1-4   Immunofluorescence photomicrograph of IgG staining of glomeruli from the renal biopsy of a patient with infective endocarditis and renal involvement. Magnification $\times$ 122. (Photograph courtesy of Richard Hong, University of Wisconsin.)

Figure 1-5 Endocarditis with large subepithelial deposits. Electron microscopy of renal tissue from a patient with culture-negative endocarditis showing extensive subendothelial and intramembranous deposits. Magnification × 10,000. (Reproduced with permission, R. A. Gutman, G. E. Striker, B. C. Gilliland et al., *Medicine* 51:1, 1972.)

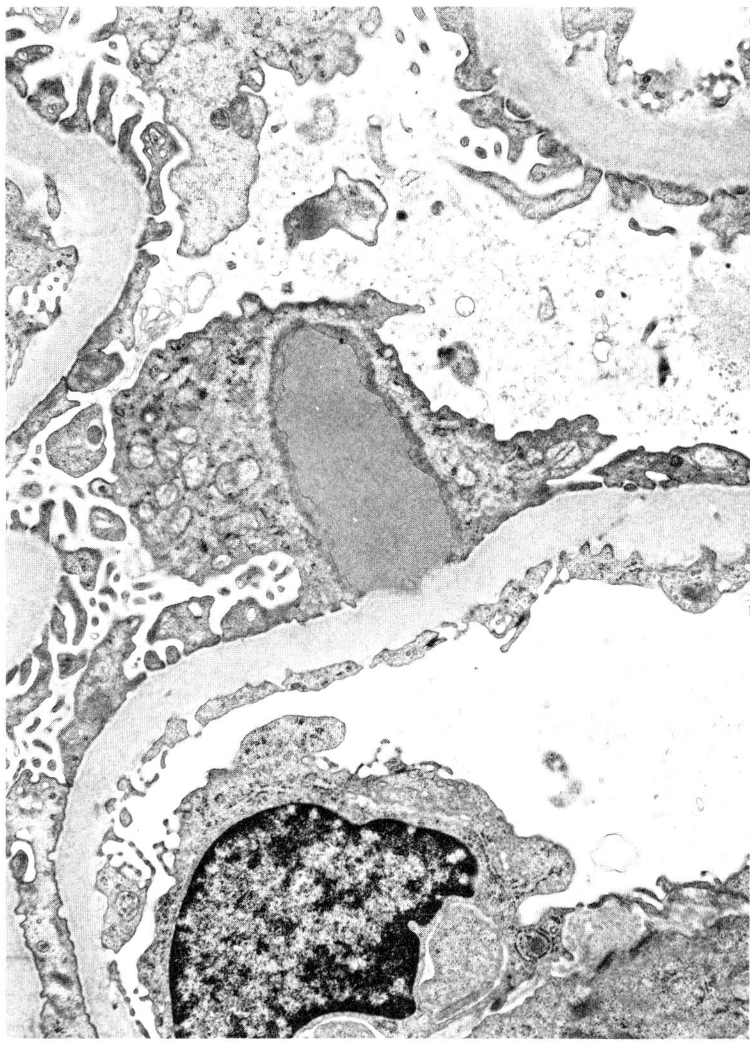

noglobulins during the course of endocarditis has been clearly documented (56–58). It is apparent from the diversity of bacterial species that have now been described in association with IE that a vast array of thymus-dependent as well as independent antigens are probably being presented to the host at risk. Since the quality and intensity of the immune response may be genetically determined and directly governed by immune-response genes (59, 60), it is clear that this aspect as well may generate considerable variability in the individual immune response.

Another feature important to a clear understanding of the relation of immune complexes to disease manifestations in both IE and shunt nephritis is related to the emerging body of knowledge now accumulating on bacterial adherence. During recent years it has become increasingly apparent that the actual stickiness or adhesiveness of individual strains of bacteria may be related to their ability to cause infections. The most convincing evidence has been provided by studies of the relative adherence of various bacteria in the case of dental caries or in IE (61, 62). Individual strains of bacteria isolated from patients with endocarditis show increased adherence or stickiness when examined in parallel with similar strains not clinically implicated in a bacterial endocarditis situation. This aspect of the general problem will require increasing attention in the future.

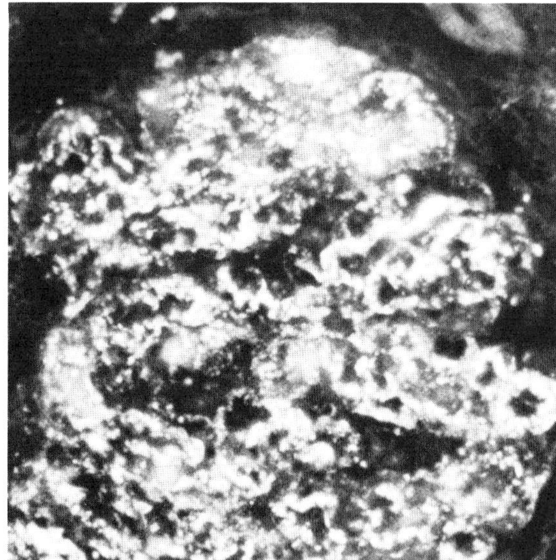

Figure 1-6 Diffuse granular deposition of properdin in the glomerulus of a patient with an infected subarachnoid-jugular shunt. Magnification × 210. (Photograph courtesy of A. F. Michael, Department of Pediatrics, University of Minnesota.)

Depending on the molecular lattice or combining ratios of antigen-antibody complexes, more or less of the potentially sticky bacterial surface or antigen might be exposed. In large complexes of Ag_2Ab_{10} or greater ratios, very little of the potentially adherent bacterial surface antigens would be available or exposed, whereas in complexes formed in low ratios of antigen to antibody (like Ag_2Ab), more potentially sticky bacterial surface antigens might be prominent. In the latter instance it is conceivable that the stickiness of antigen might then become partially responsible for the final peripheral biologic effects of such complexes.

With the availability of many parallel assay systems for the detection of antigen-antibody complexes, the original hypothesis raised concerning the presence of large quantities of circulating immune complexes in IE (37) has recently been confirmed. Reports by Bayer and associates (63) showed that 97 percent of a group of 29 patients with IE tested positive for the presence of complexes using the Raji-cell radioimmunoassay (64). Also of interest in this study were the findings of detectable elevations in circulating immune complexes in patients with right-sided IE, and decline in the quantitative levels of immune complexes in the course of successful treatment, including surgery. Notable also in this latter group of patients were extravalvular manifestations of IE —arthralgia and arthritis, splenomegaly, glomerulonephritis, and thrombocytopenia. Representative examples of serial determinations of immune complexes in patients with IE taken from the Bayer report (63) are given in Figure 1-7.

The whole question of whether peripheral manifestations of IE other than nephritis may be attributable to circulating complexes is one that has not yet been completely resolved. The early histological studies of Osler's nodes suggested intense perivascular infiltration by inflammatory cells, resembling what one might expect of an Arthus reaction where capillary or vessel wall is directly involved as the actual site of an acute antigen-antibody reaction (65, 66). More recently it has been demonstrated conclusively that etiologic bacteria often can be directly cultured or demonstrated in Gram's stains from characteristic Osler's node lesions (67, 68) where actual microabscesses in the papillary dermis may be present. Osler's nodes or emphemeral nodular lesions, usually in the skin of the hands and feet, may also be seen in typhoid fever, systemic lupus erythematosus, disseminated gonococcal infection, or marantic endocarditis (69).

This same problem of differential pathogenesis—bacterium alone or immune complex— is present in the peripheral manifestations of several important bacterial infections. In particular, one is reminded of the vasculitic skin lesions seen in some cases of gonococcal or pseudomonas sepsis. In the case of such lesions, which often resemble microinfarcts in the skin, bacteria can be demonstrated on Gram's stain; however, it is still not clear whether there are also immune complexes fixed in vivo in the lesions, which amplify the immune reaction through an acute Arthus-type reaction in small vessel walls. Most of the instances reported to date of actual microabscesses in association with Osler's node lesions have involved organisms such as *S. aureus* or candida, which are

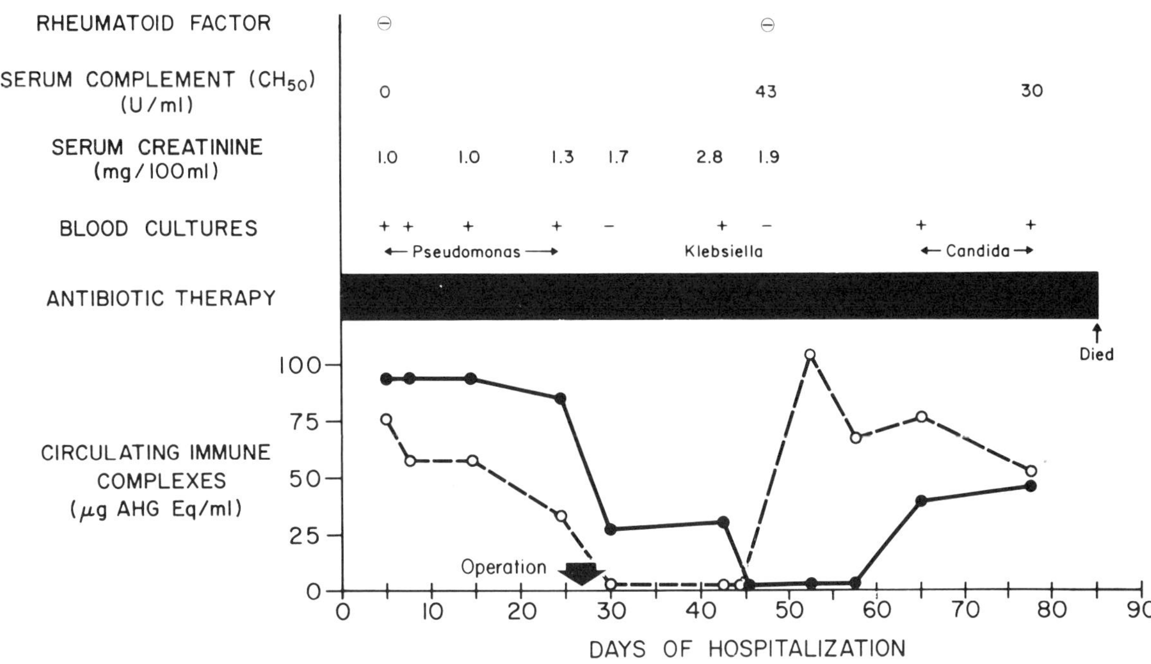

Figure 1-7 Serial studies of circulating immune complexes and other clinical parameters in a patient with infectious endocarditis. (Reproduced with permission, A. S. Bayer, A. N. Theofilopoulos, R. Eisenberg et al., *N. Engl. J. Med.* 295:1500, 1976.)

notorious for production of focal peripheral suppurative lesions in IE. Typical vasculitis lesions seen in such patients with gonococcal or pseudomonas sepsis are shown in Figures 1-8 and 1-9. The similarity of these skin lesions to those sometimes seen in association with the vasculitis of periarteritis or allergic angiitis is striking. A study of skin immunofluorescence during infective endocarditis (70) indicated that perivascular deposits of Ig and complement were often present in such patients in what appeared to be clinically normal skin, whereas control bacteremic patients without the prolonged course associated with endocarditis showed no such immune deposits. It seems clear from these and other similar observations that many of the peripheral clinical manifestations commonly associated with a variety of prolonged or particularly severe bacterial infections may be related at least in part to the local fixation of immune-complex deposits within certain tissues.

Patients with IE harbor a nidus or focus of infection, quite often with a relatively indolent and not particularly invasive or aggressive organism, and then appear to subject themselves to a subacute or chronic period of self-immunization with autologous complexes. Studies by Phair have shown that anti-γ-globulins or rheumatoid factors in sera from patients with IE often appear to show true autospecificity (71). Thus, they are best inhibited or absorbed out by autologous immune precipitates or immune complexes made from the patient's own gamma globulin and actual infecting bacterium. Recent studies by Carson and associates (72) using radioimmunoassay for both IgG and IgM rheumatoid factors have indicated that levels of these anti-γ-globulins seemed to peak later in the course of IE than did those of concurrently measured circulating complexes. The data again suggest that both IgG and IgM rheumatoid factors represent part of the host immune response to autostimulation by elevated levels of circulating immune complexes.

Since autoreactive rheumatoid factors are indeed often present and are specific or primarily directed at autologous complexes, inter-

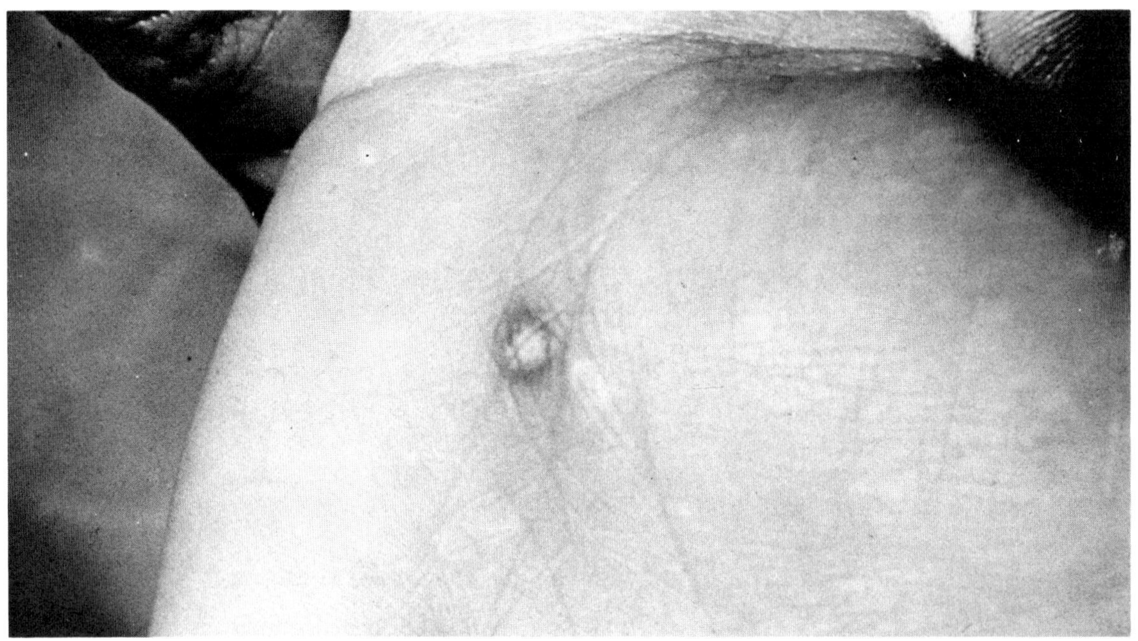

Figure 1-8 A typical circumscribed palmar lesion seen in association with gonococcal sepsis. The central purulent material in this patient yielded negative results on Gram's stain and culture.

est has centered on the possibility that they might have some physiological significance for the host. Early studies aimed at determining whether such anti-γ-globulins affected immune phagocytosis, for instance, indicated that in certain in vitro experimental systems such rheumatoid factors could block phagocytosis by interference with the binding of opsonic IgG antibody to the Fc receptor of the phagocytosing polymorph or monocyte (73). Other studies, however, appear to indicate enhancement of phagocytosis mediated by complement and rheumatoid factor (74). In the patients that I personally have studied, I have never obtained unequivocal evidence for potentiation of the immune-complex nephritis in IE by the presence of rheumatoid factor. However, in a recent large-scale survey of heterogeneous patients with a variety of renal diseases, Rossen and co-workers demonstrated what appeared to be a correlation between the degree of histological damage and the presence of tissue-bound anti-γ-globulins (75). It is not evident from the data in the Rossen study whether the method used for detecting tissue-bound rheumatoid factors was entirely comparable to

methods generally in use for detection of serum anti-γ-globulin factors. Earlier experimental evidence presented by McCormick and co-workers (76) indicated accentuation of Masugi-type nephritis in rats by passive concurrent administration of human serum or γ-globulin preparations containing rheumatoid factor activity. Thus, it is conceivable that for microvascular insults seen in areas such as the renal glomerulus or skin in IE, rheumatoid factors may intensify the basic lesions.

Potentially important to the interpretation of immune mechanisms in IE is the occurrence of so-called autoantibodies in a substantial number of patients who have been carefully studied. In addition to the presence of rheumatoid factor and immunoconglutinin (37), antinuclear antibodies and anti–smooth-muscle antibodies have been recorded in some of my own patients. One of the patients reported by Beeler and colleagues (53) actually showed a positive LE cell test as well as a low hemolytic complement level, both of which disappeared completely after successful antimicrobial treatment. Reports by Bacon and associates (77) indicated the presence of smooth-muscle anti-

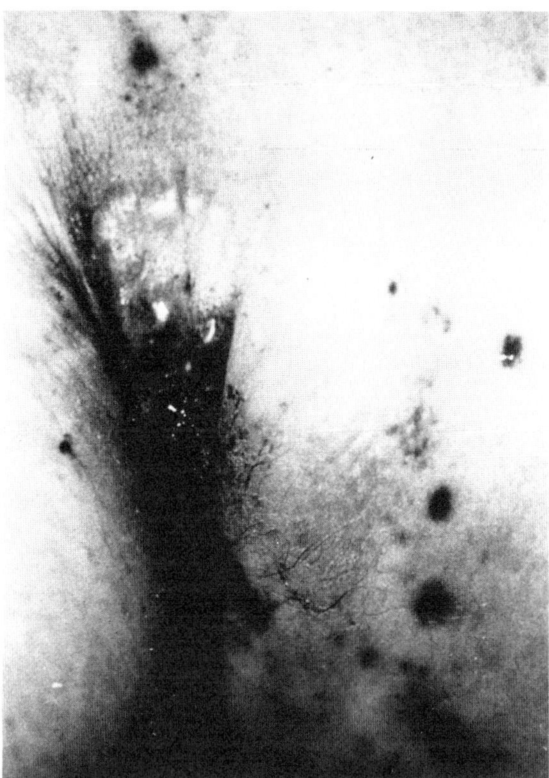

Figure 1-9 Vasculitic hemorrhagic intertriginous lesions present in a patient with pseudomonas sepsis and leukemia.

body, as well as tissue-specific antibodies directed at thyroid, skeletal muscle, or gastric parietal cells in a considerable proportion of IE patients studied. Occurrence of a variety of autoantibodies in association with a disorder presumably of known cause—namely, the infecting bacterium—should temper the opinions of those who associate the presence of autoantibody only with so-called autoimmune diseases.

Some optimism regarding the natural course of immune-complex disease in IE may be warranted because of modern approaches to treatment not available until the last few years. This is illustrated by the clinical course of a patient who was studied several years ago with severe immune-complex nephritis and uremia secondary to streptococcal endocarditis (42). The patient required dialysis support periodically for a time, but after surgery in which the damaged heart valve was replaced, enough renal reserve remained to allow virtually complete recovery. The same result was stressed by Bayer and co-workers (63), who noted a sudden disappearance of detectable circulating immune complexes in patients undergoing surgical resection of IE lesions. Thus, when the ultimate source of the immune complexes in these instances is removed by surgery, the distant lesions caused by circulating complexes may show remarkable improvement. This may be related to normal intrinsic clearing and dispersal functions of the glomerular mesangium (78) or to other processes of natural repair not yet fully understood.

A number of experimental models for the production and study of IE have been developed; these may prove extremely useful in a final clear perception of the interaction of host immune response and the particular organisms involved. It is possible to produce IE quite readily in the American opossum (*Didelphis virginiana*) using single intravenous injections of *S. viridans* or *S. aureus* (78, 79). In some instances such injections result in the production of left-sided as well as right-sided endocarditis in 100 percent of test animals. Mitral valve involvement appears to be common. The valvular lesions noted are remarkably similar to those seen in the natural disease in man. Of great interest with respect to the animal model is the fact that this particular species shows a serum electrophoretic pattern consonant with apparent marked γ-globulin deficiency. More recently, sterile endocardial platelet and fibrin vegetations induced by placement of polyethylene catheters have been used to induce an excellent model for IE (80–82). These approaches should make it possible to examine rationally the various functions of the immune system in the interactions that occur during IE.

In recent years the clinical setting in which IE is observed has changed considerably, and Watanakunakorn has pointed out quite appropriately (83) that this disease may now be regarded as a disorder sometimes resulting from medical progress. Various medical and surgical interventions are frequently found to be the precipitating factor in the actual genesis of IE. The growth of cardiac surgery and the use of prosthetic valves has made this clinical setting for IE a rather common one (84–86). These changes have also altered the types of organisms involved in the infection itself: a substantial number of patients have emerged with endocarditis caused by resistant organisms (such as candida or Gram-negative bacilli) acquired through prolonged parenteral therapy, extracorporeal devices such as the artificial kidney, the "heart-lung machine," hyperalimentation lines, or infected intravenous or arterial catheters (87–92). Thus the clinical circumstances in which IE is now frequently seen are quite different from those of 10 or 15 years ago. One of the most important aspects of this change has been the increasing proportion of patients with IE where the organisms can be clearly defined as hospital acquired (93–95). The innovations in medical practice and procedures that provide inadvertent access of bacteria or fungi to the arterial or venous circulation have altered the clinical presentation of patients currently seen with infective endocarditis. Despite these changes, the disease itself continues to present the clinician with a number of fascinating problems relating to immune interaction of the host with an established pathogen.

Marantic Endocarditis

Nonbacterial thrombotic endocarditis, or marantic endocarditis, represents an interesting but rare clinical condition that frequently simulates infective endocarditis with fever, peripheral embolic phenomena, and cardiac murmurs. It has long been associated clinically with chronic wasting disorders such as disseminated cancer (96). To date there are no reported studies concerning presence of circulating immune complexes in the sera of such individuals as identified by sensitive radioimmunoassay techniques. The valvular or endocardial vegetations in these patients are generally composed of fibrin and platelet aggregates. Since many neoplastic processes are now known to be associated with the presence of detectable circulating immune complexes, both serum and valvular lesions from patients with marantic endocardial lesions deserve immunologic study.

Pneumococcal Infection

Despite an array of effective antibiotics, the pneumococcus continues to produce an impressive morbidity and mortality in patients throughout the world. Initial studies related to natural or acquired immunity to the pneumococcus, conducted largely before the advent of antibiotics, indicated that the capsular polysaccharides are some of the most important antigens with which the host has to deal. Early work showed that immunization with specific capsular polysaccharides can prevent pneumococcal pneumonia (97, 98). The usefulness of such immunization has been reconfirmed in a number of studies using 6- and 12-valent pneumococcal capsular polysaccharide vaccines (98–100). Clear perception of the host immune response to the pneumococcus is important, since it is estimated that the current attack rate for pneumococcal pneumonia in the United States may be from 1 to 5 cases/1,000 persons per year (98), and reports of penicillin, chloramphenicol, or other antibiotic resistance have appeared (101–103). Despite the availability of effective antibiotics in the majority of instances, bacteremia develops in approximately 25 percent of all cases of pneumococcal pneumonia, with a resultant fatality of 17 to 18 percent of treated patients of all ages. The mortality in patients fifty years of age or more is over 25 percent (104). This bacterial infection still represents a serious threat, particularly when lower-numbered serotypes are involved.

As noted earlier, extensive experimental work in mice has indicated that pneumococcal polysaccharides themselves do not require T-cell help or T-cell participation in the generation of a humoral antibody immune response. These results when transposed to the clinical situation in humans are not yet clearly interpretable, since the use of capsular polysaccharide vaccines in infants under two years of age produced poor antibody responses (100). In the same study the pneumococcal vaccines showed good antibody response after two years of age. Whether this result can be interpreted as mediated by cellular mechanisms entirely unrelated to functional interactions of T helpers or T suppressors in early infancy is not yet clear. The clinical problem of pneumococcal infection in infants and children is of great practical importance, as the organism is often involved in acute otitis media. In this circumstance, when serotype-specific serum antibody was compared to that present in middle-ear fluid, the serum contained IgG and IgM antipneumococcal antibody activity whereas the ear fluid showed antibody equally distributed between immunoglobulins IgG, IgA, and IgM (105).

Studies by our group of small numbers of hospitalized persons have revealed that about 30 percent of patients with pneumococcal pneumonia showed measurable elevations of immune complexes during the first 5 to 7 days of acute illness, by either the Raji-cell radioimmunoassay or in some instances the solid-phase C1q binding technique (106). In these patients levels of complexes were well above 2 standard deviations obtained with a panel of 20 normal sera studied in parallel, but not nearly so high as those recorded in patients with infective endocarditis or systemic lupus erythematosus. There are several important aspects of the relationship between pneumococcal infection, immune complexes, and the immune system. The most important in the case of the pneumococcus is actual antigenic load. With the advent of rapid electrophoresis or electrodiffusion methods for quantifying the presence of pneumococcal antigen in cerebrospinal fluid, blood, pleural fluid, or urine, several studies have indicated a rough correlation between degree of antigenemia as measured by these techniques and mortality or morbidity (107–109).

In the study by Coonrod and Drennan (109) capsular pneumococcal polysaccharide was detected in the serum of 19 of 46 patients with pneumococcal pneumonia. Antigenemia appeared to be closely associated with bacteremia, as well as with infection by the low-numbered serotypes. Of considerable importance was the finding that even after appropriate antibiotic therapy the level of detectable pneumococcal antigen circulating in plasma declined rather slowly and could still be detected in two-thirds of the cases for 2 weeks or longer. Moreover, quantitative estimations of specific

antipneumococcal antibody indicated that circulating pneumococcal polysaccharide was associated with relative delay in the appearance of host type-specific antibody. Calculations made during this investigation showed that pneumococcal polysaccharide in the circulation was not derived solely from organisms present in the bloodstream. The studies by Frisch and colleagues (110) and Ney and Harris (111) three to four decades ago showed that pneumonia lungs removed from patients who had succumbed to pneumococcal infection contained up to 1 or 2 grams of pneumococcal polysaccharide. These early findings, together with the recent Coonrod observations, indicate that timed release of pneumococcal capsular polysaccharide can proceed in vivo long after the acute phase of the disease itself. There were, furthermore, clinical indications in the Coonrod study that antigenemia was frequently associated with a delay in resolution of the clinical disease process. In such situations it is conceivable that prolonged release of antigen could impede effective, normal clearance mechanisms by combining with and eliminating type-specific antibody.

At present it is not clear how important activation of the complement sequence is to survival of the infected host in pneumococcal infection. Studies by our group of total hemolytic complement as well as individual complement components have provided evidence for complement activation in the course of clinical pneumococcal disease (112–114). Some of this complement activation conceivably could result from direct interaction between pneumococcal cell-wall constituents and complement components, possibly without intermediate participation of specific antibody, since both pneumococcal polysaccharide and mucopeptide show potent in vitro effects in various assay systems. Another Coonrod study (115) of 25 patients with pneumococcal pneumonia showed that only 4 of these patients developed detectable levels of complement-fixing anticapsular antibody during the disease, whereas the majority showed hemagglutinating antibody activity. Most of the hemagglutinating antibody detected was sensitive to mercaptoethanol and thus probably 19S IgM.

These findings suggest that the natural antibody response in the patients studied may somehow be restricted to Ig subclasses that are inefficient in complement fixation. Similar findings have been reported previously with respect to human antibody response to the polyribophosphate capsular antigen of *Haemophilus influenzae,* type B (116), or to several other naturally occurring carbohydrates including dextran, levan, and teichoic acid (117). Thus, in pneumococcal infections the polysaccharides presented to the infected host by the pathogen may determine quality as well as subclass of immunoglobulin antibody response induced. This is interesting with respect to the whole question of the clinical or biologic significance of immune complexes generated during a number of bacterial infections.

In the small group of patients described by Rytel and associates (118) it was clear that under certain circumstances pneumococcal sepsis might be capable of directly activating the complement pathway in association with immune-complex glomerulonephritis. As is the case with many acute infections sometimes accompanied by rapid onset of intravascular coagulation, it is not yet clear what role immune complexes may play in initiation of defibrination itself.

A syndrome of rapid septic pneumococcal dissemination has also become well known in patients with previous splenectomy (119–123). The characteristic clinical features of this syndrome are rapid obtundation, shock, and death within 24 to 72 hours. One of the patients described by the Rytel group (118) fell into this category. In such circumstances Gram stains of peripheral blood buffy-coat preparations may be positive for bacteria, indicating an extremely high level of bacteremia (10^6 to 10^8 organisms/ml). This syndrome may be seen in apparently healthy, relatively normal but asplenic individuals. By the time a diagnosis has been established, many such individuals are moribund. The overwhelming sepsis syndrome in asplenic patients is frequently accompanied by leukopenia below 3,000 white blood cells per cubic millimeter of blood. Experimental study in animals has indicated that the leukopenia may result in part from granulocyte trapping in pulmonary capillaries, with granulocyte sequestration in inflammatory infiltrates or fibrin deposits within pulmonary capillaries (124). Since pneumococci do not have an abundance of extracellular toxins, they must reach relatively high levels of living organisms in the circulating blood before their constituents can activate the coagulation and complement sequence. The precise reasons for the clinical picture in asplenic patients of rapid sepsis, shock, and death, often associated with pneumococcal infection, remains incompletely understood. A number of studies have documented various immune defects in asplenic hosts; thus, clearance of certain blood-borne bacteria appears to be severely compromised (125). In some individuals there also appears to be a relative reduction in serum IgM as well as essential opsonins or leukophilic gamma globulins (126, 127). An interesting recent report attempted to assess the role of the spleen by studying the effect of splenectomy followed by autologous minced splenic tissue autotransplants on rats subsequently challenged to resist intravenous inoculation of type 25 pneumococci (128). Surprisingly, when reconstituted with autologous minced splenic tissue, such animals failed to resist the challenge. The results apparently indicate that the spleen as a whole conveys intrinsic ability to clear or modulate blood-borne pathogenic agents, such as virulent pneumococci.

These observations are of great importance in any analysis of the effects of particulate pathogenic bacteria such as pneumococci or possibly immune complexes formed between bacteria and native antibody or activated complement components in the infected host. It is not yet clear whether absence of the filtering or phagocytic function of the spleen, or perhaps loss of an effective site for trapping intermittently released boluses of immune complexes, may play an important role in the pathogenesis of the asplenic sepsis syndrome. It is also conceivable that in normal patients who have not undergone splenectomy, low levels of circulating complexes during early phases of active infection serve to mobilize important segments of the reticuloendothelial system located in the spleen (and possibly necessary for macrophage activation), outpouring of memory cells producing neutralizing or opsonic antipneumococcal antibody, or other physiologically useful acute-phase proteins. An interesting study would be careful monitoring of asplenic patients by sensitive quantitative assays for evidence of loss of control or balance in handling levels of circulating complexes. In view of the dire consequences of pneumococcal sepsis in such patients, it seems advisable that all receive prophylactic polyvalent pneumococcal vaccine (129).

Syphilis

For some time it has been known that the course of syphilis may be complicated by development of the nephrotic syndrome. In most cases recorded to date, patients have shown accompanying secondary syphilis (130–133). Careful studies by several groups have established that the nephrotic syndrome associated with secondary lues is clearly an immune-deposit disease. Granular, lumpy-bumpy immunoglobulin and complement deposits in glomeruli are accompanied by subepithelial electron-dense deposits (134, 135). In several reports distinct evidence for glomerular localization of treponemal antigen has also been furnished (136, 137), both by immunofluorescence identification of antigen using specific antisera and by elution of antitreponemal antibody from glomerular biopsy material. In all instances where precise immunochemical identification of immunoglobulin deposits has been performed, IgG has been the major Ig class present. Examples of the bright immunoglobulin fluorescence and results of elution studies performed by Gamble and Reardan (137) are shown in Figures 1-10 to 1-12.

It is of considerable interest that before the advent of effective antibiotics, when nephrosis

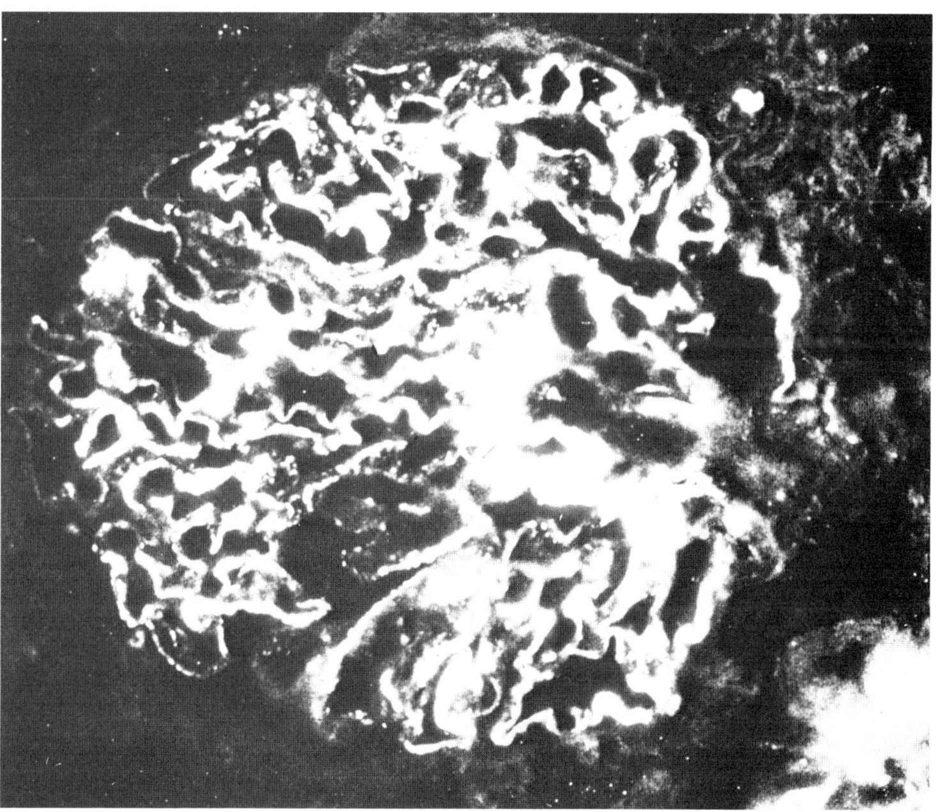

Figure 1-10 Fluorescein isothiocyanate-conjugated antihuman IgG stain, showing fine granular deposits of IgG along the glomerular capillary walls. Magnification × 285. (Reproduced with permission, C. N. Gamble and J. B. Reardan, *N. Engl. J. Med.* 292:449, 1975.)

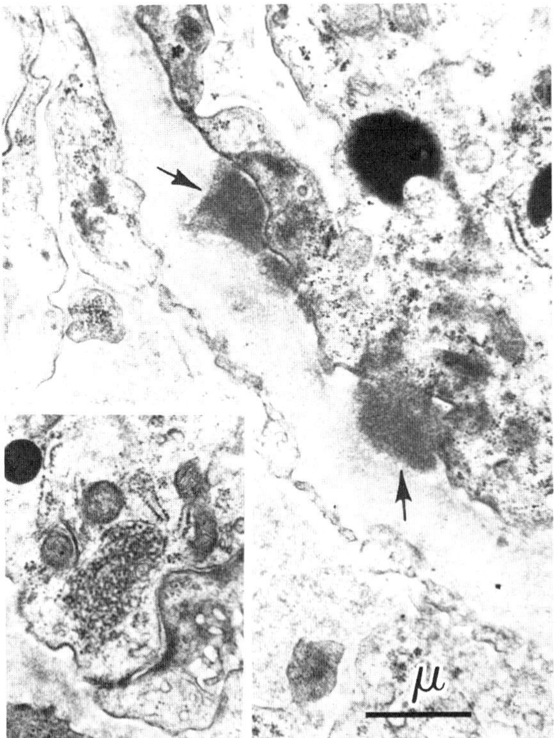

Figure 1-11 Electron micrograph of the same patient as in Figure 1-10, showing two distinct subepithelial dense deposits (*arrows*) associated with epithelial-cell foot-process fusion. The insert shows a typical tuboreticular structure of "virus-like particle" within the cytoplasm of a glomerular endothelial cell. (Reproduced with permission, C. N. Gamble and J. B. Reardan, *N. Engl. J. Med.* 292:449, 1975.)

occurred during the course of heavy-metal antisyphilitic treatment, it was regarded as a Jarisch-Herxheimer reaction localized to the kidney. In retrospect, as many of the subsequent renal-biopsy and immunofluorescence studies demonstrate, this was probably a very accurate appraisal. Studies relating changes in intravascular complement activity and antitreponemal antibody to actual Jarisch-Herxheimer reactions in 6 patients studied serially (138) indicate no pronounced interval elevation of detectable circulating immune complexes. However, depressions of total hemolytic complement, C4, C6, and C7 were observed. It was postulated that immune-complex activation of complement components was actually occurring in the extravascular compartment. This is a very important study,

since it represents one of the best documentations of in vivo antigen-antibody complex activation of complement during a severe patient reaction where quantitative estimation of circulating complexes showed no change. Also, it emphasizes the importance of the concept of potential profound clinical effects of extravascular immune-complex activation.

Studies recently conducted in our laboratory on sera from a large group of patients with both primary and secondary syphilis indicate that a considerable proportion of individuals with secondary disease (80 percent) show marked elevations well beyond normal range in circulating immune complexes by both Raji-cell and solid-phase C1q assays. Patients with primary syphilis showed a much lower incidence (25 percent) of circulating complexes. The very fact that detectable circulating complexes are present in a substantial number of patients with secondary syphilis, but that the full-blown picture of glomerulonephritis or nephrotic syndrome is relatively rare, suggests that there may be a number of host factors not yet clearly defined that modulate peripheral expression of immune-complex-mediated phenomena. In addition, it still is not clear whether the circulating complexes actually detected in patients with primary or secondary syphilis have anything to do with those that deposit in the renal glomerulus and are associated with acute or subacute glomerular injury. Definition of the immunoglobulin subclass of antibody-mediating immune-complex nephropathy, particularly in a large group of such individuals, would heighten our insight into this problem. It is conceivable that if renal biopsy were performed in conjunction with routine workup of any large series of subjects with secondary syphilis, there might be a surprising prevalence of subclinical glomerular immune-complex disease in such patients. Naturally, such a course of study would be ill advised in terms of ethical or practical considerations.

Disseminated Gonococcal Infection

Every practicing physician recognizes the marked increase seen in the United States in recent years both in gonorrheal infection

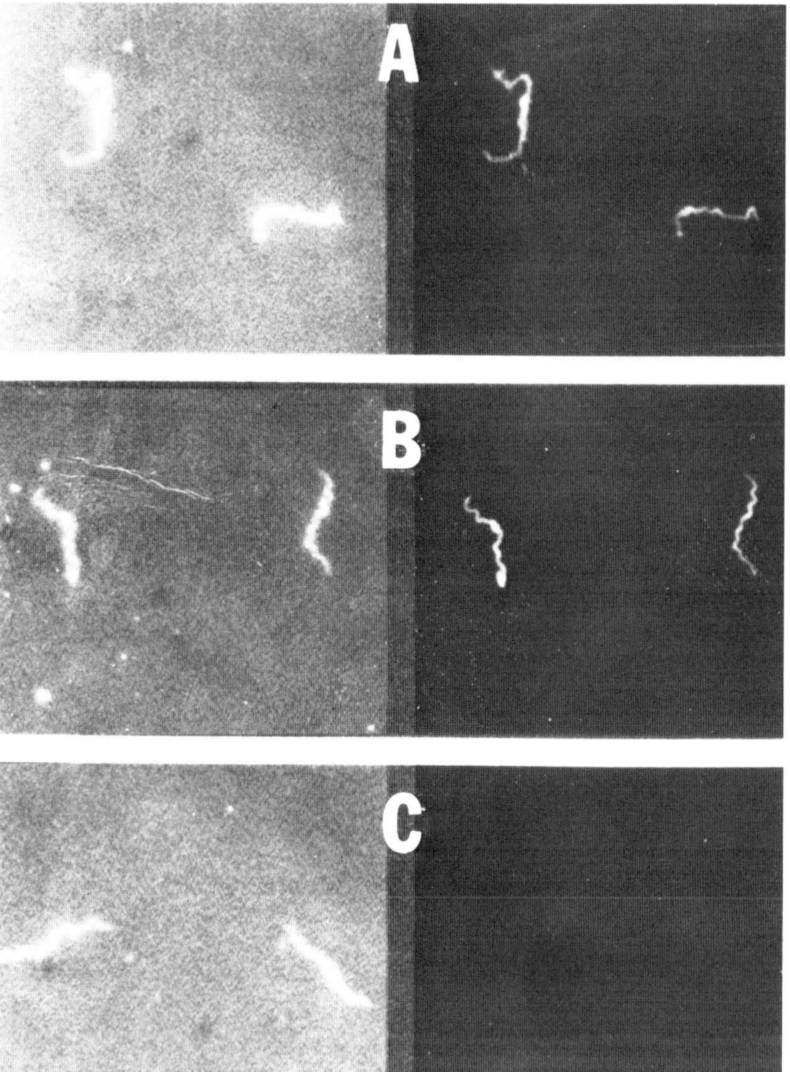

Figure 1-12 Fluorescein isothiocyanate-conjugated anti-HGG stain of *T. pallidum* substrate. Magnification × 1,045. The left-hand photographs represent tungsten dark-field examination to identify organisms; the right-hand photographs depict ultraviolet dark-field examination to define specific fluorescence. In *A* (substrate + patient's serum + anti-HGG) the positive spirochete staining on the right demonstrates the presence of antitreponemal antibody in the patient's serum. In *B* (substrate + acid citrate eluate of renal-biopsy specimen + anti-HDD) the positive spirochete staining on the right demonstrates the presence of specific antitreponemal antibody in the eluate and therefore in the glomerular immune-complex deposits. In *C* (substrate + neutral phosphate-buffered saline eluate of renal-biopsy specimen + anti-HGG) the negative spirochete staining on the right indicates that antibody was not eluted with neutral phosphate-buffered saline and that the small amount of serum present in the biopsy specimen was not responsible for the positive staining noted with the acid citrate eluate. (Reproduced with permission, C. N. Gamble and J. B. Reardan, *N. Engl. J. Med.* 292:449, 1975.)

confined to the genital tract and in its counterpart, disseminated gonorrheal infection (DGI) (139–143). The increase in patients with this disorder during the past decade has called the attention of clinicians and public health authorities to its practical importance. Many of the peripheral clinical manifestations of DGI —such as skin lesions resembling small mucopurulent infarcts, arthralgias, arthritis with synovial fluid that rarely yields positive cultures, and tenosynovitis—are similar to those seen in various connective-tissue diseases. This suggests that many of the clinical features of this illness may, as in the case of subacute bacterial endocarditis, be a peripheral manifestation of immune-complex disease. Several aspects of the clinical picture of DGI strongly suggest this possibility. Arthralgia, frank synovitis, or, more often, tendon sheath involvement are common; however, it is rare to obtain definitive bacteriologic proof of the diagnosis by synovial fluid or cutaneous lesion aspiration and direct Gram stain or culture.

Our own experience in the past eight years is that only 15 to 20 percent of synovial fluids or joint aspirations in over 50 such patients show Gram's-stain or cultural proof for the presence of *N. gonorrhoeae*. The clinical diagnosis is most often made by finding some of the characteristic microinfarcts or cutaneous lesions—often anatomically close to joints with localized synovitis (90, 91). An example of such skin lesions is shown in Figure 1-13. Fever, severe malaise, and unusual systemic complications such as pleural effusion or a perihepatitis involving Glisson's capsule and associated with mild or moderate icterus (Curtis-Fitzhugh syndrome) are also occasionally seen. The frequent synovitis without positive cultures and the skin lesions, which so often resemble microinfarcts in the fingers of patients with systemic vasculitis, have long suggested to us that a fair proportion of the systemic or peripheral manifestations of DGI may in fact be on the basis of circulating as well as tissue-fixed immune complexes. How the more unusual manifestations of perihepatitis, or even occasional urticaria (140) or pleural effusion with DGI, fit such a hypothesis is not yet clear. Experimental studies in animals (144, 145) suggest that certain types of immune complexes may show some kind of unusual physical affinity or entrapment within dense connective tissue such as tendons or cartilage. This may partially explain the frequent occurrence of tenosynovitis in the DGI syndrome.

Recent data accumulated by our group during the past two years confirm that indeed DGI is associated with a high proportion of positive reactions (76 percent) for circulating complexes during the acute illness (146). Physical studies of sera from DGI patients showing positive tests for circulating immune complexes indicated that these complexes were 19 S or

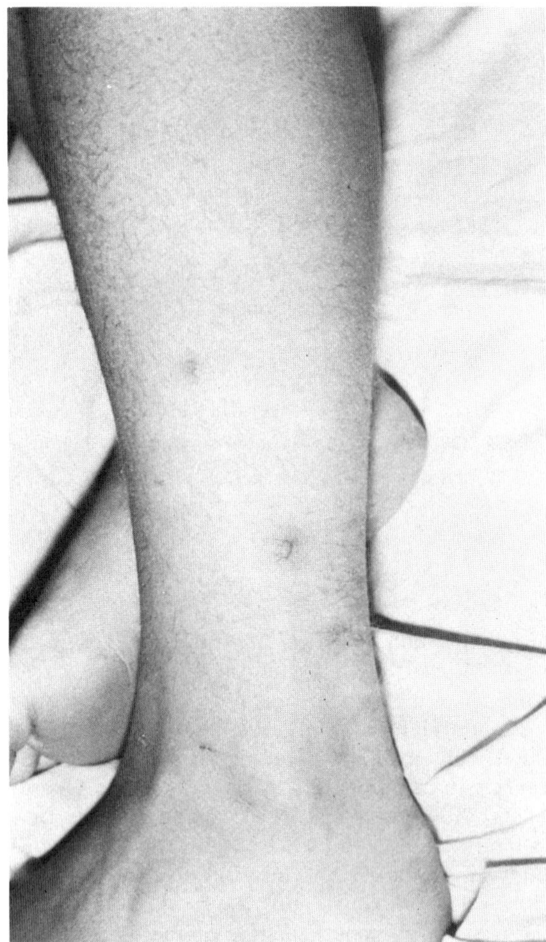

Figure 1-13   Punctate skin lesions on the leg, associated with disseminated gonococcal sepsis. The two lesions shown are located close to the ankle, which is also involved in an acute synovitis.

larger in all instances. Moreover, complement abnormalities suggestive of in vivo complement activation showed some correlation with levels of circulating complexes. Of interest was the fact that 3 of 20 control subjects studied during the acute phase of ordinary gonorrhea limited to the anogenital tract showed detectable elevations of circulating complexes as well. These findings confirm the impression we have gained in looking at many patients with heterogeneous bacterial infections, that transient moderate elevations of detectable circulating complexes are present in many common bacterial infections and are also recognized as greater in severity and quantitative amount with dissemination of the infectious process. An example of the finding of high-molecular-weight complexes in sucrose density gradient analysis of sera from DGI patients is shown in Figure 1-14.

Very little is known about host factors or elements present in the infecting bacterium that lead to DGI as opposed to gonorrhea localized to the urethra or genitourinary tract. Studies of the organisms isolated from large numbers of these patients indicate that virtually all strains isolated thus far are uniquely sensitive to penicillin but may be unusually resistant to the usual killing or bactericidal activity of serum (147, 148). Specific qualities or factors within the DGI strains that make them prone to produce disseminated infection have not yet been completely defined. A fascinating series of reports has emerged, however, which possibly implicates the complement system in the pathogenesis of DGI in some patients (149, 150). In the early reports of this association, relatively late-acting complement components (C8 and C6) were found to be either completely absent or markedly deficient functionally. In some instances such terminal complement component deficiency was not associated directly with overt infectious disease but was linked to various autoimmune disorders such as SLE (151, 152).

There is great interest in the possible association between such complement component deficiencies and the major histocompatibility region (HLA) located on chromosome 6 (153). As noted above, in most of the patients re-

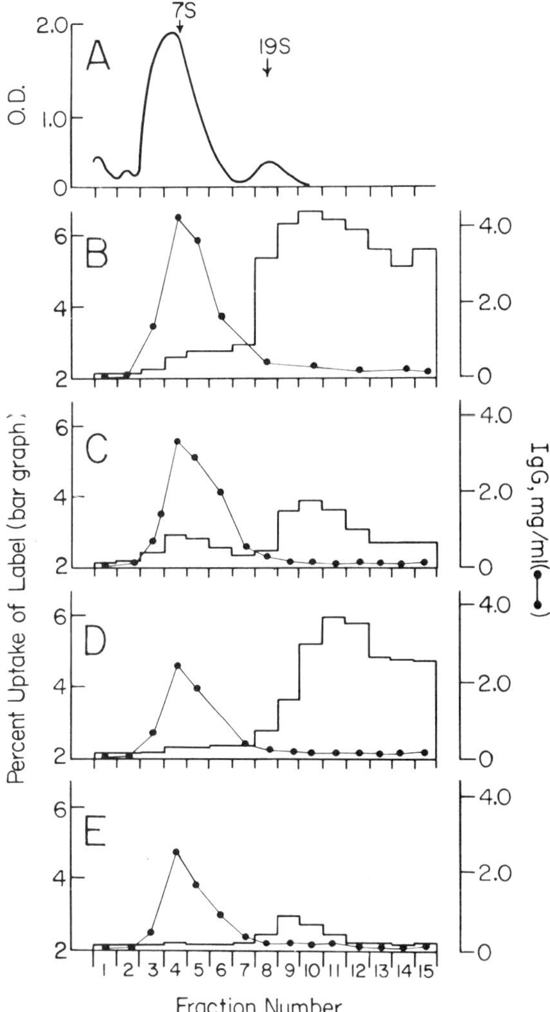

Figure 1-14 Solid-phase C1q assay for reactivity of sucrose gradient fractions obtained by ultracentrifugation of serum from 3 DGI patients and 1 normal subject: *A*, optical density (OD) pattern obtained with serum and position of 7S and 19S markers; *B*, C1qSPA positivity and IgG content of fractions of serum from patient 2; *C*, patient 1; *D*, patient 3; *E*, normal subject.

ported thus far, the defects have occurred in the terminal complement components (C6–C8). Analysis of the precise functional activity of C8 indicates that it may act primarily to effect actual terminal lysis of cell membrane, as with the membranes of bacteria (154). Of particular interest is the finding of repeated or unusually severe meningococcal as well as gonococcal infections in some patients. At present it is not clear what the terminal complement component deficiencies have to do with actual levels of circulating complexes or with the degree of bacteremia in these individuals. One could postulate that with the terminal and essential complement component (C8) missing for effective bactericidal action, antigenic mass within the infected host might increase rapidly. Although complement component C3 would undoubtedly be activated, and therefore also macrophage or other phagocytic cell receptors for activated C3d or C4 effective in reducing quantitative amounts of complexes, a functional defect in the final part of the complement sequence would allow an unusually large antigenic mass to persist in such complement-deficient patients.

Sufficient numbers of such individuals have not been studied before and after DGI or meningococcal infection, to be certain by various quantitative estimates of circulating complexes whether in fact a marked quantitative elevation in complexes does occur. This population must now be screened via sensitive immunochemical as well as functional assays for possible subtle heterozygous defects in terminal complement components. Conglutinin-like materials or ability to generate immunoconglutinin (37) should certainly be examined also in these patients. Furthermore, studies are needed to ascertain whether in fact the arthritis or arthralgia that occurs in patients with DGI may be directly correlated with detectable levels of complexes in synovial fluid at the time frank synovitis or arthritis occurs. Simultaneous serum/synovial fluid ratios to detectable immune complexes would be very helpful; to date we have not been able to obtain this sort of information from our own clinical material.

Enteric Bacterial Infections

There are scattered references in the literature to renal involvement during typhoid fever (155, 156). Indeed, Osler's textbook of medicine clearly documents the proteinuria noted in some patients during the course of the disease and attributes it to febrile proteinuria, typhoid nephritis, or posttyphoid pyelitis (157).

A report by Sitprija and colleagues (158) documents the occurrence of renal immune-complex deposition and transient proteinuria in three unselected patients with typhoid fever. Renal function in these subjects was normal, but immunofluorescence study of renal biopsies showed glomerulitis with deposition of IgG and C3, as well as Vi salmonella antigen, with specific heterologous antisera. Examples of these findings are shown in Figure 1-15*A* to *D*. A repeat renal biopsy in one patient showed rapid resolution of the mild glomerulitis and immunofluorescence findings.

The association between enteric fever, salmonella infection, and immune-complex renal disease may be correlated in certain patients with underlying schistosomal parasitic infestation, in what may be some type of mutual commensal parasitism (159–161). Farid, Higashi, and others (160, 161) have described a fascinating group of patients who show concomitant chronic *Salmonella typhi* or *S. paratyphi* enteric infection along with *S. mansoni* parasitic infestation and massive proteinuria. For therapeutic reversal of the nephrotic syndrome to take place, successful eradication of the concurrent salmonella infection appears to be essential. In some instances electron micrographs of material from these patients shows salmonella organisms in close physical contiguity to the schistosome, being actually adherent to the outer layers of the parasite (162). Whether or not an additive or combined immune response to both salmonella and schistosomal antigens is necessary for production of the type of immune complexes capable of producing immune-complex glomerular injury in this interesting syndrome is not clear. Direct demonstration of salmonella or schistosomal antigen in renal biopsies or circulating immune complexes in such patients with combined salmonella-schistosomal infections should resolve this interesting question.

Measurement of circulating immune complexes in a large group of patients studied at the Naval Medical Research Unit in Cairo, together with work of Higashi, Walker, and Tung (163), has recently indicated marked elevations of detectable circulating complexes by both solid-phase C1q and Raji-cell radioimmunoassay in the majority of a small group of such patients with salmonella enteric fevers, schistosomiasis, and nephrotic syndrome. However, parallel control observations have indicated that a considerable proportion of patients with salmonella enteric infections alone show detectable circulating complexes by the same methods.

In similar fashion we have recently completed a survey for the presence of immune complexes in the serum of children afflicted with various clinical forms of hemolytic-uremic syndrome associated with acute shigellosis in Bangladesh (164). In these children infected with Shiga-1—a particularly virulent strain of shigella—presentation in shock, hypovolemia, or with an acute leukemoid reaction is not unusual. Clinical analysis and careful pathological studies after renal biopsy or at autopsy indicate that when acute renal failure supervenes in this population of patients with shigellosis, there is no evidence by immunofluorescence of deposition of immune complexes in renal tissues. In many respects the clinical picture of acute renal failure and hypovolemic shock in children with the acute shigellosis syndrome may resemble that recognized as being associated with the dengue hemorrhagic shock syndrome where precipitous complement activation may constitute a major pathogenetic factor (165). Similar perhaps to the patients serially studied during Jarisch-Herxheimer reactions (138), important features involved in the pathogenesis of the hemolytic uremic syndrome in acute Shiga-1 syndrome, or dengue hemorrhagic shock, may be mediated by extravascular activation of complement by immune complexes fixed in tissues within the extravascular compartment. Another distinct possibility in such situations is that the bacterial lipopolysaccharides of the shiga bacillus, or even antigens related to the dengue virus itself, may conceivably be capable of direct complement activation without the mediation of any antibody at all. A number of previous experimental observations support such a mechanism (166–170).

Our own studies of children in Bangladesh with the Shiga-1 hemolytic uremic syndrome (164) have provided some fascinating data in this regard. Individual patients examined quite early in the course of the disease showed clear elevation of circulating immune complexes when fresh serum samples were assayed by two sensitive radioimmunoassay techniques (solid-phase C1q binding and Raji cell). However, parallel determinations in many patients indicated marked elevations of circulating endotoxin, presumably liberated from the acute inflammatory process within the bowel associated with the overwhelming shigellosis infection. Presence of detectable circulating immune complexes and circulating endotoxin rarely overlapped in the same patients. It appeared that the extensive and profound effects of circulating endotoxemia were more closely related to fatal outcome in such patients than actual quantitative estimations of circulating immune-complex material. This is a crucial point, since none of the patients studied at autopsy showed evidence for immune-complex deposition within the renal parenchyma or glomeruli. It thus appeared that when the host was presented with two potentially noxious reactants during a rapidly progressive and often fatal enteric infection—namely, potent Gram-negative bacterial lipopolysaccharide endotoxin and circulating immune complexes —the most telling effects in terms of a fatal outcome appeared to be related to the profound biologic effects of the endotoxin rather than those associated with immune-complex deposition. The very fact that simultaneous presence of high levels of circulating endotoxin and complexes was rarely seen is in itself of great interest.

A number of past studies in experimental animals have emphasized the apparent adjuvant effect of lipopolysaccharides from Gram-negative bacteria. Such materials appear to be capable of markedly increasing the functional activity of the reticuloendothelial system. This may explain in part why circulating complexes per se were rarely detected when serum endotoxin levels were elevated. It seems possible that endotoxin was able to help clear circulating complexes during the acute clinical phase of the disease. This general problem is significant in a number of other human disease states such as ulcerative colitis or inflammatory bowel

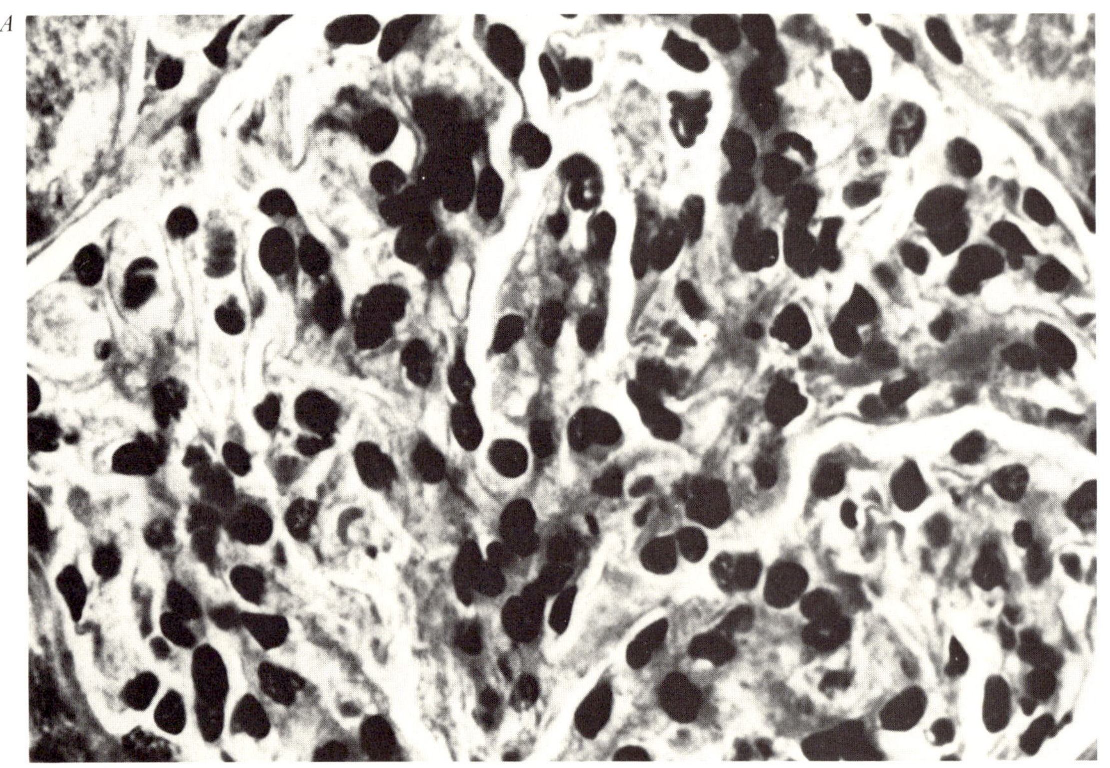

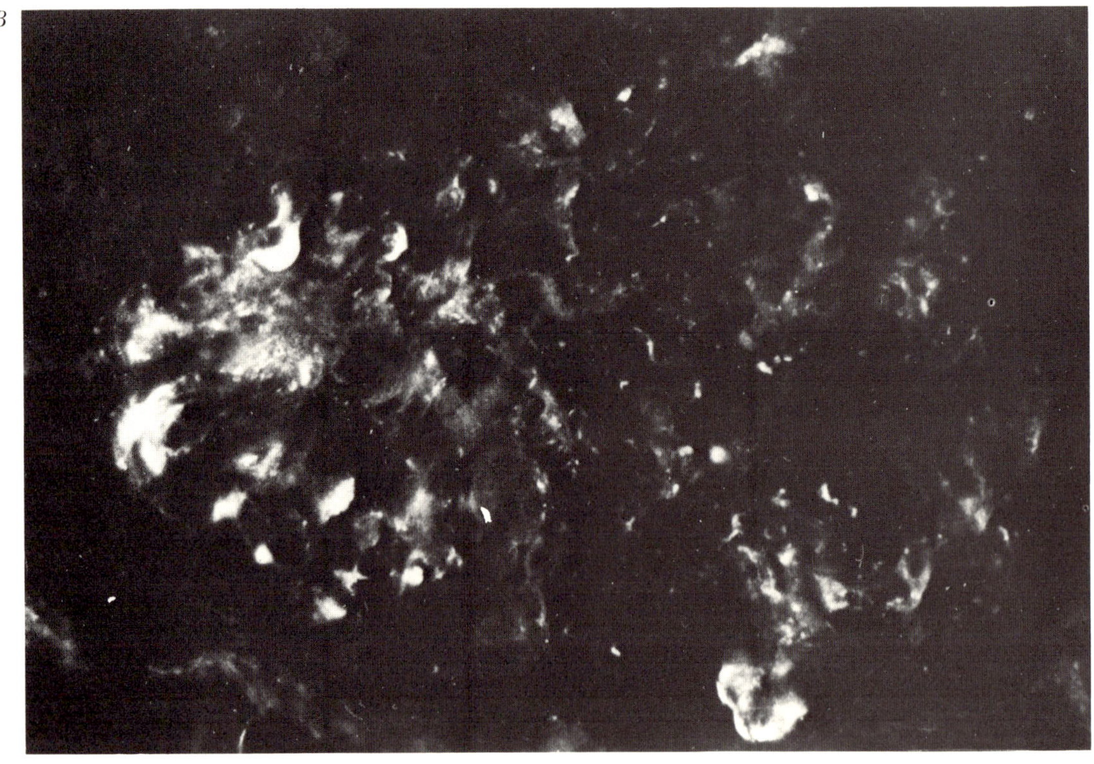

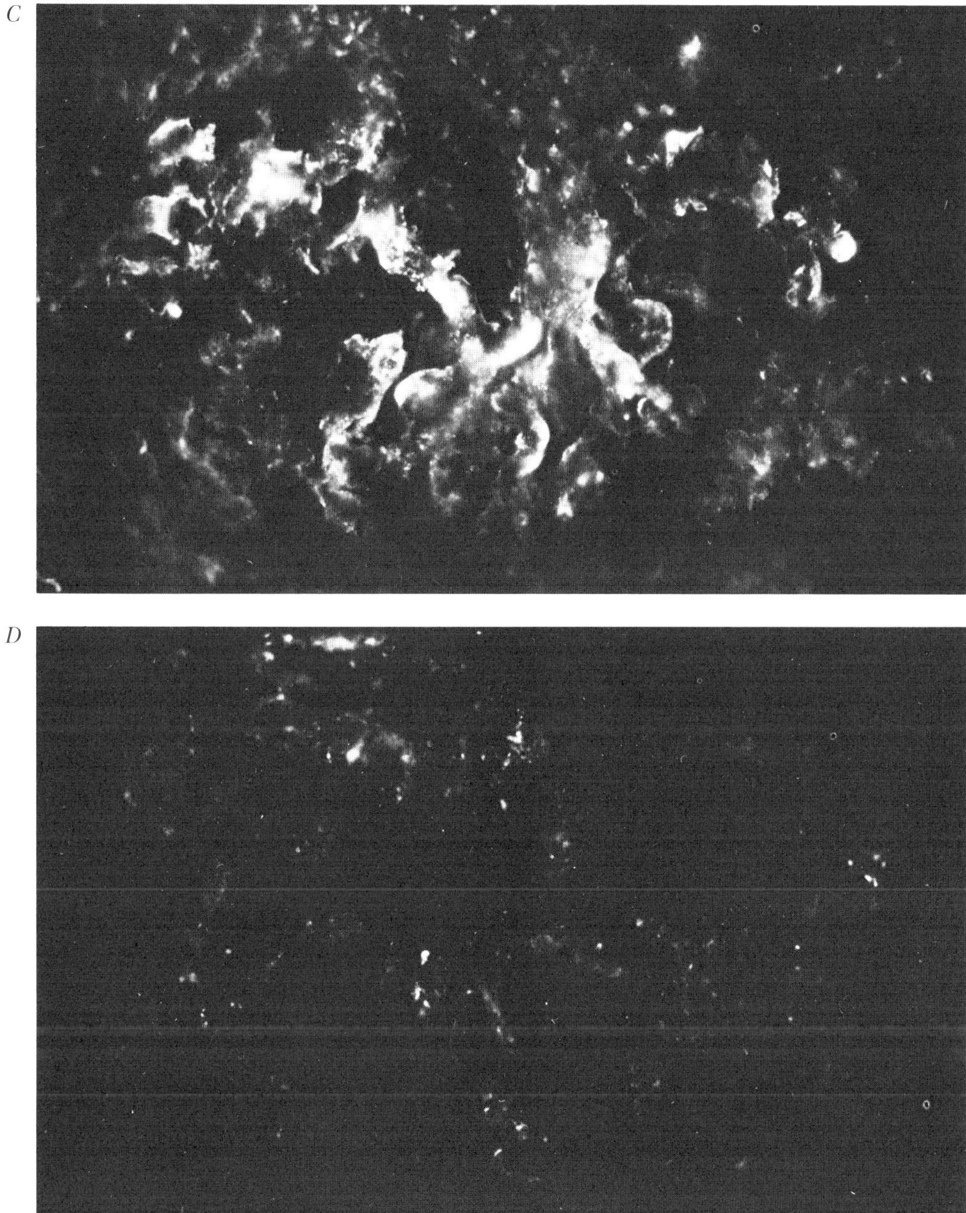

Figure 1-15 *A*, renal biopsy sample from a patient with glomerulitis and typhoid fever, showing enlargement of the glomerulus with proliferation of mesangial cells. *B*, a glomerulus from the same biopsy showing fine granular deposition of C3 in some mesangial areas. *C*, a glomerulus from the same patient, showing fine granular deposition of human IgM gamma globulin in the mesangial areas and capillary wall. *D*, granular deposition of salmonella Vi antigen along with glomerular capillary wall. All photos, magnification × 252. (Reproduced with permission, V. Sitprija, V. Pipantanagul, V. Boonpucknavig et al., *Ann. Intern. Med.* 81:210, 1974.)

disease, where circulating immune complexes have been implicated in pathogenesis of part of the central disease process itself as well as with distant peripheral manifestations such as iritis or arthritis (171–175).

Leprosy

Next to bacterial endocarditis, leprosy has perhaps the greatest fascination among bacterial infections, for those interested in the interplay between the immune system of the host and the infecting agent. Leprosy itself varies between the clearly lepromatous, deep-seated, indolent, but progressive infection of skin, nerves, and parenchymatous tissue on the one hand to the tuberculoid variety characterized by patches of sensory skin loss, nerve involvement, and a more scattered, less deeply invasive course. Typical lepromatous disease is usually accompanied by a tremendous host antigenic load, with literally billions of acid-fast bacilli in the tissues. An example of extensive lepromatous skin and soft-tissue involvement is shown in Figure 1-16. In this form of the disorder the lepromin or Mitsuda skin test, which serves as a parameter of delayed-type hypersensitivity, is generally negative. On the other hand, in the tuberculoid form of the disease bacteria are more sparsely distributed in the tissues and the lepromin skin test is usually positive. There are intermediate forms of the disease, which form a spectrum between the complete and opposite poles of lepromatous (LL) and tuberculoid (TT). These have been defined in the widely recognized classification scheme of Ridley and Jopling (176).

During lepromatous disease in some patients an acute flare of disease activity and hyperacute patient response is seen; this is termed *erythema nodosum leprosum* (ENL). This phase of the disease is accompanied by extensive erythema nodosum lesions, high fever, proteinuria, and acute systemic toxicity. Some parts of the ENL clinical picture are quite similar to those present in serum sickness or the experimental Arthus reaction (177, 178). In some instances tissue deposits of immunoglobulins and C3 as well as mycobacterial antigens have been recorded by immunofluorescence in ENL lesions

(179). Several reports have presented evidence for the presence of detectable circulating immune complexes in the serum of patients with leprosy, primarily through use of C1q binding methods (180–183). Strong evidence for presence of both circulating complexes as well as extravascular complement activation has recently been presented (183). In these studies quantitative levels of C3d were compared with C1q binding activity, and no direct correlation was found to exist. Levels of C3d were measured to differentiate the increased synthetic rate of the parent C3 molecule masking hypercatabolism. Principles important to such an analysis are illustrated diagrammatically in Figure 1-17.

Compared to the findings of other groups (182, 183), our own studies related to leprosy (184) have not revealed as high an incidence of complexes detectable either by C1q binding or Raji-cell assay. Quantitative levels of complexes

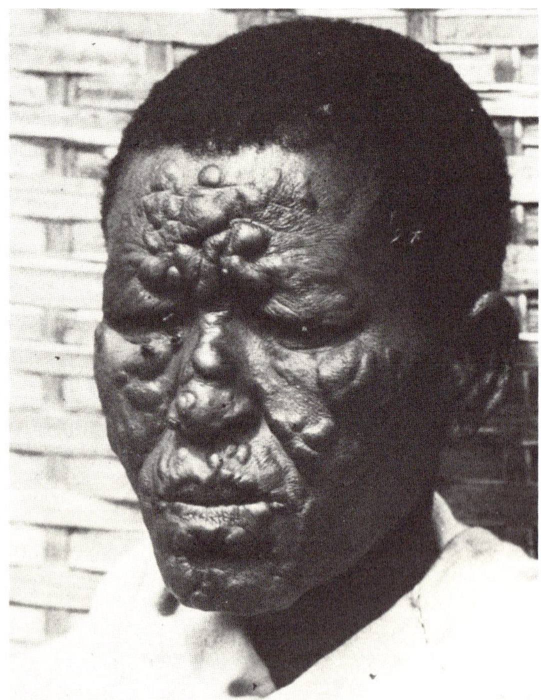

Figure 1-16 Typical lepromatous leprosy involving the facial folds and producing the classical leonine facies. (Photograph courtesy of Göran Kronvall and R. St.C. Barnetson.)

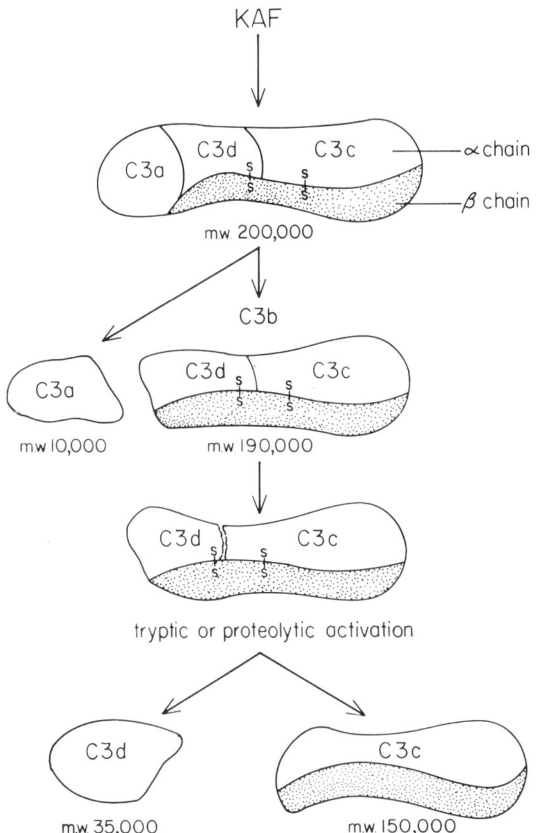

Figure 1-17 Activation of C3, resulting in fragmentation of the native molecule into C3b and C3a; C3b is then cleaved by C3b inactivator into C3c and C3d. KAF refers to conglutinin activating factor. Quantitation of C3d can be performed by a two-step procedure, which utilizes initial C3 and C3c precipitation with polyethylene glycol and subsequent single radial diffusion quantitation using anti-C3d antiserum.

in serum samples were elevated in some patients but not nearly so high as those simultaneously recorded in sera from patients with SLE (184). It is our feeling that if complexes play a basic role in the pathogenesis of disease manifestations such as ENL, they probably do so by activation of various inflammatory mechanisms outside the vascular compartment.

In some cases of leprosy peripheral manifestations of immune complexes may pervade the actual clinical presentation of the patient and initial confusion with a connective-tissue disease is possible. A patient with lepromatous leprosy presenting with polyarthritis, myositis, and actual immune-complex glomerulonephritis was described by Iveson and associates (185). Multisystem involvement and muscle tenderness raised the possibility of a diffuse vasculitis or periarteritis nodosa, and subsequent muscle biopsy and identification of *Mycobacterium leprae* on Ziehl-Neelsen staining established the real diagnosis. Granular staining of glomeruli for both IgG and IgM, as well as the presence of a mixed cryoglobulin in the serum, were also recorded in this patient.

Autoantibodies in Infections

The presence of various serum autoantibodies, particularly in lepromatous leprosy, has been recognized for some time. Lupus cell tests, tests for antinuclear and antithyroid antibody, and rheumatoid factors all may be positive. These findings appear to parallel those in other chronic bacterial infections where heavy antigenic load accompanies long duration of disease. A representative list of some of the autoantibodies recorded thus far is shown in Table 1-1.

It is well known that autoantibody formation may be present in a broad variety of other human infections, including a number of viral infections, and also in association with a number of parasitic diseases (192). Several reasons may be postulated to explain this particular association, but all will have to satisfy the observed facts—namely, that most of the autoantibodies thus far described represent a variety of antigens localized within cells. Thus a mechanism must be invoked that not only explains their occurrence in a wide variety of infectious disorders, but also elucidates why such apparently self-directed factors pick out antigens often sequestered within cellular confines. The prime exception to this general rule, of course, is the situation encountered with rheumatoid factors, which apparently are capable of reacting with native or partially altered autologous immunoglobulins.

One of the most attractive explanations, advanced by Grabar (193), relates to the teleological hypothesis that autoantibodies probably serve a scavenger function and aid in disposal

Table 1-1 Bacterial infections associated with production of autoantibody.

Bacterial infection	Type of autoantibody	Reference
Syphilis	Rheumatoid factor	Peltier and Christian (186)
Lepromatous leprosy	Rheumatoid factor	Cathcart et al. (187)
	Antinuclear antibody	Petchclai et al.
	Antithyroglobulin antibody	(188)
	Antibodies to testicular germinal cells	Wall et al. (189)
Tuberculosis	Rheumatoid factor	Singer et al. (190)
	Antinuclear antibody	Seligmann et al. (191)
Subacute bacterial endocarditis	Rheumatoid factor	Williams et al. (37)
	Antinuclear antibody	Bacon et al. (77)
	Anti–smooth muscle	
	Anti–parietal cell	

or metabolism of tissue components that are undergoing normal involutional damage or disposal. This hypothesis has a great deal of appeal from several standpoints and may eventually explain many of the observed phenomena. Worthy of particular note are the types of antigens thus far implicated in autoantibody formation after bacterial, viral, or parasitic infection: among these are nuclear and DNA antigens, smooth-muscle antibody-reactive antigens, thyroid microsomal or thyroglobulin antigens, and various cytoplasmic antigens such as Sm or RNA protein, or antigens localized within mitochondria. The intracellular localization of many of these suggests that during the infectious process an immune response, perhaps related to autologous tissue damage, occurs. The antigens are then exposed to the immunologic machinery involved in an immune reaction in such a way as to initiate reactivity. An attractive explanation in the past has been to ascribe this reactivity to intrinsic tissue damage and extrusion of intracellular materials through autolysis or destruction of cell confines. This may in fact be reasonable in the case of anti-DNA or antinuclear antibodies in association with disorders such as leprosy, where massive chronic tissue damage occurs constantly. Moreover, the documentation now being marshaled for the presence of significant

quantities of circulating or fixed immune complexes in diseases such as infective endocarditis, malaria, or leprosy would make it seem likely that such complexes themselves could serve as the original immunogen to initiate rheumatoid factor production.

However, a second and more attractive hypothesis, related to what are called polyclonal B-cell activators, has recently been presented by several groups (194–198). It has been shown that a variety of bacterial as well as other antigens related to mycoplasmae or other organisms such as PPD (199) or malarial parasites (198) are capable of induction of a polyclonal antibody response in experimental animals. Also included among these polyclonal B-cell activators are the lipopolysaccharides (LPS) of *E. coli*. These polyclonal activators are capable of inducing synthesis of antibodies directed at self determinants (15, 195–197). The mechanism involved presupposes that tolerance or central lack of response to self-antigens is a fundamental property of T cells, but that unresponsiveness to thymus-dependent antigens in B cells is mediated only by blockage of the Ig receptors and not by inactivation or elimination of self-reactive B cells. Thus, under the influence of a variety of different bacterial, mycoplasmal, viral, or parasitic polyclonal B-cell activators, self-reactive B lymphocytes are induced to divide and proliferate, thereby producing immunoglobulin products directed against autologous antigens.

This sort of explanation is attractive in explaining the triggering of autoantibody production during infections where the infectious agents themselves may contain polyclonal B-cell activators (including mycobacteria such as *M. leprae* or *M. tuberculosis* as well as a variety of bacterial and parasitic antigens). A recent report, moreover, suggests that mitogens derived from *Nocardia* may also act as polyclonal B-cell activators (200). In vitro experiments with both normal and NZB mice emphasize that a population of self-reacting B lymphocytes is present in such animals, which can under proper conditions be activated to produce autoreactive antibodies to polyriboadenylic acid as well as to nucleic acids (201). The whole concept of self-reactive lymphocytes potentially being present among the normal population is one of great interest. In the work by Bankhurst and colleagues (202, 203) all normal people tested showed a low but significant level of antigen-binding cells capable of binding two potential autoantigens—native DNA and thyroglobulin. Incidental activation of these self-reactive antigen-binding cells may be a primary feature of some autoimmune diseases such as SLE, and it could conceivably be driven by the ongoing presence of something like a polyclonal B-cell activator, with subsequent intrinsic loss of control mechanisms.

Meningococcal Infections

Infection with the meningococcus has always been a much-feared clinical event. Symptoms progress rapidly, and a significant proportion of patients present with a fulminating illness and in vivo evidence for various manifestations of microvascular injury, including purpuric rash, adrenal hemorrhage, or renal cortical necrosis. A number of the clinical manifestations of meningococcal sepsis may be related to immune-complex–mediated phenomena. An example of a typical purpuric skin lesion seen with this disorder is shown in Figure 1-18.

Several studies have emphasized the potential importance of circulating complexes in pa-

tients with meningococcal disease (204–206). More than five years ago studies by Greenwood and co-workers (206) provided direct evidence for tissue immune-complex deposition by means of immunofluorescence techniques. Patients with meningococcal sepsis were studied serially for levels of both circulating meningococcal antigen and antibody with relation to the various clinical manifestations of their disease. An example of these findings is shown in Figure 1-19. As detectable circulating antigen fell, the clinical features of skin lesions and arthritis with episcleritis became evident. Moreover, studies of synovial fluid leukocytes showed globular deposits staining for IgM, IgG, C3, and meningococcal antigen within both mononuclear and polymorphonuclear cells from such fluids. Direct examination of skin lesions from the same patients also showed IgM, C3, and meningococcal antigen immune-complex deposits. These studies provided evidence for in vivo tissue deposition of elements of immune complexes during meningococcal sepsis. Of great interest was the fact that attempts to isolate immune complexes from serum at the time that cutaneous lesions

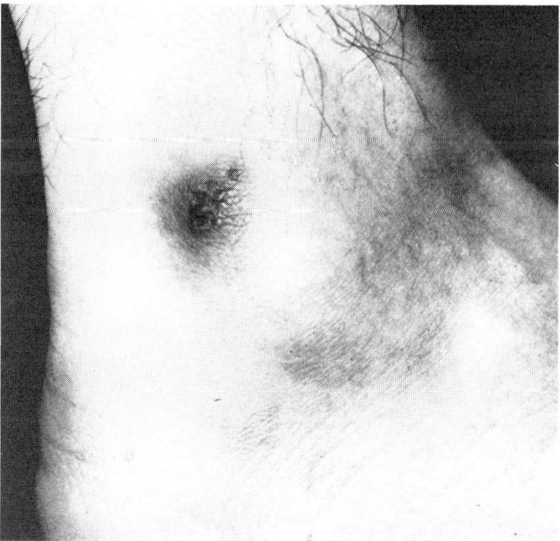

Figure 1-18 Purpuric skin lesion noted in a twenty-one-year-old man with meningococcal sepsis and sudden onset of headache, stiff neck, and obtundation. Spinal fluid examined at the time of hospitalization showed 12 white cells, the majority of which were lymphocytes.

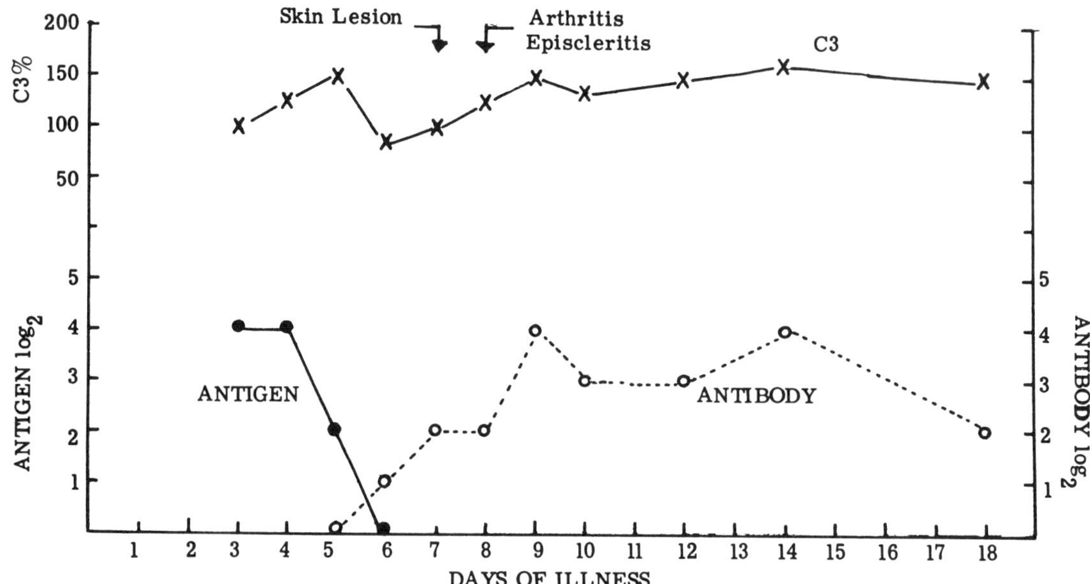

Figure 1-19 Serial estimations of meningococcal antigen (●—●), antibody (○ · · · ○), and C3 (×—×) in a patient with meningococcal sepsis, and their relation to the appearance of arthritis and cuta- neous vascular lesions. (Reproduced with permis- sion, B. M. Greenwood, H. C. Whittle, and A. D. M. Bryceson, *Br. Med. J.* 2:737, 1973.)

or arthritis were first detected resulted in no clear evidence for detection of circulating meningococcal antigen, using gel filtration to obtain macroglobulin high-molecular-weight serum fractions, dissociation of the latter at acid pH, and countercurrent electrophoresis (206).

Our group has recently encountered similar difficulty in detecting gonococcal antigen within similar serum fractions from patients with gonococcemia and concurrently positive tests for circulating immune complexes. This is an important practical problem and may be in- terpreted in several ways. First, although serum fractions positive for immune com- plexes may indeed contain antigen derived from the parent infecting organism (meningo- coccus or gonococcus), the antigen portion of the immune complex may be obscured by ex- cess antibody. This interpretation may apply to antigen-antibody complexes composed of high ratios of antibody to antigen ($Ag_2\ Ab_{10}$). Sec- ondly, direct identification of bacterial antigen within circulating immune complexes may depend on having the correct heterologous an- tibody specificity. Thus the antisera raised in other species against well-defined meningococ-

cal or gonococcal antigens may recognize anti- genic determinants that are not physically in- tact or complete in the state in which they are combined with autologous antibody in vivo. Fi- nally, there is a distinct possibility that in cer- tain situations where clear evidence for circu- lating immune complexes is present—at least with a number of the sensitive immunochemi- cal or radioimmunoassay procedures currently available—the materials giving positive reac- tions for antigen-antibody complexes may in fact contain *no* extrinsic bacterial antigen at all. In such instances the complexes may be derived from antibody originally directed at determinants on the infecting bacterium to- gether with autologous anti-idiotypic antibody itself. This question must remain open until a number of more sophisticated approaches to precise antigen identification within putative complexes in a number of well-defined human disease states have been fully explored.

Miscellaneous Bacterial Infections

A number of other serious bacterial infections of man may also be directly or indirectly linked to immune complex phenomena. In some instances, however, the evidence supporting such a link is still tenuous or poorly defined. Among the most prominent types of infections, which recently have assumed more and more practical importance for the practicing physician, are those caused by pseudomonas organisms, particularly *Pseudomonas aeruginosa*. With the advent of modern chemotherapy and immunosuppression, particularly in leukopenic patients, infections caused by this group of organisms have become a major clinical therapeutic problem. Pseudomonas infections have also long been recognized as the most prominent invader in seriously burned patients (207, 208). The recovery of pseudomonas organisms on culture from burned patients increases progressively with time after the burn injury. In the absence of topical antimicrobial therapy, by the end of the third week, 70 percent of burn wounds are colonized by pseudomonas species (209).

The pseudomonas group of organisms is considerably different from many of the other bacterial pathogens discussed above, in that its virulence appears to depend on a wide variety of extracellular toxins and other substances that contribute to pathogenicity. Considerable progress has been achieved in attempts to identify and understand the effects of these extracellular toxic products. Among the best characterized are the pseudomonas exotoxins, which produce a shock syndrome in experimental animals quite distinct from that induced by the endotoxins of Gram-negative organisms. Purified pseudomonas exotoxin inhibits protein synthesis both in vivo and in vitro (209, 210). The toxin acts at the molecular level by blocking the activity of mammalian elongation factor 2 (211, 212). Studies by Pollack and associates (213) indicate that the exotoxin may actually produce an immune response during natural infections. Other humoral antibodies that may play a part in resistance to pseudomonas infection have been identified as IgG and IgM opsonins capable of facilitating ingestion and killing of organisms by phagocytic cells such as monocytes or polymorphonuclear leukocytes (214, 215).

The clinical problems encountered in leukopenic or burned patients have recently been approached in a number of ways, including granulocyte transfusions, immunization with heptavalent lipopolysaccharide preparations, or the use of other antigen preparations (216). There is no clear body of present evidence to support an important pathogenic role for circulating or tissue-fixed immune complexes in the various syndromes associated with pseudomonas infections. A recent review of 75 patients with *P. aeruginosa* bacteremia (217) indicated that this complication appears to be most common in the sixth to eighth decades of life. About a third of the patients in this series had concomitant neoplastic disease, and the remainder showed complex medical-surgical problems. All of the 20 patients autopsied showed pseudomonas bronchopneumonia.

Patients with cystic fibrosis show repeated life-threatening infections often caused by pseudomonas species (218). These patients often demonstrate an impressive array of precipitating serum antibodies to various pseudomonas-derived bacterial antigens. In addition, studies of sputum show IgA, IgG, and IgM antipseudomonas antibody demonstrable by immunofluorescence in most cystic fibrosis patients (219), which suggests that immunoglobulins sufficient for opsonization and preparation for phagocytosis are present in sputum and tracheobronchial secretions. There is, however, fragmentary evidence that impairment of cell-mediated immune responses may be defective in cystic fibrosis. Lymphocyte responsiveness to *P. aeruginosa*, for instance, was noted to be impaired in advanced disease (220). In cystic fibrosis patients with chronic respiratory tract colonization with pseudomonas species, most of the elements necessary for apparent immune-complex–mediated disposal of the organisms appear to be present; however, the patients repeatedly sustain life-threatening infections. Clearly there must be other, possibly nonimmune, control processes that are defective in such patients. To date there are few published studies to relate immune-complex–mediated reactions to pseudomonas infection.

Haemophilus infections pose an important clinical problem, particularly during infancy and early childhood. The introduction of rapid, specific methods that employ variations on the general countercurrent immunoelectrophoresis techniques have markedly improved early diagnosis and treatment of bacterial meningitis in infants caused by *Haemophilus influenzae* type b infections (221–224). There is little in the way of direct evidence yet that such infections are mediated by immune-complex phenomena.

A number of other important bacterial infections will not be discussed in detail here, since there are still very few data that relate the occurrence of local or circulating immune complexes to pathogenesis of various disease manifestations. The role of group A streptococcal infections in the pathogenesis of acute glomerulonephritis and acute rheumatic fever is dealt with in Chapters 7 and 12.

Bilateral Symmetrical Gangrene

One of the most dramatic complications of acute bacterial infection is seen in patients with bilateral symmetrical gangrene, usually associated with staphylococcal or mixed anaerobic streptococcal and staphylococcal infection (225–227). As yet there is no clear understanding of the initiating events and various pathogenetic mechanisms that lead to the development of this clinical syndrome. Examples of the dramatic presentation sometimes seen are shown in Figure 1-20. The patient shown had no evidence for the conventional profile of intravascular coagulation. Initial radial diffusion measurements of C3 and C4 were markedly depressed, suggesting intense in vivo complement activation. The disease picture was associated initially with a staphylococcal-streptococcal cellulitis. The dramatic clinical manifestations of this syndrome, known as *purpura fulminans,* can be explained in several ways. Certain strains of the Gram-positive organisms usually implicated in this disorder may produce particularly potent extracellular products, which initiate the vasculitic process in terminal digits, ears, or extremities. It is also possible that massive release of circulating immune complexes may somehow be involved in pathogenesis, particularly since the organisms implicated represent relatively common types toward which the average normal subject must show some baseline humoral antibody. Such a

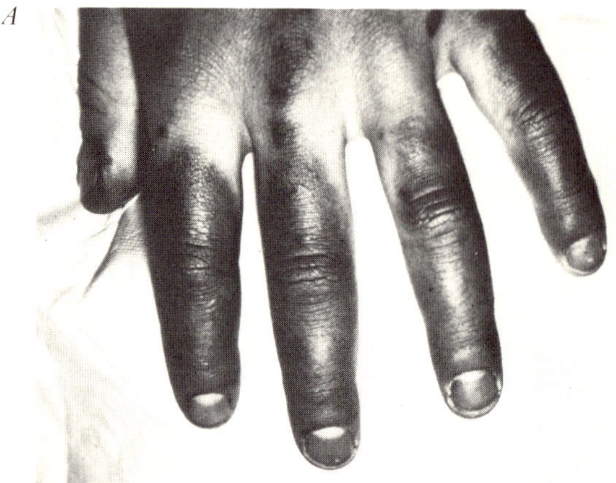

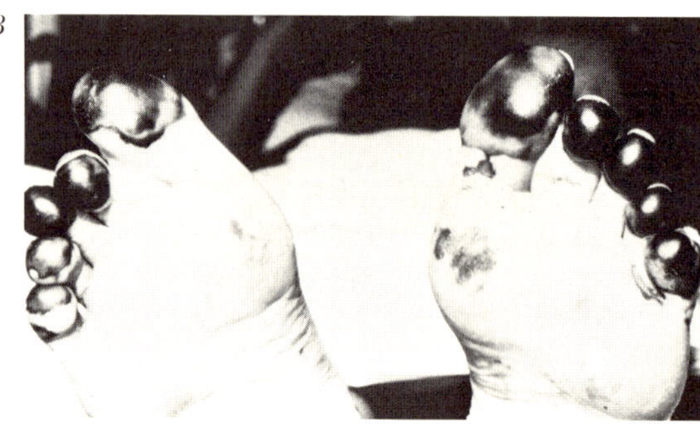

Figure 1-20 Bilateral symmetrical gangrene in the hands (*A*) and feet (*B*) of a twenty-nine-year-old man with combined staphylococcal and streptococcal cellulitis and sepsis, accompanied by subsequent development of acrocyanosis progressing to gangrene. (Photographs courtesy of George Matula, San Francisco.)

possibility is at present based only on speculation; there are no published data to support such a hypothesis. Patients with severe or overwhelming sepsis who present with bilateral symmetrical gangrene or *purpura fulminans* are often profoundly ill, hypotensive, and moribund. The extensive necrotic or rapidly progressive terminal extremity changes are similar to those seen in the Schwartzman reaction.

To date, the precise pathogenesis of this clinical picture is not clearly understood. The actual syndrome itself is not confined to overwhelming staphylococcal or combined streptococcal-staphylococcal sepsis, but has also been described in association with profound heart failure, myocardial infarction, or pulmonary embolism (228–230). Thus many features may relate to intense peripheral vasocon-striction after central pump failure or to exaggerated autonomic reflex mechanisms.

References

1. Bauer, D. C., and Stavitsky, A. B. On the different molecular forms of antibody synthesized by rabbits during the early response to a single injection of protein and cellular antigens. *Proc. Natl. Acad. Sci. USA* 47:1667, 1961.

2. Uhr, J. W., and Finkelstein, M. S. The kinetics of antibody formation, sec. 3. In *Progress in Allergy,* vol. 10, p. 43. S. Karger, New York, 1967.

3. Nossal, G. J. V., Ada, G. L., and Austin, C. M. Antigens in immunity. II. Immunogenic properties of flagella, polymerized flagellin and flagellin in the primary response. *Aust. J. Exp. Biol. Med. Sci.* 42:283, 1964.

4. Siskind, G. W., Dunn, P., and Walker, J. G. Studies on the control of antibody synthesis. II. Effect of antigen dose and of suppression by passive antibody on the affinity of antibody synthesized. *J. Exp. Med.* 127:55, 1968.

5. Walker, J. G., and Siskind, G. W. Studies on the control of antibody synthesis. Effect of antibody affinity upon its ability to suppress antibody formation. *Immunology* 14:21, 1968.

6. Siskind, G. W., and Benacerraf, B. Cell selection by antigen in the immune response. *Adv. Immunol.* 10:1, 1969.

7. Rowley, D. A., and Fitch, F. W. Clonal selection and inhibition of the primary antibody response by antibody. In B. Cinader, ed., *Regulation of the Antibody Response,* p. 127. Charles C Thomas, Springfield, Ill., 1968.

8. Wigzell, H. Antibody synthesis at the cellular level. Antibody-induced suppression of 7 S antibody synthesis. *J. Exp. Med.* 124:953, 1966.

9. Tomasi, T. B., Jr., Tan, E. M., Solomon, A., et al. Characteristics of an immune system common to certain external secretions. *J. Exp. Med.* 121:101, 1965.

10. Crabbé, P. A., and Heremans, J. F. Lack of gamma A-immunoglobulin in serum of patients with steatorrhoea. *Gut* 7:119, 1966.

11. Brandtzaeg, P., Fjellanger, I., and Gjeruldsen, S. T. Localization of immunoglobulins in human nasal mucosa. *Immunochemistry* 4:57, 1967.

12. Tomasi, T. B., Jr. Human immunoglobulin A. *N. Engl. J. Med.* 279:1327, 1968.

13. Tomasi, T. B., Jr., and Bienenstock, J. Secretory immunoglobulins. *Adv. Immunol.* 9:1, 1968.

14. Lichtenstein, L. M., Gewurz, H., Adkinson, N. F., Jr., et al. Interactions of the complement system with endotoxic lipopolysaccharide: the generation of an anaphylatoxin. *Immunology* 16:327, 1969.

15. Biberfeld, G., and Gronowicz, E. Mycoplasma pneumoniae is a polyclonal B-cell activator. *Nature* 261:238, 1976.

16. Parish, C. R., and Ada, G. L. The tolerance inducing properties in rats of bacterial flagellin cleaved at the methionine residues. *Immunology* 17:153, 1969.

17. Ada, G. L., Nossal, G. J. V., and Austin, C. M. Studies on the nature of immunogenicity employing soluble and particulate bacterial proteins. In J. Sterzl, Ed., *Molecular and Cellular Basis of Antibody Formation,* p. 31. Czechoslovak Academy of Science, Prague, 1965.

18. Torrigiani, G., and Roitt, I. M. The enhancement of 19 S antibody production by particulate antigen. *J. Exp. Med.* 122:18, 1965.

19. Kimball, J. W., Pappenheimer, A. M., Jr., and Jaton, J. C. The response in rabbits to prolonged immunization with type III pneumococci. *J. Immunol.* 106:1177, 1971.

20. Pincus, J. H., Jaton, J. C., Bloch, K. J. et al. Antibodies to type III and type VIII pneumococcal polysaccharides: evidence for restricted structural heterogeneity in hyperimmunized rabbits. *J. Immunol.* 104:1143, 1970.

21. Osterland, C. K., Miller, E. J., Karakawa, W. W., et al. Characteristics of streptococcal group-specific antibody isolated from hyperimmune rabbits. *J. Exp. Med.* 123:599, 1966.

22. Davies, A. J. S., Carter, R. L., Leuchars, E., et al. The morphology of immune reactions in normal, thymectomized and reconstituted mice. III. Response to bacterial antigens: salmonellar flagellar antigen and pneumococcal polysaccharide. *Immunology* 19:945, 1970.

23. Howard, J. G., Christie, G. H., Courtenay, B. M., et al. Studies on immunological paralysis. VI. Thymic-independence of tolerance and immunity to type III pneumococcal polysaccharide. *Cell. Immunol.* 2:614, 1971.

24. Gershon, R. K., Cohen, P., Hencin, R., et al. Suppressor T cells. *J. Immunol.* 108:586, 1972.

25. Yoshinaga, M., Yoshinaga, A., and Waksman, B. H. Regulation of lymphocyte responses *in vitro.* I. Regulatory effect of macrophages and thy-

mus-dependent (T) cells on the response of thymus-independent (B) lymphocytes to endotoxin. *J. Exp. Med.* 136:956, 1972.

26. Opitz, H. G., Niethammer, D., Lemke, H., et al. Inhibition of ³H-thymidine incorporation of lymphocytes by a soluble factor from macrophages. *Cell. Immunol.* 16:379, 1975.

27. Calderon, J., Williams, R. T., and Unanue, E. R. An inhibitor of cell proliferation released by cultures of macrophages. *Proc. Natl. Acad. Sci. USA* 71:4273, 1974.

28. Miller, T. E., Scott, L., Simpson, G., et al. Depression of the T-lymphocyte response to phytohaemagglutinin by renal cells. *Clin. Exp. Immunol.* 24:492, 1976.

29. Osler, W. Chronic infectious endocarditis. *Q. J. Med.* 2:219, 1909.

30. Horder, T. J. Infective endocarditis. With an analysis of 150 cases and with special reference to the chronic form of the disease. *Q. J. Med.* 2:289, 1909.

31. Billings, F. Chronic infectious endocarditis. *Arch. Intern. Med.* 4:409, 1909.

32. Major, R. H. Clinical and bacteriological studies on endocarditis lenta. *Bull. Johns Hopkins Hosp.* 23:326, 1912.

33. Baehr, G. Renal complications of endocarditis. *Trans. Assoc. Am. Physicians* 46:87, 1931.

34. Villarreal, H., and Sokoloff, L. The occurrence of renal insufficiency in subacute bacterial endocarditis. *Am. J. Med. Sci.* 220:655, 1950.

35. Kerr, A. *Subacute Bacterial Endocarditis.* Charles C Thomas, Springfield, Ill., 1955.

36. Bain, R. C., Edwards, J. E., Scheifley, C. H., et al. Right-sided bacterial endocarditis and endarteritis. A clinical and pathologic study. *Am. J. Med.* 24:98, 1958.

37. Williams, R. C., Jr., and Kunkel, H. G. Rheumatoid factor, complement, and conglutinin aberrations in patients with subacute bacterial endocarditis. *J. Clin. Invest.* 41:666, 1962.

38. Gutman, R. A., Striker, G. E., Gilliland, B. C., et al. The immune complex glomerulonephritis of bacterial endocarditis. *Medicine* 51:1, 1972.

39. Levy, R. L., and Hong, R. The immune nature of subacute bacterial endocarditis (SBE) nephritis. *Am. J. Med.* 54:645, 1973.

40. Keslin, M. H., Messner, R. P., and Williams, R. C., Jr. Glomerulonephritis with subacute bacterial endocarditis. Immunofluorescent studies. *Arch. Intern. Med.* 132:578, 1973.

41. Boulton-Jones, J. M., Sissons, J. G. P., Evans, D. J., et al. Renal lesions of subacute infective endocarditis. *Br. Med. J.* 2:11, 1974.

42. Perez, G. O., Rothfield, N., and Williams, R. C., Jr. Immune-complex nephritis in bacterial endocarditis. *Arch. Intern. Med.* 136:334, 1976.

43. Arnold, S. B., Valone, J. A., Askenase, P. W., et al. Diffuse glomerulonephritis in rabbits with *Streptococcus viridans* endocarditis. *Lab. Invest.* 32:681, 1975.

44. Roberts, W. C., and Rabson, A. S. Focal glomerular lesions in fungal endocarditis. *Ann. Intern. Med.* 56:610, 1962.

45. Helpern, M., and Trubek, M. Necrotizing arteritis and subacute glomerulonephritis in gonococcic endocarditis. Toxic origin of periarteritis nodosa. *Arch. Pathol.* 15:35, 1933.

46. Tu, W. H., Shearn, M. A., and Lee, J. C. Acute diffuse glomerulonephritis in acute staphylococcal endocarditis. *Ann. Intern. Med.* 71:335, 1969.

47. Holt, R. The classification of staphylococci from colonized ventriculoatrial shunts. *J. Clin. Pathol.* 22:475, 1969.

48. Black, J. A., Challacombe, D. N., and Ockenden, B. G. Nephrotic syndrome associated with bacteraemia after shunt operations for hydrocephalus. *Lancet* 2:921, 1965.

49. Stickler, G. B., Shin, M. H., Burke, E. C., et al. Diffuse glomerulonephritis associated with infected ventriculoatrial shunt. *N. Engl. J. Med.* 279:1077, 1968.

50. McKenzie, S. A., and Hayden, K. Two cases of "shunt nephritis." *Pediatrics* 54:806, 1974.

51. Dobrin, R. S., Day, N. K., Quie, P. G., et al. The role of complement, immunoglobulin and bacterial antigen in coagulase-negative staphylococcal shunt nephritis. *Am. J. Med.* 59:660, 1975.

52. Kaufman, D. B., and McIntosh, R. The pathogenesis of the renal lesion in a patient with streptococcal disease, infected ventriculoatrial shunt, cryoglobulinemia and nephritis. *Am. J. Med.* 50:262, 1971.

53. Beeler, B. A., Crowder, J. G., Smith, J. W., et al. Propionibacterium acnes: pathogen in central nervous system shunt infection. Report of three cases including immune complex glomerulonephritis. *Am. J. Med.* 61:935, 1976.

54. Beeson, P. B., Brannon, E. S., and Warren, J. V. Observations on the sites of removal of bacteria from the blood in patients with bacterial endocarditis. *J. Exp. Med.* 81:9, 1945.

55. Werner, A. S., Cobbs, C. G., Kaye, D., et al. Studies on the bacteremia of bacterial endocarditis. *J.A.M.A.* 202:199, 1967.

56. Lunn, J. S., and Bunn, P. A. Immunoglobulin responses to bacterial endocarditis. *Antimicrob. Agents Chemother.* 5:50, 1965.

57. Laxdal, T., Messner, R. P., Williams, R. C., Jr., et al. Opsonic, agglutinating, and complement-fixing antibodies in patients with subacute bacterial endocarditis. *J. Lab. Clin. Med.* 71:638, 1968.

58. Williams, R. C., Jr. Subacute bacterial endocarditis as an immune disease. *Hosp. Prac.* 6:111, 1971.

59. McDevitt, H. O., and Benacerraf, B. Genetic control of specific immune responses. *Adv. Immunol.* 11:31, 1969.

60. Shreffler, D. C., and David, C. S. The H_2 major histocompatibility complex and the I immune response region: genetic variation, function and organization. *Adv. Immunol.* 20:125, 1975.

61. Mukasa, H., and Slade, H. D. Mechanism of adherence of *Streptococcus mutans* to smooth surfaces. I. Roles of insoluble dextran-levan synthetase enzymes and cell wall polysaccharide antigen in plaque formation. *Infect. Immun.* 8:555, 1973.

62. Gould, K., Ramirez-Ronda, C. H., Holmes, R. K., et al. Adherence of bacteria to heart valves *in vitro*. *J. Clin. Invest.* 56:1364, 1975.

63. Bayer, A. S., Theofilopoulos, A. N., Eisenberg, R., et al. Circulating immune complexes in infective endocarditis. *N. Engl. J. Med.* 295:1500, 1976.

64. Theofilopoulos, A. N., Wilson, C. B. and Dixon, F. J. The Raji cell radioimmune assay for detecting immune complexes in human sera. *J. Clin. Invest.* 57:169, 1976.

65. Von Gemmingen, G. R., and Winkelmann, R. K. Osler's node of subacute bacterial endocarditis. Focal necrotizing vasculitis of the glomus body. *Arch. Dermatol.* 95:91, 1967.

66. Lian, C., Nicolau, S., and Poincloux, P. Histopathologie du nodule d'Osler. Etude sur l'endothéliite de l'endocardite maligne à évolution lente. *Presse Med.* 37:497, 1929.

67. Alpert, J. S., Krous, H. F., Dalen, J. E., et al. Pathogenesis of Osler's nodes. *Ann. Intern. Med.* 85:471, 1976.

68. Petersdorf, R. G. Immune complexes in infective endocarditis. *N. Engl. J. Med.* 295:1534, 1976.

69. Puklin, J. E., Balis, G. A., and Bentley, D. W. Culture of an Osler's node. A diagnostic tool. *Arch. Intern. Med.* 127:296, 1971.

70. Lowenstein, M. B., Urman, J. D., Abeles, M., et al. Skin immunofluorescence in infective endocarditis. *J.A.M.A.* 238:1163, 1977.

71. Phair, J. P., Klippel, J., and MacKenzie, M. R. Antiglobulins in endocarditis. *Infect. Immun.* 5:24, 1972.

72. Carson, D. A., Bayer, A. S., Eisenberg, R. A., et al. IgG rheumatoid factor in subacute bacterial endocarditis: relationship to IgM rheumatoid factor and circulating immune complexes. *Clin. Exp. Immunol.* 31:100, 1978.

73. Messner, R. P., Laxdal, T., Quie, P. G., et al. Serum opsonin, bacteria, and polymorphonuclear leukocyte interactions in subacute bacterial endocarditis. Anti-γ-globulin factors and their interaction with specific opsonins. *J. Clin. Invest.* 47:1109, 1968.

74. McDuffie, F. C., and Brumfield, H. W. Effect of rheumatoid factor on complement-mediated phagocytosis. *J. Clin. Invest.* 51:3007, 1972.

75. Rossen, R. D., Reisberg, M. A., Sharp, J. T., et al. Antiglobulins and glomerulonephritis. Classification of patients by the reactivity of their sera and renal tissue with aggregated and native human IgG. *J. Clin. Invest.* 56:427, 1975.

76. McCormick, J. N., Day, J., Morris, C. J., et al. The potentiating effect of rheumatoid arthritis serum in the immediate phase of nephrotoxic nephritis. *Clin. Exp. Immunol.* 4:17, 1969.

77. Bacon, P. A., Davidson, C., and Smith, B. Antibodies to candida and autoantibodies in subacute bacterial endocarditis. *Q. J. Med.* 43:537, 1974.

78. Sherwood, B. F., Rowlands, D. T., Jr., Vakilzadeh, J., et al. Experimental bacterial endocarditis in the opossum (Didelphis virginiana). III. Comparison of spontaneously occurring endocarditis with that induced experimentally by pyogenic bacteria and fungi. *Am. J. Pathol.* 64:513, 1971.

79. Rowlands, D. T., Jr. Animal models for human disease: bacterial endocarditis in the opossum (Didelphis virginiana). *Comp. Pathol. Bull.* 11:2, 1970.

80. Garrison, P. K., and Freedman, L. R. Experimental endocarditis. I. Staphylococcal endocarditis in rabbits resulting from placement of a polyethylene catheter in the right side of the heart. *Yale J. Biol. Med.* 42:394, 1970.

81. Durack, D. T., and Beeson, P. B. Experimental bacterial endocarditis. I. Colonization of a sterile vegetation. *Br. J. Exp. Pathol.* 53:44, 1972.

82. Durack, D. T., Beeson, P. B., and Petersdorf, R. G. Experimental bacterial endocarditis. III. Production and progress of the disease in rabbits. *Br. J. Exp. Pathol.* 54:142, 1973.

83. Watanakunakorn, C. Infective endocarditis as a result of medical progress. *Am. J. Med.* 64:917, 1978.

84. Denton, C., Pappas, E. G., Uricchio, J. F., et al. Bacterial endocarditis following cardiac surgery. *Circulation* 15:525, 1957.

85. Cherubin, C. E., and Neu, H. C. Infective endocarditis at the Presbyterian Hospital in New

York City from 1938–1967. *Am. J. Med.* 51:83, 1971.

86. Quenzer, R. W., Edwards, L. D., and Levin, S. A comparative study of 48 host valve and 24 prosthetic valve endocarditis cases. *Am. Heart J.* 92:15, 1976.

87. Harrell, E. R., and Thompson, G. R. Systemic candidiasis (moniliasis) complicating treatment of bacterial endocarditis, with review of the literature and report of apparent cure of one case with parenteral mycostatin. *Ann. Intern. Med.* 49:207, 1958.

88. Bentley, D. W., and Lepper, M. H. Septicemia related to indwelling venous catheter. *J.A.M.A.* 206:1749, 1968.

89. Leonard, A., Raij, L., and Shapiro, F. L. Bacterial endocarditis in regularly dialyzed patients. *Kidney Int.* 4:407, 1973.

90. Greene, J. F., Jr., and Cummings, K. C. Septic endocarditis and parenteral feeding. *J.A.M.A.* 225:315, 1973.

91. Gazzaniga, A. B., Mir-Sepasi, M. H., Jefferies, M. R., et al. Candida endocarditis complicating glucose total intravenous nutrition. *Ann. Surg.* 179:902, 1974.

92. Greene, J. F., Jr., Fitzwater, J. E., and Clemmer, T. P. Septic endocarditis and indwelling pulmonary artery catheters. *J.A.M.A.* 233:891, 1975.

93. Watanakunakorn, C., and Baird, I. M. Staphylococcus aureus bacteremia and endocarditis associated with a removable infected intravenous device. *Am. J. Med.* 63:253, 1977.

94. Nolan, C. M., and Beaty, H. N. Staphylococcus aureus bacteremia. Current clinical patterns. *Am. J. Med.* 60:495, 1976.

95. Pelletier, L. L., Jr., and Petersdorf, R. G. Infective endocarditis: a review of 125 cases from the University of Washington Hospitals, 1963–72. *Medicine* (Baltimore) 56:287, 1977.

96. MacDonald, R. A. and Robbins, S. L. The significance of non-bacterial thrombotic endocarditis: an autopsy and clinical study of 78 cases. *Ann. Intern. Med.* 46:255, 1957.

97. MacLeod, C. M., Hodges, R. G., Heidelberger, M., et al. Prevention of pneumococcal pneumonia by immunization with specific capsular polysaccharides. *J. Exp. Med.* 82:445, 1945.

98. Austrian, R. Random gleanings from a life with the pneumococcus. *J. Infect. Dis.* 131:474, 1975.

99. Smit, P., Oberholzer, D., Hayden-Smith, S., et al. Protective efficacy of pneumococcal polysaccharide vaccines. *J.A.M.A.* 238:2613, 1977.

100. Borgoño, J. M., McLean, A. A., Vella, P. P., et al. Vaccination and revaccination with polyvalent pneumococcal polysaccharide vaccines in adults and infants. *Proc. Soc. Exp. Biol. Med.* 157:148, 1978.

101. Hansman, D., Glasgow, H., Sturt, J., et al. Increased resistance to penicillin of pneumococci isolated from man. *N. Engl. J. Med.* 284:175, 1971.

102. Appelbaum, P. C., Scragg, J. N., Bowen. A. J., et al. Streptococcus pneumoniae resistant to penicillin and chloramphenicol. *Lancet* 2:995, 1977.

103. Dixon, J. M. S., Lipinski, A. E., and Graham, M. E. P. Detection and prevalence of pneumococci with increased resistance to penicillin. *Can. Med. Assoc. J.* 117:1159, 1977.

104. Austrian, R., and Gold, J. Pneumococcal bacteremia with especial reference to bacteremic pneumococcal pneumonia. *Ann. Intern. Med.* 60:759, 1964.

105. Sloyer, J. L., Jr., Howie, V. M., Ploussard, J. H., et al. Immune response to acute otitis media in children. I. Serotypes isolated and serum and middle ear fluid antibody in pneumococcal otitis media. *Infect. Immun.* 9:1028, 1974.

106. Tung, K. S. K., Reed, W. P., and Williams, R. C., Jr. Circulating immune complexes during acute pneumococcal infection. Unpublished observations, 1977.

107. Coonrod, J. D., and Rytel, M. W. Detection of type-specific pneumococcal antigens by counterimmunoelectrophoresis. II. Etiologic diagnosis of pneumococcal pneumonia. *J. Lab. Clin. Med.* 81:778, 1973.

108. Kenny, G. E., Wentworth, B. B., Beasley, R. P., et al. Correlation of circulating capsular polysaccharide with bacteremia in pneumococcal pneumonia. *Infect. Immun.* 6:431, 1972.

109. Coonrod, J. D., and Drennan, D. P. Pneumococcal pneumonia: capsular polysaccharide antigenemia and antibody responses. *Ann. Intern. Med.* 84:254, 1976.

110. Frisch, A. W., Tripp, J. T., Barrett, C. D., Jr., et al. The specific polysaccharide content of pneumonic lungs. *J. Exp. Med.* 76:505, 1942.

111. Ney, R. N., and Harris, A. H. Viable pneumococci and pneumococcic specific soluble substance in the lungs from cases of lobar pneumonia. *Am. J. Pathol.* 13:749, 1937.

112. Reed, W. P., Davidson, M. S., and Williams, R. C., Jr. Complement system in pneumococcal infections. *Infect. Immun.* 13:1120, 1976.

113. Dhingra, R. K., Williams, R. C., Jr., and Reed, W. P. Effects of pneumococcal mucopeptide and capsular polysaccharide on phagocytosis. *Infect. Immun.* 15:169, 1977.

114. Stephens, C. G., Williams, R. C., Jr., and Reed, W. P. Classical and alternative complement

pathway activation by pneumococci. *Infect. Immun.* 17:296, 1977.

115. Coonrod, J. D., and Rylko-Bauer, B. Complement-fixing antibody response in pneumococcal pneumonia. *Infect. Immun.* 18:617, 1977.

116. Johnston, R. B., Jr., Anderson, P., Rosen, F. S., et al. Characterization of human antibody to polyribophosphate, the capsular antigen of Hemophilus influenzae, Type B. *Clin. Immunol. Immunopathol.* 1:234, 1973.

117. Yount, W. J., Dorner, M. M., Kunkel, H. G., et al. Studies on human antibodies. VI. Selective variations in subgroup composition and genetic markers. *J. Exp. Med.* 127:633, 1968.

118. Rytel, M. W., Dee, T. H., Ferstenfeld, J. E., et al. Possible pathogenetic role of capsular antigens in fulminant pneumococcal disease with disseminated intravascular coagulation (DIC). *Am. J. Med.* 57:889, 1974.

119. King, H., and Schumacker, H. B., Jr. Splenic studies. I. Susceptibility to infection after splenectomy performed in infancy. *Ann. Surg.* 136:239, 1952.

120. Eraklis, A. J., Kevy, S. V., Diamond, L. K., et al. Hazard of overwhelming infection after splenectomy in childhood. *N. Engl. J. Med.* 276:1225, 1967.

121. Bisno, A. L., and Freeman, J. C. The syndrome of asplenia, pneumococcal sepsis and disseminated intravascular coagulation. *Ann. Intern. Med.* 72:389, 1970.

122. Torres, J., and Bisno, A. L. Hyposplenism and pneumococcemia: visualization of *Diplococcus pneumoniae* in the peripheral blood smear. *Am. J. Med.* 55:851, 1973.

123. Agger, W. A., and Overholt, E. L. Pneumococcal sepsis with disseminated intravascular coagulation in an asplenic woman: case report. *Milit. Med.* 143:40, 1978.

124. Dalldorf, F. G., Pate, D. H., and Langdell, R. D. Pulmonary capillary thrombosis in experimental pneumococcal septicemia. *Arch. Pathol.* 85:149, 1968.

125. Ellis, E. F., and Smith, R. T. The role of the spleen in immunity. With special reference to the post-splenectomy problem in infants. *Pediatrics* 37:111, 1966.

126. Claret, I., Morales, L., and Montaner, A. Immunological studies in the postsplenectomy syndrome. *J. Pediatr. Surg.* 10:59, 1975.

127. Likhite, V. V. Opsonin and leukophilic γ-globulin in chronically splenectomized rats with and without heterotropic autotransplanted splenic tissue. *Nature* 253:742, 1975.

128. Schwartz, A. D., Goldthorn, J. F., Winkelstein, J. A., et al. Lack of protective effect of autotransplanted splenic tissue to pneumococcal challenge. *Blood* 51:475, 1978.

129. Moore, G. E. Pneumococcal vaccination after splenectomy. *N. Engl. J. Med.* 298:797, 1978.

130. Robins, D. E., and Ladd, A. T. Acute syphilitic nephrosis. Case report and review of the literature. *Am. J. Med.* 32:817, 1962.

131. Thomas, E. W., and Schur, M. Clinical nephropathies in early syphilis. *Arch. Intern. Med.* 78:679, 1946.

132. Patton, E. W., and Corlette, M. B. Three cases of acute syphilitic nephrosis in adults. *Ann. Intern. Med.* 14:1975, 1941.

133. Barr, J. H., Jr., Cole, H. N., Driver, J. R., et al. Acute syphilitic nephrosis successfully treated with penicillin. *J.A.M.A.* 131:741, 1946.

134. Braunstein, G. D., Lewis, E. J., Galvanek, E. G., et al. The nephrotic syndrome associated with secondary syphilis. An immune deposit disease. *Am. J. Med.* 48:643, 1970.

135. Yuceoglu, A. M., Sagel, I., Tresser, G., et al. The glomerulopathy of congenital syphilis. A curable immune-deposit disease. *J.A.M.A.* 229:1085, 1974.

136. Tourville, D. R., Byrd, L. H., Kim, D. U., et al. Treponemal antigen in immunopathogenesis of syphilitic glomerulonephritis. *Am. J. Pathol.* 82:479, 1976.

137. Gamble, C. N., and Reardan, J. B. Immunopathogenesis of syphilitic glomerulonephritis. Elution of antitreponemal antibody from glomerular immune-complex deposits. *N. Engl. J. Med.* 292:449, 1975.

138. Fulford, K. W. M., Johnson, N., Loveday, C., et al. Changes in intra-vascular complement and antitreponemal antibody titres preceding the Jarisch-Herxheimer reaction in secondary syphilis. *Clin. Exp. Immunol.* 24:483, 1976.

139. Abu-Nassar, H., Hill, N., Fred, H. L., et al. Cutaneous manifestations of gonococcemia. A review of 14 cases. *Arch. Intern. Med.* 112:731, 1963.

140. Wheeler, J. K., Heffron, W. A., and Williams, R. C., Jr. Migratory arthralgias and cutaneous lesions as confusing initial manifestations of gonorrhea. *Am. J. Med. Sci.* 260:150, 1970.

141. Holmes, K. K., Counts, G. W., and Beaty, H. N. Disseminated gonococcal infection. *Ann. Intern. Med.* 74:979, 1971.

142. Holmes, K. K., Wiesner, P. J., and Pedersen, A. H. B. The gonococcal arthritis-dermatitis syndrome. *Ann. Intern. Med.* 75:470, 1971.

143. Handsfield, H. H. Disseminated gonococcal infection. *Clin. Obstet. Gynecol.* 18:131, 1975.

144. Cooke, T. D., Hurd, E. R., Ziff, M., et al. The pathogenesis of chronic inflammation in experimental antigen-induced arthritis. II. Preferential localization of antigen-antibody complexes to collagenous tissues. *J. Exp. Med.* 135:323, 1972.

145. Cooke, T. D., Hurd, E. R., Bienenstock, J., et al. The immunofluorescent identification of immunoglobulins and complement in rheumatoid articular collagenous tissue. *Arthritis Rheum.* 15:433, 1972.

146. Walker, L. C., Ahlin, T. D., Tung, K. S. K., et al. Circulating immune complexes in disseminated gonorrheal infection. *Ann. Intern. Med.* 89:28, 1978.

147. Wiesner, P. J., Handsfield, H. H., and Holmes, K. K. Low antibiotic resistance of gonococci causing disseminated infection. *N. Engl. J. Med.* 288:1221, 1973.

148. Schoolnik, G. K., Buchanan, T. M., and Holmes, K. K. Gonococci causing disseminated gonococcal infection are resistant to the bactericidal action of normal human sera. *J. Clin. Invest.* 58:1163, 1976.

149. Petersen, B. H., Graham, J. A., and Brooks, G. F. Human deficiency of the eighth component of complement. The requirement of C_8 for serum Neisseria gonorrheae bactericidal activity. *J. Clin. Invest.* 57:283, 1976.

150. Leddy, J. P., Frank, M. M., Gaither, T., et al. Hereditary deficiency of the sixth component of complement in man. I. Immunochemical, biologic, and family studies. *J. Clin. Invest.* 53:544, 1974.

151. Wellek, B., and Opferkuch, W. A. A case of deficiency of the seventh component of complement in man. Biological properties of a C_7-deficient serum and description of a C_7-inactivating principle. *Clin. Exp. Immunol.* 19:223, 1975.

152. Jasin, H. E. Absence of the eighth component of complement in association with systemic lupus erythematosus-like disease. *J. Clin. Invest.* 60:709, 1977.

153. Merritt, A. D., Petersen, B. H., Biegel, A. A., et al. Chromosome 6: linkage of the eighth component of complement (C_8) to the histocompatibility region (HLA). *Birth Defects* 12:331, 1976.

154. Manni, J. A., and Müller-Eberhard, H. J. The eighth component of human complement (C_8): isolation, characterization, and hemolytic efficiency. *J. Exp. Med.* 130:1145, 1969.

155. Gulati, P. D., Saxena, S. N., Gupta, P. S., et al. Changing pattern of typhoid fever. *Am. J. Med.* 45:544, 1968.

156. Faierman, D., Ross, F. A., and Seckler, S. G. Typhoid fever complicated by hepatitis, nephritis, and thrombocytopenia. *J.A.M.A.* 221:60, 1972.

157. Osler, W. Typhoid fever. In *The Principles and Practice of Medicine,* p. 26. D. Appleton & Co., New York, 1893.

158. Sitprija, V., Pipantanagul, V., Boonpucknavig, V., et al. Glomerulitis in typhoid fever. *Ann. Intern. Med.* 81:210, 1974.

159. Farid, Z., Higashi, G. I., Bassily, S., et al. Chronic salmonellosis, urinary schistosomiasis, and massive proteinuria. *Am. J. Trop. Med. Hyg.* 21:578, 1972.

160. Higashi, G. I., Farid, Z., Bassily, S., et al. Nephrotic syndrome in Schistosomiasis mansoni complicated by chronic salmonellosis. *Am. J. Trop. Med. Hyg.* 24:713, 1975.

161. Farid, Z., Higashi, G. I., Bassily, S., et al. Immune-complex disease in typhoid and paratyphoid fevers. *Ann. Intern. Med.* 83:432, 1975.

162. Higashi, G. I. Personal communication, March 1978.

163. Williams, R. C., Jr., Walker, L., Tung, K. S. K., et al. Measurement of immune complexes in salmonella infections and in patients with combined salmonella and schistosomal infection with nephrotic syndrome. In preparation, 1979.

164. Koster, F., Levin, J., Walker, L., et al. Hemolytic-uremic syndrome after shigellosis: relation to endotoxemia and circulating immune complexes. *N. Engl. J. Med.* 298:927, 1978.

165. Bokisch, V. A., Top, F. H., Jr., Russell, P. K., et al. The potential pathogenic role of complement in dengue hemorrhagic shock syndrome. *N. Engl. J. Med.* 298:996, 1973.

166. Brown, D. L., and Lachmann, P. J. The behaviour of complement and platelets in lethal endotoxin shock in rabbits. *Int. Arch. Allergy Appl. Immunol.* 45:193, 1973.

167. Gilbert, V. E., and Braude, A. I. Reduction of serum complement in rabbits after injection of endotoxin. *J. Exp. Med.* 116:477, 1962.

168. From, A. H. L., Gewurz, H., Gruninger, R. P., et al. Complement in endotoxin shock: effect of complement depletion on the early hypotensive phase. *Infect. Immun.* 2:38, 1970.

169. Morrison, D. C., and Kline, L. F. Activation of the classical and properdin pathways of complement by bacterial lipopolysaccharides (LPS). *J. Immunol.* 118:362, 1977.

170. Ulevitch, R. J., and Cochrane, C. G. Role of complement in lethal bacterial lipopolysaccharide-induced hypotensive and coagulative changes. *Infect. Immun.* 19:204, 1978.

171. Jewell, D. P., and MacLennan, I. C. M. Circulating immune complexes in inflammatory bowel disease. *Clin. Exp. Immunol.* 14:219, 1973.

172. Doe, W. F., Booth, C. C., and Brown, D. L. Evidence for complement-binding immune complexes in adult coeliac disease, Crohn's disease and ulcerative colitis. *Lancet* 1:402, 1973.

173. Hodgson, H. J. F., Potter, B. J., and Jewell, D. P. Immune complexes in ulcerative colitis and Crohn's disease. *Clin. Exp. Immunol.* 29:187, 1977.

174. Nielsen, H., Binder, V., Daugharty, H., et al. Circulating immune complexes in ulcerative colitis. I. Correlation to disease activity. *Clin. Exp. Immunol.* 31:72, 1978.

175. Nielsen, H., Hyltoft Petersen, P., and Suehag, S.-E. Circulating immune complexes in ulcerative colitis. II. Correlation with serum protein concentrations and complement conversion products. *Clin. Exp. Immunol.* 31:81, 1978.

176. Ridley, D. S., and Jopling, W. H. Classification of leprosy according to immunity. A five-group system. *Int. J. Lepr.* 34:255, 1966.

177. Waters, M. F. R., and Ridley, D. S. Necrotizing reactions in lepromatous leprosy. A clinical and histological study. *Int. J. Lepr.* 31:418, 1963.

178. Wemambu, S. N. C., Turk, J. L., Waters, M. F. R., et al. Erythema nodosum leprosum: a clinical manifestation of the Arthus phenomenon. *Lancet* 2:933 1969.

179. Bonomo, L., and Dammacco, F. Immune complex cryoglobulinaemia in lepromatous leprosy: a pathogenetic approach to some clinical features of leprosy. *Clin. Exp. Immunol.* 9:175, 1971.

180. Gelber, R. H., Drutz, D. J., Epstein, W. V., et al. Clinical correlates of C1q-precipitating substances in the sera of patients with leprosy. *Am. J. Trop. Med. Hyg.* 23:471, 1974.

181. Moran, C. J., Turk, J. L., Ryder, G., et al. Evidence for circulating immune complexes in lepromatous leprosy. *Lancet* 2:572, 1972.

182. Rojas-Espinosa, O., Mendez-Navarrete, I., and Estrada-Parra, S. Presence of C1q-reactive immune complexes in patients with leprosy. *Clin. Exp. Immunol.* 12:215, 1972.

183. Bjorvatn, B., Barnetson, R. S., Kronvall, G., et al. Immune complexes and complement hypercatabolism in patients with leprosy. *Clin. Exp. Immunol.* 26:388, 1976.

184. Tung, K. S. K., Kim, B., Bjorvatn, B., et al. Discrepancy between C1q deviation and Raji cell tests in detection of circulating immune complexes in patients with leprosy. *J. Infect. Dis.* 136:216, 1977.

185. Iveson, J. M. I., McDougall, A. C., Leathem, A. J., et al. Lepromatous leprosy presenting with polyarthritis, myositis, and immune-complex glomerulonephritis. *Br. Med. J.* 3:619, 1975.

186. Peltier, A. and Christian, C. L. The presence of the rheumatoid factor in sera from patients with syphilis. *Arthritis Rheum.* 2:1, 1959.

187. Cathcart, E. S., Williams, R. C., Jr., Ross, H., et al. The relationship of the latex fixation test to the clinical and serologic manifestations of leprosy. *Am. J. Med.* 31:758, 1961.

188. Petchclai, B., Chuthanondh, R., Rungruong, S., et al. Autoantibodies in leprosy among Thai patients. *Lancet* 1:1481, 1973.

189. Wall, J. R. and Wright, D. J. M. Antibodies against testicular germinal cells in lepromatous leprosy. *Clin. Exp. Immunol.* 17:51, 1974.

190. Singer, J. M., Plotz, C. M., Peralta, F. M., et al. The presence of anti-gamma globulin factors in sera of patients with active pulmonary tuberculosis. *Ann. Intern. Med.* 56:545, 1962.

191. Seligmann, M., Cannat, A., and Hamard, M. Studies on antinuclear antibodies. *Ann. N.Y. Acad. Sci.* 124:816, 1965.

192. Williams, R. C., Jr. Infection and autoimmunity. In *N. Talal, ed., Autoimmunity. Genetic, Immunologic, Virologic, and Clinical Aspects,* p. 457. Academic Press, New York, 1977.

193. Grabar, P. Hypothesis. Auto-antibodies and immunological theories: an analytical review. *Clin. Immunol. Immunopathol.* 4:453, 1975.

194. Biberfeld, G., and Gronowicz, E. Mycoplasma pneumoniae is a polyclonal B-cell activator. *Nature* 261:238, 1976.

195. Fournie, G. J., Lambert, P. H., and Miescher, P. A. Release of DNA in circulating blood and induction of anti-DNA antibodies after injection of bacterial lipopolysaccharides. *J. Exp. Med.* 140:1189, 1975.

196. Primi, D., Hammarström, L., Smith, C. I., et al. Characterization of self-reactive B cells by polyclonal B-cell activators. *J. Exp. Med.* 145:21, 1977.

197. Primi, D., Smith, C. I. E., Hammarström, L., et al. Evidence for the existence of self-reactive human B lymphocytes. *Clin. Exp. Immunol.* 29:316, 1977.

198. Greenwood, B. M., and Vick, R. M. Evidence for a malaria mitogen in human malaria. *Nature* 257:592, 1975.

199. Sultzer, B. M., and Nilsson, B. S. PPD tuberculin—a B-cell mitogen. *Nature (New Biol.)* 240:198, 1972.

200. Bona, C., and Cazenave, P. A. Release from maternally-induced allotypic suppression in rabbit by Nocardia water-soluble mitogen. *J. Exp. Med.* 146:881, 1977.

201. Sawada, S., Pillarisetty, R. J., Michalski, J.

P., et al. Lymphocytes binding polyriboadenylic acid and synthesizing antibodies to nucleic acids in autoimmune and normal mice. *J. Immunol.* 119:355, 1977.

202. Bankhurst, A. D., Torrigiani, G., and Allison, A. C. Lymphocytes binding human thyroglobulin in healthy people and its relevance to tolerance for autoantigens. *Lancet* 1:226, 1973.

203. Bankhurst, A. D., and Williams, R. C., Jr. Identification of DNA-binding lymphocytes in patients with systemic lupus erythematosus. *J. Clin. Invest.* 56:1378, 1975.

204. Davis, J. A. S., Peters, N., Idris, M., et al. Circulating immune complexes in a patient with meningococcal disease. *Br. Med. J.* 1:1445, 1976.

205. Greenwood, B. M., Onyewotu, I. I., and Whittle, H. C. Complement and meningococcal infection. *Br. Med. J.* 1:797, 1976.

206. Greenwood, B. M., Whittle, H. C., and Bryceson, A. D. M. Allergic complications of meningococcal disease. II. Immunological investigations. *Br. Med. J.* 2:737, 1973.

207. Tumbusch, W. T., Vogel, E. H., Jr., Butkiewicz, J. V., et al. Septicemia in burn injury. *J. Trauma* 1:22, 1961.

208. Pruitt, B. A., Jr. Infections caused by *Pseudomonas* species in patients with burns and in other surgical patients. *J. Infect. Dis.* 130:58, 1974 (suppl.).

209. Pavlovskis, O. R., and Shackelford, A. H. *Pseudomonas aeruginosa* exotoxin in mice: localization and effect on protein synthesis. *Infect. Immun.* 9:540, 1974.

210. Pavlovskis, O. R., and Gordon, F. B.: *Pseudomonas aeruginosa* exotoxin: effect on cell cultures. *J. Infect. Dis.* 125:631, 1972.

211. Iglewski, B. H., and Kabat, D. NAD-dependent inhibition of protein synthesis by *Pseudomonas aeruginosa* toxin. *Proc. Natl. Acad. Sci. USA* 72:2284, 1975.

212. Iglewski, B. H., Liu, P. V., and Kabat, D. Mechanism of action of *Pseudomonas aeruginosa* exotoxin A: adenosine diphosphate-ribosylation of mammalian elongation factor 2 *in vitro* and *in vivo*. *Infect. Immun.* 15:138, 1977.

213. Pollack, M., Callahan, L. T., III, and Taylor, N. S. Neutralizing antibody to *Pseudomonas aeruginosa* exotoxin in human sera: evidence for *in vivo* toxin production during infection. *Infect. Immun.* 14:942, 1976.

214. Bjornson, A. B., and Michael, J. G. Biological activities of rabbit immunoglobulin M and immunoglobulin G antibodies to *Pseudomonas aeruginosa*. *Infect. Immun.* 2:453, 1970.

215. Young, L. S. Role of antibody in infection due to *Pseudomonas aeruginosa*. *J. Infect. Dis.* 130:5, 1974 (suppl.).

216. Reynolds, H. Y., Levine, A. S., Wood, R. E., et al. *Pseudomonas aeruginosa* infections: persisting problems and current research to find new therapies. *Ann. Intern. Med.* 82:819, 1975.

217. Baltch, A. L., and Griffin, P. E. *Pseudomonas aeruginosa* bacteremia: a clinical study of 75 patients. *Am. J. Med. Sci.* 274:119, 1977.

218. Høiby, N. *Pseudomonas aeruginosa* infection in cystic fibrosis. Diagnostic and prognostic significance of *Pseudomonas aeruginosa* precipitins determined by means of crossed immunoelectrophoresis. A survey. *Acta Pathol. Microbiol. Scand.* 262:1, 1977 (suppl.).

219. Hann, S., and Holsclaw, D. S. Interactions of *Pseudomonas aeruginosa* with immunoglobulins and complement in sputum. *Infect. Immun.* 14:114, 1976.

220. Sorenson, R. U., Stern, R. C., and Polmar, S. H. Cellular immunity to bacteria: impairment of *in vitro* lymphocytes responses to *Pseudomonas aeruginosa* in cystic fibrosis patients. *Infect. Immun.* 18:735, 1977.

221. Shackelford, P. G., Campbell, J., and Feigin, R. D. Countercurrent immunoelectrophoresis in the evaluation of childhood infections. *J. Pediatr.* 85:478, 1974.

222. Ingram, D. L., Anderson, P., and Smith, D. H. Countercurrent immunoelectrophoresis in the diagnosis of systemic diseases caused by Hemophilus influenzae Type B. *J. Pediatr.* 81:1156, 1972.

223. Coonrod, J. D., Feigin, R. D., Wong, M. L., et al. CIE detection of bacterial antigens in meningitis. *J. Pediatr.* 90:676, 1977.

224. Pifer, L., Elliot, S., Woodard, T., et al. An improved method for detection of Hemophilus influenzae b antigen in cerebrospinal fluid. *J. Pediatr.* 92:227, 1978.

225. Henderson, W. H. Synergistic bacterial gangrene following abdominal hysterectomy. *Obstet. Gynecol.* 49:24s, 1977 (1 suppl.).

226. McGouran, R. C., and Emmerson, G. A. Symmetrical peripheral gangrene. *Br. Heart J.* 39:569, 1977.

227. Touraine, R., Baruch, J., Revuz, J., et al. La gangrène streptococcique. Importance du traitement chirurgical. *Nouv. Presse Med.* 6:247, 1977.

228. Fishberg, A. M. Redistribution of blood in heart failure. *J. Clin. Invest.* 17:510, 1938.

229. Hejtmancik, M. R., and Bruce, E. I. Symmetrical peripheral gangrene complicating pulmonary embolism. *Am. Heart J.* 45:298, 1953.

230. Cohen, H. Peripheral gangrene in a case of myocardial infarction. *Br. Med. J.* 2:1615, 1961.

CHAPTER 2

Parasitic Infections

Parasitic infestation of man and of animals involves a more commensal, less adversary setting than that encountered in the usual bacterial infection. In many instances host and parasite coexist over an extended period in a very close relationship, and this chronic association may result in a prolonged and often intense host immune response. Considerable attention has been directed to apparent shared autoantigens, which many parasites have learned to adapt from their hosts. It seems clear that the schistosomes, certainly the trypanosomes, and to a lesser extent many other parasitic forms have learned to adapt native substances and antigens derived from their host to themselves—particularly in their outer coating, which has the most direct contact with host tissues. In many ways, from a theoretic standpoint, this interface between host and parasite resembles the embryonic trophoblast and somehow seems impervious to both cell-mediated and humoral immune reactions.

At the same time there are abundant indications that a number of human parasites are capable of inducing a strong immune response during certain parts of the parasitic life cycle. In diseases such as chronic malaria, trypanosomiasis, or schistosomiasis the immune response may be characterized by hypergammaglobulinemia, activation and stimulation of major segments of the reticuloendothelial system, and peripheral sequelae of both T-cell– and B-cell–mediated immune phenomena. Examples of the latter can be recognized in the visceral manifestations of trypanosomiasis or the chronic cycles of localized liver or lung granu-

lomata in the case of *Schistosoma mansoni* infection. Thus, when one examines peripheral or localized immune reaction in the host, schistosomal granulomata are the end result of an active delayed-type hypersensitivity reaction, probably mediated for the most part by activated T cells (1–4). If animals are depleted of their T cells by either prior thymectomy or thoracic-duct drainage, the development of typical schistosomal granulomata is attenuated or even aborted.

In the case of human or experimental malaria, there is also strong indication of a profound immune response. Regardless of the visibility and appropriate nature of the immune response in such diseases as schistosomiasis and malaria, the host cannot rid itself completely of the parasite. In many respects the immune response to malarial parasites appears to be malaria antigen-specific but is often surprisingly ineffective. The same may be said of schistosomiasis and trypanosomiasis. In parasitic disorders where many intermediate forms of the parasite exist for brief periods in the host, the variety of such forms serves to complicate the question of what in effect constitutes an adequate immune response. The invading parasite is constantly changing its form, and probably its antigenic constitution. There is the general impression, particularly with respect to a disorder like malaria, that if immunity can be induced by vaccines against a key or most vulnerable form of the intricate parasitic life cycle, then effective protection may result. Chameleon-like, many parasites are capable of rapid alteration to blend with their environment, often before the host has time to mobilize an effective immune reaction.

Because of the chronicity of disease and the familiar phenomenon of relapse, the malaria parasitic infection has been the most extensively examined for evidence of antigenic variation. It is now accepted that antigenically distinct examples of parasites as monitored by challenge experiments may be present within a single malaria parasite strain. Probably central to the perplexity surrounding an effective immune response in malaria are the well-known differences in immunologic resistance of various stages of the parasite in its life cycle. Evidence for marked antigenic variation within single strains has been presented by several groups (5, 6). It seems likely that the host immune response itself may directly stimulate antigenic variation via absorbed antibody or lymphokines released during various phases of cell-mediated immune reaction.

Many techniques have been used to demonstrate various types of antiparasitic antibody. In malaria there appears to be parasite-directed as well as nonparasite-directed antibody, which functions almost like "background noise" without readily identifiable effect on the course of the infection. The degree to which hypergammaglobulinemia present in schistosomiasis or trypanosomiasis is also background noise without a clearly defined role as effective parasite-directed antibody is not at present clearly identified. It seems possible that a considerable portion of IgG antibody in many parasitic diseases may actually represent IgG anti-γ-globulin or rheumatoid factor, or possibly antibody of anti-idiotypic specificity.

In malaria as well as in other parasitic diseases that have for millennia afflicted large numbers of the world's population, important selective factors probably are responsible for changes in the quality as well as the magnitude of the immune response. There is a substantial amount of evidence that some degree of genetic resistance to human malaria may be conferred both by the sickle-cell gene and the glucose-6-phosphatase dehydrogenase (6-GPD)-deficiency gene (8–10). In the modern context it seems possible, therefore, that particular immune-response (IR) genes may be linked in some way to those selecting for a more effective natural resistance to malarial infection. Precise analysis of malarial immune functions and attention to segregation of HLA loci will be necessary to examine this question. As yet, there are no clear markers universally accepted as coded for by IR genes in man, though some linkage between Ia antigens and specific histocompatibility loci has been clearly defined in the mouse.

Besides evidence for hyperimmune response in several of the major parasitic infestations, it is important to recognize that there appears to be a complex cacophony of effects of parasitic infection on the immune response. In addition to hyperactive immunity, hypergammaglobulinemia, or accelerated cell-mediated immune response, in many parasitic disorders definite immunosuppressive features are present; several recent studies have emphasized this aspect of parasitic infestation. Adherent spleen cells show gross deficiencies as accessory or processing cells in the spleens of malaria-infected mice (11). Distinct immunosuppression on antigenic challenge with pneumococcal polysaccharide can be demonstrated in animals infected with malaria (12, 13). Studies of specific splenic function have also shown that enhanced protection or opsonization may be accompanied by a certain degree of immune suppression (14). Since splenic involvement is so prominent in many chronic parasitic infections, it may well be that splenic suppressor cells (15) may be activated as innocent bystanders and participate in a variety of modulations or depressions of the immune response. More evidence is needed to support the notion that parasitic infections such as malaria or schistosomiasis activate suppressor cells. The hypothesis is very attractive on general principles, since it may help to explain many of the seeming contradictions or discrepancies related to immune reactivity in a number of chronic parasitic infections.

One of the most interesting aspects of the role of immune complexes in parasitic diseases is possible tolerance to parasitic antigens and its effect on successive generations of infected individuals. Pertinent observations have been presented by Lewart and Mandlowitz (16), who noted that the mean diameters of schistosomal lung granulomata in mice born to infected mice were smaller than in those born to noninfected mothers. These findings raised the question of possible antenatal transfer of parasitic schistosomal antigen to the fetus or induction of partial tolerance. Thus, when such animals born to infected mothers reached adulthood and became infected, antenatal tolerogenic parasite antigen exposure might conceivably modulate or influence the quality as well as the magnitude of the immune response. It seems possible that such potential tolerogenic exposure could also influence subsequent immunoglobulin class or even avidity of antibody stimulated by reexposure and natural infection. When such tolerogenic circumstances are repeated generation after generation, there may also be positive selective factors at work enhancing natural immunity as well.

Data bearing directly on these points have been accumulated in the experimental schistosomal model, which indicated that large doses of eggs given neonatally induced tolerance, whereas low doses induced active sensitization and an appropriate immune response (17). A recent study in human infants born to mothers infected with schistosomiasis showed that a considerable proportion of such children showed delayed-type hypersensitivity to testing with intradermal schistosomal antigens (18). No precise information is yet available, however, on the influence of prenatal antigen exposure on quantity, Ig class, or avidity of antibody response—all of which may be critical factors in the actual pathogenesis of immune-complex deposition many years later in the infected adult host.

In the analysis that follows, attention is focused on three types of parasitic infection—malaria, schistosomiasis, and trypanosomiasis—since most of the information presently available relates to these parasitic disorders. By way of introduction it is also important to point out that studies of the remote effects of immune complexes in parasitic infestations have provided some of the best-developed and most fascinating examples of the importance of immune complexes in modern clinical medicine.

Malaria

The clinical association between certain forms of malaria and nephropathy was recognized quite early, even before the turn of the century (19). The relationship was so close that it prompted Giglioli to predict correctly that certain forms of renal disease would disappear in various populations after subsequent successful control of their malaria (20, 21). In studies initiated in the mid-1950s, particularly in Nigeria and Uganda, it became clear that the presentation of nephrotic syndrome among African children in these regions was slightly different from the nephrosis observed in North America or in Europe. The peak incidence of nephrotic syndrome was between age two and three years in Europe or in the United States, whereas in East Africa it occurred at age five. In addition, among affected African children a close correlation with *Plasmodium malariae* infection was noted (22–24). Early studies by Dixon (25) indicated that nephrosis in these African children was associated with deposition of immunoglobulin and complement in involved glomeruli. Subsequent studies have clearly established that an immune-complex glomerulitis is present. A rather granular pattern of deposition of IgM, IgG, IgA, and complement components as well as malarial antigen has been documented in a number of immunofluorescence studies (25–27).

Examples of typical lesions associated with *P. malariae* immune-complex glomerulopathy are shown in Figures 2-1 and 2-2. Ultrastructural analysis in many of the children afflicted with immune-complex nephrotic syndrome and moderately advanced disease showed definite electron-dense deposits, often characterized by peculiar and rather unique lacunae near such deposits, particularly in the basement membrane (28). Light microscopic studies indicated that the pathology in such patients consisted of a nonspecific membranous glomerulonephritis with progressive glomerular sclerosis and secondary tubular changes (22). Immunofluores-

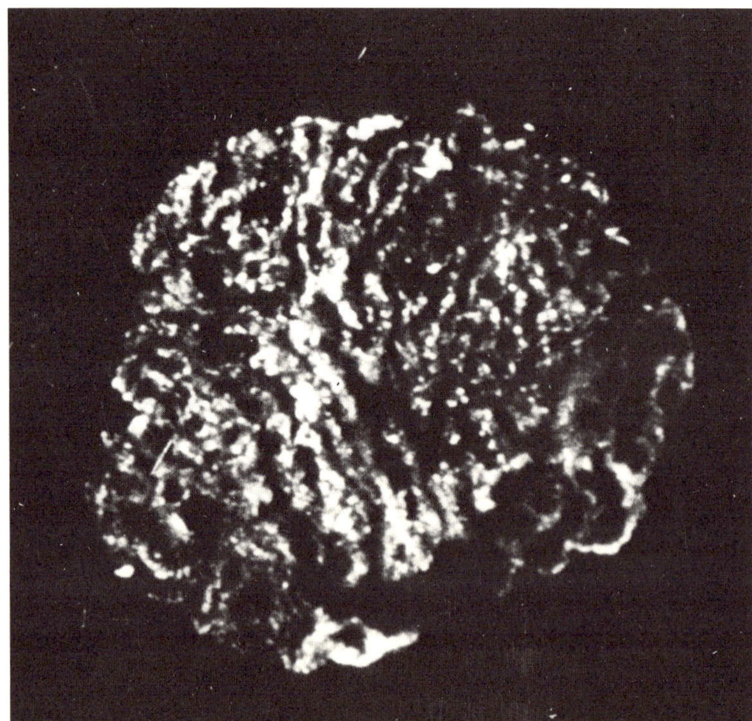

Figure 2-1 Glomerular immuno-fluorescence localization of IgG in a patient with quartan malaria and nephropathy. Punctate granular localization of immunoglobulin is present. Magnification × 300. (Photograph courtesy of V. Houba, Nairobi, Kenya.)

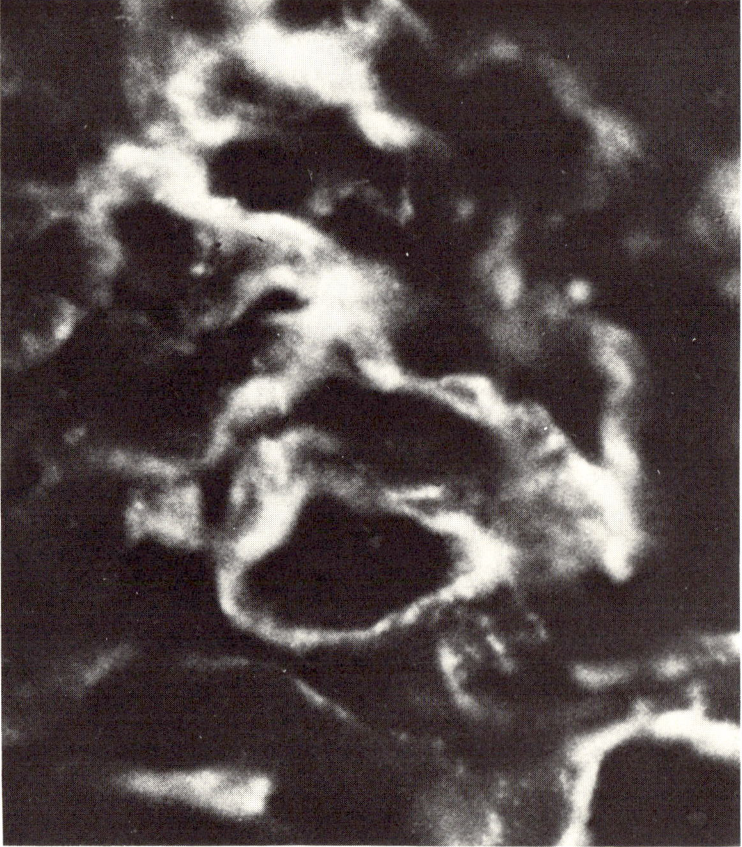

Figure 2-2 Glomerular capillary immunofluorescence localization of IgM in a patient with malarial nephropathy. Irregular immune-complex deposits in lumpy-bumpy distribution are noted. Magnification × 400. (Photograph courtesy of V. Houba, Nairobi, Kenya.)

cence demonstration of *P. malariae* antigen in *P. malariae* nephrotic syndrome is shown in Figure 2-3.

Antibody eluted from involved renal tissue showed precipitins with preparations containing *Plasmodium malariae* antigens (27). It has been known for some time that various types of malarial infection are often associated with demonstrable circulating parasitic antigens (28). However, little is yet known of the precise physical characteristics, derivation, or size of such antigens. Whether they represent only materials derived from the parasite or products of altered autologous tissue complexed with malarial antigens remains to be determined. More recent studies by Lambert and Houba have provided further direct evidence for localization of malarial antibodies in renal tissue (29, 30). IgG isolated from anti–*Plasmodium malariae* sera showed specific renal localization when labeled with ^{125}I and injected into patients with nephritis; moreover, sensitive radioimmunologic studies confirmed the presence of parasitic antigen in serum samples from acutely ill malarious subjects. The dem-

onstration of localization of labeled IgG to involved renal tissue in these reports suggests that there may be considerable renal malarial antigen not covered up or otherwise hidden by tissue-fixed immunoglobulin that is still capable of inducing accumulation of immunoglobulin in affected glomeruli. Localization of antimalarial antibody in the infected kidney was demonstrated by the same workers in *aotus* monkeys experimentally infected with *P. malariae* (29, 30). Binding of intravenously injected specific antimalarial antibody to antigens or circulating antigen-antibody complexes using radiolabeling techniques strengthens their role as mediators of renal injury. It is also possible that a phenomenon of replacement of low-affinity antibody bound in tissues by circulating high-affinity antibody may be taking place.

Studies recently summarized by Houba are helpful in interpretation of these data. In renal biopsy samples from 93 patients including 50 children and 43 adults, immunoglobulins G and M were detected in 96 percent, the third complement component in 66 percent, and *P.*

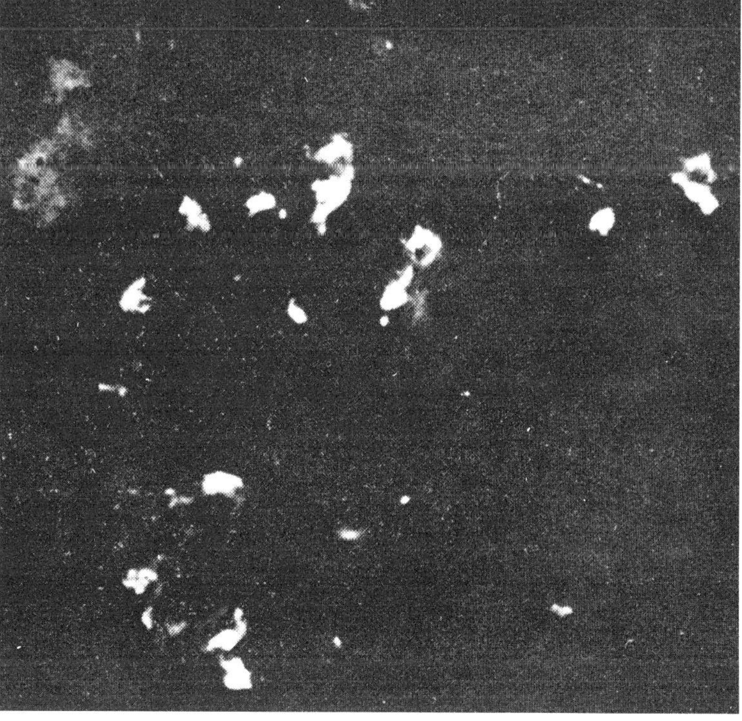

Figure 2-3 An irregular pattern of deposits, presumably malarial antigen (*P. malariae*), along glomerular capillary loops. Magnification × 350. (Reproduced with permission, P. A. Ward and J. W. Kibukamusoke, *Lancet* 1:283, 1969.)

malariae antigen in 25 percent of cases (31). A summary of these data is shown in Table 2-1. Moreover, an interesting profile of IgG H-chain subgroup deposition was noted. Coarse granular immunoglobulin deposits always showed IgG-3 alone or in combination with others, but never IgG-2. In patients with fine granular Ig deposition, a predominance of IgG-2 was noted. Moreover, tissue fixation or distribution of C3 was much more closely associated with IgM than with apparent relative quantitative amounts of IgG. Houba noted a relationship between relative response to treatment and patients who showed coarse granular or mixed granular immunofluorescence patterns of immunoglobulin deposition in renal biopsy material. These results are shown in Table 2-2.

The finding that malarial antigens tend to be localized or fixed in renal glomeruli perhaps represents an important lead in the understanding of immune-complex nephritis. These data are reminiscent of similar work recently published, which indicates a strong local affinity or primary homing of DNA for structures in the renal glomerulus (32). Thus, part of the mechanism that makes certain antigens particularly effective in initiating immune complex nephropathy may relate to their initial primary physical interaction or adherence for vulnerable sites in renal tissue. Very little attention has been directed to this aspect of pathogenesis; for such an approach to be developed with respect to malarial nephropathy, considerably more precise definition of the chemical composition and structure of the putative malarial antigens involved will be necessary.

One of the most discouraging features of the immune-complex glomerular involvement in quartan malaria is its relatively dismal prognosis—regardless of corticosteroids, immunosuppressives, or concomitant specific anti-

Table 2-1 Incidence of positive immunofluorescence staining for immunoglobulins, complement, and antigens in renal biopsies of patients with nephrotic syndrome.

| | | Immunoglobulins | | | | Comple-ment | Antigens | |
Subjects	No. examined	Total GG	IgG	IgG & IgM	IgM	C3	*P. malariae*	*P. falciparum*
Children	50	48	17	27	4	33	9[a]	0[a]
Adults	43	42	23	16	3	25	11	1
Total	93	90	40	43	7	58	20[b]	1[b]

Source: Reproduced with permission, V. Houba, *Bull. WHO* 52:199, 1975.
[a] 36 examined.
[b] 79 examined.

Table 2-2 Correlation of immunofluorescence patterns with response to treatment in nephrotic children with malaria.

| | Immunofluorescence staining | | | | | Response to treatment | | |
Pattern	Total GG	IgG	IgG & IgM	IgM	Comple-ment	Good	Fair	None
Coarse granular	19	5	2	12	16	7	3	9
Mixed granular	15	3	0	12	12	3	1	11
Fine granular	7	6	0	1	1	0	0	7
Total	41	14	2	25	29	10	4	27

Source: Reproduced with permission, V. Houba, *Bull. WHO* 52:199, 1975.

malarial therapy (22–24). The actual renal pathology is characterized by capillary-wall thickening and progressive mesangial sclerosis, with eventual total glomerular sclerosis and progressive loss of renal function. Studies conducted by Hendrickse (24) indicated that clinical features suggesting selective proteinuria rather than total or unselective urinary protein loss were generally more responsive initially to corticosteroid therapy. Whether or not selective proteinuria or relative patterns of immunofluorescence can be correlated with eventual long-term prognosis probably awaits a much more prolonged analysis.

In contrast to the situation observed with *P. malariae* nephritis and nephrotic syndrome, acute rather transient renal lesions probably also related to immune-complex disease have been described in other malarial syndromes, particularly when seen with falciparum infections (33, 34). It has been found that albuminuria during acute falciparum infection was accompanied by IgM, as well as by glomerular complement deposition along glomerular basement membranes and mesangial areas. Malarial antigen has also been observed in such patients, by the immunofluorescence technique (34). In these acute studies the interval between first febrile reaction and the time of renal biopsy was quite short, 6 to 23 days. Histological examination showed expansion of mesangial areas and hyperplasia of endothelial cells. Glomerular basement membranes were thickened, and electron-dense deposits were recorded. It was concluded that many such lesions actually cleared relatively rapidly and that in most instances the glomerular pathology was entirely reversible; changes were not detected in renal biopsies obtained 30 to 40 days after onset.

Experimental models for the study of malaria immune-complex nephropathy in mice have also provided interesting insights into several features of the disease. Studies using *P. berghei Yoelii* induced brisk parasitemia, and circulating antibody became detectable after seven days, at which time serum C3 levels decreased. Early renal lesions in this experimental mouse model were localized to the mesangium with later, more widespread involvement

of subepithelial portions of glomerular capillary loops (35). In the course of the experimental malarial nephropathy, as in the human counterpart with *P. malariae,* treatment with corticosteroids, immunosuppressive agents, anticoagulants, antiplatelet agents, and indomethacin did not arrest or significantly alter deposition of immune complexes. By contrast, when antigenemia was significantly reduced or eliminated, the progress to glomerulonephritis was prevented (35). Other studies using a mouse malaria model have directly correlated appearance of soluble malarial antigen with progression of the nephritis (36). In most such studies, however, immune sera have been used as sources for antibody to malarial or parasite-related antigen, and no complete physicochemical characterization of such antigens has yet been provided. It is not clear, for instance, that precipitin reactions developing between sera from immune animals and acute serum associated with peak parasitemia might not be 7 S IgG rheumatoid factor reacting with autologous immune complexes in the acute serum.

Several additional aspects of malaria may also be related to mechanisms induced by immune complexes. A rare condition known as malarial lung has been recognized by clinicians for some time. It is most often characterized by rapid onset of acute pulmonary edema during falciparum malaria (37). The condition is associated with acute pulmonary insufficiency and interstitial edema in the absence of cardiac failure. There is some evidence that this complication may be ushered in by disseminated intravascular coagulation (38), but other studies have suggested microcirculatory pulmonary dysfunction, blood element clumping, or an acute hypersensitivity reaction (37, 39). No immunopathologic data are present as yet to help define the etiology. Successful treatment has recently been reported by means of intermittent positive-pressure ventilation (40).

There is some indication that adsorption of malaria-induced serum antigen onto red cells may in fact induce adsorption of immune complexes and mediate anemia itself in acute malaria infections of chickens (41). If confirmed in other experimental models and other species, such a mechanism might explain the actual anemia of malaria on the basis of erythrocyte-adsorbed autologous immune complexes. More work is needed to examine this possibility in greater detail.

Finally, with respect to the relationship between immune complexes and malaria, there are many questions still unanswered. It is not clear why immune complexes are trapped in glomeruli primarily in *P. malariae* infections, in contrast to infections caused by *P. falciparum* or other forms of malaria. Immunofluorescence studies have shown malaria antigens in glomerular lesions (31); however, malarial parasites themselves are rarely noted in the specific lesions (42). Glomerular malarial immune-complex trapping could possibly be initiated by other factors, such as the physical nature of malarial antigens themselves or local release of enzymes by parasites or parasitized tissues. The propensity for chronic and often progressive renal involvement to be associated with *P. malariae* infections may indeed be related to a more prolonged or sustained-action release of antigens. *P. malariae* merozoites recycle in hepatic cells and are capable of perpetuating infection for very long periods of time. The particular type of sustained antigen release associated with *P. malariae* infection may be most compatible with production of the right size or physical properties of immune complexes most likely to lodge in vulnerable glomeruli. As yet no data are available on this particular question.

Another parameter that has probably not received enough attention in this respect are possible differences in affinity of the antimalarial antibodies primarily responsible for immune-complex deposition. Evidence has been put forward by several groups to indicate that low-affinity antibodies are perhaps most often associated with renal deposition or progressive immune-complex damage (43–45). Observations by Houba and co-workers are relevant to this point, since it was found that immunoglobulins were eluted from renal tissue at two different pH levels—pH 5.5 to 6.0 and below pH 3.0 (31). More work is needed before the exact role of antibody affinity can be elucidated in the immune-complex disease associated with malaria. The persistence and progression of

glomerular lesions, particularly in *P. malariae* infection, is poorly understood. To postulate a constant or unremitting supply of malarial parasitic antigen as the most likely explanation is probably a gross oversimplification; detection of such antigen clearly decreases with duration of disease, and progression is not favorably affected by intensive antimalarial treatment. It has been suggested that the malarial infection may initiate a self-perpetuating autoimmune process, by producing either altered tissue-antigenic components or material changed by enzymes somehow unique to the parasites themselves. There is also the remote possibility that materials within certain forms of the malarial parasite cross-react directly with autologous tissues, thereby inducing chronic ongoing autoimmune reactivity.

One of the conditions often described as affiliated with malaria is the so-called tropical splenomegaly syndrome (46, 47). This disorder is associated in some patients with considerable cryoglobulinemia or serum cryoprecipitates. It can also be associated with a depression in serum complement activity (48) and marked hypergammaglobulinemia. Although not specifically relegated to malaria as the sole or unique etiologic agent, in many populations tropical splenomegaly and chronic malarial infection appear to be related. Often an improvement is noted after prolonged malarial prophylaxis. There are reports documenting the presence of IgM, IgG, IgA, and C3 on erythrocytes from patients with tropical splenomegaly syndrome by means of sensitive enzymatic autoagglutinin or autoantibody methods (49); however, more work is needed to establish the influence, if any, of immune complexes adsorbed to erythrocytes in pathogenesis of the clinical picture.

Schistosomiasis

Schistosomes have been an important source of human morbidity and mortality in the world for at least five thousand years, with evidence of schistosomal infection demonstrated in the mummified remains of Egyptian monarchs. The schistosome itself appears to possess a unique method of evasion of host immune response by virtue of its evolution of a trilamellar outer membrane or membranocalyx. Studies by Wilson and Barnes have shown a remarkably rapid turnover of the tegumental membranocalyx of *Schistosoma mansoni* with a half-life of 2 to 3 hours (50). The outer surface or skin of the worm thus appears to be bounded or made up of a trilayered membrane that is constantly being replaced by the organism. Additional observations indicate that rate of turnover of membranocalyx may be accelerated in the presence of antischistosomal antibody adsorbed to the membranocalyx surface.

This constant turnover of outer membrane is a convenient method of escaping effective immune recognition and elimination by the host. It also may serve to provide continuous parenteral infusion of surface antigens constantly being extruded or eliminated from the membranocalyx. Such infusion has great theoretical importance in terms of induction of tolerance or as a continual source of parasitic antigens capable of inducing immune-complex formation. Figure 2-4 illustrates immunocytochemical localization of IgG on the surface of a schistosome worm.

Another property of schistosomal parasites is their ability to adsorb directly into their outer membranes various host glycoproteins or polysaccharides of immense biological importance. Studies by several groups have shown quite convincingly that *S. mansoni* can rapidly adsorb blood-group-like substances, serum proteins, and perhaps other cell surface materials such as Ia, HLA, or similar structural membrane constituents (51–55). Certain materials such as Lewis blood group substance are known to exist in plasma as glycolipids and may be capable of directly adhering to parasitic membrances (56). Whether or not the same type of mechanism is capable of transferring HLA or Ia cell surface antigens to the parasite membrane has not yet been unambiguously demonstrated. Despite the ingenious ways in which schistosomes evade host immune responses, there are clear indications that an immune reactivity is indeed initiated.

The most widely studied immune-complex disease associated with schistosomiasis is that seen in patients with *S. mansoni* infection. Early reports of glomerulosclerosis, mesangial thickening, and glomerulonephritis occurring in association with *S. mansoni* (57, 58) indicated that there was renal involvement in a certain proportion of subjects with hepatosplenic schistosomiasis. Later immunofluorescence and ultrastructural studies showed glomerular deposits of IgG and IgM as well as electron-dense deposits in these patients (59, 60). Experimental studies of *S. mansoni* in animals have also provided evidence for Ig, C, and parasite-related antigens in kidney material from infected mice and hamsters (61, 62). Moreover, reports have been published that describe nephrotic syndrome in association with *S. haematobium* infections (63), although the strong correlation with this type of schistosome has not been confirmed in subsequent followup studies (64, 65).

Several recent reports emphasize important aspects of the immune-complex nephropathy associated with schistosomiasis. The presence of schistosomal antigens in the blood, body fluids, and urine of afflicted hosts has been demonstrated by many workers both in patients and in experimental animals (66–72). A patient studied in detail by Falcão and Gould had progressed to a chronic uremic stage so severe that it necessitated a renal transplant (73). When this individual was later treated with an effective antischistosomal agent—niridazole—he experienced a transient relapse of renal dysfunction accompanied by proteinuria and a precipitious fall in serum complement. Thus, release of worm antigen reinduced immune-complex nephropathy in the transplanted kidney. In this particular instance, renal biopsy showed Ig, C3, and specific schistosomal worm antigen in the mesangium of the transplanted kidney. Representative illustrations from this carefully studied patient are shown in Figure 2-5.

Schistosomal antigen has also been detected in renal glomeruli by Hoshino-Shimuzi and colleagues (74). Material from 12 kidneys studied postmortem as well as via biopsy specimens showed glomerular localization of IgM, IgG, IgA, IgE, C3, and fibrin in most samples. *S. mansoni* antigen was found in two cases with proliferative nephritis. Renal eluates stained

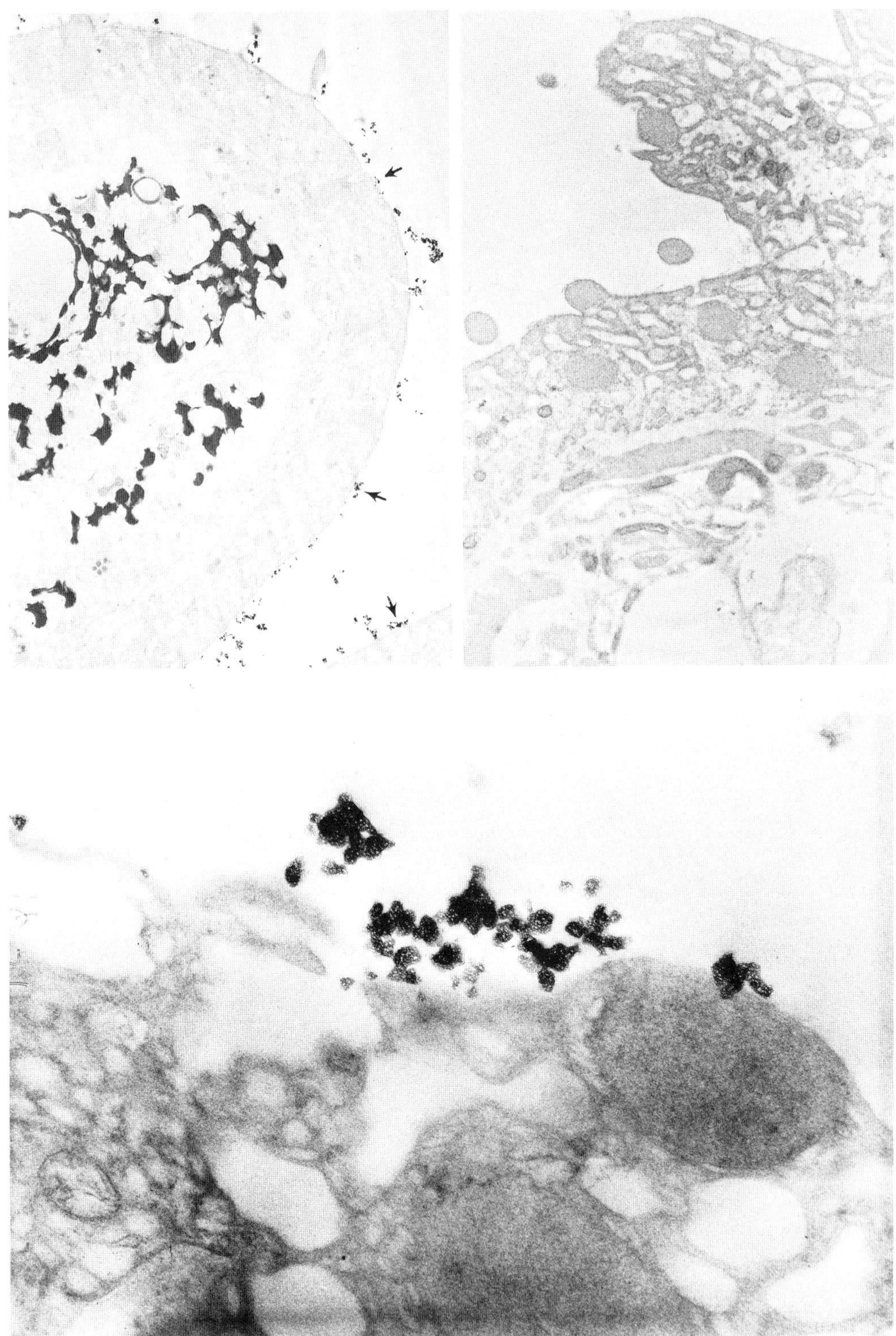

Figure 2-4 Immunocytochemical localization of IgG on the surface of *S. mansoni*. Magnifications above, × 10,000; below, × 40,000. (Reproduced with permission, W. M. Kemp and R. T. Damien, *J. Parasitology* 62:830, 1976.)

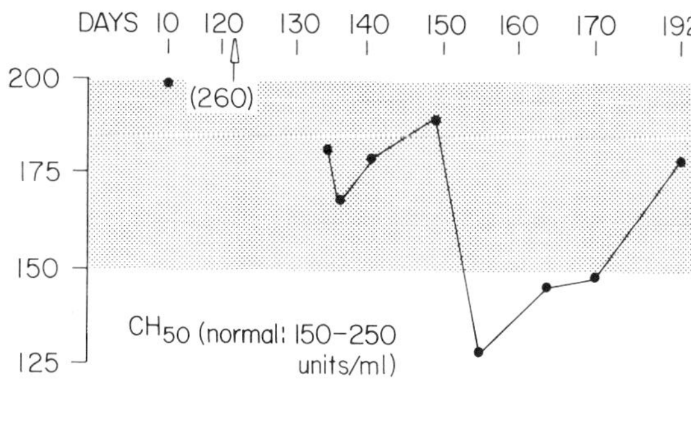
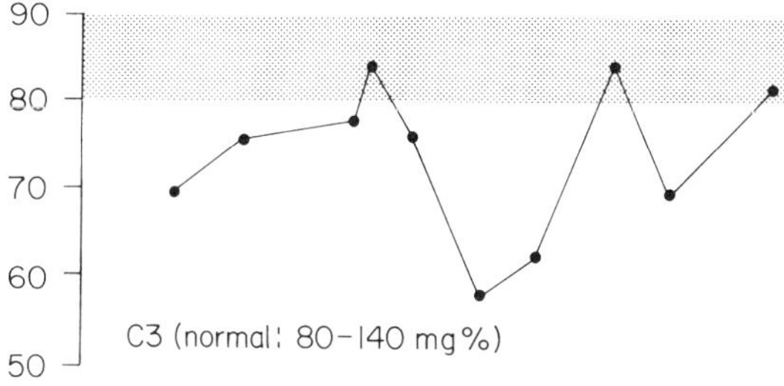
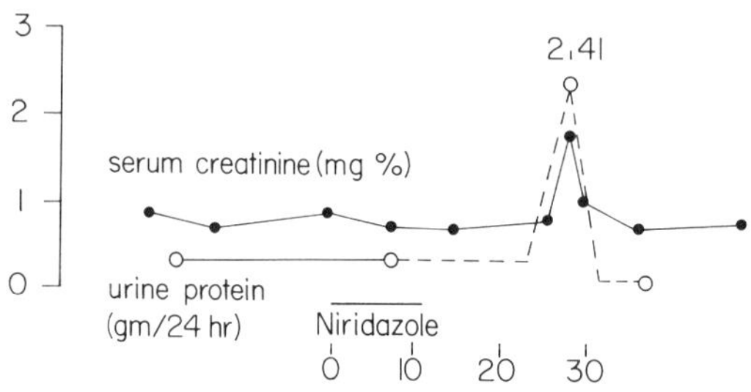

Figure 2-5 Serial serum levels of CH 50 and C3 before and after renal transplantation, with a depression of each before overt manifestations of acute schistosomal nephropathy on the twenty-eighth day after the start of niridazole therapy. Normal levels of C1q, C4, and C3PA were found with each determination. (Reproduced with permission, H. A. Falcão and D. B. Gould, *Ann. Intern. Med.* 83:148, 1975.)

schistosomal worm digestive tract strongly and gave weak reactions with schistosomal integument. These studies, which indicate preferential renal localization of schistosomal antigen concentrated in the gut of the worm, are of interest because other studies have confirmed the schistosomal gut derivation of this antigen, characterized as one that circulates in plasma or blood (75, 76). The punctate granular immunofluorescent localization of schistosomal antigen within renal glomeruli as well as the staining of worm gut antigens by kidney eluates are shown in Figure 2-6.

Studies by Bout and associates using several parallel methods showed detectable immune complexes in more than 60 percent of 65 subjects infected with *S. mansoni* (71). Actual quantitative levels were noted to be higher in patients with a mild rather than hepatosplenic form of the disease. The technique of precipitation of serum with polyethylene glycol allowed separation of antigen-antibody complexes from free parasite antigen in serum. IgE was detected in immune complexes precipitated by this method. At present, there is no body of evidence to suggest that IgE-antigen complexes participate actively in renal immune-complex injury.

A primate experimental model in baboons infected with *S. mansoni* indicated development of mild immune-complex glomerular lesions in 62 of 103 animals during infection (77). Adult worm as well as soluble egg antigen, together with IgM, IgG, and C3, were detected by immunofluorescence in most of the severe lesions. Mild lesions characterized by focal deposits of IgM were considered not to be associated with loss of renal function. However, the severe glomerular lesions were often characterized by intense IgG, complement, and parasite antigen deposition within glomerular capillary vessels. In some experimental animals in this prospective study, glomerular antigen deposition alone raised the possibility that such deposits were occurring first and that subsequent renal binding of antibody and complement might follow as a second step in the genesis of immune-complex lesions.

Schistosomiasis occurs in areas of the world that are also subject to a host of other enteric infections and fevers. The findings of Bassily and co-workers are significant in this regard (78). As mentioned in Chapter 1, these workers have described nephrotic syndrome in patients with double infections involving *Salmonella paratyphi A* and *S. mansoni*. The former was cultured from blood and urine in all patients. Histological examination of renal biopsy material showed enlarged glomeruli and increased cellularity with polymorphonuclear in-

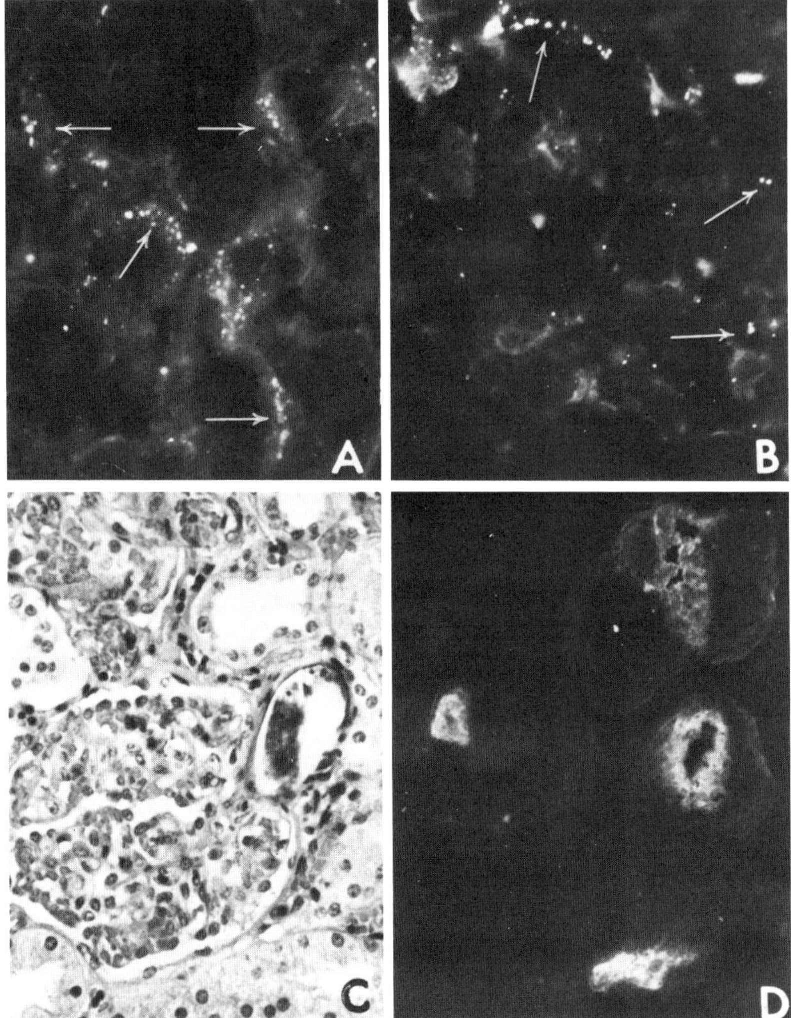

Figure 2-6 *A*, schistosomal antigen granules demonstrated by direct immunofluorescence along the mesangium and walls of glomerular loops. Necropsy specimen, magnification × 475. *B*, similar distribution of antigen granules in part of the glomerulus of a patient undergoing renal biopsy. *C*, a kidney exhibiting proliferative glomerulitis. A viable egg of *S. mansoni* is seen impacted at the afferent artery. H&E × 190. *D*, fluorescent staining of the digestive tract of adult *S. mansoni* worms after treatment with eluates of kidney-fixed antibodies and antihuman IgG conjugate. Magnification × 76. (Reproduced with permission, S. Hoshino-Shimizu, T. de Brito, H. Y. Kanamura et al., *Trans. R. Soc. Trop. Med. Hyg.* 70:492, 1976.)

filtrates and occasional crescents. Immunofluorescence studies showed diffuse staining for IgG and IgM but no evidence for *Salmonella paratyphi* antigen in the kidney lesions. All patients had resolution or improvement of their nephrotic syndrome, however, only after effective treatment of their salmonella infection.

Finally, there is considerable evidence that chronic schistosomal infection in both man and experimental animals is associated with presence of circulating immune complexes. The area in the body that has received the most attention in this regard is the kidney; very little is known about how such circulating immune complexes affect the actual microenvironment around the worm or its eggs and other intermediate forms. However, there is considerable evidence that under certain circumstances immune complexes themselves may play a direct role in immunosuppression (79, 80). Whether this effect is mediated by blockage of Fc receptors on immunocompetent cells or by direct activation of suppressor cells is not yet known.

A few unusual complications of schistosomal infections may also be related to damage by immune complexes either circulating or fixed to cells. Several series of cases with apparent schistosomal involvement of the spinal cord have been reported (81–84). In most, no clear evidence has been presented for mediation of neurologic damage by immune complexes; however, biopsies in some cases have shown granulomata as well as the histological picture of a necrotizing myelitis. Since ova are sometimes seen in biopsy material from such patients, it may be that a localized delayed-type hypersensitivity mechanism is directly involved in pathogenesis.

Trypanosomiasis

Infection with trypanosomes is now recognized as a serious problem on three continents—Africa, the Americas, and Asia. In many ways trypanosomiasis resembles malaria and schistosomiasis; it is able to persist in the host and produce chronic, often debilitating, illness, perhaps partially through evasion of effective immune response on the part of the host, and to a certain extent through a modulated combination of immunostimulation followed later by immunosuppression.

Early studies by Taliaferro indicated that two types of humoral immune response were present during the first phase of experimental infection in rats (85, 86). Initially, an antibody termed "ablastin" appeared, which was not dependent in vitro on complement activation and which was capable of inhibiting reproduction of parasitic forms. After the ablastin response converted rapidly reproducing trypanosomes to a population of monomorphic adults, the second type of antibody produced was trypanocidal, and parasitic forms were often eliminated (86, 87). More recent studies indicate

that specific resistance to trypanosomes can be transferred in mice by B lymphocytes and immune serum, more readily than by T cells (88).

However, the precise role of T cells in mediating protection against the disease is not clear. Nude mice that are congenitally athymic showed ready susceptibility to infection with consistent and prolonged elevations of parasitemia (89). In these animals infected with *Trypanosoma musculi,* thymic reconstitution restored an effective immune response. Similar results relating to T-cell deprivation and accelerating the infection have been recorded by others (90).

The role of the complement system in experimental infection of mice has been studied extensively by Jarvinen and Dalmasso (91, 92). During experimental infection of normal rats with *T. lewisi,* a striking fall in both total hemolytic complement and C4 hemolytic activities occurred. Levels of C3 were also reduced. Actual functional levels of total complement and C4 were reduced to less than 10 percent of preinfection levels—regardless of actual numbers of parasites. Degree of complement consumption, however, did correlate with amount of parasitemia, as shown in Figure 2-7. When parasitemia was eliminated, normal levels of complement activity returned. Subsequent studies indicated that parasitemia was associated with rapid consumption and activation of the early-acting complement components with lesser degrees of activation or recruitment of the alternative complement pathway. Despite these findings, it was found that complement per se did not appear to play a major role in elimination of the experimental infection.

Recently, Greenwood and Whittle have studied similar phenomena in African patients with Gambian sleeping sickness (93). Low levels of C3, C4, and factor B were found in serum samples from most patients with both early and advanced trypanosomiasis. The C3 levels increased after antitrypanosomal therapy. Marked elevations of IgM were recorded, as had previously been the case in tropical splenomegaly syndrome (94). In addition, cryoglobulins containing mainly IgM and C3 were found in most sera. It was hypothesized that high-molecular-weight immune complexes composed

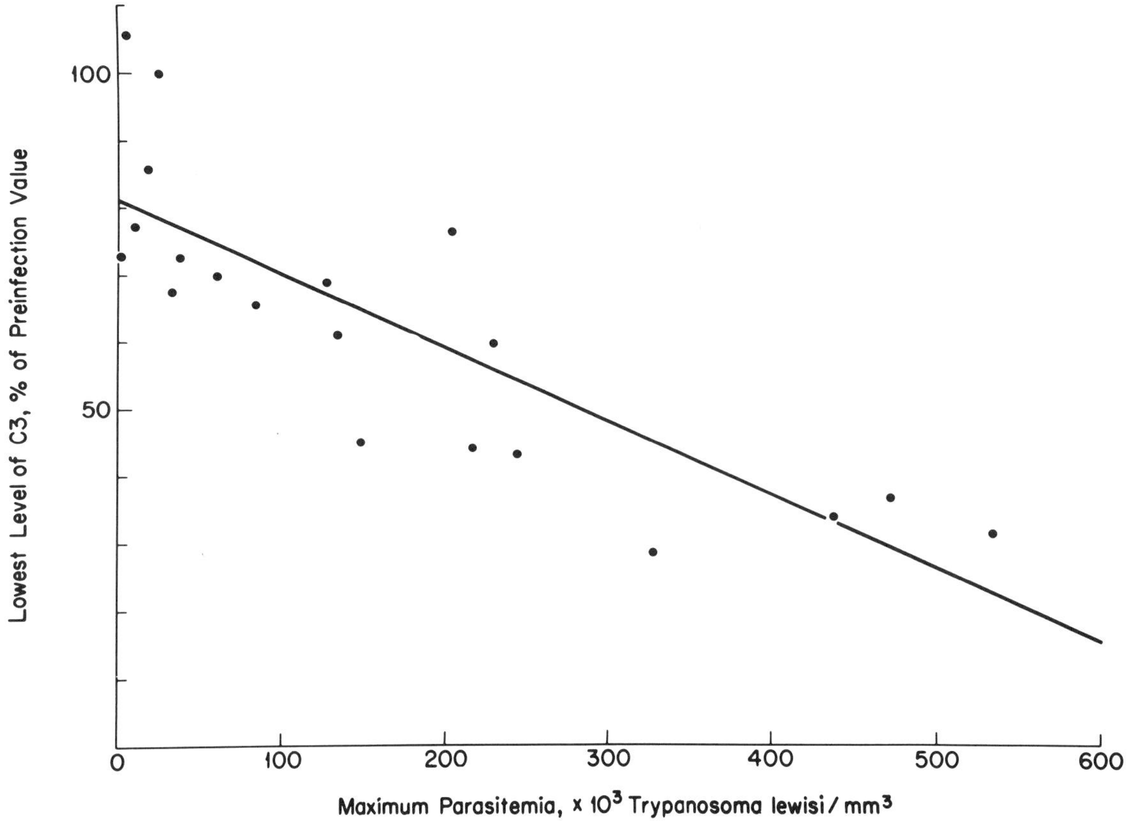

Figure 2-7   The relation of C3 to parasitemia in experimental trypanosomiasis of rats. (Reproduced with permission, J. A. Jarvinen and A. P. Dalmasso, *Infect. Immun.* 14:894, 1976.)

of IgM and activated complement components might be responsible for depression of complement in this disorder. Examples of quantitative changes in C3 and factor B of the alternate pathway in these patients are shown in Figure 2-8. Greenwood and Whittle noted that the patients studied showed no peripheral evidence of immune-complex disease—in particular, no proteinuria, clinical renal involvement, iritis, or peripheral vasculitis. They attributed this to the absence of smaller complexes—or at least of complexes capable of limited persistence— within the circulation and production of such discrete phenomena.

It is of great interest that patients with advanced forms of *T. gambiense* infection and central nervous system involvement show advanced pathological changes in cerebral vessels as well as in the meninges (95). The meninges themselves are thickened and show extensive infiltration with lymphocytes, plasma cells, and morular cells. The chronic mononuclear infiltration also extends into perivascular spaces; vascular damage, as well as brain infiltration with mononuclear cells, is common. Studies of cerebrospinal fluid (CSF) lymphocytes from patients with sleeping sickness showed that 5 percent were plasma cells, but that most of the CSF lymphocytes were B cells (96) in contrast to the usual conditions where the few lymphocytes present in normal CSF are felt to be T cells (97–99). In view of the elevation of IgM and B cells in CSF, it seems likely that some of the central nervous system tissue damage seen with this disease is mediated by local formation of immune complexes. Much more must still be learned concerning mechanisms that may act to localize immune complexes within the central nervous system.

As will be discussed in Chapter 5, evidence has now accumulated for a well-defined receptor for the activated third complement component in normal human glomeruli (100–102). Several factors could operate in a situation such as sleeping sickness to influence fixation or localization of immune complexes in the meningovascular areas. First, the parasites themselves or their antigenic residue may somehow have a unique physical predilection that initiates adherence in these anatomical areas. Thus, a local immune response mediated largely by B cells within the central nervous system and modulated via IgM antitrypanosomal antibody could produce local antibody capable of tissue deposition as part of immune complexes in situ in the central nervous system itself. Secondly, it is possible that the presence of the parasitic forms in the brain, or closely juxtaposed to meningovascular areas, somehow induces formation or expression of receptors capable of binding circulating as well as locally produced complexes. The precise problem involved in understanding the mechanism of central nervous system immune-complex–mediated phenomena, important in relating immune-complex phenomena to many clinical events, will recur repeatedly in subsequent discussions.

A great deal of experimental work has dealt with attempts to understand the role of cell-mediated immunity in various forms of trypanosomiasis. Early descriptions of the disease as seen in South American or Chagas' disease emphasized both the acute and the chronic form of the disorder (103–105). The etiologic agent causing the disease, *T. cruzi*, produces widespread infections in man and animals and is capable of parasitizing a variety of cell types including those of the myocardium. Characteristic features of the basic pathological process in this disease are accumulations of lymphocytes and macrophages within specific lesions (104); consequently, there have been a number of investigations on the role of cell-mediated immunity in this disorder. Many studies have

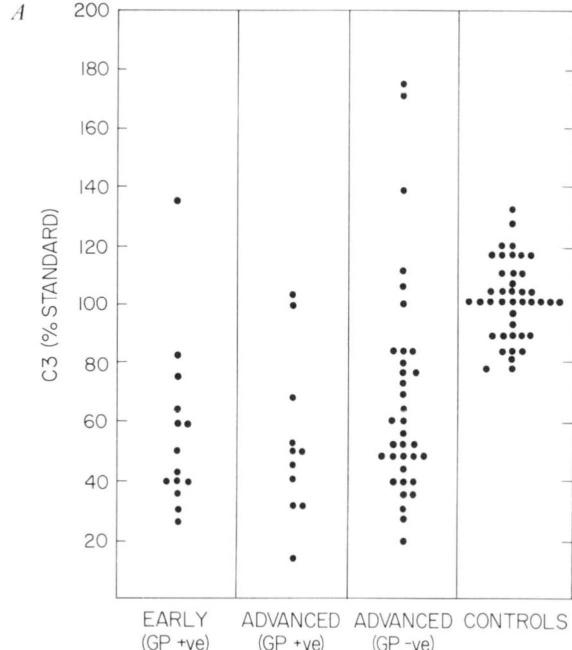

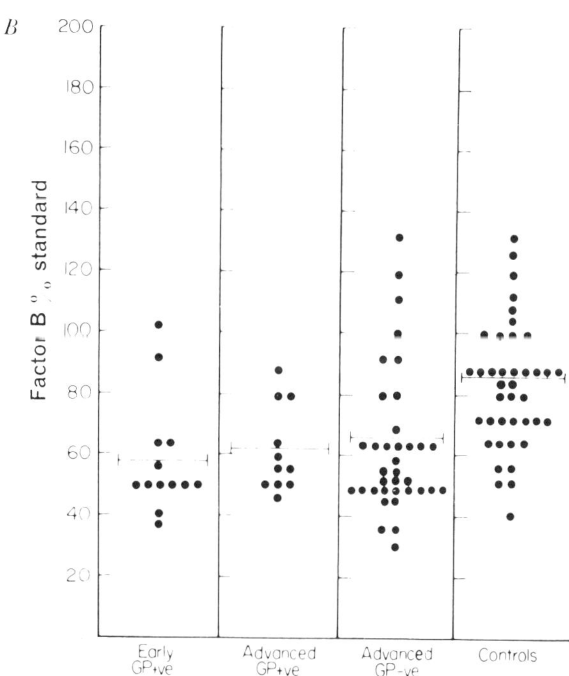

Figure 2-8 The mean and distribution of serum C3 levels (*A*) and serum factor B levels (*B*) in 60 patients with Gambian sleeping sickness and in 40 controls. GP = gland puncture. (Reproduced with permission, B. M. Greenwood and H. C. Whittle, *Clin. Exp. Immunol.* 24:133, 1976.)

provided evidence for delayed-type hypersensitivity toward antigens associated with the causative organism in this disease (106–108). As yet, there is no clear understanding of precisely how the several arms of the immune response interact or possibly negate one another during long-term human infection.

In several experimental animal models, Williams and associates (109, 110) have reported that activation of macrophages was capable of producing a marked increment in effective resistance to the intracellular multiplication of *T. cruzi.* Similar studies by Hoff showed no clear evidence for cross immunity in mice immunized with *T. cruzi* or BCG (111). Other groups of workers have provided evidence for specific immunity in animals afforded by prior immunization with avirulent or cross-reacting strains of trypanosomes (112, 113). Rabbits chronically infected with *T. cruzi,* as well as those immunized with various subcellar antigens prepared from *T. cruzi,* demonstrated intense cell-mediated immune reactions; however, immune sera and sensitized lymphocytes from either chronically infected or immunized animals did not have any effect on the infective trypomastigote forms of *T. cruzi* in vitro (104, 114).

Fascinating observations by Santos-Buch and Teixeira (114) have indicated that lymphocytes from rabbits sensitized either by *T. cruzi* infection or immunization with *T. cruzi* lysosome preparations were capable of destroying both parasitized and nonparasitized heart cells in vitro. Some increment in destruction of target heart cells was observed with parasitized heart cells, but destruction of nonparasitized normal heart cells was also recorded. These experimental results indicate the very ultimate in molecular mimicry by the parasite, for receptors on actively immunized lymphocytes appear to be cross reacting with antigens present on normal heart cells (114). Acute Chagas' disease represents an infection distributed in many organs—with lesions probably being related to the intracellular location of *T. cruzi* organisms (115). However, the chronic, slowly progressive form of Chagas' disease in humans is characterized by a diffuse myocarditis with persistent lymphocytic infiltration of myofibers in the absence of demonstrable parasites in situ. It has therefore been suggested repeatedly by several groups that Chagas' myocarditis may in fact result from an autoimmune or allergic state of the host (104, 114, 116).

It has long been recognized that trypanosomiasis, like malaria and schistosomiasis, is capable somehow of evading or effectively circumventing the immune response. One mechanism that has been identified in the African salivarian trypanosome infections of man and animals is antigenic variation. In these infections successive waves of blood parasitemia are characterized by a novel variant-specific glycoprotein antigen that does not react with antibodies induced against preceding waves of variants (117, 118), a feature that has important implications with respect to the formation of immune complexes in the host. If the primary antigen associated with the parasite, then, has a mechanism whereby it can change its immunodominant antigens rapidly with each fresh new wave of parasites, antibodies formed to preceding waves of antigen or even residual fragments of such antigens will necessarily be of low affinity. This is true in any short-lived immune response. In general, the length of the immune stimulus bears a direct relationship to the avidity of the antibody produced. If the postulates of Soothill and Steward (44) are correct, this sort of situation would be predestined to be that most likely to be associated with immune-complex disease. If low-affinity antibodies with low total-binding constants are capable of forming antigen-antibody lattices of such a magnitude as not to be cleared immediately by one passage through the circulation, then short antigenic bursts of stimulation such as are afforded by a particular parasite strain capable of extremely rapid antigenic variation should be most liable to induce immune-complex phenomena. Experimental confirmation of such a hypothesis is certainly now feasible.

Several other mechanisms pertinent to the discussion of general immunounresponsiveness in trypanosomiasis have also been suggested. Infections in animals and man are known to be associated with a marked increase in IgM. Furthermore, careful studies have shown that a large proportion of such IgM may indeed be "background noise" not specifically directed at antigens relevant to the infecting parasite (119–122). Recent related studies by Hudson and colleagues (123) are also of interest: they showed that mice infected with *T. brucei brucei* caused a progressive increase in plaque-forming cells producing antibodies to sheep red blood cells and in particular to cells coated with a highly substituted hapten (TNP). Such background responses have been ascribed in the past to a possible polyclonal B-cell activation such as that produced by lipopolysaccharide (124, 125). A subsequent relative immunosuppression is thought to result from B-cell clonal exhaustion and premature depletion of B cells capable of responding to the appropriate parasitic antigens.

The concept of immunoacceleration via the polyclonal B-cell activator mechanism has been explored experimentally by Mansfield and co-workers (126). Extracts of *T. brucei* and *T. congolense* were incubated with nonimmune lymphocytes of mice, rats, guinea pigs, and rabbits. The antigens failed to alter plant-mitogen–induced lymphocyte responses and were not by themselves mitogenic. Mild stimulation of lymphocytes from rabbit peripheral blood and spleen was recorded. In these experiments the extracts used did not function in the fashion of typical polyclonal activators; however, it is conceivable that artifically prepared extracts of parasites are different in terms of the repertoire of antigens they contain from those associated with the natural infection.

The concept of polyclonal B-cell activation as an impetus not only toward hypergammaglobulinemia but also toward autoantibody formation is supported by several interesting observations with regard to trypanosomiasis. Production of anti-γ-globulins is common (120); other autoantibodies, particularly against various intracellular antigens (one present in normal liver tissue) have been described by a number of workers (127, 128). It is important here to point out the recent descriptions by Cossio and co-workers (129) of a gamma-globulin factor present in the serum of patients with Chagas' disease, which reacts with endocardium and plasma membrane of striated muscle and endothelial cells (129, 130). This antibody may be the humoral counterpart of the self-reacting lymphocytes found in experimental Chagas' cardiomyopathy by Santos-Buch and colleagues (114, 115). Recent evidence indicates that this antibody can interact with living tissue as monitored in the isolated rat atrial appendage (131). Presence of the antibody in medium produced significant increases in frequency of contractions, an effect that could be blocked by pretreatment with β-adrenergic blocking agents but not with alpha blockers or histamine. It was suggested that this so-called EVI antibody (129–131) might be acting as a β-adrenergic agonist at the myocardial cell plasma membrane (131). If this work is confirmed and extended, it may represent a situation analogous to antibodies to acetylcholine receptors in patients with myasthenia gravis (132–134) or to insulin receptors in some rare instances of diabetes associated with hypergammaglobulinemia and acanthosis nigricans (135–137). Thus, immune complexes deposited in vivo in the course of Chagas' disease may interfere in an immune blockade of normal cardiac muscle fiber function. Examples of typical lesions seen in the myocarditis associated with cardiac involvement in trypanosomiasis (138) are shown in Figures 2-9 and 2-10. Reaction of the EVI antibody with cardiac tissues is shown in Figures 2-11 and 2-12 (139).

Enlargement of the spleen is common in both experimental and human trypanosomal infections. Evidence has now accumulated that this may be directly related to relative immunosuppression in the disorder itself. Evidence supporting stimulation or augmentation of suppressor T-cell mechanisms during experimental trypanosomal infection has been provided by several groups (140–142). In the report by Albright and associates (142) it was observed that serum as well as trypanosomal antigen preparations produced a certain amount of immunodepression in vitro. These findings may indicate that immune complexes themselves are capable of selectively defusing the immune response. As will be discussed in subsequent sections, there is already a con-

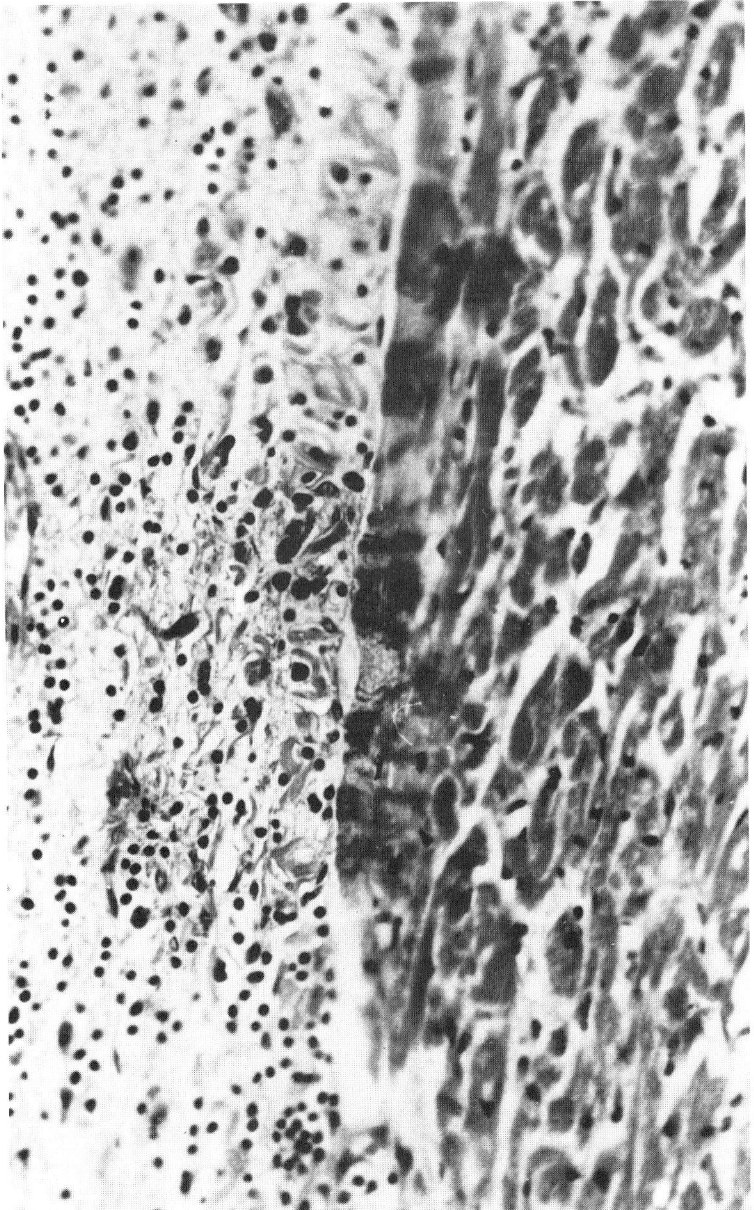

Figure 2-9 Parietal endocarditis and myocarditis in human African trypanosomiasis. Superficial myocytolysis is evident, with contraction bands and edematous and fibrous thickening of the endocardium and chronic cellular infiltration, H&E × 87. (Reproduced with permission, A. Poltera, J. N. Cox, and R. Owor, *Br. Heart J.* 38:827, 1976.)

siderable body of experimental evidence on the negative feedback effects of immune complexes on immune reactivity in a number of experimental situations.

An early observation by Ingram and Soltys (143) indicated that immunoconglutinin was markedly elevated in animals infected with *T. brucei*. Immunoconglutinin is considered to be an antibody to altered portions of the third complement component. Findings of substan-

tial immunoconglutinin elevation in trypanosomiasis are seen as evidence that immune complexes are released in significant amounts during various phases of the infection.

Studies by Nagle and co-workers (144) and Lambert and Houba (29) have documented immune-complex nephritis in both experimental animals and patients with trypanosomal infection. Moreover, there is evidence for a disseminated vasculitis in the course of the

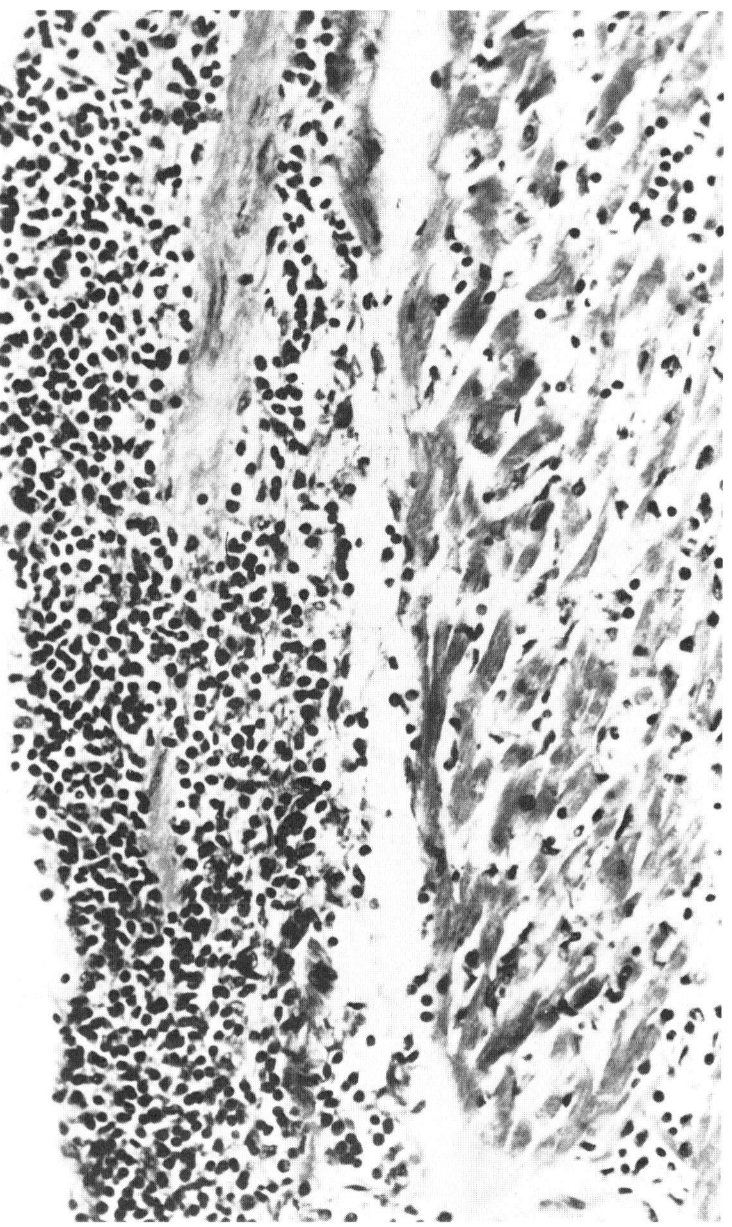

Figure 2-10 Linear dense infiltration with fragmentation of muscle fiber, which leads eventually to granuloma formation. H&E × 87. (Reproduced with permission, A. Poltera, J. N. Cox, and R. Owor, *Br. Heart J.* 38:827, 1976.)

disease with extensive lesions in brain and heart. Immunofluorescence studies in monkeys showed granular deposits of IgM, C3, and properdin (144). The Lambert and Houba studies in experimental mice demonstrated a high degree of parasitemia as well as renal mesangial proliferation and glomerular basement membrane thickening. Ultrastructural analysis showed electron-dense deposits and IgG, IgM, and C3 deposition by immunofluorescence.

Early immunofluorescence deposits were noted in renal mesangial areas, and later were recorded in capillary loops. Trypanosomal antigens also were identified by immunofluorescence in this study.

Of interest relative to antigenic variation is the fact that the trypanosomal antigens identified in glomeruli were those of the parasites in their initial wave of infection and were not related to parasitic antigens circulating at the

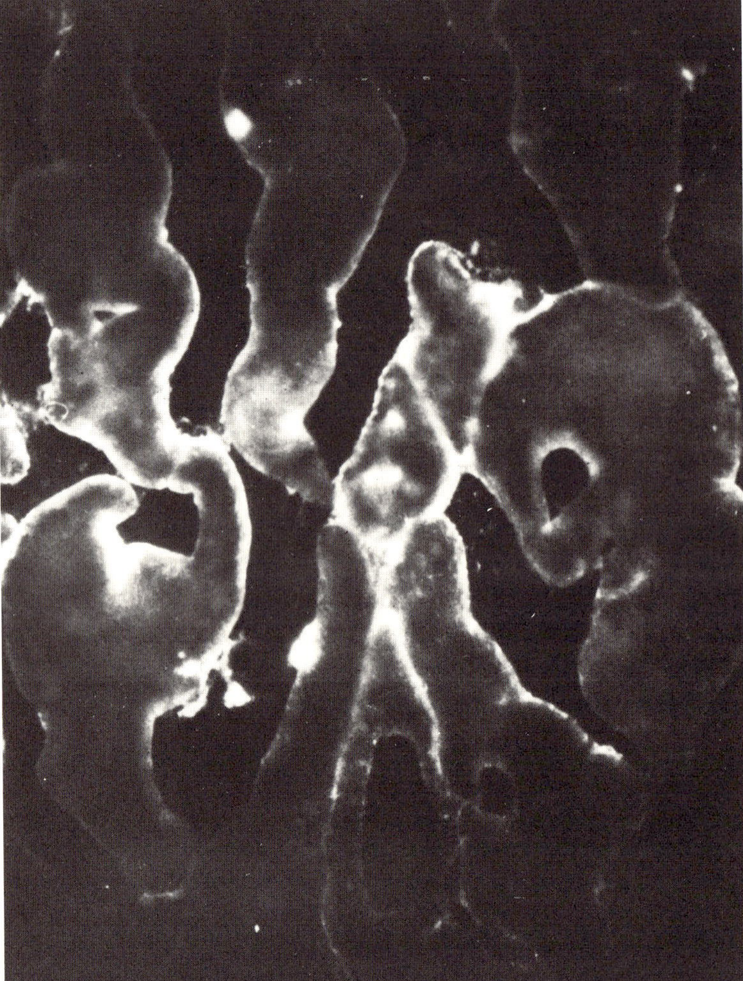

Figure 2-11 EVI antibody in a chagasic patient, demonstrated by direct immunofluorescence test. A myocardial section through the left ventricle of a patient with Chagas' disease has been treated with fluorescein-labeled goat γ-globulin anti-human γ-globulin. Positive staining for human γ-globulin is present in the sarcolemmal area. Magnification × 250. (Reproduced with permission, P. M. Cossio, R. P. Laguens, E. Kreutzer et al., *Am. J. Pathol.* 86: 533, 1977.)

time the animals were killed. These findings indicated immediate localization or some type of sequestration of early parasitic antigen in the glomerulus. The same data might also be compatible with an ongoing process of local immune-complex formation at sites of eventual localization of trypanosomal material during initial phases of parasitemia. Lambert and Houba also studied heart lesions in experimental mice and were able to identify degenerating as well as intact trypanosomes in relatively early lesions (29). These findings suggest that local formation of immune complexes within cardiac lesions may be taking place with tissue fixation of such complexes, particularly in the continued presence of antibody excess. In addition, these authors demonstrated granular deposits of immunoglobulins in the choroid plexus and in perivascular areas of brains in 10 percent of their infected mice. As noted above, similar mechanisms may be operative in producing meningoencephalitic infiltrations in sleeping sickness.

Studies of human biopsy and autopsy material have documented various forms of renal involvement in the course of visceral leishmaniasis (145–147). Clinical studies have shown that this is usually mild; it is associated with moderate proteinuria and hematuria, but usually does not progress to full-blown nephrotic syndrome (148). A study reported by de Brito and co-workers (149) showed glo-

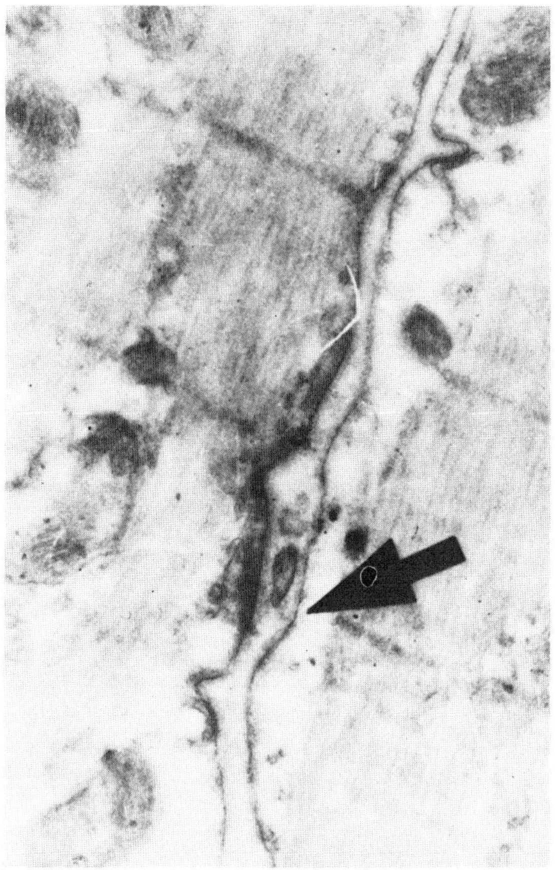

Figure 2-12 Electron micrograph of two ventricular myocardial cells after incubation with peroxidase-labeled antihuman γ-globulin. The plasmalemma (*arrow*) shows a positive reaction for enzyme, indicating the presence of bound autologous γ-globulin. Magnification × 10,500. (Reproduced with permission, P. M. Cossio, R. P. Laguens, E. Kreutzer et al., *Am. J. Pathol.* 86:533, 1977.)

merular involvement with mesangial cell proliferation and fibrillar thickening of axial regions. Deposits of immunoglobulins G and M were recorded along with C3—mostly in a mesangial pattern. The immunofluorescence pattern was granular and resembled that previously seen in association with schistosomiasis. In this particular study attempts to demonstrate antigen using staining with heterologous antitrypanosomal antibody were unsuccessful. The pattern of histologic and immunofluorescence studies in these patients suggests that during active trypanosomal infection, rela-

tively large insoluble aggregates are formed, which are then rapidly shunted to renal mesangial cells. Since these areas of the glomerulus are most efficient at removal of foreign materials, no progressive glomerular deposition is present and the renal lesion is usually mild. On the other hand, there appear to be intrinsic features of the disease itself that make myocardial and meningovascular involvement progressive and severe. The work of Lambert and Houba in experimental mice (29) would suggest that this may well be modulated or somehow influenced by extravascular immune-complex deposition both in the myocardium and the central nervous system.

Other Parasitic Disorders

Other parasitic diseases undoubtedly are influenced to a large extent by various pathological or physiological phenomena mediated by immune complexes. Parasites such as *E. histolytica*, which are confined principally to the enteric distribution in their initial phase, have not been extensively studied. Regional localization of the behavior of immune complexes within various portions of the portal circulation has not been performed. This is an important aspect, which in turn may be related to a precise interpretation of what effects other types of complexes originating within the bowel may have on local sites draining directly from the gut or in more distant tissues. Some of the deep-seated complications of amebiasis such as amebic abscess of the liver or lung are probably governed or influenced by local deposition of immune complexes, or possibly even by receptors for complexes in various target tissues. It is also not clear to what extent many of the peripheral manifestations of other parasitic infections may be determined by immune-complex phenomena. The fever, urticaria, generalized myositis, and soft-tissue edema associated with trichinosis, for instance, have always been attributed to direct invasion of affected tissue by worms prior to encystment. However, there are many aspects of these symptoms that occur at a time after initial invasion of the gut of the host approximately right for local immune-complex–mediated phenomena. A report by Géniteau and colleagues (150) has documented elevation of circulating complexes in six trichinosis patients one month after infection. Serial studies in several patients showed a fall of complexes as symptoms subsided. No evidence for extensive in vivo complement activation was obtained in this study.

It is also possible that the presence of detectable elevations of circulating complexes among active trichinosis patients represents an epiphenomenon in no way related to the local cutaneous or soft-tissue pathological process. Of interest, however, is an isolated case report of glomerulonephritis occurring in association with trichinosis (151); unfortunately no immunofluorescence data are available in this particular instance. Similar correlations may eventually become clear in the case of other peripheral manifestations of parasitic infections such as filariasis or nematode infections.

General Features of Parasitic Disease

One of the most striking findings in parasitic infection is eosinophilia. Although not a feature of all parasitic disorders, it is common enough to be singled out as perhaps one of the most general features of such infections (152). In recent years eosinophilia has become associated with the IgE immunoglobulin system and various other allergic manifestations. Early work pointed to a relationship between various types of sensitization and eosinophilic response (153). In addition, antigen-antibody reactions in vitro were shown to be associated with phagocytosis by eosinophils (154). Work by Basten and Beeson (155) has indicated that functioning T cells are necessary somehow to produce an eosinophil response. In animals depleted of T cells or T-cell precursors by various experimental maneuvers, subsequent challenge with trichina parasitic infestation did not induce an eosinophilia. Recently specific antieosinophilic sera have been produced that have greatly facilitated study of the specific role of this cell type in various immune reactions (156, 157). Furthermore, evidence has been accumulated that the eosinophil may be capable of functioning as a specific killer cell in

systems where parasitic forms are sensitized by immune IgG antibody (158, 159).

Eosinophils have for some time been associated with immune complexes. Fifteen years ago Litt showed that immune complexes were ingested or taken up by eosinophils during the induction of experimental eosinophilia (160, 161). The findings of Butterworth and associates (158, 159) that immune complexes or specific antibody affixed to vulnerable forms of the schistosome parasite generate direct antibody-mediated killing in the antibody-mediated cytotoxicity mechanism (Figure 2-13) may be of fundamental importance in understanding some of the protective immune phenomena in a wide range of parasitic infections. This basic system has now been studied in a number of different variations. It is clear that the killer cells mediating lysis of antibody-coated target cells may comprise a broad variety of cell types including lymphocytes, polymorphonuclear leukocytes, monocytes, and macrophages (162–169). That eosinophils can also mediate such reactions in the presence of IgG antibody fixed to target cells indicates that such cells must of necessity possess intrinsic Fc receptors capable of reacting with tissue-directed immune complexes. One of the puzzling aspects of the killer-cell-mediated lysis of

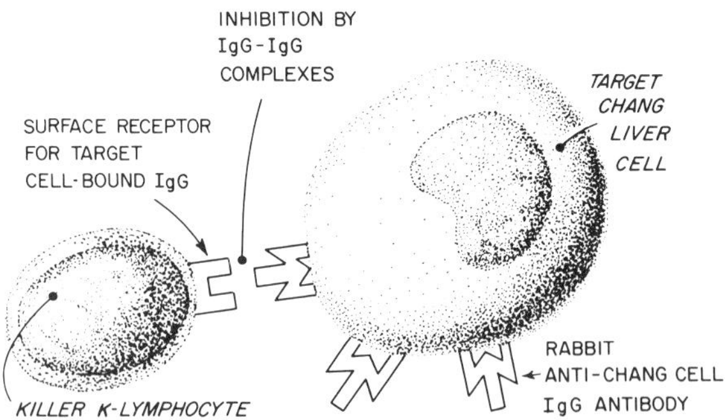

Figure 2-13   A typical mechanism involved in antibody-mediated cytotoxicity. The killer cell (here a killer lymphocyte) interacts with a target cell (Chang cell) sensitized with IgG antibody. The killer cell itself may vary in different experimental systems from a lymphocyte to a polymorphonuclear leukocyte, monocyte, or macrophage. Eosinophils may also function as killer cells in this system.

target cells as studied in the numerous test systems employed to date has been the precise identity of the killer cells involved. Recent evidence points to the fact that various cells known to function as K-cells in the so-called antibody-mediated cytotoxicity system may also contain elements of the membrane attack system of complement on their surfaces (170, 171).

Another general feature of many parasitic infections is their association with generation of large amounts of homocytotrophic antibody or IgE in the infected host. As will be discussed in Chapter 9, there is very little evidence that IgE-containing complexes participate directly in the tissue damage associated with these same parasitic infestations, except by sensitization of tissue mast cells or basophils and subsequent release of mediators such as histamine.

In the beginning of this chapter attention was directed to the theoretical difficulties involved in any study of the immune response to a number of common human parasites. The features of antigenic variation, associated intrinsic immunosuppression through activation of suppressor-cell mechanisms, or background-noise antibody apparently relatively ineffective in affording protective immunity are common to many parasitic diseases such as malaria, schistosomiasis, or trypanosomiasis. Nevertheless, the prospects for possible eventual vaccine protection against such a disease as malaria have improved as insight into specific features of the immune response has increased. By choosing extracellular forms in the life cycle of malarial parasites such as merozoites, researchers have developed vaccines that have proved effective in protection against lethal *P. knowlesi* malaria in the rhesus monkey (172). In addition, merozoite vaccination has protected douroucouli monkeys against *P. falciparum,* the most virulent of the human malarias (173, 174). One of the most significant recent breakthroughs has been the continuous in vitro cultivation of erythrocytic forms of *P. falciparum* (175); this technique could pave the way for a uniform or controllable source of merozoite antigen suitable for human vaccination trials. It remains to be seen whether practical implementation will afford eventual protective vaccination programs for large segments of the world population still at risk. Finally, it is clear that precise knowledge of the influence of immune complexes in the evolution of host-immune reactivity to the spectrum of important human parasites will be necessary in evaluating peripheral as well as primary effects of infestation in individual patients.

References

1. Domingo, E. O., Cowan, R. B. T., and Warren, K. S. The inhibition of granuloma formation around *Schistosoma mansoni* eggs. *Am. J. Trop. Med. Hyg.* 16:284, 1967.

2. Bloch, E. H., Wahab, M. F. A., and Warren, K. S. *In vivo* microscopic observations of the pathogenesis and pathophysiology of hepatosplenic schistosomiasis in the mouse liver. *Am. J. Trop. Med. Hyg.* 21:546, 1972.

3. Mahmoud, A. A. F., Mandel, M. A., Warren, K. S., et al. Niridazole. II. A potent long-acting suppressant of cellular hypersensitivity. *J. Immunol.* 114:279, 1975.

4. Mahmoud, A. A. F., and Warren, K. S. Anti-inflammatory effects of tartar emetic and Niridazole: suppression of schistosome egg granuloma. *J. Immunol.* 112:222, 1974.

5. Brown, K. N., and Brown, I. N. Immunity to malaria: antigenic variation in chronic infections of *Plasmodium knowlesi. Nature* 208:1286, 1965.

6. Voller, A., and Rossan, R. N. Immunological studies on simian malaria. III. Immunity to challenge and antigenic variation in *P. knowlesi. Trans. R. Soc. Trop. Med. Hyg.* 63:507, 1969.

7. Brown, I. N. Immunological aspects of malarial infection. *Adv. Immunol* 11:267, 1969.

8. Allison, A. C. Parasitological reviews. Malaria in carriers of the sickle-cell trait and in newborn children. *Exp. Parasitol.* 6:418, 1957.

9. Edington, G. M., and Watson-Williams, E. J. Sickling, haemoglobin C, glucose-6-phosphate dehydrogenase deficiency and malaria in western Nigeria. In J. H. P. Jonxis, ed., *Abnormal Haemoglobins in Africa,* p. 393. Oxford University Press, New York, 1965.

10. Gilles, H. M., Fletcher, K. A., Hendrickse,

R. G., et al. Glucose-6-phosphate dehydrogenase deficiency, sickling and malaria in African children. *Lancet* 1:138, 1967.

11. Warren, H. S., and Weidanz, W. P. Malarial immunodepression *in vitro:* adherent spleen cells are functionally defective as accessory cells in the response to horse erythrocytes. *Eur. J. Immunol.* 6:816, 1976.

12. McBride, J. S., Michlem, H. S., and Ure, J. M. Immunosuppression in murine malaria. I. Response to type III pneumococcal polysaccharide. *Immunology* 32:635, 1977.

13. Wedderburn, N., and Dracott, B. N. The immune response to type III pneumococcal polysaccharide in mice with malaria. *Clin. Exp. Immunol.* 28:130, 1977.

14. Wyler, D. J., Miller, L. H., and Schmidt, L. H. Spleen function in quartan malaria (due to *Plasmodium inui*) evidence for both protective and suppressive roles in host defense. *J. Infect. Dis.* 135:86, 1977.

15. Folch, H., and Waksman, B. H. The splenic suppressor cell. I. Activity of thymus dependent adherent cells: changes with age and stress. *J. Immunol.* 113:127, 1974.

16. Lewart, R. M., and Mandlowitz, S. Schistosomiasis: prenatal induction of tolerance to antigens. *Nature* 224:1029, 1969.

17. Hang, L. M., Boros, D. L., and Warren, K. S. Induction of immunological hyporesponsiveness to granulomatous hypersensitivity in *Schistosoma mansoni* infections. *J. Infect. Dis.* 130:515, 1974.

18. Camus, D., Carlier, Y., Bina, J. C., et al. Sensitization to *Schistosoma mansoni* antigens in uninfected children born to infected mothers. *J. Infect. Dis.* 134:405, 1976.

19. Atkinson, I. E. Bright's disease of malarial origin. *Am. J. Med. Sci.* 88:149, 1884.

20. Giglioli, G. Malaria and renal disease, with special reference to British Guiana. I. Introduction. *Ann. Trop. Med. Parasitol.* 56:101, 1962.

21. Giglioli, G. Malaria and renal disease, with special reference to British Guiana. II. The effect of malaria eradication on the incidence of renal disease in British Guiana. *Ann. Trop. Med. Parasitol.* 56:225, 1962.

22. Gilles, H. M., and Hendrickse, R. G. Nephrosis in Nigerian children. Role of *Plasmodium malariae* and effect of antimalarial treatment. *Br. Med. J.* 2:27, 1963.

23. Kibukamusoke, J. W., Hutt, M. S. R., and Wilks, N. E. The nephrotic syndrome in Uganda and its association with quartan malaria. *Q. J. Med.* 36:393, 1967.

24. Hendrickse, R. G. The quartan malarial nephrotic syndrome. *Adv. Nephrol.* 6:229, 1976.

25. Dixon, F. J. Comment on immunopathology. *Milit. Med.* 131:1233, 1966 (suppl.).

26. Allison, A. C., Hendrickse, R. G., Edington, G. M., et al. Immune complexes in the nephrotic syndrome of African children. *Lancet* 1:1232, 1969.

27. Ward, P. A., and Kibukamusoke, J. W. Evidence for soluble immune complexes in the pathogenesis of the glomerulonephritis of quartan malaria. *Lancet* 1:283, 1969.

28. McGregor, I. A., Turner, M. W., Williams, K., et al. Soluble antigens in the blood of African patients with severe *Plasmodium falciparum* malaria. *Lancet* 1:881, 1968.

29. Lambert, P. H., and Houba, V. Immune complexes in parasitic diseases. In L. Brent and J. Holborow, eds., *Progress in Immunology II,* vol. 5, p. 57. North-Holland Publishing Company, Amsterdam, 1974.

30. Houba, V., Lambert, P. H., Voller, A., et al. Clinical and experimental investigation of immune complexes in malaria. *Clin. Immunol. Immunopathol.* 6:1, 1976.

31. Houba, V. Immunopathology of nephropathies associated with malaria. *Bull. WHO* 52:199, 1975.

32. Izui, S., Lambert, P. H., and Miescher, P. A. *In vitro* demonstration of a particular affinity of glomerular basement membrane and collagen for DNA. A possible basis for a local formation of DNA-anti-DNA complexes in systemic lupus erythematosus. *J. Exp. Med.* 144:428, 1976.

33. Berger, M., Birch, L. M., and Conte, N. F. The nephrotic syndrome secondary to acute glomerulonephritis during falciparum malaria. *Ann. Intern. Med.* 67:1163, 1967.

34. Bhamarapravati, N., Boonpucknavig, S., Boonpucknavig, V., et al. Glomerular changes in acute *Plasmodium falciparum* infection. An immunopathologic study. *Arch. Pathol.* 96:289, 1973.

35. George, C. R. P., Parbtani, A., and Cameron, J. S. Mouse malaria nephrology. *J. Pathol.* 120:235, 1976.

36. Boonpucknavig, S., Wongsawang, S., Boonpucknavig, V., et al. Serum-soluble malarial antigens and immune complex nephritis in *Plasmodium berghei* infected mice. *J. Trop. Med. Hyg.* 79:116, 1976.

37. Brooks, M. H., Kiel, F. W., Sheehy, T. W., et al. Acute pulmonary edema in falciparum malaria: a clinicopathological correlation. *N. Engl. J. Med.* 279:732 1968.

38. Dungagupta, S., Srichaikal, T., Nitiyanaut, P., et al. Acute pulmonary insufficiency in falci-

parum malaria: survey of 12 cases with evidence of disseminated intravascular coagulation. *Am. J. Trop. Med. Hyg.* 23:551, 1974.

39. Godard, J. E., and Hansen, R. A. Interstitial pulmonary edema in acute malaria. Report of a case. *Radiology* 101:523, 1971.

40. Marks, S. M., Holland, S., and Gelfand, M. Malarial lung: report of a case from Africa successfully treated with intermittent positive pressure ventilation. *Am. J. Trop. Med. Hyg.* 26:179, 1977.

41. Soni, J. L., and Cox, H. W. Pathogenesis of acute avian malaria. III. Antigen and antibody complexes as a mediator of anemia in acute *Plasmodium gallinaceum* infections of chickens. *Am. J. Trop. Med. Hyg.* 24:423, 1975.

42. Ward, P. A., and Conran, P. B. Immunopathologic studies of simian malaria. *Milit. Med.* 131:1225, 1966 (suppl.).

43. Christian, C. L. The character of non-precipitating antibodies. *Immunology* 18:457, 1970.

44. Soothill, J. F., and Steward, M. W. The immunopathological significance of the heterogeneity of antibody affinity. *Clin. Exp. Immunol.* 9:193, 1971.

45. Steward, M. W., and Voller, A. The effect of malaria on the relative affinity of mouse antiprotein antibody. *Br. J. Exp. Pathol.* 54:198, 1973.

46. Musgrave, E. W., Wherry, W. B., and Wooley, P. G. Tropical splenomegaly. *Bull. Johns Hopkins Hosp.* 17:28, 1906.

47. McIntosh, J. F. Cryptogenetic splenomegaly (Banti's disease). A review and report of cases from North China. *Chin. Med. J.* 46:992, 1932.

48. Ziegler, J. L., and Stuiver, P. C. Tropical splenomegaly syndrome in Rwandan kindred in Uganda. *Br. Med. J.* 3:79, 1972.

49. Ssebabi, E. C. T., Jagne, J. G. M., Nzaro, E., et al. Tropical splenomegaly syndrome: an immune complex disease. *East Afr. Med. J.* 52:680, 1975.

50. Wilson, R. A., and Barnes, P. E. The formation and turnover of the membranocalyx on the tegument of *Schistosoma mansoni*. *Parasitology* 74:61, 1977.

51. Clegg, J. A. The schistosome surface in relation to parasitism. In A. E. R. Taylor and R. Muller, eds., *Functional Aspects of Parasite Surfaces.* Symposium of the British Society for Parasitology, vol. 10, p. 23. Blackwell Press, Oxford and London, 1972.

52. Damian, R. T., Greene, N. D., and Hubbard, W. J. Occurrence of mouse α_2 macroglobulin antigenic determinants on *Schistosoma mansoni* adults, with evidence on their nature. *J. Parasitol.* 59:64, 1973.

53. Goldring, O. L., Clegg, J. A., Smithers, S.

R., et al. Acquisition of human blood group antigens by *Schistosoma mansoni*. *Clin. Exp. Immunol.* 26:181, 1976.

54. Smithers, S. R., Terry, R. J., and Hockley, D. J. Host antigens in schistosomiasis. *Proc. R. Soc. Lond. (Biol.)* 171:483, 1969.

55. Clegg, J. A., Smithers, S. R., and Terry, R. J. Host antigens associated with schistosomes: observations on their attachment and their nature. *Parasitology* 61:87, 1970.

56. Marcus, D. M., and Cass, L. E. Glyco-sphingolipids with Lewis blood group activity; uptake by human erythrocytes. *Science* 164:553, 1969.

57. Andrade, Z. A., and deQueiroz, A. C. Lesões renais na esquistossomose hepatesplênica. *Rev. Inst. Med. Trop. Sao Paulo* 10:36, 1968.

58. Andrade, Z. A., Andrade, S. A., and Sadgursky, M. Renal changes in patients with hepatosplenic schistosomiasis. *Am. J. Trop. Med. Hyg.* 20:77, 1971.

59. daSilva, L. C., deBrito, T., Camargo, M. E., et al. Kidney biopsy in the hepatosplenic form of infection with *Schistosoma mansoni* in man. *Bull. WHO* 42:907, 1970.

60. Queroz, F. P., Brito, E., Martinelli, R., et al. Nephrotic syndrome in patients with *Schistosoma mansoni* infection. *Am. J. Trop. Med. Hyg.* 22:622, 1973.

61. Hillyer, G. V., and Lewert, R. M. Studies on renal pathology in hamsters infected with *Schistosoma mansoni* and *S. japonicum*. *Am. J. Trop. Med. Hyg.* 23:404, 1974.

62. Andrade, Z. A., and Susin, M. Renal changes in mice infected with *Schistosoma mansoni*. *Am. J. Trop. Med. Hyg.* 23:400, 1974.

63. Barsoum, R. S., Bassily, S., Baligh, O. K., et al. Renal disease in hepatosplenic schistosomiasis: a clinicopathological study. *Trans. R. Soc. Trop. Med. Hyg.* 71:387, 1977.

64. Smith, J. H., Kamel, I. A., Elwi, A., et al. A quantitative postmortem analysis of urinary schistosomiasis in Egypt. I. Pathology and pathogenesis. *Am. J. Trop. Med. Hyg.* 23:1054, 1974.

65. Sadgursky, M., Andrade, Z. A., Danner, R., et al. Absence of schistosomal glomerulopathy in *Schistosoma haematobium* infection in man. *Trans. R. Soc. Trop. Med. Hyg.* 70:322, 1976.

66. Moriearty, P. L., and Brito, E. Elution of renal antischistosome antibodies in human schistosomiasis mansoni. *Am. J. Trop. Med. Hyg.* 26:717, 1977.

67. Berggren, W. L., and Weller, T. H. Immunoelectrophoretic demonstration of specific circulating antigen in animals infected with *Schistosoma mansoni*. *Am. J. Trop. Med. Hyg.* 16:606, 1967.

68. Okabe, K., and Akusawa, M. Antigenic substance in urine of rabbits infected with *Schistosoma japonicum. Kurume Med. J.* 18:51, 1971.

69. Okabe, K., and Tanaka, T. Urine precipitin reaction for Schistosomiasis japonica. *Kurume Med. J.* 8:24, 1961.

70. Nash, T. E., Prescott, B., and Neva, F. A. The characteristics of a circulating antigen in schistosomiasis. *J. Immunol.* 112:1500, 1974.

71. Bout, D., Santoro, F., Carlier, Y., et al. Circulating immune complexes in schistosomiasis. *Immunology* 33:17, 1977.

72. Madwar, M. A., and Voller, A. Circulating soluble antigens and antibody in schistosomiasis. *Br. Med. J.* 1:435, 1975.

73. Falcão, H. A., and Gould, D. B. Immune complex nephropathy in schistosomiasis. *Ann. Intern. Med.* 83:148, 1975.

74. Hoshino-Shimizu, S., deBrito, T., Kanamura, H. Y., et al. Human schistosomiasis: *Schistosoma mansoni* antigen detection in renal glomeruli. *Trans. R. Soc. Trop. Med. Hyg.* 70:492, 1976.

75. von Lichtenberg, F., Bawden, M. P., and Shealey, S. H. Origin of circulating antigen from the schistosome gut. An immunofluorescent study. *Am. J. Trop. Med. Hyg.* 23:1088, 1974.

76. Nash, T. E. Localization of the circulating antigen within the gut of *Schistosoma mansoni. Am. J. Trop. Med. Hyg.* 23:1085, 1974.

77. Houba, V., Sturrock, R. F., and Butterworth, A. E. Kidney lesions in baboons infected with *Schistosoma mansoni. Clin. Exp. Immunol.* 30:439, 1977.

78. Bassily, S., Farid, Z., Barsoum, R. S., et al. Renal biopsy in Schistosoma-salmonella associated nephrotic syndrome. *J. Trop. Med. Hyg.* 79:256, 1976.

79. Gorczynski, R. M., Kilburn, D. G., Knight, R. A., et al. Nonspecific and specific immunosuppression in tumour-bearing mice by soluble immune complexes. *Nature* 254:141, 1975.

80. Wilson, R. J. M. Parasites in the immunized host: mechanisms of survival. In *Ciba Foundation Symposium,* vol. 25, p. 185. Associated Scientific Publishers, Elsevier–Excerpta Medica–North Holland, 1974.

81. Wakefield, G. S., Carroll, J. D., and Speed, D. E. Schistosomiasis of the spinal cord. *Brain* 85:535, 1962.

82. Bird, A. V. Acute spinal schistosomiasis. *Neurology (Minneap.)* 14:647, 1964.

83. Lechtenberg, R., and Vaida, G. A. Schistosomiasis of the spinal cord. *Neurology (Minneap.)* 27:55, 1977.

84. Cohen, J., Capildeo, R., Rose, F.C., et al. Schistosomal myelopathy. *Br. Med. J.* 1:1258, 1977.

85. Taliaferro, W. H. A reaction product in infections with *Trypanosoma lewisi* which inhibits the reproduction of the trypanosomes. *J. Exp. Med.* 39:171, 1924.

86. Taliaferro, W. H. Trypanocidal and reproduction-inhibiting antibodies to *Trypanosoma lewisi* in rats and rabbits. *Am. J. Hyg.* 16:32, 1932.

87. D'Alesandro, P. A. Electrophoretic and ultracentrifugal studies of antibodies to *Trypanosoma lewisi. J. Infect. Dis.* 105:76, 1959.

88. Campbell, G. H., and Phillips, S. M. Adoptive transfer of variant-specific resistance to *Trypanosoma rhodesiense* with B lymphocytes and serum. *Infect. Immun.* 14:1144, 1976.

89. Rank, R. G., Roberts, D. W., and Weidanz, W. P. Chronic infection with *Trypanosoma musculi* in congenitally athymic nude mice. *Infect. Immun.* 16:715, 1977.

90. Viens, P., Targett, G. A. T., Leuchers, E., et al. The immunological response of CBA mice to *Trypanosoma musculi.* I. Initial control of the infection and the effect of T-cell deprivation. *Clin. Exp. Immunol.* 16:279, 1974.

91. Jarvinen, J. A., and Dalmasso, A. P. Complement in experimental *Trypanosoma lewisi* infections of rats. *Infect. Immun.* 14:894, 1976.

92. Jarvinen, J. A., and Dalmasso, A. P. *Trypanosoma musculi* infections in normocomplementemic C5-deficient, and C3-depleted mice. *Infect. Immun.* 16:557, 1977.

93. Greenwood, B. M., and Whittle, H. C. Complement activation in patients with Gambian sleeping sickness. *Clin. Exp. Immunol.* 24:133, 1976.

94. Ziegler, J. L. Cryoglobulinaemia in tropical splenomegaly syndrome. *Clin. Exp. Immunol.* 15:65, 1973.

95. Mott, F. W. Histological observations on sleeping sickness and other trypanosome infections. *Rep. Sleep Sick. Comm. R. Soc.* 7:3, 1906.

96. Greenwood, B. M., Whittle, H. C., Oduloju, K. O., et al. Lymphocytic infiltration of the brain in sleeping sickness. *Br. Med. J.* 2:1291, 1976.

97. Manconi, D. E., Zaccheo, D., Bugiani, O., et al. T and B lymphocytes in normal cerebrospinal fluid. *N. Engl. J. Med.* 294:49, 1976.

98. Gangji, D., Collard-Ronge, E., Balleriauz-Waha, D., et al. T-lymphocytes in cerebrospinal fluid. *N. Engl. J. Med.* 294:902, 1976.

99. Naess, A. Demonstration of T lymphocytes in cerebrospinal fluid. *Scand. J. Immunol.* 5:165, 1976.

100. Gelfand, M. C., Frank, M. M., and Green,

I. A receptor for the third component of complement in the human renal glomerulus. *J. Exp. Med.* 142:1029, 1975.

101. Shin, M. L., Gelfand, M. C., Nagle, R. B., et al. Localization of receptors for activated complement on visceral epithelial cells of the human renal glomerulus. *J. Immunol.* 118:869, 1977.

102. Burkholder, P. M., Oberley, T. D., Barber, T. A., et al. Immune adherence in renal glomeruli. Complement receptor sites on glomerular capillary epithelial cells. *Am. J. Pathol.* 86:635, 1977.

103. Chagas, C. Nova trypanosomiaze humana: estudos sobre a morfolojia e o ciclo evolutivo do *Schizotrypanum cruzi n. gen., n. sp.,* ajente etiolojico de nova entidade morbida do homem. *Mem. Inst. Oswaldo Cruz* 1:159, 1909.

104. Torres, C. M. Patogenia de la miocarditis crónica en la enfermedad de Chagas. *Sociedad Argentina de Patología Regional del Norte,* Quinta Reunión, 2:902, 1930.

105. Chagas, C. Estado actual da trypanosomiase americana. *Rev. Biol. e Hyg.* 5:58, 1934.

106. Tschudi, E. I., Anziano, D. F., and Dalmasso, A. P. Lymphocyte transformation in Chagas' disease, *Infect. Immun.* 6:905, 1972.

107. Gonzales Cappa, S. M., Schmunis, G. A., Traversa, O. C., et al. Complement fixation tests, skin tests, and experimental immunization with antigens of *Trypanosoma cruzi* prepared under pressure. *Am. J. Trop. Med. Hyg.* 17:709, 1968.

108. Yanofsky, J. F., and Albado, E. Humoral and cellular responses to *Trypanosoma cruzi* infection. *J. Immunol.* 109:1159, 1972.

109. Williams, D. M., and Remington, J. S. Effect of human monocytes and macrophages on *Trypanosoma cruzi. Immunology* 32.19, 1977.

110. Williams, D. M., Sawyer, S., and Remington, J. S. Role of activated macrophages in resistance of mice to infection with *Trypanosoma cruzi. J. Infect. Dis.* 134:610, 1976.

111. Hoff, R. J. Killing *in vitro* of *Trypanosoma cruzi* by macrophages from mice immunized with *T. cruzi* or BCG and absence of cross immunity on challenge *in vivo. J. Exp. Med.* 142:299, 1975.

112. Marr, J. S., and Pike, E. H. The protection of mice by "Corpus Christi" strain *Trypanosoma cruzi* when challenged with "Brasil" strain. *J. Parasitol.* 53:657, 1967.

113. Seah, S., and Marsden, P. D. The protection of mice against a virulent strain of *Trypanosoma cruzi* by previous inoculation with an avirulent strain. *Ann. Trop. Med. Parasitol.* 63:211, 1969.

114. Santos-Buch, C. A., and Teixeira, A. R. L. The immunology of experimental Chagas' disease.

III. Rejection of allogeneic heart cells *in vitro. J. Exp. Med.* 140:38, 1974.

115. Teixeira, A. R. L., Roters, F. A., and Mott, K. E. Acute Chagas' disease. *Gaz. Med. Bahia* 3:176, 1970.

116. Teixeira, A. R. L., Teixeira, M. L., and Santos-Buch, C. A. The immunology of experimental Chagas' disease. IV. Production of lesions in rabbits similar to those of chronic Chagas' disease in man. *Am. J. Pathol.* 80:163, 1975.

117. Vickerman, K., and Luckins, A. G. Localization of variable antigens on the surface coat of *Trypanosoma brucei* using ferritin conjugated antibody. *Nature* 224:1125, 1969.

118. Cross, G. A. M. Identification, purification and properties of clone-specific glycoprotein antigens constituting the surface coat of *Trypanosoma brucei. Parasitology* 71:393, 1975.

119. Houba, V., and Allison, A. C. M-antiglobulins (rheumatoid-factor-like globulins) and other gamma globulins in relation to tropical parasitic infections. *Lancet* 1:848, 1966.

120. Houba, V., Brown, K. N., and Allison, A. C. Heterophile antibodies, M-antiglobulins and immunoglobulins in experimental trypanosomiasis. *Clin. Exp. Immunol.* 4:113, 1969.

121. Freeman, T., Smithers, S. R., Targett, G. A. T., et al. Specificity of immunoglobulin G in rhesus monkeys infected with *Schistosoma mansoni, Plasmodium knowlesi,* and *Trypanosoma brucei. J. Infect. Dis.* 121:401, 1970.

122. Hudson, K. M., Freeman, J. C., Byner, C., et al. Immunodepression in experimental African trypanosomiasis. *Trans. R. Soc. Trop. Med. Hyg.* 69:273, 1975.

123. Hudson, K. M., Byner, C., Freeman, J., et al. Immunodepression, high IgM levels and evasion of the immune response in murine trypanosomiasis. *Nature* 264:256, 1976.

124. Coutinho, A., and Moller, G. Thymus-independent B-cell induction and paralysis. *Adv. Immunol.* 21:113, 1975.

125. Zauderer, M., and Askonas, B. A. Several proliferative phases precede maturation of IgG-secreting cells in mitogen-stimulated cultures. *Nature* 260:611, 1976.

126. Mansfield, J. M., Craig, S. A., and Stelzer, G. T. Lymphocyte function in experimental African trypanosomiasis: mitogenic effects of trypanosome extracts *in vitro. Infect. Immun.* 14:976, 1976.

127. Mansfield, J. M., and Kreier, J. P. Autoimmunity in experimental *Trypanosoma congolense* infections of rabbits. *Infect. Immun.* 5:648, 1972.

128. Seed, J. R., and Gam, A. A. The presence

of antibody to a normal rabbit liver antigen in rabbits infected with *Trypanosoma gambiense*. *J. Parasitol.* 53:946, 1967.

129. Cossio, P. M., Diez, C., Szarfman, A., et al. Chagasic cardiopathy: demonstration of a serum gamma globulin factor which reacts with endocardium and vascular structures. *Circulation* 49:13, 1974.

130. Cossio, P. M., Laguens, R. P., Diez, C., et al. Chagasic cardiopathy: antibodies reacting with plasma membrane of striated muscle and endothelial cells. *Circulation* 50:1252, 1974.

131. Sterin-Borda, L., Cossio, P. M., Gimeno, M. F., et al. Effect of chagasic sera on the rat isolated atrial preparation: immunological, morphological and functional aspects. *Cardiovasc. Res.* 10:613, 1976.

132. Richman, D. P., Patrick, J., and Arnason, B. G. W. Cellular immunity in myasthenia gravis. Response to purified acetylcholine receptor and autologous thymocytes. *N. Engl. J. Med.* 294:694, 1976.

133. Appel, S. H., Almon, R. R., and Levy, N. Acetylcholine receptor antibodies in myasthenia gravis. *N. Engl. J. Med.* 293:760, 1975.

134. Patrick, J., and Lindstrom, J. Autoimmune response to acetylcholine receptor. *Science* 180:871, 1973.

135. Flier, J. S., Kahn, C. R., Roth, J., et al. Antibodies that impair insulin receptor binding in an unusual diabetic syndrome with severe insulin resistance. *Science* 190:63, 1975.

136. Kahn, C. R., Flier, J. S., Bar, R. S., et al. The syndromes of insulin resistance and acanthosis nigricans. Insulin-receptor disorders in man. *N. Engl. J. Med.* 294:739, 1976.

137. Bruce, D. H., Bernard, W., and Blackard, W. G. Spontaneous disappearance of insulin-resistant diabetes mellitus in a patient with a collagen disease: a case report, with review of the literature for conditions associated with insulin resistance. *Am. J. Med.* 48:268, 1970.

138. Poltera, A. A., Cox, J. N., and Owor, R. Pancarditis affecting the conducting system and all valves in human African trypanosomiasis. *Br. Heart J.* 38:827, 1976.

139. Cossio, P. M., Laguens, R. P., Kreutzer, E., et al. Chagasic cardiopathy. I. Immunopathologic and morphologic studies in myocardial biopsies. *Am. J. Pathol.* 86:533, 1977.

140. Jayawardena, A. N., and Waksman, B. H. Suppressor cells in experimental trypanosomiasis. *Nature* 265:539, 1977.

141. Ackerman, S. B., and Seed, J. R. Immunodepression during *Trypanosoma brucei gambiense* infections in the field vole, *Microtus montanus. Clin. Exp. Immunol.* 25:152, 1976.

142. Albright, J. F., Albright, J. W., and Dwanic, D. G. Trypanosome-induced splenomegaly and suppression of mouse spleen cell responses to antigen and mitogens. *J. Reticuloendothel. Soc.* 21:21, 1977.

143. Ingram, D. G., and Soltys, M. A. Immunity in trypanosomiasis. IV. Immunoconglutinin in animals infected with *Trypanosoma brucei. Parasitology* 50:231, 1960.

144. Nagle, R. B., Ward, P. A., Lindsley, H. B., et al. Experimental infections with African trypanosomes. VI. Glomerulonephritis involving the alternate pathway of complement activation. *Am. J. Trop. Med. Hyg.* 23:15, 1974.

145. Uebel, H. Über einneisstoffwechselstörungen bei infantiler visceraler Leishmaniose unter besonderer Berücksichtigung der pathologisch anatomischen Veränderungen. *Z. Tropenmed. u. Parasitol.* 2:327, 1951.

146. Bogliolo, L. Nova contribuicão ao conhecimento de anatomia patológica de leishmaniose visceral. A propósito de um caso brasileiro e com especial referência a fibrose hepática leishmaniótica. *Hospital (Rio de Janeiro)* 50:393, 1956.

147. De Paolo, D., and Silva, J. R. Histopathologie der Kala-Azar. *Ergeb. Allg. Pathol. Path. Anat.* 39:1, 1966.

148. Most, H., and Lavietes, P. H. Kala azar in American military personnel. *Medicine* 26:221, 1947.

149. deBrito, T., Hoshino-Shimizu, S., Neto, V. Amato, et al. Glomerular involvement in human Kala-azar. A light, immunofluorescent, and electron microscopic study based on kidney biopsies. *Am. J. Trop. Med. Hyg.* 24:9, 1975.

150. Géniteau, M., Verroust, P. J., Smith, M. D., et al. Circulating immune complexes in six patients with trichinosis. *Clin. Exp. Immunol.* 30:141, 1977.

151. Schoenfeld, M. R., and Edis, G. T. Trichinosis and glomerulonephritis. *Arch. Pathol.* 84:625, 1967.

152. Samter, M., and Czarny, D. Secondary cells involved in the allergic reaction: eosinophils, basophils, neutrophils. In M. Samter, ed., *Immunological Diseases,* ed. 2, p. 375. Little, Brown and Co. Boston, 1971.

153. Samter, M. The response of eosinophils in the guinea pig to sensitization, anaphylaxis and various drugs. *Blood* 4:217, 1949.

154. Archer, G. T., and Bosworth, N. Phagocytosis by eosinophils following antigen-antibody reac-

tions *in vitro. Aust. J. Exp. Biol. Med. Sci.* 39:157, 1961.

155. Basten, A., and Beeson, P. B. Mechanism of eosinophilia. II. Role of the lymphocyte. *J. Exp. Med.* 131:1288, 1970.

156. Mahmoud, A. A. F., Warren., K. S., and Boros, D. L. Production of a rabbit anti-mouse eosinophil serum with no cross-reactivity to neutrophils. *J. Exp. Med.* 137:1526, 1973.

157. Mahmoud, A. A. F., Warren, K. S., and Peters, P. A. A role for the eosinophil in acquired resistance to *Schistosoma mansoni* infection as determined by antieosinophil serum. *J. Exp. Med.* 142:805, 1975.

158. Butterworth, A. E., Sturrock, R. F., Houba, V., et al. Antibody-dependent cell-mediated damage to schistosomula *in vitro. Nature* 252:503, 1974.

159. Butterworth, A. E., David, J. R., Franks, D., et al. Antibody-dependent eosinophil-mediated damage to ^{51}Cr-labeled schistosomula of *Schistosoma mansoni:* damage by purified eosinophils. *J. Exp. Med.* 145:136, 1977.

160. Litt, M. Studies in experimental eosinophilia. VI. Uptake of immune complexes by eosinophils. *J. Cell. Biol.* 23:355, 1964.

161. Litt, M. Eosinophils and antigen-antibody reactions. *Ann. N.Y. Acad. Sci.* 116:964, 1964.

162. Greenberg, A. H., Hudson, L., Shen, L., et al. Antibody-dependent cell-mediated cytotoxicity due to a "null" lymphoid cell. *Nature (New Biol.)* 242:111, 1973.

163. Wisloff, F., and Froland, S. S. Antibody-dependent lymphocyte-mediated cytotoxicity in man: no requirement for lymphocytes with membrane-bound immunoglobulin. *Scand. J. Immunol.* 2:151, 1973.

164. Greenberg, A. H., Shen, L., and Roitt, I. M. Characterization of the antibody-dependent cytotoxic cell. A non phagocytic monocyte? *Clin. Exp. Immunol.* 15:251, 1973.

165. Pollack, S. B., Nelson, K., and Grausz, J. D. Killer cells from murine spleen: effectors of antibody-dependent cellular cytotoxicity. *Transplant. Proc.* 7:477, 1975 (suppl.).

166. Perlmann, P., Perlmann, H., and Wigzell, H. Lymphocyte mediated cytotoxicity *in vitro.* Induction and inhibition by humoral antibody and nature of effector cells. *Transplant. Rev.* 13:91, 1972.

167. Van Boxel, J. A., Stobo, J. D., Paul, W. E., et al. Antibody-dependent lymphoid cell-mediated cytotoxicity; no requirement for thymus-derived lymphocytes. *Science* 175:194, 1972.

168. Zighelboim, J., and Gale, R. P. Interspecies variability in antibody-dependent cellular cytotoxicity (ADDC). *J. Immunol.* 113:1145, 1974.

169. Perlmann, P., Perlmann, H., Larsson, A., et al. Antibody-dependent cytolytic effector lymphocytes (K cells) in human blood. *J. Reticuloendothel. Soc.* 17:241, 1975.

170. Sundsmo, J. S., Kolb, W. P., and Müller-Eberhard, H. J. Reactions of human peripheral blood lymphocytes with C5b-9 complement complex-specific antibodies. In D. O. Lucas, ed., *Regulatory Mechanisms in Leukocyte Activation,* p. 359. Proceedings of the 11th Leukocyte Culture Conference. Academic Press, New York, 1977.

171. Curd, J. G., Sundsmo, J. S., Kolb, W. P., et al. Neoantigen of the membrane attack complex of human complement. *Arthritis Rheum.* 21:177, 1978.

172. Mitchell, G. H., Butcher, G. A., and Cohen S. Merozoite vaccination against *Plasmodium knowlesi* malaria. *Immunology* 29:397, 1975.

173. Mitchell, G. H., Richards, W. H. G., Butcher, G. A., et al. Merozoite vaccination of douroucouli monkeys against falciparum malaria. *Lancet* 1:1335, 1977.

174. Siddiqui, W. A. An effective immunization of experimental monkeys against a human malaria parasite, *Plasmodium falciparum. Science* 197:388, 1977.

175. Trager, W., and Jensen, J. B. Human malaria parasites in continuous culture. *Science* 193:673, 1976.

CHAPTER 3

Viral Infections

The problem of immune complexes as related to viral infections is a broad one and an area where the fragmentary knowledge accumulated in humans is not so complete as that which has been developed in animal models. It seems possible that a great many diseases of unknown etiology may be intertwined with viral etiology or viral effects. Most provocative are studies that indicate integration of various parts of the viral genomes' coding for C-type viral constituents in normal cells (1, 2). Perhaps also of basic importance to this problem is the suggestion that viral products or receptors for viruses may be of some intrinsic importance to function of the immune system as cell-to-cell receptors (3) and thus may conceivably contribute to survival. It is held that many (if not all) mammalian cells have genomes for potential expression of materials originally derived as segments of genetic information from C-type viruses intercalated within their own DNA sequences. Expression of such intrinsic C-type viral genomes can be brought out by various external stimuli—for instance, irradiation or mitogen stimulation by concanavalin A or pokeweed (2). It is fascinating to consider that certain of these genomes have been retained during evolution because they may in some way have provided survival advantage through coding for cell surface proteins, which function as useful receptors. Modern concepts related to virus expression and viral influences on various gene products have found it expedient to query in many systems what is and is not actually self. These questions are applicable to many of the concepts involved in autoimmunity.

The present discussion will deal with a few representative human viral diseases, in conjunction with a survey of phenomena mediated by viral immune complexes in specific clinical situations. In Chapter 13 a number of experimental viral infections and their relevance to immune complexes are analyzed.

Infectious Mononucleosis

Infectious mononucleosis is a disorder that has always been viewed in a special aura of relationships to the immune system (4). Even before clear recognition of the importance of Epstein-Barr (EB) virus in its pathogenesis, (5–7), the clinical presentation and multiplicity of systemic complications such as myocarditis, thrombocytopenia, cryoglobulinemia, pericarditis, hepatitis, aseptic meningitis, and occasionally serum-sickness-like manifestations of arthralgias or urticaria suggested that a diffuse vascular process was directly involved in the disease itself. Occasional patients have been reported in whom clinical evidence for renal involvement or an immune-complex–mediated glomerulonephritis was present in association with the usual clinical syndrome (8–18). In the average patient clinical evidence for renal disease is rare, but histological abnormalities are probably relatively common.

Varying types of renal involvement associated with infectious mononucleosis have been documented. Thus the patient described by Wallace and colleages (16) showed 6.5 grams of proteinuria per day and histological evidence for thickening of glomerular basement membranes with electron-dense deposits and lowering of serum C3, whereas the patient reported in elegant detail by Andres and co-workers (17) died of Gram-negative sepsis complicating infectious mononucleosis with jaundice, oliguria, and renal failure. In this latter case careful studies of renal tissue showed granular mesangial deposits of IgM and C3 along with electron-dense mesangial deposits on electron microscopy. Conventional microscopy showed the presence of interstitial lymphoid infiltrates and moderate mesangial cell proliferation. Eluates from postmortem renal material in this patient showed Paul-Bunnell heterophil antibodies as well as heterophil antigen. However, staining of renal tissue with heterologous antibody to EB virus antigens was negative, and it appeared that immune complexes comprised of IgM antibody, C3, and heterophil antigen were definitely involved in the immune-complex nephritis documented in this fatal case.

These findings represent well-founded evidence that heterophil antigens may be directly related to key peripheral manifestations of immune-complex phenomena in infectious mononucleosis. Actually, very little is known about the precise role that heterophil antigens play in the normal homeostatic mechanism. These antigens have occasionally been described in association with several unusual forms of lymphoma or leukemia. Studies by Peters showed presence of heterophil antigen in the cytoplasm of tubular and glomerular cells in 12 of 13 patients with infectious mononucleosis (14). All of these patients showed patchy interstitial lymphoid infiltrates. The exact relation of the heterophil antigens to the EB virus and the clinical syndrome has not been completely elucidated (19).

Several studies have documented the frequent occurrence of antilymphocyte antibodies during the clinical evolution of infectious mononucleosis (20, 21). Since antibodies to lymphocytic determinants have been detected in cryoprecipitates of many sera of infectious mononucleosis as well as systemic lupus erythematosus, it seems possible that such cryoproteins may represent antigen-antibody complexes, which may participate somehow in the mediation of peripheral or localized disease manifestations. At present there is no informa-

tion available on antilymphocyte or other cell-directed specificities of circulating antibodies or tissue eluates from patients with transient glomerulonephritis or arthralgias and cutaneous evidence for a vasculitic process.

The studies reported by Andres and colleagues (17) indicate a predominant mesangial distribution of IgM and C3 immunofluorescence in glomeruli affected in infectious mononucleosis. This particular pattern was previously identified by Germuth and Rodriguez (22) as typical for high-molecular-weight IgM antibody-immune deposits. It seems likely that large aggregates containing combined IgM antibodies and their respective antigens may be rapidly shunted to the mesangium and localize there instead of at more vulnerable glomerular loops or near basement membranes.

Infectious mononucleosis is sometimes associated with hematologic complications that include severe thrombocytopenia and in some cases hemolytic anemia. A number of reports document the occurrence of occasional instances of severe thrombocytopenia (23–27). In several instances antiplatelet antibodies have been reported (27, 28). Since it is now clear that platelets themselves have receptors for the Fc portion of IgG, some instances of thrombocytopenia associated with infectious mononucleosis may be accentuated by adsorption of complexes to such intrinsic platelet Fc receptors, as well as by direct mediation of antiplatelet antibodies themselves.

The occasional patient who develops a hemolytic syndrome during infectious mononucleosis presents difficult therapeutic and diagnostic problems. Cold-reacting antibodies or cold agglutinins with anti-i or mixed specificities have been implicated in the hemolytic anemias associated with infectious mononucleosis (29–34). Significant hemolytic anemia in classic infectious mononucleosis is uncommon; it occurs in perhaps 0.5 to 1.0 percent of cases. It is not clear how antibodies to autologous red-cell determinants are actually generated in this disease. Several possibilities have been suggested. First, it is conceivable that the viral infection itself stimulates self-reactive or forbidden clones in a manner analogous to the concept of polyclonal B-cell activation discussed in Chapters 1 and 2 (35). Another possibility is that generation of cold-reacting antierythrocyte antibodies during infectious mononucleosis represents a cross reaction between human erythrocyte antigens and material intrinsic to EB virus or perhaps membrane proteins coded for by part of the EB viral genome (36). The precise mechanism whereby hemolysis is induced in infectious mononucleosis is felt to represent activation of an autologous immune complex on the surface of the red cell (31, 32), with 7S antibody actually reacting with determinants on the erythrocyte surface and cold-reacting 7S IgG or 19S IgM anti-γ-globulin factor reacting in turn with this complex. This interpretation, though attractive, has not been uniformly borne out, since the study by Wilkinson and associates (33) did not in fact provide support for such a mechanism in a series of three carefully studied patients. These authors found patients with moderately severe hemolytic syndromes who did not show detectable IgG anti-i or anti-autologous erythrocyte antibody.

Interaction of 7S coating antibody and 7S IgG or 19S IgM cold-reactive rheumatoid factor raises the interesting problem of whether or not such a system is capable of activating the conventional or alternate complement pathway (37–40). Support for direct complement activation by rheumatoid factor reacting with antigen-antibody complexes or by blockade of effective complement activation has been provided by in vitro systems, which depend largely on varying the immunologic reactants and individual assay systems employed. In practical terms a considerable proportion of patients with infectious mononucleosis actually develop anti-i cold agglutinins, but only occasionally do patients appear to manufacture anti-i antibody of sufficient thermal amplitude—±30° C—and high enough avidity or titer to mediate in vivo hemolysis. Originally it was felt that clinically apparent hemolysis might occur when circulating erythrocytes reached peripheral capillary beds, such as in the extremities where the thermal requirement of the anti-i antibody was met. Subsequent activation of complement might then rapidly complete the process through the well-defined complement membrane attack mechanisms.

A number of reports have emphasized the common occurrence of neurological manifestations in the course of infectious mononucleosis. It has been estimated from several large series that approximately 2 percent of patients with the disease show some type of neurological involvement (41, 42). A wide variety of clinical syndromes has been described, ranging from aseptic meningitis to stupor, chorea, or occasionally focal neurological deficits such as unilateral sensorineural deafness (42–44). The mechanisms involved in producing a number of these lesions are unknown, and a variety of minor pathological changes have been recorded within central nervous system (CNS) tissues. Such descriptions have included the presence of atypical inflammatory cells around small blood vessels, occasional degenerative changes of ganglion cells in the cerebrum, brain stem nuclei or Purkinje cells, and mononuclear meningeal infiltration (45). To what extent viral invasion of CNS tissues is involved in such pathology is not clear. The possibility remains, however, that some of the neuropathological localization present when certain areas are preferentially affected hinges on the fact that the viral infection itself actually induces changes in cell membranes or membrane structures, which then may act to attract or fix locally produced or circulating immune complexes in certain anatomical locations.

To date there are few hard data relative to quantitation of circulating immune complexes during infectious mononucleosis. One report by Wands and co-workers (46) documents the presence of circulating cryoprotein immune complexes in a patient with infectious mononucleosis and urticarial rash. In this case evidence for the cryoprecipitates as elements of an immune complex was provided by the presence of IgG, IgM, and IgA as well as C3, C4, C5, and EB virus antibody and antigen in the isolated cryoglobulin. The C3PA component of the alternate complement pathway was detected in acute serum, but not after recovery in this particular instance. The immunochemical profile of the cryoprotein in this patient is shown in Table 3-1. Figure 3-1 shows the ultrastructural identification of viral particles within the cryoprotein complex in the same patient. Parallel clinical observations indicated that the

Table 3-1 Characterization of the cryoprotein immune complexes in infectious mononucleosis.

	Clinical			Cryoprotein complex									Whole serum	
Symptom	Day of study	SGOT (IU)	Bili-rubin (mg/ 100 ml)	TP[a]	C3	C4	C5	IgG	IgM	IgA	EB virus antibody titer[b]	Beef red blood cell titer	EB virus anti-body titer	Beef red blood cell titer
Pharyngitis	1	256	9.4	7.4	+	+	+	+	+	+	1:50	1:160	>1:400	>1:5120
Rash	5	ND[c]	ND	5.2	0	0	0	+	+	+	ND	ND	ND	ND
	9	130	7.2	3.4	0	0	0	+	+	+	ND	ND	ND	ND
	18	ND	ND	2.2	0	0	0	0	+	0	ND	ND	ND	ND
	53	29	0.4	0	0	0	0	0	0	0	0	0	1:400	1:160

IgG subtypes in the cryoprotein immune complexes on first day of study:

IgG-1[d]	IgG-2	IgG-3	IgG-4
1.60	0.10	0.108	0

Source: Reproduced with permission, J. R. Wands, J. L. Perrotto, and K. J. Isselbacher, *Am. J. Med.* 60:269, 1976.

[a] Cryoprecipitable protein concentration (mg/ml) was calculated as the amount of protein measured in the cryoprecipitate redissolved in 0.5 ml of the same BSA-containing buffer minus the amount of protein measured in 0.5 ml of the same BSA-containing buffer when no cryoprecipitate was detectable.

[b] IFA (measured by P. M. Feorino, Viral Oncology Branch, Communicable Disease Center, Atlanta, Georgia).

[c] ND = not determined.

[d] Concentration expressed as mg/ml.

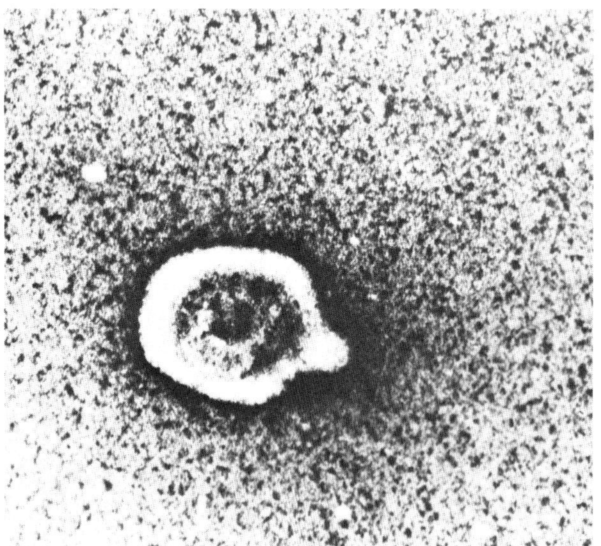

Figure 3-1 Phosphotungstic acid stain of a cryo-protein immune complex. A viral particle with dense outer core and apparent central nucleoid is evident. Magnification × 213,000. (Reproduced with permission, J. R. Wands, J. L. Perrotto, and K. J. Issel-bacher, *Am. J. Med.* 60:269, 1976.)

extensive urticarial rash in this case was related to the presence of cryoglobulin in the serum, but no direct study of skin biopsy material was performed. Previous study by Kaplan (47) of cryoglobulins from patients with infectious mononucleosis had shown the presence of multiple classes of immunoglobulin as well as several types of autoantibody including antinuclear antibody and rheumatoid factor. Thus a multiplicity of materials other than specific EB virus capsid antigen and antibody may participate somehow in the local effects of materials that precipitate as cryoglobulins in such sera.

Serum complement profiles in a series of 34 patients studied by Charlesworth provided evidence for both classical and alternate pathway activation (48). In one patient glomerulonephritis occurred during infectious mononucleosis; renal biopsy indicated alternate complement pathway activation, with properdin demonstrated by immunofluorescence in glomerular material.

The whole problem of EB virus infection and host immune response is a fascinating one that continues to present provocative interrela-

tionships. It is not obvious, for instance, why EB virus produces infectious mononucleosis in adolescents of relatively high socioeconomic class, whereas in Africa it is clearly associated with Burkitt's lymphoma (49). Epidemiologic data are currently being collected that bear directly on this interesting question. Whether the clinical difference in expression of lymphoma in African children or young adults and infectious mononucleosis results from differences in initial peak incidence of EB virus exposure during normal growth and development, or possibly to distinct variation in other environmental factors affecting the immune system such as concomitant malarial infection, remains to be determined (50). It seems likely that many of the clinical features of the infectious mononucleosis syndrome may be related somehow to expressions of cell-mediated immunity. Osborn and co-workers have recently reported that patients with infectious mononucleosis show peripheral blood lymphocytes that are directly toxic to target lymphoid cells containing EB virus (51). Many of the direct pathological observations in the disease itself have emphasized the occurrence of mononuclear cell infiltrates in various tissues (8, 17). There is also recent evidence for a relative depression of some areas of cell-mediated immunity in the course of the disease (52). In many ways the group of disorders now clearly associated with EB virus infections represents a rich ongoing opportunity for the study of a number of important human diseases.

Landry-Guillain-Barré Syndrome

The Landry-Guillain-Barré syndrome of acute polyneuritis is usually characterized by an initial prodrome of what appears to be a viral illness, followed by progressive and sometimes increasingly severe peripheral nervous system involvement with motor weakness of arms, legs, and respiratory muscles and autonomic nervous system abnormalities (53). There are many aspects of this clinical syndrome which suggest that an abnormal, perhaps self-directed immune response may be involved in pathogenesis. Perivascular infiltrates in many of the affected peripheral nerves are present;

patients may show the presence of complement-fixing antibodies to antigens present in peripheral nerves; and there is evidence of cell-mediated immune response to peripheral nerve antigens as indicated by lymphocyte transformation or migration inhibition studies (54–57). Many antecedent viral infections have been implicated in the initiation of the acute syndrome—varicella, influenza A, parainfluenza 3, mumps, herpes, or even infections with EB virus itself (58–61). The timing of the illness and onset in the second phase of any immune response possibly directed at the original infecting viral agent is such that an allergic reaction associated with the initial stimulus—infecting or otherwise—seems likely. In the United States during 1977, a wave of Guillain-Barré patients seen in temporal association with administration of the A/New Jersey/76 killed-influenza vaccination program raised questions about initial or parallel immune stimuli in afflicted individuals. In this regard secondary allergic reactions subsequent to initial viral infection have highlighted some fascinating possibilities of interplay of various immunologic effects. For some time it has been recognized that certain viral infections result in intense but temporary immunosuppression (62–64). Skin-test reactivity and other manifestations of delayed-type hypersensitivity are markedly reduced after influenza infection. The basic sequence of events is unknown, but there is now substantial evidence that certain viral infections can concurrently produce a profound alteration of either a primary or secondary immune response. Therefore, it is conceivable that secondary postviral effects might in some way alter either antibody affinity or the qualities of antibodies being produced in such a way as to promote immune-complex formation or low-affinity antibodies capable of extended persistence in the circulation. The current rapid development of precise methods of assessing cellular and humoral antibody immune reponse may eventually help to elucidate these still unresolved questions.

Experimental allergic neuritis (EAN) can be induced in laboratory animals upon injection of peripheral nervous system antigens along with complete Freund's adjuvant (65–67).

Since EAN can be transferred with lymphoid cells, it seems clear that a considerable portion of the underlying pathology in patients must relate to mechanisms mediated directly by sensitized lymphocytes rather than to processes involved with circulating complexes.

There are several observations, however, that appear to link Landry-Guillain-Barré syndrome with mechanisms involved in the handling of immune complexes. A number of patients with Landry-Guillain-Barré involvement and nephrotic syndrome (68–70) have now been recorded. In one carefully studied case granular glomerular deposits of IgG and IgM, along with subepithelial electron-dense glomerular deposits, were present (70). Representative histological and immunofluorescence studies from this particular patient are shown in Figures 3-2 and 3-3.

We have recently had the opportunity to study a small group of sera from 4 patients with Landry-Guillain-Barré syndrome, using the solid-phase C1q radioimmunoassay as well as the Raji-cell test. Serum samples obtained during the acute illness showed no significant elevations of circulating immune complexes; however, it seems likely that other modulating factors perhaps related to individual patients' immune response genes or actual load of antigens released at a critical time during the clinical illness may play an important part in determining which patients are affected by localized immune-complex deposition. Assays of circulating immune complexes in patients with Landry-Guillain-Barré syndrome have also been recorded by Tachovsky and associates (71), using the sensitive Raji-cell radioimmunoassay technique. In these patients 45 percent of a group of individuals with active Guillain-Barré showed detectable elevations of circulating immune-complex material.

The precise antigenic components of CNS or other tissues to which individual patients may be sensitized is not yet completely clear, although the experimental data available thus far indicate that complexes detected in this clinical situation may be relatively small and not of extremely high molecular weight (71). An understanding of one of the most prominent clinical features of the disorder might be

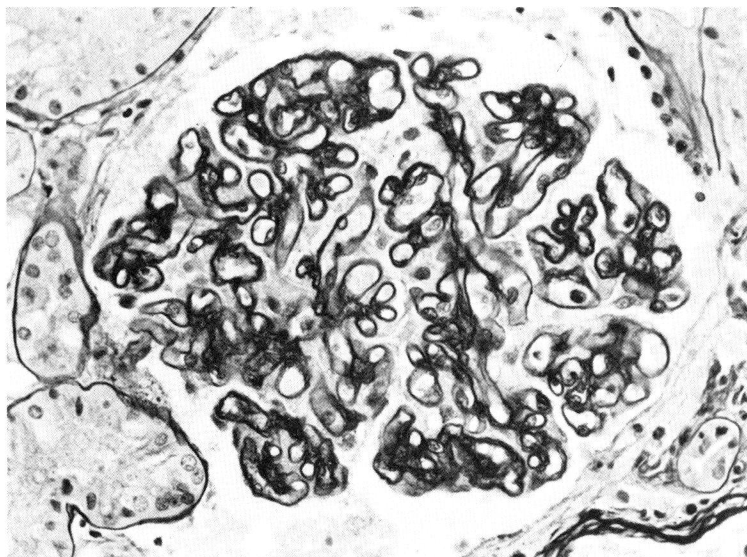

A

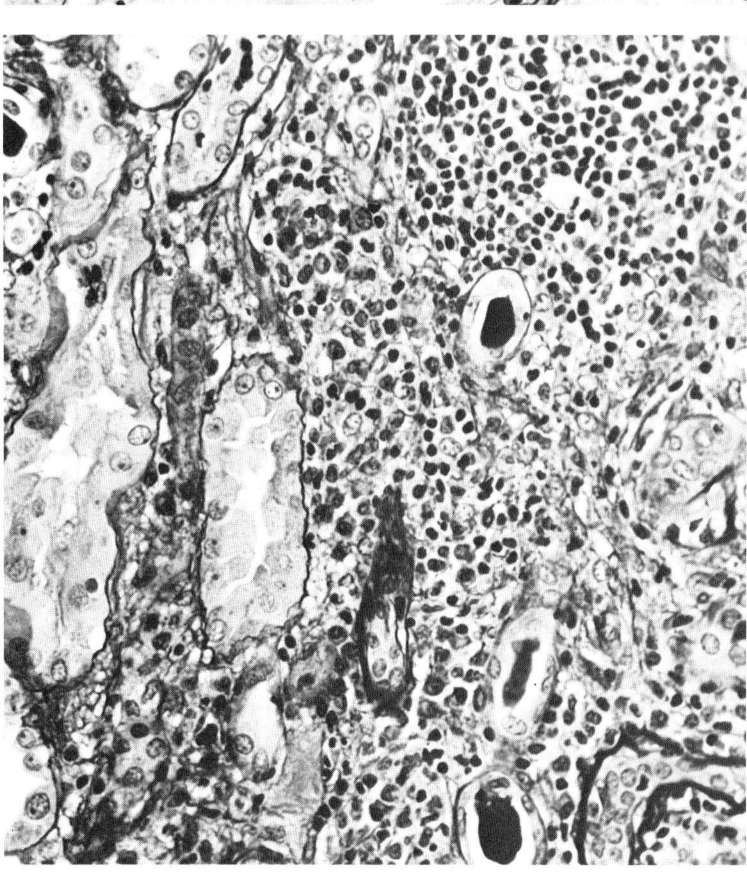

B

Figure 3-2   *A*, glomerulus showing diffuse moderate basement membrane thickening in a patient with Landry-Guillain-Barré syndrome and immune-complex nephritis. Periodic-acid/Schiff, magnification × 250. *B*, a typical field from the renal cortex of the same patient; focal chronic cellular infiltrate and tubular atrophy are evident. P.A.S. × 250. (Reproduced with permission, P. O. Behan, L. M. Lowenstein, M. Stiliphant et al., *Lancet* 1:850, 1973.)

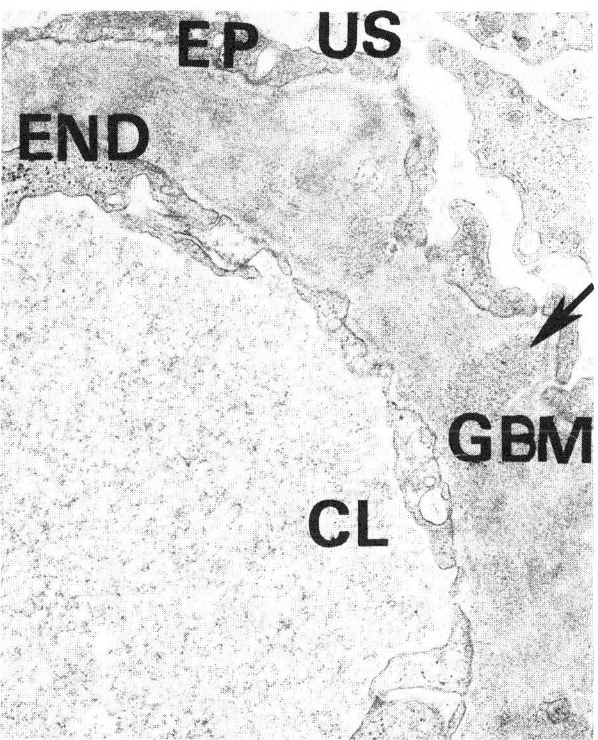

Figure 3-3 *A*, electron micrograph of glomerular subepithelial deposits in a patient with Landry-Guillain-Barré syndrome and immune-complex nephritis. END = endothelial cell; EP = epithelial cell; US = urinary space; CL = capillary lumen; GBM = glomerular basement membrane. *B*, immunofluorescence study of the same patient, showing diffuse finely granular immune deposits of IgG along the basement membrane. Magnification × 475. (Reproduced with permission, P. O. Behan, L. M. Lowenstein, M. Stiliphant et al., *Lancet* 1:850, 1973.)

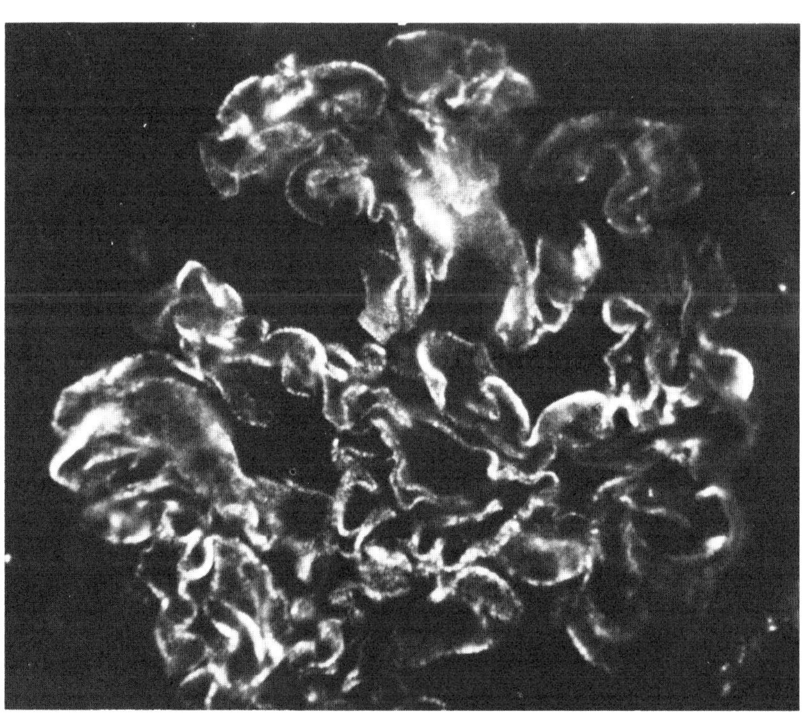

forthcoming if more were actually known about possible trapping or filtering systems within portions of the CNS. Patients with Landry-Guillain-Barré characteristically show marked elevations of cerebrospinal fluid protein with little in the way of concomitant inflammatory cells in the cerebrospinal fluid (CSF). It is conceivable that local deposition of immune complexes within the choroid plexus or other organ systems directly involved with spinal fluid production may somehow be responsible for the CSF abnormality represented by high protein and low cell counts. Serial studies of individual patients as well as more definitive identification of the specific antigens involved are now needed in affected patients. It is also clear that exceptional, still poorly understood factors must be operative in patients who develop Landry-Guillain-Barré syndrome, since the viruses that have been implicated are common and yet the full-blown clinical syndrome itself is quite rare.

Viral Hepatitis

Viral hepatitis is undoubtedly one of the most common infectious diseases in our society. Development of a system whereby virus and viral products could be recognized by serological and eventually by radioimmunoassay techniques represented a tremendous step forward in understanding this disease (72). Moreover, recognition of several distinct types of hepatitis virus based initially on clinical differences and, later, on serological and immunologic classification as hepatitis B, hepatitis A, and more recently non-A and non-B varieties has furthered understanding of this general group of disorders. Apart from the usual clinical presentation of fever, anorexia, jaundice, dark urine, and gradual resolution recognized in the usual or typical case of viral hepatitis, there is now a group of syndromes or variations on a single theme associated with viral hepatitis which has made it one of the most variegated and interesting clinical examples of immune-complex disorders. In this regard viral hepatitis associated with hepatitis B viral infection in current clinical medicine can be likened to syphilis in the last century as the great imitator.

In 1970 a group of patients described by Gocke and co-workers (73) presented with a spectrum of multisystem manifestations of polyarteritis nodosa. In these patients clear evidence was found for vasculitis and vascular damage mediated by immune complexes comprised of hepatitis B antigen and its homologous antibody. These patients showed arthritis, frequent renal involvement, and clinical presentation characterized by necrotizing vasculitis involving multiple organ systems. Immunofluorescence study of tissues obtained at biopsy or autopsy showed widespread vascular deposition of Ig and complement. A similar distribution of staining for hepatitis B antigen was detected. Physical and immunochemical studies of sera from this patient group provided evidence that complexes detectable in such samples were of relatively high molecular weight. Characteristic immunofluorescence findings in this group of patients are shown in Figure 3-4. Electron microscopic examination of ultracentrifuged pellets from serum of these patients showed clusters of hepatitis-B–related particles as shown in Figure 3-5. The Gocke group found evidence for underlying hepatitis B infection and associated immune-complex disease in 30 percent of all patients with necrotizing vasculitis seen over a period of several years. Similar patients since have been reported and carefully studied by many other groups of workers (74, 75). A fascinating report by Levo and co-workers (76) summarizes findings in a group of patients with essential mixed cryoglobulinemia.

Three of 25 serum samples from such patients contained hepatitis B antigen and 12 showed presence of anti–hepatitis B antibody. However, when the cryoprecipitates in these same patients were examined, 74 percent were positive either for hepatitis B Ag or its antibody. Electron microscopic study of four cryoprecipitates showed structures that resembled the 20-nm and 27-nm spheres, tubules, and Dane particles of hepatitis B infection. Examples of these findings are shown in Figure 3-6. The data are of interest, since the clinical presentation of essential mixed cryoglobulinemia often resembles that of periarteritis nodosa, rheumatoid vasculitis, or systemic lupus erythematosus (77, 78).

Long-term follow-up of the patients origi-

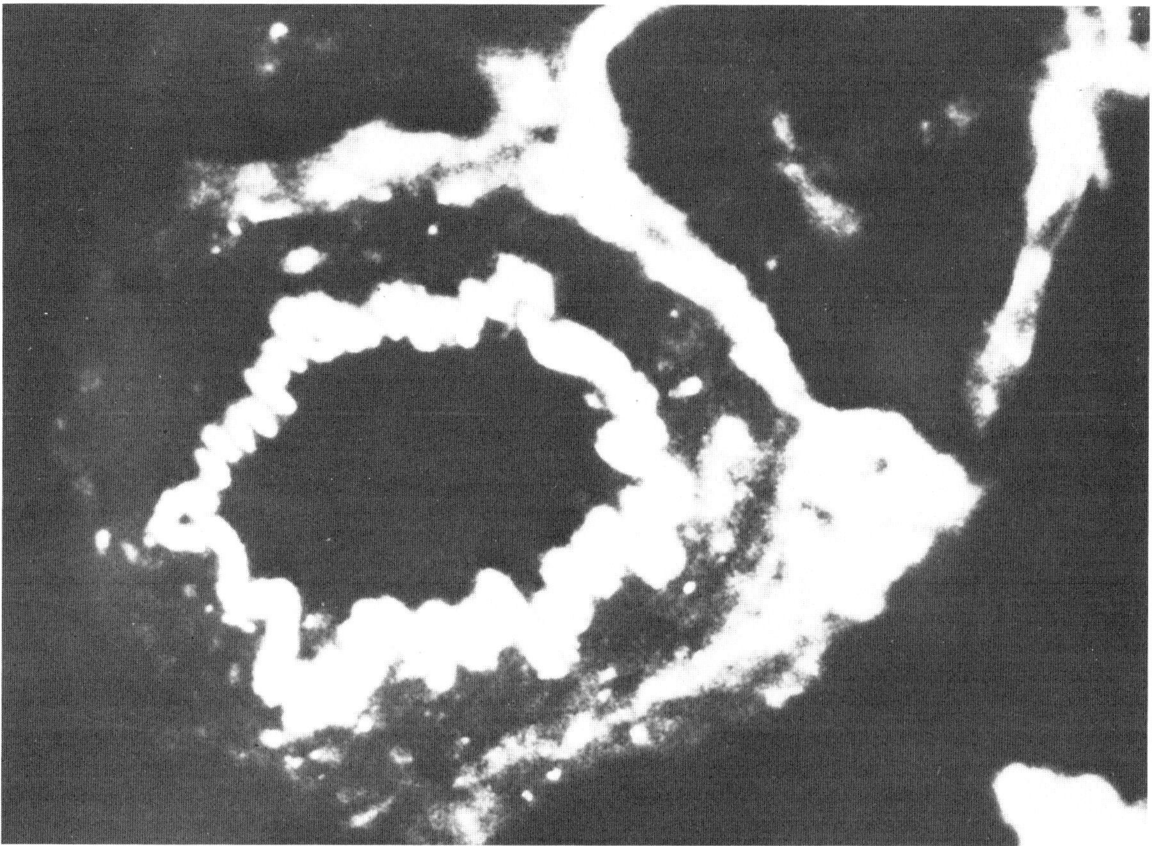

Figure 3-4 Immunofluorescent staining of muscle tissue from a patient with a clinical picture of polyarteritis nodosa associated with hepatitis B infection. Fluorescent deposits in the blood-vessel wall (IgM) are distributed along the elastic membrane. Original magnification × 250. (Reproduced with permission, D. J. Gocke, K. Hsu, C. Morgan et al., *Lancet* 2:1149, 1970.)

nally described by Gocke and associates (73) has provided useful additional data (79). The patients studied ranged in age from twenty-six to sixty-three, with an average age of forty-seven. Two patients presented with the clinical picture of chronic active hepatitis for two to three years before development of any manifestations of vasculitis. After initial presentation as mild acute hepatitis, 3 patients progressed to a series of vasculitic complications. In 2 patients chronic liver disease later dominated the clinical picture, and in 4 cases, after an initial period of three to eight months of active vasculitis, recovery ensued. This long-term follow-up information is useful, in that it indicates a broad range of possible clinical courses and patterns of disease associated with hepatitis B viral infection.

The group of patients with chronic hepatitis B infection and clearcut manifestations of apparent chronic polyarteritis represents a very difficult practical problem. It is not clear precisely what features lead to the production of the complete clinical syndrome. The initial vascular damage may result somehow from the presence of virus within vessel tissues or vascular endothelium. Alternatively, it could result from chronic or subacute accumulations of waves of immune complexes in vulnerable capillary beds. If continued vasculitis were indeed related to persistence of hepatitis B antigen within the circulation, it might make some sense to attempt to remove or artificially to reverse such continuous antigenemia. In such instances an affinity column or some device capable of efficiently removing antigen from the circulating intravascular volume would seem plausible. Several groups have actually made

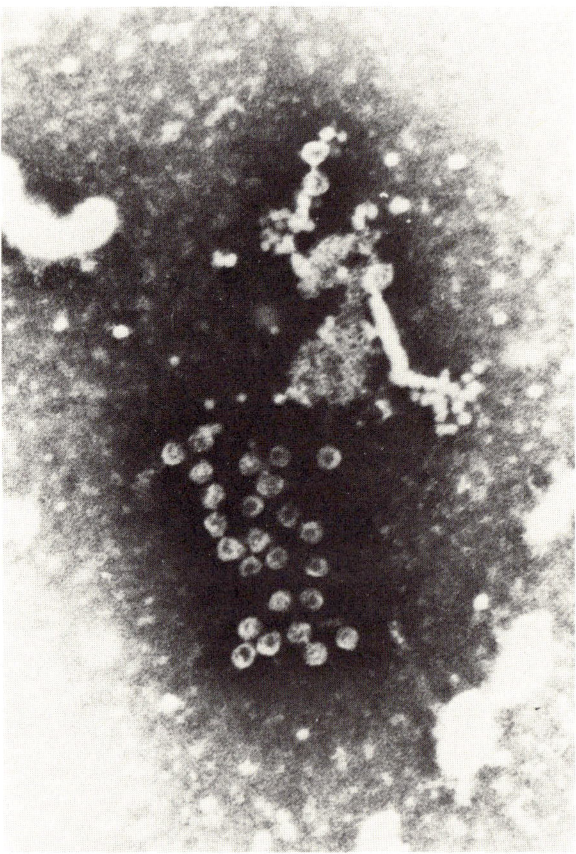

Figure 3-5 Electron micrograph of a negatively stained preparation of serum pellet from a patient with hepatitis B and diffuse vasculitis. Clusters of the characteristic 20 and 40 μm particles commonly associated with the Au or hepatitis B antigen are seen. Magnification × 62,500. (Reproduced with permission, D. J. Gocke, K. Hsu, C. Morgan et al., *Lancet* 2:1149, 1970.)

considerable progress technically in the development of a process that could be utilized for such a therapeutic approach. Experimental systems using both antigen and antibody affixed to extracorporeal immunoabsorbent columns have shown considerable promise (80–86). Moreover, by means of such techniques it might be possible to devise specific immunoabsorbent columns bound to materials known to have high intrinsic affinity for immune complexes (conglutinin, immunoconglutinin, rheumatoid factors, or even C1q). A number of other changes, including activation of leuko-

cyte complement receptors, occur in the course of such extracorporeal techniques (87–89). These are discussed in Chapter 5.

Acute and Chronic Viral Hepatitis

For a considerable time it has been recognized that 15 to 20 percent of patients with viral hepatitis manifest peripheral signs, possibly mediated by immune-complex phenomena. Thus, icteric acute viral hepatitis is sometimes preceded or accompanied by a serum-sickness-like clinical picture with arthralgias, frank arthritis and synovitis, rash, urticaria, and occasionally hematuria and proteinuria (90–93). At times we have had the distinct impression that this clinical presentation as an early manifestation of viral hepatitis appears to be more common with a particular wave of cases or local epidemic. Whether it eventually will be related to antigenic differences in infecting strains remains to be determined. The clinical symptom complex of skin eruption, urticarial rash, and arthralgias or frank polyarthritis may be present for several weeks before the onset of obvious hepatitis itself and usually disappears by the time overt jaundice is noted. There are occasional patients in whom the early symptoms and clinical picture of the serum-sickness–hepatitis equivalent closely resemble rheumatoid arthritis. In such individuals a clear differentiation cannot be established until clinical evidence of jaundice and hepatic dysfunction later supervene.

The first recognition of the relation of polyarthritis to hepatitis is reported in the writings of Sir Robert Graves, an Irish physician of the nineteenth century (94). Subsequently, it was recorded by several groups of observers in Europe and elsewhere, as well as in the United States (95–99), but was not clearly defined until the early '70s when the association was studied in detail by several different groups of investigators (91–93, 100–102). The study by Alpert and colleagues (92) included 18 patients who were examined during various phases of acute viral hepatitis. Actually one of the authors of that paper himself provided the first case; he noted rather acute onset of angioneurotic edema involving the soles of the feet, which progressed rapidly to an urti-

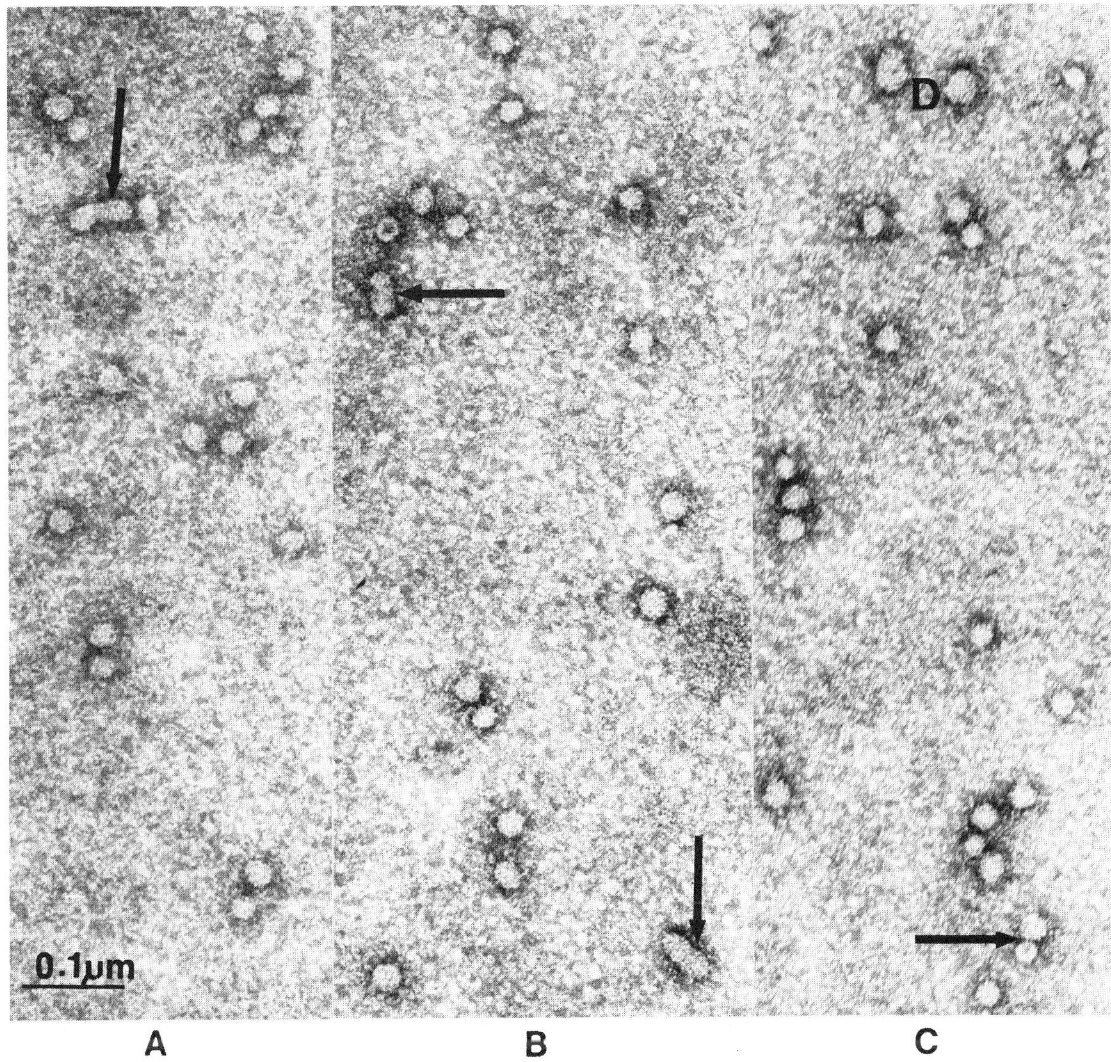

Figure 3-6 Representative sample of particles found in one of the cryoprecipitates from a patient with essential mixed cryoglobulinemia in which 27-nm size dominated. In *A* and *B* arrows indicate tubular structures; a doughnut-shaped particle is seen at the top of *B*. In *C* the arrow points to juxtaposed 20-nm particles, and *D* labels Dane particles. Magnification × 120,000. (Reproduced with permission, Y. Levo, P. D. Gorevic, H. J. Kassab et al., *N. Engl. J. Med.* 296:1501, 1977.)

carial eruption. This was followed by progressively more severe morning stiffness and arthralgias, particularly in the proximal interphalangeal joints (PIP) of the hands. These symptoms abated only with the clinical onset of jaundice. A representation of the evolution of clinical features of this syndrome is shown in Figure 3-7. In this study the most frequently affected joints were PIP areas, whereas in the cases recorded by Fernandez and McCarty (93) there was progressive involvement of many joints including ankles, hands, and in one instance lumbosacral spine.

Observations that favored an immune-complex–mediated synovitis during viral hepatitis included serial studies by Alpert and colleagues (92) of hemolytic complement as well as various complement components. Nine pa-

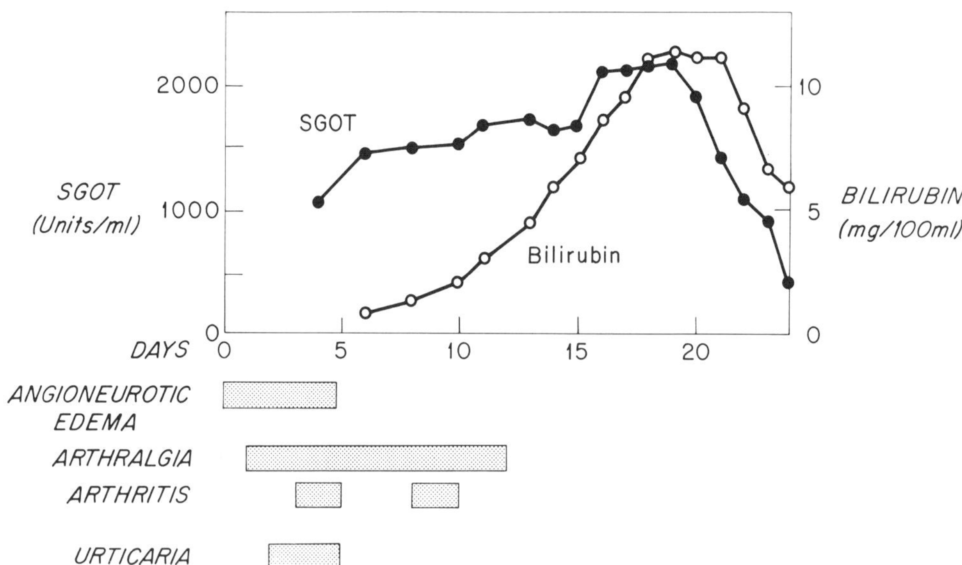

Figure 3-7 Serial clinical observations in a patient with viral hepatitis showing serum sickness prodromata. (Reproduced with permission, E. Alpert, K. J. Isselbacher, and P. H. Schur, *N. Engl. J. Med.* 285:185, 1971.)

tients in this study were examined during the acute phase of joint symptoms. Total hemolytic complement and C4 were depressed, and levels of C3 were moderately depressed as well. It was also demonstrated that low total serum complement levels were present in patients with high titers of hepatitis-associated antigen. Correlations of onset of joint and skin symptoms and changes in complement profiles suggested that local deposition of immune complexes was involved. Representative changes in complement and complement components among patients during the course of hepatitis-B–associated arthritis are shown in Figures 3-8 and 3-9.

Studies of patients observed by Fernandez (93) and Onion (91) and their colleagues indicated that when synovial fluids were examined, a type I or noninflammatory type of fluid was observed with 1 to 2,000 cells/mm³. Direct comparisons of serum and synovial fluid complement activity in one study (91) indicated marked relative depression in synovial fluid as compared to simultaneously studied serum. No direct examination of such synovial fluids for immune complexes was reported;

however, with the current availability of sensitive methods for detection of immune complexes such as the Raji-cell and solid-phase C1q assays, reexamination of this particular syndrome would seem to be in order. The size and molecular characteristics of any complexes detected directly within synovial fluid itself should be of particular interest.

It is significant perhaps that a number of clinical observations in viral hepatitis suggest that a situation analogous to acute serum sickness may indeed be occurring. Several early observations clearly established that hepatitis viral antigen-antibody complexes were capable of direct complement fixation (102, 103) and were vividly depicted in ultrastructural studies as immune conglomerates (104). The serial studies recorded in many reports, both of abrupt fall in complement levels and antigenemia followed by subsequent rise in antibody to hepatitis viral antigens, emphasize the remarkably close parallel this particular clinical syndrome bears to the serum sickness model initially studied in animals (105). An example of these reciprocal changes is shown in Figure 3-9.

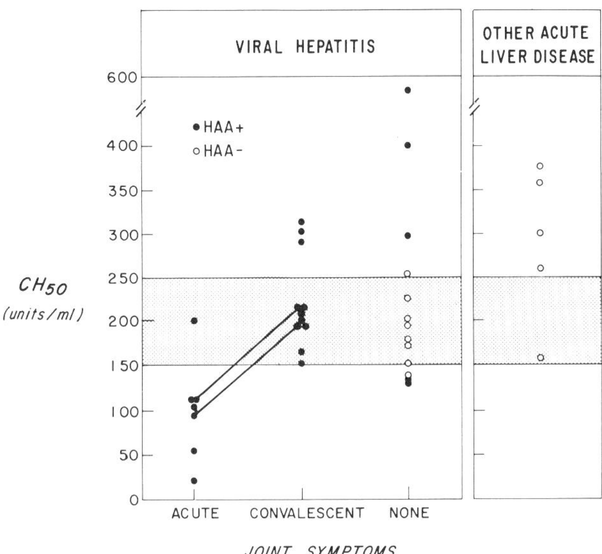

Figure 3-8 CH 50 levels in patients with acute hepatitis. (Reproduced with permission, E. Alpert, K. J. Isselbacher, and P. H. Schur, *N. Engl. J. Med.* 285:185, 1971.)

Further studies of the immune complexes themselves have utilized cryoproteins or cryoprecipitates from patients with acute viral hepatitis (106). Cryoprecipitating materials from patients with arthritis contained IgA and C3, C4, C5, as well as IgG and IgM. The IgG H-chain subgroups noted in these cryoglobulins were IgG1 and IgG3, the types known to fix complement most effectively. It was also shown that the cryoprecipitable proteins isolated from patients with active arthritis associated with hepatitis B infection were capable of converting C3PA to C3A in vitro; this observation supports the notion that immune complexes associated with hepatitis B could activate both conventional and alternative complement pathways. The finding of IgA in cryoprotein precipitates only from patients with arthritis is of interest, since naturally occurring polymeric forms of IgA are felt not to be very effective activators of the complement system (107).

In view of the reports by Levo and associates (76) indicating a high degree of correlation between hepatitis B surface antigen and the cryoprecipitates found in mixed cryoglobulinemia of unknown etiology, a careful examination of all cryoprecipitates from multiple clini-

cal syndromes must now be undertaken. It is not clear what physical or immunochemical factors are necessary for cryoprecipitation in vitro. The phenomenon itself was first described by Lerner and Watson in 1947 (108). Various materials including complement components, DNA, rheumatoid factors, and monoclonal proteins have been noted in cryoglobulin precipitates recorded in the connective tissue diseases as well as in numerous other clinical associations (109). Undoubtedly there are physical factors that relate to cryoprecipitation of sera when cooled to 4° C and are as yet unknown or incompletely defined. The fortuitous recognition that many such cryoprecipitates might indeed represent relatively cold-insoluble immune complexes is a finding of potentially great practical importance.

Peripheral manifestations of cryoproteins in a patient with chronic active hepatitis were described by Farivar and associates (110). In this particular patient the cryoprotein contained

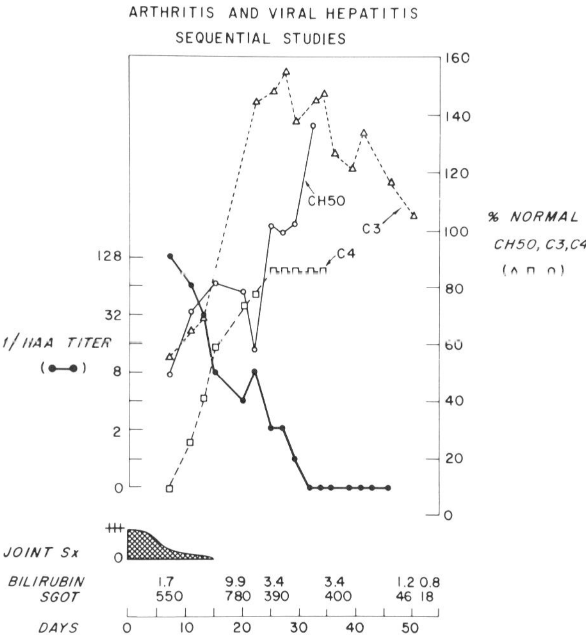

Figure 3-9 Changes in CH 50, C3, and C4 serum concentration and HBAg (HAA) titers during the course of HBAg-related arthritis and viral hepatitis. (Reproduced with permission, E. Alpert, P. H. Schur, and K. J. Isselbacher, *N. Engl. J. Med.* 287:103, 1972.)

IgM, IgG, and hepatitis B surface antigen. The virus-related antigen was identified by ultra-structural as well as immunofluorescence studies in the walls of small arteries and veins. The patient showed evidence of severe peripheral neuropathy, and it was postulated that the cryoprotein may have played some role in the pathogenesis of the neuropathy either through induction of a microvasculitis activating the complement system with subsequent inflammatory destruction and impedance to nerve function, or by depositing in vessels and causing progressive impedance to blood flow in small capillary networks as well as arterioles supplying the nerve structures. Severe neuropathy has been recognized as a complication of cryoglobulinemia in the past (78, 111), most commonly in essential mixed cryoglobulin syndromes. From a clinical standpoint it is important that the peripheral manifestations of cryoproteins are often recognized when they affect organ systems of obvious clinical vulnerability where symptoms or physiological sequelae rapidly make themselves known. Thus cryoprotein activation of intrinsic complement systems or vascular occlusion in other relatively silent clinical areas may not be associated with frank clinical symptomatology, but it may be equally important in the pathogenesis of unrecognized underlying disease.

The presence of circulating as well as tissue-localizing immune complexes in the course of acute viral hepatitis is a biological phenomenon of great interest. The following are the immediate and subacute results of activation of the conventional as well as alternate complement pathways: (1) inflammatory response mediated by increased vascular permeability and chemotactic attraction of inflammatory cells including polymorphonuclear leukocytes, monocytes, macrophages, and lymphocytes; (2) viral neutralization; (3) immune adherence promoting phagocytosis; and (4) alteration in cell membranes, leading to lysis of tissues. It seems likely that all of these separate phenomena are occurring in various stages of the evolution of acute viral hepatitis. Some may be involved in local tissue destruction, or cell death of hepatocytes; others may be protective, helping the body eventually to clear excess phagocytosed

materials. It is not yet understood which specific factors are the most important in determining what precipitates the various peripheral manifestations of immune-complex localization or activation.

*Renal Disease Associated
with Hepatitis Virus Persistence*

A number of reports have documented the association of chronic progressive renal disease and hepatitis B viral infection. Histological studies of renal tissues in such patients have usually shown a spectrum of morphological changes ranging from chronic membranous glomerulonephritis or membranoproliferative nephritis to focal and epimembranous lesions (112–116). Morphology in liver biopsies from most patients in this category has shown chronic active or chronic persistent hepatitis. Evidence for either chronic hepatitis B antigenemia or persistence of hepatitis B viral expression in liver tissue has been a common feature. Convincing documentation of antigen-antibody complexes in the glomerular lesions has been presented in several carefully studied patients (114, 116), including immunofluorescent and ultrastructural demonstration of hepattis B viral materials or antigens in the renal lesions themselves. Examples of these findings are shown in Figures 3-10 to 3-12. In the patients with predominant renal manifestations of chronic immune-complex disease, there have in some instances been initial prodomata or clinical characteristics of a more generalized vasculitis. In the patient studied by Kohler and co-workers (116) circulating complexes containing both hepatitis B antigen and antibody were noted to be concentrated in serum cryoprecipitates; the clinical value of knowing where to look in establishing the presence of definable immune-complex phenomena is again emphasized.

The variation of the renal morphological spectrum from chronic membranous to focal or epimembranous changes is important, particularly when one considers renal histological lesions and ultimate interpretations or prognosis ascribed to various histological types of renal disease, presently of unknown etiology. Since in chronic hepatitis-B–type infection it is

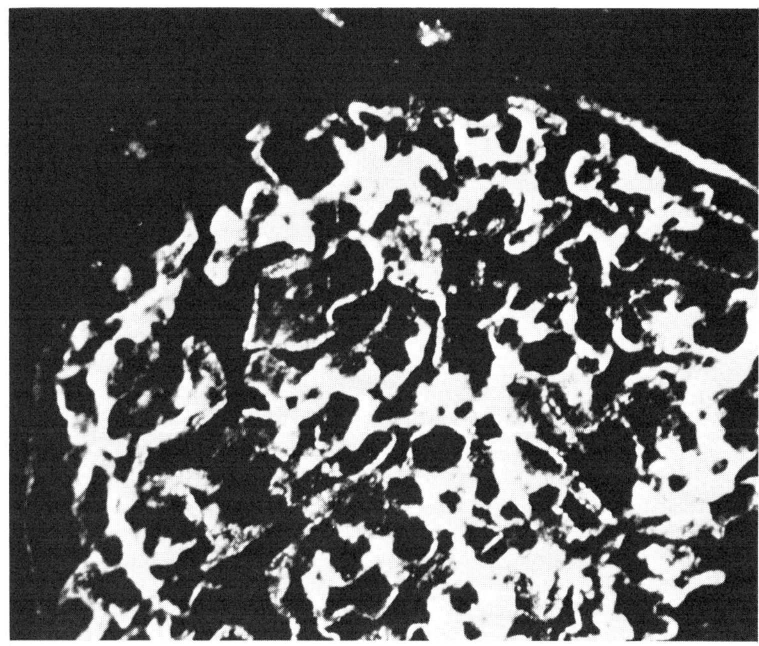

Figure 3-10 Indirect immunofluorescent staining of hepatitis B antigen in glomerulus from a patient with chronic hepatitis B and renal insufficiency. Granular and extensive distribution of hepatitis B antigen is evident in the glomerular basement membrane as well as in some mesangial areas. Magnification × 400.

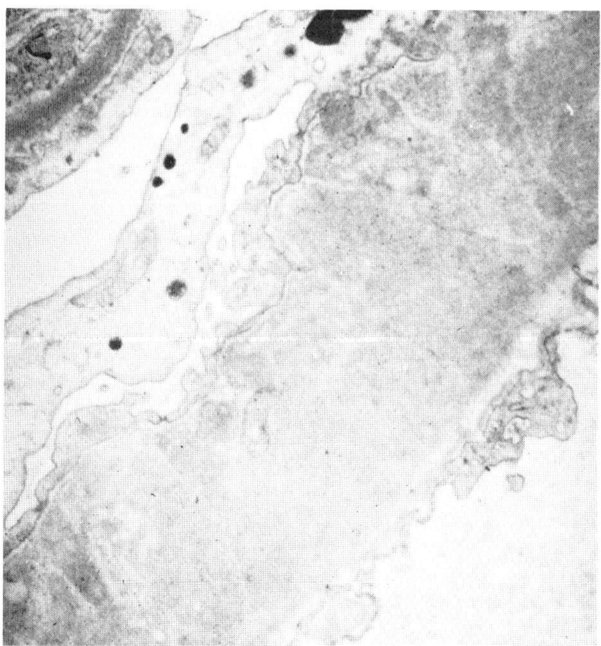

Figure 3-11 Massive electron-dense deposits on the glomerular basement membrane of a young patient with hepatitis B viral persistence and immune-deposit disease. (Electron micrograph courtesy of Peter Kohler, Denver.)

clear that a broad variety of reactive patterns may be induced, no meaningful order can be expected in classifying chronic renal disease of unknown cause until the offending antigens can be identified with certainty.

Another aspect of great significance to the basic biologic question raised by these patients relates to the underlying mechanisms for viral persistence, and inability of individual patients afflicted with chronic hepatitis B viral infection to clear themselves of the infection despite evidence for a vigorous humoral immune response against antigens induced by the infecting virus. In chronic hepatitis B viral infection, there is evidence that the absence of a coordinated and effective cell-mediated arm of the immune response is somehow essential to perpetuation and progression of the ongoing immune-complex disorder (116–118). It is difficult to predict what long-term effects would be produced, for instance, in such individuals treated with therapy designed to stimulate their cellular immunity and to help mobilize a universal immune response. If agents such as levamisole or transfer factor are effective in

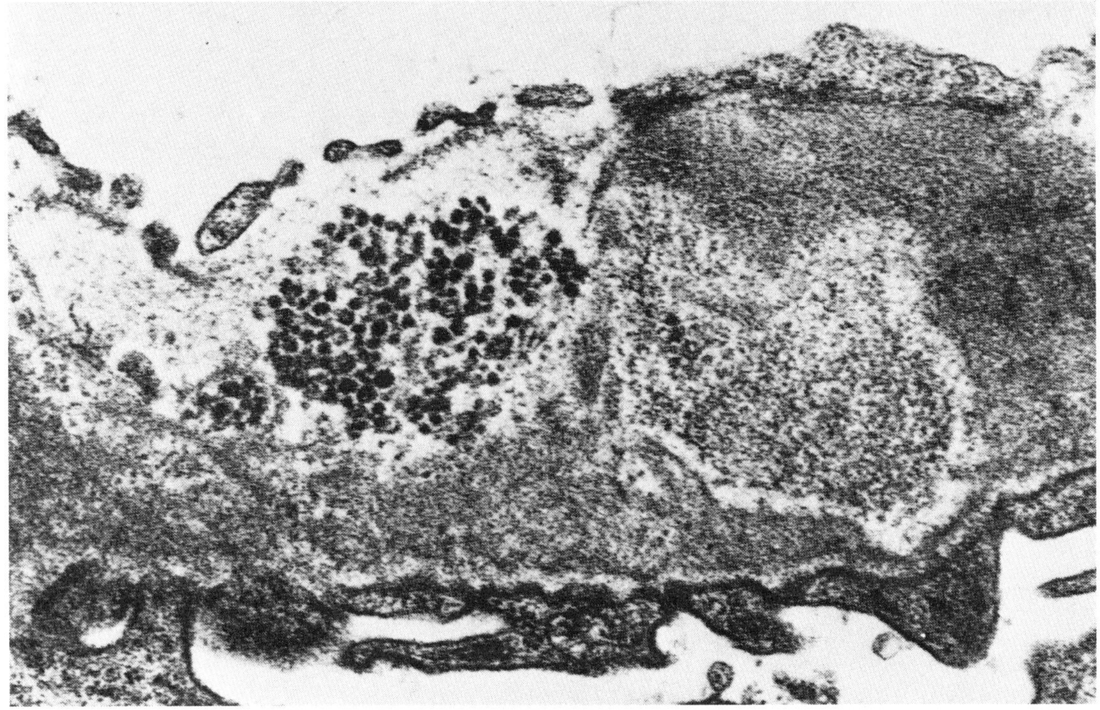

Figure 3-12 Peripheral electron-dense deposits showing discrete finely granular deposits and a more electron-dense deposit composed of 300 to 500 Å spherical particles. Original magnification × 27,500.

(Reproduced with permission, M. R. Knieser, E. H. Jenis, D. T. Lowenthal et al., *Arch. Pathol.* 97:193, 1974. Copyright 1974, American Medical Association.)

restoring the immune response, they could by their combined effects actually increase humoral reactivity and accelerate the ongoing immune-complex disorder. Thus immunostimulating drugs or protocols might conceivably induce activation of helper T cells and thereby augment an outpouring of antibody capable of forming additional potentially deleterious immune complexes. A group of patients with chronic hepatitis B infection has in fact been treated with transfer factor, as discussed by Kohler and co-workers (119). Long-term effectiveness of this therapeutic approach remains to be determined.

Determination of circulating complexes in chronic hepatitis B infection has been performed by a number of groups with a variety of methods. Visualization by electron microscopy (104), complement fixation (103), and radioimmunoassay (120) have yielded positive results. As already noted, studies of cryoglobu-

lins or cryoprecipitates have provided positive identification in a number of laboratories (119, 121). Recently, three parallel techniques have been assayed for detection of immune complexes in this disorder: the ^{125}I-C1q binding assay, complement fixation, and optical density measurements of a 3-percent polyethylene glycol precipitate of serum (122). The last method followed by addition of ^{125}I-C1q labeled hepatitis B Ag proved more sensitive than conventional radioimmunoassay.

Serum immune complexes from patients with acute hepatitis B infection have been studied in detail by Theofilopoulos and colleagues (123). They found complexes in 63.1 percent of patients with acute viral hepatitis positive for hepatitis B antigen; in 40 percent of patients with hepatitis B−negative acute hepatitis; and in 13.5 percent of asymptomatic carriers of hepatitis B virus. A summary of the data compiled in this study is given in Table

3-2. The complexes identified were of high molecular weight and were localized in 19 S or larger fractions of sucrose gradient separations. Further serial studies are needed to ascertain whether fluctuation in amounts, or differences in molecular size of complexes in the various types of sequelae to hepatitis B virus infection, can in fact be more closely related to differences in individual clinical presentation.

Immune Complexes in Hepatic Tissue

It has become apparent that tissue-fixed immune complexes may eventually provide direct insight into the process of ongoing liver cell injury associated with chronic active hepatitis. Cell-mediated immune reactions have frequently been implicated or suggested as part of the process that may be involved in such injury or in gradual progression to hepatocyte death and fibrosis (124, 125). Cell-mediated immune reactions to liver-specific protein antigens can be demonstrated in patients with both chronic active hepatitis and cryptogenic cirrhosis. The incidence of positive reactivity in HB_s Ag-positive and HB_s Ag-negative cases is similar (124). An example of the infiltrates dominated by lymphocytes, occasional plasma cells, and potentially immunocompetent cells that have suggested a chronic immunologic reaction is shown in Figure 3-13. The intrinsic presence of hepatitis B antigens or products of the virus is difficult to relate to demonstrable presence or absence of the virus.

Early studies by Edgington and Ritt (126) and by Nowoslawski and co-workers (127) showed immunoglobulins and complement distributed along sinusoidal walls and actually within hepatocytes or Kupffer cells of patients with HB_s Ag-positive hepatitis. In addition, C1q complement component was found in hepatic cell nucleoli of HB_s Ag-positive patients (126). IgG antibodies capable of in vitro complement fixation with hepatitis B antigen present in liver cell nuclei were later recorded by several groups (128–130), and extensions of these findings have been published by Gerber and associates (131) in studies of patients with chronic active hepatitis, viral hepatitis, and massive hepatic necrosis. In 11 cases with chronic active hepatitis a granular pattern of immunofluorescence using specific antihepatitis B antibody with specificity for the core antigen (HB_c) was detected in many hepatocyte nuclei, with 50 percent or more nuclei positive in 9 of the 11 patients. Parallel staining with reagents specific for IgG showed similar patterns. Cytoplasm of a few hepatocytes from 9 patients with chronic active hepatitis also contained HB_s Ag, but no immunoglobulins or complement could be identified. Representative immunofluorescent identification of hepatitis B core antigen in hepatic cell nuclei from this study is shown in Figure 3-14. In direct contrast, hepatic tissue from 10 patients with acute viral hepatitis or massive necrosis showed HB antigen in only a few scattered nuclei, and immunoglobulins and complement were not

Table 3-2 Raji-cell radioimmunoassay for immune complexes in patients with acute hepatitis with HB_s Ag, acute hepatitis without HB_s Ag, and in asymptomatic carriers of HB_s Ag.

Diagnosis	No. of cases	No. positive	Percent positive	AHG (μg eg/ml) Mean	Range
Acute hepatitis with HB_s Ag	19	12	63.1	68	24–212
Acute hepatitis without HB_s Ag	15	6	40	62	24–155
Asymptomatic carriers of HB_s Ag	59	8	13.5	55	24–100

Source: Reproduced with permission, A. N. Theofilopoulos, C. B. Wilson, and F. J. Dixon, *J. Clin. Invest.* 57:169, 1976.

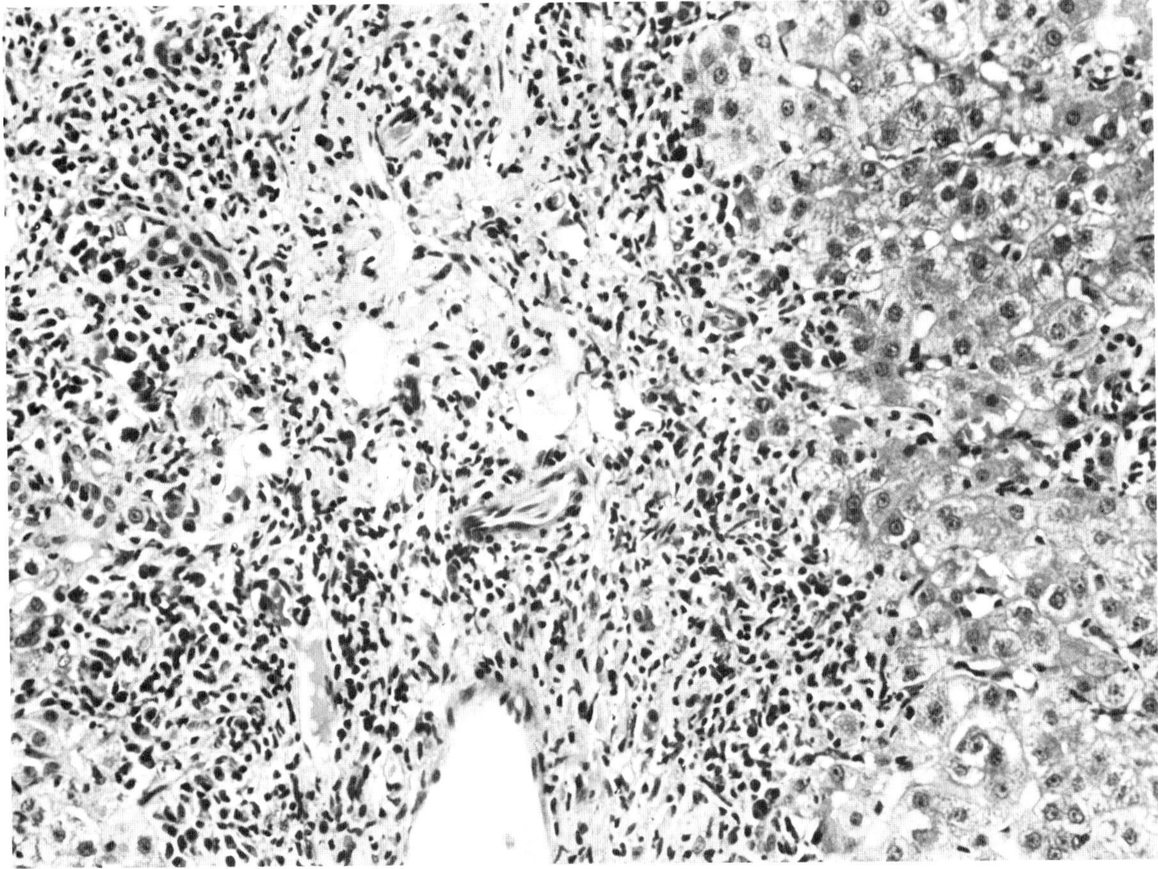

Figure 3-13 Typical hepatic cellular infiltrate in a patient with chronic active hepatitis. H&E × 230. (Photomicrograph courtesy of P. J. Scheuer, Royal Free Hospital, London.)

identified. Specificity of staining reactions in these studies was confirmed by appropriate absorption and blocking experiments. Elution of IgG by treatment with acidic citrate buffers suggested that HB antigens, IgG, and complement were present primarily in nuclear material of hepatocytes involved in chronic active hepatitis. Intranuclear immunoglobulin was not found in specimens that did not show HB antigens in the same distribution. Studies using incubation of sections with fresh human serum followed by fluorescein-conjugated antisera to C3 showed the capacity of hepatic nuclear immune complexes to fix complement; however, no direct evidence for in vivo complement fixation was obtained. Electron microscopic observations also indicated aggregates of 20-nm to 25-nm intranuclear hepatitis-B-related core particles in association with electron-dense material reacting with peroxidase-conjugated antihuman IgG.

These findings provide further direct evidence for intranuclear immune complexes of IgG and HB antigen in a large proportion of patients with chronic active hepatitis. In the past it has generally been assumed that immunoglobulins do not cross membranes of viable cells; the presence of IgG and complement within nuclear structures in hepatocytes of such patients then becomes difficult to explain. It is conceivable that intranuclear residence of hepatitis B virus might actually alter local cellular membrane permeability characteristics. In this context, in vivo binding of immunoglobulin to nuclei within skin (132) and kidney (133) has been demonstrated in patients with systemic lupus erythematosus.

Similar studies concentrating primarily on

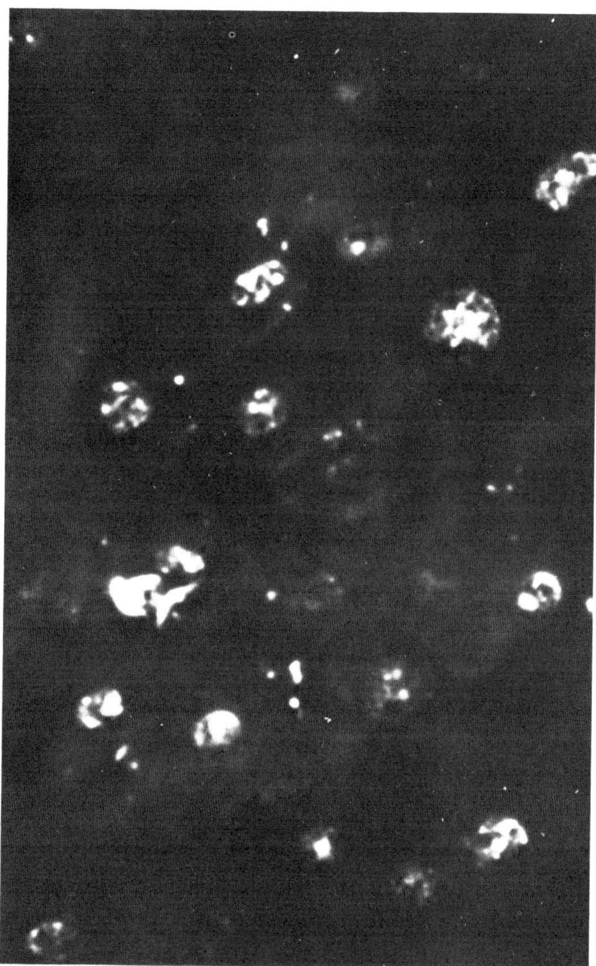

Figure 3-14 Hepatitis B core antigen present in granular distribution in many hepatocyte nuclei in chronic active hepatitis. Fluoresceinated anti-BHc × 400. (Reproduced with permission, M. A. Gerber, E. Sarno, and S. J. Vernace, *N. Engl. J. Med.* 294:922, 1976.)

localization of hepatitis B on liver cell surfaces have recently been recorded by Alberti and co-workers (134). During acute hepatitis B, surface antigen or HB_s Ag was noted on cell membranes of hepatocytes during the early phase of the disease process but not during the recovery period. These findings could be compatible with the concept that immune reactivity to HB_s Ag-positive hepatocytes might be involved in in vivo lysis of such cells and hepatic necrosis during the acute phase of the illness. The presence of viral antigen in the membranes of such acutely involved cells, together with evolution of antibody to HB antigen during acute viral hepatitis, suggests that a mechanism involving antibody-mediated cytotoxicity might be involved in liver cell damage during the evolution of acute viral hepatitis, or possibly at some stage of chronic active hepatitis.

Antibody-mediated cytotoxicity has been shown to function via so-called killer or K cells bearing an Fc receptor. As noted in Chapter 2, precise definition of K cells is still rather controversial; however, most groups working with such systems agree that K cells have an Fc receptor. Pertinent to this is a report by Thomson and co-workers (135), which shows in vitro cytotoxicity to rabbit liver cells with lymphocytes from patients with chronic active hepatitis. Cytotoxicity in this particular assay system was not T-cell mediated and appeared to be a function of K cells. An extension of this general concept has recently been suggested by a report showing enhancement of HB_s Ab production during fulminant viral hepatitis B (136). Several previous studies had suggested overproduction of HB_s Ab during particularly fulminant or severe viral hepatitis (104, 137). In the study by Woolf and colleagues clearance and production of HB_s Ab was examined in two groups of patients with viral hepatitis— fulminant and noncomplicated. Clearance of HB_s-specific antibody was significantly higher in the fulminant group; in addition, 41 percent of the patients with fulminant hepatitis showed HB_s Ab on hospital admission; none of the uncomplicated subjects did. The authors postulated that since marked enhancement or delayed clearance of antibody was present in fulminant disease, such antibody presumably was present in higher concentration in portal blood and might participate in a local Arthus-type reaction within the sinusoids of the liver. Such a reaction would involve formation of an acute antigen-antibody complex within vessel walls and is generally associated with acute necrosis, ischemia, and intense inflammation as described in the original experimental models (138). Figure 3-15 shows an example of the deposition within the vessel wall of antigen associated with an acute inflammatory reaction when such vessel-fixed antigen meets circulat-

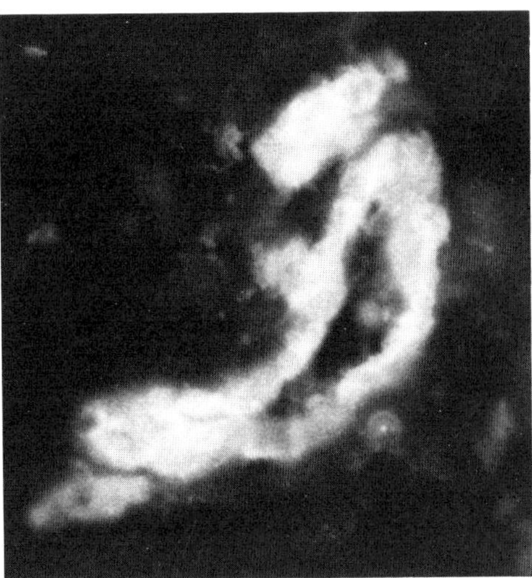

Figure 3-15   Immunofluorescent demonstration of the fixation of antigen (BSA) within a small blood vessel in an experimental acute Arthus reaction. Magnification × 300, staining with fluorescein-labeled goat antibovine serum albumin. Conventional H&E stain showed an intense infiltration of the blood-vessel wall by polymorphonuclear leukocytes.

ing antibody. Once the acute Arthus reaction is established, attempts at modulation through immunosuppressive therapy or corticosteroids are likely to fail. It has long been recognized that the use of corticosteroids in fulminant hepatitis tends to be disappointing.

Fulminant hepatitis may be more prominent in female patients (136), whereas in other clinical conditions associated with hepatitis B infection (such as HB_s Ag-positive chronic active hepatitis or the healthy carrier state, as well as uncomplicated hepatitis B viral hepatitis) the opposite sex ratio holds (139). Female predominance is the case in other presumed autoimmune conditions such as thyroiditis, systemic lupus erythematosus, and lupoid hepatitis. It has been repeatedly established in animal studies that females surpass males in relative quantitative amounts of immune responsiveness. This may have a direct bearing on the findings discussed above regarding specific HB Ab reactivity during acute fulminant hepatitis B infections.

Genetic Factors

A great deal of interest has centered on the association of selected histocompatibility antigens of the HLA system with specific disease states. The most striking recent examples relate to observations that document high correlation of HLA-B27 with anklylosing spondylitis (140, 141) and Reiter's syndrome (142, 143), as well as A1 and B8 in celiac syndrome (144, 145), and of A1 and B8 with chronic active hepatitis (146). The original observations related to hepatitis B virus infection—expression of detectable "Australia antigen" (HB_s Ag) in the blood of patients and various other human populations—was felt to relate to genetic polymorphism itself (147). A study of hepatitis B surface antigenemia was conducted in an attempt to relate occurrence of persistent HB_s Ag with HLA B locus markers in patients from a renal transplant center (148). This group of patients was selected because of the well-known persistence of antigenemia in patients with chronic renal disease undergoing maintenance dialysis or subsequent transplantation (149, 150). A significant association among Bw15, Bw17, Bw35, and HB_s antigenemia was demonstrated (148). One possible explanation is that HLA antigenic determinants, present as they are on the surfaces of cell membranes, may be in an ideal position to influence recognition of HB_s Ag as similar to "self" antigens and thus make the host unable to mount an effective inactivating immune response against the virus itself.

A Marker for Immune Complexes?

Since the original observations and unfolding of the hepatitis B antigen story (72), analysis of the antigenic structure of materials associated with hepatitis B virus has revealed considerable antigenic complexity and heterogeneity. Hepatitis B surface antigen or HB_s Ag, and some of the particles originally described by Dane and associates (151), show a diameter of approximately 42 nm and contain an inner core of material (HB core antigen) encompassing DNA. In 1972 a new complex of antigens was described by Magnius and Espmark (152), which they referred to collectively as "e antigen." This group of antigens (e Ag) is distinct from HB$_s$ Ag and shows different immunological and physical chemical properties (153). It is also a marker for HB virus infection, with a persistence somehow related to chronic liver disease (154). Recent elegant studies directed at clear definition of e antigen have revealed—surprisingly—that the antigen itself is an immunoglobulin (155). The studies indicate that e antigen shows the physical and immunochemical properties of a 7S IgG immunoglobulin of the IgG-4 H-chain subclass. Thus the presence of e antigen may indeed be the final denouement in our perception of the role of immune complexes in the disease itself.

Neurath and Strick (155) have postulated that the e antigen itself, being antibody, is directed at HB virus determinants and thus blocks other antibodies, possibly by steric hindrance from closely juxtaposed strategic viral antigens. Moreover, particular significance may be related to the finding that e antigen represents IgG molecules of the IgG-4 subclass, only a very small fraction (1 to 2 percent) of all IgG molecules present in the organism (156). It has been shown that unlike other IgG molecules, this particular IgG subclass does not react with C1q, the initial complement component, nor does it bind to macrophages. Thus if complement activation is blocked by the very nature of the autologous immune response, the natural first line of defense against invading virus may be critically impaired, and the presence of e antigen may then be considered as a blocking antibody, which facilitates viral persistence and chronicity of disease.

The concept of e antigen as an antibody somehow blocking effective host defenses is a novel one. Physical-chemical studies have revealed that it may exist as a polymeric form of IgG—being either dimeric or of a higher polymeric structure (155, 157). If e antigen represents a type of self-reacting rheumatoid factor or an antibody specific for hepatitis B determinants plus anti-IgG, we would have further insight into its association with viral persistence.

There are several other well-documented examples of what are felt to be self-associating rheumatoid factors—largely from the serum of patients with hyperviscosity syndrome and rheumatoid arthritis (158, 159). Very little is yet known concerning the exact physiological significance of this interesting class of self-associating 7S IgG rheumatoid factors. Whether they are in themselves modulators of the immune response or whether they act to effectively circumvent natural host mechanisms of defense remains to be determined. The problem is discussed in detail in Chapter 7.

The final vista of the relationship between hepatitis B viral infection and human disease has probably not yet been elucidated. Reports of an association with polymyalgia rheumatica (160) and infantile papular acrodermatitis (161), for example, have appeared. To examine the evolution of the understanding of hepatitis B infection and the importance of circulating as well as tissue-fixed immune complexes related to the original viral infection is a lesson in itself (162). The whole hepatitis B virus story emphasizes the signal importance of being able to recognize antigen in conjunction with some of the overt immune-complex–related clinical lesions with which it is associated.

Subacute Sclerosing Panencephalitis

Subacute sclerosing panencephalitis (SSPE) is a rare degenerative disease of the central nervous system that occurs principally in young children and adolescents. The clinical picture is one of insidious onset of mental deterioration, motor dysfunction, and inexorable progression to convulsions, coma, and death. In approximately 10 percent of cases the course is rapid; death takes place within three months. In about 80 percent of cases the more typical subacute but relentless disease terminates fatally after one to three years, and in the remaining 10 percent of patients the disease may run a more protracted course of four to eight years. Spontaneous clinical remissions, or even what appear to be periods of temporary clinical improvement, are well documented in occasional patients (163–165).

The neuropathological changes found in the

disease were first described in 1933 by Dawson (166), but it was not until many years later that a relation to measles was recognized. A virus with many of the biological properties of measles has now been isolated from brain tissues of many patients with SSPE (167–169). Moreover, the disease is characterized by the presence of marked elevations in humoral antibody response to measles virus antigens both in the blood and in the cerebrospinal fluid (CSF) (170–172). Anti-measles antibodies in blood and CSF show definite evidence of oligoclonal restriction—thus, instead of appearing as a broad heterogeneous smear of immunoglobulins of diverse electrophoretic mobilities such as is present in normal immunoglobulin, electrophoretic patterns of CSF as well as blood show multiple monoclonal or homogeneous populations of antibody molecules (173–176). Examples of the remarkable oligoclonal restriction or several homogeneous populations of immunoglobulin G antibodies are shown in Figure 3-16. Elution and fractionation studies

have documented that these restricted oligoclonal antibody populations represent antibodies directed against diverse structural antigenic components of measles virus (174, 175, 177). Careful absorption studies have indicated that the great majority of oligoclonal antibodies detected on electrophoresis of CSF are indeed antibodies directed at measles virus antigens (178). Although there is no extensive evidence of accompanying autoantibody formation, studies by Ma and colleagues (179) have shown that when CSF from an SSPE patient was absorbed with measles virus and subsequently incubated with the brain homogenate from the same individual, an additional 10 to 15 percent of IgG was removed.

The occurrence of oligoclonal antibodies of markedly restricted electrophoretic mobility in serum and CSF from patients with SSPE is reminiscent of the homogenous antibodies that have been produced after experimental hyperimmunization with various streptococcal or pneumococcal polysaccharides or bacterial vaccines (180–182). The exact mechanisms controlling production of single or multiple M components or relative oligoclonality in these experimental models have not been completely defined, but it would appear that relative structural restriction of polysaccharide antigenic determinants, genetic influences, and prolonged immunization are probably essential factors. Genetic factors may actually play a major role, since some strains of rabbits immunized with streptococcal variant organisms produce oligoclonal restricted antibodies in much higher proportion than others; this characteristic can be bred for and selected out among individual rabbit progeny (180). The occurrence of oligoclonal restriction particularly within SSPE CSF suggests that the infected host picks out a limited set of antigenic determinants on the measles virus and focuses a prolonged and uniform response on this limited antigenic repertoire. Since there are many features of SSPE that suggest immunologic imbalance—particularly exaggerated humoral responses in the face of depressed cellular immunity—it is also possible that oligoclonal antimeasles antibody production is the result of uneven activation of normal suppressor-cell

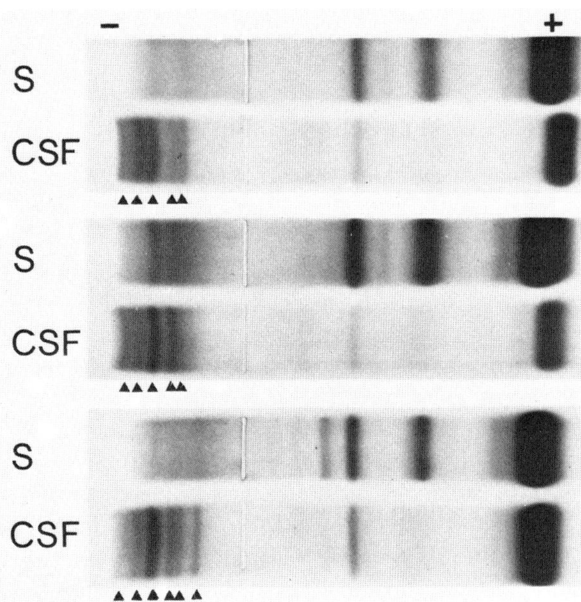

Figure 3-16 Serum and concentrated cerebrospinal fluid (CSF) from a patient with SSPE at various stages of the disease. A number of oligoclonal γ-globulin bands are present in the CSF. Similar restriction is faintly noted in parallel serum samples. (Photograph courtesy of Bodvar Vandvik, Oslo.)

control mechanisms, which effectively suppress some clones of antibody-forming cells but do not act on a few that manage to proliferate in uncontrolled fashion.

Fortunately, SSPE is a relatively rare disease with an estimated prevalence of 0.45 cases per million population. Epidemiologic studies of 350 clinically confirmed cases of SSPE recorded in the U.S. National Registry (183) showed that 292 of these patients gave a previous history of measles, while of the remaining 58 patients, 40 had received live attenuated measles vaccine. In those with a definite clinical history of measles, the initial measles infection in nearly half occurred before the age of two years. The mean interval between measles infection and SSPE was 7 years. No consistent relation between live measles vaccination and onset of SSPE was observed. Examination of data obtained from American and other national registries indicates that the prevalence of the disorder appears to be slowly decreasing. Its most prominent clinical features are given below:

Onset: Often slow or intermittent.
Course: Rapid, with death in three months (10 percent). Slowly progressive (classic form), with death in 1 to 3 years (80 percent). Slow, with death in 4 to 8 years (10 percent).
Population affected: Children and teenagers.
Laboratory findings: Marked elevation of measles antibodies in serum and CSF. Antimeasles antibodies, principally IgG; CSF shows oligoclonal immunoglobulins. Electroencephalographic changes characteristic. Brain biopsy—diagnostic histopathologic picture; measles virus and viral antigen demonstrable.

As noted above, a large body of clinical and experimental data have accumulated that directly link measles virus with SSPE (184). After recovery of virus from the brains of SSPE patients, viral infection has been successfully transferred to dogs, calves, and laboratory rodents (185–187). More recently, virus from SSPE patients has been successfully transferred to rhesus monkeys, where it caused a chronic progressive encephalitis in spite of preexisting measles immunity and a vigorous secondary antibody response in serum (188). Previous to this report by Albrecht and co-workers, study of the disease

had been hampered by lack of a reproducible primate model. One aspect of great interest in the Albrecht studies was the apparent absence of demonstrable lytic complement in the CSF throughout the experimental infection.

SSPE appears to be a viral disease principally of the central nervous system, where there is now abundant evidence for participation of immune complexes in much of the pathological process. Several investigators have also reported immune complexes of measles viral antigens and antibodies in renal basement membranes and in peripheral tissues in patients with SSPE (189–191). In the patient studied by Dayan and Stokes (189) granular deposits of IgG were noted in 10 to 15 percent of all glomeruli, along with C3 and particulate measles antigen. Moreover, studies of both serum and CSF have demonstrated the presence of measles virus–antibody complexes in patients with SSPE (192, 193). In these instances it was found that brain cells cultured from a patient with SSPE were lysed by the patient's own serum and that the lysis was dependent on the presence of autologous antimeasles antibody and complement. A fluorescence photomicrograph of the cultured brain cells from this patient binding rabbit antibody to measles virus antigen is shown in Figure 3-17. Immune complexes present in the serum were demonstrated by the addition of ^{125}I-labeled C3 to CSF or serum and subsequent ultracentrifugal separation. This technique identified a considerable proportion of material in the patient's CSF, which reacted with labeled C3 (presumably since it presented immune complexes).

One of the central enigmas with respect to the pathogenesis of ongoing cell destruction and progression of SSPE relates to the marked enhancement of humoral antibody response to measles virus antigens in the face of what appears to be a depression of cellular immunity. Years ago Burnet postulated that a specific defect in cell-mediated immunity somehow induced by the persistence of the measles virus actually allowed unbridled humoral antibody response in the face of defective cellular mechanisms generally capable of eventual virus elimination (194). There does indeed appear

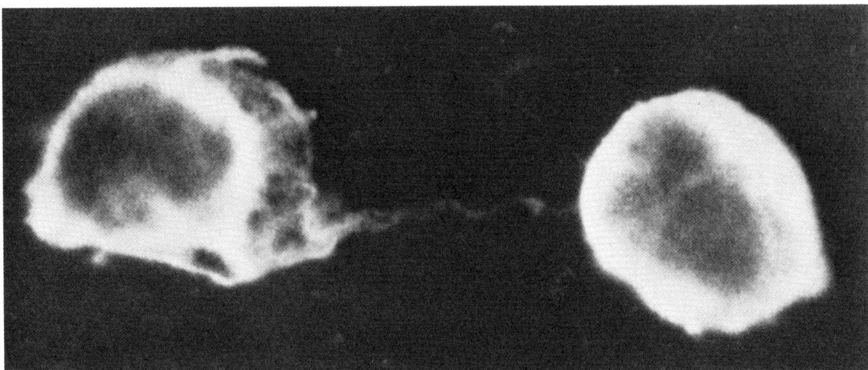

Figure 3-17 A fluorescence photomicrograph of cultured brain cells from a patient with SSPE. The cells were stained by the direct immunofluorescence technique, with rabbit antibody to measles virus conjugated to fluorescein isothiocyanate. Measles virus antigen is present in these cells. (Reproduced with permission, M. B. A. Oldstone, V. A. Bokisch, F. J. Dixon et al., *Clin. Immunol. Immunopathol.* 4:52, 1975.)

to be some degree of imbalance between humoral and cellular immunity in SSPE, but complete subversion of the cellular phase is contradicted by a number of experimental findings. Kreth and associates, for instance, were able to show cell-mediated cytotoxicity against measles virus in SSPE in vitro (195). In favor of some degree of depression in the cell-mediated immune system are studies by Ahmed and co-workers (196), which indicate that blocking factors may somehow be responsible for failure of the immune system to eliminate the measles virus. In three different assays they noted that plasma or CSF from SSPE patients was capable of blocking the inhibition of macrophage migration, lymphocyte transformation, and release of lymphotoxin usually noted when measles virus is mixed with sensitized cells. Preliminary characterization of the blocking factors involved showed that they were present in the exclusion or high-molecular-weight fractions of Sephadex G-200 gel filtration separations and could be removed by using antibody to human C3. These observations appear to be consistent with the presence of high-molecular-weight immune complexes binding C3.

A simple explanation for the humoral-cellular immune imbalance in SSPE is not yet at hand. Recent reports that focus on the killing of cells that express measles antigen (197–199)

using killer or K cells from patients with SSPE indicate that killing of virus-infected target cells was enhanced by SSPE serum or CSF and that the killing effect appeared to be related to measles antibody concentrations. Moreover, it was found that cells bearing Fc or C3 receptors appeared to be most important in killing of allogeneic measles-virus-infected target cells. Cytotoxic reactions were inhibited by Fab fragments of IgG that contained antimeasles antibodies, and the killing of infected target cells did not require histocompatibility of the cytotoxic killer peripheral blood lymphocytes with the target cell. Furthermore, killing was not enhanced by a histocompatibility fit (199). No blocking of killing was recorded when sera from SSPE patients were introduced into the test system. These data, together with the previous studies of Oldstone and co-workers (192), indicate that the ingredients for the killing of autologous cells infected with measles virus are present in patients with SSPE. The changes in cellular immunity may not be determined by blocking factors or primary measles-induced T-cell defects; it seems possible instead that anti-measles antibody may actually be capable of cellular modulation whereby viral antigen is constantly cleared or partially altered on infected cell surfaces. This mechanism may be in turn influenced by defective virus production. Absence of stable measles viral antigen in such situations is very similar to the situation discussed in Chapter 2, where cell-surface antigens during trypanosomiasis are constantly modulated by antibodies.

The problems involved in a final understanding of the pathogenesis of continuing cellular damage in SSPE are extremely important; in this disease the agent has been identified, the presence of antigen, virus, and local immune complexes within the central nervous system has been documented, and an experimental model using autologous cultured brain cells and putative sensitized lymphoid cells and humoral factors can be studied. In many respects the problems underlying the understanding of SSPE persistence are very similar to those encountered with the hepatitis B virus. Further observations on each should provide final clear insight into the mechanisms of basic pathogenesis. Once again the intimate association of immune complexes fixed to cell membranes or cell nuclei appears to be directly related to disease pathogenesis.

Finally, several experimental lines of evidence have been presented which indicate that with respect to SSPE all that appears to be measles may not be exactly the same. There have been scattered lines of evidence in the past that measles virus isolated from the brains of patients with SSPE may in fact be slightly different from the usual strains of measles virus (200–202). Recent experiments directed at clarifying this important point have been reported by Hall and ter Meulen (203), who demonstrated by hybridization and RNA homology studies that virus isolated from SSPE contains all of the genetic information present in measles virus, but that it also contains an additional 10 percent of genetic material. The authors speculate that this may indicate that the actual SSPE agent represents a recombination of measles virus with another still unknown virus. Such recombination, if it occurs, would involve the intact genome of measles virus and a defective second virus genome. Such recombination of defective and complete viral genomes to yield a stable recombinant capable of viral persistence has now been well documented in work with the vesicular stomatitis virus (204, 205). The concept of the SSPE agent as a possible recombinant of measles virus and a second defective virus could explain minor antigenic differences noted in the past between SSPE strains and measles virus. Furthermore, it could provide an explanation for the rarity of the disorder itself even though it is associated with a common virus infection. Confirmation and extension of such avenues of investigation is needed. The applicability to comparable problems encountered in other experimental systems such as NZB mouse disease or human SLE is obvious.

At present no effective treatment for SSPE has been established. Many forms of therapy directed at restoration of normal immunologic balance or altered immune responses have been undertaken. These include immunosuppression, courses of transfer factor, leukophoresis, and use of putative antiviral agents such as Isoprinosine[R], but to date no definite positive responses have been recorded. This in itself is a paradox. The agent—or at least the general type of agent—has been identified. Many of the abnormalities related to the disorder are known. Yet there still is no effective therapy.

Dengue and the Hemorrhagic Shock Syndrome

Dengue hemorrhagic fever is caused by a group B arbovirus infection transmitted by the *Aedes aegypti* mosquito. The clinical disease is endemic in urban portions of Southeast Asia and afflicts primarily children four to twelve years of age, most commonly during the rainy season. A major medical complication is the acute shock syndrome, which is seen in 10 percent of hospitalized patients.

Marked antigenic cross-reactivity is present among the four known types of dengue virus. A mechanism that has been postulated for initiation of the shock syndrome is recall or anamnestic antibody response cross-reacting with the actual infecting strain sufficiently to stimulate nonprotective antiviral antibody and early production of antigen-antibody complexes (206). Careful studies of 127 dengue patients in Thailand by Bokisch and co-workers (207) documented profound and rapid changes in complement proteins in temporal association with the onset of dengue shock syndrome among 49 of these patients. In severe cases C3 and C5 were rapidly reduced to 20 to 40 percent of normal, and evidence for defibrination as manifested by the appearance of fibrin split products and thrombocytopenia provided evidence for concomitant intravascular coagulation. Metabolic studies of radiolabeled C3 and C1q showed marked acceleration of fractional catabolic rates, particularly during shock. These studies provided substantial support for the concept that complement activation and precipitous complement consumption may play a crucial role in initiating the shock syndrome. In addition, they indicate that activation of the complement cascade may be important during certain disease states in initiating a second and much more harmful amplification—namely, the coagulation process. Similar mechanisms have been invoked for intravascular coagulation that occurs during pneumococcal or Gram-negative sepsis (Chapter 1). Strong experimental support for the functional interdependence of the complement and coagulation systems has been provided by Zimmerman and Müller-Eberhard (208).

It seems likely that the elegant studies of acute in vivo decomplementation and shock conducted on the dengue fever patients may be analogous to a number of other more common infectious disease states. Intravascular coagulation has now been recorded with a wide variety of septic conditions ranging from staphylococcal sepsis and endotoxemia in immunosuppressed hosts to miliary tuberculosis or fungal infections. It is possible that many such conditions are initiated, or at least partially initiated, by reactivity between C1q—the first complement component—and either nonprotective antibody or circulating lipopolysaccharide and other bacteria antigens capable of initiating complement activation and perhaps coagulation mechanisms simultaneously. Several other rapidly progressive infectious disease states often associated with diffuse vasculitic features and septic shock come to mind; fulminant rickettsial infection, overwhelming staphylococcal sepsis, or meningococcemia.

With newer and more readily available methods of immune-complex determination and complement component estimation, the exact role played by immune complexes may soon be clarified.

Lyme Arthritis and the Erythema Chronicum Migrans Syndrome

During the past five years a relatively new disorder has become clinically apparent in eastern Connecticut. It occurs largely in summer and early fall and is characterized by onset with red cutaneous macules or papules that expand to form large concentric rings. The illness is also accompanied by fever, myalgias, and monarticular or oligoarticular arthritis, which may be present 4 days to 22 weeks after onset. Several patients have reported being bitten by ticks at the site of the initial skin lesions 4 to 20 days before onset (209–211).

The clinical entity was originally recognized because of what appeared to be rather close geographic clustering of many cases. About three-quarters of cases recognized thus far have occurred in children, and brief but recurrent episodes of an asymmetric oligoarticular swelling and pain in large joints, particularly the knee, have been noted. In some patients clinical evidence has demonstrated myocardial conduction abnormalities, as well as development of cryoglobulin precipitates in serum. Although extensive attempts to culture synovium and synovial fluid as well as other patient material have produced no specific identifiable agent, it appears likely that patients afflicted with Lyme arthritis most probably suffer from infection by an arthropod-borne virus. Typical skin lesions, described as *erythema chronicum migrans,* are shown in Figure 3-18. Histologic examination of such lesions has shown heavy mononuclear cell infiltrations around blood vessels, and edema in papillary dermis as well as intracellular and extracellular edema. The initial clinical presentation in many subjects has clearly suggested an infectious process with fever, generalized adenopathy, splenomegaly, occasional malar rash, and rarely periorbital edema (211). Most patients have shown an ele-

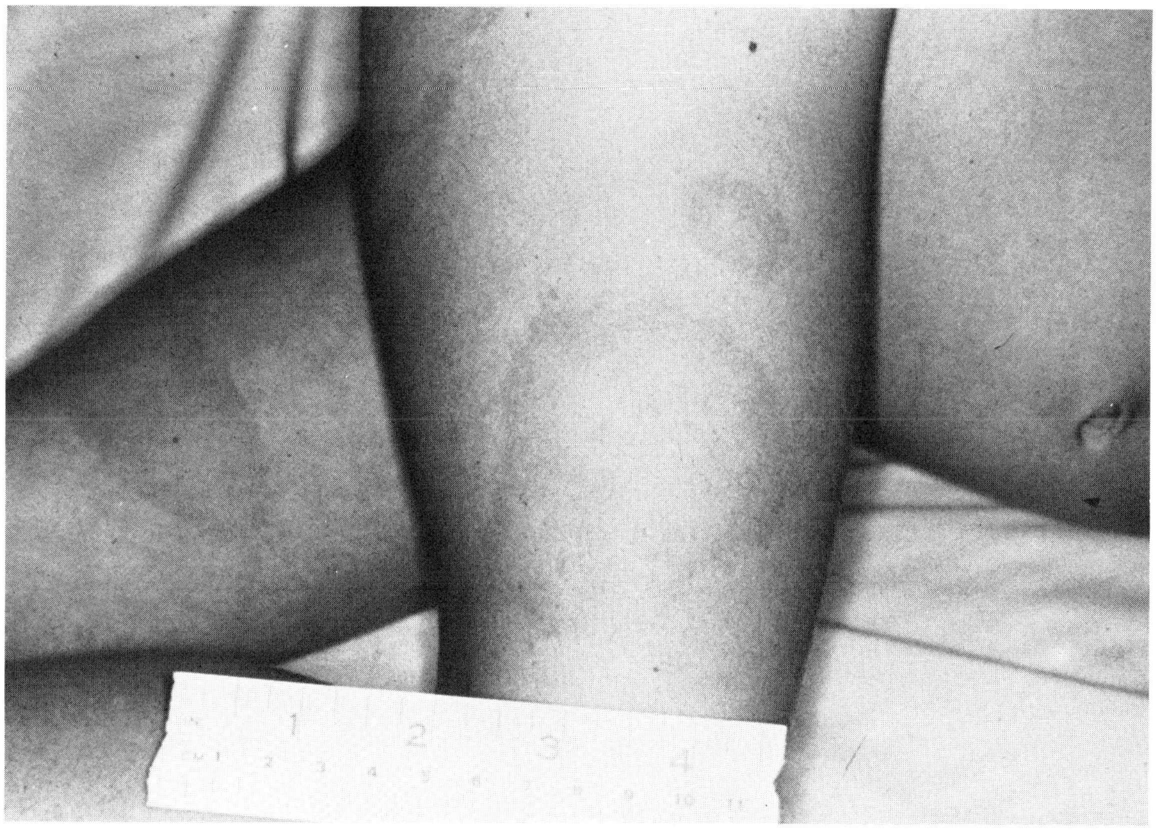

Figure 3-18 Skin lesions typical of *erythema chronicum migrans* associated with Lyme arthritis. (Reproduced with permission, A. C. Steere, S. E. Malawista, J. A. Hardin et al., *Ann. Intern. Med.* 86:685, 1977.)

vation of sedimentation rate and some elevation of serum IgM above 250 mg/dl.

Clinical examinations have revealed an interesting evolution of the disease with respect to joint symptomatology. Most patients appear to suffer from repeated attacks of arthritis usually separated by one- to ten-week periods of remission. A profile of joint involvement recorded in Steere's studies (211) is shown in Figure 3-19. Serum complement level was not uniform during attacks and complement levels were noted to increase, decrease, or remain constant in serial studies of individual patients. Two patients in the group showed 1:160 and 1:320 titers of serum rheumatoid factors. Joint fluid analyses have generally shown median leukocyte counts of 24,240 cells/mm³ (predominantly granulocytes); joint-fluid complement levels have not shown relative depression with respect to serum levels.

From the clinical descriptions of patients studied to date, it is apparent that this disease is difficult in its early stages to differentiate from juvenile or adult rheumatoid arthritis. A helpful finding in some patients in whom the diagnosis is still in doubt after reasonable follow-up is the development of antinuclear antibodies or iridocyclitis—positive in approximately 25 percent of patients with pauciarticular juvenile rheumatoid arthritis (212). In most patients with Lyme arthritis the disorder follows a relapsing but slowly improving course and appears to subside after 6 to 24 months of followup. Long-term sequelae in such patients are not yet known.

The skin lesions of *erythema chronicum migrans* have been observed in Europe, Scandinavia, Russia, and the United States (213–215). In the past these lesions have been associated most commonly with tick bites, but a clear defi-

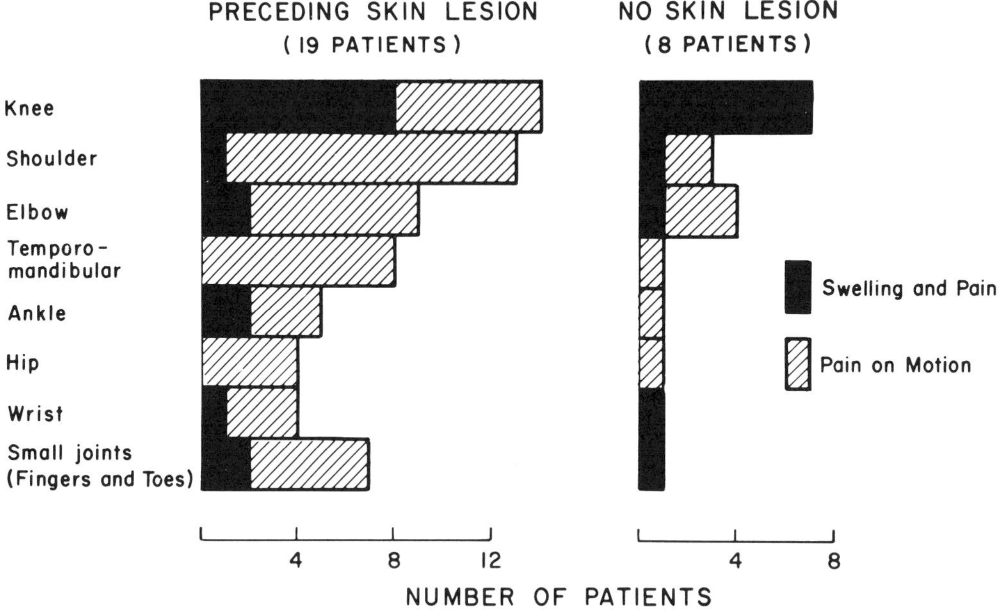

Figure 3-19 The joints affected by swelling and pain and by pain on motion, in patients with and without *erythema chronicum migrans.* The involved joints are similar in the two groups. (Reproduced with permission, A. C. Steere, S. E. Melawista, J. A. Hardin et al., *Ann. Intern. Med.* 86:685, 1977.)

nition of the causative infectious agent—either rickettsial or viral—has not been presented (216–221).

A discussion of Lyme arthritis has been included in this chapter because the illness, although not yet identified as definitely viral in etiology, is clearly associated with the presence of immune complexes. Serial serum samples recently examined by us in collaboration with Hardin and colleagues (222) have shown marked elevations of immune complexes during clinical illness. The serum cryoglobulins frequently noted in patients with Lyme arthritis, although they do not appear to correlate directly with the presence of detectable circulating immune complexes, are of interest; in many ways their occurrence resembles similar phenomena in other infectious disease states, such as subacute bacterial endocarditis, infectious mononucleosis, or chronic hepatitis B viral infection. Studies of the cryoglobulins from patients with Lyme arthritis have shown presence of predominant IgM, with trace amounts of IgG and C3 and C4.

There are many viral diseases that have now been directly related either to circulating or tissue-bound immune-complex phenomena. It seems most likely that the exact role of immune complexes in the future will be clarified by the study of viral illnesses, where broad knowledge of the actual agent and a battery of sensitive reagents capable of detecting various antigenic components of immune complexes are readily available. The antigenic heterogeneity of the hepatitis B virus or the studies of RNA hybridization techniques involving measles virus and RNA from SSPE strains hold the most immediate promise for success. One cannot examine the whole clinical profile of diseases related to hepatitis B or measles-like agents without perceiving that further insight into the basic disease processes associated with these agents will be immediately helpful in unraveling immune-complex diseases of still unknown etiology, such as systemic lupus erythematosus or rheumatoid arthritis.

References

1. Callahan, R., Benveniste, R. E., Lieber, M. M., et al. Nucleic acid homology of murine Type-C viral genes. *J. Virol.* 14:1394, 1974.

2. Wecker, E., Schimpl, A., and Hünig, T. Expression of MuLV GP71-like antigen in normal mouse spleen cells induced by antigenic stimulation. *Nature* 269:598, 1977.

3. Moroni, C., and Schumann, G. Are endogenous C-type viruses involved in the immune system? *Nature* 269:600, 1977.

4. Dameshek, W. Speculations on the nature of infectious mononucleosis. In R. L. Carter and H. G. Penman, eds., *Infectious Mononucleosis,* p. 225. Blackwell Scientific Publications, Oxford, 1969.

5. Henle, W., and Henle, G. Epstein-Barr virus and infectious mononucleosis. *N. Engl. J. Med.* 288:263, 1973.

6. Miller, G., Niederman, J. C., and Andrews, L. Prolonged oropharyngeal excretion of Epstein-Barr virus after infectious mononucleosis. *N. Engl. J. Med.* 288:229, 1973.

7. Joncas, J. H. Clinical significance of the EB herpesvirus infection in man. *Prog. Med. Virol.* 14:200, 1972.

8. Ziegler, E. E. Infectious mononucleosis, report of a fatal case with autopsy. *Arch. Pathol.* 37:196, 1944.

9. Thompson, W. T., Jr., and Pitt, C. Frank hematuria as a manifestation of infectious mononucleosis. *Ann. Intern. Med.* 33:1274, 1950.

10. Taub, E. A. Renal lesions, gross hematuria and marrow granulomas in infectious mononucleosis. *J.A.M.A.* 195:1153, 1966.

11. Tennant, F. S. The glomerulonephritis of infectious mononucleosis. *Tex. Rep. Biol. Med.* 26:603, 1968.

12. Brun, C., Madsen, S., and Olsen, S. Infectious mononucleosis with hepatic and renal involvement. *Scand. J. Gastroenterol. Suppl.* 7:89, 1970.

13. Peters, J. H., Flume, J., and Fuccillo, D. Nephritis in infectious mononucleosis. *Clin. Res.* 10:254, 1962.

14. Peters, J. H. Heterophile reactive antigens in infectious mononucleosis. *Science* 157:1200, 1967.

15. Editorial. Nephritis in infectious mononucleosis. *Lancet* 1:647, 1973.

16. Wallace, M., Leet, G., and Rothwell, P. Immune complex-mediated glomerulonephritis with infectious mononucleosis. *Aust. N.Z. J. Med.* 4:192, 1974.

17. Andres, G. A., Kano, K., Elwood, C., et al. Immune deposit nephritis in infectious mono-nucleosis. *Int. Arch. Allergy Appl. Immunol.* 52:136, 1976.

18. Lowery, T. A., Rutsky, E. A., Hartley, M. W., et al. Renal failure in infectious mononucleosis. *South. Med. J.* 69:1212, 1976.

19. Malavé, I., and Milgrom, F. Heterophile antigen detected by infectious mononucleosis sera on lymphoid cells. *Int. Arch. Allergy Appl. Immunol.* 44:601, 1973.

20. Thomas, D. B., and Phillips, B. Membrane antigens specific for human lymphoid cells in the dividing phase. *J. Exp. Med.* 138:64, 1973.

21. Mottironi, V. D., and Terasaki, P. I. Lymphocytotoxins in disease. I. Infectious mononucleosis, rubella and measles. In P. I. Terasaki, ed., *Histocompatibility Testing,* p. 301. Williams & Wilkins Co., Baltimore, 1970.

22. Germuth, F. G., and Rodriquez, E. Immune complex deposit glomerular disease. In *Immunopathology of the Renal Glomerulus,* pp. 21, 38. Little, Brown and Co., Boston, 1973.

23. Magner, W., and Brooks, E. F. Infectious mononucleosis with acute thrombopenic purpura. *Can. Med. Assoc. J.* 47:35, 1942.

24. Grossman, L. A., and Wolff, S. M. Acute thrombocytopenic purpura in infectious mononucleosis. *J.A.M.A.* 171:2208, 1959.

25. Radel, E. G., and Schorr, J. B. Thrombocytopenic purpura with infectious mononucleosis: report of two cases and a review of the literature. *J. Pediatr.* 63:46, 1963.

26. Smith, D. S., Abell, J. D., and Cast, I. P. Auto-immune hemolytic anemia and thrombocytopenia complicating infectious mononucleosis. *Br. Med. J.* 1:1210, 1963.

27. Krishnamurthy, M., Lee, C. K., and Dosik, H. Infectious mononucleosis and severe thrombocytopenia. *Am. J. Med. Sci.* 272:221, 1976.

28. Karpatkin, S., Strick, N., Karpatkin, M. B., et al. Cumulative experience in the detection of anti-platelet antibody in 234 patients with idiopathic thrombocytopenic purpura; systemic lupus erythematosus and other clinical disorders. *Am. J. Med.* 52:776, 1972.

29. Jenkins, W. J., Koster, H. G., Marsh, W. L., et al. Infectious mononucleosis: an unsuspected source of anti-i. *Br. J. Haematol.* 11:480, 1965.

30. Rosenfield, R. E., Schmidt, P. J., Calvo, R. C., et al. Anti-i, a frequent cold agglutinin in infectious mononucleosis. *Vox Sang.* 10:631, 1965.

31. Capra, J. D., Dowling, P., Cook, S., et al. An incomplete cold-reactive γG antibody with i specific-

ity in infectious mononucleosis. *Vox Sang.* 16:10, 1969.

32. Goldberg, L. S., and Barnett, E. V. The role of rheumatoid (antiglobulin) factors in hemolytic anemia. *Ann. N.Y. Acad. Sci.* 168:122, 1969.

33. Wilkinson, L. S., Petz, L. D., and Garratty, G. Reappraisal of the role of anti-i in haemolytic anaemia in infectious mononucleosis. *Br. J. Haematol.* 25:715, 1973.

34. Horwitz, C. A., Moulds, J., Henle, W., et al. Cold agglutinins in infectious mononucleosis and heterophil-antibody-negative mononucleosis-like syndromes. *Blood* 50:195, 1977.

35. Coutinho, A., and Möller, G. Thymus-independent B-cell induction and paralysis. *Adv. Immunol.* 21:114, 1975.

36. Roelcke, D. A review: cold agglutination. Antibodies and antigens. *Clin. Immunol. Immunopathol.* 2:266, 1974.

37. Notkins, A. L. Infectious virus-antibody complexes: interaction with anti-immunoglobulins, complement, and rheumatoid factor. *J. Exp. Med.* 134:41s, 1971.

38. Kissmeyer-Nielsen, F., Svejgaard, A., Kjerbye, K. E., et al. Blocking effect of rheumatoid factor on complement fixation by thrombocyte isoantibodies. *Vox Sang.* 12:199, 1967.

39. Romeyn, J. A., and Bowman, D. M. Inhibition of complementary lysis by rheumatoid sera. *Nature* 216:180, 1967.

40. Schmid, F. R., Roitt, I. M., and Rocha, M. J. Complement fixation by a two-component antibody system: immunoglobulin G and immunoglobulin M antiglobulin (rheumatoid factor). Paradoxical effect related to immunoglobulin G concentration. *J. Exp. Med.* 132:673, 1970.

41. Hafström, T. Neurological complications of mononucleosis. *Acta Neurol. Scand. (Suppl.)* 39:69, 1963.

42. Silverstein A., Steinberg, G., and Nathanson, M. Nervous system involvement in infectious mononucleosis. The heralding and/or major manifestation. *Arch. Neurol.* 26:353, 1972.

43. Friedland, R., and Yahr, M. D. Meningoencephalopathy secondary to infectious mononucleosis. Unusual presentation with stupor and chorea. *Arch. Neurol.* 34:186, 1977.

44. Petheram, I. S. Severe haemolysis and unilateral sensorineural deafness in infectious mononucleosis. *Practitioner* 217:945, 1976.

45. Sworn, M. J., and Urich, J. Acute encephalitis in infectious mononucleosis. *J. Pathol.* 100:201, 1970.

46. Wands, J. R., Perrotto, J. L., and Issel-

bacher, K. J. Circulating immune complexes and complement sequence activation in infectious mononucleosis. *Am. J. Med.* 60:269, 1976.

47. Kaplan, M. E. Cryoglobulinemia in infectious mononucleosis: Quantitation and characterization of the cryoproteins. *J. Lab. Clin. Med.* 71:754, 1968.

48. Charlesworth, J. A., Pussell, B. A., Roy, L. P., et al. The complement system in infectious mononucleosis. *Aust. N.Z. J. Med.* 7:23, 1977.

49. Henle, W., and Henle, G. In P. M. Biggs, G. de-Thé, and L. N. Payne, eds., *Oncogenesis and Herpesviruses*, p. 269. I.A.R.C. Scientific Publication no. 2, Lyon, 1972.

50. de-Thé, G. Is Burkitt's lymphoma related to perinatal infection by Epstein-Barr virus? *Lancet* 1:335, 1977.

51. Osborn, D. C., Fox, R. A., Fernandez, L. A., et al. Cytotoxic lymphocytes in infectious mononucleosis. *Can. Med. Assoc. J.* 115:1118, 1976.

52. Mangi, R. J., Niederman, J. C., Kelleher, J. E., et al. Depression of cell-mediated immunity during acute infectious mononucleosis. *N. Engl. J. Med.* 291:1149, 1974.

53. Wiederholt, W. C., Mulder, D. W., and Lambert, E. H. The Landry-Guillain-Barré-Strohl syndrome or polyradiculoneuropathy: Historical review, report on 97 patients, and present concepts. *Mayo Clin. Proc.* 39:427, 1964.

54. Melnick, S. C. Thirty-eight cases of the Guillain-Barré syndrome: an immunological study. *Br. Med. J.* 1:368, 1963.

55. Knowles, M., Saunders, M., Currie, S., et al. Lymphocyte transformation in the Guillain-Barré syndrome. *Lancet* 2:1168, 1969.

56. Rocklin, R. E., Sheremata, W. A., Feldman, R. G., et al. The Guillain-Barré syndrome and multiple sclerosis. *In vitro* cellular responses to nervous-tissue antigens. *N. Engl. J. Med.* 284:803, 1971.

57. Behan, P. O., Behan, W. M. H., Feldman, R. G., et al. Cell-mediated hypersensitivity to neural antigens. Occurrence in human patients and nonhuman primates with neurological diseases. *Arch. Neurol.* 27:145, 1972.

58. Rhodes, A. J., and Van Rooyen, C. E. Group A coxsackievirus. In *Textbook of Virology*, ed. 5., p. 585. Williams & Wilkins Co., Baltimore, 1968.

59. Novak, M., Filipova, V., and Kulkova, H. *Cas. Lek. Cesk.* 114:1352, 1975.

60. Callaghan, N., Flaherty, T., and McGarry, J. D. Landry-Guillain-Barré syndrome associated with recent herpes virus hominis infection. *Ir. Med. J.* 67:541, 1974.

61. Grose, C., Henle, W., Henle, G., et al. Pri-

mary Epstein-Barr-virus infections in acute neurologic diseases. *N. Engl. J. Med.* 292:392, 1975.

62. Von Pirquet, C. Das Verhalten der Kutanen Tuberkulin-reaktion während der Masern. *Dtsch. Med. Wochenschr.* 34:1297, 1908.

63. Bech, V. Measles epidemics in Greenland. *Am. J. Dis. Child.* 103:252, 1962.

64. Nalbant, J. P. The effect of contagious diseases on pulmonary tuberculosis and on the tuberculin reaction in children. *Am. Rev. Tuber.* 36:773, 1937.

65. Waksman, B. H., and Adams, R. D. Allergic neuritis: an experimental disease of rabbits induced by the injection of peripheral nervous tissue and adjuvants. *J. Exp. Med.* 102:213, 1955.

66. Waksman, B. H., and Adams, R. D. A comparative study of experimental allergic neuritis in the rabbit, guinea pig and mouse. *J. Neuropathol. Exp. Neurol.* 15:293, 1956.

67. Abramsky, O., Teitelbaum, D., and Arnon, R. Experimental allergic neuritis induced by a basic neuritogenic protein (P_1L) of human peripheral nerve origin. *Eur. J. Immunol.* 7:213, 1977.

68. Faber, V., and Balslov, J. T. Immunofluorescent studies of renal biopsies in acute polyradiculitis. *Acta Pathol. Microbiol. Scand. (A)* 78:655, 1970.

69. Whitaker, J. N., Dowling, P. C., and Cook, S. D. Immunofluorescent studies of the kidney in human neurologic disorders. *J. Neuropathol. Exp. Neurol.* 30:129, 1971 (abstract).

70. Behan, P. O., Lowenstein, L. M., Stilmant, M., et al. Landry-Guillain-Barré-Strohl syndrome and immune-complex nephritis. *Lancet* 1:850, 1973.

71. Tachovsky, T. G., Lisak, R. P., Koprowski, H., et al. Circulating immune complexes in multiple sclerosis and other neurological diseases. *Lancet* 2:997, 1976.

72. Blumberg, B. S. Australia antigen and the biology of hepatitis B. *Science* 197:17, 1977.

73. Gocke, D. J., Hsu, K., Morgan, C., et al. Association between polyarteritis and Australia antigen. *Lancet* 2:1149, 1970.

74. Prince, A. M., and Trepo, C. Role of immune complexes involving SH antigen in pathogenesis of chronic active hepatitis and polyarteritis nodosa. *Lancet* 1:1309, 1971.

75. Gocke, D. J., Hsu, K., Morgan C., et al. Vasculitis in association with Australia antigen. *J. Exp. Med.* 134:330s, 1971.

76. Levo, Y., Gorevic, P. D., Kassab, H. J., et al. Association between hepatitis B virus and essential mixed cryoglobulinemia. *N. Engl. J. Med.* 296:1501, 1977.

77. Meltzer, M., Franklin, E. C., Elias, K., et al. Cryoglobulinemia—a clinical and laboratory study. II. Cryoglobulins with rheumatoid factor activity. *Am. J. Med.* 40:837, 1966.

78. Brouet, J-C., Clauvel, J. P., Danon, F., et al. Biologic and clinical significance of cryoglobulins: a report of 86 cases. *Am. J. Med.* 57:775, 1974.

79. Sergent, J. S., Lockshin, M. D., Christian, C. L. et al. Vasculitis with hepatitis B antigenemia. Long-term observations in nine patients. *Medicine* 55:1, 1976.

80. Schenkein, I., Bystryn, J. C., and Uhr, J. W. Specific removal of *in vivo* antibody by extracorporeal circulation over an immumoadsorbent in gel. *J. Clin. Invest.* 50:1864, 1971.

81. Lyle, L. R., Parker, B. M., and Parker, C. W. The use of protein-substituted nylon catheters for selective immunoadsorption *in vivo.* *J. Immunol.* 113:517, 1974.

82. Terman, D. S., Stewart, I., Robinette, J., et al. Specific removal of DNA antibody *in vivo* with an extracorporeal immunoadsorbent. *Clin. Exp. Immunol.* 24:231, 1976.

83. Terman, D. S., Tavel, T., Petty, D., et al. Specific removal of bovine serum albumin (BSA) antibodies *in vivo* by extracorporeal circulation over BSA immobilized on nylon microcapsules. *J. Immunol.* 116:1337, 1976.

84. Terman, D. S., Tavel, A., Tavel, T., et al. Degradation of circulating DNA by extracorporeal circulation over nuclease immobilized on nylon microcapsules. *J. Clin. Invest.,* 57:1201, 1976.

85. Terman, D. S., Ogden, D., and Petty, D. Removal of circulating antigen and immune complexes with immunoreactive collodion membranes. *F.E.B.S. Lett.* 68:89, 1976.

86. Terman, D. S., Tavel, T., Petty, D., et al. Specific removal of antibody by extracorporeal circulation over antigen immobilized in collodion-charcoal. *Clin. Exp. Immunol.* 28:180, 1977.

87. Craddock, P. R., Fehr, J., Brigham, K., et al. Complement and leukocyte-mediated pulmonary dysfunction in hemodialysis. *N. Engl. J. Med.* 296:769, 1977.

88. Craddock, P. R., Fehr, J., Dalmasso, A. P., et al. Hemodialysis leukopenia: pulmonary vascular leukostasis resulting from complement activation by dialyzer cellophane membranes. *J. Clin. Invest.* 59:879, 1977.

89. Fehr, J., and Jacob, H. S. *In vitro* granulocyte adherence and *in vivo* margination: two associated complement-dependent functions. Studies based on the acute neutropenia of filtration leukophoresis. *J. Exp. Med.* 146:641, 1977.

90. Mirick, G. S., and Shank, R. E. An epidemic of serum hepatitis studied under controlled conditions. *Trans. Am. Clin. Climatol. Assoc.* 71:176, 1959.

91. Onion, D. K., Crumpacker, C. S., and Gilliland, B. C. Arthritis of hepatitis associated with Australia antigen. *Ann. Intern. Med.* 75:29, 1971.

92. Alpert, E., Isselbacher, K. J., and Schur, P. H. The pathogenesis of arthritis associated with viral hepatitis. Complement-component studies. *N. Engl. J. Med.* 285:185, 1971.

93. Fernandez, R., and McCarty, D. J. The arthritis of viral hepatitis. *Ann. Intern. Med.* 74:207, 1971.

94. Graves, R. J. In *A System of Clinical Medicine,* P. 564. Fannin and Company, Dublin, 1843.

95. Klemola, E., and Törmä, S. Arthralgia and arthritis caused by infectious hepatitis. *Ann. Med. Intern. (Fenn.)* 38:161, 1949.

96. Martini, G. A. Über polyarthritis im Vorstadium der Inokulationshepatitis. *Dtsch. Med. Wochenschr.* 75:1464, 1950.

97. Crespi, B. P., Tomás-Escúe, A., and Rotés, J. El síndrome articular de la hepatitis vírica ictérica. *Rev. Esp. Reum. Enferm. Osteoartic.* 11:189, 1966.

98. Gue, T. B., and Bonner, W. M. Jr. Articular manifestations of infectious hepatitis. *J. S.C. Med. Assoc.* 63:279, 1977.

99. National Communicable Disease Center. Polyarthritis and viral hepatitis: a report of three cases with this relatively unusual association, and review of the literature. In *Hepatitis Surveillance Report No. 28,* p. 20. Atlanta, Jan. 31, 1968.

100. Ljunggren, B., and Möller, H. Hepatitis presenting as transient urticaria. *Acta Derm. Venereol. (Stockh.)* 51:295, 1971.

101. Stevens, D. P., Walker, J., Crum, E., et al. Anicteric hepatitis presenting as polyarthritis. *J.A.M.A.* 220:687, 1972.

102. Shulman, N. R., and Barker, L. F. Viruslike antigen, antibody, and antigen-antibody complexes in hepatitis measured by complement fixation. *Science* 165:304, 1969.

103. Almeida, J. D., and Waterson, A. P. Immune complexes in hepatitis. *Lancet* 2:983, 1963.

104. Gocke, D. J., Hsu, K., Morgan, C., et al. Vasculitis in association with Australia antigen. *J. Exp. Med.* 134:330 S, 1971.

105. Alpert, E., Schur, P. H., and Isselbacher, K. J. Sequential changes of serum complement in HAA related arthritis. *N. Engl. J. Med.* 287:103, 1972.

106. Wands, J. R., Mann, E., Alpert, E., et al. The pathogenesis of arthritis associated with acute hepatitis-B surface antigen-positive hepatitis complement activation and characterization of circulating immune complexes. *J. Clin. Invest.* 55:930, 1975.

107. Müller-Eberhard, H. J. Chemistry and reaction mechanisms of complement. *Adv. Immunol.* 8:1, 1968.

108. Lerner, A. B., and Watson, C. J. Studies of cryoglobulins. I. Unusual purpura associated with the presence of a high concentration of cryoglobulin (cold precipitable serum globulin). *Am. J. Med. Sci.* 214:410, 1947.

109. Grey, H. M., and Kohler, P. F. Cryoimmunoglobulins. *Semin. Hematol.* 10:87, 1973.

110. Farivar, M., Wands, J. R., Benson, G. D., et al. Cryoprotein complexes and peripheral neuropathy in a patient with chronic active hepatitis. *Gastroenterology* 71:490, 1976.

111. Logothetis, J., Kennedy, W. R., Ellington, A., et al. Cryoglobulinemic neuropathy. Incidence and clinical characteristics. *Arch. Neurol.* 19:389, 1968.

112. Combes, B., Stastny, P., Shorey, J., et al. Glomerulonephritis with deposition of Australia antigen-antibody complexes in glomerular basement membrane. *Lancet* 2:234, 1971.

113. Myers, B. D., Griffel, B., Naveh, D., et al. Membrano-proliferative glomerulonephritis associated with persistent viral hepatitis. *Am. J. Clin. Pathol.* 60:222, 1973.

114. Knieser, M. R., Jenis, E. H., Lowenthal, D. T., et al. Pathogenesis of renal disease associated with viral hepatitis. *Arch. Pathol.* 97:193, 1974.

115. Eknoyan, G., Györkey, F., Dichoso, C., et al. Renal morphological and immunological changes associated with acute viral hepatitis. *Kidney Int.* 1:413, 1972.

116. Kohler, P. F., Cronin, R. E., Hammond, W. S., et al. Chronic membranous glomerulonephritis caused by hepatitis B antigen-antibody immune complexes. *Ann. Intern. Med.* 81:448, 1974.

117. Dudley, F. J., Fox, R. A., and Sherlock, S. Cellular immunity and hepatitis-associated Australia antigen liver disease. *Lancet* 1:723, 1972.

118. Dudley, F. J., Scheuer, P. J., and Sherlock, S. Natural history of hepatitis-associated antigen-positive chronic liver disease. *Lancet* 2:1388, 1972.

119. Kohler, P. F., Trembath, J., Merrill, D. A., et al. Immunotherapy with antibody, lymphocytes and transfer factor in chronic hepatitis B. *Clin. Immunol. Immunopathol.* 2:465, 1974.

120. Coller, J. A., Millman, I., Halbherr, T. C., et al. Radioimmunoprecipitation assay for Australia antigen, antibody, and antigen-antibody complexes. *Proc. Soc. Exp. Biol. Med.* 138:249, 1971.

121. Wands, J. R., Alpert, E., and Isselbacher, K. J. Arthritis associated with chronic active hepatitis: complement activation and characterization of circulating immune complexes. *Gastroenterology* 69:1286, 1975.

122. Santoro, F., Wattre, P., Dessaint, J-P., et al. Hepatitis B circulating immune complexes. Characterization by radioimmunoprecipitation—PEG Assay (RIPEGA) *J. Immunol. Methods* 15:201, 1977.

123. Theofilopoulos, A. N., Wilson, C. B., and Dixon, F. J. The Raji cell radio-immune assay for detecting immune complexes in human sera. *J. Clin. Invest.* 57:169, 1976.

124. Meyer zum Büschenfelde, K. H., Knolle, J., and Berger, J. Cellulare Immunreaktione gegenüber homologen leberspezifischen Antigenen (HLP) bei chronischen Leberentzundungen. *Klin. Wochenschr.* 52:246, 1974.

125. Reed., W. D., Lee, W. M., Eddleston, A. L. W. F., et al. Cell-mediated immunity to hepatitis B antigen in antigen-negative active chronic hepatitis. *Gut* 15:341, 1974.

126. Edgington, T. S., and Ritt, D. J. Intrahepatic expression of serum hepatitis virus-associated antigens. *J. Exp. Med.* 134:871, 1971.

127. Nowoslawski, A., Krawczyński, K., Brzosko, W. J., et al. Tissue localization of Australia antigen immune complexes in acute and chronic hepatitis and liver cirrhosis. *Am. J. Pathol.* 68:31, 1972.

128. Gerber, M. A., Brodin, A., Steinberg, D., et al. Periarteritis nodosa, Australia antigen and lymphatic leukemia. *N. Engl. J. Med.* 286:14, 1972.

129. Hadziyannis, S., Gerber, M. A., Vissoulis, C., et al. Cytoplasmic hepatitis B antigen in "ground-glass" hepatocytes of carriers. *Arch. Pathol.* 96:327, 1973.

130. ten Kate, F. J. W., Feltkamp-Vroom, T., Helder, A. W., et al. Demonstration of HB antigens in liver tissue. *Digestion* 10:305, 1974.

131. Gerber, M. A., Sarno, E., and Vernace, S. J. Immune complexes in hepatocytic nuclei of HB Ag-positive chronic hepatitis. *N. Engl. J. Med.* 294:922, 1976.

132. Tan, E. M., and Kunkel, H. G. An immunofluorescent study of the skin lesions in systemic lupus erythematosus. *Arthritis Rheum.* 9:37, 1966.

133. Paronetto, F., and Koffler, D. Immunofluorescent localization of immunoglobulins, complement, and fibrinogen in human diseases. I. Systemic lupus erythematosus. *J. Clin. Invest.* 44:1657, 1965.

134. Alberti, A., Realdi, G., Tremolada, F., et al. Liver cell surface localization of hepatitis B antigen and of immunoglobulins in acute and chronic hepatitis and in liver cirrhosis. *Clin. Exp. Immunol.* 25:396, 1976.

135. Thomson, A. D., Cochrane, M. A. G., McFarlane, I. G., et al. Lymphocyte cytotoxicity to isolated hepatocytes in chronic active hepatitis. *Nature* 252:721, 1974.

136. Woolf, I. L., El Sheikh, N., Cullens, H., et al. Enhanced Hbs Ab production in pathogenesis of fulminant viral hepatitis Type B. *Br. Med. J.* 2:669, 1976.

137. Trepo, C. G., Robert, D., Motin, J., et al. Hepatitis B antigen (HBs Ag) and/or antibodies (anti-HBs and anti-HBc) in fulminant hepatitis: pathogenic and prognostic significance. *Gut* 17:10, 1976.

138. Arthus, M. Injections répétées de sérum de cheval chez le lapin. *C.R. Soc. Biol. (Paris)* 55:817, 1903.

139. Blumberg, B. S., Sutnick, A. I., London, W. T., et al. Sex distribution of Australia antigen. *Arch. Intern. Med.* 130:227, 1972.

140. Caffrey, M. F. P., and James, D. C. O. Human lymphocyte antigen association in ankylosing spondylitis. *Nature* 242:121, 1973.

141. Schlosstein, L., Terasaki, P. I., Bluestone, R., et al. High association of an HL-A antigen, W27, with ankylosing spondylitis. *N. Engl. J. Med.* 288:704, 1973.

142. Brewerton, D. A., Caffrey, M., Nicholls, A., et al. Reiter's disease and HL-A 27. *Lancet* 2:996, 1973.

143. Morris, R., Metzger, A. L., Bluestone, R., et al. HL-A W27—a clue to the diagnosis and pathogenesis of Reiter's syndrome. *N. Engl. J. Med.* 290:554, 1974.

144. Stokes, P. L., Asquith, P., Holmes, G. K. T., et al. Histocompatibility antigens associated with adult celiac disease. *Lancet* 2:162, 1972.

145. Falchuk, Z. M., Rogentine, G. N., and Strober, W. Predominance of histocompatibility antigen HL-A8 in patients with gluten-sensitive enteropathy. *J. Clin. Invest.* 51:1602, 1972.

146. Mackay, I. R., and Morris, P. J. Association of autoimmune active chronic hepatitis with HL-A1,-8. *Lancet* 2:793, 1972.

147. Blumberg, B. S., Friedlander, J. S., Woodside, A., et al. Hepatitis and Australia antigen: autosomal recessive inheritance of susceptibility to infection in humans. *Proc. Natl. Acad. Sci. USA* 62:1108, 1969.

148. Hillis, W. D., Hillis, A., Bias, W. B., et al. Associations of hepatitis B surface antigenemia with

HLA locus B specificities. *N. Engl. J. Med.* 296:1310, 1977.

149. Szmuness, W., Prince, A. M., Grady, G. F., et al. Hepatitis B infection: a point-prevalence study in 15 U.S. hemodialysis centers. *J.A.M.A.* 227:901, 1974.

150. Pirson, Y., Alexandre, G. P. J., and van Ypersele de Strihou, C. Long-term effect of HBs antigenemia on patient survival after renal transplantation. *N. Engl. J. Med.* 296:194, 1977.

151. Dane, D. S., Cameron, C. H., and Briggs, M. Virus-like particles in serum of patients with Australia-antigen-associated hepatitis. *Lancet* 1:695, 1970.

152. Magnius, L. O., and Espmark, J. A. New specificities in Australia antigen positive sera distinct from the Le Bouvier determinants. *J. Immunol.* 109:1017, 1972.

153. Magnius, L. O. Characterization of a new antigen-antibody system associated with hepatitis B. *Clin. Exp. Immunol.* 20:209, 1975.

154. McAuliffe, V. J., Purcell, R. H., and Le Bouvier, G. L. e: A third hepatitis B antigen? *N. Engl. J. Med.* 294:779, 1976.

155. Neurath, A. R., and Strick, N. Host specificity of a serum marker for hepatitis B: evidence that "e antigen" has the properties of an immunoglobulin. *Proc. Natl. Acad. Sci. USA* 74:1702, 1977.

156. Natvig, J. B., and Kunkel, H. G. Human immunoglobulins: classes, subclasses, genetic variants and idiotypes. *Adv. Immunol.* 16:1, 1973.

157. Neurath, A. R., and Strick, N. e/anti-e in hepatitis B, an antibody/anti-antibody system. *Lancet* 1:146, 1977.

158. Schrohenloher, R. E. Characterization of the γ-globulin complexes present in certain sera having high titers of anti-γ globulin activity. *J. Clin. Invest.* 45:501, 1966.

159. Pope, R. M., Teller, D. C., and Mannik, M. The molecular basis of self-association of antibodies to IgG (Rheumatoid factors) in rheumatoid arthritis (IgG rheumatoid factor/ultracentrifugal analysis). *Proc. Natl. Acad. Sci. USA* 71:517, 1974.

160. Bacon, P. A., Doherty, S. M., and Zuckerman, A. J. Hepatitis-B antibody in polymyalgia rheumatica. *Lancet* 2:476, 1975.

161. Gianotti, F. Papular acrodermatitis of childhood: an Australia antigen disease. *Arch. Dis. Child.* 48:794, 1973.

162. London, W. T. Hepatitis B virus and antigen-antibody complex diseases. *N. Engl. J. Med.* 296:1528, 1977.

163. Jabbour, J. T., Duenas, D. A., Sever, J. L., et al. Epidemiology of subacute sclerosing panencephalitis (SSPE). *J.A.M.A.* 220:959, 1972.

164. Landau, W. M., and Luse, S. A. Relapsing inclusion encephalitis (Dawson type) of eight years' duration. *Neurology* 8:669, 1958.

165. Cobb, W. A., and Morgan-Hughes, J. A. Non-fatal subacute sclerosing leucoencephalitis. *J. Neurol. Neurosurg. Psychiatry* 31:115, 1968.

166. Dawson, J. R., Jr. Cellular inclusions in cerebral lesions of lethargic encephalitis. *Am. J. Pathol.* 9:7, 1933.

167. Horta-Barbosa, L., Fuccillo, D. A., Sever, J. L., et al. Subacute sclerosing panencephalitis: isolation of measles virus from a brain biopsy. *Nature* 221:974, 1969.

168. Payne, F. E., Baublis, J. V., and Itabashi, H. H. Isolation of measles virus from cell cultures of brain from a patient with subacute sclerosing panencephalitis. *N. Engl. J. Med.* 281:585, 1969.

169. Barbanti-Brodano, G., Oyanagi, S., Katz, S., et al. Presence of two different viral agents in brain cells of patients with subacute sclerosing panencephalitis. *Proc. Soc. Exp. Biol. Med.* 134:230, 1970.

170. Connolly, J. H., Allen, I. V., Hurwitz, L. J., et al. Measles-virus and antigen in subacute sclerosing panencephalitis. *Lancet* 1:542, 1967.

171. Cutler, R. W. P., Merler, E., and Hammarstad, J. P. Production of antibody by the central nervous system in subacute sclerosing panencephalitis II. *Neurology* 18:129, 1968.

172. Connolly, J. H., Haire, M., and Hadden, D. S. M. Measles immunoglobulins in subacute sclerosing panencephalitis. *Br. Med. J.* 1:23, 1971.

173. Vandvik, B., and Norrby, E. Oligoclonal IgG antibody response in the central nervous system to different measles virus antigens in subacute sclerosing panencephalitis. *Proc. Natl. Acad. Sci. USA* 70:1060, 1973.

174. Norrby, E., and Vandvik, B. Relationship between measles virus-specific antibody activities and oligoclonal IgG in the central nervous system of patients with subacute sclerosing panencephalitis and multiple sclerosis. *Med. Microbiol. Immunol. (Berl.)* 162:63, 1975.

175. Mehta, P. D., Kane, A., and Thormar, H. Relationship between homogenous IgG fractions and measles virus antibody activities in subacute sclerosing panencephalitis brain. *J. Immunol.* 117:2053, 1976.

176. Mehta, P. D., Kane, A., and Thormar, H. Quantitation of measles virus-specific immunoglobulins in serum, CSF, and brain extract from patients with subacute sclerosing panencephalitis. *J. Immunol.* 118:2254, 1977.

177. Vandvik, B. Immunopathological aspects in the pathogenesis of subacute sclerosing panencephalitis with special reference to the significance of the immune-response in the central nervous-system. *Ann. Clin. Res.* 5:308, 1973.

178. Vandvik, B., Norrby, E., Nordal, H. J., et al. Oligoclonal measles virus-specific IgG antibodies isolated from cerebrospinal fluids, brain extracts, and sera from patients with subacute sclerosing panencephalitis and multiple sclerosis. *Scand. J. Immunol.* 5:979, 1976.

179. Ma, B. I., Tourtellotte, W. W., Brandes, D. W., et al. Quantitation of measles and brain specific IgG in subacute sclerosing panencephalitis (SSPE) cerebrospinal fluid (CSF). *Fed. Proc.* 35:391, 1976.

180. Eichmann, K., Lackland, H., Hood, L., et al. Induction of rabbit antibody with molecular uniformity after immunization with group C streptococci. *J. Exp. Med.* 131:207, 1970.

181. Miller, E. J., Osterland, C. K., Davie, J. M., et al. Electrophoretic analysis of polypeptide chains isolated from antibodies in the serum of immunized rabbits. *J. Immunol.* 98:710, 1967.

182. Kimball, J. W., Pappenheimer, A. M., Jr., and Jaton, J. C. The response in rabbits to prolonged immunization with type III pneumococci. *J. Immunol.* 106:1177, 1971.

183. Modlin, J. F., Jabbour, J. T., Witte, J. J., et al. Epidemiologic studies of measles, measles vaccine, and subacute sclerosing panencephalitis. *Pediatrics* 59:505, 1977.

184. Zeman, W., and Kolar, O. Reflections on the etiology and pathogenesis of subacute sclerosing panencephalitis. *Neurology (Minneap.)* 18, pt 2:1, 1968.

185. Katz, M., Käckell, Y. M., Müller, D., et al. Immunohistological, microscopical, and neurochemical studies on encephalitides. VII. Subacute sclerosing panencephalitis. Susceptibility of dogs to the virus, and characterization of host response. *Acta Neuropathol. (Berl.)* 25:81, 1973.

186. Johnson, K. P., and Norrby, E. Subacute sclerosing panencephalitis (SSPE) agent in hamsters. III. Induction of defective measles infection in hamster brain. *Exp. Mol. Pathol.* 21:166, 1974.

187. Thein, P., Mayr, A., ter Meulen, V., et al. Subacute sclerosing panencephalitis. Transmission of the virus to calves and lambs. *Arch. Neurol.* 27:540, 1972.

188. Albrecht, P., Burnstein, T., Klutch, M. J., et al. Subacute sclerosing panencephalitis: experimental infection in primates. *Science* 195:64, 1977.

189. Dayan, A. D., and Stokes, M. I. Immune complexes and visceral deposits of measles antigens in subacute sclerosing panencephalitis. *Br. Med. J.* 2:374, 1972.

190. Phillips, P. E. Immune complexes in subacute sclerosing panencephalitis. *N. Engl. J. Med.* 286:949, 1972.

191. Whitaker, J. N., and Engel, W. K. Vascular deposits of immunoglobulin and complement in idiopathic inflammatory myopathy. *N. Engl. J. Med.* 286:333, 1972.

192. Oldstone, M. B. A., Bokisch, V. A., Dixon, F. J., et al. Subacute sclerosing panencephalitis: destruction of human brain cells by antibody and complement in an autologous system. *Clin. Immunol. Immunopathol.* 4:52, 1975.

193. Perrin, L. H., and Oldstone, M. B. A. The formation and fate of virus antigen-antibody complexes. *J. Immunol.* 118:316, 1977.

194. Burnet, F. M. Measles as an index of immunological function. *Lancet* 2:610, 1968.

195. Kreth, W. H., Käckell, M. Y., and ter Meulen, V. Demonstration of *in vitro* lymphocyte-mediated cytotoxicity against measles virus in SSPE. *J. Immunol.* 114:1042, 1975.

196. Ahmed, A., Strong, D. M., Sell, K. W., et al. Demonstration of a blocking factor in the plasma and spinal fluid of patients with subacute sclerosing panencephalitis. I. Partial characterization. *J. Exp. Med.* 139:902, 1974.

197. Kreth, H. W., and ter Meulen, V. Cell-mediated cytotoxicity against measles virus in SSPE. I. Enhancement by antibody. *J. Immunol.* 118:291, 1977.

198. Kreth, H. W., and Wiegand, G. Cell-mediated cytotoxicity against measles virus in SSPE. II. Analysis of cytotoxic effector cells. *J. Immunol.* 118:296, 1977.

199. Perrin, L. H., Tishon, A., and Oldstone, M. B. A. Immunologic injury in measles virus infection. III. Presence and characterization of human cytotoxic lymphocytes. *J. Immunol.* 118:282, 1977.

200. Payne, F. E., and Baublis, J. V. Measles virus and subacute sclerosing panencephalitis. In M. Pollard, ed., *Perspectives in Virology*, vol. 7, p. 179. Academic Press, New York, 1971.

201. ter Meulen, V., Katz, M., Käckell, Y. M., et al. Subacute sclerosing panencephalitis: *in-vitro* characterization of viruses isolated from brain cells in culture. *J. Infect. Dis.* 126:11, 1972.

202. Katz, M. Measles and central nervous system disease. A critical appraisal. *Med. Microbiol. Immunol. (Berl.)* 160:247, 1974.

203. Hall, W. W., and ter Meulen, V. RNA homology between subacute sclerosing panencephalitis and measles viruses. *Nature* 264:474, 1976.

204. Lazzarini, R. A., Weber, G. H., Johnson, L. D., et al. Covalently linked message and anti-message (genomic) RNA from a defective vesicular stomatitis virus particle. *J. Mol. Biol.* 97:289, 1975.

205. Holland, J. J. Slow, inapparent and recurrent viruses. *Sci. Am.* 230 (2):33, 1974.

206. Russell, P. K. Immunopathologic mechanisms in the dengue shock syndrome. In B. Amos, ed., *Progress in Immunology,* p. 831. Academic Press, New York, 1971.

207. Bokisch, V. A., Top, F. A., Russell, P. K., et al. The potential pathogenic role of complement in dengue hemorrhagic shock syndrome. *N. Engl. J. Med.* 289:996, 1973.

208. Zimmerman, T. S., and Müller-Eberhard, H. J. Blood coagulation initiation by a complement-mediated pathway. *J. Exp. Med.* 134:1601, 1971.

209. Steere, A. C., Malawista, S. E., Snydman, D. R., et al. A cluster of arthritis in children and adults in Lyme, Connecticut. *Arthritis Rheum.* 19:824, 1977 (abstract).

210. Steere, A. C., Malawista, S. E., Snydman, D. R., et al. Lyme arthritis: an epidemic of oligoarticular arthritis in children and adults in three Connecticut communities. *Arthritis Rheum.* 20:7, 1977.

211. Steere, A. C., Malawista, S. E., Hardin, J. A., et al. Erythema chronicum migrans and Lyme arthritis. The enlarging clinical spectrum. *Ann. Intern. Med.* 86:685, 1977.

212. Schaller, J., and Wedgewood, R. J. Juvenile rheumatoid arthritis: a review. *Pediatrics* 50:940, 1972.

213. Magazanik, S. S., and Pagodina, V. V. On erythematosus reactions of the skin in tick-borne encephalitis (in Russian with English summary). *Klin. Med. (Mosk.)* 38 (2, 9):59, 1960.

214. Scrimenti, R. J. Erythema chronicum migrans. *Arch. Dermatol.* 102:104, 1970.

215. Mast, W. E., and Burrows, W. M., Jr. Erythema chronicum migrans in the United States. *J.A.M.A.* 236:859, 1976.

216. Dalsgaard-Nielsen, T., and Kierkegaard, A. Allergic meningitis and chronic erythema migrans. Afzelii after bite by Ixodes reduvius. *Acta Allergol. (Kbh)* 1:388, 1948.

217. Hard, S. Erythema chronicum migrans (Afzelii) associated with mosquito bite. *Acta Derm. Venereol. (Stockh.)* 46:473, 1966.

218. Sonck, C. E. Erythema chronicum migrans with multiple lesions. *Acta Derm. Venereol. (Stockh.)* 45:34, 1965.

219. Binder, E., Doepfmer, R., and Hornstein, O. Übertragung des Erythema chronicum migrans von Mensch zu Mensch in zwei Passagen. *Klin. Wochenschr.* 33:727, 1955.

220. Wagner, L., Susens, G., Heiss, L., et al. Erythema chronicum migrans: a possibly infectious disease imported from northern Europe. *West J. Med.* 124:503, 1976.

221. Weber, K. Erythema-chronicum-migrans-Meningitis-eine bakterielle. Infektionskrankheit? (Letter.) *Munch. Med. Wochenschr.* 117:1358, 1975.

222. Hardin, J. A., Walker, L. C., Trumble, T. C., et al. Circulating immune complexes in Lyme arthritis: detection by ^{125}I-C1q binding. C1q solid phase and Raji cell assays. *J. Clin. Invest.* 63:468, 1979.

CHAPTER 4

Physical and Immunochemical Considerations

Fundamental to an understanding of the role of immune complexes in disease states is a clear perception of the factors that govern formation, ability to circulate, and biologic consequences within the body proper. Many features of the basic antigen-antibody reaction contribute to produce a heterogeneous range of combinations, some of which are beneficial and easily handled by natural disposal mechanisms and others of which are potentially harmful. This chapter deals principally with what is known about the physical, chemical, and immunologic factors that govern or contribute to the formation of immune complexes in health and disease. Chapter 5 will deal with features notable in the body as a whole, or associated with particular disease states, that seem to function to provoke immunologic injury or important pathogenetic sequelae.

Basic Immunologic Aspects

Foreign antigens introduced into the body provoke a natural immune response, since they are immediately recognized by the host as extra-self. The formation of immune complexes is a natural sequel to the humoral immune response. Thus when foreign antigen is injected, inhaled, ingested, or otherwise absorbed, it is rapidly sequestered by elements of the body normally programmed to clear extraneous materials. In the lungs these are alveolar macrophages or polymorphonuclear cells (PMNs) circulating through capillaries or lymphatics; in the skin and subcutaneous tissues, phagocytic cells such as macrophages, mono-

cytes, or PMNs rapidly ingest such foreign materials.

The monocyte system itself derives from a pool of cells arising primarily within the bone marrow; it shows a remarkable degree of versatility as well as a built-in capacity for amplification in terms of sheer numbers. Quantitative assessment of fixed, circulating, and reserve pools of monocytes has been elegantly defined in a series of experiments utilizing labeling and tracing of precursor cells and their progeny (1–5). Diversification for specific functions in various anatomic locations is apparent, since alveolar macrophages, for example, show different morphological and functional capacities from macrophages in blood or fixed phagocytic cells within the reticuloendothelial system.

Monocytes and macrophages recently have received considerable attention as important constituents of the immune system. Under various experimental conditions they can achieve a supranormal state or become activated (6–8). This occurs in the local microenvironment of inflammatory foci. Once activated, they alter their basic metabolic setting, tend to spread out on surfaces, and show ruffled or undulating cell-membrane margins. Once activated, macrophages may participate directly in various aspects of inflammation or the immune response as primary effector cells capable, for instance, of killing bacteria or bystander tumor cells. Activated or "angry" macrophages may play a central role in many phases of the immune response (9–11).

In the gastrointestinal tract, molecules cross epithelial surfaces largely within the absorptive areas of the gut—including oral mucosa, stomach, duodenum, small bowel, and to a lesser extent colon—and undergo either assimilation and breakdown to basic constituents or (if undigestible) phagocytosis by macrophages and fixed phagocytic cells of the reticuloendothelial system draining various levels of the gastrointestinal tract. These built-in systems of foreign material removal are located largely in areas drained by the portal system of the liver and spleen, of which the Kupffer cells are an important subpopulation. Between this first line of defense and the systemic circulation, primary components of the immune system are conveniently located to serve as a major amplification system for the normal, fundamentally protective immune response. Thus in the lung alveolar macrophages, being mobile and specially adapted to this site, take foreign materials to regional lymph nodes in the hilum or mediastinum. In the extremities, connective tissue, subcutaneous tissues, or skin the natural first line of amplification is again the regional lymph node. Within the gastrointestinal tract there are normally scattered lymphoid collections such as Peyer's patches, appendix, or more distant regional lymph nodes in retroperitoneal and intraabdominal locations; these again serve as first- or second-line amplifiers and major traffic centers in the primary generation of a local immune response.

Very little is known about the primary immune traffic or direct stimulus that may occur within the central nervous system. Selective interference of passage of materials from blood to cerebrospinal fluid for years has been called the blood-brain barrier (12–15). Yet it is clear that many small molecules (such as some drugs, oxygen, glucose, and various metabolites) pass rapidly into cells of the central nervous system and readily cross the blood-brain threshold. In many instances an active transport system appears to be involved (15). No local or fixed system of lymphoid aggregates is present within the brain or spinal cord, and in many ways this makes the understanding of immune reactions within these particular confines more interesting but perhaps more complex. From neuropathological studies the monocytes and astrocytes of the central nervous system have been identified as being related to scavenger activity, and thus these cells could process putative antigens. Monoclonal or oligoclonal restriction of IgG components within the CSF (as in SSPE, discussed in Chapter 3) is a striking example of important immune reactions within the central nervous system.

It is also clear that lymphocytic meningeal or intracerebral infiltration frequently occurs in response to acute immunologic injury or infection, as in viral encephalitis or tuberculous meningitis. The primary source of lymphoid elements infiltrating these areas of the central nervous system is an important area for exploration. Basic mechanisms involved in calling forth a local immunologic defense reaction to sites located within the central nervous system proper need better definition. Some of the naturally occurring infectious disease states related to acute and chronic inflammatory reactions within the brain (such as African trypanosomiasis or sleeping sickness, discussed in Chapter 2) may provide answers to these questions. Certainly in clinical conditions such as tuberculous meningitis, cerebral abscess, or possibly in primary brain neoplasms themselves, local production and fixation of immune complexes to tissue elements may be of fundamental importance in basic pathogenesis.

Much evidence has now accumulated to indicate that the gut and what has been termed the gut-associated lymphoid tissue (GALT) reacts in a way that is unique and distinct from the rest of the body (16–19). Primary processing of antigens crossing the gut epithelial absorptive surfaces occurs in the regional lymphoid apparatus associated with the gut itself. Local immune responses appear in many ways to be restricted and delimited from the systemic circulation. The proximity of the spleen to the GALT is probably of fundamental importance, and there is now support for the view that the GALT functions autonomously, in many ways independent of other extraneous immunologic controls. The development of a unique type of immunoglobulin (secretory IgA) protecting mucosal and other secretory systems underscores the distinctive character of immune reactions within this system (20, 21).

Several examples of the independence of

immune reactions within the gut have been demonstrated in experiments directed at homing of lymphocytes to gut-associated lymphoid elements. Gowans and Knight noted that blast cells found in the thoracic duct homed to the gut, suggesting that this might reflect prior sensitization of cells to antigens present there (22). However, homing of cells to gut mucosa may not be dependent on antigens alone, for Griscelli and co-workers noted that homing and return of mesenteric node blastic cells to gut lymphoid tissue occurred as readily in germ-free as in normal animals (23). The characteristic compartmentalization of gut-associated lymphoid cellular responses and the unique secretory IgA antibody product make immune responses within the secretory systems quite distinct from generalized or systemic immune reactions. Local lymphocyte traffic, homing to GALT tissues and probable direct feedback, and a certain degree of control by pools of amplifier, precursor, or suppressor cells in the spleen may also be significant (20–23).

Any immune response requires antigen processing and subsequent presentation of processed antigenic material to reactive cells of the immune system. Antigen processing occurs to a great extent in various phagocytic cells—largely monocytes and macrophages (24–26). These cells are relatively radioresistant and appear to be uniquely capable of degrading large molecules of protein, carbohydrate, or lipopolysaccharide through their rich assortment of lysosomal enzymes. A considerable body of experimental data has now been mustered which favors the concept that the actual antigenic message or signal may be transmitted from macrophage to immunocyte or immunologically competent cell in the form of an informational polynucleotide molecule or even antigen-message-bearing RNA (25–27). Whether this is the case with all antigens remains to be determined, but the general consensus favors the concept that processed antigen is presented to the immunocytes by macrophages in a form capable of directly initiating an immune response. The studies of Unanue (28, 29) have indicated that macrophages are capable of presenting antigens in

such a way as to focus significant antigenicity; it may well be that in many instances actual antigenic determinants rather than messenger RNA are transferred to the immunocyte after having been focused near the macrophage membrane (30, 31). It is important to stress that most of the antigen handled by macrophages is destroyed and that immune recognition appears to be limited largely to conformational antigenic determinants present on the native molecule or its fragments (32). Continued study of the immunologic functions of macrophages (29, 33) is essential for perception of the fundamental changes that accompany many diseases characterized by immune-complex disposition. For during various phases of their evolution disorders such as infective endocarditis, lepromatous leprosy, and schistosomiasis are often accompanied by marked hypertrophy of the reticuloendothelial system and striking prolonged monocytosis.

The next step in the sequence is thought to be presentation of processed antigen to various antigen-binding cells or immunocytes capable of binding antigen, or possibly of receiving its RNA messenger molecules to initiate an immune response. Antigen-binding cells have receptors that are capable of recognizing or receiving these discrete messages. In most of the animal and human studies bearing on this matter, antigen-binding cells appear to be B cells with surface immunoglobulins or Fc receptors capable of interaction with complexed antigen, however, T cells also are capable of antigen binding (34–36). The elegant studies of Ada and co-workers (35, 36) have shown that immune response to a particular antigen can be completely negated in groups of experimental animals by "kamikaze" experiments in which antigen-binding cells are totally destroyed by giving highly radiolabeled antigen, which then binds to antigen-binding cells and kills them. Subsequent challenge of such animals with the same antigen does not induce detectable antigen-binding cells nor any evidence for an immune response.

Humoral Responses

For the generation of humoral antibody responses to many types of foreign antigens, a cooperative effort between B cells derived from the bone marrow and T cells originating in the thymus is necessary. As noted above, B cells show surface immunoglobulin and are felt to represent elemental precursors of antibody-forming plasma cells. T cells do not show readily detectable surface immunoglobulin but possess cell-surface characteristics distinct from B cells and also show a capacity for the same sort of precise immunologic specificity as antibodies. This latter feature reinforces the concept that T cells must indeed bear some variety of specific antigen receptor. No known mechanism for adaptability to the wide range of potential antigens in the environment other than something akin to the antibody combining site has yet been described; therefore the absence of identifiable immunoglobulin on antigen-specific or immunologically committed T cells remains an intriguing puzzle. Recent work directed at the very heart of this question suggests, in fact, that the antigen-specific receptor unit on T cells may have something very similar to an antibody combining site without the structural skeleton or backbone of the whole immunoglobulin molecule (37–39). Final definition of the molecular size and precise physical makeup of such antigen receptors on T cells remains elusive.

One of the most interesting features of our knowledge concerning initiation of the immune response is that some variety of initial antigen-binding cells appears to be required. This basic concept is in line with the original clonal selection theory of Burnet (40). It appears that the host has antigen-binding cells already preformed and preprogrammed for all the antigens it will encounter during its lifetime. Initiation of an immune response to a particular antigen thus may involve merely selective triggering within the repertoire of antigen-binding cells already on hand. Extension of this concept to its logical conclusion suggests that all so-called autoantibodies arise by triggering of original antigen-binding cells capable of reacting with self-antigens—a hypothesis somewhat at variance with the concept of clonal deletion originally proposed by Burnet, since the body contains a repertoire of self-reactive antigen-binding cells capable of activation or stimulation under the proper circum-

stances (41–43). This fundamental concept is particularly important in considering many of the autoantibody responses noted during various hyperimmune infections or parasitic disease states and already alluded to in the discussion of bacterial and parasitic infections.

Antigens have been rather arbitrarily divided into those which appear to require T-cell–B-cell cooperation to achieve a maximal immune response and those in which T-cell help does not appear essential (44, 45). It is well established in many experimental animals as well as in man that B cells bearing surface immunoglobulin or receptors for immune complexes differentiate into plasmablasts and later plasma cells, making humoral immunoglobulins of a single defined specificity in the presence of antigen itself, antigen complexed with antibody, or some form of antigenic message from macrophages. On the other hand, it is also well known that under many circumstances addition of T cells to B cells preprogrammed or already stimulated by antigen results in what is termed T-cell help. In other words, T cells have the capacity to confer help or amplification to an ongoing humoral antibody response being carried out by B cells (45). Exactly how this assistance is given is not yet clear, but soluble components—antigen-specific as well as nonspecific amplifiers—have now been described in a number of experimental systems. Of great current interest is the concept that antigen-specific helper factors must in some way contain recognitive units with the fine specificity or capacity for immunologic discrimination for particular antigens above all others *and* in addition carry what are termed Ia antigens (46–49). Antigen-specific help, then, appears to be a property of relatively low-molecular-weight molecules of 60,000 to 80,000 Daltons, which bear Ia antigens as well as recognition units capable of specific interaction with antigens they are programmed to help. Similar antigen-specific–Ia-antigen complexes also have been described for suppressor factors. The Ia antigens represent cell-surface molecules similar to HLA antigens, inherited as alleles coded for by genetic regions directly linked to the HLA system (48, 49).

Many antigens implicated in various disease

states show cooperative effects between T cells and B cells in production of a maximal humoral immune response. On the other hand, as previously noted, there is a separate and important group of antigens that does not per se require T-cell help. These antigens have been designated as T independent; many of them are characterized by uniform repeating monomeric units of antigen arranged in close physical proximity on large molecules (45). Examples of clearly defined T-independent antigens of fundamental pathological importance are the dextrans and pneumococcal or streptococcal polysaccharides, as well as certain antigenic moieties on biologically potent lipopolysaccharides or endotoxins (44, 45, 50–52).

The humoral immune response thus far has been described as entry of antigen, antigen processing, antigenic message preparation, and finally delivery of the antigenic message to an antigen-binding cell—most often a B cell which differentiates into a plasma cell, making antibody with primary specificity for the original antigenic message. B-cell differentiation and output can be markedly amplified or increased through antigen-specific or nonspecific T-cell help. Beyond the concept of antigen-binding cells differentiating to humoral antibody cells, a considerable amount of evidence now exists that receptors for immune complexes on B cells activated by adsorbed complexes may also cause differentiation and division of antibody-forming cells (53–56) The sequence of events involved in antigenic stimulation is shown in Figure 4-1.

An important aspect of the initiation of the immune response is that some of the original antigen-binding cells are T cells. These become programmed toward a cellular immune response that is in its own right antigen specific. Some of the antigen-primed T cells appear to be relatively long-lived and may function as memory cells capable of responding much later to secondary antigenic challenge.

Cell-Mediated Immunity

Cell-mediated immune responses can be measured in the laboratory by stimulation of division of lymphocytes or by engendering capacity for direct sensitization of such cells to the original antigen. In more practical terms, cell-

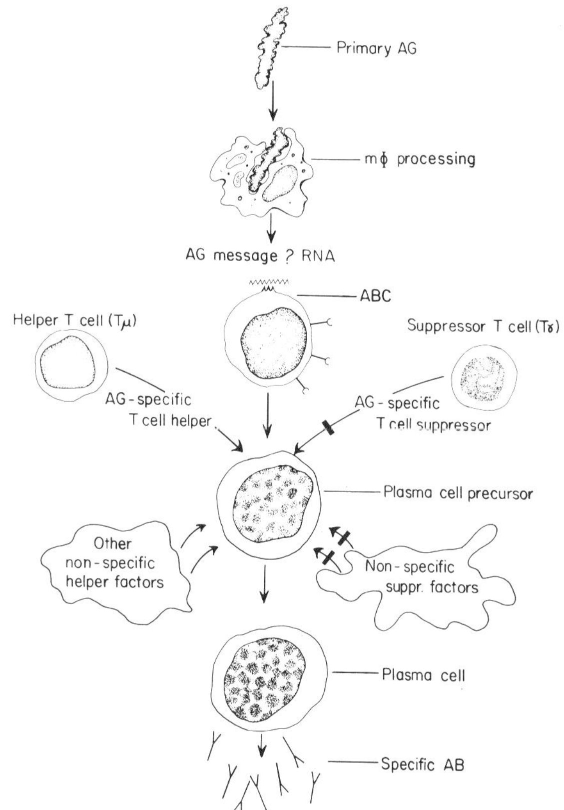

Figure 4-1 General features of the humoral immune response in man, from processing of primary antigen to secretion of humoral antibody by plasma cell. ABC refers to antigen-binding cell; helper T cells show receptors for Fc of IgM and are called Tμ; suppressor T cells show receptors for Fc of IgG and are designated Tγ; mΦ refers to macrophages.

mediated immune reactions include the capacity of sensitized T lymphocytes to directly kill other cells bearing the original antigen, or to release humoral substances called lymphokines capable of further amplification of either killing or other essential aspects of the inflammatory response. Cell-mediated immunity in the past has been most directly associated with clinical phenomena such as the delayed-type hypersensitivity tuberculin reaction, rejection of homografts, or lymphocyte-mediated killing of certain tumors. Although T cells are most directly involved in carrying out the functions of cell-mediated immunity, it has become increasingly clear that the final effector in many cell-mediated reactions may be low-molecular-weight molecules or products of lymphocytes, which constitute the T cells' "magic bullets." A partial catalog of such lymphokines appears below, and a brief analysis of some of the physical and chemical properties of four of the most extensively characterized lymphokines is given in Table 4-1.

Mediators affecting macrophages
   (*a*) Macrophage-inhibiting factors (MIF)
   (*b*) Macrophage-activating factors (MAF)
   (*c*) Macrophage-specific chemotactic factors
Mediators affecting neutrophils
   (*a*) Leukocyte-inhibiting factors (LIF)
   (*b*) PMN-specific chemotactic factors
Mediators affecting lymphocytes
   (*a*) Mitogenic factors
   (*b*) Antibody-enhancing factors
   (*c*) Antibody-suppressive factors
   (*d*) Lymphocyte-specific chemotactic factors
Mediators affecting basophils
   (*a*) Basophil-specific chemotactic factors
Mediators affecting other cell types
   (*a*) Cytotoxic or cytolytic factors
   (*b*) Immune interferon (?) produced by monocytes
   (*c*) Osteoclast-stimulating factors
   (*d*) Colony-stimulating factors
   (*e*) Procoagulant factors

Modulation of the Immune Response

One further aspect of the immune response must be mentioned, and this relates to current concepts of suppressor-cell function. We have dealt with B-cell and T-cell activation and with T-cell help in amplifying the output of humoral antibody by B cells differentiating to plasma cells. A great deal of experimental work suggests the existence of a regulatory mechanism—namely, the suppressor cell—that acts as a type of built-in immunostat. Suppressor cells have been described in a number of experimental and clinical conditions as modulators or brakes on the immune response (57–61). To assign suppressor-cell function to only one group or class of cells would be premature at the present time, since such activity has been associated with adherent cells, macrophages, T cells, and other less well-defined mononuclear cell populations (57–65). However, one concept that has been popularized primarily by Waldmann and co-workers (66) in experiments using cells from patients with adult-acquired agammaglobulinemia is that suppressor cells do indeed modulate or markedly decrease certain humoral immune reactions. These studies stand as a landmark in pointing up the possible physiological significance of suppressor cells to the humoral antibody response. In many of these patients normal proportions and absolute numbers of B cells bearing immunoglobulin or surface Fc receptors are noted in the peripheral blood, yet there is virtually no detectable circulating humoral antibody of the IgG, IgA, or IgM class. Waldmann and associates showed in co-culture experiments that T cells from some patients with acquired agammaglobulinemia were capable of suppressing synthesis of immunoglobulin by two unrelated donor lymphocytes in a nonblocked mixed lymphocyte reaction stimulated

Table 4-1 Comparative physical and chemical properties of four representative lymphokines.

Feature	Macrophage-inhibiting factor	Leukocyte-inhibiting factor	Lymphocyte chemotactic factor	Lymphotoxin
Heat, 56°C, 30 minutes	Stable	Stable	Stable	Stable
Sepharose gel filtration size	25,000	68,000	125,000	90,000
Electrophoretic mobility	Albumin	Albumin	Albumin	Postalbumin
Behavior on isopycnic centrifugation	Like protein	Like protein		Like protein
Chymotryptic digestion	Sensitive	Sensitive		Sensitive
Neuraminidase treatment	Resistant	Resistant		

additionally by pokeweed mitogen. This may not be the general mechanism for depression of serum immunoglobulin levels in such patients, but it was the first convincing demonstration in a human system of T-cell suppression of human B-cell Ig synthesis. A clear understanding of these concepts is important to the discussion in the chapters to follow of immune complexes, their processing, and their abnormal consequences.

To date suppressor cells have been most extensively characterized as belonging either to a subset of T cells or, in some other situations, as adherent cells probably related to macrophages (57–65). Exactly how suppressor cells express their negative or modulating effects is not yet entirely clear. Suppressor T-cell subsets have been elegantly characterized using alloantisera in several murine systems. Mouse strains lacking certain antigenic determinants on their T cells are immunized with T cells from another mouse strain. Such intraspecies immunizations—called alloimmunizations—tend to accentuate subtle differences among antigens within the same species, which would not be recognized by heteroimmunizations across different species lines. Using these reagents and series of functional assays, Cantor and Boyse (67) have defined mouse lymphocytes bearing the Ly2 and 3 determinants as being suppressor cells and cells bearing Ly1 as helper cells. No parallel reagents are yet available for use in human systems; however, considerable evidence has been presented that human suppressor T cells may bear Fc receptors for IgG (Tγ), and helper cells may bear Fc receptors for IgM (Tμ) (68) as markers for these particular subsets.

Additional evidence has been presented by several groups that suppressor-cell activity in some systems may function through the mediation of adherent cells, which appear to be monocytes or macrophages. Recent data from our laboratory indicate that such effects may be mediated by prostaglandins of the E series in some systems involving assay of lymphocyte responsiveness from normal subjects as well as patients with Hodgkin's disease (69, 70). It seems likely that a number of mechanisms involving suppressor cells functioning as T cells,

macrophages, or perhaps other intermediary cells will be more completely defined as work in this general area expands. A recent study has extended morphological and histochemical studies of human T- cell subpopulations (71). This report indicated that Tμ (or presumably helper T cells) generally show features of small or medium-sized lymphocytes and distinctive cytoplasmic accumulations of nonspecific acid esterase activity identified by histochemical techniques. By contrast, Tγ suppressor cells show a more complex system of cytoplasmic organelles, numerous surface villous projections, and distinct cytoplasmic vesicles. Representative illustrations of the cytochemical and electron microscopic differences in appearance of these two major human T-cell functional subclasses are shown in Figures 4-2 and 4-3.

A great deal of work recently has focused on both antigen-specific and nonspecific suppressor-cell factors. Experimental data from several laboratories appear to support the concept that in certain instances antigen-specific suppressor factors are released, which are capable of reacting directly with antigen-activated cells in a way that suggests a high degree of immunologic specificity. Such antigen-specific suppressive factors, as in the case of similar factors producing help, appear to bear specificity similar to that seen with the antibody combining site and in addition show presence of Ia antigens (72, 73). Other nonspecific suppressor factors linked directly with products of the immune response, including materials such as interferon or lymphotoxin (74–76), have also shown general suppressive qualities. It is clear that considerably more must be learned about suppressive mechanisms, since they may indeed represent a built-in regulator capable of affecting the course of immune-complex disorders. Modulation of the humoral as well as the cellular immune response by suppressor cells and by helper cells and other nonspecific suppressor or helper factors is shown diagrammatically in Figure 4-4. It is important to point out that helper-cell and suppressor-cell effects are directed not only at the cells making humoral antibody but also at cells involved in cell-mediated responses.

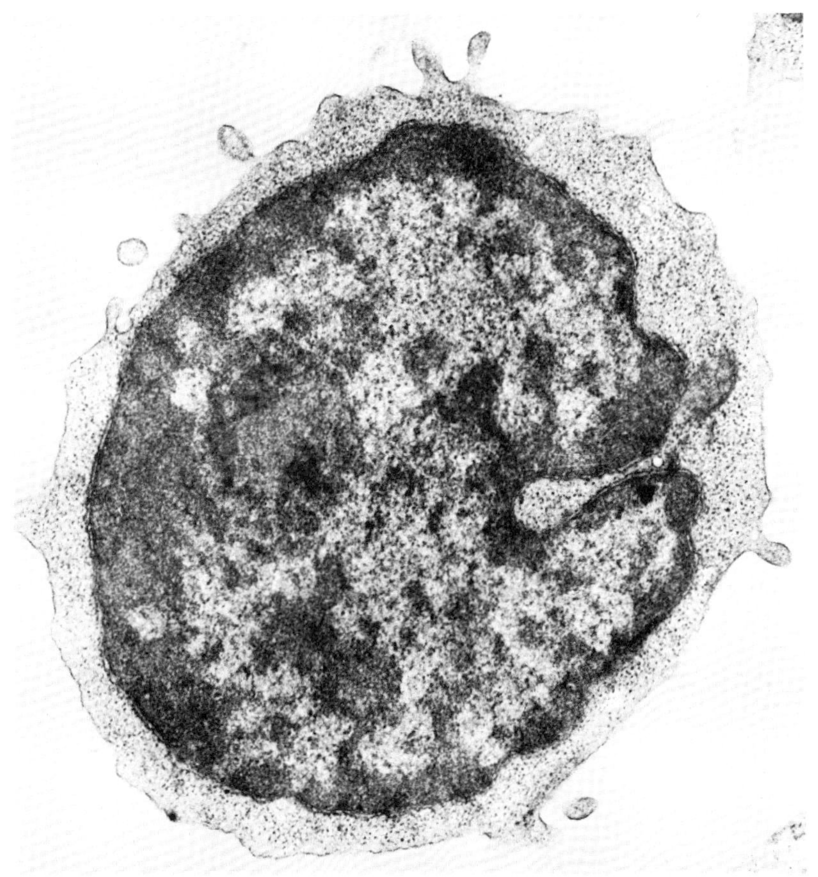

Figure 4-2 *A*, electron microscopic features of a Tμ cell (presumed human helper T cell). The nucleus with a single deep indentation shows marginated heterochromatin and a prominent nucleolus. The cytoplasm, with the exception of monoribosomes, appears devoid of the common cytoplasmic organelles. The cell surface is relatively smooth, with isolated, short microvillous projections. Magnification × 20,000. *B*, nonspecific acid esterase (ANAE) activity in Tμ (helper) T-cell subpopulations. Most of the specifically isolated Tμ cells show one or two large cytoplasmic spots of ANAE positivity. Occasional cells show a small dispersed dot of esterase activity (arrow), and some appear to be ANAE-negative. The insert at the lower right corner shows intense ANAE activity of a macrophage. Magnification × 1,250. (Reproduced with permission, C. E. Grossi, S. R. Webb, A. Zicca et al., *J. Exp. Med.* 147:1405, 1978.)

A

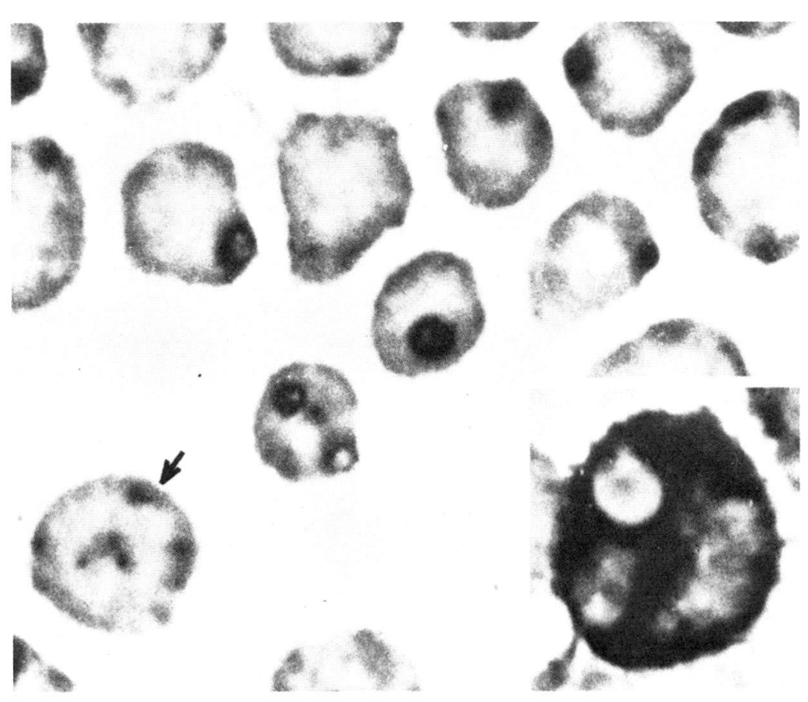

B

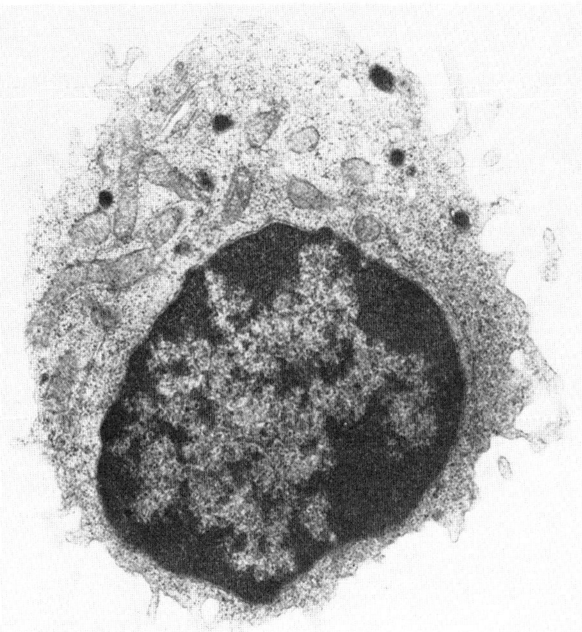

Figure 4-3 Fine structural features of Tγ (suppressor cells). In comparison with Tμ cells, the cytoplasm is more extensive and contains numerous mitochondria, profiles of rough endoplasmic reticulum, and Golgian cisternae. Several electron-dense granules are scattered throughout the cytoplasm. Acid esterase stains of Tγ cells are mainly negative. A few cells show small granules dispersed within the cytoplasm. Magnification × 12,300. (Reproduced with permission, C. E. Grossi, S. R. Webb, A. Zicca et al., *J. Exp. Med.* 147:1405, 1978.)

Quantitative Aspects of Immune-Complex Formation

Nowhere in the realm of basic biology has the application of careful quantitative studies of the immune response and of the interaction of antigen and antibody molecules proved more enlightening than in the area of immune-complex formation. Physical as well as immunochemical aspects of the reactants have added to the complexity of their intrinsic interactions; clear insight into all the circumstances governing how the body deals with immune complexes presents a challenging problem. However, a great deal has already been learned relative to understanding of the biologic behavior and significance of immune-complex formation. The discussion that

follows will attempt to stress the most clearly understood elements of the problem.

One of the fundamental aspects of the formation of antigen-antibody complexes is the quality and quantity of reactants. Early pioneering studies by Heidelberger and Kendall (77–81) utilizing quantitative precipitin curves described a variety of interactions between well-defined antigens and antibodies. It was found, for instance, that rabbit antisera raised

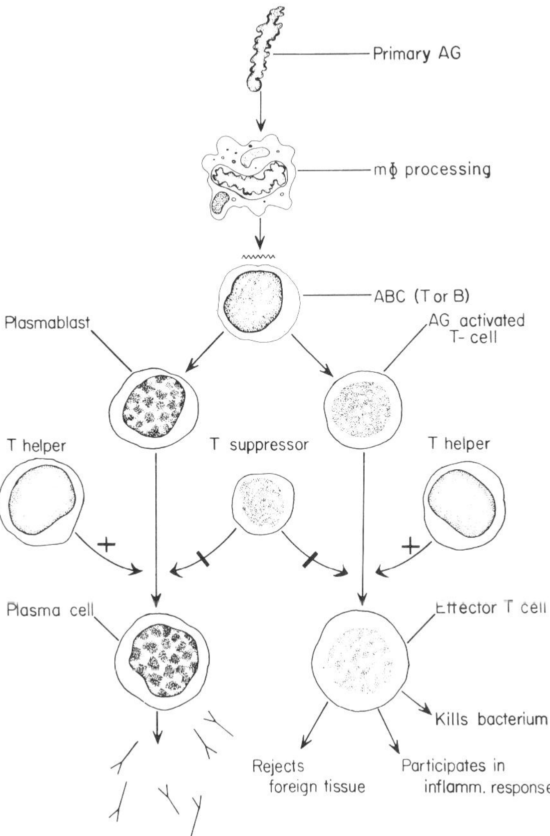

Figure 4-4 Modulating effects of helper and suppressor cells on both humoral and cell-mediated immunity. ABC represents antigen-binding cells. Φ refers to processing cells such as macrophages. It is not clear whether the same population of cells functions as helper or suppressor for both cell-mediated and humoral immune responses. Soluble helper or suppressor factors (not shown in this simplified scheme) also are important in final modulation of the immune response.

against polysaccharide or protein antigens showed rather sharp or limited precipitin curves, whereas those formed between similar antigens and horse antisera showed entirely different quantitative precipitating relationships. Although limited somewhat by its emphasis on the precipitability of various sorts of antigen-antibody ratios, the precipitin curve is extremely useful as a model in understanding the physical features important in antigen-antibody interactions. A representative quantitative precipitin curve is shown in Figure 4-5. In this graph the amount of immune precipitate (vertical axis) is shown when increasing amounts of protein antigen (horizontal axis) are added to equal volumes of serum containing specific antibody. An immune precipitate formed in slight antibody excess or at the zone of equivalence can be dissolved either partially or completely by additional amounts of antigen, producing soluble complexes in the zone of antigen excess. This type of experiment can be performed in vitro by taking an immune precipitate at the equivalence point and actually adding further antigen. In time the immune precipitate is completely dissolved and a solution of soluble antigen-antibody complexes results. This particular concept is essential for clear understanding of the pathogenesis of various clinical and experimental phenomena

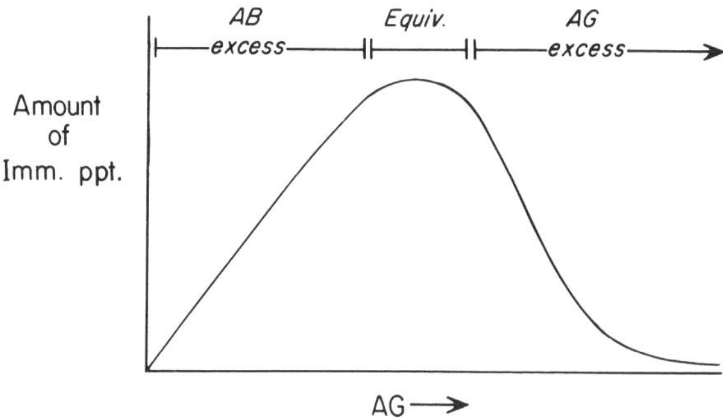

Figure 4-5 The amounts of immune precipitate formed between a rabbit-BSA antibody and BSA antigen. The rising slope of the curve to the left is designated as the area of antibody excess, the equivalence zone occurs at the peak of the curve, and the zone of antigen excess is to the right. In this plot a constant amount of anti-BSA antibody is added to increasing quantities of antigen.

associated with immune-complex disorders. Thus, when the situation exists in vitro so as to provide optimal ratios of antigen and antibody largely in the zone of antigen excess, soluble immune complexes are formed that are capable of either circulation in the plasma or tissue deposition.

Several important corollaries follow from this type of quantitative relationship between precipitating and soluble complexes. When immune complexes settle out of solution or precipitate, they do so because the physical-chemical forces that hold them in solution are overcome. The most common molecular pattern of immune complexes which precipitate is that of large aggregates of multiple antigen and antibody molecules cross-linked by bivalent doubly reacting IgG antibody molecules. Theoretical schemata for descriptions of various sorts of antigen-antibody complexes have generally been based on calculations involving IgG molecules possessing two identical combining sites. Similar schemes might be proposed for monomeric IgA, but they may not be applicable for IgM antibody molecules, which are composed of pentameric structures having multiple binding sites. Since IgM molecules of 900,000 molecular weight are about 5.6 times as large as IgG molecules, the behavior of immune complexes composed of IgG and of IgM understandably is quite different. Moreover, the spider-like pentameric structure of IgM molecules evident under the electron microscope, as well as their physical behavior during ultracentrifugation, suggest that these molecules behave entirely differently than do those of the smaller bivalent IgG. In similar fashion IgG molecules of 160,000 M.W. reacting with large, rather asymmetric structures such as branched chain polysaccharides may not form cross-linkages between antigens as readily as they do between symmetrical or smaller polysaccharide, protein, or polypeptide antigens.

Some of these fundamental physical considerations are illustrated graphically in Figure 4-6, which shows various types of antigen-antibody complexes composed of varying ratios of IgG antibody to antigen. From sequence and physical data currently available, it has become clear that as few as several mono-

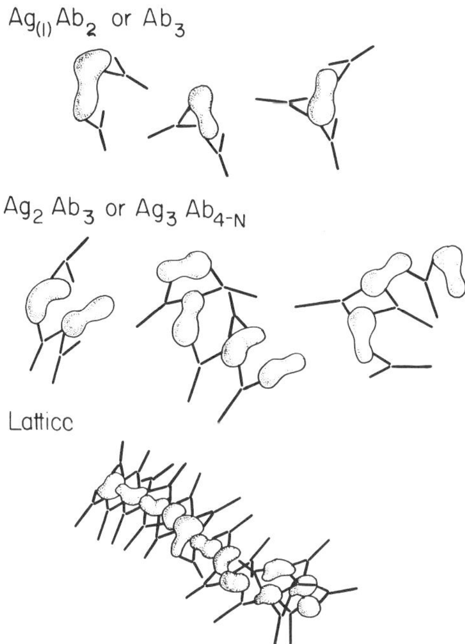

Figure 4-6 Different molecular ratios of immune complexes formed between antigen (Ag) and IgG antibody molecules (Ab). The lattice or network formed by large conglomerates is the most efficient in complement activation.

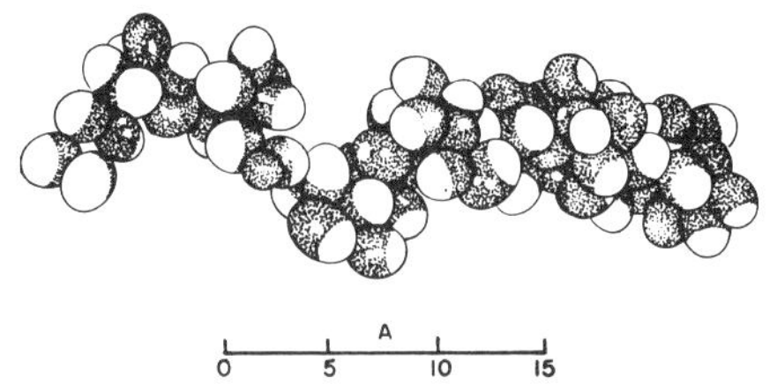

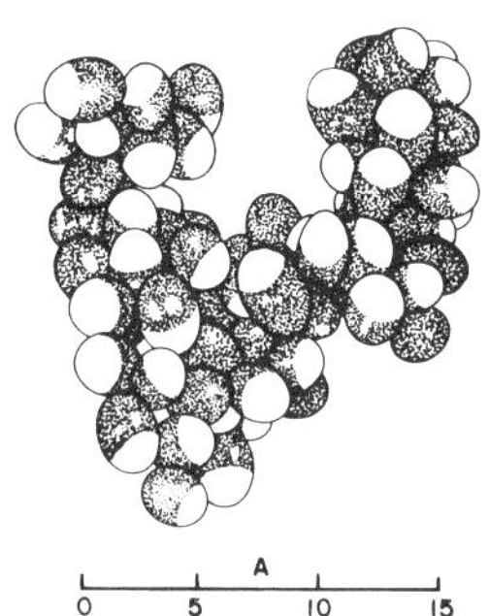

Figure 4-7 Extended and compact models of an antigenic determinant on a sugar moiety. (Adapted from E. A. Kabat, *J. Cell. Comp. Physiol.* 50 (1):97, 1957, suppl.)

saccharide units may constitute dominant antigenic determinants on large repetitive polysaccharide structures (82–84). Molecular models of this type of restricted antigenic determinant, exemplified in the elegant studies of Kabat, are shown in Figure 4-7. Using highly characterized antibodies to dextran, a repeating polysaccharide polymer, Kabat characterized the three-dimensional limits for antibody-binding sites on specific monosaccharides linked in predictive fashion (84). The same can be said of complex globular or asymmetric proteins, where particular immunodominant regions of the antigen molecule provide most of the antigenic determinants reacting with a heterogeneous pool of antibody molecules.

As emphasized by the work of Sela (32), in many protein or polymeric antigens conformation or the three-dimensional shape of the molecules may determine important antigenic sites where reactive antibodies tend to cluster. The same is apparently true of complex branched polysaccharide or lipopolysac-

charides such as are illustrated in Figure 4-8. The physical parameters that appear to be of most fundamental importance in the actual expression of antigenic moieties interacting with bivalent IgG or pentavalent IgM antibodies involve the distribution of dominant antigenic determinants along the antigen molecule itself. Conversely, it has long been recognized that the smaller the molecule the less antigenic it becomes. Viewed in its simplest terms, this may result from a physical lack of significant immunodominant antigenic determinants within a limited area or from the absence of a sufficient variety of conformational antigens. It may also relate to the fact that smaller molecules of 5,000 Daltons or less are more easily ingested and completely degraded by macrophage phagocytic lysosomal enzymatic systems, so that small antigens literally disappear and

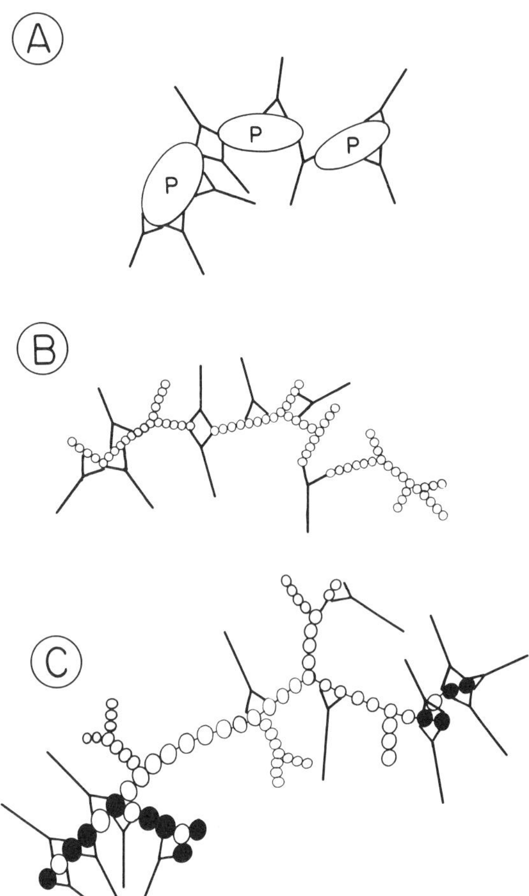

Figure 4-8 Various types of antigens as represented on small protein (*A*), branched polysaccharides (*B*), or more complex polysaccharide or lipopolysaccharide materials (*C*), where certain immunodominant groups constitute the major antigenic determinants.

are no longer available in any recognizably foreign form to react with immunocytes.

Several other aspects of physical interaction between antigen and antibody molecules follow as logical corollaries from these principles. Most antigen-antibody complexes formed in the zone of antibody excess are by definition composed of complexes such as $AgAb_2$ or $AgAb_3$. Beyond the zone of equivalence immune complexes are more likely to be comprised of larger, more complex associations such as Ag_2Ab_2, Ag_2Ab_3, or Ag_3Ab_4 (as shown in Figure 4-6). When the sheer physical size

and conglomeration of such immune complexes outweighs the natural ionic and hydrophobic forces actually at the surface of the respective molecules interacting with one another, slow precipitation occurs. Thus an immune precipitate has generally been visualized as a latticework of antigen-antibody complexes held together by the network of multivalent antibodies and limited in its tightness of lattice or fit primarily by physical qualities, internal rotatory elasticity, or size of the antigen molecules making up the immune complex lattices.

It is quite obvious from a close examination of these molecular models that several physical features of immune-complex formation bear directly on their biologic behavior. First, the tail end or Fc portion of immunoglobulin G and also of IgM is known to be involved in complement fixation. When the antibody combining sites of multiple antibody molecules combine directly with their respective antigens, various physical changes occur in the remainder of the immunoglobulin molecule, probably to a large extent through what is called an allosteric effect. This type of change is usually envisaged as a sort of alteration in shape or alignment at one end of the molecule, induced by activation or engagement at the other. An analogy might be that of a clown's hat, which frequently flies off after he has been kicked in the seat of the pants. Fixation or activation of complement is felt to be initiated by interaction of allosterically altered Fc portions of IgG molecules whose combining sites have been engaged or fixed to antigen. Furthermore, proximity of respective Fc IgG domains one to another appears to be an important factor in effectively triggering the complement cascade. This is illustrated by the diagram in Figure 4-9. It is clear that antigenic determinants located at distant intervals from one another along the topography of the antigen proper are not close enough to put two Fc ends of reacting antibodies into enough proximity to form structures capable of efficient activation of complement. This is an important basic point, and one on which a great deal more information needs to be developed before a precise physical explanation for the behavior of certain general sub-

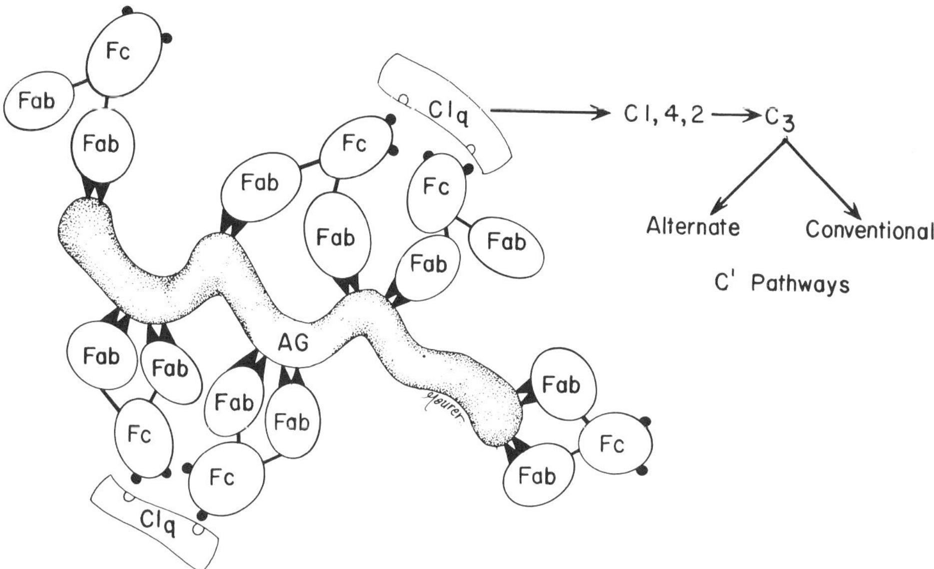

Figure 4-9 A long, asymmetric antigen (Ag) reacting with a number of 7S IgG antibody molecules. When the combining site of the antibodies reacts with closely spaced antigenic determinants, their respective Fc portions are closely enough juxtaposed to produce efficient activation of the complement pathway. This diagram may be an oversimplification, since it is not certain that C1q, the initially reacting complement component, can always react with two Fc structures. However, conglomeration of complement-activating Fc regions is capable of producing enough activated C1q molecules to initiate the complement cascade.

classes of antigens in many disease states can be set forth. Important also is the fact that many antigens occurring naturally in bacterial glycoproteins or polysaccharides are composed of repeating immunodominant simple sugar moieties or conformational determinants on surface proteins, which in many ways load the dice toward effective immunologic amplification through close approximation of antigenic structures. An example of the importance of repeating simple antigenic units can be seen in the chemical structure of the peptidoglycan of group A or group C streptococci, or in the monotonously repetitive units of several simple sugars in the type III pneumococcal polysaccharides, shown in Figure 4-10.

Immunoglobulin Class and Diversity

The eventual handling by the host of immune complexes formed during infection, tissue breakdown, injury, or neoplastic proliferation is determined in part by what type of immunoglobulin antibody has been produced and, in turn, by the particular characteristics and unique properties of the antibody molecules involved. As alluded to earlier, IgG molecules are probably the most efficient in terms of forming lattices or immune complexes with a variety of antigens. For some biologic purposes (such as cell killing after fixation to membrane antigens), however, IgM molecules appear to be most efficient. In the native monomeric state commonly present in serum, IgA (molecular weight 180,000 to 200,000) is not active in complement activation but may function to activate complement when aggregated or polymerized (85, 86). Immunoglobulin G has been shown to be comprised of four distinct IgG subclasses on the basis of genetically determined variable sequences within heavy chains (87, 88). These H-chain subgroups show considerable variability in their immunochemical structure, numbers of intrachain disulfide bonds, and most importantly in their ability to activate complement. For example, IgG-1 and

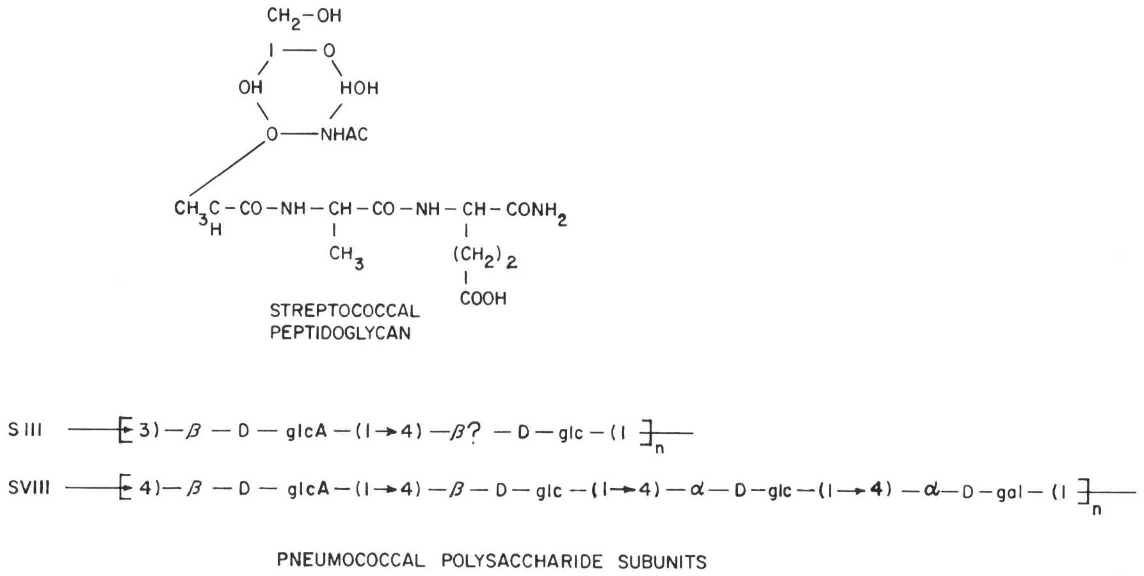

$$
\begin{array}{c}
CH_2-OH \\
\mid\text{---}O \\
OH \qquad HOH \\
O\text{---}NHAC \\
\end{array}
$$

$$CH_3\underset{H}{C}-CO-NH-CH-CO-NH-CH-CONH_2$$

$$\qquad\qquad\qquad CH_3 \qquad\qquad (CH_2)_2$$

$$\qquad\qquad\qquad\qquad\qquad\qquad\qquad COOH$$

STREPTOCOCCAL
PEPTIDOGLYCAN

S III ——$[$3$)-\beta-D-glcA-(1\to4)-\beta?-D-glc-(1]_n$——

SVIII ——$[$4$)-\beta-D-glcA-(1\to4)-\beta-D-glc-(1\to4)-\alpha-D-glc-(1\to4)-\alpha-D-gal-(1]_n$——

PNEUMOCOCCAL POLYSACCHARIDE SUBUNITS

Figure 4-10 Representation of the simple immuno-dominant sugar moieties contained in several well-characterized bacterial antigens.

IgG-3 are effective in complement fixation, IgG-2 less so, and IgG-4 least effective (87–89). Differences in H-chain subgroup composition related to immune-complex deposition have now been documented in several clinical disorders including systemic lupus nephritis and in several other disease states (90, 91). Some patients with hypergammaglobulinemic purpura appear to have high proportions of serum IgG-3, which may be correlated with a tendency to form self-associating IgG-IgG complexes sedimenting as 11 S to 17 S immunoglobulin polymers on analytical ultracentrifugation (92).

The predilection for certain types of IgG antibodies to occur among selected or restricted IgG subclasses is not yet understood. Individuals immunized with various bacterial polysaccharides such as levan or dextran may show almost monoclonal restriction of antibody to one H-chain subgroup (88). It has been repeatedly observed that anti-factor VIII antibodies occurring in some patients with factor VIII deficiency or hemophilia, or antibodies to other coagulation factors such as factor IX, are apparently often restricted to the IgG-4 H-chain subgroup (93, 94). The remarkable mono-clonal restriction of one such antibody described in detail by Pike and co-workers (95) was illustrated by the fact that the antibody itself appeared to contain molecules of IgG-4 with lambda chains only. The occurrence of antibodies to factors VIII and IX as monoclonal IgG-4 products is of theoretical interest; IgG-4 does not bind to C1q (96), and thus immune complexes composed of antibody of this particular subclass do not fix complement. Immunization with complex multideterminant antigens such as blood group substances, diphtheria, or tetanus toxoids usually produces a heterogeneous mixture of antibodies in which the IgG-4 subgroup occurs in minor proportions (97). Moreover, as noted in Chapter 3, e antigen associated with chronic active hepatitis or persistence of hepatitis B antigen appears to be an antibody restricted to the IgG-4 subclass (98). Very little is known about what induces selective expression of IgG subgroup antibodies during a specific immune response. It seems likely that genetic factors in the host as well as still undefined features of the particular antigens themselves may determine H-chain subgroup expression in a diverse spectrum of immune responses. The clinical and pathological importance of the quality—for instance, IgG H-chain subgroup—of antibodies participating in the formation of immune complexes is obvious, since immune complexes made up of IgG-4 or IgG-2 molecules would be much less likely to activate the complement system than those characterized by high proportions of IgG-1 or IgG-3. There is assuredly some degree of controversy about the validity of data showing differential reactivity of various H-chain subgroups with Fc receptors on various types of cells involved in the immune response. As observed by Dickler (99), when individual myeloma proteins are utilized as aggregates binding to Fc receptors on test cells, variability in the individual native degree of aggregability for each myeloma protein makes clear-cut differentiation of true subclass specificity extremely difficult. Various degrees of reactivity for Fc receptors on macrophages or other mononuclear cells have been suggested for members of the four IgG subclasses. Thus higher reactivity for IgG-1 and IgG-3 with Fc receptors on such cells has been noted than for IgG-2 or IgG-4 (100, 101).

Clinical serial studies bearing on this particular point have been performed by Puritz and co-workers (102). These observations were made on patients with SLE nephritis and included immunohistological studies of IgG subclass variation within renal biopsy material, correlated with in vivo and in vitro ability of IgG antibody to fix complement on frozen sections of affected glomeruli. A close parallel between active clinical nephritis and IgG deposition involving IgG-1 and IgG-3 was recorded. Differential reactivity with certain IgG H-chain subgroups and not others would allow H-chain subgroup IgG molecules of low preferential Fc receptor reactivity to escape entrapment and allow them to continue in the general circulation for longer periods of time.

Immune complexes containing IgA antibodies show a unique pattern of behavior, since many such complexes are probably derived from contact with antigen on secretory surfaces. From experimental studies in animals and man it appears that a large proportion of polymeric IgA, and certainly the IgA associated with secretory piece, are derived from

mucosal or other secretory surfaces. The physiology of secretory IgA—in particular the role of secretory piece—has not yet been fully elucidated. Secretory IgA proteins are composed of heavy and light chains plus two additional structural components, J chains and secretory piece. Simplified molecular models of the three main immunoglobulins—IgG, IgA, and IgM—are shown in Figure 4-11. The exact role of the 60,000 M.W. secretory piece in the IgA molecule has not been established, but the secretory piece appears to be synthesized in epithelial cells entirely distinct from the plasma cells involved in the manufacture of heavy and light chains making up the IgA molecule. An important physical feature also associated with the IgA class of immunoglobulin is their tendency to occur in polymeric form. This charac-

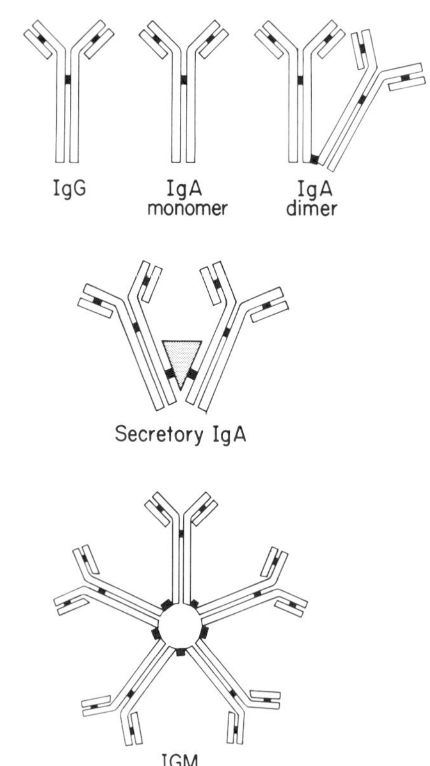

Figure 4-11 Structural diagrams of IgG and IgA monomer and dimer, which are present in serum. Secretory IgA consists of a dimer of two IgA molecules attached to 60,000 M.W. secretory piece (SP). The large 900,000 M.W. IgM molecule is shown below.

teristic apparently depends on the ready formation of intermolecular linkages between individual molecules attributed to noncovalent forces.

Whether or not the polymeric aspects of IgA molecules are directly pertinent to the problems of immune-complex deposition is still not clear, but an interesting condition associated with aggregation of IgA in glomeruli of some patients (Berger's syndrome) may conceivably relate to this feature (103, 104). The clinical entity is discussed in detail in Chapter 12. A good deal of experimental and clinical data point to the secretory IgA system as a natural barrier to antigens that never are allowed to reach the first way station of the immune system in the gut or other exposed surfaces. Thus patients with various severe immunodeficiencies show high levels of antibody to a number of antigens commonly present in foods (105, 106); presumably they lack sufficient protective secretory IgA to complex with and eliminate the protein antigens that cross the absorptive surfaces. In many ways the efficient complexing of secretory IgA to gut-localized potential antigens therefore represents, a protective, surveillance arrangement. When such local immune complexes are not formed, the secretory shield is bridged and an immune response is rapidly generated.

In some instances the immune response may be harmful. This question has been approached directly in a series of elegant experiments by André and colleagues (107). Oral immunization of rats with human serum albumin significantly impaired subsequent oral absorption of albumin administered via the intragastric route. When antigen was administered together with intestinal secretions of rats immunized by the intragastric route, a marked decrease in intestinal absorption of test doses of antigen was again observed. Furthermore, secretory IgA antibodies can effectively prevent bacteria from adhering to epithelial cells (108); such a function would limit local bacterial colonization and penetration of mucosa.

The problems related to abnormal functioning of the protective secretory system are emphasized in some of the interesting immune derangements found in chronic liver disease.

In patients with cirrhosis or chronic inflammatory processes in the liver, hypergammaglobulinemia is often noted. A primary dysfunction in the ability of the liver and fixed areas of the reticuloendothelial system to clear antigens from the portal circulation has been proposed as one of the principal causes of hypergammaglobulinemia associated with chronic hepatic disease (109, 110). The marked decrements in cell-mediated immune reactivity in many patients with cirrhosis could arise through loss of normal humoral and cellular control mechanisms and increased splenic T-cell suppressor activation through maldistribution of antigen, or antigenic signals directly to the spleen itself (111–113).

Immune complexes containing IgA generally are not considered as potentially dangerous to the host as those composed of IgG— first, because of the low probability of complement pathway activation and second, because complexes containing multiple molecules of IgA are large and normally are cleared rapidly by the reticuloendothelial system. On the other hand, it is evident that IgA molecules have the unique property of forming complexes with other proteins. These protein-protein interactions or associations (with albumin, alpha globulins, or other substances) do not appear to occur because of antigen-antibody interaction (114, 115). It is conceivable, nevertheless, that such nonimmunologic complexes containing either monomeric or polymeric IgA may be directly involved in some disease processes. Wherever IgA appears to constitute a major immunoglobulin in sites where immune complexes are suspect, such nonspecific protein-protein interactions should be considered. This is particularly true of Berger's disease and IgA nephropathy, which in many instances has been clinically associated with antecedent respiratory or streptococcal infections (103, 104).

Since IgA of the secretory type is intimately involved in protection of mucosal surfaces, it appears to have increased ability to resist proteolytic or degradative enzymes present within many areas of the gastrointestinal tract (116–118). Like IgG, IgA can be divided into two major H-chain subgroups, IgA-1 and IgA-2; the IgA-2 subclass normally present in a minor population of serum IgA molecules is increased proportionately in secretory IgA. This relative increase in IgA-2 within secretions may reflect evolutionary pressures, as IgA-2 is more resistant to proteolysis by bacterial IgA proteases present in normal gut flora (119).

The Fc portion of IgA does not in fact mediate many of the basic effector functions of other immunoglobulins after they have complexed with their respective antigens. For instance, immune-complexed IgA is not active in complement fixation, anaphylaxis, chemotaxis, or cytophilic reactions. This lack of participation in potentially destructive or inflammation-directed aspects of antibody complexed with its antigen may also have physiological importance, for local damaging effects of immune complexes comprised of IgA antibody are usually not present during disease states.

Immune complexes of IgM and antigen tend to be very large; on a molecular basis in comparison with IgG, they show marked efficiency in complement fixation and in direct membrane damage to cells to which they are affixed. An anomalous clinical example of complexes customarily containing large proportions of IgM can be seen in patients with mixed cryoglobulinemia. Such mixed cryo-globulins normally are composed of a mono-clonal IgM anti-γ-globulin, capable of reacting with autologous IgG. Patients with the mixed cryoglobulin syndrome show a number of clinical associations with diffuse peripheral vasculitis and may show progressive immune-complex glomerulopathy (120, 121). There are very few clinical data available on IgM immune complexes and tissue pathology. However, as will be discussed in Chapter 7 dealing with systemic lupus erythematosus (SLE) and the connective-tissue diseases, clinical evidence for acceleration of the immune-complex glomerular lesions in SLE nephritis has been obtained where IgM rheumatoid factors are detected by immunofluorescence or elution studies in affected glomeruli (122). The contribution of this variety of anti-immunoglobulin to tissue injury or acceleration of inflammatory responses in a variety of clinical conditions has not been completely explored. An example of the possible role of anti-idiotypic or unique-determinant-specific anti-immunoglobulins in glomerular injury is shown in Figure 4-12. Piggy-back anti-idiotype or anti-γ-globulin may indeed be capable of further complement fixation or activation, or alternatively of protection of original autologous immune complex from natural dissolution by normal body disposal mechanisms.

Effect of Size of Complex

Central to our understanding of clinical immune-complex phenomena is the influence of size. Two basic problems are apparent: first, the physical size of the complexes themselves, and second, the particular antigens involved. In a series of carefully monitored experiments immune complexes of particular size and well-defined combining ratios were passively infused into experimental animals by Mannik, Arend, and co-workers (123–126). Using a labeled relatively stable protein antigen such as human serum albumin, these researchers found that complexes of 19S or larger were rapidly removed from the circulation, whereas intermediate-sized complexes of approximately 11S had a slower disappearance curve. Representative results from this series of experiments are shown in Figures 4-13 and 4-14. Size distribution of preformed complexes was

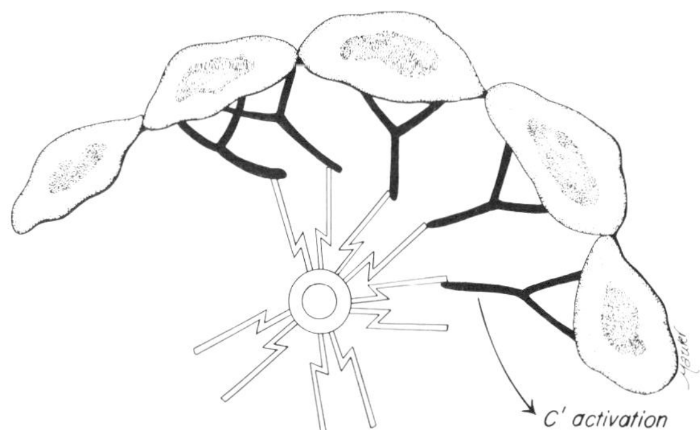

Figure 4-12 Diagrammatic representation of IgG molecules fixed to tissue sites reacting with IgM rheumatoid factor, showing primary reactivity with altered determinants on fixed autologous IgG antibody. This process may result in additional amplification by activation of complement.

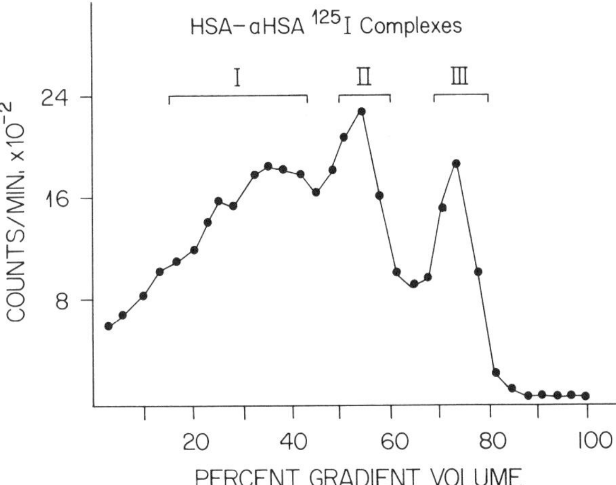

Figure 4-13 Density gradient ultracentrifugation pattern of HSA–anti-HSA ^{125}I complexes prepared at five-fold antigen excess. A gradient of 10 to 30 percent sucrose and a SW41Ti rotor were used; the top of the gradient is represented by 100 percent of gradient volume. Pool I represents complexes greater than 11 S that range from 14 S to 22 S; pool II, 11 S complexes; and pool III, unbound 6.6 S antibodies. (Reproduced with permission, M. Mannik, W. P. Arend, A. P. Hall et al., *J. Exp. Med.* 133:713, 1971.)

determined after separation in linear sucrose gradient ultracentrifugation. Gradient separation of labeled HSA–anti-HSA ^{125}I complexes used in these passive infusion experiments is shown in Figure 4-13. Complement-fixing ability of preformed ^{125}I-labeled complexes was determined in parallel. The antigens used were human serum albumin (molecular weight 67,000) and isolated 19 S human IgM, molecular weight 900,000. Molecular weights of intermediate 11 S HSA–anti-HSA complexes were estimated at 357,000 Daltons. From the data in Figure 4-14 it can be seen that 11 S immune complexes of 357,000 M.W. composed of HSA-anti-HSA were still detectable in the circulation 40 hours after passive infusion. Experiments using human IgM as antigen complexed to rabbit 7 S anti-human IgM showed surprising persistence of total complexes in the circulation at 40 hours and beyond. Reduction and alkylation of anti-IgM antibodies resulted in longer persistence of complexes in the circulation than complexes formed of native unre-

duced antibody. Representative results of these experiments are shown in Figure 4-15.

It was also found that temporary decomplementation of experimental animals receiving passively infused immune complexes did not appreciably affect the disappearance of circulating complexes after intravascular administration (124, 127, 128). Yet there was some evidence that if the conformation or stability of the antibody molecules making up immune complexes was disturbed, as by reduction of interchain disulfide bonds, host recipient handling and removal of the passively administered labeled complexes was altered and they

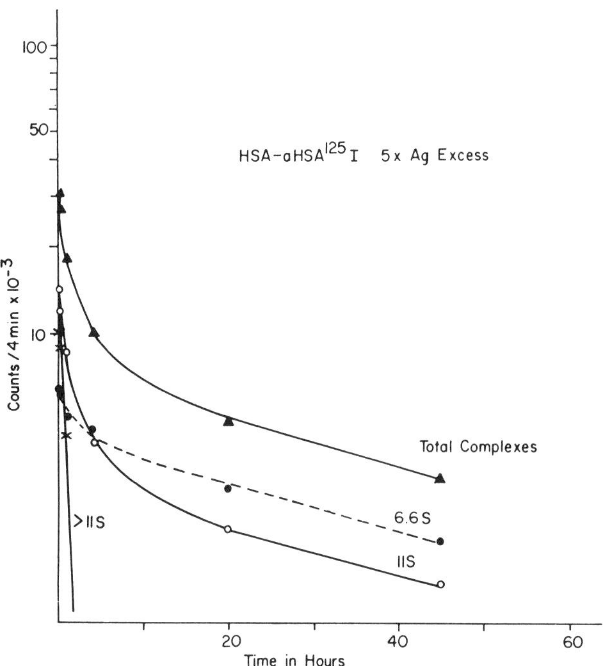

Figure 4-14 Disappearance curves of the individual components of HSA–anti-HSA ^{125}I complexes prepared at five-fold antigen excess. The counts per 4 minutes remaining under the >11 S and 11 S complexes and the 6.6 S peak on density gradient ultracentrifugation were estimated for six bleedings and plotted against time. The >11 S complexes (×—×) disappeared quickly as one exponential component, whereas the 11 S complexes (O—O) and the 6.6 S antibodies (●---●) had two exponential components. (Reproduced with permission, M. Mannik, W. P. Arend, A. P. Hall et al., *J. Exp. Med.* 133:713, 1971.)

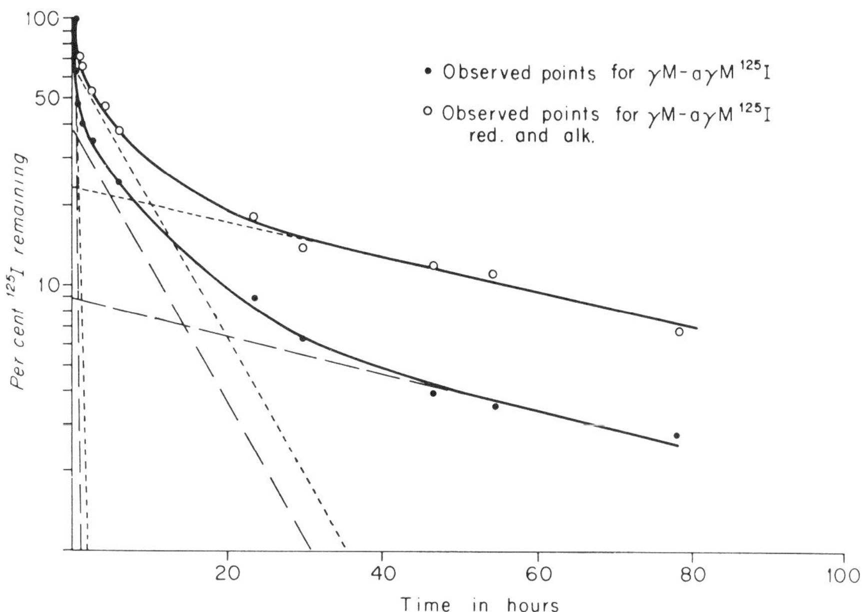

Figure 4-15 Disappearance of γM–anti-γM¹²⁵I (aγM) and γM–anti-γM¹²⁵I reduced and alkylated complexes from the circulation of rabbits. The solid circles (●) and the open circles (○) indicate the experimentally observed points for the disappearance of γM–anti-γM¹²⁵I and γM–anti-γM¹²⁵I reduced and alkylated complexes respectively; the solid lines indicate the curves fitted to these points by computer. The larger broken lines (———) indicate the three exponential components that compose the curve for the γM–anti-γM¹²⁵I complexes, and the smaller broken lines (---) indicate the three exponential components that make up the curve for the γM–anti-γM¹²⁵I reduced and alkylated complexes. (Reproduced with permission, M. Mannik, W. P. Arend, A. P. Hall et al., *J. Exp. Med.* 133:713, 1971.)

were cleared much more slowly. It is clear from this work that a considerable fraction of large complexes of 1,000,000 M.W. or more did not pass more than perhaps once or twice through portions of the circulation, whereas complexes of intermediate size had a longer half-life—in some instances from 12 to 20 hours. The absence of a detectable effect of decomplementation was surprising, but appeared to indicate that tissue-fixed receptors specific for characteristics on complexes other than affixed or activated complement components were of primary importance.

The experiments showing alteration of immune-complex disposal after reduction of inter-H-chain disulfides can also be interpreted as indicating that physical compactness and perhaps shape of circulating complexes may be of fundamental importance in their biologic behavior. The use of complexes formed with reduced and alkylated antibodies was associated with prolonged circulation of complexes composed of more than two antigens and two antibody molecules ($>Ag_2Ab_2$); markedly increased glomerular deposition was recorded (127, 128). Simultaneously the hepatic clearance of such reduced and alkylated complexes was markedly diminished. Ultrastructural studies showed that the sequence of glomerular deposition was first in endothelial cell fenestrae and subendothelial spaces, followed later in mesangial matrix between individual mesangial cells. Moreover, complexes containing reduced and alkylated antibody showed marked persistence in glomerular sites, whereas complexes formed with intact antibody were cleared more rapidly. These findings are illustrated in Figures 4-16 and 4-17. Persistence of circulating complexes composed of reduced immunoglobulins did not appear to correlate with activation of intrinsic complement mechanisms, since such re-

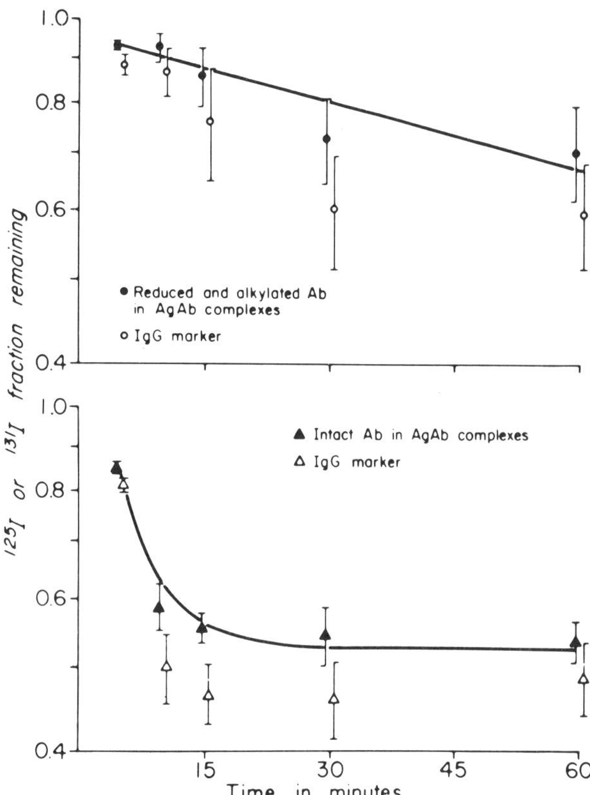

Figure 4-16 Disappearance of normal rabbit IgG marker protein administered simultaneously with either AgAb reduced and alkylated (*top*) or AgAb (*bottom*). The mean ± 1 standard deviation fraction of the injected marker or complexes remaining was plotted. Linear and curvilinear regression lines were fitted by computer to the disappearance of AgAb reduced and alkylated and AgAb, respectively. The disappearance of marker protein approximated the disappearance of complexes in each group and therefore was slower in mice receiving AgAb reduced and alkylated than in mice receiving AgAb. (Reproduced with permission, A. O. Haakenstad and M. Mannik, *Lab. Invest.* 35:283, 1976.)

duction and alkylation is known to impair normal complement sequence activation.

From the clinical standpoint there is at present only fragmentary evidence on the size and shape of complexes occurring during various disease states. Observations on a number of patients followed by our laboratory and others appear to relate high-molecular-weight complexes with glomerular injury and progressive immune deposit disease, particularly in the

case of SLE or in patients with renal disease and persistence of hepatitis B antigen. This particular point was carefully studied in the in vivo serum sickness model in rabbits by Cochrane and co-workers (129, 130): vascular damage in renal, muscular, or cardiac arterioles was closely related to the appearance of intermediate- and higher-molecular-weight immune complexes in the circulation. The influence of other factors modulating local permeability to complexes was probably another area of basic importance. Physical factors related to variation in flow probably are also relevant in determining actual sites of deposition of circulating immune complexes, since arterial lesions in acute immune complex disease of rabbits occur most often at the entrance of coronary arteries and at branches or bifurcations of the aorta (130). Local tissue factors and host response, which relate most directly to immune-complex deposition, are explored in Chapter 5.

In any discussion of physical factors and size of complexes it is appropriate to point out the significance of physical features of the antigens involved. This aspect has recently been emphasized by studies reported by Izui and colleagues with respect to the intrinsic affinity of DNA for collagen-like structures in the glomerular basement membrane (131). Their work has demonstrated the marked tendency of DNA itself, without any complexed or adherent antibody, to bind to collagen structures present in glomerular basement membrane materials. It is possible, then, that certain high-molecular-weight antigens may by themselves deposit in vulnerable capillary beds and subsequently accumulate conglomerations of antibody after being initially fixed within critical areas. Locally deposited immune complexes might accumulate under such circumstances, as by a local affinity column of fixed antigen constantly pulling out antibody molecules of higher and higher affinity.

Along the same lines, more insight is needed into the importance and immunochemical characteristics of different classes of antigens as related to the immune reaction they induce and their possible secondary or adjuvant effects. Small antigens such as simple chemical

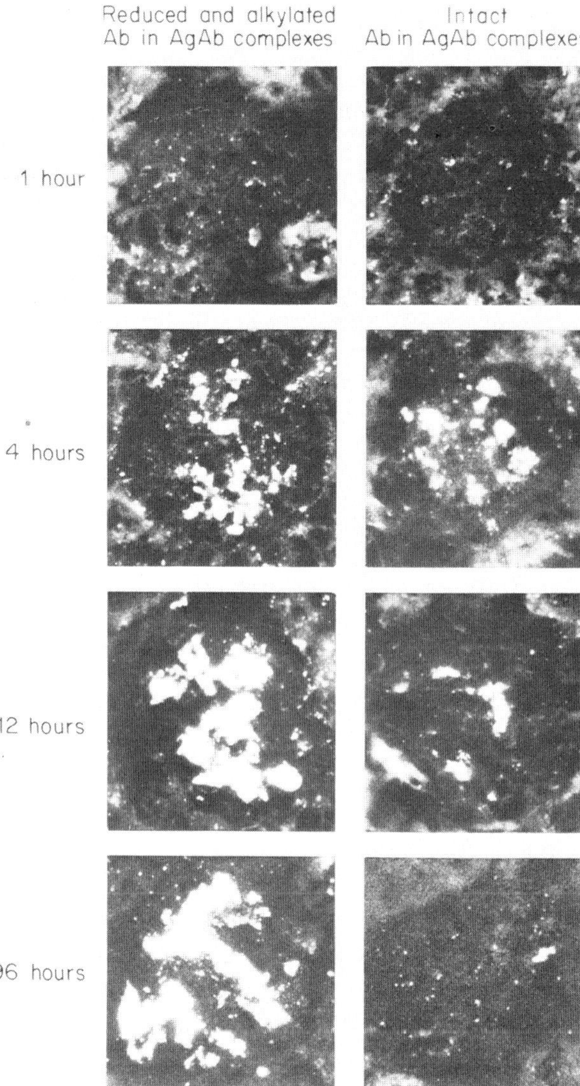

Figure 4-17 Glomerular deposition of rabbit immune complexes by immunofluorescence microscopy (magnification × 320). Representative glomeruli, stained with fluorescein-conjugated goat antirabbit IgG, were exposed and developed for the same length of time. The deposits were greater in intensity and persisted longer following the administration of AgAb reduced and alkylated complexes than following the administration of AgAb complexes. (Reproduced with permission, A. O. Haakenstad and M. Mannik, *Lab Invest.* 35:283, 1976.)

compounds or molecules of molecular weight 5,000 to 10,000 tend not to be very antigenic. In certain circumstances, however, when small antigens are physically complexed to larger so-called carrier molecules, they achieve potent antigenicity. One of the most familiar clinical examples of this phenomenon results in sensitization to quinidine and quinidine purpura where the complex between the drug and the presumptive carrier or affixed serum protein (probably albumin) produces antibodies cross-reacting directly with determinants on the patient's own autologous blood platelets. In most instances humoral antibody or B-cell-derived immune responses are directed principally at the small haptenic determinants, whereas T-cell-mediated cellular immune reactions are produced against the carrier molecules. Therapeutic manipulation of this particular circumstance, therefore, seems feasible and promising if binding to carrier molecules can in some way be avoided. As yet there are no clinical examples of such situations where potentially harmful hapten-specific humoral antibody responses have been successfully subverted by either desensitization to carrier determinants or maneuvers aimed at preventing binding of haptens to potential carriers.

The immunochemical qualities of certain types of substances render them particularly good antigens in eliciting humoral antibody responses. High-molecular-weight proteins—in particular, those that have been either aggregated or conglomerated—are potent antigens. Studies by Biro and García (132) showed that the relative antigenicity of such molecules as heterologous globulins could be markedly reduced if the preparations were freed of aggregated materials by ultracentrifugation before being used for immunization. Other antigens, including tubercle bacilli or Gram-negative bacteria containing lipopolysaccharide endotoxins, show an antigenic capacity far beyond what might be expected on a milligram-for-milligram basis. As noted in Chapter 1, such materials possess intrinsic adjuvant effects that boost both the humoral and the cellular immune response. Adjuvant effects necessarily will exert a marked augmenting effect on subsequent formation of immune complexes as more and more antigen is slowly released over time. In general, foreign molecules capable of resisting phagocytic vacuolar enzymatic degradation and persistent for extended periods are known to be associated with a heightened immune response. Particularly with regard to bacterial or tumor immune reactions, if memory cells are present in the organism challenged for the second time or repeatedly with a particular antigen, the recall or anamestic response is most likely to be one resulting in immediate rather than delayed production of IgG antibodies.

Antibody Affinity

No discussion of the quantitative and physical properties important in immune complex disorders would be complete without mention of antibody affinity. Its exact role in the pathogenesis of various complications of immune complex disease is controversial. Relative energies of binding between antigens and pools of antibody can be expressed quantitatively as K values or as binding constants. There are essentially two schools of thought on the importance of high- or low-affinity antibodies in the generation of peripheral manifestations of immune disorders. A series of observations by Lightfoot and colleagues (133), using chronic immunization to produce immune-complex nephropathy in rabbits, indicated that antibodies possessing relatively low binding constants affixed to their respective antigens in such a way as to be associated with prolonged retention in plasma as circulating immune complexes. Such low-avidity antibodies would of necessity not be as likely to form larger and larger lattices capable of rapid clearing by the fixed phagocytic disposal systems of the body.

In like manner, studies by Steward and co-workers (134–138) indicated that low-affinity antibodies existing as limited member complexes were most likely to be associated with immune complex nephritis. This viewpoint was supported by determinations of both quantitative amounts and avidity of anti-DNA antibody in the serum of New Zealand black/white (NZB/W F1) hybrid mice. The Steward studies have shown an interesting age

and sex variation in avidity or relative binding constants among NZB/W mice as they grow older and the manifestations of immune complex disease become more pronounced. In mice of both sexes, avidity of anti-DNA increased with age until five months; thereafter affinity of antibody fell. Female mice consistently showed lower avidity than males, which was felt to be consistent with the increased severity of renal immune-complex tissue deposition in the female NZB/W F1. It appeared that time of onset, temporal development, and clinical severity could in this murine model be directly correlated with the avidity of anti-DNA antibody produced.

Contrary data, particularly related to the nephropathy associated with systemic lupus erythematosus, indicate that high-affinity antibodies are the population most concentrated within the renal lesions themselves. Through direct examination of glomerular eluates Winfield and co-workers (139) found a direct correlation between high-DNA and antinuclear antigen-binding antibody in materials eluted from glomerular lesions and the presence of significant or progressive nephropathy in individual patients. Avidity of DNA antibody in serum cyroprecipitates and in glomerular eluates was studied concurrently. Glomerular eluates were prepared by treating isolated glomeruli from SLE kidneys with deoxyribonuclease, followed by concentration of the glomerular eluate using 50-percent saturated ammonium sulfate. Estimation of anti-DNA avidity utilized the Farr assay. The relative mean serum anti-nDNA avidity in patients with active glomerulonephritis was 0.29 ± 0.04, whereas the mean avidity of anti-nDNA serum antibodies in SLE patients without clinical evidence of renal disease was significantly higher, 1.09 ± 0.21 ($p < 0.001$).

These findings in a sense parallel those of Steward in the murine NZB/W model. However, when attention was focused on SLE glomerular eluates, the avidity of anti-nDNA antibody was more than ten-fold higher (3.51 ± 1.21) than that in serum. In one patient studied during a phase of active SLE nephritis proceeding to terminal renal failure and death, anti-nDNA in serum was 0.25 but avidity of

IgG eluted from the kidneys after death was 4.20. The relative avidity of anti-nDNA in cryoprecipitates from serum of patients with SLE did *not* in many instances appear to be different from that present in serum. A summary of these data is given in Table 4-2.

Pertinent to the basic question raised by these studies is the finding that anti-nDNA of intermediate activity was noted in sera of patients with active SLE who did not show clinical evidence for active glomerulonephritis. Since anti-nDNA antibodies in glomerular eluates were found to have ten times as high an avidity for nDNA as those in serum, it would appear that high-avidity antibodies are quickly removed from the circulation and presumably actively deposit in tissue lesions. The data presented by Winfield and co-workers (139) are not in agreement with previous studies in which the slopes of DNA binding curves were utilized to examine anti-DNA avidity and its relation to SLE nephritis (140); however, binding curves in the latter study may have combined data on binding to nDNA with those of partially denatured DNA antigens. Active SLE nephritis is most often associated with relative excess of anti-nDNA antibody, a finding that is precisely the opposite from that associated with the classic serum sickness model of immune complex disease (129). Thus it appears that SLE nephritis associated with immune-complex renal injury and nDNA–anti-nDNA complexes in the kidney may occur in the anti-

body excess zone of the curve (Figure 4-5), whereas the chronic serum sickness model is most often associated with immune-complex deposition in the zone of antigen excess where soluble immune complexes are most frequent. A direct explanation for these paradoxical findings may be provided by the work of Izui (131), in that the putative primary antigen— nDNA itself—may have an unusual tendency to bind first to collagen-like molecules in the glomerular basement membrane. Thus an ongoing local immune complex accumulation might be steadily piling up in the face of apparent antibody excess in the serum.

The strong affinity between DNA and collagen might also help to explain the presence of DNA–anti-DNA complex deposition in the skin during the clinical course of SLE (141, 142). Previous observations of DNA binding to C1q, the first component of complement, are pertinent in this regard, since it has been established that C1q contains polypeptide chains similar to collagen (143) and is also affected by digestion with collagenase (144). The mechanism of binding in these instances may be related to forces between the highly negatively charged DNA molecules and the basically charged sites on collagen, glomerular basement membranes, or C1q.

It is important to point out that if high-avidity anti-nDNA antibodies are important in establishing the glomerular lesion in SLE, basic underlying factors determining K values or

Table 4-2 Avidity of anti-nDNA antibodies in SLE cryoprecipitates (comparison with serum avidity).

		Relative avidity	
Patient	Clinical status	Cryoprecipitate	Serum
1	Active; no nephritis	0.38	—[a]
2	Active nephritis	0.46	0.51
3	Active nephritis	0.85	0.14
4	Active; no nephritis	0.86	0.51
5	Active; no nephritis	1.00	1.00
	Mean ± SEM	0.71 ± 0.12	0.54 ± 0.18

Source: Reproduced with permission, J. B. Winfield, J. Faiferman, and D. Koffler, *J. Clin. Invest.* 59:90, 1977.

[a] Serum $ABC_{nDNA} < 0.5$ μg/ml.

binding constants of antibodies need to be better understood or more clearly defined in terms of what process in the disease creates a sudden or gradual rise in antibody binding avidity. It has long been known that avidity of antibodies produced in any B-cell response increases with passage of time after initial antigenic challenge. In addition, with each anamnestic response, antibody avidity increases. Cyclical variation of antibody avidity can also be shown in some experimental systems. Most of the available evidence appears to relate persistence of antigen to increasing avidity or higher and higher binding constants of the antibodies produced.

A fascinating biologic phenomenon might be added as a caveat to any discussion related to antibody avidity or specificity of binding. This has been emphasized by Michaelides and Eisen in what they have described as "strange" cross-reactions between menadione or vitamin K_3 and seemingly unrelated 2,2-dinitrophenyl ligands binding myeloma proteins, as well as cross-reactions involving conventional antibodies (145). The chemical basis for cross-reactions within the same antibody combining site has also been extensively explored by Richards and associates (146). These observations emphasize what any chemist looking at the antigen-antibody reaction would predict—namely, that cross-reactions between seemingly unrelated structures may occur and that great caution should be exercised before assigning primary reactivity to any individual antibody.

Finally, the most important quantitative and physical features of immune complexes relate to the size and chemical properties of specific antigens, the immunoglobulin class and subclass of antibodies produced, and the size and shape of the immune complexes themselves. Although clinical correlations and data are not yet complete, it appears that antigen-antibody complexes comprised of at least Ag_2Ab_2 or greater are most often associated with serious clinical pathologic sequelae. IgG antibodies have been most often linked to peripheral manifestations of immune-complex phenomena. High-affinity antibodies of extremely firm binding avidity may be most important in local fixation to sites of immune injury, and direct localizing factors involving interactions of certain antigens themselves with target tissues may also affect the local deposition of immune-complex injury. The following chapter will deal with the host factors felt to be important in mediation and expression of tissue injury in immune-complex disorders.

References

1. Volkman, A., and Gowans, J. L. The origin of macrophages from bone marrow in the rat. *Br. J. Exp. Pathol.* 46:62, 1965.

2. van Furth, R., and Cohn, A. A. The origin and kinetics of mononuclear phagocytes. *J. Exp. Med.* 128:415, 1968.

3. van Furth, R., and Diesselhoff-den Dulk, M. M. C. The kinetics of promonocytes and monocytes in the bone marrow. *J. Exp. Med.* 132:813, 1970.

4. van Furth, R., Diesselhoff-den Dulk, M. M. C., and Mattie, H. Quantitative study on the production and kinetics of mononuclear phagocytes during an acute inflammatory reaction. *J. Exp. Med.* 138:1314, 1973.

5. Thompson, J., and van Furth, R. The effect of glucocorticosteroids on the proliferation and kinetics of promonocytes and monocytes of the bone marrow. *J. Exp. Med.* 137:10, 1973.

6. Mackaness, G. B. Lymphocyte-macrophage interaction. In I. H. Lepow and P. A. Ward, eds., *Inflammation: Mechanisms and Control*, p. 163. Academic Press, New York, 1972.

7. Mackaness, G. B. The influence of immunologically committed lymphoid cells on macrophage activity *in vivo*. *J. Exp. Med.* 129:973, 1969.

8. Nathan, C. F., Karnovsky, M. L., and David, J. R. Alterations of macrophage functions by mediators from lymphocytes. *J. Exp. Med.* 133:1356, 1971.

9. Bianco, C., Griffin, F. M., Jr., and Silverstein, S. C. Studies of the macrophage complement receptor. Alteration of receptor function upon macrophage activation. *J. Exp. Med.* 141:1278, 1975.

10. Gallily, R. The killing capacity of immune macrophages. In R. van Furth, ed., *Mononuclear Phagocytes in Immunity, Infection and Pathology*, p. 895 Blackwell Scientific Publications, Oxford, 1975.

11. Hibbs, J. B., Jr., Lambert, L. H., Jr., and Remington, J. S. Possible role of macrophage me-

diated nonspecific cytotoxicity in tumour resistance. *Nature (New Biol.)* 235:48, 1972.

12. Wisse, B. L., and Taxdal, D. R. Studies of the blood-brain barrier utilizing hematoporphyrin. *Brain Res.* 4:387, 1967.

13. Davson, H., Kleeman, C. R., and Levin, E. Quantitative studies of the passage of different substances out of the cerebrospinal fluid. *J. Physiol. (Lond.)* 161:126, 1962.

14. Bakay, L. Basic aspects of brain tumour localization by radioactive substances. A review of current concepts. *J. Neurosurg.* 27:239, 1967.

15. Dobbing, J. The blood-brain barrier. *Physiol. Rev.* 41:130, 1961.

16. Guy-Grand, D., Griscelli, C., and Vassalli, P. The gut-associated lymphoid system: nature and properties of the large dividing cells. *Eur. J. Immunol.* 4:435, 1974.

17. Joel, D. D., Hess, M. W., and Cottier, H. Magnitude and pattern of thymic lymphocyte migration in neonatal mice. *J. Exp. Med.* 135:907, 1972.

18. Crabbé, P. A., Nash, D. R., Bazin, H., et al. Antibodies of the IgA type in intestinal plasma cells of germfree mice after oral or parenteral immunization with ferritin. *J. Exp. Med.* 130:723, 1969.

19. Lawton, A. R., Self, K. S., Royal, S. A., et al. Ontogeny of B-lymphocytes in the human fetus. *Clin. Immunol. Immunopathol.* 1:84, 1972.

20. Tomasi, T. B., Jr., Tan, E. M., Solomon, A., et al. Characteristics of an immune system common to certain external secretions. *J. Exp. Med.* 121:101, 1965.

21. Lamm, M. E. Cellular aspects of immunoglobulin A. *Adv. Immunol.* 22:223, 1976.

22. Gowans, J. L., and Knight, E. J. The route of re-circulation of lymphocytes in the rat. *Proc. R. Soc. Lond. (Biol.)* 159:257, 1964.

23. Griscelli, C., Vassalli, P., and McCluskey, R. T. The distribution of large dividing lymph node cells in syngeneic recipient rats after intravenous injection. *J. Exp. Med.* 130:1427, 1969.

24. Gallily, R., and Feldman, M. The role of macrophages in the induction of antibody in X-irradiated animals. *Immunology* 12:197, 1967.

25. Fishman, M., and Adler, F. L. Antibody formation initiated *in vitro*. II. Antibody synthesis in X-irradiated recipients of diffusion chambers containing nucleic acid derived from macrophages incubated with antigen. *J. Exp. Med.* 117:595, 1963.

26. Fishman, M., Hammerstrom, R. A., and Bond, V. P. *In vitro* transfer of macrophage RNA to lymph node cells. *Nature* 198:549, 1963.

27. Gottlieb, A. A., Glisin, V. R., and Doty, P. Studies on macrophage RNA involved in antibody production. *Proc. Natl. Acad. Sci. USA* 57:1849, 1967.

28. Unanue, E. R. Thymus dependency of the immune response to hemocyanin: an evaluation of the role of macrophages in thymectomized mice. *J. Immunol.* 105:1339, 1970.

29. Unanue, E. R. The regulatory role of macrophages in antigenic stimulation. *Adv. Immunol.* 15:95, 1972.

30. Unanue, E. R., and Cerottini, J-C. The immunogenicity of antigen bound to the plasma membrane of macrophages. *J. Exp. Med.* 131:711, 1970.

31. Unanue, E. R. The regulation of the immune response by macrophages. In R. van Furth, ed., *Mononuclear Phagocytes in Immunity, Infection and Pathology,* p. 721. Blackwell Scientific Publications, Oxford, 1975.

32. Sela, M. Immunological studies with synthetic polypeptides. *Adv. Immunol.* 5:29, 1966.

33. Cohn, Z. A. The structure and function of monocytes and macrophages. *Adv. Immunol.* 9:163, 1968.

34. Hämmerling, G. J., and McDevitt, H. O. Antigen binding T and B lymphocytes. I. Differences in cellular specificity and influence of metabolic activity on interaction of antigen with T and B cells. *J. Immunol.* 112:1726, 1974.

35. Ada, G. L. Antigen-binding cells in tolerance and immunity. *Transplant. Rev.* 5:105, 1970.

36. Ada, G. L., and Byrt, P. Specific inactivation of antigen-reactive cells with ^{125}I-labelled antigen. *Nature* 222:1291, 1969.

37. Binz, H., and Wigzell, H. Shared idiotypic determinants on B and T lymphocytes reactive against the same antigenic determinants. II. Determination of frequency and characteristics of idiotypic T and B lymphocytes in normal rats using direct visualization. *J. Exp. Med.* 142:1218, 1975.

38. Binz, H., and Wigzell, H. Shared idiotypic determinants on B and T lymphocytes reactive against the same antigenic determinants. I. Demonstration of similar or identical idiotypes on IgG molecules and T-cell receptors with specificity for the same alloantigens. *J. Exp. Med.* 142:197, 1975.

39. Binz, H., and Wigzell, H. Antigen-binding, idiotypic T-lymphocyte receptors. *Contemp. Top. Mol. Immunobiol.* 7:113, 1977.

40. Burnet, F. M. In *The Clonal Selection Theory of Acquired Immunity.* Vanderbilt University Press, Nashville, Tenn. 1959.

41. Bankhurst, A. D., Torrigiani, G., and Allison, A. C. Lymphocytes binding human thyroglobulin in healthy people and its relevance to tolerance for autoantigens. *Lancet* 1:226, 1973.

42. Roberts, I. M., Whittingham, S., and

Mackay, I. R. Tolerance to an auto-antigen-thyroglobulin. Antigen-binding lymphocytes in thymus and blood in health and autoimmune disease. *Lancet* 2:936, 1973.

43. Bankhurst, A. D., and Williams, R. C., Jr. Identification of DNA-binding lymphocytes in patients with systemic lupus erythematosus. *J. Clin. Invest.* 56:1378, 1975.

44. Möller, G., and Michael, G. Frequency of antigen-sensitive cells to thymus-independent antigens. *Cell. Immunol.* 2:309, 1971.

45. Coutinho, A., and Möller, G. Thymus-independent B-cell induction and paralysis. *Adv. Immunol.* 21:113, 1975.

46. Taussig, M. J., Mozes, E., and Isac, R. Antigen-specific thymus cell factors in the genetic control of the immune response to poly-(tyrosyl, glutamyl)-poly-D, L-alanyl--poly-lysyl. *J. Exp. Med.* 140:301, 1974.

47. Schwartz, B. D., Paul, W. E., and Shevach, E. M. Guinea-pig Ia antigens: functional significance and chemical characterization. *Transplant. Rev.* 30:174, 1976.

48. Klein, J. Genetic control of immune response. In *Biology of the Mouse Histocompatibility-2 Complex,* p. 411. Springer-Verlag, New York, 1975.

49. Frelinger, J. A., Niederhuber, J. E., and Shreffler, D. C. Effects of anti-Ia sera on mitogenic responses. III. Mapping the genes controlling the expression of Ia determinants on concanavalin-A reactive cells to the I-J subregion of the H-2 gene complex. *J. Exp. Med.* 144:1141, 1976.

50. Haber, E. Antibodies of restricted heterogeneity for structural study. *Fed. Proc.* 29:66, 1970.

51. Braun, D. G., Kjems, E., and Cramer, M. A rabbit family of restricted high responders to the streptococcal group A-variant polysaccharide. Selective breeding narrows the isoelectric focusing spectra of dominant clones. *J. Exp. Med.* 138:645, 1973.

52. Möller, G. Triggering mechanisms for cellular recognition. In R. T. Smith and M. Landy, eds., *Immune Surveillance,* p. 85. Academic Press, New York, 1970.

53. Basten, A., Miller, J. F. A. P., Sprent, J., et al. A receptor for antibody on B lymphocytes. I. Method of detection and functional significance. *J. Exp. Med.* 135:610, 1972.

54. Paraskevas, F., Lee, S. T., Orr, K. B., et al. A receptor for Fc on mouse B-lymphocytes. *J. Immunol.* 108:1319, 1972.

55. Yoshida, T. O., and Andersson, B. Evidence for a receptor recognizing antigen complexed immunoglobulin on the surface of activated mouse thymus lymphocytes. *Scand. J. Immunol.* 1:401, 1972.

56. Berman, M. A., and Weigle, W. O. B-lymphocyte activation by the Fc region of IgG. *J. Exp. Med.* 146:241, 1977.

57. Gershon, R. K., and Kondo, K. Infectious immunological tolerance. *Immunology* 21:903, 1971.

58. Herzenberg, L. A., Okumura, K., and Metzler, C. M. Regulation of immunoglobulin and antibody production by allotype suppressor T cells in mice. *Transplant. Rev.* 27:57, 1975.

59. Baker, P. J., Stashak, P. W., Amsbaugh, D. F., et al. Regulation of the antibody response to type III pneumococcal polysaccharide. IV. Role of suppressor T cells in the development of low-dose paralysis. *J. Immunol.* 112:2020, 1974.

60. Rich, S. S., and Rich, R. R. Regulatory mechanisms in cell-mediated immune responses. I. Regulation of mixed lymphocyte reactions by alloantigen-activated thymus-derived lymphocytes. *J. Exp. Med.* 140:1588, 1974.

61. Kapp, J. A., Pierce, C. W., Schlossman, S., et al. Genetic control of immune response *in vitro.* V. Stimulation of suppressor T cells in nonresponder mice by the terpolymer L-glutamic acid^{60}-L-alanine^{30}-L-tyrosine^{10} (GAT). *J. Exp. Med.* 140:648, 1974.

62. Folch, H., and Waksman, B. H. Regulation of lymphocyte responses *in vitro.* V. Suppressor activity of adherent and nonadherent rat lymphoid cells. *Cell. Immunol.* 9:12, 1973.

63. Katz, S. I., Parker, D., Turk, J. L. B-cell suppression of delayed hypersensitivity reactions. *Nature* 251:550, 1974.

64. Keller, R. Major changes in lymphocyte proliferation evoked by activated macrophages. *Cell. Immunol.* 17:542, 1975.

65. Twomey, J. J., Laughter, A. H., Farrow, S., et al. Hodgkin's disease. An immunodepleting and immunosuppressive disorder. *J. Clin. Invest.* 56:467, 1975.

66. Waldmann, T. A., Durm, M., Broder, S., et al. Role of suppressor T cells in pathogenesis of common variable hypogammaglobulinaemia. *Lancet* 2:609, 1974.

67. Cantor, H., and Boyse, E. A. Functional subclasses of T lymphocytes bearing different Ly antigens. I. The generation of functionally distinct T-cell subclasses is a differentiative process independent of antigen. *J. Exp. Med.* 141:1376, 1975.

68. Moretta, L., Webb, S. R., Grossi, C. E., et al. Functional analysis of two human T-cell subpopulations: help and suppression of B-cell responses by T cells bearing receptors for IgM or IgG. *J. Exp. Med.* 146:184, 1977.

69. Goodwin, J. S., Bankhurst, A. D., and Messner, R. P. Suppression of human T-cell mito-

genesis by prostaglandin: existence of a prostaglandin producing suppressor cell. *J. Exp. Med.* 146:1719, 1977.

70. Goodwin, J. S., Messner, R. P., Bankhurst, A. D., et al. Prostaglandin producing suppressor cells in Hodgkin's disease. *N. Engl. J. Med.* 297:963, 1977.

71. Grossi, C. E., Webb, S. R., Zicca, A., et al. Morphological and histochemical analyses of two human T-cell subpopulations bearing receptors for IgM or IgG. *J. Exp. Med.* 147:1405, 1978.

72. Tada, T., Taniguchi, M., and Takemori, T. Properties of primed suppressor T cells and their products. *Transplant. Rev.* 26:106, 1975.

73. Tada, T., Taniguchi, M., and David, C. S. Properties of the antigen-specific suppressive T-cell factor in the regulation of antibody response of the mouse. IV. Special subregion assignment of the gene(s) that codes for the suppressive T-cell factor in the H-2 histocompatibility complex. *J. Exp. Med.* 144:713, 1976.

74. Paucker, K., Dalton, B. J., Törmä, E. T., et al. Biological properties of human leukocyte interferon components. *J. Gen. Virol.* 35:341, 1977.

75. Finlay, G. J., Booth, R. J., and Marbrook, J. Interferon-induced antibody suppression: a selective effect on high density, late responding precursor cells. *Eur. J. Immunol.* 7:123, 1977.

76. Williams, R. C., Jr., and Korsmeyer, S. J. Studies of human lymphocyte interactions with emphasis on soluble suppressor activity. *Clin. Immunol. Immunopathol.* 9:335, 1978.

77. Heidelberger, M. Quantitative absolute methods in the study of antigen-antibody reactions. *Bacteriol. Rev.* 3:49, 1939.

78. Heidelberger, M., and Kendall, F. E. A quantitative study of the precipitin reaction between type III pneumococcus polysaccharide and purified homologous antibody. *J. Exp. Med.* 50:809, 1929.

79. Heidelberger, M., and Kendall, F. E. The precipitin reaction between type III pneumococcus polysaccharide and homologous antibody. II. Conditions for quantitative precipitation of antibody in horse sera. *J. Exp. Med.* 61:559, 1935.

80. Heidelberger, M., and Kendall, F. E. Quantitative studies on antibody purification. IV. The dissociation of precipitates formed by pneumococcus specific polysaccharides and homologous antibodies. *J. Exp. Med.* 64:161, 1936.

81. Kimball, J. W., Pappenheimer, A. M., Jr., and Jaton, J. C. The response in rabbits to prolonged immunization with type III pneumococci. *J. Immunol.* 106:1177, 1971.

82. Kabat, E. A. Some configurational requirements and dimensions of the combining site on an antibody to a naturally occurring antigen. *J. Am. Chem. Soc.* 76:3709, 1954.

83. Kabat, E. A. Heterogeneity in extent of the combining regions of human antidextran. *J. Immunol.* 77:377, 1956.

84. Kabat, E. A. The upper limit for the size of the human antidextran combining site. *J. Immunol.* 84:82, 1960.

85. Götze, O., and Müller-Eberhard, H. J. The C3-activator system: an alternate pathway of complement activation. *J. Exp. Med.* 134:90s, 1971.

86. Colten, H. R., and Bienenstock, J. Lack of C3-activation through classical or alternate pathways by human secretory IgA anti blood group A antibody. *Adv. Exp. Med. Biol.* 45:305, 1974.

87. Natvig, J. B., Kunkel, H. G., Yount, W. J., et al. Further studies on the γG-heavy chain gene complexes, with particular reference to the genetic markers Gm(g) and Gm(n). *J. Exp. Med.* 128:763, 1968.

88. Natvig, J. B., and Kunkel, H. G. Human immunoglobulins: classes, subclasses, genetic variants, and idiotypes. *Adv. Immunol.* 16:1, 1973.

89. Ishizaka, T., Ishizaka, K., Salmon, S., et al. Biologic activities of aggregated γ-globulin. VIII. Aggregated immunoglobulins of different classes. *J. Immunol.* 99:82, 1967.

90. Lewis, E. J., Busch, G. J., and Schur, P. H. Gamma G globulin subgroup composition of the glomerular deposits in human renal diseases. *J. Clin. Invest.* 49:1103, 1970.

91. Kacaki, J. N., Callerame, M. L., Blomgren, S. E., et al. Immunoglobulin G subclasses of antinuclear antibodies and renal deposits. Comparison of systemic lupus erythematosus, drug-induced lupus and rheumatoid arthritis. *Arthritis Rheum.* 14:276, 1971.

92. Capra, J. D., and Kunkel, H. G. Aggregation of γG3 proteins: relevance to the hyperviscosity syndrome. *J. Clin. Invest.* 49:610, 1970.

93. Andersen, B. R., and Terry, W. D. Gamma G4-globulin antibody causing inhibition of clotting Factor VIII. *Nature,* 217:174, 1968.

94. Robboy, S. J., Lewis, E. J., Schur, P. H., et al. Circulating anticoagulants to Factor VIII. Immunochemical studies and clinical response to factor VIII concentrates. *Am. J. Med.* 49:742, 1970.

95. Pike, I. M., Yount, W. J., Puritz, E. M., et al. Immunochemical characterization of a monoclonal γG4, λ human antibody to Factor IX. *Blood* 40:1, 1972.

96. Augener, W., Grey, H. M., Cooper, N. R., et al. The reaction of monomeric and aggregated

immunoglobulins with C1. *Immunochemistry* 8:1011, 1971.

97. Yount, W. J., Dorner, M. M., Kunkel, H. G., et al. Studies on human antibodies. VI. Selective variations in subgroup composition and genetic markers. *J. Exp. Med.* 127:633, 1968.

98. Neurath, A. R., and Strick, N. Host specificity of a serum marker for hepatitis B: evidence that "e antigen" has the properties of an immunoglobulin. *Proc. Natl. Acad. Sci. USA* 74:1702, 1977.

99. Dickler, H. B. Lymphocyte receptors for immunoglobulin. *Adv. Immunol.* 24:167, 1976.

100. Larsson, A., Perlmann, P., and Natvig, J. B. Cytotoxicity of human lymphocytes induced by rabbit antibodies to chicken erythrocytes. Inhibition by normal IgG and by human myeloma proteins of different IgG subclasses. *Immunology* 25:675, 1973.

101. MacLennan, I. C. M., Howard, A., Gotch, F. M., et al. Effector activating determinants on IgG. I. The distribution and factors influencing the display of complement, neutrophil and cytotoxic B-cell determinants on human IgG subclasses. *Immunology* 25:459, 1973.

102. Puritz, E. M., Yount, W. J., Newell, M., et al. Immunoglobulin classes and IgG subclasses of human antinuclear antibodies. A correlation of complement fixation and the nephritis of systemic lupus erythematosus. *Clin. Immunol. Immunopathol.* 2:98, 1973.

103. Berger, J. IgA glomerular deposits in renal disease. *Transplant. Proc.* 1:939, 1969.

104. Zimmerman, S. W., and Burkholder, P. M. Immunoglobulin A nephropathy. *Arch. Intern. Med.* 135:1217, 1975.

105. Buckley, R. H., and Dees, S. C. Correlation of milk precipitins with IgA deficiency. *N. Engl. J. Med.* 281:465, 1969.

106. Butler, J. E., and Oskvig, R. Cancer, autoimmunity and IgA-deficiency related by a common antigen-antibody system. *Nature* 249:830, 1974.

107. André, C., Lambert, R., Bazin, H., et al. Interference of oral immunization with the intestinal absorption of heterologous albumin. *Eur. J. Immunol.* 4:701, 1974.

108. Williams, R. C., Jr., and Gibbons, R. J. Inhibition of bacterial adherence by secretory immunoglobulin A: a mechanism of antigen disposal. *Science* 177:697, 1972.

109. Triger, D. R., Alp, M. H., and Wright, R. Bacterial and dietary antibodies in liver disease. *Lancet* 1:60, 1972.

110. Bjørneboe, M., Prytz, H., and Orskov, F. Antibodies to intestinal microbes in serum of patients with cirrhosis of the liver. *Lancet* 1:58, 1972.

111. Thomas, H. C., MacSween, R. N. M., and White, R. G. The role of the liver in controlling the immunogenicity of commensal bacteria in the gut. *Lancet* 1:1288, 1973.

112. Thomas, H. C., Singer, C. R. J., Tilney, N. L., et al. The immune response in cirrhotic rats. Antigen distribution, humoral immunity, cell-mediated immunity and splenic suppressor cell activity. *Clin. Exp. Immunol.* 26:574, 1976.

113. Fox, R. A., James, D. G., Scheuer, P. J., et al. Impaired delayed hypersensitivity in primary biliary cirrhosis. *Lancet* 1:959, 1969.

114. Mannik, M. Binding of albumin to gamma-A-myeloma proteins and Waldenström macroglobulins by disulfide bonds. *J. Immunol.* 99:899, 1967.

115. Tomasi, T. B., Jr., and Hauptman, S. P. The binding of α-1 antitrypsin to human IgA. *J. Immunol.* 112:2274, 1974.

116. Shim, B. S., Kang, Y. S., Kim, W. J., et al. Self-protective activity of colostral IgA against tryptic digestion. *Nature* 222:787, 1969.

117. Brown, W. R., Newcomb, R. W., and Ishizaka, K. Proteolytic degradation of exocrine and serum immunoglobulins. *J. Clin. Invest.* 49:1374, 1970.

118. Haneberg, B. Immunoglobulins in feces from infants fed human or bovine milk. *Scand. J. Immunol.* 3:191, 1974.

119. Plaut, A. G., Wistar, R., Jr., and Capra, J. D. Differential susceptibility of human IgA immunoglobulins to streptococcal IgA protease. *J. Clin. Invest.* 54:1295, 1974.

120. Meltzer, M., and Franklin, E. C. Cryoglobulinemia. A study of 29 patients. I. IgG and IgM cryoglobulins and factors affecting cryoprecipitability. *Am. J. Med.* 40:828, 1966.

121. Verroust, P., Mery, J-P., Morel-Maroger, L., et al. Glomerular lesions in monoclonal gammopathies and mixed essential cryoglobulinemias IgG-IgM. *Adv. Nephrol.* 1:161, 1971.

122. Koffler, D., Schur, P. H., and Kunkel, H. G. Immunological studies concerning the nephritis of systemic lupus erythematosus. *J. Exp. Med.* 126:607, 1967.

123. Mannik, M., Arend, W. P., Hall, A. P., et al. Studies on antigen-antibody complexes. I. Elimination of soluble complexes from rabbit circulation. *J. Exp. Med.* 133:713, 1971.

124. Mannik, M., and Arend, W. P. Fate of preformed immune complexes in rabbits and rhesus monkeys. *J. Exp. Med.* 134:19s, 1971.

125. Arend, W. P., and Mannik, M. *In vitro* adherence of soluble immune complexes to macrophages. *J. Exp. Med.* 136:514, 1972.

126. Arend, W. P., and Mannik, M. Studies on antigen-antibody complexes. II. Quantification of tissue uptake of soluble complexes in normal and complement-depleted rabbits. *J. Immunol.* 107:63, 1971.

127. Haakenstad, A. O., and Mannik, M. The disappearance kinetics of soluble immune complexes prepared with reduced and alkylated antibodies and with intact antibodies in mice. *Lab. Invest.* 35:283, 1976.

128. Haakenstad, A. O., Striker, G. E., and Mannik, M. The glomerular deposition of soluble immune complexes prepared with reduced and alkylated antibodies and with intact antibodies in mice. *Lab. Invest.* 35:293, 1976.

129. Cochrane, C. G., and Hawkins, D. Studies on circulating immune complexes. III. Factors governing the ability of circulating complexes to localize in blood vessels. *J. Exp. Med.* 127:137, 1968.

130. Cochrane, C. G., and Koffler, D. Immune complex disease in experimental animals and man. *Adv. Immunol.* 16:185, 1973.

131. Izui, S., Lambert, P. H., and Miescher, P. A. *In vitro* demonstration of a particular affinity of glomerular basement membrane and collagen for DNA. A possible basis for a local formation of DNA-anti-DNA complexes in systemic lupus erythematosus. *J. Exp. Med.* 144:428, 1976.

132. Biro, C. E., and García, G. The antigenicity of aggregated and aggregate-free human gamma-globulin for rabbits. *Immunology* 8:411, 1965.

133. Lightfoot, R. W., Jr., Drusin, R. E., and Christian, C. L. Properties of soluble immune complexes. *J. Immunol.* 105:1493, 1970.

134. Steward, M. W., Glass, D. N., Maini, R. N., et al. Role of low avidity antibody to native DNA in human and murine lupus syndrome. *J. Rheumatol.* 1:75, 1974 (abstract).

135. Steward, M. W., Gaze, S. E., and Petty, R. E. Low affinity antibody production in mice—a form of immunological tolerance? *Eur. J. Immunol.* 4:751, 1974.

136. Steward, M. W., and Petty, R. E. The antigen-binding characteristics of antibody pools of different relative affinity. *Immunology* 23:881, 1972.

137. Steward, M. W., Petty, R. E., and Soothill, K. F. Low affinity antibody—its possible immunopathologic significance. *Int. Arch. Allergy Appl. Immunol.* 45:176, 1973.

138. Steward, M. W., Katz, F. E., and West, N. J. The role of low affinity antibody in immune complex disease. The quantity of anti-DNA antibodies in NZB/W F1 hybrid mice. *Clin. Exp. Immunol.* 21:121, 1975.

139. Winfield, J. B., Faiferman, I., and Koffler, D. Avidity of anti-DNA antibodies in serum and IgG glomerular eluates from patients with systemic lupus erythematosus. Association of high avidity antinative DNA antibody with glomerulonephritis. *J. Clin. Invest.* 59:90, 1977.

140. Gershwin, M. E., and Steinberg, A. D. Qualitative characteristics of anti-DNA antibodies in lupus nephritis. *Arthritis Rheum.* 17:947, 1974.

141. Tan, E. M., and Kunkel, H. G. An immunofluorescent study of the skin lesions in systemic lupus erythematosus. *Arthritis Rheum.* 9:37, 1966.

142. Landry, M., and Sams, W. M., Jr. Systemic lupus erythematosus. Studies of the antibodies bound to skin. *J. Clin. Invest.* 52:1871, 1973.

143. Yonemasu, K., Stroud, R. M., Niedermeier, W., et al. Chemical studies on C1q; a modulator of immunoglobulin biology. *Biochem. Biophys. Res. Commun.* 43:1388, 1971.

144. Knobel, H. R., Heusser, C., Rodrick, M. L., et al. Enzymatic digestion of the first component of human complement (C1q). *J. Immunol.* 112:2094, 1974.

145. Michaelides, M. D., and Eisen, H. N. The strange cross reaction of menadione (vitamin K3) and 2,4-dinitrophenyl ligands with a myeloma protein and some conventional antibodies. *J. Exp. Med.* 140:687, 1974.

146. Richards, F. F., Amzel, L. M., Konigsberg, W. H., et al. Polyfunctional antibody combining regions. In E. E. Sercarz, A. R. Williamson, and C. F. Fox, eds., *The Immune System: Genes, Receptors, Signals,* p. 53. Academic Press, New York, 1974.

CHAPTER 5

Host Factors: The Core of the Problem

The occurrence of immune complexes in plasma and in tissues during many disease states is clearly a normal biological phenomenon. How the host deals with such complexes, and its mechanisms for removal or clearing of both tissue-fixed complexes and those that circulate, constitute the most important aspects of the subject. The discussion in this chapter focuses directly on these host factors.

Genetic Aspects

One of the most important areas in modern clinical immunology relates to the genetic factors within the host that govern or control response to antigen. No longer can one regard a streptococcal or pneumococcal infection on the one hand or a malignant melanoma on the other as a universal signal, nor can one consider patients confronted with such diverse antigens as a homogeneous pool of response.

The basic importance of genetic control over the immune response was originally recognized in the 1960s when multiple inbred strains of animals were challenged with uniform well-characterized antigens such as those made up of dinitrophenyl (DNP), poly-*L*-lysine (PLL), or other repeating polymeric linkages of simple amino acids (1–3). The results obtained were extraordinary. Some inbred strains produced quite high levels of humoral antibody or cell-mediated reactions to test antigens; these animals were termed responders. Other strains showed very little if any detectable immune reactivity and were labeled nonresponders for the particular antigen involved. Still other

strains fell somewhere between these two poles, with an intermediate gradation of either humoral or cellular responsiveness. The most important aspect of these differences in immune response is the relationship between cell-surface recognition units such as H-2 or HLA antigens and quantitative genetic differences in individual immune response (4–6). This perception led to recognition of what are now called immune response, or IR, genes (7). Currently these genes are more accurately defined in the mouse than they are in man. They occur in close proximity on the chromosome for genes coding for the cell-surface antigen recognition units known as H-2 determinants (Figure 5-1) and correspond to HLA antigens in man. Largely through use of synthetic well-defined antigens and manipulations involving backcrosses and studies of progeny in responder and nonresponder strains of experimental animals, an outline of the linkage between IR genes and immune responses has begun to emerge in recent years. A simplified map or schema of the H-2 or HLA system and proposed relative general locations of IR genes in the mouse as well as in man are shown in Figure 5-1. Currently it is felt that, in humans, genetically determined cell-surface determinants classified according to what is called the HLA-D typing system are probably most closely related to IR genes. This system utilizes cell-surface antigen typing on the basis of reactivity in mixed leukocyte culture reactions or with well-defined antisera that appear to recognize such specificities.

There are now a number of clinical exam-

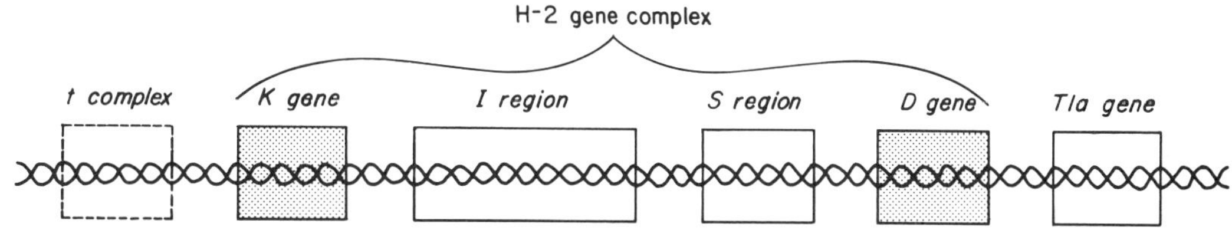

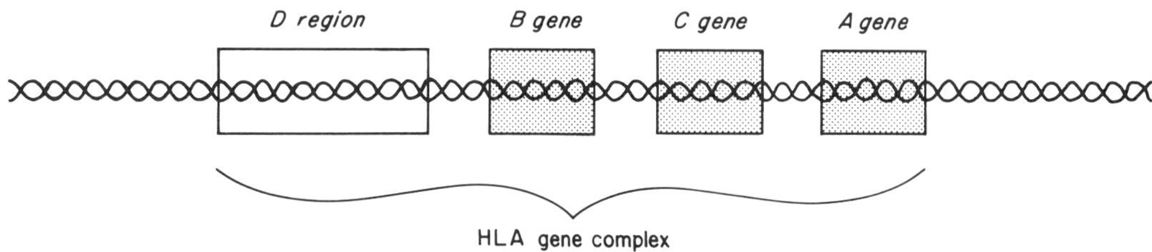

Figure 5-1 Spatial map for mouse chromosome 17 and human chromosome 6.

ples of what appear to be HLA-linked disease associations (7, 8) including ankylosing spondylitis (9), chronic active hepatitis (10), multiple sclerosis (11), psoriasis (12), adult coeliac disease (13), gluten sensitive enteropathy (14), and others. Since human populations are for the most part outbred, heterogeneous, and more difficult to study than the inbred strains of mice and guinea pigs originally used in definition of the antigen-specific immune response gene concept, many of the relationships between HLA, HLA-B, or HLA-D typing and specific human disorders still must be clarified.

Some fascinating speculations have evolved concerning the underlying reasons for an apparent relation between histocompatibility cell-surface antigens and well-defined human disease states. In the case of diseases like hepatitis B or subacute sclerosing encephalitis (SSPE), known to be associated with specific viral etiology, it has been suggested that the physical structures making up the surface glycoprotein moieties of certain HLA antigens might in fact be cell-surface receptors through which the virus enters the cell. To date there has been no clear-cut experimental confirmation of such a hypothesis. A general impression of what HLA or H-2 antigens are like in relation to the cell-membrane lipid bilayer is shown in Figure 5-2. In diseases of unknown etiology, including rheumatoid arthritis or systemic lupus erythematosus, genetically determined cell-surface HLA and other antigenic relationships require better definition; infectious agents, if present, must be identified before such a hypothesis can be adequately tested. Histocompatibility associations with rheumatoid arthritis, revealed by the work of Stastny (15, 16), appear very promising in defining a relationship between disease occurrence and the presence of the cell-surface structures identified in a relatively large portion of the individual patients studied. Previous observations on the nonstimulation in mixed lymphocyte cultures of individual nonrelated subjects with rheumatoid arthritis (17, 18) have provided useful background; ordinary HLA typing had shown no clear association with rheumatoid disease (19,

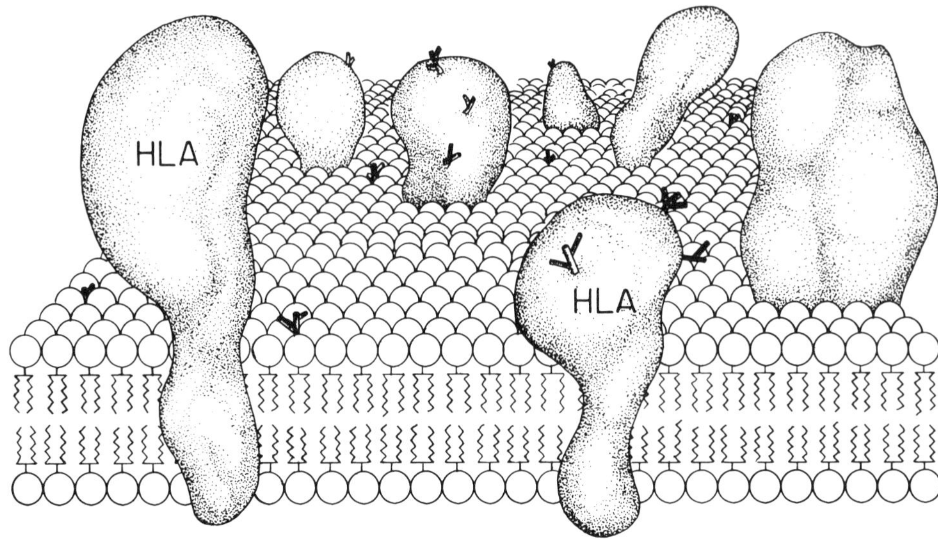

Figure 5-2   The major histocompatibility antigens, shown schematically as part of a large number of proteins present in the cell-membrane lipid bilayer. In the case of the HLA antigens, one portion ex-tends inside the cell, where it can interact with cyto-plasmic proteins; the other part extends out and is capable of interacting with other cells.

20). Recently, however, rapid development of HLA-D typing systems has greatly expanded our understanding. Striking HLA-D type associations have been observed with several connective-tissue diseases. Studies by Reinersten and colleagues (21) have indicated that both HLA-DRw2 and HLA-DRw3 were increased in systemic lupus erythematosus. The typing systems employed reagents reacting with Ia-like determinants expressed principally on B cells. In addition, such B-cell alloantigen differences have been documented with similar techniques in rheumatoid arthritis and systemic lupus erythematosus (22). The new B-cell human alloantigens are defined by Ia phenotypes designated as HLA-DR (23). Work in this area is expanding rapidly. Most recently, an association of a new B-cell alloantigen with susceptibility to rheumatic fever has been recorded (24).

One of the most important points in HLA disease association is that genetic control of the immune response is recognized at many different levels. Genetic variability in capacity to produce antibodies of high or low avidity is an example of control at multiple levels in both the afferent and efferent arms of the immune response.

An ever increasing number of diverse observations are being made relative to deficiency of individual complement components and the occurrence of so-called autoimmune disorders (25–28). Prominent in the clinical data among such patients is the high frequency of diseases (such as SLE, glomerulonephritis, or mixed connective-tissue disease syndromes) where the tissue lesions are directly related to immune-complex deposition. It is particularly interesting that potential linkage, or at least a genetic explanation for the association between various complement component deficiencies and autoimmune disease, has been recognized. Most striking in the complement deficiencies associated with SLE has been the finding of homozygous and heterozygous C-2 deficiency (25, 27). In addition, SLE-like syndromes have been recorded in patients with defects of the terminal complement complex (C5–9) (29, 30). Direct experimental data linking HLA determinants with C-2 deficiency in several interesting families have been presented, using typing systems that detect determinants now recognized as belonging to LD or HLD loci (31, 32).

Additional studies have focused on the relationship between genetic control of complement and HLA or H-2 in man or mouse respectively (33–36). Since an intact complement system appears to be important in various aspects of virus neutralization (37, 38), association of complement component deficiencies with a variety of syndromes similar to SLE might be used as evidence for a viral etiology of the disease itself. The most compelling direct evidence for possible viral involvement in SLE, however, has come from the studies related to C-type RNA viruses (39–43). Linkage of hypocomplementemic states to a number of apparent immune-complex–mediated autoimmune disorders is intriguing. The association of hypocomplementemic nephritis and membranoproliferative glomerulonephritis, and similar direct associations between hypocomplementemic nephritis and lipodystrophy, have recently become apparent (44–46). It has been postulated that selected defects in the complement cascade enhance repeated, perhaps subclinical, infectious episodes and greatly augment exposure to cyclic release of circulating immune complexes. Whether increased intrinsic susceptibility to many types of infection can actually be related to an increased propensity to develop an autoimmune response needs considerably more documentation. In particular, instead of being causally related, both complement defects and autoimmune reactivities could be the result themselves of some other causative factor. As noted in Chapter 4, when experimental animals passively infused with immune complexes were decomplemented, no profound changes were recorded in the handling of immune complexes within the animal model.

Histocompatibility Fit for Cell-to-Cell Interaction

The factors that have been defined regarding genetic influence on specific types of immune response will probably turn out to be among the most important host features determining the extent and severity of many clinical immune-complex–mediated phenomena. One relevant feature of the general question of cell-surface recognition structures and genetic linkage has been the particular requirements for direct cell-mediated killing of cells infected by virus. Products of the major histocompati-

bility complex apparently are important as potential target structures in T-lymphocyte–mediated killing of target cells infected with virus. Thus, sensitized T cells appear to be capable of killing virus-infected cells only if both killer T cell and target cell are similar at either the K or the D region (Figure 5-1) of the major histocompatibility complex (47–50). It has recently been shown that human virus-infected target cells lacking HLA antigens resist specific T-lymphocyte cytolysis (51), and that H-2/viral protein complexes may exist on cells. This could explain the HLA or H-2 restriction of cytotoxicity in such systems (52). A graphic representation of the restriction in H-2 or HLA loci between effector killer cell and target cells in virus infections or tumor immune reactions is shown in Figure 5-3. Genetic factors modulating specific immune responses are operative at a number of different levels: it would be an oversimplification to dwell on the concept of high and low responders in humoral antibody responses as the most pertinent or central to the problem of immune-complex disease. There are undoubtedly separate genetic controls that affect macrophage antigen processing, levels of humoral antibody production, and subsequent avidity of antibodies produced. The Zinkernagel-Doherty phenomenon (47–50) is a dramatic example of genetic

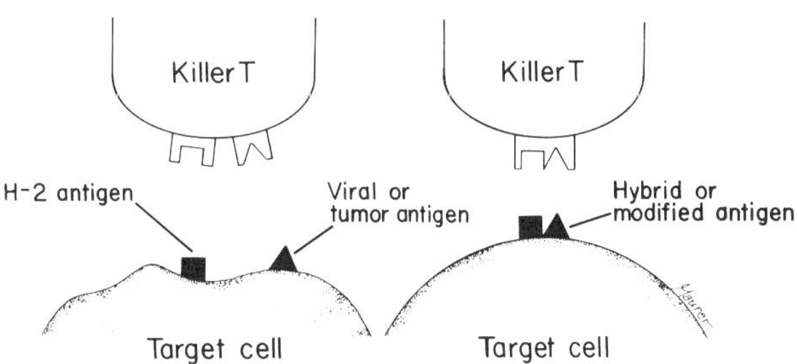

Figure 5-3 Two possible ways in which "histocompatibility fit" may be involved in immune T-cell–mediated killing of target cells. In the left-hand example, separate receptors for histocompatibility structures (H-2) and viral or tumor antigen are shown; on the right a single interaction involving a hybrid target antigen (viral protein closely opposed to histocompatibility-related structure) is diagrammed.

control at an entirely different level. Finally, it seems likely that other, still undefined, genetically determined mechanisms can influence not only actual immune-complex deposition but also dissolution or natural clearance mechanisms of the body proper.

The Serum Sickness Model

The sequential events involved in the generation of tissue lesions and the pathological manifestations of immune-complex disease are nowhere better illustrated than in the acute experimental model provided by one-shot serum sickness, or the model of chronic serum sickness in which more prolonged or repetitive antigenic challenge is necessary (53, 54). In the acute experimental immune-complex model, a well-defined single foreign protein antigen such as bovine serum albumin (BSA) is administered intravenously to rabbits. If such an antigen is first labeled with ^{125}I, its equilibration phase in plasma followed by normal catabolism and later rapid immune elimination can be shown graphically in the familiar profile illustrated in Figure 5-4. During the phase of im-

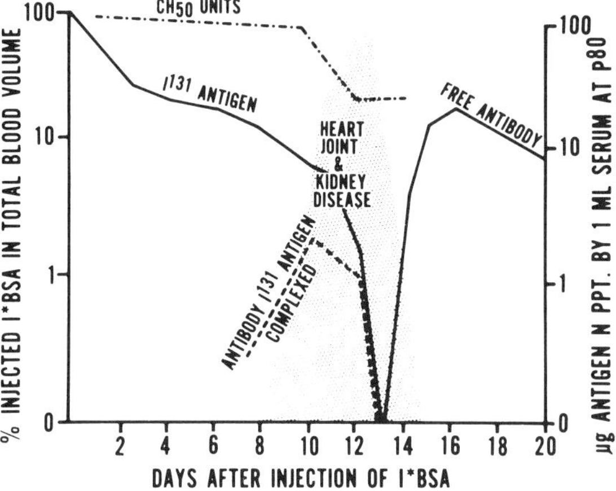

Figure 5-4 Elimination of bovine serum albumin ^{131}I antigen from the circulation of a typical rabbit, showing the appearance of immune complexes in the circulation and the development of lesions. Free antibody was measured by precipitation. (Reproduced with permission, C. G. Cochrane and D. Koffler, *Adv. Immunol.* 16:185, 1973.)

mune elimination of antigen, complexes composed of antigen and antibodies can be detected within the circulation, and at this time the acute lesions of immune-complex disease are seen in glomeruli, joints, and myocardial vessels of the experimental animals. The glomerular lesions in animals afflicted with immune-complex lesions during acute serum sickness are associated with endothelial swelling and marked proteinuria. An example of the glomerular edema and swelling seen in the acute phase of experimental serum sickness is shown in Figure 5-5. Immunofluorescence microscopic monitoring of the lesions shows antigen, host γ-globulin, and complement (C3) in granular deposits along the glomerular basement membrane and in small vessels elsewhere. The granular appearance of acute immune-deposit disease is illustrated in Figure 5-6 and has become one of the hallmarks of acute immune-complex deposition and injury. Electron microscopic examination shows little more than swelling and slight edema of vascular endothelial cells.

The acute phase of serum sickness is also marked by an arteritis, which begins as a mild proliferation or deposition in glomerular intimal endothelial cells and usually becomes apparent during the initial immune elimination of antigen (Table 5-1). Neutrophils (PMNs) entering the lesions are prominent and lysosomal enzymes released by such phagocytic cells rapidly degrade underlying vascular membranes, including internal elastic laminae and later portions of the vessel media and adventitia. Often this is immediately followed by the appearance of characteristic fibrinoid necrosis within arterial walls. At this stage immunofluorescence techniques are capable of identifying immunoglobulin, C3, and antigen within the arterial wall lesion. However, in very short order phagocytic cells engulf such complexes and in several days they are no longer detectable. The evanescence of sequential changes during this phase of acute immune-complex-mediated arteritis is important in any consideration of similar lesions seen during acute vasculitis in the human, since rapid histological change and phagocytic removal of immune-complex materials from inflamed vessel

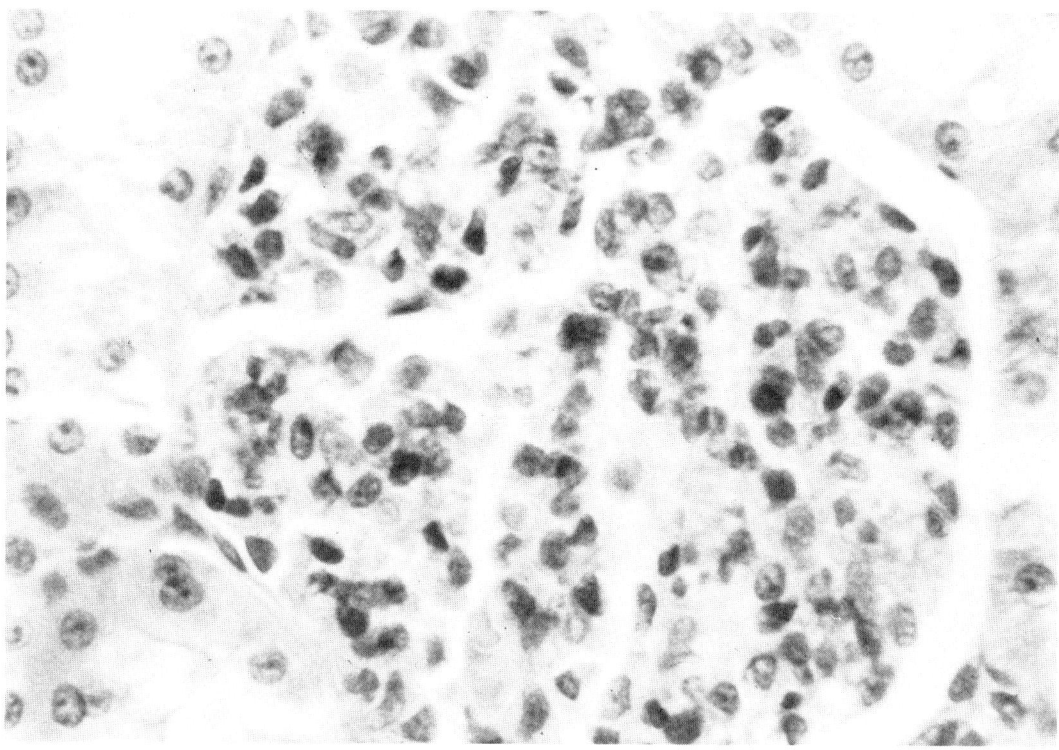

Figure 5-5 Histological changes in the glomerulus of a rabbit with experimental serum sickness. Extensive swelling of the entire glomerulus is present. Magnification × 350. (Photograph courtesy of C. B. Wilson, Scripps Research Foundation, La Jolla, California.)

walls may make precise definition of evolving lesions difficult. This is especially true if histological specimens are inadvertently timed so as to miss such evolution.

The sequential development of vascular and glomerular injury in the acute serum sickness model involves in vivo deposition of immune complexes with concomitant marked depression in circulating complement levels. Abrupt falls in total hemolytic complement (CH 50) in acute one-shot serum sickness are reminders of the fact that low serum complement activity is often noted during the active phase of systemic lupus erythematosus, in the evolution of acute poststreptococcal glomerulonephritis, or in the dengue virus shock syndrome. However, sudden falls in serum complement, particularly as noted in such rapidly changing clinical situations, require caution in interpretation; they are also profoundly influenced by changes in rates of catabolism or of

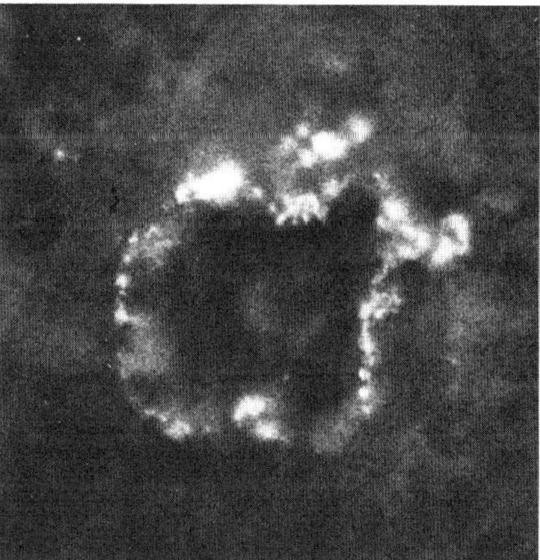

Figure 5-6 Granular deposition of BSA antigen in a small blood vessel of the myocardium during the acute phase of one-shot serum sickness. The distribution of host IgG and complement in parallel studies were similar. Magnification × 275. (Photograph courtesy of C. G. Cochrane, Scripps Research Foundation, La Jolla, California.)

Table 5-1 Relation between sedimentation characteristics of circulating immune complexes and development of actual lesions in serum sickness. The data are from C. G. Cochrane and D. Hawkins, *J. Exp. Med.* 127:137, 1968.

No. of rabbits	Average amount of BSA − ^{131}I bound to globulin (%)[a]	Pattern of BSA − ^{131}I sedimentation	Number of glomerular lesions	Total amount of proteinuria (mg)	Maximum complement depletion (%)
9	43.3	Heavy (19 S or greater)	2.3 +	567	78
5	41.6	Light (< 19 S)	0 to ±	0	67

[a] Percent BSA bound to globulins precipitated by ammonium sulfate at 50-percent saturation.

synthesis of individual complement components during the respective disease states.

Neutrophils are an essential feature of the acute serum sickness arteritic lesion. If animals are experimentally depleted of neutrophils before acute serum sickness induction, no arteritis can be detected, although glomerular injury does not seem to be substantially affected (53, 55, 56). This is an important point and one that is basic to the pathogenesis of the Arthus reaction, since PMNs constitute essential cellular components in this situation—which represents an acute in vivo reaction between antigen and antibody within vascular walls. The role of PMNs in eliciting the basic inflammatory response of the Arthus reaction has been carefully documented by several groups (57–60). It seems possible therefore that immunosuppressive therapy that in any way interferes with granulocyte or granulocytic precursor mobilization will affect the vasculitic phase of acute serum sickness injury, and an intact polymorphonuclear leukocyte inflammatory response appears to be necessary for full development of the arteritis.

The Arthus-type reaction, occurring as it does within the walls of small blood vessels, may represent a model for many phenomena seen during commonly recognized clinical circumstances. This has been previously alluded to in Chapter 1 in connection with the skin lesions of gonococcal sepsis or in similar cutaneous lesions such as Osler's nodes in subacute bacterial endocarditis. Many of the peripheral lesions of acute disseminated gonococcal infection or even secondary syphilis may in fact reflect an acute local vascular reaction between foreign antigens fixed in tissues and circulating host antibodies. Moreover, during the acute phase of hypersensitivity angiitis it seems possible that local vascular deposition of antigen-antibody complexes may be involved in the initial phase of vascular inflammation or injury. The enigma in such cases of course arises when one has to explain continued progression, eventual fibrosis, or aneurysmal change associated with chronic inflammation within vessels where immunofluorescence techniques no longer show detectable evidence of immunoglobulin or activated complement components. Arthus-type reactions may also be involved in such widely diverse disease manifestations as the rash of viral xanthemata (including measles or chickenpox) or in the evanescent erythema marginatum associated with disorders like acute rheumatic fever. Something akin to the Arthus phenomenon has been invoked as a possible explanation for the initial arterial lesion of erythema nodosum.

Some quantitative estimates of the molecular amounts of antigen and antibody required to produce acute glomerular injury have been provided by the experiments of Wilson and Dixon (61). On the assumption that each kidney has 200,000 glomeruli (62), it was estimated that at the height of disease 1 to 35 μg of BSA was bound to rabbit kidney, along with 1.3×10^9 molecules of antibody complexed to antigen per glomerulus. Such quantitative data fit well with the observed immunofluorescence and ultrastructural distribution of antigen-antibody deposits.

Complement as well as neutrophils appear to be of importance in the acute serum sickness injury model. If complement in experimental animals is depleted using cobra venom factor or other experimental techniques, marked diminution or arteritis is noted, although glomerular injury appears to remain relatively unaffected (63).

Chronic Experimental Immune-Complex Disease

Chronic experimental immune-complex disease, originally described and developed as a model for the understanding of chronic glomerulonephritis, has also provided a useful basis for insight into the chronic lesions associated with other disorders related to prolonged immune-complex injury. The classic chronic serum sickness model as originally developed in the rabbit (63, 64) involved daily injections of animals with a variety of heterologous protein antigens. The amounts of antigen given appeared to be critical; for lesions to develop, a daily state of antigen excess was necessary after each injection (63). As defined in the relationships expressed by the quantitative precipitin curve (Chapter 4), a chronic remitting state of antigen excess would provide daily infusions of soluble complexes. This model generally was noted to produce glomerulonephritis but not arteritis. Moreover, if amounts of antigen were given that were too small—that is, still in the zone of antibody excess—then no substantial quantities of soluble complexes were induced and no subacute or chronic glomerulonephritis was noted. Animals without a significant antibody response did not develop disease, while rabbits showing weak responses required much longer intervals of repeated injections before chronic glomerulonephritis was noted. It follows that some degree of humoral immune response must be present to invoke peripheral or localized tissue injury attributable to immune-complex–mediated phenomena. It is therefore obvious that lesions that could be ascribed to modulation through immune complexes are not seen in patients receiving high doses of immunosuppressive drugs—for instance, in acute leukemia—unless some quantity of prior circulating antibody to tumor-specific or other antigen is present.

If soluble immune complexes represent the sine qua non of acute immune-complex injury, it seems logical to attempt therapeutic intervention during such a phase in acute clinical situations. This has indeed been attempted with considerable vigor and some degree of success in the case of disorders such as myasthenia gravis, systemic lupus, Goodpasture's syndrome, or rapidly progressive glomerulonephritis. The therapeutic benefit of such procedures may in fact be serendipitous and result from inadvertent activation of intrinsic host mechanisms of immune-complex removal by the lungs, as will be discussed later in this chapter.

The possible importance of relative degrees of immune deficiency has been emphasized by Peters and Lachmann (65), who point out that chronic glomerulonephritis is difficult to induce in animals making too strong an immune response, since chronic antigen administration only results in more and more rapid elimination of antigen. In order to produce chronic immune-complex disease the animal must make just enough antibody to remain in the zone of antigen excess but not so much that all injected antigen is immediately eliminated. Obviously the balance between helper and suppressor influence during such an ongoing humoral immune response raises interesting problems. The murine model provided by NZB/W mouse disease, characterized as it is by humoral hyperresponsiveness and apparent T-cell deficiency, has been highly instructive in this respect. It is discussed in detail in Chapter 12.

In animals with full-blown chronic immune-complex glomerulonephritis, the disease progresses to uremia and eventual fatal outcome much in the manner of human chronic glomerulonephritis. Chronic changes progress from thickening of glomerular capillaries without proliferation, to proliferation, to glomerular sclerosis, then to final obliteration. In some animals with heightened immune responsiveness PMN accumulations may be accompanied by proliferation and swelling of glomerular endothelial cells and subsequent crescent formation by epithelial cells present in Bowman's space. Immunofluorescence studies frequently show large deposits of antigen, host IgG, and C3 along glomerular basement membranes localized primarily along the external surfaces. Quantitative studies aimed at estimation of actual injected antigen remaining in the kidneys after clinical onset of proteinuria revealed 47 ± 18 μg at onset, increasing to 600 ± 73 μg as the chronic lesions progressed (61). The amount of antigen deposited in glomeruli rose by a factor of ten when established chronic disease developed; however, such deposition of antigen still represented only 0.5 percent of the amount of antigen injected. As immune deposits grew, the normal glomerular mesangial clearing mechanisms intrinsic to disposal of such materials became overloaded and could not clear additional deposits as they formed and were sequestered in individual glomeruli. During the phase of chronic established immune-complex disease, electron-dense immune deposits in and around the external aspects of glomerular basement membranes were characteristic. As in all chronic models of immune-complex disease, the key requirement was for sufficient quantities of injected antigen each day to ensure removal of antibodies from circulation and promotion of bursts of circulating soluble complexes. Once a chronic glomerular deposition of immune complexes had been successfully established, injection of marked excess of antigen—that is, ten- to forty-fold excess—was capable of dramatically reversing the underlying process of immune-complex injury (66). This was true because complexes after deposition were apparently capable of in vivo solubilization in the zone of antigen excess. In this type of study heavy γ-globulin deposits decreased and slowly disappeared when high levels of antigen administration were continued. In other studies conducted by Wilson and Dixon (61), although deposition of complexes showed regression as determined by serial immunofluorescence,

proteinuria did not completely disappear presumably as a result of previous irreversible glomerular injury.

Host Factors Affecting Immune-Complex Deposition

When immune complexes circulate, they may undergo one of two types of disposition—either they are engulfed and cleared by phagocytic reticuloendothelial or monocytic cells, or they are deposited in vascular structures and potentially result in immune-complex–mediated tissue injury. The early studies of Benacerraf and co-workers (67) indicated that some type of active process was required for immune-complex tissue deposition. When mice were injected intravenously with colloidal carbon and then given several vasoactive substances such as histamine, serotonin, epinephrine, or preformed immune complexes, carbon deposition was noted in the intimal layers of large arteries, the endocardium of the heart, and the walls of various venules. It was suggested that the immune complexes themselves might liberate vasoactive amines in vivo and result in particulate carbon deposition. Moreover, the careful studies of Cochrane and colleagues (55, 68–70) have shown that circulating-complex deposition can be induced by simultaneous infusion of agents that cause liberation of mast-cell vasoactive amines. Pretreatment with antihistamines prevented released histamine from influencing vascular basement membrane (69–73). These findings (Table 5-2) suggest either filtration or perhaps active transport across such limiting membranes.

In the initial studies of this particular process by Kniker and Cochrane (68) complexes of various sizes were prepared in vitro, and it was found that only complexes of 19S or greater became entrapped. Large proteins such as crab hemocyanin (7×10^6 Daltons) or aggregates of IgG (>19S) also deposited in such membranes. During these experiments additional evidence for local factors was obtained, in that immune-complex deposition was often directly associated with conditions favoring local increased vascular permeability.

Table 5-2 Incidence and severity of serum sickness lesions in treated and control rabbits. The data are from W. T. Kniker and C. G. Cochrane, *J. Exp. Med.* 127:119, 1968.

Lesions	Rabbits treated with antihistamine and antiserotonin (% positive)	Control rabbits (% positive)	
		Platelet depletion	
	(11 rabbits)	(16 rabbits)	(10 rabbits)
Coronary artery			
Endothelial proliferation	9	44	90
Medial necrosis	9	19	80
Glomeruli			
Immunofluorescent deposits	0 to +	0 to +	+ to ++
Endothelial swelling and proliferation	1.0	1.7	2.2

Thus agents that blocked vasoactive amines markedly diminished local immune-complex deposition. This was also illustrated when animals were depleted of platelets—a high natural reservoir of vasoactive substances.

Subsequent studies have provided additional evidence that long-term treatment with antagonists of vasoactive amines such as chlorpheniramine or methysergide reduces deposition of immune complexes in chronic immune-complex-mediated experimental glomerulonephritis (74, 75). It was shown by Chused and Tarpley (76) that administration of methysergide, a serotonin antagonist, ameliorated naturally occurring immune-complex nephritis in NZB/W mice. When administration of the drug was begun early in life, experimental animals showed less proteinuria and renal pathology than did untreated controls. Cyproheptadine, an antagonist of both serotonin and histamine, also has been shown to delay onset of proteinuria in the NZB/W model. However, attempts to alter the course of autologous immune-complex nephritis with this agent in rats were unsuccessful even when used in combination with powerful anti-inflammatory or immunosuppressive agents (77).

A complex local series of events is probably involved in the exact process of immune-complex deposition. During experimental or clinical conditions associated with immune-complex injury, increased vascular permeability may occur as a result of release of vasoactive materials in key areas within the microvascular circulation. For instance, in the case of pneumococcal sepsis or Gram-negative bacteremia, potent cell-wall or extracellular bacterial products may be capable of marked amplification of the process. It is also conceivable that factors directly associated with other infectious agents such as the measles virus, hepatitis B antigens, circulating gonococci, or even various tumor products can activate local tissue release of potent vasoactive substances. Careful studies directed at this area may eventually explain tissue distribution of lesions under diverse conditions.

In the face of marked increased local permeability, large macromolecular complexes are held up and deposited at limiting vascular membranes and an inflammatory response rapidly ensues. This sequence of events is summarized diagrammatically in Figure 5-7.

Other Potential Mechanisms of Local Tissue Deposition

One of the most likely sources of local buildup or widespread distribution of vasoactive amines has always been alleged to be blood platelets, which are rich in histamine and serotonin. A number of experimental approaches

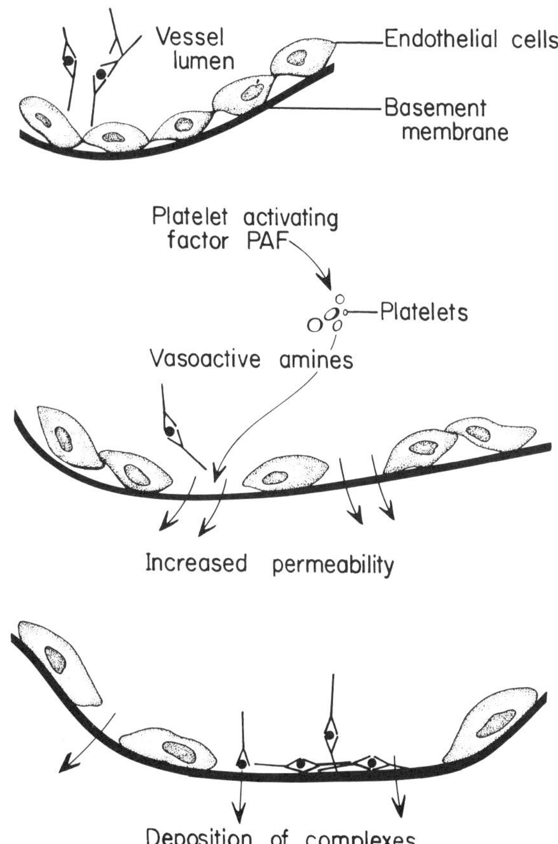

Figure 5-7 Possible ways in which vasoactive amines may influence deposition of immune complexes.

aimed at elucidating this potential mechanism have been conducted. Rabbit platelets are known to be capable of amine release in the presence of immune complexes and plasma (78–82). The reaction is markedly increased under conditions of antibody excess, and in some experimental models complement activity has also been shown to be necessary for vasoactive-amine release. Immune complexes studied by Henson and Cochrane (83, 84) in C6-deficient rabbit plasma failed to release histamine and serotonin, but release was restored upon addition of C3. The potential importance of cell interactions was emphasized in studies using C6-deficient plasma, where platelets and immune complexes were capable of amine release if neutrophils were also added (83).

A further mechanism involving cellular interaction has been described in which sensitized PMNs and platelets showed active amine release in the presence of antigen (85, 86). In this particular reaction plasma or antibody was apparently not required, and the reactive cell capable of direct histamine release was defined as a basophil (87). Later studies have defined basophilic release of active amines with sensitization by IgE (88), since leukocyte-platelet reactions could be elicited with purified anti-IgE. Sensitized basophils released platelet-activating factor, which bound rapidly to albumin and initiated platelet clumping as well as vasoactive amine release.

As discussed in Chapter 4, an intact complement system does not appear to be necessary for actual deposition of immune complexes. Initial experiments to explore this question were performed by Cochrane and co-workers, using depletion of C3 and terminal complement components with cobra venom factor (89). These studies provided clear evidence for glomerular immune-complex deposition despite functional complement depletion. Arterioles were mildly affected, but with complement effectively absent, PMN accumulation did not occur and no arteritis was observed. These findings were extended by Mannik and co-workers, who found that prior depletion of complement in animals passively infused with soluble complexes did not significantly affect immune-complex deposition either (90, 91). The fact that an intact complement mechanism was not essential for immune-complex deposition was surprising and of potential clinical importance: several disease situations exist where low levels of circulating complement are present (as in nephrotic syndrome, acute glomerulonephritis, or poststreptococcal glomerulonephritis) and continuation of immune-complex–mediated tissue destruction ensues.

Tissue Factors Affecting Immune-Complex Deposition

One of the most interesting recent developments relative to tissue localization of circulating or locally formed immune complexes has been the demonstration that certain tissues— notably normal human glomeruli—contain potential receptors for immune complexes. This phenomenon was first described by Gelfand and colleagues (92–94), who used erythrocytes sensitized with antibody and activated complement components. Ultrastructural studies directed at precise localization of such glomerular immune-complex receptors have indicated that they occur on the visceral epithelial cells of the renal capillary and that they react with activated components of C3 or C3b.

Demonstration of such receptors via the scanning electron microscope is shown in Figure 5-8, taken from studies by Burkholder and

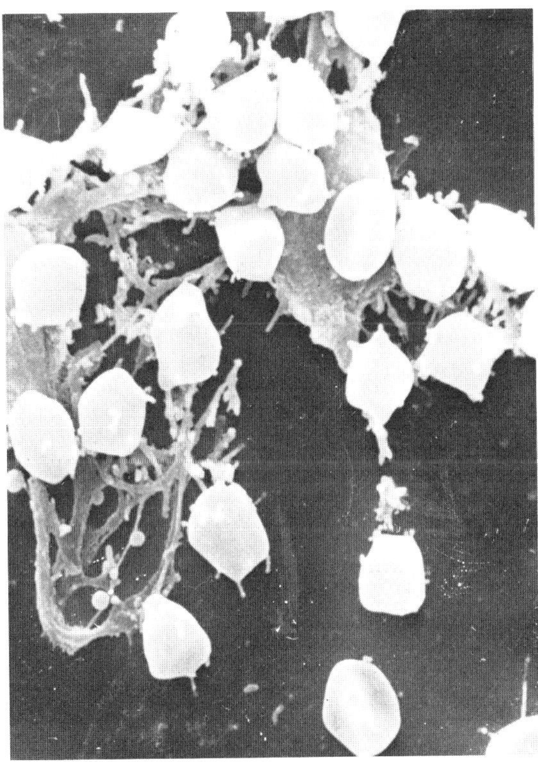

Figure 5-8 Scanning electron microscopy of human glomerular epithelial cells maintained in culture on a cover slip and incubated with sheep cells sensitized with antibody and activated complement components. Foot processes are strongly positive for immune adherence. (Reproduced with permission, P. M. Burkholder, T. D. Oberley, T. A. Barber et al., *Am. J. Pathol.* 86:635, 1977.)

associates (95). It can be seen that indicator sheep erythrocytes, sensitized with IgM antibody and activated C3, bind to the glomerular tuft. The receptor appeared to consist of structures actually binding the activated form of bound C3. In addition, human tissues that showed prior in vivo deposition of IgG and C3 in the form of immune complexes showed no in vitro residual activity of the tissue receptors (93, 94). Thus, renal biopsy specimens obtained from patients with granular immune glomerular deposits showed no further in vitro C3b receptor activity, presumably because of steric hindrance or saturation by the immune deposits already present.

Patients with membranous glomerulonephritis, as well as poststreptococcal glomerulonephritis where immune complexes are usually noted on the subepithelial sides of glomerular capillaries (96), were studied—also patients with SLE who showed both subepithelial and subendothelial deposits (97). A summary of the data of Shin and colleagues (94) is given in Table 5-3. In this instance patients with primarily mesangial immune deposits showed preservation of tissue glomerular C3 or C3b receptor sites. Patients with various forms of immune-complex renal disease have also been studied by Sobel and associates (98). Using a similar method of assay, these workers reported C3b receptor activity to be normal in patients with membranous glomerulonephritis and moderately decreased with mesangial deposition. The reason for the discrepancy between the findings recorded in several of these reports (93–95, 98) is not yet clear.

One technical difficulty recognized by Shin and co-workers in using the scanning electron-microscopic technique (94) was that exposure of potential sites for C3b receptor activity on endothelial sides of glomerular capillaries was not completely adequate; the method itself tended to expose the epithelial sides of glomerular structures most readily. Interesting as they are, these observations still do not explain the predominant subendothelial glomerular localization of immune complexes in many types of immune-complex disease. Shin has suggested some degree of mobility of C3b receptors, whereby such structures might be

Table 5-3 Correlation between complement-binding activity and pattern and location of immunoglobulin and C3 in human renal glomerulus.

Group no.	Case no.	Light microscopic and clinical diagnosis	C3 binding activity	Pattern of glomerular C3 and Ig deposits
1	1	Membranous GN,[a] idiopathic	0	Diffuse granular deposition along capillary wall
	2	Membranous GN, idiopathic	0	
	3	Proliferative GN (SLE)[b]	0	
	4	Proliferative GN (poststreptococcal)	0	
2	5	Diffuse proliferative GN (anti-GBM[c] disease)	3+	Diffuse, smooth, linear deposits along capillary wall
	6	Focal proliferative GN (malignant lymphosarcoma)	2+	
	7	Diffuse proliferative GN (rapidly progressive GN)	2 to 3+	
3	8	Focal proliferative GN (Berger's disease)	3 to 4+	Diffuse mesangial deposition of C3, IgA, and IgG
	9	Focal proliferative GN (Berger's disease)	2+	
	10	Focal proliferative GN	2 to 3+	
4	11	Minimal change lesion	3+	No deposits
	12	Minimal change lesion	3+	

Source: Reproduced with permission, M. L. Shin, M. C. Gelfand, R. B. Nagle et al., *J. Immunol.* 118:869, 1977.

[a] GN = glomerulonephritis.
[b] SLE = systemic lupus erythematosus.
[c] GBM = glomerular basement membrane.

reactive at the base or membrane side of the epithelial cell as well as along its outermost margins. However, no experimental support for such a hypothesis is currently available. Beyond the reservations already discussed relevant to the general applicability of the concept of C3b glomerular receptors in various forms of renal disease, thus far such receptors have only been described in human glomeruli (95, 99). No similar receptor has been identified in other species tested by Moran and co-workers (99), including mouse, rat, guinea pig, rabbit, and even rhesus monkey. The absence of the receptor, or lack of easy demonstration of this structure in glomeruli of rabbits where acute and chronic serum sickness induced by immune-complex disease is well established, raises serious doubts about its relevance or importance.

It is notable that in several reports that have emerged since the original observations (92, 93) inverse correlation between histological or immunologic glomerular evidence for immune-complex disease and actual demonstrability in vitro in such C3b receptor sites has not been confirmed (95, 99). The studies of Moran and co-workers (99) have been of interest in that they reported a loss of in vitro assayable C3b receptor in kidney biopsy specimens where concurrent immunofluorescence techniques showed no evidence for in vivo C3 deposition. Such findings could signify that immunofluorescence had failed to detect small amounts of C3b sufficient to block the in vitro tissue detection system, or that epithelial-cell damage might obscure one type of manifestation but not the other. This study indicated that with clinical improvement in general condition as well as in renal function, detectable C3b receptors returned as monitored in repeat follow-up renal biopsy material. Moreover, epithelial crescents showed no detectable C3b receptor activity, perhaps supporting the general view that crescents are formed by proliferation of the epithelial cells of Bowman's space.

One of the most intriguing aspects of the finding of built-in immune-complex receptors within the glomerulus relates to the question of what primary role these structures actually serve. It is difficult to believe that a structure like the glomerulus, unambiguously shown to be extremely vulnerable to immune-complex deposition and subsequent chronic injury, would be furnished by nature with built-in receptors that lead to its own destruction. Alternatively, it seems possible that C3b receptors on the epithelial side of the glomerular capillary might serve some other, possibly unrelated physiological function in body economy. It is conceivable that, as Gelfand and co-workers suggest (93), naturally occurring C3b receptors serve as a second line of defense in clearing the body of complexes (the spleen being the primary organ site for ordinary immune-complex disposal). Moreover, studies focusing on the kinetics of complement component half-life and disappearance have emphasized the extremely short half-life of C3 in the circulation (100). Alarçon-Segovia has recently suggested that the C3b receptor situated on the outside or epithelial surface of the glomerulus may function to regulate intrarenal hormonal control of blood flow or actually handle critical electrolytes, possibly through the renin or prostaglandin system (101). At present there is little direct experimental evidence to support such a possibility. Possible alternative functions of the glomerular C3b receptor certainly need to be explored before it is arbitrarily assigned a built-in self-destruct mechanism.

Fc Receptors

The finding of naturally occurring receptors for immune complexes within structures of the glomerular epithelial cell arouses other interesting speculation related to the broad field of cell surface receptors in general, and in particular whether similar structures are located in other portions of the body, which therefore become more vulnerable to immune-complex deposition. Findings in clinical disorders like SLE with central nervous system involvement, or in various human or animal viral infections of the central nervous system such as subacute sclerosing panencephalitis or lymphocytic choriomeningitis, raise the question whether C3b receptors or something akin to them may be present within specific areas of the nervous system. Observations by Atkins and colleagues (102) concerning the immunofluorescence localization of IgG and C3 within the choroid plexus during active SLE and similar findings in experimental animal virus infections by Lampert and Oldstone (103, 104) indicate the possibility that some sort of receptor for immune complexes may be present either in the choroid plexus itself or in other vulnerable structures within the central nervous system.

Recent observations in our laboratory (105) indicate that receptors for Fc of IgG are in fact present within human choroid plexus tissues. Costa and co-workers (106) have demonstrated that infection of cells with herpes virus induces the cells to form cell surface structures capable of functioning as Fc receptors. Uninfected cells showed no evidence of Fc receptors, whereas after viral infection strong binding to materials containing complexed IgG was noted. A recent study by Cooper and associates (107), aimed at clearer definition of the chemical constitution of Fc receptors on cell surfaces, showed that Fc receptors on cells were diverse in that distinctly separable molecules were capable of binding native IgG independently of IgG complexed to antigen. If the work of the Costa group is viewed as indicating that many viruses may be capable of inducing the expression of active cell surface receptors, then more attention must be directed to basic pathogenetic mechanisms in a wide variety of diseases including the spontaneously occurring NZB/W C-type virus-related disorder of mice, chronic human glomerulonephritis, or even SLE itself. It also seems possible that Fc receptors, if actually capable of being programmed by viral infection of a cell, could function to localize tissue immune-complex distribution in diseases such as

Burkitt's lymphoma, persistent hepatitis virus B infection, or subacute sclerosing panencephalitis.

The potential importance of Fc receptors to a fundamental understanding of tissue immunopathology is underscored in a recent report of Gelfand and colleagues (108), who demonstrated IgG Fc-receptor binding sites in the renal interstitium of man and in a variety of other species, through adherence of IgG-coated sheep or human red blood cells to frozen sections of renal tissue. Reagent erythrocytes coated with the F(ab)′₂ fragment of IgG (devoid of course of Fc) were not bound to tissues. The presence of such receptors within the kidney interstitium may play a role in the interstitial immune-complex injury known to occur in systemic lupus erythematosus and in Sjögren's syndrome (see Chapter 12). It is also possible that similar Fc receptors occur in other body tissues that may be involved in immune-complex injury. One of the most obvious possibilities is the eye, which has not been systematically examined.

The complexity of cell-surface materials involved in the binding of soluble immune complexes has been extensively reviewed by Dickler (109). Lymphocytes, monocytes, macrophages, and PMNs all contain well-defined structures capable of binding the Fc portion of IgG either in native form or as part of antigen-antibody complexes. It is not clear, for instance, that Fc receptors reacting with IgG or IgG antibody complexed to antigen constitute the same or similar structures on these heterogeneous cells. Moreover, reactions that appear to be dependent on interaction of various cells with structures on the Fc portion of IgG have been described in a number of cell types that do not per se have a direct relation to the immune system, such as reticulum cells in normal liver (110), or in some instances to skeletal muscle and central nervous tissue (111, 112). In addition, specific Fc receptors have also been described for malignant tissues (110) and in the placenta (113, 114). From much of the in vitro as well as the in vivo work it seems obvious that receptors must play an important role in the tissue fixation of circulating immune complexes. The studies of Mannik and co-

workers (90, 91) have indicated that Fc receptor mechanisms can be surfeited or overcome by excessive loading, either by passive infusion or by hyperimmunization procedures. Precise definition of the molecular heterogeneity of cell surface Fc receptors has been directly approached in only a few studies (115). Furthermore, endogenous receptors for various antigens themselves may be most directly involved in the localization or clearing of immune complexes by fixed phagocytic cells of the reticuloendothelial system, or endothelial cells of the microcirculation repeatedly involved clinically in immune-complex–mediated lesions.

Tissue Saturation and Kinetics of Removal

Experimental studies have established that the reticuloendothelial system (RES) of the liver probably is principally involved in clearing of passively administered immune complexes to animals (116). Moreover, reports by Mannik and co-workers (90, 91, 117) established that passive infusion of preformed immune complexes comprising more than two antigen and antibody molecules (Ag_2Ab_2) was rapidly cleared by the liver. Furthermore, when the phagocytic disposal system of the RES was saturated, immune-complex retention within the circulation and deposition was markedly accelerated (118). In this study passively administered soluble human serum albumin (HSA) complexes with anti-HSA were examined in mice. Complexes with molecular composition greater than Ag_2Ab or larger than 11S were preferentially cleared by the hepatic RES. When the dose of complexes was raised, demonstrable RES saturation occurred, particularly with AgAb complexes of greater than two antigen and two antibody molecules; and the time of persistence of complexes >11S was markedly prolonged. Graphical analysis of these results is shown in Figure 5-9.

Previous studies had demonstrated a finite number of Fc receptors on available surfaces of functional macrophages (119, 120), and these receptors appeared capable of preferential trapping and removal of complexes of 11S and above. It is also possible that in various

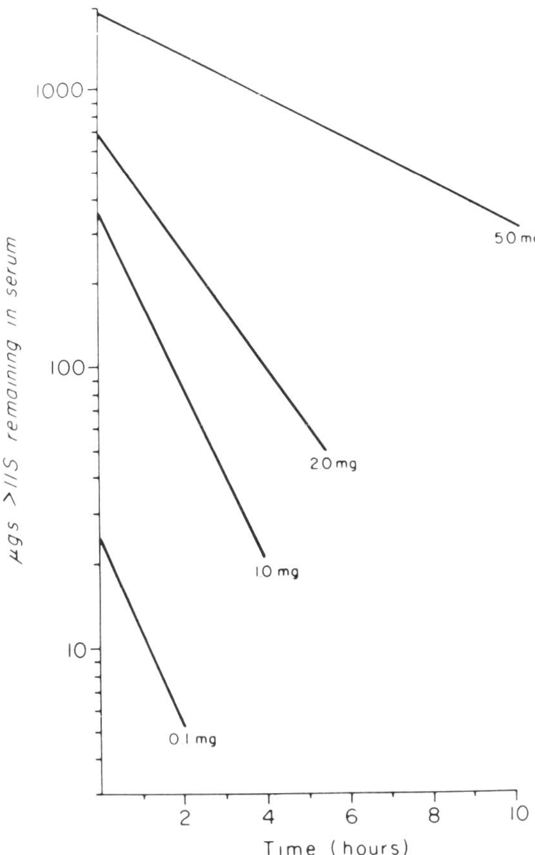

Figure 5-9 A semilog plot comparing the regression lines after transformation to micrograms of >11S complexes. The slope (reflecting the clearance rate) becomes less as the dose is increased. (Reproduced with permission, A. O. Haakenstad and M. Mannik, *J. Immunol.* 112:1939, 1974.)

clinical situations other physiological changes within the functional macrophage system (such as injury or death from previously ingested microorganisms capable of intracellular persistence, like the leprosy bacillus or the staphylococcus) may further impair phagocytic or removal capabilities. The saturation kinetics of removal of immune complexes passively administered to animals treated with corticosteroids was studied by Haakenstad and coworkers (121), who noted marked retardation of immune-complex disposal in cortisone-treated mice. The half-life of complexes $>Ag_2Ab$ was prolonged from 1.93 hours in controls to 4.71 hours in cortisone-treated ani-

mals, whereas the half-life of Ag_2Ab_2 complexes remained unchanged. Prolongation of half-life and diminished RES clearing of immune complexes in corticosteroid-treated mice was also associated in this study with a marked increment in glomerular immune-complex deposition.

These findings are of interest in view of the frequent use of steroids in the treatment of a variety of immune-complex disorders including SLE or rapidly progressive glomerulonephritis. A representative disappearance curve from the above study is shown in Figure 5-10. The reason for depression of clearance of complexes in cortisone-treated animals was presumed to be marked slowing and impairment of phagocytic efficiency within the fixed RES. Corticosteroid effects on the clearance of colloidal or particulate materials have in the past been ascribed to their effects on the mononuclear phagocyte system (122, 123). Moreover, the phagocytic activity of inflammatory macrophages and PMNs has been observed to

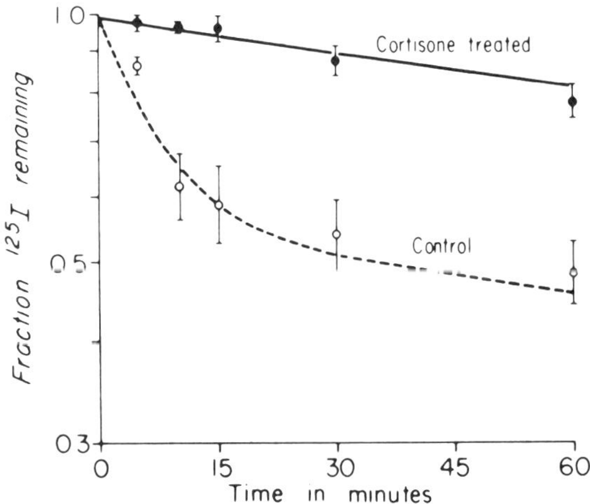

Figure 5-10 A plot of the disappearance during the first hour of HSA-^{125}I anti-HSA complexes containing 2.9 mg of antibodies from the circulation of cortisone-treated and control mice. The curves represent the best fit obtained by either two-component or three-component computer analyses of all the mean data (± 1 S.D.) for cortisone-treated and control mice. The rapid clearance phase is absent in cortisone-treated mice. (Reproduced with permission, A. O. Haakenstad, J. B. Case, and M. Mannik, *J. Immunol.* 114:1153, 1975.)

be suppressed in both patients and animals receiving corticosteroids (124, 125). Thus it might be expected that large doses of corticosteroids administered during overwhelming infections might significantly affect immune-complex removal.

The concept that the RES has a fixed threshold for ability to dispose of circulating immune complexes is extremely important in its applications to clinical medicine. It may be a crucial factor in the ultimate peripheral effects of circulating complexes in such disorders as schistosomiasis or malaria (Chapter 2) or in the immune-complex–mediated phenomena seen in SLE or infective endocarditis. Other pharmacological agents beside corticosteroids may profoundly alter the disposal of certain types of complexes. Considerably more work is needed to define such potentially important effects before specific therapy can be designed. Little direct evidence is currently available, for instance, on the effects of such agents as beta-blockers or propranolol used in the treatment of thyrotoxicosis or hypertension or on other potent pharmacological agents such as dopamine, now frequently used for maintenance of blood pressure in acutely ill hypotensive subjects with a variety of vascular or infectious complications.

Several recent studies have materially increased our understanding of the physiological importance of both tissue Fc receptor function and the reticuloendothelial system. Research by Frank and colleagues (126) appeared to show defective Fc receptor function in patients with systemic lupus erythematosus. These assays involved measurements of the clearance of IgG-sensitized, ^{51}Cr-labeled erythrocytes by splenic macrophage membrane receptors in 15 untreated patients. Fc-specific clearance rates were abnormal in 13 of the 15 patients and markedly prolonged as compared to controls. These prolonged clearance rates of the IgG-sensitized erythrocytes correlated both with immune-complex levels as measured by C1q-binding assays and with disease activity. The studies pointed to a defect in Fc receptor function in patients with active SLE, which could lead to extended circulation of immune complexes and significantly contribute to tissue

deposition and tissue damage. The precise reason for the defective Fc receptor function is unknown, but it seems possible that saturation of fixed-tissue macrophage Fc receptors by endogenously deposited complexes may be involved. Clearance methods employing labeled IgG-coated erythrocytes focus principally on splenic and hepatic reticuloendothelial system receptor function.

The effects of reversal of impaired splenic function in patients with nephritis or vasculitis by plasma exchange or plasmapheresis have been documented by Lockwood and colleagues (127). A reversible blockade of the splenic component of reticuloendothelial (RES) function existed in 14 of 15 patients treated with plasma exchange either alone or in combination with corticosteroids and cytotoxic agents. Reversal of the RES blockade after plasma exchange was demonstrated in 3 patients within 48 hours. Again in serial studies, an inverse correlation was noted between splenic function and the levels of circulating complexes as detected by a C1q-binding assay. These studies reemphasize the central importance of RES function during clinical immune-complex disease.

Endogenous Mechanisms for Immune-Complex Removal

The fixed and circulating segments of the RES constitute the first line of defense against circulating particulate materials or smaller aggregates such as circulating immune complexes. On the other hand, another highly tuned mechanism for immune-complex removal has recently been described by Miller, Czop, and their co-workers (128, 129) that involves activation of the complement system. Rather than being essential for immune-complex dissemination or deposition, the complement system seems to be uniquely designed for rapid and efficient dissolution of immune complexes, particularly those distributed on various body surfaces as insoluble precipitates. Miller and Nussenzweig (128) have demonstrated that antigen-antibody aggregates are solubilized when incubated with fresh serum at 37° C yielding relatively small molecular weight complexes containing antigen, antibody, and complement. Although this process did not require the presence of calcium ions, a requirement for magnesium ions was definitely established, suggesting activation of the alternate (properdin) complement pathway. After solubilization most of the immune complexes were smaller than 19S and appeared to contain antigenic determinants of C3. Furthermore, it was observed that the immunoglobulin class and the avidity of antibodies present in immune precipitates subjected to slow dissolution through the natural action of complement affected the speed and efficiency of the reaction (129). Studies concerning the precise mechanism involved in such solubilization also indicated that Fab fragments of antibody directed at the IgG present in the precipitate were capable of in vitro immune-complex dissolution. These findings suggested that processes capable of spatial separation of portions of the immune precipitates were capable of forcing the original components apart and disturbing otherwise rigid antigen-antibody lattices in the original immune precipitate.

Studies by Czop and Nussenzweig (129) have examined the basic mechanism involved in immune-complex solubilization through the properdin or alternate complement cascade. Their data indicated that such complement solubilizing activity was not a function of enzymatic proteolysis of antibody within the antigen-antibody lattice but probably depended on interdigitation of fragments of C3 (C3b and C4b) into the original immune lattice. If C3b and C4b are capable of inserting themselves into relatively stable immune precipitates, their binding to components of the lattice itself must be on the basis of nonspecific short-range— perhaps hydrophobic—bonds. Both of these complement fragments are relatively high in molecular weight (175,000 to 200,000 Daltons) and show short periods of activation before becoming inactive.

If proven to be a universal or even common phenomenon in vivo, these findings have great relevance to the biologic effects of insoluble antigen-antibody complexes present in various tissue sites such as capillary microvasculature or glomeruli. If insoluble deposits are constantly being solubilized by intercalation or insertion of C3b and C3d fragments, therapeutic use of this particular mechanism seems feasible, particularly in clinical situations where immune-complex deposition occurs in the presence of hypocomplementemic states (as in active SLE). From a theoretical standpoint therapeutic administration of materials rich in certain C3 components capable of inducing immune-complex solubilization might be highly beneficial. It is conceivable that part of the immediate benefit observed in patients with SLE after plasmapheresis is not the result of the physical removal of large quantities of anti-DNA antibody or immune complexes alone, but also of their incidental replacement by normal plasma components containing an excess of C3 sufficient to generate fresh C3d and C3b available for tissue-deposited immune-complex solubilization. The mechanisms involved in such a process are shown diagrammatically in Figure 5-11.

One of the experimental models that bears a close resemblance to rheumatoid arthritis is that developed by Dumonde and Glynn involving intraarticular injection of antigen into animals previously immunized with a foreign protein antigen (130, 131). This model of subacute or chronic synovitis requires not only prior sensitization with extraneous antigen but also the presence of delayed-type hypersensitivity, presumably mediated by T cells in the experimental animal. Several features have been recognized that bear on the signal importance of local persistence of antigen in the joints and juxtaposed dense connective tissues. These features emphasize the role of local tissue mechanisms that may dramatically influence reactions mediated by immune complexes.

A surprising feature of the experimental model developed by Dumonde and Glynn was the persistence for 2 to 6 months of inflammatory reaction in joints after only a single intraarticular antigen challenge. In many instances such inflammatory synovitis lasted for many months, suggesting retention of antigen within the local confines of the joint regardless of presumed natural phagocytic removal mechanisms. Subsequent elegant immuno-

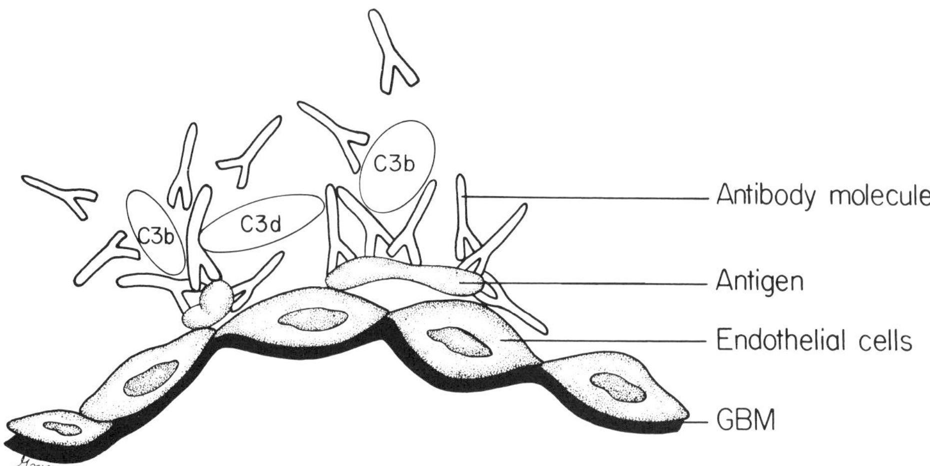

Figure 5-11 Dispersal of antigen-antibody complexes deposited in microvascular regions of the kidney on endothelial cells by interdigitation of large C3 fragments (C3b and C3d). Whether or not such a process occurs in vivo has not yet been established.

fluorescence and elution studies by Cooke and co-workers (132) using this experimental model have provided an explanation. They demonstrated that antigen becomes localized in cartilage and dense ligamentous connective tissues of the joint and initiates a durable immune-complex–mediated synovitis. Protein antigens labeled with ^{125}I were utilized and showed marked persistence as radioactivity localized to avascular dense collagenous tissues —such as tendons or ligaments of experimental animals. Examples of radioautographic localization obtained is shown in Figure 5-12.

It was postulated that antigen binding to such structures was in part a function of their avascular nature. A major proportion of retained antigen was present in patchy distribution within the superficial layers of the articular surfaces of affected joints, including menisci and articular cartilage. Localization of injected antigen to avascular, collagenous tissues provided a reasonable explanation for the slow elimination rates of radiolabeled antigen after only a single injection and the prolonged persistence of an active inflammatory synovitis. Furthermore, elution studies indicated binding of labeled antigen to collagen fibrils rather than to the interfibrillar matrix. Of particular significance was the finding of immunoglobulin and C3 bound within dense collagenous tissues in similar distribution to and presumably complexed with antigen. This model, therefore, presents a striking example of the tremendous local inflammatory potential of antigen-antibody complexes retained in certain tissues because of particular local factors preventing or markedly affecting their gradual natural elimination. One cannot help but wonder whether similar as yet undefined mechanisms are at work in the persistence of measles virus or measles virus antigen, within the central nervous system tissues involved by subacute sclerosing panencephalitis or even in the etiology of disorders like multiple sclerosis, rheumatoid arthritis, or regional ileitis.

The specific role of antibody in the induction of antigen-antibody complexes in collagenous tissues has been further investigated by Jasin (133). Over 20 times more antigen was irreversibly retained in dense collagenous tissues of previously immunized rabbits than was present or retained in nonimmunized controls. Under these circumstances antigen retention seemed to be dependent on prior delayed-type sensitivity to the antigen utilized. These findings are of great interest in that they point out how discrete tissue factors may profoundly influence the localization and entrapment of immune complexes. It may well be that a similar mechanism pertains to other well-devel-

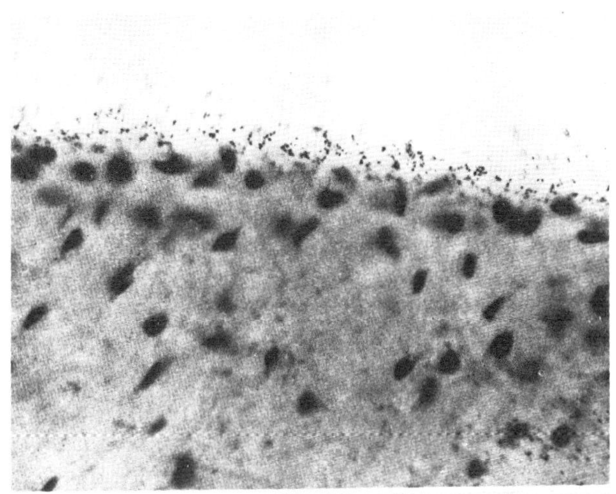

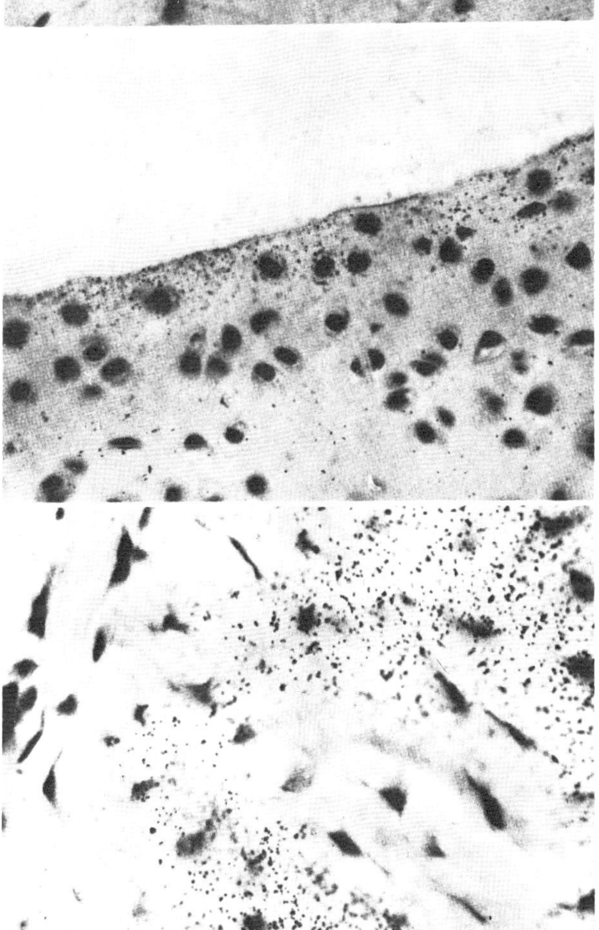

Figure 5-12 *Above,* radioautograph of meniscus from a rabbit with synovitis induced 4 weeks previously with 2.5 mg of EA-^{125}I. The cartilage appears relatively normal and there is thick clustering of silver grains in the surface layers. *Middle,* radioautograph of articular cartilage from a rabbit with synovitis induced 4 weeks previously by intraarticular (IA) injection of 2.5 mg of BSA-^{125}I. The silver grains are localized at the surface in a patchy distribution. *Below,* radioautograph of IA ligament, stained with H&E, from a rabbit with synovitis induced 2 weeks previously by IA injection of 2.5 mg of BSA-^{125}I. Radioactivity is found dispersed throughout the ligament. All magnifications × 250. (Reproduced with permission, T. D. Cooke, E. R. Hurd, M. Ziff et al., *J. Exp. Med.* 135:323, 1972.)

oped clinical human conditions such as rheumatoid disease or even the synovitis associated with disseminated gonococcal infection. Prior sensitization or immune response with presence of antibody may be necessary before vascular dissemination of antigen sets off the chronic or acute synovitis. Recently we have been impressed, for instance, with the frequency of prior gonococcal infection in the clinical evolution of synovitis and arthritis associated with disseminated gonorrhea. A substantial proportion (about 30 percent) of patients with the synovial reaction so often seen in this syndrome give a history of prior gonococcal infection. Moreover, if initial urethral or other gonorrheal infection was contracted days or weeks before the onset of synovitis, an amnestic or even primary antibody response could precipitate intraarticular complex deposition, retention within dense ligamentous structures, and an acute or subacute synovitis of much the same pattern as that noted in the Dumonde-Glynn model. It is possible, moreover, that similar mechanisms play a role in the tissue lesions of other heterogeneous disorders such as infective endocarditis and some of the immune-complex lesions associated with this disease. As mentioned in Chapter 1, there is experimental evidence in rabbits that the nephritis of experimental infective endocarditis is much easier to induce in animals previously immunized with the particular organism involved (134). Moreover, the dense immunoglobulin and complement deposits seen in the basal layers of the skin in SLE may also be an example of local trapping within the dense collagenous tissues of immune complexes. Whether such localizing features operate through immunologic reactions between antigens and collagenous fibrils or whether they represent simple ion exchange or chemical binding reactions has not yet been determined.

In an opposite vein, certain well-defined local circumstances may work to deter and impede immune-complex formation. Perhaps the most extensively studied of such phenomena is the impedance to intestinal absorption of antigens provided by prior immunization (135–138). Certain proteins consumed in food penetrate the normal mucosal barrier and pass to the general systemic circulation, thereby contributing to the pathogenesis of various disease states (139, 140). It is clear from a number of studies comparing oral and parenteral immunization procedures that prior immunization effectively hinders absorption on subsequent repeat oral or intestinal challenge. When in vitro absorption of preformed immune complexes was compared, using rat jejunal and ileal gut sacs (138), it was found that complexes prepared in two-fold antibody excess were absorbed in significantly smaller amounts than antigen alone, whereas complexes prepared in fifty-fold antigen excess were absorbed in amounts equal to those of antigens not bound to antibody. Complexes formed in antibody excess appeared to stimulate secretion of mucus; they became engulfed and were thereafter associated with the mucus fraction, presumably being excluded from any process of pinocytosis and subsequent absorption. The effectiveness of the mucosal barrier mechanism in protecting the organism from constant overstimulation through antigens absorbed in the gastrointestinal tract is an example of the benefits of local immune-complex formation as a normal defense process. The absence of complement activation by antigen-antibody complexes composed of IgA may also act as an impediment to induction of potentially harmful inflammatory reactions. Such local processes, similar to that extensively studied by Walker and co-workers in the gut (135–138), may also be at work in secretory IgA systems bathing the tracheobronchial tree, perineum, or other mucosal surfaces.

Cellular Effects of Immobilized Immune Complexes

Several rather special biologic effects have recently been described that relate to the influence of antigen-antibody complexes immobilized on surfaces. Rabinovitch and colleagues (141) have reported that ingestion, but not attachment, of erythrocytes sensitized with IgG antibody was inhibited if macrophages were first exposed to glass- or plastic-bound immune complexes composed of bovine serum albumin (BSA) and anti-BSA. By contrast, interaction and ingestion of red blood cells sensitized with antibody and complement was not affected—nor was phagocytic ingestion of latex particles, yeast cells, or glutaraldehyde-treated erythrocytes influenced in any way. These experiments indicated a selective ability of immune complexes spread on a surface to interact with macrophage Fc receptors in such a way as to block macrophage ingestion capacity. From a practical standpoint these findings indicate that surface-associated complexes in the body proper are more protected from phagocytic macrophage ingestion than those circulating freely in the blood or lymph. The blockade or saturation of the RES observed by previous workers (118) may be partially explained by this mechanism.

A different series of experiments on the biologic behavior of immobilized antigen-antibody complexes reported by Ryan and colleagues (142) indicated that antigen-antibody complexes immobilized on plastic surfaces were able to inhibit B-cell proliferation in the face of stimulants usually capable of profound direct B-cell activation. In order to produce significant inhibition, such complexes required interaction through an intact Fc portion of their IgG molecules. Complexes prepared with IgA antibody or with IgG molecules devoid of Fc portions did not inhibit B-cell proliferation. Furthermore, rather dramatic differences in inhibition were recorded when immobilized complexes were compared to those in solution or suspension: only the immobilized complexes showed clearcut inhibitory effects. The Ryan group suggested several possible explanations for their results. They felt that the lattice of immobilized complexes might be more effective in binding to Fc receptors on B cells and that subsequently such receptors were capped or polarized on the cell surface before being internalized. An alternative explanation suggested that complexes immobilized on a surface present a repeating lattice of IgG molecules to B-cell Fc receptors capable of triggering an "off" signal for the cells either by a capping process or by changing intracellular ratios of cAMP and cGMP (143). In the experimental system where B-cell mitogenesis by potent B-cell stimulators such as lipopolysaccharide was blocked, it seems possible that part of the blocking effect may have been mediated through Fc receptors on macrophages present in the system. Thus, lipopolysaccharide B-cell mitogen contacts macrophages first and is then transferred in some form to lymphocytes (144). It is conceivable that the blockade of B-cell triggering occurs at the level previously demonstrated by Rabinovitch and co-workers (141). From a broad biologic viewpoint the finding that immobilized immune complexes may be capable of defusing or shutting off further B-cell proliferation represents one of the basic feedback control systems within the immune response. There has been no extensive exploration of whether such mechanisms are functionally operative in hyperimmune situations, where a tremendous load of immune complexes is constantly presented to the host —as in the case of malaria, schistosomiasis, or trypanosomiasis.

Physical Measures and the Patient

Any discussion of immune complexes and their importance in clinical medicine that emphasizes host factors should focus at some point on the patient. Granted that circulating and tissue-fixed complexes are capable of inducing a train of events leading on the one hand to acute vasculitis or on the other to glomerular deposition, injury, and finally obliterative sclerosis, the major clinical problem confronting the physician is how to prevent

such sequelae. One direct approach presently in vogue is the use of massive plasma exchanges or plasmapheresis (145–148). Encouraged by reports that levels of rhesus isoantibody in pregnant women could be substantially reduced by plasmapheresis (145), Verrier-Jones and colleagues (147) used this method in 8 patients with SLE. Removal of 5 to 8 liters of plasma weekly in 4 subjects with low C3, high levels of anticomplementary activity, high DNA binding, and positive C1q precipitin tests for presence of immune complexes produced what was judged to be striking clinical improvement in some individuals. Volumes of plasma removed during this study were replaced by human plasma-protein fraction and fresh-frozen plasma. The clinical course in one of their patients is shown in Figure 5-13. During successive rounds of plasmapheresis C3 and C4 levels increased, anticomplementary activity and C1q precipitins disappeared, and maintenance levels of corticosteroid could be reduced. In other patients who reportedly did not show peripheral manifestations of immune-complex disease, no benefit from plasmaphersis was recorded. In these studies, the anticomplementary activity in serum fell rapidly; it was found in high-molecular-weight exclusion (>19S) fractions from Sephadex G-200 gel filtration separations of plasma. The suggestion was made that these high-molecular-weight fractions normally cleared rapidly by the RES were only detectable in the patients studied because of functional RES and phagocytic blockade.

Plasma exchange together with immunosuppression was also reported by Lockwood and associates (146) in 9 patients with fulminating immune-complex crescentic nephritis. Five of these patients showed early and quick improvement from rapidly progressive renal failure. By means of the C1q deviation test to assess presence of circulating complexes, positive results were obtained in 5 patients before treatment; these disappeared after plasmapheresis and immunosuppressive therapy. In 3 patients temporary withdrawal of plasma exchange was followed by reappearance of detectable circulating complexes; in the other 2 patients there was subsequent deterioration of renal func-

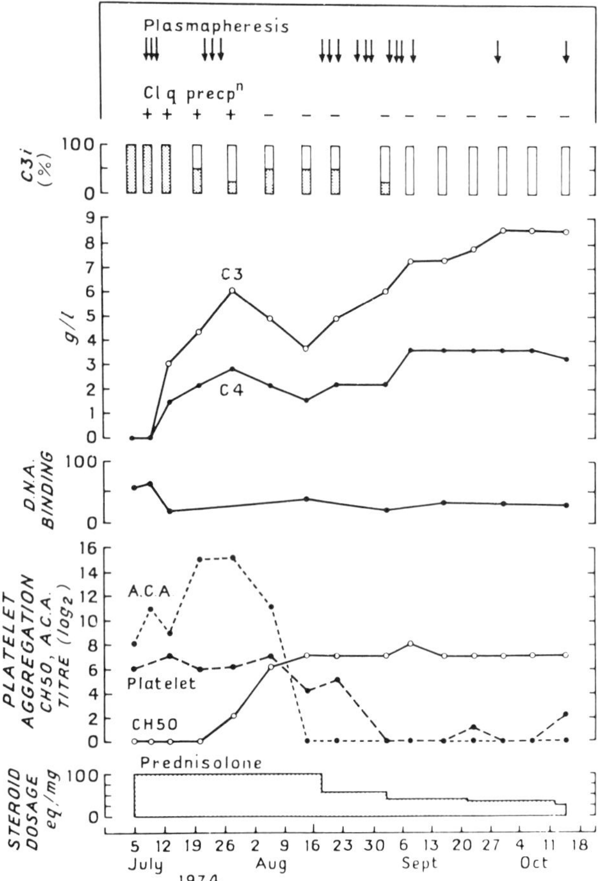

Figure 5-13 The clinical course of a patient with SLE treated by plasmapheresis. (Reproduced with permission, T. Verrier Jones, R. C. Bucknall, R. H. Cumming et al., *Lancet* 1:709, 1976.)

tion. The rationale for plasma exchange in these patients was that removal of circulating complexes as well as depletion of inflammatory mediators generated from both the complement and the coagulation system was intended, yet their plasma was replaced with normal fresh plasma or plasma components. These patients were plasmapheresed or exchanged with a cell separator. Final interpretation of the clinical results of this study is somewhat beclouded by the interplay of potent immunosuppressive therapy and plasmapheresis. Though clinical and laboratory parameters appeared to change significantly when immunosuppressive drugs were maintained unchanged and plasmapheresis was discontinued,

it is hard to sort out precisely which agent caused which reaction, since more than two forms of therapy were used simultaneously.

The technique of plasmapheresis has also been used in the treatment of Goodpasture's syndrome (149). Improvement in renal function was recorded in some of these patients, and pulmonary hemorrhage was said to have been rapidly controlled in 5 patients in whom it was the presenting problem. In this instance plasma exchange was accompanied by volume replacement with plasma-protein fraction, which involved substantial depletion of complement and fibrinogen as well. Since immunologic injury of tissue can be directly attributed to the presence of circulating antiglomerular basement membrane antibody in Goodpasture's syndrome, massive attempts at removal of circulating antibody through plasmapheresis seem entirely logical.

Initial success has also been recorded with plasma exchange in myasthenia gravis to deplete the antibodies to acetylcholine receptor that apparently are directly involved in genesis and continuation of the disease (150–152). Myasthenia patients treated with plasmapheresis showed considerable improvement, with unequivocal recovery from muscle weakness and general fatigability (153). In reverse manner, it has been shown that reinfusion of γ-globulin fractions of plasma or lymph from patients with myasthenia causes an exacerbation of their symptoms (154). It is not difficult to envision that plasmapheresis and removal of anti-acetylcholine receptor antibody might improve basic neuromuscular transmission mechanisms by allowing expression of new receptors, which are constantly being synthesized to function without the impedance of antibody. Massive antibody removal could profoundly alter the equilibrium between receptor and residual bound γ-globulins. Thus far circulating immune complexes have not been directly implicated in the pathogenesis of myasthenia.

A disorder falling somewhat in between SLE and myasthenia with respect to precise concepts of pathogenesis is thrombotic thrombocytopenic purpura (TTP), where primary clinical features include a microangiopathic hemolytic anemia, thrombocytopenia, fever, neurological symptoms, and renal abnormalities. The basic pathological finding in TTP is extensive intravascular hyalin thrombi. Fatal outcome occurs in a majority of patients described in the current literature. A recent report has appeared citing the apparent benefit of plasmapheresis in 2 patients treated (155). These therapeutic attempts were based on favorable results after exchange transfusions (156) in the same patients. To our knowledge no measurements of circulating immune complexes before and after plasmapheresis therapy for TTP have yet been reported, and the mechanism behind apparent clinical improvement has not been clarified.

The precise steps that take place in plasmapheresis therapy deserve careful scrutiny. We became interested in the physical and possibly serendipitous aspects of such measures as plasmapheresis or even hemodialysis therapy on the basis of clinical observations of 2 patients during acute hemodialysis for, in one case, SLE with rapidly deteriorating renal failure and, in the other, acute rapidly progressive glomerulonephritis. Both patients had serial determinations of immune complexes before and after hemodialysis, and both showed dramatic falls in detectable circulating complexes immediately after initiation of conventional coil hemodialysis (157). A representative clinical course on one of the patients is shown in Figure 5-14.

Of great interest in a third patient with SLE and similar dramatic clinical improvement in both active SLE nephritis and marked elevations of circulating complexes, was the clinical finding that approximately 3 to 4 hours after completion of dialysis and removal of 3 to 4 pounds of body fluid, pulmonary edema would repeatedly ensue. This sequence of events was puzzling at the time, but in retrospect it may have reflected pulmonary disposal of immune complexes trapped by neutrophils whose C3 receptors had been activated serendipitously by passage over the plastic dialysis membranes (151). Although we have no direct proof for this hypothesis, these clinical observations may indicate that some of the positive features or clinical improvement in patients following either dialysis or plasmapheresis are

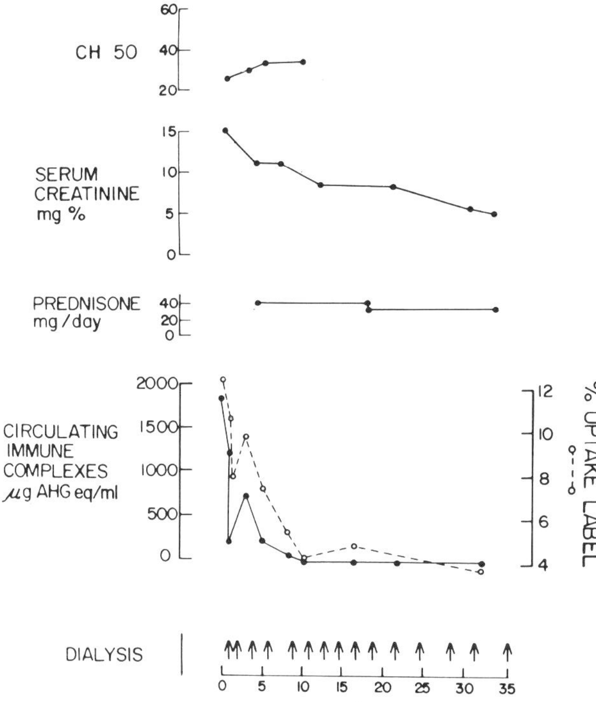

Figure 5-14 Serial determination of serum complement (CH 50), creatinine, and circulating immune complexes in a patient with rapidly progressive glomerulonephritis, before and after hemodialysis. Changes in circulating immune complexes are depicted for the Raji-cell radioimmunoassay (O--O) and the C1q solid-phase radioimmunoassay. (Reproduced with permission, T. D. Ahlin, K. S. K. Tung, L. Walker et al., *Am. J. Med.* 64:672, 1978.)

related to blood elements being passed over plastic surfaces more than the actual removal of complexes in the discarded plasma. In the case of our patient with SLE who showed dramatic improvement in clinical signs of active lupus nephritis as well as renal function after dialysis, careful examination of the coils used in the first several dialysis procedures showed no evidence of trapped DNA or γ-globulins, but rather millions of adherent PMNs and mononuclear cells stuck to the dialysis membrane.

Since plasmapheresis was suggested to be beneficial in a number of immune-complex disorders, it was reasonable to examine recent reports on the subject by Craddock, Jacob, and co-workers (158–160). Their studies have demonstrated that when blood elements come into contact with plastic surfaces, neutrophil C3 receptors become activated and many neutrophils become sticky and lodge quickly in the lungs. This sequence actually is profound enough to produce significant impairment of pulmonary gas exchange. The functional contribution of the alternate complement pathway appears to be important in this reaction. It seems likely that the same mechanism may occur during plasmapheresis, where blood is passed over various surfaces as components are separated and then reinfused into the patients. It seems possible that contact with the plastic makes granulocytes sticky; after lodging in the lung they are then able to act transiently as a splint for more directly vulnerable tissues such as the kidney and actually function to remove immune complex directly. It is conceivable that immune-complex elimination occurs principally in the lungs and other parts of the RES, and not externally by removal of plasma.

It is very important to remain critical of the concept that plasmapheresis or removal of toxic products in plasma has anything to do with the apparent clinical improvement in patients with either rapidly progressive glomerulonephritis or SLE. A common feature among many of the patients in whom improvement has been reported is that after plasmapheresis, they are given volume replacement with plasma fractions or fresh-frozen plasma. In view of the experiments of Nussenzweig and co-workers showing that the intact complement system and in particular the alternate or properdin pathway are capable of dissolution of immune precipitates (128, 129), it seems possible that the fresh normal plasma given to patients with SLE after the "therapy" of plasmapheresis may actually be one of the beneficial items in the entire process. The striking resolution of peripheral manifestations of the vasculitis of SLE in some patients is consonant with this view. Moreover, the observations of Frank and colleagues (126) and Lockwood and co-workers (127) concerning the abnormalities of RES function and improvement in the latter after plasma exchange are also pertinent.

Particular caution, including a number of control observations, is needed before the precise sequence of events is understood relating to gross physical measures like plasmapheresis or plasma exchange. Attention has been directed particularly by Terman and associates (161–164) to the practical possibility of removing circulating antigen or antibody by passage over an extracorporeal affinity column or immunoabsorbent affixed to collodion membranes or charcoal nylon microspheres. The schema of an apparatus used for removal of anti-BSA in actively immunized dogs is shown in Figure 5-15. During this study (164) levels of antibody binding to labeled BSA antigen gradually returned to the same approximate level or degree of binding capacity as before active immunoabsorption, suggesting perhaps (as have many previous studies) that the level of specific antibody released is controlled by quantitative amounts of circulating antibody.

More specific attention to the application of these techniques for elimination of either circulating DNA or anti-DNA antibody has also been explored by Terman and his colleagues (165, 166). They have examined the feasibility of removal of free DNA or DNA bound to antigen-antibody complexes by reactions with nuclease immobilized on nylon microspheres or, in the case of antibody, by an extracorporeal immunoabsorbent of DNA-cellulose incorporated into agar gel. Rabbits actively immunized with methylated bovine serum albumin conjugated to single-stranded DNA showed significant falls in anti-DNA antibody when whole blood was passed over such immunoabsorbent columns. Little release of ^{125}I DNA to blood and tissues was observed, and immunoabsorbent columns showed no appreciable accumulation of thrombotic material or cellular debris. The same approach has been applied in experimental animals to remove circulating antibodies to glomerular basement membrane (GBM) (167). Again, this method seemed capable of specific antibody removal without appreciable release of free GBM antibody, as measured by labeled GBM antigen incorporated into the immunoabsorbent.

Removal of circulating tumor antigens from cancer patients has been reported by Langvad and co-workers (168). In their work F(ab')$_2$ fragments were isolated from hypernephroma

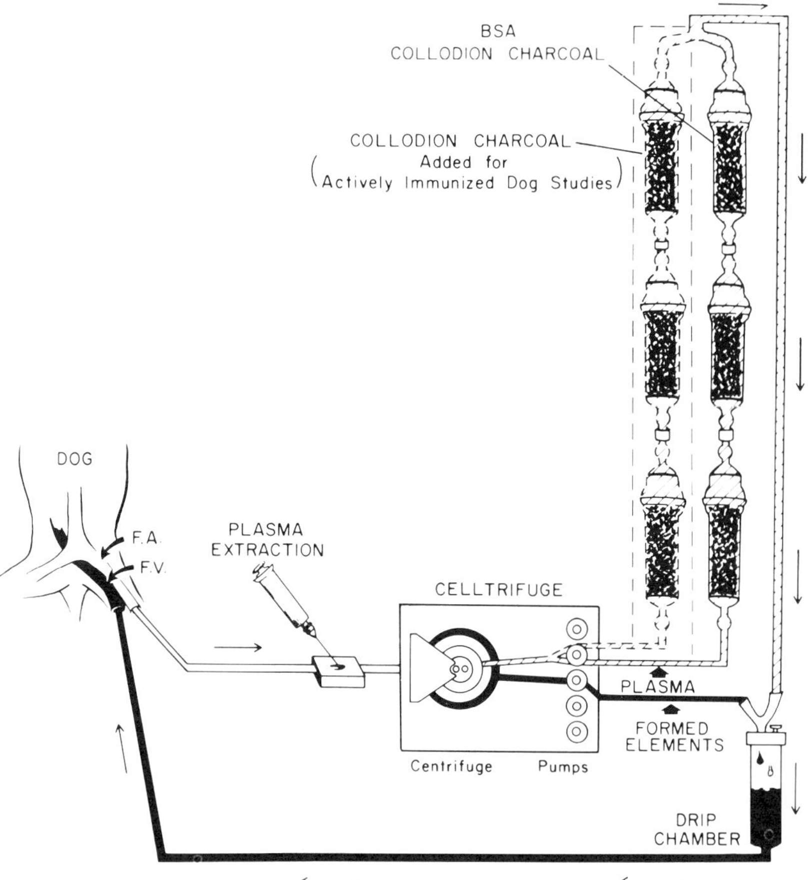

Figure 5-15 Schematic representation of an extracorporeal circulation system. A control system was employed in actively immunized dog perfusion studies in order to compare the uptake of passively infused I-labeled anti-BSA on BSA collodion charcoal with that on control collodion charcoal. (Reproduced with permission, D. S. Terman, T. Tavel, D. Petty et al, *Clin Exp Immunol* 28:180, 1977.)

patients to prepare the immunoabsorbent connected to the patients through an arteriovenous shunt. Three distinct proteins not detectable in normal human serum were found in the eluate from the extracorporeal immunoabsorbent apparatus. Most interesting was the finding that large amounts of C9, C3 activator, and C3 were also isolated in the immunoabsorbent chamber; this indicates that in vitro extracorporeal antigen-antibody reactions had occurred. However, we must remember the studies by Craddock, Jacob, and co-workers in which activation of C3 occurred merely on contact with plastic surfaces. The approach suggested by the Langvad group (168) seems particularly important in view of recent reports of large amounts of what appear to be immune complexes in the plasma of patients with various forms of acute leukemia (169), particularly those with an unfavorable prognosis. The problem of immune complexes or blocking factors in tumor immunity is discussed in depth in Chapter 8. The general approach appears to be promising, although more clinical observations are necessary before application of methods involving either specific removal of antigen or antibody or more general measures including plasmapheresis can be seriously entertained. Caution is necessary, since all extracorporeal manipulations of plasma or whole blood—particularly if they involve passage of blood over plastic surfaces—

probably will invoke the Craddock phenomenon and increased stickiness of white blood cells, transient pulmonary dysfunction, and other possible serendipitous effects.

Despite the lack of clear insight into precisely what is happening during plasmapheresis or plasma exchange therapy, we have seen that this approach has proved beneficial in a number of critical clinical situations. The studies by Lockwood and colleagues (127) have demonstrated that intensive plasmapheresis procedures may improve reticuloendothelial system function. Precisely how this comes about is not clear and the phenomenon reemphasizes the complexity of effects to be anticipated in patients undergoing these procedures.

The host reaction to immune complexes is essentially the core of the problem, with primary responsiveness of the host the final result of genetic controls at many levels. Probably more important than size, shape, or other intrinsic properties of immune complexes are host factors, which either impede or facilitate deposition. The natural clearance mechanisms afforded by the RES can be saturated or overloaded; when this occurs, tissue deposition and injury are most likely to occur. There are probably natural features, particularly in the alternate complement pathway, that modulate immune-complex dissolution. Physical approaches (including plasmapheresis, plasma exchange, or extracorporeal specific immunoabsorption) may afford great benefit in certain clinical conditions, but great caution is called for in specifying a cause-and-effect relationship.

References

1. Levine, B. B., Ojeda, A., and Benacerraf, B. Studies on artificial antigens. III. The genetic control of the immune response to hapten-poly-L-lysine conjugates in guinea pigs. *J. Exp. Med.* 118:953, 1963.

2. Levine, B. B., and Benacerraf, B. Genetic control in guinea pigs of immune response to conjugates of haptens and poly-L-lysine. *Science* 147:517, 1965.

3. McDevitt, H. O., and Sela, M. Genetic control of the antibody response. I. Demonstration of determinant-specific differences in response to synthetic polypeptide antigens in two strains of inbred mice. *J. Exp. Med.* 122:517, 1965.

4. McDevitt, H. O., and Tyan, M. L. Genetic control of the antibody response in inbred mice. Transfer of response by spleen cells and linkage to the major histocompatibility (H-2) locus. *J. Exp. Med.* 128:1, 1968.

5. Ellman, L., Green, I., and Benacerraf, B. Effect of gene dose on the immune response to a 2,-4-dinitrophenyl glutamic acid lysine copolymer. *Nature* 227:1140, 1970.

6. Bluestein, H. G., Green, I., and Benacerraf, B. Specific immune response genes of the guinea pig. I. Dominant genetic control of immune responsiveness to copolymers of L-glutamic acid and L-alanine and L-glutamic acid and L-tyrosine. *J. Exp. Med.* 134:458, 1971.

7. Gasser, D. L., and Silvers, W. K. Genetic determinants of immunological responsiveness. *Adv. Immunol.* 18:1, 1974.

8. Svejgaard, A., Platz, P., Ryder, L. P., et al. HL-A and disease associations—a survey. *Transplant. Rev.* 22:3, 1975.

9. Schlosstein, L., Terasaki, P. I., Bluestone, R., et al. High association of an HL-A antigen, W27, with ankylosing spondylitis. *N. Engl. J. Med.* 288:704, 1973.

10. Mackay, I. R., and Morris, P. J. Association of autoimmune active chronic hepatitis with HL-A1, 8. *Lancet* 2:793, 1972.

11. Jersild, C., Svejgaard, A., and Fog, T. HL-A antigens and multiple sclerosis. *Lancet* 1:1240, 1972.

12. Russell, T. J., Schultes, L. M., and Kuban, D. J. Histocompatibility (HL-A) antigens associated with psoriasis. *N. Engl. J. Med.* 287:738, 1972.

13. Stokes, P. L., Asquith, P., Holmes, G. K. T., et al. Histocompatibility antigens associated with adult coeliac disease. *Lancet* 2:162, 1972.

14. Falchuk, Z. M., Rogentine, G. N., and Strober, W. Predominance of histocompatibility antigen HL-A8 in patients with gluten-sensitive enteropathy. *J. Clin. Invest.* 51:1602, 1972.

15. Stastny, P. Mixed lymphocyte culture typing cells from patients with rheumatoid arthritis. *Tissue Antigens* 4:471, 1974.

16. Stastny, P. Mixed lymphocyte cultures in rheumatoid arthritis. *J. Clin. Invest.* 57:1148, 1976.

17. Astorga, G. P., and Williams, R. C., Jr. Al-

tered reactivity in mixed lymphocyte culture of lymphocytes from patients with rheumatoid arthritis. *Arthritis Rheum.* 12:547, 1969.

18. Hedberg, H., Källén, B., Löw, B., et al. Impaired mixed leucocyte reaction in some different diseases, notably multiple sclerosis and various arthritides. *Clin. Exp. Immunol.* 9:201, 1971.

19. Lies, R. B., Messner, R. P., and Troup, G. M. Histocompatibility antigens and rheumatoid arthritis. *Arthritis Rheum.* 15:524, 1972.

20. Seignalet, J., Clot, J., Sany, J., et al. HL-A antigens in rheumatoid arthritis. *Vox Sang.* 23:468, 1972.

21. Reinertsen, J. L., Klippel, J. H., Johnson, A. H., et al. B lymphocyte alloantigens associated with systemic lupus erythematosus. *N. Engl. J. Med.* 299:515, 1978.

22. Gibofsky, A., Winchester, R. J., Patarroyo, M., et al. Disease associations of the Ia-like human alloantigens. Contrasting patterns in rheumatoid arthritis and systemic lupus erythematosus. *J. Exp. Med.* 148:1728, 1978.

23. WHO-IUIS Terminology Committee. Nomenclature for factors of the HLA system. In W. Bodmer and R. Batchelor, eds., *Histocompatibility Testing,* p. 14. Munksgaard, Copenhagen, 1977.

24. Patarroyo, M. E., Winchester, R. J., Vejerano, A., et al. Association of a B-cell alloantigen with susceptibility to rheumatic fever. *Nature* 278:173, 1979.

25. Stroud, R. M. Genetic abnormalities of the complement system of man associated with disease. *Transplant. Proc.* 6:59, 1974.

26. Polley, M. J., and Bearn, A. G. Genetic aspects of diseases of complement: an explosion. *Am. J. Med.* 58:105, 1975.

27. Glass, D., Raum, D., Gibson, D. S., et al. Inherited deficiency of the second component of complement. Rheumatic disease associations. *J. Clin. Invest.* 58:853, 1976.

28. Rosenfeld, S. I., Kelly, M. E., and Leddy, J. P. Hereditary deficiency of the fifth component of complement in man. I. Clinical, immunochemical, and family studies. *J. Clin. Invest.* 57:1626, 1976.

29. Boyer, J. T., Gall, E. P., Norman, M. E., et al. Hereditary deficiency of the seventh component of complement. *J. Clin. Invest.* 56:905, 1975.

30. Jasin, H. E. Absence of the eighth component of complement in association with systemic lupus erythematosus-like disease. *J. Clin. Invest.* 60:709, 1977.

31. Fu, S. M., Stern, R., Kunkel, H. G., et al. Mixed lymphocyte culture determinants and C2 de-

ficiency: LD-7a associated with C2 deficiency in four families. *J. Exp. Med.* 142:495, 1975.

32. Kohler, P. F. Inherited complement deficiencies and systemic lupus erythematosus: an immunogenetic puzzle. *Ann. Intern. Med.* 82:420, 1975.

33. Démant, P., Capková, J., Hinzová, E., et al. The role of the histocompatibility-2-linked Ss-Slp region in the control of mouse complement. *Proc. Natl. Acad. Sci. USA* 70:863, 1973.

34. Ferreira, A., and Nussenzweig, V. Genetic linkage between serum levels of the third component of complement and the H-2 complex. *J. Exp. Med.* 141:513, 1975.

35. Fu, S. M., Kunkel, H. G., Brusman, H. P., et al. Evidence for linkage between HL-A histocompatibility genes and those involved in the synthesis of the second component of complement. *J. Exp. Med.* 140:1108, 1974.

36. Day, N. K., L'Esperance, R., Good, R. A., et al. Hereditary C2 deficiency: genetic studies and association with the HL-A system. *J. Exp. Med.* 141:1464, 1975.

37. Daniels, C. A., Borsos, T., Rapp, H. J., et al. Neutralization of sensitized virus by purified components of complement. *Proc. Natl. Acad. Sci. USA* 65:528, 1970.

38. Cooper, N. R., Jensen, F. C., Welsh, R. M., Jr., et al. Lysis of RNA tumor viruses by human serum: direct antibody-independent triggering of the classical complement pathway. *J. Exp. Med.* 144:970, 1976.

39. Christian, C. L. Editorial. Systemic lupus erythematosus and type C-RNA viruses. *N. Engl. J. Med.* 295:501, 1976.

40. Mellors, R. C., and Mellors, J. W. Antigen related to mammalian type-C-RNA viral p30 proteins is located in renal glomeruli in human systemic lupus erythematosus. *Proc. Natl. Acad. Sci. USA* 73:233, 1976.

41. Lewis, R. M., Tannenberg, W., Smith, C., et al. C-type viruses in systemic lupus erythematosus. *Nature* 252:78, 1974.

42. Strand, M., and August, J. T. Type-C RNA virus gene expression in human tissue. *J. Virol.* 14:1584, 1974.

43. Phillips, P. E. Type C oncornavirus studies in systemic lupus erythematosus. *Arthritis Rheum.* 21:S76, 1978.

44. West, C. D., Winter, S., Forristal, J., et al. Evidence for *in vivo* breakdown of β_{1C}-globulin in hypocomplementemic glomerulonephritis. *J. Clin. Invest.* 46:539, 1967.

45. Bennet, W. M., Bardana, E. J., Wuepper, K., et al. Partial lipodystrophy, C3 nephritic factor

and clinically inapparent mesangiocapillary glomerulonephritis. *Am. J. Med.* 62:757, 1977.

46. Reichel, W., Köbberling, J., Fischbach, H., et al. Membranoproliferative glomerulonephritis with partial lipodystrophy. Discordant occurrence in identical twins. *Klin. Wochenschr.* 54:75, 1976.

47. Zinkernagel, R. M., and Doherty, P. C. Restriction of *in vitro* T cell-mediated cytotoxicity in lymphocytic choriomeningitis within a syngeneic or semiallogeneic system. *Nature* 248:701, 1974.

48. Koszinowski, U., and Ertl, H. Lysis mediated by T cells and restricted by H-2 antigen of target cells infected with vaccinia virus. *Nature* 255:552, 1975.

49. Doherty, P. C., and Zinkernagel, R. M. T-cell-mediated immunopathology in viral infections. *Transplant. Rev.* 19:89, 1974.

50. Schrader, J. W., and Edelman, G. M. Participation of the H-2 antigens of tumor cells in their lysis by syngeneic T cells. *J. Exp. Med.* 143:601, 1976.

51. Tursz, T., Fridman, W. H., Senik, A., et al. Human virus-infected target cells lacking HLA antigens resist specific T-lymphocyte cytolysis. *Nature* 269:806, 1977.

52. Blank, K. J., and Lilly, F. Evidence for an H-2/viral protein complex on the cell surface as the basis for the H-2 restriction of cytotoxicity. *Nature* 269:808, 1977.

53. Cochrane, C. G., and Koffler, D. Immune complex disease in experimental animals and man. *Adv. Immunol.* 16:185, 1973.

54. Unanue, E. R., and Dixon, F. J. Experimental glomerulonephritis: immunological events and pathogenetic mechanisms. *Adv. Immunol.* 6:1, 1967.

55. Kniker, W. T., and Cochrane, C. G. Pathogenic factors in vascular lesions of experimental serum sickness. *J. Exp. Med.* 122:83, 1965.

56. Cochrane, C. G., Unanue, E. R., and Dixon, F. J. A role of polymorphonuclear leukocytes and complement in nephrotoxic nephritis. *J. Exp. Med.* 122:99, 1965.

57. Stetson, C. A., Jr. Similarities in the mechanisms determining the Arthus and Schwartzman phenomena. *J. Exp. Med.* 94:347, 1951.

58. Humphrey, J. H. The mechanism of Arthus reactions. I. The role of polymorphonuclear leucocytes and other factors in reversed passive Arthus reactions in rabbits. *Br. J. Exp. Pathol.* 36:268, 1955.

59. Humphrey, J. H. The mechanism of Arthus reactions. II. The role of polymorphonuclear leucocytes and platelets in reversed passive reactions in the guinea-pig. *Br. J. Exp. Pathol.* 36:283, 1955.

60. Cochrane, C. G., Weigle, W. O., and Dixon, F. J. The role of polymorphonuclear leukocytes in the initiation and cessation of the Arthus vasculitis. *J. Exp. Med.* 110:481, 1959.

61. Wilson, C. B., and Dixon, F. J. Antigen quantitation in experimental immune complex glomerulonephritis. I. Acute serum sickness. *J. Immunol.* 105:279, 1970.

62. Smith, H. W. Comparative physiology of the kidney. In *The Kidney: Structure and Function in Health and Disease,* p. 567. Oxford University Press, New York, 1951.

63. Dixon, F. J., Feldman, J. D., Vazquez, J. J. Experimental glomerulonephritis. The pathogenesis of a laboratory model resembling the spectrum of human glomerulonephritis. *J. Exp. Med.* 113:899, 1961.

64. Germuth, F. G., Jr., Senterfit, L. B., Pollack, A. D. Immune complex disease. I. Experimental acute and chronic glomerulonephritis. *Johns Hopkins Med. J.* 120:225, 1967.

65. Peters, D. K., and Lachmann, P. J. Immunity deficiency in pathogenesis of glomerulonephritis. *Lancet* 1:58, 1974.

66. Valdes, A. J., Senterfit, L. B., Pollack, A. D., et al. The effect of antigen excess on chronic immune complex glomerulonephritis. *Johns Hopkins Med. J.* 124:9, 1969.

67. Benacerraf, B., McCluskey, R. T., and Patras, D. Localization of colloidal substances in vascular endothelium: A mechanism of tissue damage. I. Factors causing the pathologic deposition of colloidal carbon. *Am. J. Pathol.* 35:75, 1959.

68. Kniker, W. T., and Cochrane, C. G. The localization of circulating immune complexes in experimental serum sickness. The role of vasoactive amines and hydrodynamic forces. *J. Exp. Med.* 127:119, 1968.

69. Cochrane, C. G. Studies on the localization of antigen-antibody complexes and other macromolecules in vessels. I. Structural studies. *J. Exp. Med.* 118:489, 1963.

70. Cochrane, C. G. Studies on the localization of antigen-antibody complexes and other macromolecules in vessels. II. Pathogenetic and pharmacodynamic studies. *J. Exp. Med.* 118:503, 1963.

71. Alksne, J. F. The passage of colloidal particles across the dermal capillary wall under the influence of histamine. *Q. J. Exp. Physiol.* 44:51, 1959.

72. Majno, G., and Palade, G. E. Studies on inflammation. I. The effect of histamine and serotonin on vascular permeability: an electron microscopic study. *J. Biophys. Biochem. Cytol.* 11:571, 1961.

73. Peterson, R. D. A., and Good, R. A. Mor-

phology of vascular permeability. I. Passive cutaneous anaphylaxis. *Lab. Invest.* 11:507, 1962.

74. Kniker, W. T. The role of vasoactive amines in the pathogenesis of complex-induced chronic glomerulonephritis. *Fed. Proc.* 27:409, 1968.

75. Kniker, W. T. Modulation of the inflammatory response *in vivo:* prevention or amelioration of immune complex disease. In I. H. Lepow and P. A. Ward, eds., *Inflammation: Mechanisms and Control,* p. 335. Academic Press, New York, 1972.

76. Chused, T. M., and Tarpley, T. M., Jr. Antagonism of vasoactive amines in NZB/W glomerulonephritis. I. Beneficial effect of methysergide. *Proc. Soc. Exp. Biol. Med.* 144:281, 1973.

77. Kupor, L. R., Lowance, D. C., and McPhaul, J. J., Jr. Single and multiple drug therapy in autologous immune complex nephritis in rats. *J. Lab. Clin. Med.* 87:27, 1976.

78. Humphrey, J. H., and Jaques, R. The release of histamine and 5-hydroxy-tryptamine (serotonin) from platelets by antigen-antibody reactions (*in vitro*). *J. Physiol. (Lond.)* 128:9, 1955.

79. Barbaro, J. F. The release of histamine from rabbit platelets by means of antigen-antibody precipitates. I. The participation of the immune complex in histamine release. *J. Immunol.* 86:369, 1961.

80. Gocke, D. J., and Osler, A. G. *In vitro* damage of rabbit platelets by an unrelated antigen-antibody reaction. I. General characteristics of the reaction. *J. Immunol.* 94:236, 1965.

81. Bryant, R., and Des Prez, R. Mechanisms of immunologically-induced rabbit platelet injury. *Clin. Res.* 16:318, 1968.

82. Henson, P. M. The adherence of leucocytes and platelets induced by fixed IgG antibody or complement. *Immunology* 16:107, 1969.

83. Henson, P. M., and Cochrane, C. G. Immunological induction of increased vascular permeability. II. Two mechanisms of histamine release from rabbit platelets involving complement. *J. Exp. Med.* 129:167, 1969.

84. Henson, P. M., and Cochrane, C. G. In H. Z. Movat, ed., *Cellular and Humoral Mechanisms in Anaphylaxis and Allergy,* p. 129. Karger, Basel, 1969.

85. Schoenbechler, M. J., and Sadun, E. H. *In vitro* histamine release from blood cellular elements of rabbits infected with *Schistosoma mansoni. Proc. Soc. Exp. Biol. Med.* 127:601, 1968.

86. Siraganian, R. P., Secchi, A. G., and Osler, A. G. In K. F. Austen and E. L. Becker, eds., *Biochemistry of the Acute Allergic Reactions,* p. 215. Blackwell Press, Oxford, 1968.

87. Siraganian, R. P., and Osler, A. G. Destruction of rabbit platelets in the allergic response of sensitized leukocytes. II. Evidence for basophil involvement. *J. Immunol.* 106:1252, 1971.

88. Benveniste, J., and Henson, P. M. Leukocyte-dependent mechanism of histamine release from rabbit platelets: transfer of responsible antibody. *Fed. Proc.* 30:2568, 1971.

89. Cochrane, C. G., Müller-Eberhard, H. J., and Aikin, B. S. Depletion of plasma complement *in vivo* by a protein of cobra venom: its effect on various immunologic reactions. *J. Immunol.* 105:55, 1970.

90. Mannik, M., and Arend, W. P. Fate of preformed immune complexes in rabbits and rhesus monkeys. *J. Exp. Med.* 134:19s, 1971.

91. Arend, W. P., and Mannik, M. Studies on antigen-antibody complexes. II. Quantification of tissue uptake of soluble complexes in normal and complement-depleted rabbits. *J. Immunol.* 107:63, 1971.

92. Gelfand, M. C., Frank, M. M., and Green, I. A receptor for the third component of complement in the human renal glomerulus. *J. Exp. Med.* 142:1029, 1975.

93. Gelfand, M. C., Shin, M. L., Nagle, R. B., et al. The glomerular complement receptor in immunologically mediated renal glomerular injury. *N. Engl. J. Med.* 295:10, 1976.

94. Shin, M. L., Gelfand, M. C., Nagle, R. B., et al. Localization of receptors for activated complement on visceral epithelial cells of the human renal glomerulus. *J. Immunol.* 118:869, 1977.

95. Burkholder, P. M., Oberley, T. D., Barber, T. A., et al. Immune adherence in renal glomeruli. Complement receptor sites on glomerular capillary epithelial cells. *Am. J. Pathol.* 86:635, 1977.

96. Heptinstall, R. H. Pathology of acute glomerulonephritis. In M. B. Strauss and L. G. Welt, eds., *Diseases of the Kidney,* ed. 2, vol. 1, p. 405. Little, Brown and Co., Boston, 1971.

97. Grishman, E., Porush, J. G., Lee, S. L., et al. Renal biopsies in lupus nephritis. Correlation of electron microscopic findings with clinical course. *Nephron* 10:25, 1973.

98. Sobel, A. T., Gabay, Y. E., and Lagrue, G. Analysis of glomerular complement receptors in various types of glomerulonephritis. *Clin. Immunol. Immunopathol.* 6:94, 1976.

99. Moran, J., Colasanti, G., Amos, N., et al. C3b receptors in glomerular disease. *Clin. Exp. Immunol.* 28:212, 1977.

100. Alper, C. A., and Rosen, F. S. Studies of the *in vivo* behavior of human C′3 in normal subjects and patients. *J. Clin. Invest.* 46:2021, 1967.

101. Alarçon-Segovia, D. Receptors for the third component of complement in the human glomerulus. *J. Rheumatol.* 3:327, 1976.

102. Atkins, C., Kondon, J., Jr., Quismorio, F., et al. The choroid plexus in systemic lupus erythematosus. *Ann. Intern. Med.* 76:65, 1972.

103. Lampert, P. W., and Oldstone, M. B. A. Pathology of the choroid plexus in spontaneous immune complex disease and chronic viral infections. *Virchows Arch. (Pathol. Anat.)* 363:21, 1974.

104. Lampert, P. W., and Oldstone, M. B. A. Host immunoglobulin G and complement deposits in the choroid plexus during spontaneous immune complex disease. *Science* 180:408, 1973.

105. Williams, R. C., Jr., Husby, G., Wedege, E., et al. Sydenham's chorea, antineuronal antibodies, circulating immune complexes and the choroid plexus Fc receptor. In B. Schwabe, ed., *Menarini Foundation and World Health Organization Symposium on Immunopathology of Central Nervous System.* Basel, forthcoming.

106. Costa, J., Rabson, A. S., Yee, C., et al. Immunoglobulin binding to herpes virus-induced Fc receptors inhibits virus growth. *Nature* 269:251, 1977.

107. Cooper, S. M., Sambray, Y., and Friou, G. J. Isolation of separate Fc receptors for IgG complexed to antigen and native IgG from a murine leukaemia. *Nature* 270:253, 1977.

108. Gelfand, M. C., Frank, M. M., Green, I., et al. Binding sites for immune complexes containing IgG in the renal interstitium. *Clin. Immunol. Immunopathol.* 13:19, 1979.

109. Dickler, H. B. Lymphocyte receptors for immunoglobulin. *Adv. Immunol.* 24:167, 1976.

110. Tönder, O., Morse, P. A., Jr., and Humphrey, L. J. Similarities of Fc receptors in human malignant tissue and normal lymphoid tissue. *J. Immunol.* 113:1162, 1974.

111. Aarli, J. A., and Tönder, O. Fc binding of IgG to skeletal muscle tissue. *Int. Arch. Allergy Appl. Immunol.* 47:273, 1974.

112. Aarli, J. A., Aparicio, S. R., Lumsden, C. E., et al. Binding of normal human IgG to myelin sheaths, glia, and neurons. *Immunology* 28:171, 1975.

113. Johnson, P. M., Trenchev, P., and Faulk, W. P. Immunological studies of human placentae. Binding of complexed immunoglobulin by stromal endothelial cells. *Clin. Exp. Immunol.* 22:133, 1975.

114. Matre, R., Tönder, O., and Endresen, C. Fc receptors in human placenta. *Scand. J. Immunol.* 4:741, 1975.

115. Rask, L., Klarkeskog, L., Ostberg, L., et al. Isolation and properties of a murine spleen cell Fc receptor. *Nature* 257:231, 1975.

116. Benacerraf, B., Sebestyen, M., and Cooper, N. S. The clearance of antigen-antibody complexes from the blood by the reticulo-endothelial system. *J. Immunol.* 82:131, 1959.

117. Mannik, M., Arend, W. P., Hall, A. P., et al. Studies on antigen-antibody complexes. I. Elimination of soluble complexes from rabbit circulation. *J. Exp. Med.* 133:713, 1971.

118. Haakenstad, A. O., and Mannik, M. Saturation of the reticuloendothelial system with soluble immune complexes. *J. Immunol.* 112:1939, 1974.

119. Phillips-Quagliata, J. M., Levine, B. B., Quagliata, F., et al. Mechanisms underlying binding of immune complexes to macrophages. *J. Exp. Med.* 133:589, 1971.

120. Arend, W. P., and Mannik, M. The macrophage receptor for IgG: number and affinity of binding sites. *J. Immunol.* 110:1455, 1973.

121. Haakenstad, A. O., Case, J. B., and Mannik, M. Effect of cortisone on the disappearance kinetics and tissue localization of soluble immune complexes. *J. Immunol.* 114:1153, 1975.

122. Nicol, T., Vernon-Roberts, B., and Quantock, D. C. The influence of various hormones on the reticulo-endothelial system: endocrine control of body defense. *J. Endocrinol.* 33:365, 1965.

123. Vernon-Roberts, B., and Jessop, J. D. Effects of gold and prednisolone on inflammation and phagocytosis in the rat. *Ann. Rheum. Dis.* 31:536, 1972.

124. Jessop, J. D., Vernon-Roberts, B., and Harris, J. Effects of gold salts and prednisolone on inflammatory cells. I. Phagocytic activity of macrophages and polymorphs in inflammatory exudates studied by a 'skin window' technique in rheumatoid and control patients. *Ann. Rheum. Dis.* 32:294, 1973.

125. Vernon-Roberts, B., Jessop, J. D., and Doré, J. Effects of gold salts and prednisolone on inflammatory cells. II. Suppression of inflammation and phagocytosis in the rat. *Ann. Rheum. Dis.* 32:301, 1973.

126. Frank, M. M., Hamburger, M. I., Lawley, T. J., et al. Defective reticuloendothelial system Fc-receptor function in systemic lupus erythematosus. *New Engl. J. Med.* 300:518, 1979.

127. Lockwood, C. M., Worlledge, S., Nicholas, A., et al. Reversal of impaired splenic function in patients with nephritis or vasculitis (or both) by plasma exchange. *New Engl. J. Med.* 300:524, 1979.

128. Miller, G. W., and Nussenzweig, V. A new complement function: solubilization of antigen-anti-

body aggregates. *Proc. Natl. Acad. Sci. USA* 72:418, 1975.

129. Czop, J., and Nussenzweig, V. Studies on the mechanism of solubilization of immune precipitates by serum. *J. Exp. Med.* 143:615, 1976.

130. Dumonde, D. C., and Glynn, L. E. The production of arthritis in rabbits by an immunological reaction to fibrin. *Br. J. Exp. Pathol.* 43:373, 1962.

131. Glynn, L. E. The chronicity of inflammation and its significance in rheumatoid arthritis. *Ann. Rheum. Dis.* 27:105, 1968.

132. Cooke, T. D., Hurd, E. R., Ziff, M., et al. The pathogenesis of chronic inflammation in experimental antigen-induced arthritis. II. Preferential localization of antigen-antibody complexes to collagenous tissues. *J. Exp. Med.* 135:323, 1972.

133. Jasin, H. E. Mechanism of trapping of immune complexes in joint collagenous tissues. *Clin. Exp. Immunol.* 22:473, 1975.

134. Arnold, S. B., Valone, J. A., Askenase, P. W., et al. Diffuse glomerulonephritis in rabbits with *Streptococcus viridans* endocarditis. *Lab. Invest.* 32:681, 1975.

135. Walker, W. A., Isselbacher, K. J., and Bloch, K. J. Intestinal uptake of macromolecules: effect of oral immunization. *Science* 177:608, 1972.

136. Walker, W. A., Isselbacher, K. J., and Bloch, K. J. Intestinal uptake of macromolecules. II. Effect of parenteral immunization. *J. Immunol.* 111:221, 1973.

137. Walker, W. A., Wu, M., Isselbacher, K. J., et al. Intestinal uptake of macromolecules. III. Studies on the mechanism by which immunization interferes with antigen uptake. *J. Immunol.* 115:854, 1975.

138. Walker, W. A., Abel, S. N., Wu, M., et al. Intestinal uptake of macromolecules. V. Comparison of the *in vitro* uptake by rat small intestine of antigen-antibody complexes prepared in antibody or antigen excess. *J. Immunol.* 117:1028, 1976.

139. Bernstein, I. D., and Ovary, Z. Absorption of antigens from the gastrointestinal tract. *Int. Arch. Allergy Appl. Immunol.* 33:521, 1968.

140. Walker, W. A., and Isselbacher, K. J. Uptake and transport of macromolecules by the intestine. Possible role in clinical disorders. *Gastroenterology* 67:531, 1974.

141. Rabinovitch, M., Manejias, R. E., and Nussenzweig, V. Selective phagocytic paralysis induced by immobilized immune complexes. *J. Exp. Med.* 142:827, 1975.

142. Ryan, J. L., Arbeit, R. D., Dickler, H. B., et al. Inhibition of lymphocyte mitogenesis by immobilized antigen-antibody complexes. *J. Exp. Med.* 142:814, 1975.

143. Watson, J. The influence of intracellular levels of cyclic nucleotides on cell proliferation and the induction of antibody synthesis. *J. Exp. Med.* 141:97, 1975.

144. Bona, C., Anteunis, A., Robineaux, R., et al. Transfer of antigenic macromolecules form macrophages to lymphocytes. I. Autoradiographic and quantitative study of ^{14}C endotoxin and ^{125}I hemocyanin transfer. *Immunology* 23:799, 1972.

145. Fraser, I. D., Bothamley, J. E., Bennett, M. O., et al. Intensive antenatal plasmapheresis in severe rhesus isoimmunization. *Lancet.* 1:6, 1976.

146. Lockwood, C. M., Pinching, A. J., Sweny, P., et al. Plasma-exchange and immuno-suppression in the treatment of fulminating immune-complex crescentic nephritis. *Lancet* 1:63, 1977.

147. Verrier-Jones, J., Bucknall, R. C., Cumming, R. H., et al. Plasmapheresis in the management of acute systemic lupus erythematosus? *Lancet* 1:709, 1976.

148. Editorial. Plasma-exchange in nephritis. *Lancet* 1:83, 1977.

149. Lockwood, C. M., Pearson, T. A., Rees, A. J., et al. Immunosuppression and plasma-exchange in the treatment of Goodpasture's syndrome. *Lancet* 1:711, 1976.

150. Almon, R. R., Andrew, C. G., and Appel, S. H. Serum globulin in myasthenia gravis: inhibition of α-bungarotoxin binding to acetylcholine receptors. *Science* 186:55, 1974.

151. Aharonov, A., Tarrab-Hazdai, R., Abramsky, O., et al. Humoral antibodies to acetylcholine receptor in patients with myasthenia gravis. *Lancet* 2:340, 1975.

152. Lindstrom, J. M., Lennon, V. A., Seybold, M. E., et al. Experimental autoimmune myasthenia gravis and myasthenia gravis: biochemical and immunochemical aspects. *Ann. N.Y. Acad. Sci.* 274:254, 1976.

153. Pinching, A. J., Peters, D. K., and Davis, J. N. Remission of myasthenia gravis following plasma-exchange. *Lancet* 2:1373, 1976.

154. Lefvert, A. K., and Bergström, K. Effect of lymph IgG from patients with myasthenia gravis on cholinergic receptors. *Eur. J. Clin. Invest.* 6:334, 1976 (abstract).

155. Bukowski, R. M., King, J. W., and Hewlett, J. S. Plasmapheresis in the treatment of thrombotic thrombocytopenic purpura. *Blood* 50:413, 1977.

156. Bukowski, R. M., Hewlett, J. S., Harris, J. W., et al. Exchange transfusions in the treatment of

thrombotic thrombocytopenic purpura. *Semin. Hematol.* 13:219, 1976.

157. Ahlin, T. D., Tung, K. S. K., Walker, L., et al. Decrease in circulating immune complexes during hemodialysis. *Am. J. Med.* 64:672, 1978.

158. Craddock, P. R., Fehr, J., Dalmasso, A. P., et al. Hemodialysis leukopenia: pulmonary vascular leukostasis resulting from complement activation by dialyzer cellophane membranes. *J. Clin. Invest.* 59:879, 1977.

159. Craddock, P. R., Fehr, J., Brigham, K. L., et al. Complement and leukocyte-mediated pulmonary dysfunction in hemodialysis. *N. Engl. J. Med.* 296:769, 1977.

160. Fehr, J., and Jacob, H. S. *In vitro* granulocyte adherence and *in vivo* margination: two associated complement-dependent functions. Studies based on the acute neutropenia of filtration leukophoresis. *J. Exp. Med.* 146:641, 1977.

161. Terman, D. S., Ogden, D., and Petty, D. Removal of circulating antigen and immune complexes with immunoreactive collodion membranes. *F.E.B.S. Lett.* 68:89, 1976.

162. Terman, D. S., Petty, D., Ogden, D., et al. Specific extraction of antigen *in vivo* by extracorporeal circulation over antibody immobilized in collodion-charcoal. *J. Immunol.* 117:1971, 1976.

163. Terman, D. S., Tavel, T., Petty, D., et al. Specific removal of bovine serum albumin (BSA) antibodies *in vivo* by extracorporeal circulation over BSA immobilized on nylon microcapsules. *J. Immunol.* 116:1337, 1976.

164. Terman, D. S., Tavel, T., Petty, D., et al. Specific removal of antibody by extracorporeal circulation over antigen immobilized in collodion-charcoal. *Clin. Exp. Immunol.* 28:180, 1977.

165. Terman, D. S., Tavel, A., Tavel, T., et al. Degradation of circulating DNA by extracorporeal circulation over nuclease immobilized on nylon microcapsules. *J. Clin. Invest.* 57:1201, 1976.

166. Terman, D. S., Stewart, I., Robinette, J., et al. Specific removal of DNA antibodies *in vivo* with an extracorporeal immuno-adsorbent. *Clin. Exp. Immunol.* 24:231, 1976.

167. Terman, D. S., Durante, D., Buffaloe, G., et al. Attenuation of canine nephrotoxic glomerulonephritis with an extracorporeal immunoadsorbent. *Scand. J. Immunol.* 6:195, 1977.

168. Langvad, E., Hydén, H., Wolf, H., et al. Extracorporeal immunoadsorption of circulating specific serum factors in cancer patients. *Br. J. Cancer* 32:680, 1975.

169. Carpentier, N. A., Lange, G. T., Fiere, D. M., et al. Clinical relevance of circulating immune complexes in human leukemia. Association in acute leukemia of the presence of immune complexes with unfavorable prognosis. *J. Clin. Invest.* 60:874, 1977.

CHAPTER 6

Methods of Detection

For the practicing physician it is all well and good to speculate on how immune complexes cause important biologic phenomena or certain tissue lesions, but most important of all it is vital to know how to detect them. Then, if immune complexes are in fact present, what clinical implications can be drawn? For a number of years immune complexes were alluded to in a broad, vague sense but rarely defined—certainly not actually measured. Recently the tide has turned, and during the past decade a number of methods have been introduced to detect the presence of complexes. A mass of new information has almost overwhelmed us with the variety of clinical circumstances in which circulating immune complexes have been measured: everything from the postprandial state or normal pregnancy to disseminated cancer or systemic lupus erythematosus (1–3)

As methods for detection of circulating complexes have become more sensitive and more sophisticated, what appear to be slight or even moderate elevations of complexes in the serum or plasma of normal subjects are being detected perhaps 10 to 15 percent of the time in any large random sample from otherwise healthy individuals. Thus one of the key questions yet to be settled is what should be considered a reasonable normal range, and secondarily, of course, what is indeed abnormal? Numerical values or quantity of circulating complexes defining abnormality are not entirely accurate or even perhaps meaningful in absolute terms; as discussed in Chapter 5, when complete prior saturation of the RES clearing system is present, mild elevations of

detectable circulating complexes become significant and potentially toxic in some disorders. Such elevations accompanied by RES saturation may rapidly result in glomerular or other forms of microvascular injury. Evaluation of the significance of quantitative measurements of immune complexes in various clinical conditions requires precise knowledge of the degree of saturation and saturation kinetics of the available reticuloendothelial system receptors at a given time, plus quantitative amount, size, and intrinsic properties of the complexes being measured. This is illustrated in Figure 6-1. Although precise methods for quantitating amounts of complexes as well as their size and heterogeneity are currently available, a simple and accurate method for measuring RES or phagocytic cell saturation that is suitable for serial clinical studies has not yet been popularized. It is conceivable that future modification of existing methods utilizing uptake of radiolabeled colloidal materials or macroaggregates of albumin might be combined with immune-complex determinations to provide useful data in a number of clinical circumstances. However, labeled albumin aggregates or other such materials may not reflect tissue handling of immune complexes very accurately, since Fc receptors or C3 receptors show fine degrees of specificity for conformational or other structural determinants not present on unrelated colloidal or macroaggregated materials. In addition, possible natural in vivo pathways of immune-complex dissolution by insertion of C3b or C3d into complex matrices may vary during acute illness.

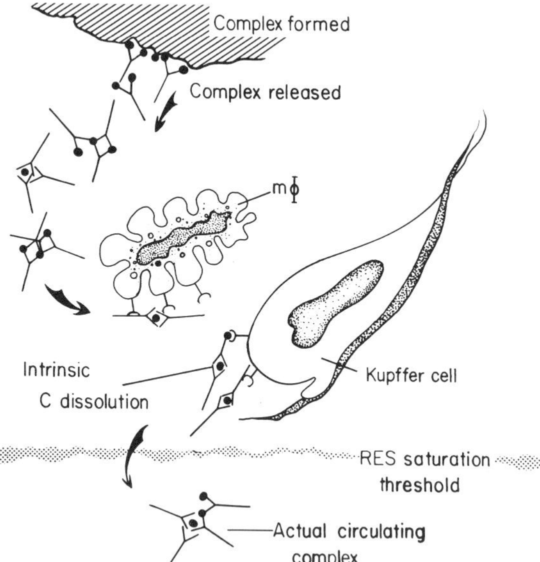

Figure 6-1 Diagram of the various compartments and kinetics involved in detection of circulating immune complexes. What actually circulates as an immune complex may depend on a number of intrinsic variables including normal RES disposal mechanisms, intrinsic ability of activated complement components to induce complex dissolution, and relative saturation of the reticuloendothelial system. Φ represents macrophages of the RES.

Much of the intricacy involved in measuring immune complexes in blood, plasma, or other body fluids derives from the fact that many of the methods utilized depend on both the size and physicochemical qualities of the complexes. Some methods are better at detecting large complexes; others are capable of detecting complexes whether or not complement activation has occurred. As an illustration of this, if circulating immune complexes are larger than 11 to 19S, they are most readily detected by such assays as the Raji-cell test, whereas smaller 9 to 11S complexes are best assayed by an alternative technique that employs binding to ^{125}I-labeled C1q, the first component of complement. In the same vein, certain assay techniques depend on the ability of immune complexes to activate the complement system; if there are circulating complexes composed of IgG or IgA antibodies which for physical or structural reasons do not activate the complement cascade, then a negative result may well

be recorded even in the presence of noncomplement-fixing complexes. Perhaps currently there is not as much interest in noncomplement-fixing immune complexes, since such aggregates are generally not associated with recognizable untoward peripheral clinical effects. However, the failure to detect a broad spectrum of both complement-fixing and noncomplement-fixing immune complexes represents a clear deficiency in contemporary methods.

In the discussions that follow, it will be apparent that in many situations a panel of simultaneous tests is useful. It would be impractical for the clinician to be required to assimilate three different results each time he orders a hemoglobin. To a certain extent diversity of possibilities provided by one clinical test result is already present, as with the isoenzymes of LDH or transaminase. Unfortunately, we are far from the stage of rapid simple assays that will provide the kinds of information useful in interpreting the kind of two- or three-compartmental problem shown in Figure 6-1. Criteria are needed for proof that materials causing positive reactions in the various in vivo tests currently being used are indeed immune complexes. Rather than being a euphemism, this statement is meant to point out that materials containing immunoglobulins and activated complement components that produce positive Raji-cell, C1q, or conglutinin binding also contain recognizable *antigen*. Surprisingly, pertinent data are very sparse. Materials considered to be immune complexes because of their relative increment in molecular weight or change in sedimentation behavior and positive reactivities in many biological test systems cannot indeed be considered proven to be immune complexes unless antigen of some kind is eventually identified.

This point is particularly significant because of the well-documented capacity of IgG molecules to form self-reactive molecules of rheumatoid factor, or more precisely molecules of 7S anti-γ-globulin that react with one another. Studies of so-called intermediate complexes were first initiated by Kunkel and associates (4) in rheumatoid arthritis, and subsequent observations by Schrohenloher (5) and a number of other workers (6–10) have reemphasized their importance. In a variety of hypergammaglobulinemic states, self-associating anti-γ-globulin factors have now been characterized (9, 10). Most recently the relationship of IgG-IgG complexes to syndromes related to high plasma viscosity and severe mixed connective-tissue disease, Sjögren's syndrome, or rheumatoid arthritis has also been stressed (11–13). Thus some materials producing positive results for immune complexes in certain test systems may conceivably be self-associated IgG anti-γ-globulins, and not by strict definition antigen-antibody complexes (unless one considers native gamma globulin an antigen in these particular circumstances). We should insist that eventually in all clinical disorders where it is claimed that circulating immune complexes are present, the *antigen* must be unequivocally identified. If strict adherence to this criterion is followed, much future confusion should be avoided as more and more clinical disorders are examined, particularly in relation to the alleged presence of true immune complexes.

Review of Current Methods

No single method is yet considered ideal for the detection and estimation of immune complexes in various disease states. Actually, one of the most long established and widely accepted indications for their presence is the finding of granular or lumpy-bumpy deposits of immunoglobulin and complement in histological and immunofluorescence studies of renal glomeruli. One cannot perform renal biopsy on every patient suspected of having immune-complex manifestations, but it probably is fair to state that direct immunofluorescence and electron microscopic study of glomeruli has already established a granular, lumpy-bumpy immunoglobulin and C3 pattern of immune-complex deposition in a wide variety of human and animal disease states. Immunofluorescence study of tissues for Ig and complement deposits long preceded the introduction of ultrasensitive radioimmunoassay techniques, which are used today in the study of a number of disorders.

Thus the human glomerulus is one of the most sensitive detectors currently available. Its status has come about first by recognition of the types of immunofluorescence patterns and ultrastructural changes thoroughly studied during the evolution of experimental "one-shot" or chronic serum sickness disease in animals, as well as a series of careful observations of human disease states such as systemic lupus where actual in vivo tissue deposition of immune complexes has now been convincingly demonstrated (as will be discussed in detail in Chapter 7). It is fair to state that granular or lumpy glomerular basement membrane immune deposits are accepted by most pathologists and clinical immunologists as resulting from immune-complex etiology. A partial listing of the wide variety of clinical conditions in which immune complexes have been directly demonstrated by immunofluorescent techniques is given below:

Infections: Poststreptococcal glomerulonephritis
Subacute bacterial endocarditis
Secondary syphilis
Pneumococcal sepsis
Typhoid fever
Lepromatous leprosy
Ventricular shunt infection
Infectious mononucleosis
Subacute sclerosing encephalitis
Landry-Guillain-Barré syndrome
Hepatitis B infection
Quartan malaria
Schistosomiasis (with or without salmonella infection)
Trypanosomiasis

Neoplasms: Hepatoma
Lymphoma and Hodgkin's disease
Acute leukemia
Hypernephroma
Carcinoma of the colon
Bronchogenic carcinoma
Burkitt's lymphoma

Connective-tissue disorders: Systemic lupus erythematosus
Periarteritis nodosa
Chronic glomerulonephritis

Miscellaneous: Acute or subacute thyroiditis
Vinyl chloride poisoning
Chronic liver disease (?)
Mixed cryoglobulinemias
Berger's disease or IgA nephropathy (?)
Rapidly progressive glomerulonephritis
Sickle cell anemia

No such list can be complete, for new disease states are constantly being added to the roster.

An important caveat to holding forth the human glomerulus as a sensitive indicator of immune-complex disease emerges from the results of Germuth and colleagues (14), who showed that chronic glomerular changes can develop in experimental animals with a modification of the usual course of serum sickness whereby no immunofluorescence evidence of immune deposits can be detected, even in the face of continued tissue injury and progression of lesions. In these studies tissue lesions were attributed to a state of induced borderline antigen excess, where soluble complexes were apparently capable somehow of initiating tissue damage.

Anticomplementary Activity of Serum

Over a period of years it was recognized that certain sera showing marked elevation of gamma globulin produced what were called anticomplementary effects when tested for complement fixation with a variety of well-defined antigens (15, 16). This characteristic was often attributed to aggregates or self-associating polymeric forms of IgG present in the sera. More recently the anticomplementary effect of such sera has been revived as a possible means of detecting immune complexes (17, 18). In its present state this method is insensitive and cannot accurately differentiate between complement fixation by self-associating IgG molecules or autologous aggregates coming out of solution in vitro after blood has been collected and true immune complexes determined to be present. High levels of anticomplementary activity are often detected in serum samples of patients with multiple myeloma or hypergammaglobulinemia, for instance, because of intrinsic gamma-globulin aggregate formation. Such aggregation may occur rapidly even after overnight storage at 4° C. Despite its shortcomings, anticomplementary activity still turns up in a number of clinical reports as an assay for presumed immune complexes.

Platelet Aggregation

Aggregation of human platelets in vitro has been shown in several model systems to be a sensitive indicator for complexes composed of IgG (19–21). However, IgM components with anti-IgG activity or rheumatoid factors are capable of inhibiting platelet aggregation induced either by immune complexes containing IgG or by heat-aggregated human IgG (22). This test has been used to detect the presence of circulating immune complexes in *Mycoplasma pneumoniae* infections (23), sarcoidosis (24), and rubella (25). The actual procedure in which platelets are aggregated apparently is not based on cross-linking of the platelets by complexes but results from changes induced by the complexes in the intrinsic aggregability of the platelets. The platelets used must be viable, since surface alterations induced by contact with complexes depend on alteration of platelet metabolism. Like the Raji-cell test discussed below, the reaction is most sensitive to large complexes. An unfortunate feature is the apparent capacity of IgM rheumatoid factor to produce inhibition. The necessity for a continuous supply of viable platelets is limiting for some laboratories, particularly since the cost of such materials can be considerable if fresh viable platelets are used daily or several times a week. These technical limitations have probably produced some curtailment in use of the platelet aggregation test as a method to detect immune complexes in various biological samples.

Methods Using C1q

One of the most widely used methods currently applied to the detection of immune complexes is based on the binding of the first complement component C1q to IgG-1, IgG-2, IgG-3, and IgM. This binding is greatly enhanced by aggregation or minor degrees of lattice formation of these immunoglobulins, but under proper conditions soluble complexes will bind and can be precipitated (26–28). Reaction of C1q with aggregated immunoglobulins or immune complexes sometimes can be demonstrated in gel diffusion (Figure 6-2). Reduction and alkylation of immunoglobulins, which is known to destroy their complement-activating properties, in addition eliminates the precipitin reaction with C1q; this is illustrated also in Figure 6-2.

The precipitin reaction between C1q and immune complexes was first used to detect the latter in various sera and pathological fluids from patients with rheumatoid arthritis and other connective-tissue diseases (29, 30). During initial studies of the C1q reaction, it became apparent that C1q produced precipitating reactions with materials quite different from immune complexes, including DNA and endotoxin as well as low-molecular-weight serum materials associated with an SLE-related syndrome (32–34). The exact identity of these low-molecular-weight materials has not yet been completely defined. Irrelevant C1q bind-

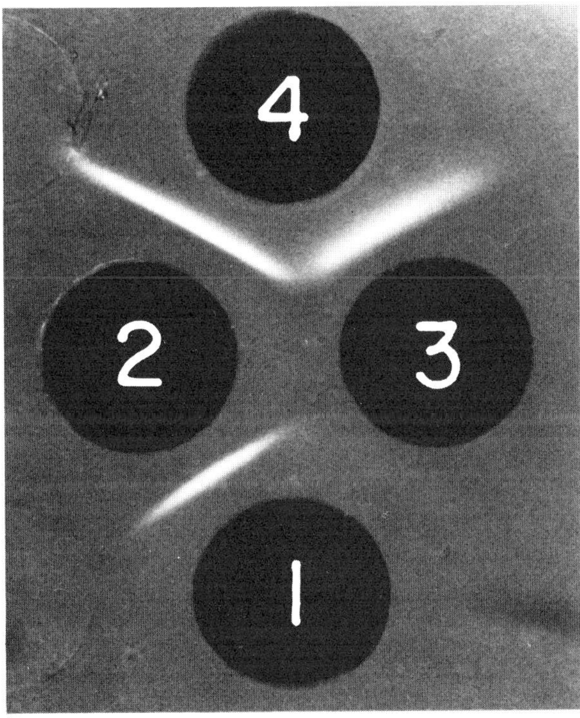

Figure 6-2 Immune diffusion reactions in agarose gel showing well 1 (C1q); well 2 (aggregated IgG); well 3 (reduced and alkylated aggregated IgG); and well 4 (monoclonal rheumatoid factor). A clear precipitin reaction between C1q in well 1 and IgG aggregate in well 2 is noted. (Reproduced with permission, V. Agnello, R. J. Winchester, and H. G. Kunkel, *Immunology* 19:909, 1970.)

ing makes interpretation of test results difficult in the case of infections or other conditions where such molecules might be present even in trace amounts in plasma or serum. This was recognized quite early by Sobel and co-workers (35), in a modification of C1q binding termed the C1q deviation test, which markedly increased sensitivity of the reaction. The procedure utilized inhibition of radiolabeled C1q binding to sensitized sheep erythrocytes by C1q reactive materials in test sera. A number of different test procedures have subsequently been introduced, all of which essentially are based on C1q binding to immunoglobulins in immune complexes.

One widely used procedure is that developed by Nydegger and associates (36), which utilizes binding to ^{125}I-labeled C1q. It was found to be highly reproducible and sensitive, detecting as little as 3 to 5 μg% of complexes in test sera. Later the procedure was modified so that test sera did not require heat inactivation before addition to labeled C1q reagent (37). (There had been concern that heat inactivation of some serum samples at 56° C for 30 to 45 minutes might inadvertently induce aggregates of IgG, which would then register as complexes in the test.) The modification utilized a mixture of test serum with EDTA to prevent integration of ^{125}I-C1q into the intrinsic C1qrs complex. In addition, 2.5 percent polyethylene glycol was added to precipitate C1q bound to macromolecular complexes, presumably reducing the competitive effects of intrinsic C1q and other possible interfering substances such as DNA or bacterial polysaccharide. This modification may be particularly useful in detecting circulating complexes in sera of SLE patients where interfering substances such as DNA might be present. The sensitivity of this test was such that 2.5 μg/ml of aggregated γ-globulin were detected when added to normal human serum. The possible artifact introduced by preheating or inactivating test serum samples is an important technical consideration that surprisingly has been ignored by a number of groups using C1q binding for estimation of circulating immune complexes. Figure 6-3 gives a graphical analysis of the differences in C1q binding ac-

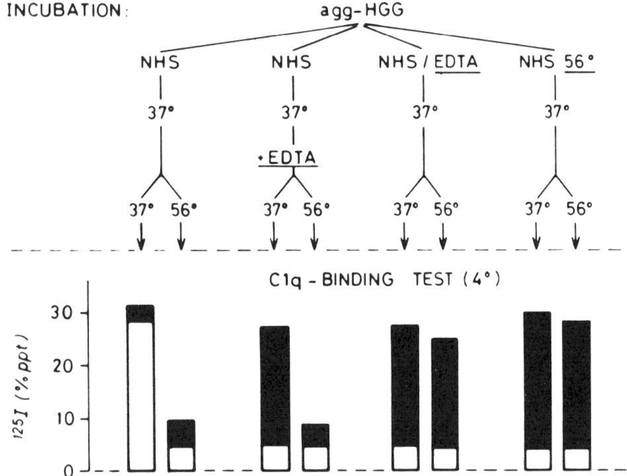

Figure 6-3 Effect of heat inactivation of C1q binding. The lower part of the graph represents C1q binding activity of various serum samples containing aggregated human gamma globulin and prepared as outlined in the upper part of the graph. ■ = specific C1q binding, □ = C1q binding activity of controls without addition of aggregated human IgG. (Reproduced with permission, R. H. Zubler, G. Lange, P. H. Lambert et al., *J. Immunol.* 116:232, 1976.)

tivity under different circumstances of serum treatment.

Another extremely useful variation on the general theme of C1q binding has been introduced by Hay and co-workers (38). Their method utilizes C1q made insoluble and bound on the surfaces of plastic tubes in what is called a solid-phase radioimmunoassay. With the C1q bound to the plastic tube surfaces, test material is introduced and then washed off the inside of the tube. Immune complexes bind to the C1q fixed to the tube and are detected by subsequent addition of ^{125}I-labeled rabbit antihuman IgG specific for the Fc portion of human IgG. A quantitative standard curve is constructed by addition of aggregates of human IgG. The basic principles of this method are shown diagrammatically in Figure 6-4. It is important to point out that this solid-phase C1q-binding radioimmunoassay, as well as the C1q method devised by the Nydegger group (36), are based on the relative availability of human C1q, which can be rapidly purified in most laboratories by the technique of Yonemasu and Stroud (39). Their method, now employed in many laboratories throughout the

world, makes use of C1q binding either in liquid phase, or after polyethylene glycol precipitation, or in the solid-phase assay methods. Our own experience with Hay's solid-phase assay has been very good; it is one of the routine procedures we now utilize for immune-complex determinations in clinical samples.

It must be pointed out, however, that there is still no single test that seems completely ideal for immune-complex assays. Complexes comprised of IgG4 molecules, for instance, do not bind to C1q. Immune complexes composed of immunoglobulin molecules that do not bind complement, such as IgA, are not detected either. The C1q binding test does appear to be useful in detecting a large spectrum of antigen-antibody complexes in terms of size. In our experience it seems slightly more sensitive in detecting 9 to 11 S complexes than does the Raji-cell test. Furthermore, C1q binding of immune complexes does not seem to be appreciably affected by the presence of various concentrations of sucrose, which makes the test useful for assaying complex size after separation of test serum samples over sucrose gradients by preparative ultracentrifugation.

Tests Employing Immune-Complex Receptors on Cells

A number of cellular tests have been studied and a few recommended for clinical use in the

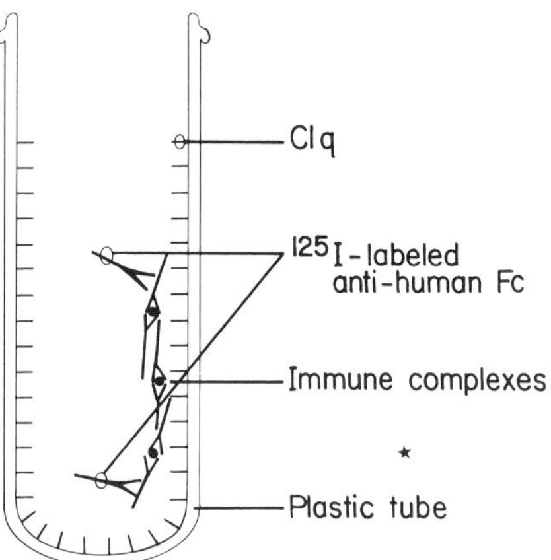

Figure 6-4 Graphic representation of the general principles involved in solid-phase C1q assay for immune complexes.

detection of immune complexes in pathological human serum. One method introduced by Onyewotu and co-workers (40, 41) utilized macrophages harvested from guinea pigs three to five days after intraperitoneal injection with sterile liquid parafin. Macrophages were pretested with gamma globulin—presumably to block surface receptors—and then test serum was added to macrophages along with labeled human IgG aggregates. Uptake of aggregates was measured by counting radioactivity associated with the guinea pig macrophages after washing. This test was devised on the principle of competitive inhibition; in other words, inhibition of guinea pig macrophage uptake of labeled IgG aggregates was judged to result from presence of immune complexes in test samples. Test samples were inactivated at 56° C before assay, a procedure which, as noted above, may itself introduce aggregation of autologous γ-globulins, particularly in hypergammaglobulinemic sera. The guinea pig macrophage uptake assay has been utilized in studies of various subgroups of patients with rheumatoid arthritis, both with and without cutaneous vasculitis (41). About half the sera tested from patients with vasculitis showed enhancement rather than inhibition of labeled IgG aggregate uptake—the reverse of what had been observed in sera from patients with SLE. This enhancement was attributed to the presence of rheumatoid factor in the sera. No studies were reported on possible effects on the guinea pig system of antilymphocyte antibodies undoubtedly also present in many of the SLE patients. Enhancement of uptake in the presence of anti-γ-globulins reported in this particular assay system makes its use problematical. Extensive applicability seems unlikely, since many of the conditions in which clinical assessment of immune complexes is important are themselves associated with the occurrence of detectable serum anti-γ-globulins.

Raji-Cell Test

The Raji-cell test was first described by Theofilopoulos and colleagues in 1974 (42, 43). The Raji cell line, originally derived from a patient with Burkitt's lymphoma, was selected after tests had been conducted on a number of similar available cell lines. The Raji cell itself lacks intrinsic surface membrane immunoglobulin but shows clear evidence of receptors for Fc of IgG, C3b, and C3d. It was found that cell surface Fc receptors for IgG could be inhibited by preincubation with gamma globulin, with the receptors for activated C3 subsequently allowed to serve as the primary binding phenomenon for immune-complex detection. Patterns of immune complexes binding to such Raji cells were first detected by immunoflourescence. A typical example is shown in Figure 6-5. Later this method was adapted for radioimmunoassay, using inhibition of labeled IgG aggregates and a suitable standard curve or by using labeled antihuman IgG (44).

In general, the assay is quite sensitive, being capable of detecting 5 to 10 μg/ml of aggregates or immune complexes; it is also highly reproducible and does not appear to be significantly affected by presence of either anti-γ-globulins or antilymphocyte antibodies (there is still some disagreement on the latter point). Much attention has been directed at this particular part of the assay, since many of

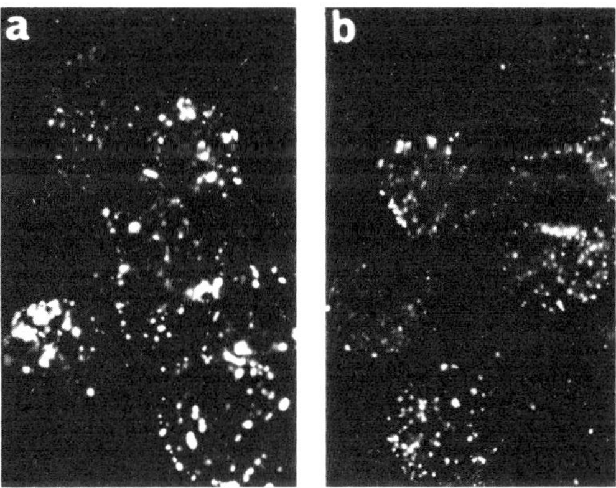

Figure 6-5 Immunofluorescence staining patterns of Raji cells carrying fluorescein-labeled aggregated human γ-globulin or fluorescein-labeled 7S IgG. Magnification × 400. (*a*), aggregated human γ-globulin-bearing Raji cells, with many large, irregular granules of IgG visible on the cell surface. (*b*), 7S IgG-bearing Raji cells, with fine granules of IgG evenly distributed on the cell surface. (Reproduced with permission, A. N. Theofilopoulos, C. B. Wilson, V. A. Bokisch et al., *J. Exp. Med.* 140:1230, 1974.)

the diseases in which serial immune-complex determinations would be useful are disorders such as SLE, known to be accompanied by the presence of antibodies to lymphocytes (45, 46). In this regard, it was important to be sure that immunoglobulin binding to such lymphoid cell lines as the Raji did not in reality represent inadvertent binding of antilymphocyte antibody, instead of adherence of immune complexes to C3b and C3d receptors. A diagrammatic representation of the principles basic to the Raji-cell test is given in Figure 6-6.

An essential feature for proper application of the Raji-cell test is maintenance of the cell line in continuous culture and a uniform, viable state. It is essential to use the Raji cells immediately after their growth phase, while a high degree of viability and preservation of cell surface structures is still present. If cells are allowed to stand or are used too long after their initial growth phase, the proportions of nonviable cells increase and in the test system will show a relatively high background by nonspecific absorption. Another important feature for reproducibility and day-to-day standardization originally emphasized by Theofilopoulos and associates (44) is the use of uniformly standardized IgG aggregates, made fresh each day and cleared in the centrifuge at

1,500 g for 15 minutes immediately before use to remove large insoluble aggregates, or stored in small aliquots at $-70°$ C for not more than one month.

A further refinement to ensure uniformity is to prepare aggregates and size them by means of overnight sucrose gradient ultracentrifugation or gel filtration, saving 11 to 18 S fractions for comparison with those of 19 S and above. This technique is particularly useful in the assay of immune complexes of unknown size in test sera, but it requires calibration or size estimates of the different fractions through independent molecular-size markers. We have found the solid-phase C1q test of the Hay group (38) most readily adaptable to studies of immune complexes occurring in various pathologic sera separated by sucrose gradient ultracentrifugation or other physical techniques; we have found it technically difficult to apply the Raji method to gel filtration or sucrose gradient fractions.

The Raji-cell test has one other distinct theoretical advantage related to the problem of antigen identification. Direct immunofluorescent localization or identification of bacterial, viral, or other antigen should theoretically also be possible using heterologous antisera or $F(ab')_2$ fragments of antibody to presumed antigen studied in paralled with C3 or Ig on surfaces of test Raji cells. To date we have found this particular approach to be exceedingly difficult for reasons that are not yet clear. There is also no unambiguous reason why the solid-phase C1q radioimmunoassay cannot be utilized with the same end in mind. Thus, after complexes have been fixed to the solid-phase C1q lining the plastic tubes, heterologous specific antibody or $F(ab')_2$ fragments of the latter could be used to identify concurrent presence of putative antigens in the immune complexes fixed on the solid-phase C1q coating. As mentioned earlier, there are surprisingly few data directed specifically at the important point of identifying what constitutes antigen in complexes in many diverse states. Indeed, the question arises whether the 11 to 19 S "complexes" being detected in many systems may in fact be self-associating anti-γ-globulins composed only of 7 S IgG.

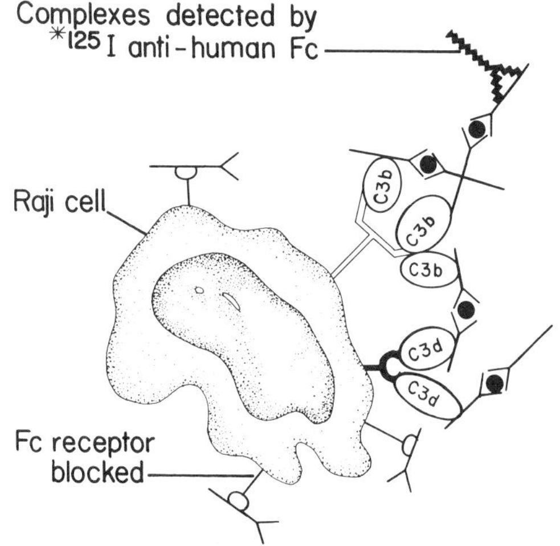

Figure 6-6 Principles of the Raji-cell test for detection of immune complexes.

Use of Conglutinin

Bovine conglutinin (K) seems to be a potentially ideal reagent for identification of immune complexes. This material, which occurs naturally in bovine serum, is known to show avid reactions for fixed C3d (47, 48). The distinct advantage of a test using conglutinin fixed in a solid-phase assay is that this method does not appear to be directly influenced by potential interference by DNA, endotoxins, bacterial polysaccharides, heparin, or anti–cell-surface-membrane antibodies. Solid-phase conglutinin assays have recently been introduced by two groups (49, 50). In one method, that of Eisenberg and co-workers (49), the bovine conglutinin was fixed on the inside of plastic tubes, much as in the solid-phase C1q assay, and showed highly specific binding to immune complexes or aggregates of human IgG. The assay appeared to show preferential reactivity for relatively large complexes and was minimally influenced by monomeric IgG. However, high ionic strength, calcium chelation, and aceto-amido sugars produced some inhibition of the reactions.

Parallel Raji-cell and conglutinin-binding assays for immune complexes in the serial serum samples collected from a patient with Candida infectious endocarditis are shown in Figure 6-7, taken from the Eisenberg study. Similar parallel studies of patients with SLE using the two methods showed only 21-percent positivity in SLE by conglutinin or K-binding solid-phase assay, and 62-percent positivity in the Raji-cell test. It is conceivable that in this instance the Raji-cell test is influenced by the presence of anti–cell-directed or antilymphocyte antibodies. Alternatively, complexes detected by the K-binding test may bear relatively more fixed C3d, essential for conglutinin binding, whereas the complexes binding to Raji cells may have a majority of the complement components affixed to them in the form of C3b.

This particular study is a good demonstration that perhaps no single test is capable of detecting or quantitating all members of a broad spectrum of different types of immune complexes. During a 1976 World Health Organization conference on methods of detection of immune complexes, a comparison of many

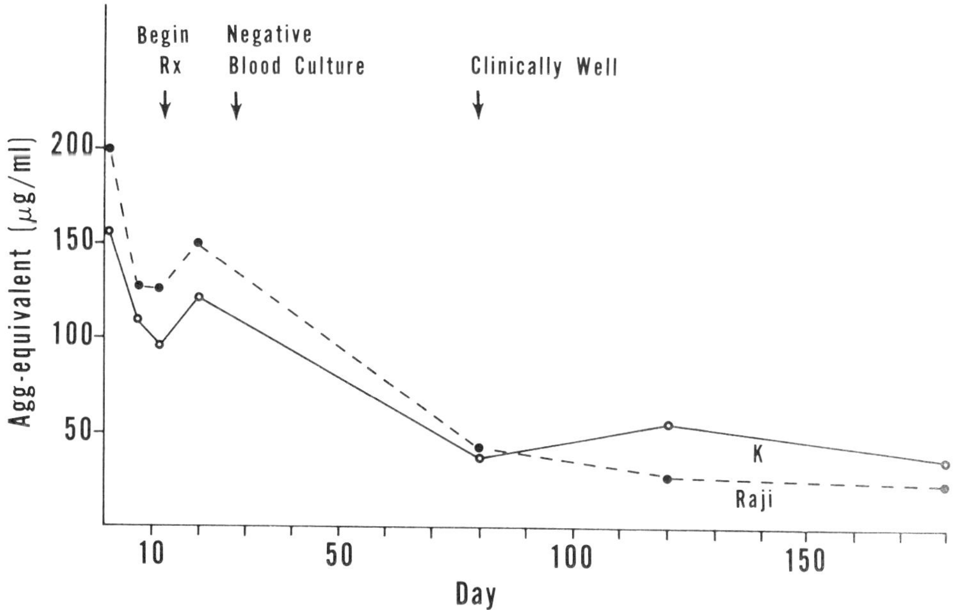

Figure 6-7 Parallel determinations of circulating immune complexes in a patient with Candida endocarditis, using the Raji-cell and conglutinin-binding (K) methods. (Reproduced with permission, R. A. Eisenberg, A. N. Theofilopoulos, and F. J. Dixon, *J. Immunol.* 118:1428, 1977.)

parallel methods for detecting immune complexes was made, utilizing serial or concurrent data collected from a number of primary laboratories in many parts of the world. After an analysis of the data presented, it was clear that in a variety of conditions (including various parasitic infections, SLE, and cancer) when a number of methods were compared, there were discrepancies in both sensitivity and positivity. The cumulative results of this study have now been published (51). It is currently recommended that at least two and possibly three methods be used concurrently and in parallel for immune-complex detection in any clinical series of subjects studied. We use a modification of the solid-phase C1q radioimmunoassay originally devised by Hay and associates (38) and, in parallel, the radioimmunoassay Raji-cell technique described by Theofilopoulos and co-workers (44). The combination is still not completely ideal, as it does not detect non-complement-fixing complexes or those primarily composed of IgA antibodies.

A further modification of the solid-phase conglutinin-binding assay was introduced by Casali and co-workers (50), with the use of enzyme-conjugated anti-immunoglobulin antibody. This particular method has great appeal. It is rapid and utilizes an enzymatic reaction product to measure the reaction of anti-immunoglobulin antibody to immunoglobulin in the complexes bound to conglutinin coated as the solid-phase reagent to the tube. In this particular modification the advantage for widespread laboratory use is that a radioactive element counter is not required. A colorimetric reaction for measurement of the enzyme product is utilized for complex quantitation.

A diagrammatic representation of this solid-phase enzyme immunoassay, similar to the ELISA assay originally described by Engvall and Perlmann (51), is shown in Figure 6-8. Using this method, the Casali group (50) found that complexes of large size, such as those formed in antigen excess, were more efficiently bound than those of smaller size. The exceptional stability of bovine conglutinin, which allows for long-term storage, and the excellent reproducibility of this technique are

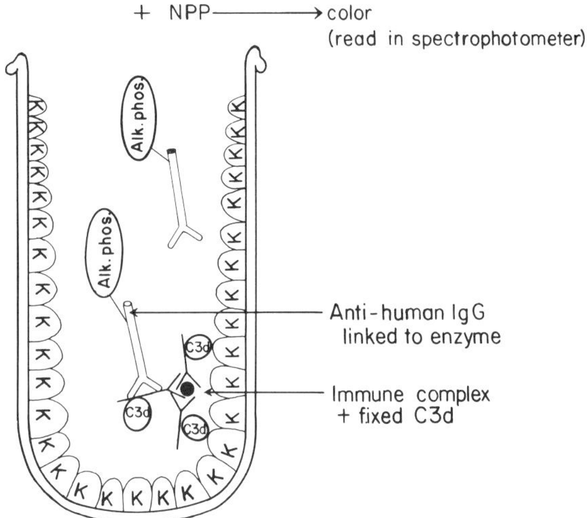

Figure 6-8   Solid-phase ELISA assay for immune complexes. Bovine conglutinin (K) is bound to the plastic tube and in turn reacts with activated C3d affixed to immune complexes. Antihuman IgG linked to alkaline phosphatase is subsequently added, and when the chemical reagent NPP is added, a color develops and can be related by parallel standard curves to the amounts of complexes bound.

distinct advantages. In addition, long-term cultivation and the care necessary to maintain cell lines such as the Raji are not required. One theoretical disadvantage is that the assay might be disturbed when antigens containing large quantities of aceto-amido sugar moieties are present, since such sugars as n-acetyl-o-glucosamine can competitively inhibit binding of conglutinin (K) to fixed C3d (47). The K-binding test also can be used to detect complexes containing IgM; IgA complexes would require some activation of complement perhaps through the alternative complement pathway (52, 53), because fixed C3d is necessary for the reaction. Finally, the K-binding methods compare favorably with the Raji-cell radioimmunoassay or the various methods employing C1q binding in that they are capable of detecting aggregated IgG to levels of 3 μg/ml in undiluted human serum (50). Correlation of three tests used to detect immune complexes in the sera of patients with acute and chronic leukemia from the Casali study (50) is shown in Table 6-1.

Table 6-1 Correlation of three tests in human leukemia.

Patient groups	Test	Mean value[a] (± 1 s.d.)	t[b]	Percent positive	Correlation between all 3 tests, W[c]
Acute leukemia	KgB	8.4 ± 12.6	2.23∫	50	
(n = 16)	Raji-cell RIA	21.1 ± 24.5	2.45∫	56	0.58∫
	^{125}I-labeled C1q BA	4.1 ± 6.8	2.28∫	38	
Chronic leukemia	KgB	4.9 ± 5.7	1.71	50	
(n = 8)	Raji-cell RIA	11.2 ± 12.6	1.17	25	0.70∫
	^{125}I-labeled C1q BA	1.4 ± 2.1	1.44	13	
Total	KgB	7.2 ± 10.7	2.65∫	50	
(n = 24)	Raji-cell RIA	17.8 ± 21.4	2.64∫	46	0.49∫
	^{125}I-labeled C1q BA	3.2 ± 5.7	2.48∫	29	

Source: Reproduced with permission, P. Casali, A. Bossus, A. Nicole et al., *Clin. Exp. Immunol.* 29:342, 1977.

[a] The mean values ± 1 s.d. for the group of healthy donors (n = 30) were as follows: KgB, 1.4 ± 0.8 (AHG μg ea/ml); Raji-cell RIA, 5.5 ± 3.2 (AHG μg eq/min); ^{125}I-labeled C1q BA, 0.2 ± 1.4 (percent of specific ^{125}I-labeled C1q precipitated).

[b] The discrimination between patient groups and the group of healthy donors was assayed by the Student's t-test (for populations with unequal variances).

[c] W = Kendall's coefficient of concordance. All the values within normal range are given the same rank order.

∫ $p < 0.05$.

Rheumatoid Factors

The use of IgM rheumatoid factors for detection of immune complexes represents one of the earliest approaches to the characterization of materials present in sera and synovial fluids from patients with rheumatoid arthritis, SLE, and other connective tissue diseases (7, 32–39). Monoclonal rheumatoid factors in particular have received considerable attention, since many react preferentially with complexed immunoglobulins but not with monomeric subunits or native IgG. One distinct advantage in the use of monoclonal IgM rheumatoid factors is that they may be capable of detecting both complement-fixing and noncomplement-fixing complexes over a wide range of molecular size. This principle has been adapted to several radioimmunoassay procedures (54, 55) and appears to offer a precise assay system when used with carefully standardized techniques. In the study reported by Gabriel and Agnello (55) initial heating of the serum to inactivate complement was not required, and complexes were detected by inhibition of binding of ^{125}I-labeled monoclonal IgM rheumatoid factor to insolubilized IgG linked to Sepharose beads. This assay was most useful in detecting complexes containing human or rabbit IgG because of the inherent specificity present in most of these human IgM monoclonal anti-γ-globulins. A sensitivity of 0.5 μg/ml for human aggregates was demonstrated. However, some degree of interference by monomeric IgG was observed, particularly in sera with high levels of IgG (55).

Widespread use of monoclonal rheumatoid factors for immune-complex detection will undoubtedly be limited by availability of such reagents in the routine clinical laboratory and perhaps by difficulties related to standardization among various laboratories. Another problem is inherent in each individual monoclonal rheumatoid factor employed; each may have unique specificities against particular γ-globulin conformational determinants, which may not be shared by similar but nonidentical monoclonal IgM anti-immunoglobulins. On the other hand, by using such naturally occurring anti-immunoglobulin reagents, it is theoretically possible to detect immune complexes composed primarily of IgA. In addition, monoclonal IgM rheumatoid factors show great sensitivity for immune complexes of relatively low molecular weight (9 to 11 S) and probably are more sensitive in this regard than the Raji-cell radioimmunoassay technique.

A further modification of the general principle utilized in rheumatoid factor assays has recently been introduced by Lurhuma and associates (56). Human rheumatoid factors from several sources as well as C1q were compared in inhibition reactions using Ig-coated particles. This particular assay appeared to be extremely sensitive; in some sera, inhibition of particle agglutination by C1q could only be demonstrated after endogenous rheumatoid-factor–like agglutinizing activity was absorbed out with insolubilized IgG. Whether or not such a system provides an accurate semiquantitative method for estimation of immune complexes remains to be seen. One inherent problem, similar to that discussed in relation to the use of monoclonal rheumatoid factors introduced by Agnello and co-workers (7, 29, 32), is the differing specificities of individual preparations or lots of rheumatoid factor. In comparison with the precision and well-defined accuracy of such methods as the K-binding or C1q-binding tests discussed above, the latter are more available to the average laboratory and still afford accurate and quantitative estimations of the presence of various types of complexes.

Identification of Antigen

One of the key problems already mentioned in this chapter relates to identification of antigen within presumed antigen-antibody complexes. We have been vexed on several occasions by inability to detect antigen directly using immunofluorescence and heterologous antigen-specific antibodies on the Raji-cell surface, where IgG and C3 components of presumed complexes are also easily identified. A possible explanation for these difficulties may be that antigens in circulating immune complexes are relatively buried or covered up by a variety of other immunologic reactants, including af-

fixed immunoglobulin molecules or adherent activated complement components (Figure 6-9).

One approach, suggested by Milgrom and associates (57), may be of considerable use in particular circumstances where tissues are available and there is already some insight into the putative antigens involved. This procedure has been applied in immune-complex nephritis where kidney tissues were minced, washed, and soaked in an agarose or agar plate. Separation of immune complexes was achieved by electrophoresis at 56° C and antibody was readily detected thereafter by means of anti-IgG antisera and high-velocity electrophoresis (58). After initial electrophoresis in the case of lupus kidney material, it was noted that additional counterimmunoelectrophoresis was necessary to identify DNA in the immune deposits. These studies emphasize the difficulties in antigen identification both in tissue deposits and within circulating immune aggregates.

Similar approaches have been tried, particularly in the case of sera from patients with SLE, using DNase digestion in an attempt to dissociate antibody from its complexed antigen. Reports of increase in residual DNA binding capacity after presumed enzymatic digestion of complexed antigen (59) have suggested this as another possible indirect way of identifying antigens; however, the general method has not proved to be very reproducible, and considerably more direct approaches are needed. One that appears to hold great promise employs in-

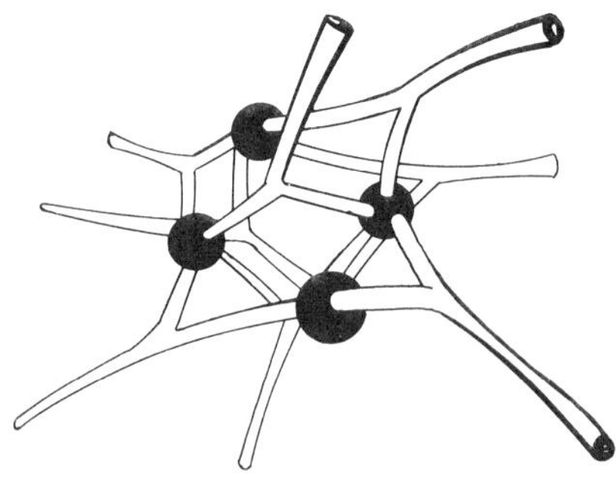

Figure 6-9   Antigen molecules (●) relatively buried or covered up by IgG antibody molecules in an immune complex.

itial concentration of immune complexes themselves, obtained from positive sera by precipitation with polyethylene glycol, and subsequent radiolabeling of this material followed by analysis on SDS polyacrylamide gels. Bands related to putative antigen can then be distinguished from those of the constituent heavy and light chains of immune-complex immunoglobulins.

Cryoglobulins and Cryoprecipitation

For some time the phenomenon of cryoprecipitation of materials out of solution in serum has been linked to possible presence of immune complexes. The original recognition of cryoprecipitation was recorded some years ago by Wintrobe and Buell and later by Lerner and colleagues (60, 61). A good deal of attention was focused initially on the physical properties and temperature amplitude of cryoprecipitates found in serum, as well as their relation to monoclonal M components in the serum itself. Cryoglobulins that occurred in the presence of IgM, IgA, or IgG M components were described, plus those formed by complexes between IgM and IgG (62). Other cold-precipitable plasma proteins distinct from immunoglobulins have been recognized and include cryofibrinogens, C-reactive protein-albumin complexes, a heparin-precipitable protein apparently related to fibrinogen, and a nonclotting component of Cohn fraction I-1 from normal pooled serum (63). Precipitation of cryoglobulins out of solution in serum kept at 4° C may not be as unusual as originally thought, particularly when 50-ml aliquots of blood are studied. In one survey mixed IgM-IgG cryoprecipitates were detected in 25 of 49 normal sera, and in 16 of these mixed cryoprecipitates rheumatoid-factor activity was detected (64). Quantitative amounts of cryoprecipitate recorded in normal sera during this study varied between 10 and 80 μg/ml. Thus, trace amounts of cryoprecipitate are frequently noted in normal serum samples.

If plasma is examined instead of serum, a considerable precipitate, usually composed of fibrinogen-related materials, is noted after storage at 4° C for a period of several days.

Many physical and chemical factors are capable of modulating the cryoprecipitation of immunoglobulins. Among these are pH, ionic strength, protein concentration, and temperature range. For some time cryoglobulins were regarded as unusual phenomena that appeared to be related to peculiar features of certain monoclonal or polyclonal immunoglobulins. Experiments conducted by Zinneman and colleagues (65) indicated that the IgG in cryoglobulins lacked sialic acid. Whether this deficiency is a property of all cryoimmunoglobulin IgG proteins has not been elucidated. Rather than being an odd experiment of nature, cryoglobulinemia may be a model for similar occurrences in immune complexes associated with disease of still obscure or unknown etiology. One of the intriguing aspects of many carefully studied cryoglobulins is that anti-γ-globulin or rheumatoid-factor–like activity has been found in a large proportion. That this is the case in the mixed cryoglobulinemia syndrome is quite easy to demonstrate from the monoclonal IgM M component from such cryoprecipitates.

Distinct anti-IgG antibody activity has been described in human monoclonal IgG cryoglobulins as well (66). When the actual binding forces between the monoclonal IgM rheumatoid-factor component and the autologous IgG have been measured, as reported by Stone and Metzger (67), relatively low values of 5.4 to 6.9 $\times$ 10^4 liters/m were recorded. This binding value is quite low compared with the equilibrium constants of 10^6 to 10^8 commonly observed in rabbit hapten-antihapten systems (68).

The frequent occurrence of anti-γ-globulin reactivities in many cryoglobulin components remains a feature of great interest. In view of the relatively low binding constants for what is felt to be their primary antigen—namely, structures on the Fc portion of human IgG—one must wonder whether the reactivity for human IgG actually represents a cross-reaction of antibody directed initially at some other undefined antigen. The studies conducted by Eisen, Richards, and their co-workers (69–71) on "strange" cross-reactions, or possible polyfunctional antibody combining sites, are noteworthy when one considers the evidence that has accumulated regarding cryoglobulin precipitates and specific disease states, such as poststreptococcal glomerulonephritis, persistent hepatitis B infection, or infective endocarditis. While specific antibodies have been sought with relation to the disease state, very little evidence has accumulated to date for such antibodies being concentrated or enriched in cryoglobulin precipitates; in a remarkable number of instances, antibody activity showing rheumatoid-factor–like reactions has been found (72, 73). In a patient with distinct serum cryoglobulins in association with acute poststreptococcal glomerulonephritis (74) or in the instance of cryoglobulins found in renal disease presumed to be the result of deposition of staphylococcal-antigen-antibody complexes (75), no evidence for selective concentration of antibacterial antibodies was detected. More recently, similar studies in patients with infective endocarditis by Hurwitz and co-workers (76) showed no apparent selective concentrations of antibacterial antibodies in cryoglobulin precipitates. On the other hand, the finding of hepatitis-B related viral material in serum cryoprecipitates provides some evidence for presence of presumptive antigen in cryoprecipitates (77). In addition, concentration of anti-DNA and DNA has been convincingly demonstrated in cryoprecipitates from patients with SLE (78).

Despite some difficulty in being able to identify known antigen or enrichment of specific antibody, cryoprecipitates (particularly those in the form of mixed cryoglobulins) are felt by many to represent relatively insoluble antigen-antibody complexes. Support for this view can be detected from early studies showing many constituents within such mixed cryoglobulin precipitates that were presumed to be derived from immune complexes, including rheumatoid factors and the C1q component of complement (79–81).

The biologic properties of cryoglobulins from selected sera have also been studied by McIntosh and associates (82, 83). When injected intradermally into guinea pigs, cryoglobulins from patients with poststreptococcal nephritis caused a local inflammatory re-

sponse. When infused intravenously into rabbits, they produced a mild nephritis presumably distinct from that caused by other foreign proteins. These experiments might be explained on the basis of local activation of the inflammatory mechanisms if such cryoglobulin precipitates contained aggregated IgG material; however, their potential biologic importance is suggested in the demonstration by Whitsed and Penney (84) that purpuric cutaneous lesions in a patient with IgA-IgG cryoglobulinemia could be produced in the same patient by intradermal injection of minute amounts of his own cryoglobulin.

At present it is reasonable to suggest that the occurrence of cryoglobulins in various disorders is suggestive evidence that immune complexes are present. Factors governing the quantitative estimation and analysis of cryoglobulin precipitates have been critically reviewed by Weisman and Zvaifler (85), with particular attention to clinical significance in the vasculitis of rheumatoid arthritis. These authors very properly pointed out that conditions of the cryoglobulin determinations had varied considerably from one laboratory to another, so that comparisons of many of the data in the literature are not valid. The conditions suggested by Weisman and Zvaifler were 72-hour incubation of serum sample at 4° C, resuspension of cryoprecipitate to a final volume of 1 ml per 5 ml of starting serum, and expression of all protein amounts as concentration per final 1 ml of solution.

To anyone who has actually worked with cryoprecipitates, the sequence of procedure and careful analytic technique offered by Weisman and Zvaifler will be extremely useful. If cryoglobulins are left to stand at 4° C for too long (over 72 hours or up to a week) they are quite difficult to resolubilize and reactive components of most interest to the clinician or clinical immunologist are irreversibly lost through aggregation or denaturation. Loss of antibody activity in the face of extreme changes in pH encountered during efforts to resolubilize cryoprecipitates is also appropriately discussed. It is evident that if formation of cryoglobulins is to be utilized as a rough index for the presence of circulating complexes, some degree of uniformity and standardization of the procedure must be established.

Detection by Changes in Size or Molecular Behavior

One of the earliest suggestions that changes in size of reactants might be involved in the formation of immune complexes was in the initial description and interaction of 19 S IgM rheumatoid factor (86, 87). Sera from patients with rheumatoid arthritis showed presence of high-molecular weight IgM anti-γ-globulins capable of forming 22 S complexes with autologous or native 7 S IgG. A variety of later studies extended this reactivity to other antigen-antibody complexes by showing the heterogeneity of reactions between IgM anti-γ-globulins and many antigenic sites on 7 S IgG itself.

Work on the 7 S IgG rheumatoid factors was initiated when it was found that so-called intermediate complexes observed during analytical ultracentrifugation of various hypergamma-globulinemic sera (4, 5) could be dissociated by treatment with acidic buffers. The intermediate complexes occurring in these sera showed dramatic shifts in molecular size and appearance during analytical ultracentrifugal analysis, so that it was recognized quite early that immune complexes might produce rather major alterations in the physical profile and behavior of individual reactants. An example of the physical behavior of such self-associating IgG rheumatoid factors or anti-γ-globulins present as 11 S complexes in a patient with hyperviscosity syndrome is shown in Figure 6-10.

Many of the changes in molecular weight of immune reactants in various disease states are not as gross or obvious as was suggested in the initial analytical ultracentrifuge studies of 19 S and 7 S anti-γ-globulins. Actually, ultracentrifugal determination is a rather crude method of analysis of ordinary serum samples for immune complexes, since the concentration of reactants must be high in order for the peaks to be adequately visualized (0.5 to 2.0 mg/ml), and only major degrees of association or disassociation are apparent during an analytic run. The advantage of ultracentrifugal analysis is,

of course, that certain mass types of reactions or complexes can be directly visualized during the course of the experiment. However, changes in apparent molecular size and distribution of reactants have provided useful information under a number of conditions to support the impression that an immune-complex reaction has indeed occurred. In some instances this has involved positive findings for complex reactive material in a size distribution larger than that expected within the normal serum profile. Material such as C3, normally appearing in lower-molecular-weight regions in serum separation profiles, may be detected in high-molecular-weight distributions, for instance—presumably as part of an antigen-antibody complex binding activated C3. Figure 6-11 shows sample data where size distribution changes after various methods of physical separation of serum fractions have indicated probable presence of complexes.

In the serum samples from patients with hepatitis B infection studied by Theofilopoulos and colleagues (44), the HB_s antigen occurred in 7 to 8 S distribution in the serum of the carrier, but was found in association with C3 in high-molecular-weight fractions from serum samples collected from a patient with acute hepatitis B. The finding of a distribution shift of both antigen and bound C3 (presumably) in this serum supported the fact that high-molecular-weight immune complexes containing both HB_s-Ag and activated C3 were present in this sample. Similarly, in a study by Hodgson and co-workers (89), a shift toward what was felt to be anticomplementary activity in regions of serum gel filtration associated with high-molecular-weight IgG was used as presumptive evidence for the presence of immune complexes in these fractions. One of the problems inherent in analysis of changes in size distribution of reactants in serum samples separated by gel filtration, sucrose gradient ultracentrifugation, or other physical techniques is the distinct possibility of in vitro formation of aggregates of IgG after the fractionation procedures have been completed. Nevertheless, changes in physical behavior and size distribution of individual reactants supporting the presence of immune complexes represent important evi-

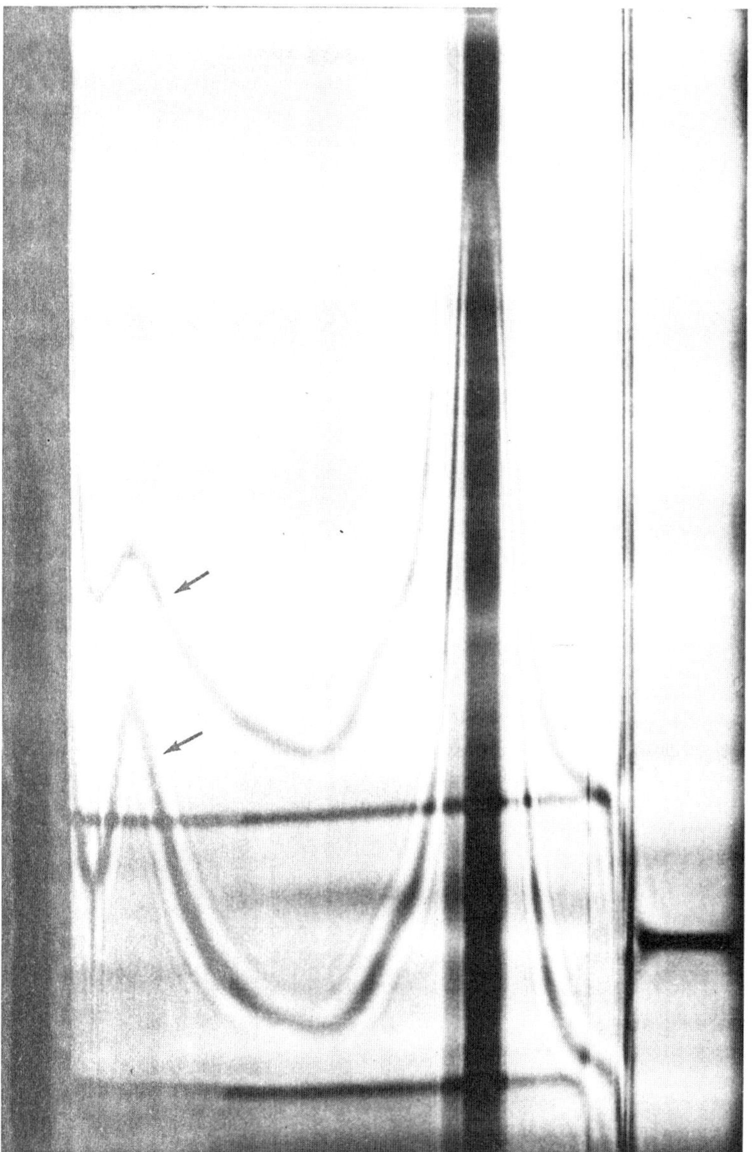

Figure 6-10 The ultracentrifugal pattern of serum samples with large quantities of 9 to 17S intermediate complexes. Direction of sedimentation is from right to left. The serum in the upper frame shows the smaller quantity of intermediate complexes, marked by arrows.

dence for their presence in various assay situations.

Miscellaneous Assays

One method suggested by the work of Jewell and MacLennan (90) involved inhibition of antibody-dependent cell-mediated cytotoxicity, or the so-called K-cell system. In this assay inhibition of killing of target cells by killer cells was measured and related to the presence of aggregates or immune complexes in an in vitro system. The rationale of this method is shown diagramatically in Figure 6-12. The same approach has recently been utilized by Feldmann and co-workers (91) in an attempt to measure immune complexes in patients with autoimmune and connective-tissue diseases. Our own experience (92, 93) indicates that the test may be influenced directly or indirectly by the presence of anti-γ-globulin factors and by simultaneous presence of antibodies to lymphocytes.

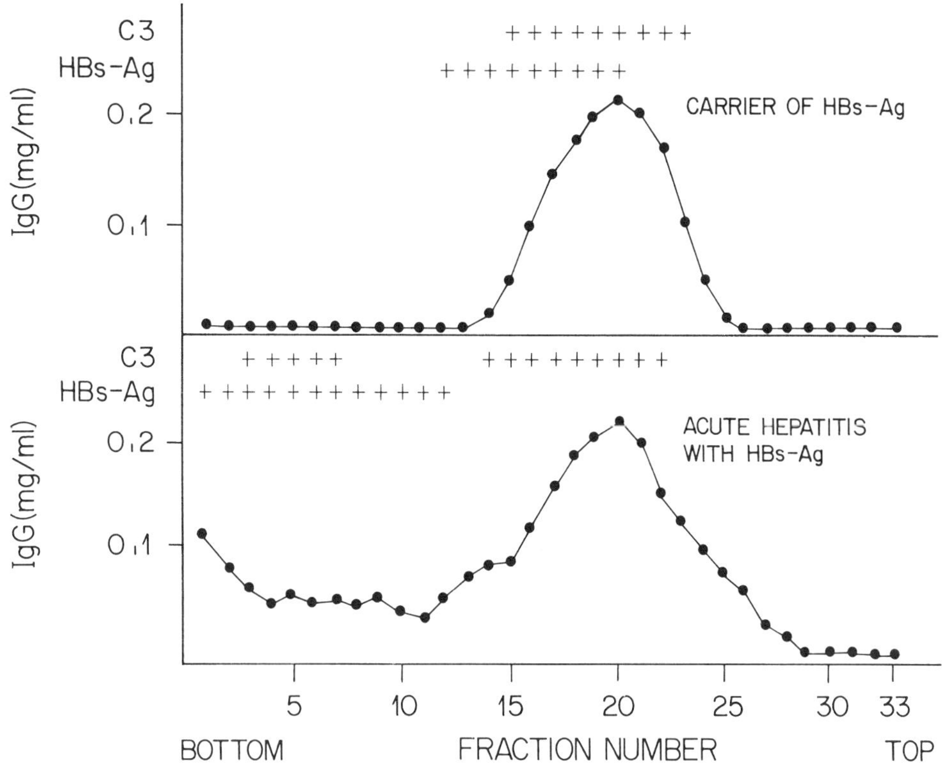

Figure 6-11 Sucrose density gradient fractionation of sera from an asymptomatic carrier of HG_s-Ag negative for immune complexes (*above*) and a patient with acute hepatitis and HB_s-Ag having immune complexes (*below*). Fractions in which C3 and HB_s-Ag were detected are shown (+) at the top of each panel. The distribution of IgG in each fraction is also indicated (●—●). (Reproduced with permission, A. N. Theofilopoulos, C. B. Wilson, and F. J. Dixon, *J. Clin. Invest.* 57:169, 1976.)

The latter may bind directly with the lymphoid K cell, or anti-γ-globulins may react either with the immune complexes present in the test serum or with the IgG used to sensitize the labeled target cells. The problem of inference by antibodies to lymphocytes was particularly troublesome in the case of sera from patients with SLE (92). Assay by inhibition of cell-mediated cytotoxicity is therefore fraught with difficulty, both in interpretation and in standardization, and it is not recommended for routine use.

It has long been recognized that protein A of the staphylococcus shows the capacity for binding to immunoglobulins—particularly IgG of IgG-1, 2, and 4 H-chain subclasses (94–96). There is recent additional evidence that binding may occur with subgroups of IgA and IgM (97, 98). However, IgG appears to be the major immunoglobulin class participating in the reaction. The binding of protein A occurs through an interaction of the staphylococcal protein and the Fc portion of gamma globulins. No protein A is bound to pepsin-digested IgG; the reaction is particularly convenient because it does not involve reactivity with F(ab′)_2 areas involved in the antibody combining regions.

Immune-complex assays utilizing the specific reactivity between Fc of IgG and protein A have recently been described by Farrell and associates (99). Their test utilized solid-phase C1q and ^{32}P-labeled, protein A–rich *Staphylococcus aureus* organisms as an indicator system. The assay detected high-molecular-weight IgG aggregates (19 to 25 S) at concentrations down to 8 μg/ml. Initial results with this particular assay showed that identification of complexes depended on both the degree of IgG polymer-

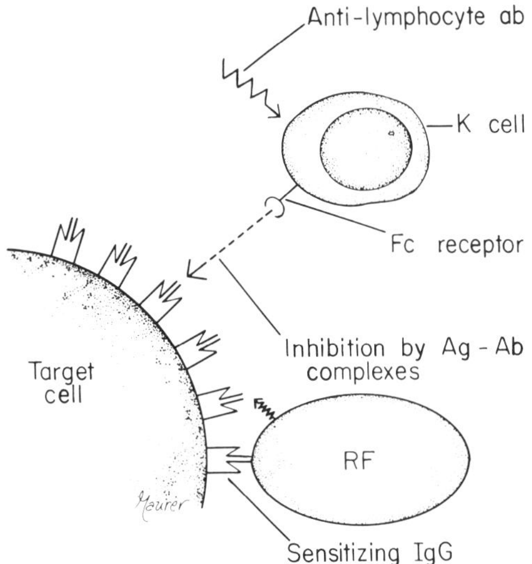

Figure 6-12 An antibody-mediated lymphocytoxicity system, mediated by the killer K-cell bearing Fc receptors. Inhibition of this reaction may be induced by antigen-antibody complexes reacting with K-cell Fc receptors. The reaction may also be blocked if rheumatoid factor (RF) is present, since the latter can react directly with the IgG coating the sensitized target cell.

ization and the molar ratios achieved between C1q linked to the polystyrene assay tubes and the reactive IgG polymers. Thus when C1q was present in very high concentration, a decrease in binding index was recorded. The sensitivity of the assay system was also affected to a certain extent by the age of the ^{32}P-labeled bacterial cells used as indicator reagent, since some elution or loss of radioactivity was noted after storage for several weeks. Despite these potential problems, the use of protein A either as a Coombs-type reagent or in other aspects of the assay of immune complexes holds great promise. Ease of use and avidity of binding of protein A for IgG, particularly in polymeric form, are positive features. One disadvantage inherent in the reaction itself is absence of reactivity with the monomers or aggregates of the IgG-3 H-chain subclass (96). However, the protein A method has recently been adapted by McDougal and associates for assay of clinical samples (100). Because of the capacity of protein A to bind to IgG through multipoint attachment, complexed IgG was favored over monomeric

IgG binding. This particular adaptation was not complement dependent, but was affected by presence of rheumatoid factors.

A new method that shows considerable promise has been described by Levinsky and Soothill (101), using heterologous IgM antibody made in rabbits against specific human IgG, IgA, or IgM immunoglobulins. The specific immunoglobulins were then coated on latex particles, and the rabbit IgM agglutinating antibodies were used in a direct agglutination reaction. Immune complexes were tested for their ability to inhibit this reaction; of interest was the finding that monomeric immunoglobulins did not produce inhibition. Semiquantitative estimates of immune complexes were made by electronically counting residual unagglutinated latex particles, indicating that automation and therefore rapid assays might be feasible. In addition, a method of linking antigens to latex particles was introduced via DNP coupling. Decomplementation was achieved using EDTA–sigma cell–IgG adsorption previously employed with other methods. During the studies by Lurhuma and co-workers (56), it had been noted that C1q from fresh normal sera was capable of inhibiting IgG-coated latex agglutination by rheumatoid factor. The C1q released after incubation of serum with EDTA agglutinated such particles, but after absorption with IgG-coated sigma cell, no agglutination was observed. The method proposed by Levinsky was said to be capable of removing intrinsic rheumatoid factor that might result in false positive agglutination. One feature that is still a possible deficiency in this system is that removal of rheumatoid factor in any serum containing immune complexes may actually absorb out complexes bound to such rheumatoid factor. Wider experience and application are necessary before any final judgment of the eventual applicability of this technique can be made.

Immune complexes presumably composed of IgA were detected in the Levinsky study, in the serum from a patient with Henoch-Schönlein nephritis. In this instance gel filtration of serum fractions showed IgA-containing complexes in the 2.5 to 4.0×10^6 and the 4.0 to 8.0×10^6 molecular weight ranges. This test appears to satisfy many requirements of a rapid, reproducible assay capable of adaptability for testing immunoglobulin class, size, and intrinsic constituents of immune complexes. Further analysis and comparison with other methods currently in use will provide a definitive answer on its eventual usefulness.

Measurement by Indirect Techniques

One of the most consistent consequences of the in vivo formation of immune complexes during experimental conditions or in human disease states is activation of the complement sequence. Inhibition of complement-dependent lymphocyte rosette formation (102) has been suggested as a method for assay of immune complexes in some clinical situations. Since certain populations of normal human lymphocytes show distinct C3 receptors, inhibition of rosettes formed between cells coated with IgM antibody and activated C3 components (including C3) may be used as a measure of free activated C3 components bound to immune complexes in serum. Although such an assay could be used in conjunction with other more direct methods, it has the obvious failing of not differentiating unambiguously between free activated C3 components and those bound to antigen-antibody complexes.

Another indirect but extremely useful technique involves the measurement of total hemolytic complement (CH 50) activity of serum in conjunction with assessment of the general profile of complement component levels and hemolytic activity. Quantitative estimates in addition to direct functional assays for multiple complement components are usually beyond the technical capacity or expertise of the average clinical laboratory. On the other hand, total hemolytic complement activity as well as quantitative radial diffusion estimates of complement components such as C3, C3PA, C1, and C4 have now become technically feasible and available on a large-scale basis. Indications of generalized, conventional or alternate pathway, or alternate pathway alone, can be gained from quantitative radial diffusion measurements of complement component concentrations in serum during many acute clinical dis-

orders. It is important to recognize that quantitative depressions of levels of *antigens* detected by antisera to C3, C3PA, or C4 reflect the levels of antigenic determinants of these particular molecules in serum at a given time. Such estimates cannot be directly related to presumed levels of *functional* complement component activity. This is a very important point that cannot be emphasized strongly enough.

Many disorders associated with apparent clear-cut acute complement consumption and tissue deposition of immune-complex materials are involved with antigen-antibody reaction; however, hypercatabolism or deficiency in production of complement components must also be considered. In order to study the influence of these particular governing factors, trace-labeled purified complement components can be measured serially for disappearance or distribution between vascular and extravascular compartments, and for some indication of consumption or hypercatabolism as well as decreased synthesis. Such assays require sophisticated techniques and the availability of highly purified complement components or cofactors, and they are not feasible in the average clinical laboratory. Likewise, complement activation proceeding mostly through the properdin pathway may be associated with quantitative reduction of antigens as detected in immunochemical determinations of C3 and C3PA—to a greater extent perhaps than changes in measured antigenic concentrations of C1 or C4 (Table 6-2). However, concentrations of antigens related to C3 and as detected by antisera made in rabbits to isolated whole native C3 show varying amounts of antibodies to the important C3 breakdown products—C3b, C3d, and C3c. As mentioned in Chapter 1, useful clinical information focusing on this point can now be gained through an elegant but simple manipulation that employs polyethylene glycol precipitation to remove C3b (35,000 M.W.) and C3c (150,000 M.W.). The quantitative amounts of residual C3d (35,000 M.W.) can then be estimated with the same anti–whole C3 antiserum, provided this antiserum contains antibodies specific for determinants unique to C3d (103). Since C3 activator

Table 6-2 Complement component profiles in immune-complex disease.

Profile noted	Comment
↓ CH 50 total hemolytic C	May represent consumption or hypercatabolism by immune reactants; may also reflect isolated (inherited) C component deficiency or lack of C synthesis.
↓ C3 ↓ C1 ↓ C4 ↓ C3PA	Profile most often recognized with primarily conventional C pathway consumption.
↓ C3 C1N; C4N; ↓ C3PA	Profile associated with alternate C pathway activation.

cleaves C3b to C3c and C3d, this technique affords additional insight into whether low levels of C3 may be occurring as a feature of conventional complement pathway consumption or by consumption through the alternate pathway as well.

Studies of the possible effects of immune complexes on activation of the complement cascade have also been greatly facilitated by use of the two-dimensional agarose gel system. This particular approach has proved of great practical utility in analyzing various patterns of complement activation, for instance, in studies of synovial fluids from patients with various connective-tissue diseases (104, 105).

Analyses of CH 50, together with complement components, by simultaneous measurement of functional activity and protein content may prove helpful in an indirect assessment of apparent immune-complex activation. The study reported by Rynes and colleagues (106) on levels of complement components and properdin factors in patients with inflammatory arthritides is directly relevant. However, it was noted that protein measurements in localized body compartments often included antigenically intact, nonfunctional protein as well as native complement components. Therefore determination of complement component antigens alone, particularly by radial diffusion techniques, did not accurately reflect complement depressions. The functional significance of local body space complement levels has recently been emphasized in a study of heat-labile opsonic activity and complement levels associated with evidence of C3 breakdown products in patients with infected pleural effu-

sions (107). Hemolytic activity of complement (CH 50) and levels of C3d were measured in sera and pleural fluid samples, and in additional patients with pleural effusions of the same etiology. Effusions with positive cultures showed lower CH 50 values and higher C3d values compared to culture-negative pleural fluids. In addition, levels of immune complexes in pleural effusions as measured by the C1q binding assay were considerably higher in culture-positive effusions. Of interest was the fact that opsonic activity showed a positive correlation with CH 50 titers for all fluids tested. These results appeared to indicate that one important reason for bacterial persistence in empyema may be decreased opsonization of bacteria secondary to local complement consumption.

There has also been recent interest in the possible fundamental importance of regulatory complement proteins. In a study of renal biopsies from patients with a variety of immune-type renal diseases, Carlo and colleagues (108) demonstrated deposits of $\beta 1H$ in every instance (21 of 21 biopsies) in which C3 deposits were identified irrespective of the underlying renal disease. In no instance was $\beta 1H$ found independently of C3. Since $\beta 1H$ binds to C3 (presumably C3b) during activation of the complement system, it is possible that intrinsic local $\beta 1H$ activity may contribute substantially to the degree of local tissue destruction. The $\beta 1H$ binding to C3b accelerates the decay of alternative pathway convertases by displacing factor B (109). It is conceivable that basic alterations in control or modulating proteins such as $\beta 1H$ may ultimately play a major role in local tissue injury initiated by complexes activating the complement system.

In summary, many methods, both direct and indirect, have proved useful in identifying immune complexes in various clinical and experimental disease states. At the present time there is no single or universal method immediately suitable for identification of all sizes and all types of the immunoglobulin components that make up the wide spectrum of complexes participating in human immune reactions. Of greatest importance is what might be regarded as the mirror-image phenomenon—that is, the complexes measured in serum or circulating plasma may not be the ones that are actually producing tissue damage or those of the most fundamental importance. Many of the methods used to measure immune complexes are time consuming and intricate, or require precise attention to details of standardization and reproducibility. However, there are now several well-tested assays that show great accuracy and sensitivity. Whether or not carefully timed studies utilizing some of these assays will provide us with precise insight into the disorders associated with immune-complex–mediated lesions remains to be seen. What is happening in vulnerable microcapillary beds such as the retina, the glomerulus, or the choroid plexus may be a great deal different than what is detected as circulating complexes in serial serum samples. A summary of the methods

useful in establishing the presence of immune complexes in tissue is shown in Table 6-3, and methods for detection of circulating immune complexes are given in Table 6-4. The lists represent only a partial catalogue of recently developed procedures; new and perhaps improved techniques are constantly being introduced into the armamentarium of the clinical immunologist and practicing physician.

Demonstration of complexes deposited in tissues represents one of the most well established and widely accepted criteria for immune-complex participation in the pathogenesis of specific disease states. Beside lumpy-bumpy deposition of Ig, C components, and antigen and electron-dense deposits identified by ultrastructural studies, several other demonstrations of tissue-bound immune complexes have furnished practical assistance to their precise identification in lesions. One new technique, which has not yet been widely applied but which appears to have great promise as a rapid and direct aid for visualizing both antibody and antigen, is the use of peroxidase-conjugated antibody (110, 111) to either immunoglobulin and complement or specific antigens. The most important advantage is that this method can be utilized with tissues that have previously been fixed and embedded for routine histological examination. So often immune mechanisms are considered in a particular case after death, when frozen sections or fresh biopsy material are no longer available.

Table 6-3 Methods for detection of immune complexes in tissues.

Method	Comments
Immunofluorescence localization of immunoglobulin, C, and antigen	Lumpy-bumpy or granular distribution, particularly in glomerulus.
Electron microscopic localization	Electron-dense deposits in subepithelial distribution.
Peroxidase-conjugated antibody	Brown staining in conjunction with tissue distribution of enzyme reaction product.
Extraction of tissue by heat, elution using dissociating agents, or electrophoresis into gels	Most definitive proof of specific relative concentration of antibody as compared to serum levels.

Table 6-4 Direct methods for detection of complexes in serum or body fluids.

Method	Comments
Anticomplementary activity of serum	May be falsely positive in hyper-gammaglobulinemic sera because of *in vitro* aggregate formation.
Platelet aggregation	Requires viable platelets; aggregation not induced by actual cross-linking involving complexes; inhibited by IgM anti-IgG rheumatoid factor.
Binding to C1q	
(a) C1q precipitation in gels	Sensitive; some antigens react directly with gel and do not diffuse properly.
(b) C1q binding using ^{125}IC1q or C1q fixed in solid phase	Extremely sensitive (3 to 5 μg/ml); can be made more specific using solid-phase C1q or polyethylene glycol precipitation. C1q may react directly in *nonimmune* fasion with DNA, endotoxin, or bacterial polysaccharides.
Inhibition of uptake of ^{125}I by guinea pig macrophages	May be facilitated by anti-γ-globulins; no assurance that antilymphocyte antibodies do not interfere.
Raji cell	Sensitive (5 to 25 μg/ml), but tends to show preferential binding to larger complexes ($>$ 11 S). May be influenced by antilymphocyte antibodies. Requires continuous culture or availability of cell lines.
Binding to bovine conglutinin (K)	Extremely sensitive (5 μg/ml); requires activation of C and bound C3d; not affected by DNA, bacterial polysaccharides, or antilymphocyte antibody (may be inhibited by aceto-amido sugars).
Rheumatoid factor	Can be used as monoclonal M component in solid-phase radioimmunoassay; reacts with small as well as large complexes; does not require C activation by complexes; different RFs may show unique specificities; some inhibition by monomer IgG.
Cryoglobulin formation or cryoprecipitation	Useful as general screen. Unique and repeated association with rheumatoid factor activity. Occasionally shows specific concentration of antigen or antibody.
Bioassay	Complicated methodological procedure; unknown factors involved in results of assay.

Table 6-4 *(continued)*

Method	Comments
Changes in molecular size (gel filtration, gradient ultracentrifugation)	Simple and rapid; gives direct proof that complex has been formed; identification of antigen essential.
Complexing with protein A	Reaction rapid; influenced markedly by concentration of reactants; no reaction with IgG3 complexes or some IgA and IgM immunoglobulins.
Inhibition of agglutination of latex particles coated with immunoglobulins of known class	Using human rheumatoid factor, competition occurs with C1q; using rabbit IgM anti-immunoglobulin and prior EDTA decomplementation, procedure may have promise.

Until recently the technical problems inherent in accurate application of this technique to previously fixed and embedded tissues were significant enough that such materials were never used. But it now seems possible that peroxidase-conjugated antibody may prove extremely helpful in selected instances; more extensive application of the technique appears justified.

The evolution of a number of methods for determination of immune complexes was considered during a World Health Organization collaborative study (112). Eighteen methods for detection were compared based on interaction of immune complexes with C1q, conglutinin, rheumatoid factors, or complement or Fc receptors on cells. Certain methods clearly emerged as preferentially capable of immune-complex determination depending on the disorders tested. At present it is accurate to state that there is no single method that will suffice for assay of serum immune complexes in all clinical conditions. However, the information derived from the large number of assays included in this collaborative study has provided a good basis for comparison and analysis of future reports.

Finally, ultimate proof of the significance of immune complexes in individual lesions remains to be elucidated. If antigen and antibody can be demonstrated to be concentrated relative to serum in immune deposits within tissue, then their importance as major factors in the pathogenesis of lesions is obvious. Most of the convincing data in this regard have been derived from studies of tissue eluates using buffers or reagents that are capable of dissociating antigen-antibody complexes. Perhaps the most elegant and convincing evidence has come from the elution studies by Koffler and colleagues (113) and from Krishnan and Kaplan (114) in their research on the glomerulonephritis associated with SLE. Eluate from isolated glomeruli showed gamma-globulin components that were markedly enriched for antibodies to native DNA and to other nuclear antigens. Convincing evidence for relative enrichment of antibodies to DNA, as well as the presence of DNA antigen itself, was presented in these studies. Similar work is now needed in other disease states where immune complexes are felt to play a significant part in either pathogenesis or ultimate prognosis. In SLE nephritis, glomerular eluates are indeed quite appropriate, since many patients with this disorder die of progressive renal failure; techniques for elution of antibody from individual human glomeruli have been carefully worked out. In acute leukemia, however, where presence of circulating immune complexes has been demonstrated to have a direct bearing on prognosis (115), the problem of what tissues to elute and where to direct one's attention is more difficult.

As more and more diseases are associated with presence of immune-complex phenomena, increased understanding of possible biologic effects—beyond the microvascular circulation in the brain, glomerulus, or small peripheral arterioles—is needed. It seems possible that extravascular or third-compartment effects of immune-complex activation may be very important in a number of disease states. At the moment this particular aspect of the problem is poorly defined. What goes on outside the blood vessels, between the capillaries and the cell membranes, should be the focus of future work.

References

1. Rosenthal, M. Enhanced phagocytosis of immune complexes in pregnancy. *Clin. Exp. Immunol.* 28:189, 1977.

2. Andrews, B. S., and Penny, R. The role of immune complexes in the pathogenesis of disease. *Aust. N.Z. J. Med.* 6:591, 1976.

3. Koffler, D. Immunopathogenesis of systemic lupus erythematosus. *Ann. Rev. Med.* 25:149, 1974.

4. Kunkel, H. G., Müller-Eberhard, H. J., Fudenberg, H. H., et al. Gamma globulin complexes in rheumatoid arthritis and certain other conditions. *J. Clin. Invest.* 40:117, 1961.

5. Schrohenloher, R. E. Characterization of the γ-globulin complexes present in certain sera having high titers of anti-γ-globulin activity. *J. Clin. Invest.* 45:501, 1966.

6. Hannestad, K. Presence of aggregated γ-G-globulin in certain rheumatoid synovial effusions. *Clin. Exp. Immunol.* 2:511, 1967.

7. Winchester, R. J., Agnello, V., and Kunkel, H. G. Gamma globulin complexes in synovial fluids of patients with rheumatoid arthritis. Partial characterization and relationship to lowered complement levels. *Clin. Exp. Immunol.* 6:689, 1970.

8. Pope, R. M., Teller, D. C., and Mannik, M. The molecular basis of self-association of antibodies to IgG (rheumatoid factors) in rheumatoid arthritis. *Proc. Natl. Acad. Sci. USA* 71:517, 1974.

9. Capra, J. D., and Kunkel, H. G. Aggregation of γG3 proteins: relevance to the hyperviscosity syndrome. *J. Clin. Invest.* 49:610, 1970.

10. Capra, J. D., Winchester, R. J., and Kunkel, H. G. Hypergammaglobulinemic purpura. Studies on the unusual anti-γ-globulins characteristic of the sera of these patients. *Medicine (Baltimore)* 50:125, 1971.

11. Alarcón-Segovia, D., Fishbein, E., Abruzzo, J., et al. Serum hyperviscosity in Sjögren's syndrome interaction between IgG and IgG rheumatoid factor. *Ann. Intern. Med.* 80:35, 1974.

12. Pope, R. M., Mannik, M., Gilliland, B. C., et al. The hyperviscosity syndrome in rheumatoid arthritis due to intermediate complexes formed by self-association of IgG–rheumatoid factors. *Arthritis Rheum.* 18:97, 1975.

13. Pope, R. M., Fletcher, M. A., Mamby, A., et al. Rheumatoid arthritis associated with hyperviscosity syndrome and intermediate complex formation. *Arch. Intern. Med.* 135:281, 1975.

14. Germuth, F. G., Valdes, A. J., Taylor, J. J., et al. Fatal immune complex glomerulonephritis without deposits. *Johns Hopkins Med. J.* 136:189, 1975.

15. Williams, R. D., and Gutman, A. B. Hyperproteinemia with reversal of the albumin: globulin ratio in lymphogranuloma inguinale. *Proc. Soc. Exp. Biol. Med.* 34:91, 1936.

16. Castanedo, J. P., and Williams, R. C., Jr. Anticomplementary activity of sera from patients with connective tissue disease and normal subjects. *J. Lab. Clin. Med.* 69:217, 1967.

17. Cream, J. J. Anticomplementary sera in cutaneous vasculitis. *Br. J. Dermatol.* 89:555, 1973.

18. Verrier-Jones, J., Cumming, R. H., Bucknall, R. C., et al. Plasmapheresis in the management of acute systemic lupus erythematosus? *Lancet* 1:709, 1976.

19. Penttinen, K., Myllylä, G., Mäkelä, O., et al. Soluble antigen-antibody complexes and platelet aggregation. *Acta Pathol. Microbiol. Scand.* 77:309, 1969.

20. Penttinen, K., Vaheri, A., and Myllylä, G. Detection and characterization of immune complexes by the platelet aggregation test. I. Complexes formed *in vitro. Clin. Exp. Immunol.* 8:389, 1971.

21. Penttinen, K., Wager, O., Räsänen, J. A., et al. Platelet aggregation and cryo-IgM in the study of hepatitis and immune complex states. *Clin. Exp. Immunol.* 15:409, 1973.

22. Wager, O., Penttinen, K., Räsänen, J. A., et al. Inhibition of IgG complex-induced platelet aggregation by antiglobulin-active cryoglobulin IgM components. *Clin. Exp. Immunol.* 15:393, 1973.

23. Biberfeld, G., and Norberg, R. Circulating immune complexes in *Mycoplasma pneumoniae* infection. *J. Immunol.* 112:413, 1974.

24. Hedfors, E., and Norberg, R. Evidence for circulating immune complexes in sarcoidosis. *Clin. Exp. Immunol.* 16:493, 1974.

25. Myllylä, G., Vaheri, A., Vesikari, T., et al.

Interaction between human blood platelets, viruses, and antibodies. IV. Post-rubella thrombocytopenic purpura and platelet aggregation by rubella antigen-antibody interaction. *Clin. Exp. Immunol.* 4:323, 1969.

26. Müller-Eberhard, H. J., and Calcott, M. A. Interaction between C1q and γ-G-globulin. *Immunochemistry* 3:500, 1966 (abstract).

27. Augener, W., Grey, H. M., Cooper, N. R., et al. The reaction of monomeric and aggregated immunoglobulins with C1. *Immunochemistry* 8:1011, 1971.

28. Müller-Eberhard, H. J., and Kunkel, H. G. Isolation of a thermolabile serum protein which precipitates γ-globulin aggregates and participates in immune hemolysis. *Proc. Soc. Exp. Biol. Med.* 106:291, 1961.

29. Agnello, V., Winchester, R. J., and Kunkel, H. G. Precipitin reactions of the C1q component of complement with aggregated γ-globulin and immune complexes in gel diffusion. *Immunology* 19:909, 1970.

30. Agnello, V., Koffler, D., Eisenberg, J. W., et al. C1q precipitins in the sera of patients with systemic lupus erythematosus and other hypocomplementemic states: characterization of high and low molecular weight types. *J. Exp. Med.* 134:228s, 1971.

31. Winchester, R. J., Kunkel, H. G., Agnello, V. Occurrence of γ-globulin complexes in serum and joint fluid of rheumatoid arthritis patients: use of monoclonal rheumatoid factors as reagents for their demonstration. *J. Exp. Med.* 134:286s, 1971.

32. Agnello, V., Gabriel, A., Jr., and Tai, M. Detection of immune complexes. *J. Invest. Dermatol.* 67:339, 1976.

33. McDuffie, F. C., Sams, W. M., Maldonado, J. E., et al. Hypocomplementemia with cutaneous vasculitis and arthritis: possible immune complex syndrome. *Mayo Clin. Proc.* 48:340, 1973.

34. Oishi, M., Takano, M., Miyachi, K., et al. A case of unusual SLE related syndrome characterized by erythema multiforme, angioneurotic edema, marked hypocomplementemia and C1q precipitins of the low molecular weight type. *Int. Arch. Allergy Appl. Immunol.* 50:463, 1976.

35. Sobel, A. T., Bokisch, V. A., and Müller-Eberhard, H. J. C1q deviation test for the detection of immune complexes, aggregates of IgG, and bacterial products in human serum. *J. Exp. Med.* 142:139, 1975.

36. Nydegger, U. E., Lambert, P. H., Gerber, H., et al. Circulating immune complexes in the serum in systemic lupus erythematosus and in carriers of hepatitis B antigen. Quantitation by binding to radiolabelled C1q. *J. Clin. Invest.* 54:297, 1974.

37. Zubler, R. H., Lange, G., Lambert, P. H., et al. Detection of immune complexes in unheated sera by a modified ^{125}I-C1q binding test. Effect of heating on the binding of C1q by immune complexes and application of the test to systemic lupus erythematosus. *J. Immunol.* 116:232, 1976.

38. Hay, F. C., Nineham, L. J., and Roitt, I. M. Routine assay for the detection of immune complexes of known immunoglobulin class using solid phase C1q. *Clin. Exp. Immunol.* 24:396, 1976.

39. Yonemasu, K., and Stroud, R. M. C1q: rapid purification method for preparation of monospecific antisera and for biochemical studies. *J. Immunol.* 106:304, 1971.

40. Onyewotu, I. I., Holborow, E. J., and Johnson, G. D. Detection and radioassay of soluble circulating immune complexes using guinea pig peritoneal exudate cells. *Nature* 248:156, 1974.

41. Onyewotu, I. I., Johnson, P. M., Johnson, G. D., et al. Enhanced uptake by guinea-pig macrophages of radio-iodinated human aggregated immunoglobulin G in the presence of sera from rheumatoid patients with cutaneous vasculitis. *Clin. Exp. Immunol.* 19:267, 1975.

42. Theofilopoulos, A. N., Dixon, F. J., and Bokisch, V. Binding of soluble immune complexes to human lymphoblastoid cells. I. Characterization of receptors for IgG Fc and complement and description of the binding mechanism. *J. Exp. Med.* 140:877, 1974.

43. Theofilopoulos, A. N., Wilson, C. B., Bokisch, V. A., et al. Binding of soluble immune complexes to human lymphoblastoid cells. II. Use of Raji cells to detect circulating immune complexes in animal and human sera. *J. Exp. Med.* 140:1230, 1974.

44. Theofilopoulos, A. N., Wilson, C. B., and Dixon, F. J. The Raji cell radio-immune assay for detecting immune complexes in human sera. *J. Clin. Invest.* 57:169, 1976.

45. Winchester, R. J., Winfield, J. B., Siegal, F., et al. Analyses of lymphocytes from patients with rheumatoid arthritis and systemic lupus erythematosus. Occurrence of interfering cold-reactive anti-lymphocyte antibodies. *J. Clin. Invest.* 54:1082, 1974.

46. Winfield, J. B., Winchester, R. J., Wernet, P., et al. Nature of cold-reactive antibodies to lymphocyte surface determinants in systemic lupus erythematosus. *Arthritis Rheum.* 18:1, 1975.

47. Lachmann, P. J. Conglutinin and immunoconglutinins. *Adv. Immunol.* 6:479, 1967.

48. Lachmann, P. J., and Müller-Eberhard, H. J. The demonstration in human sera of "conglutinogen-activating factor" and its effect on the third component of complement. *J. Immunol.* 100:691, 1968.

49. Eisenberg, R. A., Theofilopoulos, A. N., and Dixon, F. J. Use of bovine conglutinin for the assay of immune complexes. *J. Immunol.* 118:1428, 1977.

50. Casali, P., Bossus, A., Nicole, A., et al. Solid-phase enzyme immunoassay or radioimmunoassay for the detection of immune complexes based on their recognition by conglutinin: conglutinin-binding test. *Clin. Exp. Immunol.* 29:342, 1977.

51. Engvall, E., and Perlmann, P. Enzyme-linked immunosorbent assay, ELISA. III. Quantitation of specific antibodies by enzyme-labeled anti-immunoglobulin in antigen-coated tubes. *J. Immunol.* 109:129, 1972.

52. Müller-Eberhard, H. J. Biochemistry of complement. In B. Amos, ed., *Progress in Immunology*, p. 553. Academic Press, New York, 1971.

53. Miller, G. W. Solubilization of IgA immune precipitates by complement. *J. Immunol.* 117:1374, 1976.

54. Cowdery, J. S., Treadwell, P. E., and Fritz, R. B. A radioimmunoassay for human antigen-antibody complexes in clinical material. *J. Immunol.* 114:5, 1975.

55. Gabriel, A., Jr., and Agnello, V. Detection of immune complexes. The use of radioimmunoassays with C1q and monoclonal rheumatoid factor. *J. Clin. Invest.* 59:990, 1977.

56. Lurhuma, A. Z., Cambiaso, C. L., Masson, P. L., et al. Detection of circulating antigen-antibody complexes by their inhibitory effect on the agglutination of IgG-coated particles by rheumatoid factor of C1q. *Clin. Exp. Immunol.* 25:212, 1976.

57. Milgrom, F., Campbell, W. A., and Andres, G. A. Antigen in immune complex nephritis. V. Recovery and identification by gel precipitation. *Immunology* 30:277, 1976.

58. Landsteiner, K., and Miller, C. P., Jr. Serological studies on the blood of the primates. II. The blood groups in anthropoid apes. *J. Exp. Med.* 42:853, 1925.

59. Stingl, G., Meingassner, J. G., Swelty, P., et al. An immunofluorescence procedure for the demonstration of antibodies to native, double-stranded DNA and of circulating DNA-anti-DNA complexes. *Clin. Immunol. Immunopathol.* 6:131, 1976.

60. Wintrobe, M. M., and Buell, M. V. Hyperproteinemia associated with multiple myeloma, with report of case in which extraordinary hyperproteinemia was associated with thrombosis of retinal veins and symptoms suggesting Raynaud's disease. *Bull. Johns Hopkins Hosp.* 52:156, 1933.

61. Lerner, A. B., Barnum, C. P., and Watson, C. J. Studies of cryoglobulins. II. The spontaneous precipitation of protein from serum at 5° C in various disease states. *Am. J. Med. Sci.* 214:416, 1947.

62. Grey, H. M., and Kohler, P. F. Cryoimmunoglobulins. *Semin. Hematol.* 10:87, 1973.

63. Putnam, F. W. In *The Plasma Proteins*, vol. 2, p. 352. Academic Press, New York, 1960.

64. Cream, J. J. Cryoglobulins in vasculitis. *Clin. Exp. Immunol.* 10:117, 1972.

65. Zinneman, H. H., Levi, D., and Seal, U. S. On the nature of cryoglobulins. *J. Immunol.* 100:594, 1968.

66. Grey, H. M., Kohler, P. F., Terry, W. D., et al. Human monoclonal γG-cryoglobulins with anti γ globulin activity. *J. Clin. Invest.* 47:1875, 1968.

67. Stone, M. J., and Metzger, H. Binding properties of a Waldenström macroglobulin antibody. *J. Biol. Chem.* 243:5977, 1968.

68. Eisen, H. N., and Siskind, G. W. Variations in affinities of antibodies during the immune response. *Biochemistry* 3:996, 1964.

69. Michaelides, M. C., and Eisen, H. N. The strange cross-reaction of menadione (vitamin K_3) and 2,4-dinitrophenyl ligands with a myeloma protein and some conventional antibodies. *J. Exp. Med.* 140:687, 1974.

70. Richards, F. F., and Konigsberg, W. H. Speculations. How specific are antibodies? *Immunochemistry* 10:545, 1973.

71. Richards, F. F., Amzel, L. M., Konigsberg, W. H., et al. Polyfunctional antibody combining regions. In E. E. Sercarz, A. R. Williamson, and C. F. Fox, eds., *The Immune System: Genes, Receptors, Signals*, p. 53. Academic Press, New York, 1974.

72. Balázs, V., and Fröhlich, M. M. Antibody activity of normal and pathological gamma globulin fractions of sera containing rheumatoid factor-cryoglobulin. *Am. J. Med. Sci.* 257:294, 1969.

73. Wager, O., Räsänen, J. A., Hagman, A., et al. Mixed cryoimmunoglobulinemia in infectious mononucleosis and Cytomegalovirus mononucleosis. *Int. Arch. Allergy Appl. Immunol.* 34:345, 1968.

74. McIntosh, R. M. Cryoproteins in post-streptococcal glomerulonephritis. *Ann. Intern. Med.* 73:857, 1970.

75. Seegal, B. C., Andres, G. A., Hsu, K. C., et al. Studies on the pathogenesis of acute and progressive glomerulonephritis in man by immuno-fluorescein and immunoferritin techniques. *Fed. Proc.* 24:100, 1965.

76. Hurwitz, D., Quismorio, F. P., and Friou, G. J. Cryoglobulinaemia in patients with infectious endocarditis. *Clin. Exp. Immunol.* 19:131, 1975.

77. Levo, Y., Gorevic, P. D., Kassab, H. J., et al. Association between hepatitis B virus and essential

mixed cryoglobulinemia. *N. Engl. J. Med.* 296:1501, 1977.

78. Winfield, J. B., Koffler, D., and Kunkel, H. G. Specific concentration of polynucleotide immune complexes in the cryoprecipitates of patients with systemic lupus erythematosus. *J. Clin. Invest.* 56:563, 1975.

79. Hanauer, L. B., and Christian, C. L. Studies of cryoproteins in systemic lupus erythematosus. *J. Clin. Invest.* 46:400, 1967.

80. Barnett, E. V., Bluestone, A., Cracchiolo, A., III, et al. Cryoglobulinemia and disease. *Ann. Intern. Med.* 73:95, 1970.

81. Christian, C. L., Hatfield, W. B., and Chase, P. H. Systemic lupus erythematosus. Cryoprecipitation of sera. *J. Clin. Invest.* 42:823, 1963.

82. McIntosh, R. M., Kulvinskas, C., and Kaufman, D. B. Cryoglobulins. II. The biological and chemical properties of cryoproteins in acute post-streptococcal glomerulonephritis. *Int. Arch. Allergy Appl. Immunol.* 41:700, 1971.

83. McIntosh, R. M., Kaufman, D. B., Kulvinskas, C., et al. Cryoglobulins. I. Studies on the nature, incidence, and clinical significance of serum cryoproteins in glomerulonephritis. *J. Lab. Clin. Med.* 75:566, 1970.

84. Whitsed, H. M., and Penny, R. IgA-IgG cryoglobulinemia with vasculitis. *Clin. Exp. Immunol.* 9:183, 1971.

85. Weisman, M., and Zvaifler, N. Cryoimmunoglobulinemia in rheumatoid arthritis. Significance in serum of patients with rheumatoid vasculitis. *J. Clin. Invest.* 56:725, 1975.

86. Franklin, E. C., Holman, H. R., Müller-Eberhard, H. J., et al. An unusual protein component of high molecular weight in the serum of certain patients with rheumatoid arthritis. *J. Exp. Med.* 105:425, 1957.

87. Franklin, E. C., Kunkel, H. G., and Ward, J. R. Clinical studies of seven patients with rheumatoid arthritis and uniquely large amounts of rheumatoid factor. *Arthritis Rheum.* 1:400, 1958.

88. Schrohenloher, R. E., Kunkel, H. G., and Tomasi, T. B. Activity of dissociated and reassociated 19 S anti-γ-globulins. *J. Exp. Med.* 120:1215, 1964.

89. Hodgson, H. J. F., Potter, B. J., and Jewell, D. P. Immune complexes in ulcerative colitis and Crohn's disease. *Clin. Exp. Immunol.* 29:187, 1977.

90. Jewell, D. P., and MacLennan, I. C. M. Circulating immune complexes in inflammatory bowel disease. *Clin. Exp. Immunol.* 14:219, 1973.

91. Feldmann, J. L., Becker, J., Moutsopoulos, H., et al. Antibody-dependent cell-mediated cytotoxicity in selected autoimmune diseases. *J. Clin. Invest.* 58:173, 1976.

92. Diaz-Jouanen, E., Bankhurst, A. D., Messner, R. P., et al. Serum and synovial fluid inhibitors of antibody-mediated lymphocytotoxicity in rheumatoid arthritis and systemic lupus erythematosus. *Arthritis Rheum.* 19:142, 1976.

93. Diaz-Jouanen, E., Bankhurst, A. D., and Williams, R. C., Jr. Antibody-mediated lymphocytotoxicity in rheumatoid arthritis and systemic lupus erythematosus. *Arthritis Rheum.* 19:133, 1976.

94. Forsgren, A., and Sjöquist, J. "Protein A" from *Staphylococcus aureus.* I. Pseudo-immune reaction with human γ-globulin. *J. Immunol.* 97:822, 1966.

95. Forsgren, A., and Sjöquist, J. "Protein A" from *Staphylococcus aureus.* III. Reaction with rabbit γ-globulin. *J. Immunol.* 99:19, 1967.

96. Kronvall, G., and Williams, R. C., Jr. Differences in anti-protein A activity among IgG subgroups. *J. Immunol.* 103:828, 1969.

97. Lind, I., Harboe, M., and Fölling, I. Protein A reactivity of two distinct groups of human monoclonal IgM. *Scand. J. Immunol.* 4:843, 1975.

98. Harboe, M., and Fölling, I. Recognition of two distinct groups of human IgM and IgA based on different binding to staphylococci. *Scand. J. Immunol.* 3:471, 1974.

99. Farrell, C., Søgaard, H., and Svehag, S. E. Detection of IgG aggregates or immune complexes using solid-phase C1q and protein A-rich *Staphylococcus aureus* as an indicator system. *Scand. J. Immunol.* 4:673, 1975.

100. McDougal, A. J. S., Redecha, P. B., Inman, R. D., et al. Binding of immunoglobulin G aggregates and immune complexes in human sera to *Staphylococci* containing protein A. *J. Clin. Invest.* 63:627, 1979.

101. Levinsky, R. J., and Soothill, J. F. A test for antigen-antibody complexes in human sera using IgM of rabbit antisera to human immunoglobulins. *Clin. Exp. Immunol.* 29:428, 1977.

102. Gluckman, J. C., Beaufils, H., and Sanchez, F. Inhibition of complement-dependent lymphocyte rosette formation by sera of patients with chronic glomerulonephritis. *Clin. Exp. Immunol.* 26:247, 1976.

103. Bjorvatn, B., Barnetson, R. S., Kronvall, G., et al. Immune complexes and complement hypercatabolism in patients with leprosy. *Clin. Exp. Immunol.* 26:388, 1976.

104. Laurell, C. B. Antigen-antibody crossed electrophoresis. *Anal. Biochem.* 10:358, 1965.

105. Bunch, T. W., Hunder, G. G., McDuffie,

F. C., et al. Synovial fluid complement determination as a diagnostic aid in inflammatory joint disease. *Mayo Clin. Proc.* 49:715, 1974.

106. Rynes, R. I., Ruddy, S., Schur, P. H., et al. Levels of complement components, properdin factors, and kininogen in patients with inflammatory arthritides. *J. Rheumatol.* 1:413, 1974.

107. Lew, P. D., Zubler, R., Vaudaux, P., et al. Decreased heat-labile opsonic activity and complement levels associated with evidence of C3 breakdown products in infected pleural effusions. *J. Clin. Invest.* 63:326, 1979.

108. Carlo, J. R., Ruddy, S., Sauter, S., et al. Deposition of β1H globulin in kidneys of patients with immune renal disease. *Arthritis Rheum.* 22:403, 1979.

109. Pangborn, M. K., Schreiber, R. D., and Müller-Eberhard, H. J. Human complement C3b inactivator: isolation, characterization and demonstration of an absolute requirement for the serum protein β1H for the cleavage of C3b and C4b in solution. *J. Exp. Med.* 146:257, 1977.

110. Nakane, P. K. Localization of hormones with the peroxidase-labeled antibody method. *Methods Enzymol.* 37:133, 1975.

111. Knowles, D. M., II, Winchester, R. J., and Kunkel, H. G. A comparison of peroxidase- and fluorochrome-conjugated antisera for the demonstration of surface and intracellular antigens. *Clin. Immunol. Immunopathol.* 7:410, 1977.

112. Lambert, P. H., Dixon, F. J., Zubler, R. H., et al. A WHO collaborative study for the evaluation of eighteen methods for detecting immune complexes in serum. *J. Clin. Lab. Immunol.* 1:1, 1978.

113. Koffler, D., Schur, P. H., and Kunkel, H. G. Immunological studies concerning the nephritis of systemic lupus erythematosus. *J. Exp. Med.* 126:607, 1967.

114. Krishnan, C., and Kaplan, M. H. Immunopathologic studies of systemic lupus erythematosus. II. Anti-nuclear reaction of γ-globulin eluted from homogenates and isolated glomeruli of kidneys from patients with lupus nephritis. *J. Clin. Invest.* 46:569, 1967.

115. Carpentier, N. A., Lange, G. T., Fiere, D. M., et al. Clinical relevance of circulating immune complexes in human leukemia. Association in acute leukemia of the presence of immune complexes with unfavorable prognosis. *J. Clin. Invest.* 60:874, 1977.

CHAPTER 7

Connective-Tissue Diseases

Much of the current impetus in relating the presence of immune complexes to various disease states had its origin in the study of connective-tissue disorders, particularly rheumatoid arthritis and systemic lupus erythematosus (SLE). Concepts of basic pathogenetic mechanisms now applied to a broad spectrum of clinical disorders ranging from infectious mononucleosis to acute leukemia have evolved as natural extensions of ideas first applied to these two connective-tissue diseases. It is appropriate, therefore, to review in some detail what is and is not yet understood concerning immune complex participation in these disease prototypes. Moreover, although the relation of fixed or circulating complexes to other connective-tissue diseases such as dermatomyositis, scleroderma, periarteritis, the mixed connective-tissue disease syndrome, or even acute rheumatic fever is much less clearly defined, it is also important to examine evidence implicating immune complexes in pathogenesis of these disorders.

Rheumatoid Arthritis

Rheumatoid arthritis is a generalized systemic disease involving diverse tissue sites including the eye, heart, lung, pleura, subcutaneous tissues, muscles, reticuloendothelial system, and the synovium and joints (1). In many instances the clinical features of rheumatoid arthritis blend imperceptibly into those of one of the other connective-tissue diseases such as SLE or scleroderma. The very fact that so many patients fall into the interstices between major

diagnostic categories suggests that there may be many similar features or overlap in the basic pathogenesis. Thus, any discussion of the disorder must from the outset consider possible mechanisms involved in generating lesions and subsequent acute and chronic inflammatory reactions within a diverse number of anatomic sites other than the joints. Several pathological features are relatively uniform, including the presence of elements of a microvasculitis and the formation of characteristic rheumatoid granuloma (2–6). Characteristic lesions are illustrated in Figure 7-1. Careful microscopic and ultrastructural studies of rheumatoid nodules have indicated that the primary event in initiating lesions may be related to an area of central segmental vascular inflammatory reaction leading to gradual evolution to the established granuloma with central necrosis, palisading monocytes, and peripheral cellular infiltrates consisting of lymphocytes and the plasma cells, as shown in Figure 7-2. Conventional and electron microscopic studies of very early rheumatoid synovial changes within the first few weeks of disease performed by Schumacher and Kitridou (7) have also emphasized that perivascular inflammatory reaction and a microvasculitis are present at the outset of disease.

Few studies have been performed relating deposition of Ig or complement in such extremely early rheumatoid lesions. At present there are no observations on the serial changes of detectable circulating immune complexes during the first few weeks of early disease. In the samples of early rheumatoid nodules or

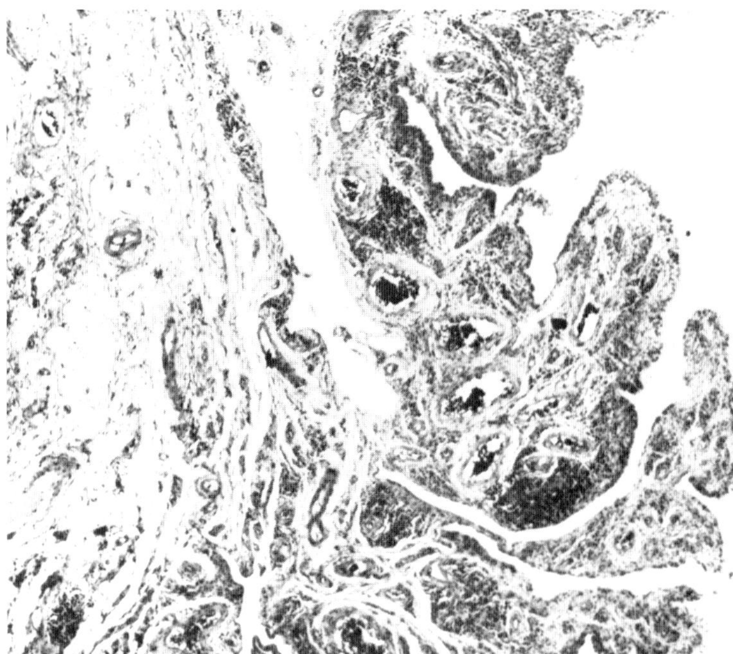

Figure 7-1 Characteristic histological involvement of active rheumatoid synovitis showing marked hypertrophy of synovial lining cells, intense infiltration of edematous synovium with mononuclear cells and lymphocytes, and perivascular collection of chronic inflammatory cells. Magnification × 75.

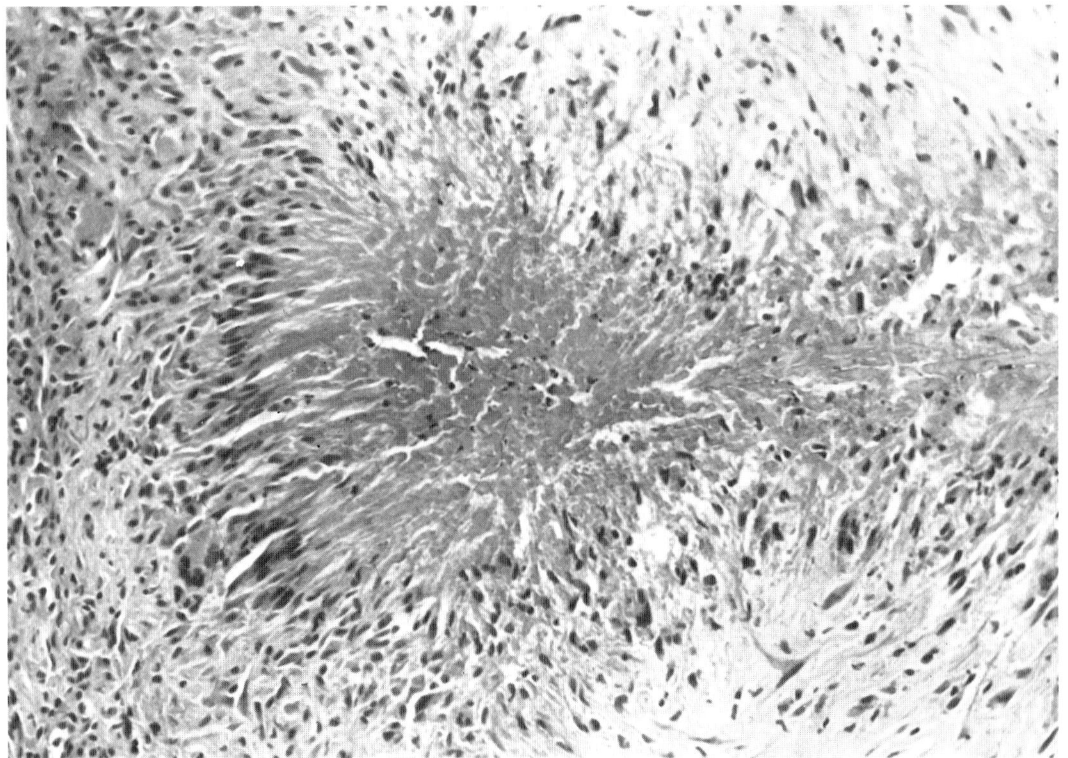

Figure 7-2 Rheumatoid nodule with central zone of necrosis, surrounded by palisading fibroblasts and monocytes with peripheral zone characterized by spotty lymphocytic infiltration. Magnification × 250.

granulomata we have examined, however, there have been impressive deposits of IgG, IgM, and C3 in the walls of arterioles and capillaries of these lesions. One of the basic difficulties in understanding the precise histological and immunologic evolution of rheumatoid lesions relates to the inability to identify an extrinsic antigen or initiating agent in this process. Many features of such lesions make antigen-antibody reaction within vessel walls a good candidate for the initial triggering event. Inspection of the histological appearance of the microvascular changes reveals interstitial edema and cellular infiltrates similar to those seen during evolution of an Arthus reaction. Recent work concerning presence of a rheumatoid-arthritis–related antigen found in certain cultured cell-line strains showing a high proportion of positive precipitating reactions with serum samples from patients with rheumatoid arthritis (8, 9) raises the question of whether a disease-specific antigen has at last been identified. In these latter studies the expression of the rheumatoid-arthritis-related antigen appears to closely parallel the presence of EB virus in cell lines used to produce the antigen. Cell lines that do not harbor EB virus do not produce the rheumatoid-arthritis-related antigen (10). Whether the antigen revealed in this particular system is related to etiology or disease initiation remains to be seen. Examples of these findings are shown in Figure 7-3.

In distinct contrast to what is seen in the early stages of rheumatoid granuloma or microvasculitis, some patients who have had an apparently ordinary clinical presentation and disease evolution over a number of months or years may subsequently show superimposition of an acute vasculitis process. Rather than the evanescent and minimal vascular process noted in early lesions, this vasculitis is often generalized and may resemble periarteritis or an accelerating vasculitis involving many visceral sites (11–19). Heart, mesenteric vessels, vessels supplying large peripheral nerves, or digital vessels may be involved and a fatal outcome may ensue despite immunosuppressive, corticosteroid, or penicillamine therapy. An example of the peripheral manifestations of rheumatoid vasculitis is shown in Figure 7-4.

We have often been impressed that minor almost subclinical manifestations of what may well be a generalized vasculitic process are frequently clinically apparent in patients with severe unremitting rheumatoid disease. Very little is known concerning the basic events involved in precipitating rheumatoid vasculitis. However, the very fact that the disease may occasionally take this turn also reinforces the idea that some type of continuing vascular injury may be implicit in subclinical form in many patients. Individuals with superimposed rheumatoid vasculitis often show marked elevations of conventional 19 S IgM rheumatoid factor, but in addition show significant increments of 7 S rheumatoid factors (20–22). Of great theoretical interest is the question of how presence of rheumatoid factors may accentuate the arteritic tissue lesions. Several observers have shown that rheumatoid factor may actually activate the complement system (23, 24). A number of animal-model experiments indicate that passive administration of serum containing high titers of rheumatoid factor is capable of markedly accelerating ongoing tissue damage mediated by immune complexes or other inflammatory foci (25–27). Plasmapheresis of patients afflicted with severe rheumatoid vasculitis can provide dramatic temporary improvement particularly in the peripheral digital manifestations of the vasculitic process. Whether this is actually caused by removal of immune complex is at present not clearly understood, as discussed in detail in Chapter 5.

When one examines the seat of the action or the pathological process under way within the rheumatoid synovium, indications suggest that local effects of immune complexes may represent initiating factors in the generation of the inflammatory process. Dissection out of whichever of a large number of parallel or concomitant phenomena is most important has thus far proven difficult. Among the potentially central factors are T lymphocytes, B cells, and plasma cells producing immunoglobulins and rheumatoid factors, activation of complement, activated macrophages, mediator molecules such as prostaglandins, lymphokines, or vasoactive amines capable of initiating actual tissue damage. Presently there is little in the way

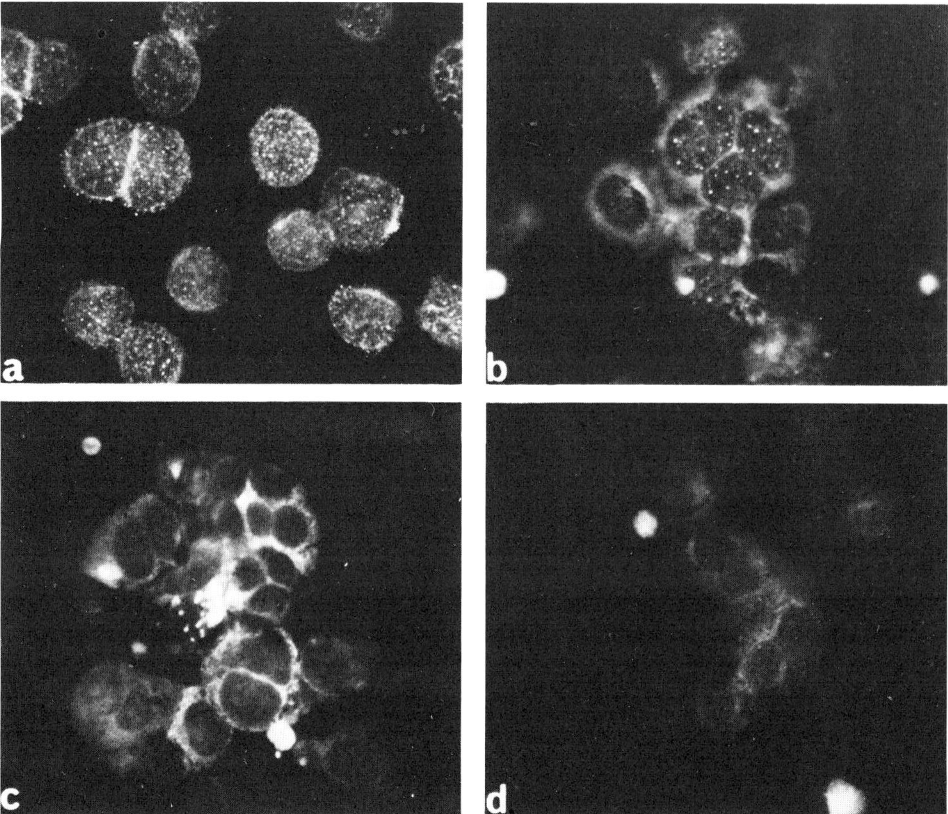

Figure 7-3 Indirect immunofluorescence to demonstrate the presence of nuclear antigen reactive with antibody in RA sera. Tissue culture cells were cytocentrifuged onto glass slides, reacted with RA serum containing antibody, and stained with fluorescein-conjugated antihuman IgG. *A*, discretely distributed finely speckled nuclear staining observed on WiL$_2$ cells; *B*, EBV-infected peripheral blood leukocytes at day 20 of culture. A few discretely distributed fine nuclear speckles were seen at this time and became more numerous after the cells transformed into continuous lines; *C*, the same EBV-infected cells (day 20) reacted with normal human serum; and *D*, a control noninfected cell culture at day 20, reacted with the same RA serum as in *B*, showing absence of nuclear staining. (Reproduced with permission, M. A. Alspaugh, F. C. Jensen, H. Rabin et al., *J. Exp. Med.* 147:1018, 1978.)

of direct evidence that T cells per se are the principal factors mediating tissue injury in rheumatoid arthritis. Indirect evidence that T cells are somehow important can be derived from the reports of Paulus and co-workers (28, 29) showing that massive depletion of lymphocytes using thoracic duct drainage produces impressive but temporary amelioration of the disease process. In similar manner, lymphokines have been shown to be capable of induction of an inflammatory synovitis when instilled into the joints of experimental animals (30), but a clear idea of what induces their formation in the first place is not yet present.

If one considers the possible factors involved in the basic rheumatoid inflammatory process, several important well-established observations suggest that a variety of types of immune complexes may be fundamental in initiating and perpetuating the underlying disease process. Fluid from patients with active rheumatoid arthritis frequently contains complexes of IgG occurring in polydisperse (8 to 17 S) form. These IgG-IgG complexes were first recognized by Hannestad using a precipitin reaction with various rheumatoid factors (31). The IgG complexes were later studied in detail by Winchester and co-workers (32–35). Much of this

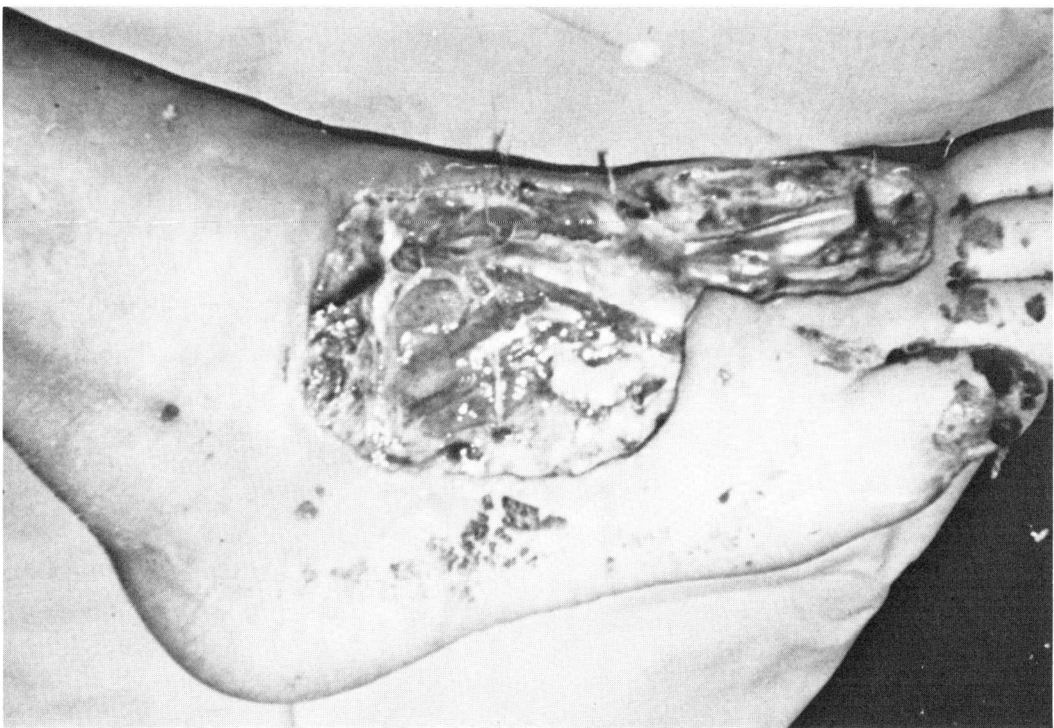

Figure 7-4 Deep penetrating dorsal ulcer of foot in patient with rheumatoid disease and superimposed peripheral vasculitis. (Photograph courtesy of J. S. Davis IV, Charlottesville, Virginia.)

material appears to represent IgG rheumatoid factors complexed with each other or with IgG-IgM. Their genesis is by no means clarified but they appear to be somehow uniquely associated with severe progressive rheumatoid disease. When IgG-IgG complexes interact with IgM rheumatoid factors, subsequent higher-molecular-weight complexes are formed that are capable of efficient activation of the complement pathway.

In patients with large amounts of synovial fluid IgG or IgG-IgM complexes, depressions of synovial complement activity are noted. That complexes of IgG-IgG rheumatoid factors or IgG-IgM plus activated complement are of more than passing interest was emphasized by the studies of Hurd and colleagues (36, 37), who showed that components of such complexes were present within phagocytic lining cells of the rheumatoid synovium and synovial fluid and that incubation of normal polymorphonuclear leukocytes with rheumatoid synovial fluid is followed by rapid phagocytosis

and ingestion of IgG and IgG-IgM plus complement complexes. Immunofluorescent visualization of this process is shown in Figure 7-5. Phagocytic lining cells, cells from rheumatoid synovial fluids, or normal polymorphonuclear leukocytes incubated with rheumatoid synovial fluid show ingestion of complexes of IgG, IgM, and complement. These data represent important evidence for assigning immune complexes a central role in the generation of the basic inflammatory process associated with the disease.

Some mention has already been made of the parts of the puzzle in rheumatoid arthritis that are as yet poorly defined. One of these is the vagary implicit in what constitutes the original antigenic stimulus that is capable of generating an ongoing and florid immune response within the involved synovium. The harder one looks at the puzzle in search of antigen, the more often one finds what appears to be evidence for both humoral and cell-mediated immunity to IgG. This vexing conundrum lies at the very

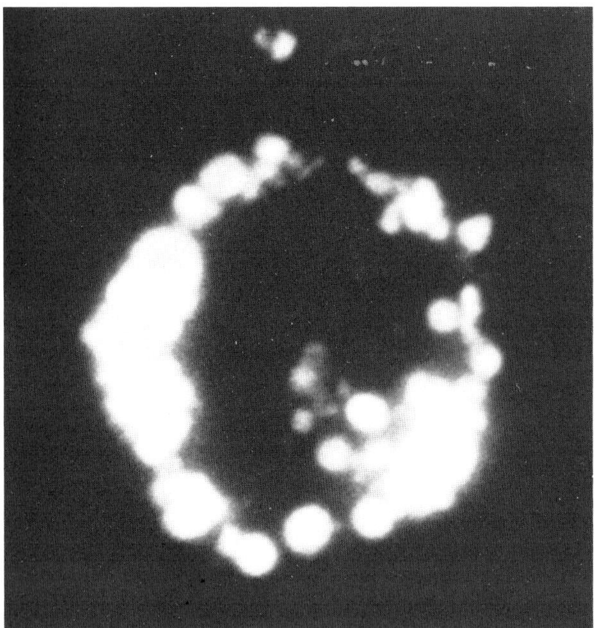

Figure 7-5 Peripheral blood neutrophil from a patient with rheumatoid arthritis and Felty's syndrome. Multiple inclusions of IgG are noted in peripheral parts of the cytoplasm. Similar intracytoplasmic inclusions containing IgG, C3, and IgM are often noted in PMNs from synovial fluid in rheumatoid arthritis. Magnification × 450. (Photograph courtesy of E. R. Hurd, Southwestern Medical School, University of Texas, Dallas.)

root of the problem. Sera and synovial fluid from diseased patients show the presence of a broad spectrum of antibodies to determinants on gamma globulins. These antibodies have now been described and extensively characterized as belonging to the IgG, IgM, and IgA classes. Within the very core of the rheumatoid synovial inflammatory process are clusters of plasma cells producing both IgM and IgG rheumatoid factors (38–40). Most if not all of the IgG manufactured within the rheumatoid synovium may possibly represent rheumatoid factor. Studies of the capacity for such tissues to produce immunoglobulin when cultured in vitro (41) have indicated a strong previous commitment toward generation of Ig that cannot be influenced by immunization procedures immediately before tissues are surgically removed from the joint. The work of Munthe

and Natvig (40) has indicated that complement-fixing intracellular complexes of IgG rheumatoid factor can be demonstrated directly within plasma cells of the rheumatoid synovium. Studies by Vaughan and co-workers have indicated that peripheral blood lymphocytes capable of in vitro manufacture of rheumatoid factors seem to parallel disease activity when a spectrum of patients are studied (42). Everywhere one looks for antigen in the disease itself, one finds evidence of cells that appear to be making antibodies to autologous IgG. Examples of synovial cells making IgG rheumatoid factor are shown in Figure 7-6. Moreover, as noted above, a considerable body of evidence has been marshaled to support rheumatoid factors complexed to various polymeric forms of IgG activating the complement sequence. All of these components can be demonstrated not only directly fixed to tissues within rheumatoid synovium but also within phagocytosing inflammatory cells of rheumatoid synovial fluids.

Regardless of these data, it is very difficult to envision gamma globulin as the primary antigen responsible for the underlying disease. Gamma globulin is a normal body component; it is hard to see how it alone can be blamed for production of the disease. What we may be seeing is the result of some other as yet unidentified antigenic stimulus. One possibility mentioned much more frequently several decades ago, when the initial studies of rheumatoid factor and its specificity were being conducted, is that apparent reactivity for autologous gamma globulins actually represents a cross-reaction between gamma globulin and something else.

When one considers the data thus far accumulated regarding the physicochemical interactions between gamma globulins and rheumatoid factors, several items of considerable interest emerge: first, the binding constants that have been measured between IgM rheumatoid factors and autologous or heterologous IgG are surprisingly low (1.5 to 5.4 × 10^4 or 10^5 l/m) (43–45) in contrast to other well-studied IgM antibodies in for instance various classic hapten-antihaptenic systems (46–47), where binding constants of 10^6 to 10^8 l/m have been recorded. Coupled with these findings

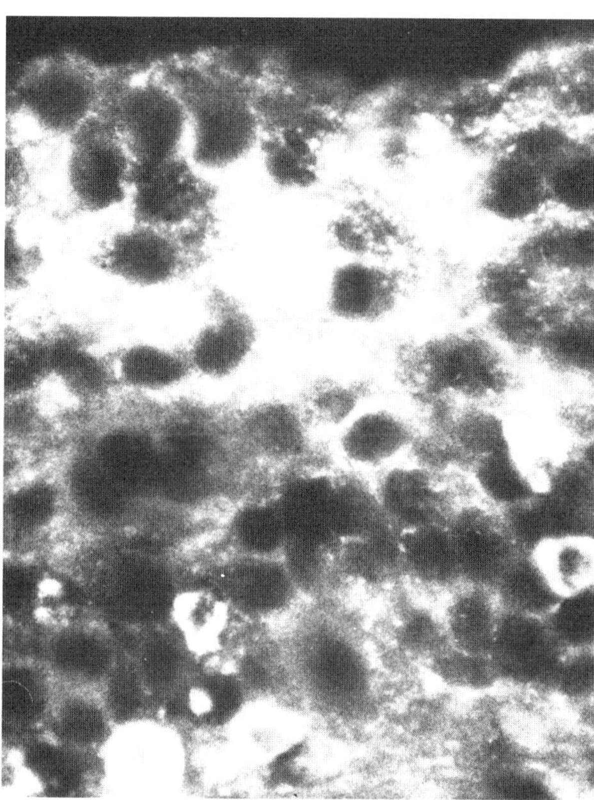

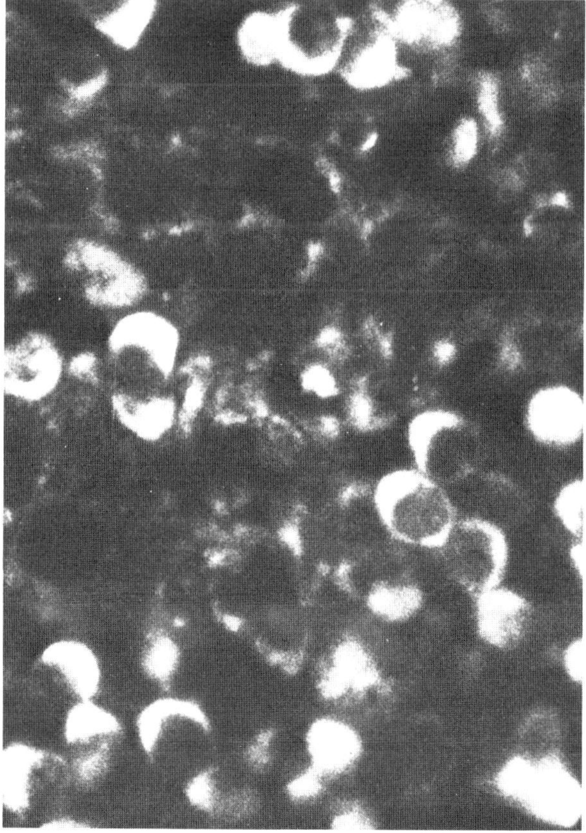

Figure 7-6 *Above,* section from rheumatoid synovial membrane stained with FITC-labeled anti-IgG. Granular deposits of IgG are localized in and between the phagocytic synovial lining cells. These deposits were shown to contain IgG-C3 complexes by double staining. Some IgG plasma cells are seen in the deeper layers. *Below,* effect of pepsin digestion on rheumatoid tissue. Rheumatoid synovial tissue stained with FITC-labeled aggregated IgG after treatment with pepsin; about one-third to one-half of the plasma cells have fixed IgG. (Reproduced with permission, E. Munthe and J. B. Natvig, *Scand. J. Immunol.* 1:217, 1972.)

one must consider the recent work of Michael-ides and Eisen directed at so-called strange reactions of various myeloma proteins with unusual ligands (DNP or vitamin K) (48). Such unexpected cross-reactions have also been studied in detail by Richards and co-workers (49, 50) and the concept developed of polyfunctional antibody combining sites. This idea emphasizes that well-characterized antibody combining sites, for instance in the case of rheumatoid factors, may show a spectrum of combining energies or partial fits for a number of conformational antigens perhaps diversely distributed in nature. Observations paralleling this general avenue of thinking are the findings of Bokisch and co-workers (51, 52), which demonstrate that certain monoclonal or highly restricted 7S IgG rheumatoid factors actually showed primary reactivity against bacterial peptidoglycans used in the primary immunization process that initially generated them. This line of argument supports the idea that instead of having primary reactivity for autologous gamma globulins, rheumatoid factors are antibodies directed at something else showing strong and diverse cross-reactivity for many sites on gamma globulins. If the primary binding energies for the antigen initiating such factors could be measured, instead of 10^4 it might well be 10^7 or 10^8. Again, this argument presupposes that such antigens entirely distinct from gamma globulin may eventually be identified. Evidence for a fascinating direct cross-reaction between rheumatoid factors reacting with IgG and nuclear antigens has recently been presented by Hannestad (53). In this study IgM molecules with demonstrable rheumatoid-factor activity for IgG could also be shown to possess antinuclear antibody reactivity. An extension of this approach may eventually uncover the basic or primary antigen in rheumatoid disease.

There is other compelling evidence that immune complexes may be at the heart of the action within the inflamed joints, as represented by in vivo consumption of complement within involved joints. The initial documentation was provided by the studies of Hedberg (54, 55) and Pekin and Zvaifler (56), who showed that hemolytic complement activity was markedly

reduced within the rheumatoid joint. As knowledge concerning the molecular biology of both the classical and the alternate complement pathways advanced, additional studies showed that both pathways were activated in rheumatoid synovial fluid (57, 58). The presence of chemotactic and biologically active C3 breakdown products within rheumatoid synovial fluid was clearly documented (59) and provided a rational explanation for the ingress of polymorphonuclear leukocytes and mononuclear cells into the areas of acute inflammatory reaction. Finally, as noted in Chapter 5, the demonstration that immune reactants might be held within dense connective-tissue structures of the joints for long periods of time because of the physical entrapment of such materials in collagenous or cartilage structures (60, 61) completed the assessment of the basic inflammatory process within the rheumatoid synovium.

A strong case can now be made for the basic or central precipitating role of immune complexes in the rheumatoid process. Phagocytosis of immune-complex reactants by PMNs seems to be facilitated by the presence of both rheumatoid factors and complexes within synovial fluid. Once ingested, phagocytosed complexes are capable of setting off degranulation of the cell lysosomal apparatus and release of potentially toxic lysosomal materials like tissue cathepsins and collagenases. Continued local manufacture of IgG rheumatoid factors within the inflamed rheumatoid synovium provides a ready source of materials feeding reactants capable of potentiating and continuing the basic process. This local sequence of events is summarized in Figure 7-7.

A clear perception of the possible effects of immune complexes on cell-mediated immunity in rheumatoid arthritis is not yet available. Originally we demonstrated that some anti-γ-globulins from sera of rheumatoid arthritic patients were capable of inducing cell division using an in vitro lymphocyte transformation system (62). At present, the possibility that the types of immune complexes found in rheumatoid synovial fluids or sera are directly involved in modulating or somehow triggering primary T-cell responses has not been completely ex-

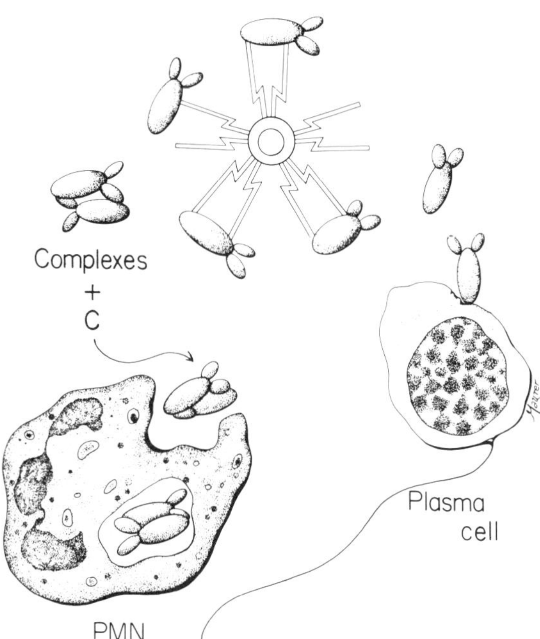

Figure 7-7 Immune complexes of Ig, some of which may be aggregates of 7S IgG rheumatoid factor produced locally within plasma cells of the rheumatoid synovium, and may react with 19S rheumatoid factor or be phagocytosed by PMNs in the local tissues creating lysosomal release and further potentiating the inflammatory reaction.

plored. A subpopulation of T cells bearing receptors for the Fc portion of IgG have been shown in an in vitro system to function as suppressor cells in the presence of immune complexes (63). Thus it is conceivable that such T cells might be activated in vivo in the presence of large local concentrations of IgG complexes in their microenvironment. No direct evidence for such an interaction is yet available. However, several interesting reports by Kinsella (64, 65) may bear on this point. Autologous lymphocytes from patients with rheumatoid arthritis showed transformation in the presence of synovial fluids (64). It seems possible that immune complexes were directly involved in this lymphocyte activation, although no studies of the physical size of the reactants were included in the initial report. Later Kinsella demonstrated enhancement of lymphocyte transformation in the presence of aggregated human IgG in rheumatoid subjects

(65), and increased lymphocyte response was only recorded in the presence of a source of complement. It was suggested that since IgG complexes similar to aggregated IgG and human complement were both available within the rheumatoid joint, such a mechanism might indeed enhance the cellular proliferation within involved synovial tissue. Beside having surface receptors for activated complement, B cells are known to be capable of activation through binding of immune complexes to Fc receptors. One could therefore construct a theoretical scheme whereby immune complexes present in rheumatoid synovial fluid might drive or amplify the system already described. Activation of B cells through Fc receptors might provide amplification of the ongoing immune plasma-cell response producing immunoglobulins with reactivity for autologous gamma globulins, therefore raising production of IgG-IgG complexes in situ. Also, if complexes can amplify T-cell proliferation, such an effect might nonspecifically increase humoral immune response through helper factor effects. Amplification of T-cell proliferation might also release more potentially harmful lymphokines capable of direct tissue injury. This complex-driven system of potential interactions is shown in Figure 7-8. It must be stressed that such a scheme is not yet completely supported by experimental data.

Rheumatoid arthritis is a systemic disease characterized by microvasculitis and granulomata in many locations. Extensive evidence for the presence of immune-complex components in capillary beds of tissues such as lung (66), synovium (67), and even vessels supplying peripheral nerves (68) has already been accumulated. There is a variety of immune complexes both free within the synovial fluid and phagocytosed in cellular infiltrates and synovial fluid cells. Whether all manifestations of the disease can be attributed to such phenomena is uncertain, but it seems obvious that they represent reactants at the very center of the action.

Measurement of Complexes
in Rheumatoid Arthritis

Immune complexes were first probably recognized as such in the sera of patients with rheu-

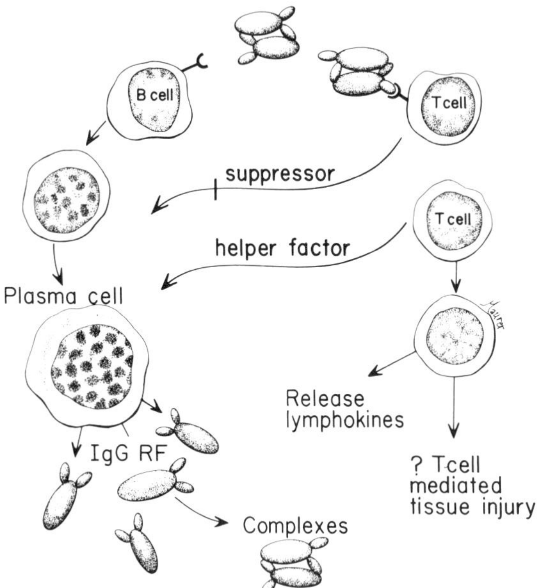

Figure 7-8 Immune complexes of IgG-IgG rheumatoid factors or, alternatively, IgG combined with an unknown antigen (*top*) react with Fc receptors on B cells or T cells. This in turn may activate humoral or cell-mediated immune mechanisms with subsequent release of more complexes again helping to drive the system.

matoid arthritis when the physical-immunochemical reactions of rheumatoid factors were described by Franklin and co-workers using direct visualization of complex formation in the analytical ultracentrifuge (69, 70), with observations of interaction between 19S IgM rheumatoid factors and autologous or isologous 7S IgG molecules. Amounts of both 19S rheumatoid factors and 22S complexes showed a rough parallel with clinical disease activity. It was later recognized that uniquely high titers of conventional 19S IgM rheumatoid factor, as measured by the standard latex fixation test, bore a relationship to disease manifestations. Patients with generalized visceral involvement showed much higher titers of serum rheumatoid factor than other patients with milder disease (71–73).

In many ways the clinical assessment of presence of rheumatoid factors was one of the earliest methods used to estimate a type of immune complex associated with the disease.

Continued clinical and laboratory refinements, however, indicated that titers of IgM rheumatoid factors alone could not always be directly related to severity of disease or clinical progress. It was noted that a variety of other complexes composed principally of 7S Ig subunits were frequently present in serum samples from a variety of patients. These intermediate or 9 to 16S complexes of IgG self-associating rheumatoid factors were also recognized as being of potential importance in the visceral and direct synovial tissue pathological process (74, 75). In effect, virtually everywhere that one looked in the rheumatoid process, one could find either what appeared to be complexes or their constituents about to form or generate. Actual measurement of quantitative amounts of complexes in sera or other body fluids in rheumatoid disease presents a problem not so much of detection as of identification of which complexes are important in understanding what is really significant to the disease process.

Technical and theoretical progress in the study of immune complexes in rheumatoid arthritis has advanced from the rather gross interactions observed initially in the analytic ultracentrifuge to the use of precipitin reactions with monoclonal rheumatoid factors or C1q and most recently to the use of radioimmunoassays employing the Raji-cell or solid phase C1q-binding techniques. All of these approaches have proven useful in generating data of practical interest in actual assessment of disease activity. As an example, it was recognized quite early in these studies that the presence of uniquely large amounts of rheumatoid factors paralleled severe extra-articular and extensive rheumatoid granulomatous tissue involvement, such as neurovascular alterations or superimposed vasculitis (72, 73). In turn the characterization of the broad range of complexes within serum and synovial fluid using the C1q-binding or precipitin assay (32–35) provided clear insight into the physical composition and potential biological importance of these materials. This research also provided a rational explanation for the previously observed marked depressions of rheumatoid synovial complement relative to complement activity within the blood. Finally, application of the newer C1q-binding or radioimmunoassay techniques to estimation of circulating complexes in rheumatoid arthritis has provided a much higher degree of sensitivity in assessing clinical progress or distinct disease profiles. Positive tests registered in the Raji-cell radioimmunoassay have shown a high degree of positivity in patients with clinical rheumatoid vasculitis (76). This is an important point, since positive results in the Raji-cell test depend on the ability of the complexes in the serum sample tested to bind to activated complement components and thereby adhere to the Raji-cell C3b receptor. Most sera from patients with rheumatoid arthritis have complexes of one sort or another. If the Raji-cell test is capable of preferentially estimating complement-activated complexes, and if such complexes correlate directly with flagrant clinical evidence of vasculitis, we may have reached a state of fine tuning or discrimination that will be extremely useful in monitoring clinical therapeutic trials and subsequent course.

Rheumatoid factors represent a broad and rather heterogeneous spectrum of anti-γ-globulins, some of which can be shown clearly to activate the complement system (23, 24, 77). It therefore becomes of considerable importance to understand exactly what may be happening in the course of rheumatoid vasculitis during which large amounts of complexes with adsorbed activated C3 are present. This does not appear to be the case in patients with an ordinary uncomplicated clinical course. Several features of the individual immune response may be unique to such clinical situations. It is conceivable that among certain individuals IgG-IgG complexes are predisposed to activate C3 because of their relative amounts of complement-fixing H-chain IgG subclasses, such as IgG-3 or IgG-1. Furthermore, local tissue factors perhaps modulated by vasoactive substances, corticosteroid therapy, or even direct complement pathway activation may also be involved. These and many other possibilities have now arisen with the availability of sensitive radioimmunoassay techniques for quantitative estimation of immune complexes in disorders such as chronic active rheumatoid

arthritis. During the past year we have monitored a group of patients with chronic uncomplicated rheumatoid arthritis, using the solid-phase C1q and the Raji-cell radioimmunoassay. We have been impressed with the frequent abrupt rises in detectable immune complexes (particularly as monitored by the solid-phase C1q test) as being predictive or occurring immediately before a clinical exacerbation of the disease (78). These observations must now be extended and further serial assays compared with clinical course before a complete evaluation of this finding can be presented.

Several recent reports have explored the practical usefulness of immune-complex detection and monitoring in rheumatoid disease, using radioimmunoassay with monoclonal rheumatoid factor (79) and ^{125}I-C1q binding (80). A high proportion of subjects studied with the C1q-binding method showed detectable complexes in both sera and synovial fluids. The C1q-binding was higher in patients who were seropositive for rheumatoid factor and was found in 10 to 34 S fractions after ultracentrifugal gradient analysis. It also appeared that DNA or DNA–anti-DNA complexes did not significantly alter C1q binding. Using radioimmunoassay and monoclonal rheumatoid factor (79), higher levels of complexes were noted in synovial fluids than in sera. No significant interference with the assay by polyclonal rheumatoid factor was observed, and presence of immune-complex material showed an inverse correlation with the level of serum C4. Another recent study extending this work utilized quantitative estimation of the C3 breakdown product C3d to investigate complement activation in rheumatoid arthritis (81). A significant correlation between C3d elevation and levels of circulating complexes measured by C1q-binding radioimmunoassay was recorded. In addition, C3d levels and C1q binding appeared to correlate with clinical activity.

Another aspect of the problem of immune-complex measurement and interpretation of physiological meaning of sensitive radioimmunoassays in patients with rheumatoid arthritis centers around the rather special situation involving catabolism or turnover of autologous gamma globulin in subjects with rheumatoid arthritis. The situation is unique in this disease, since seropositive patients have a built-in humoral immune response capable of reacting directly with their own gamma globulins. Catabolism and half-life of gamma globulin in rheumatoid arthritis has been studied by a number of investigators (82–87). Recent studies by Catalano and colleagues (88) confirm a more rapid turnover of IgG in patients with rheumatoid arthritis. In addition, faster catabolic rate and turnover was observed when autologous rather than homologous-labeled protein was studied. Increment of autologous IgG catabolism was also observed in the extravascular compartment. In this latter study differences in catabolism of labeled autologous IgG preparations could not be correlated directly with results of Raji-cell determinations for presence of detectable circulating complexes studied concurrently within the same patients. Curves of labeled gamma-globulin survival taken from this study (88) are shown in Figures 7-9 and 7-10. Periodically there have been suggestions that immunoglobulins might be intrinsically different or altered in patients with

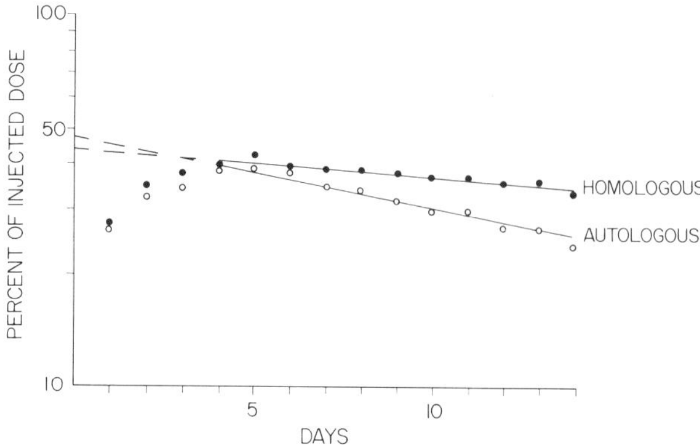

Figure 7-10   Mean curves for E autologous (○) and homologous (●) IgG in the HRAs. Derivation is by least squares analysis of mean data for days 4 to 14. The p value for slopes is < 0.001. (Reproduced with permission, M. A. Catalano, E. H. Krick, D. H. De Heer et al., *J. Clin. Invest.* 60:313, 1977.)

rheumatoid arthritis (89–91). Variations as measured by circular dichroism techniques or in galactose content for gamma globulins isolated from patients with rheumatoid arthritis have been suggested, but there is no substantial body of evidence to support this hypothesis. Certainly, if there were basic alterations in composition or conformation in all antibody molecules present in rheumatoid arthritis serum, it would be reflected eventually in how such molecules were handled as parts of immune complexes. More data in this area are needed before a final assessment can be made.

In summary, rheumatoid arthritis provides an interesting model for study of the relation of immune complexes to a particular generalized systemic disease state. The disorder itself is characterized by a remarkable variety of tissue lesions occurring both in extra-articular and articular distribution. Presence in the serum, synovial fluid, and tissues of apparent antibodies to components of gamma globulin serves as a source for the manufacture and deposition of a wide range of complexes, some of which are capable of directly activating both the classical and alternate complement pathways. Extravascular immune-complex deposition appears to be the rule; there is also evidence for phagocytosed immune-complex constituents being intrinsic to the actual in-

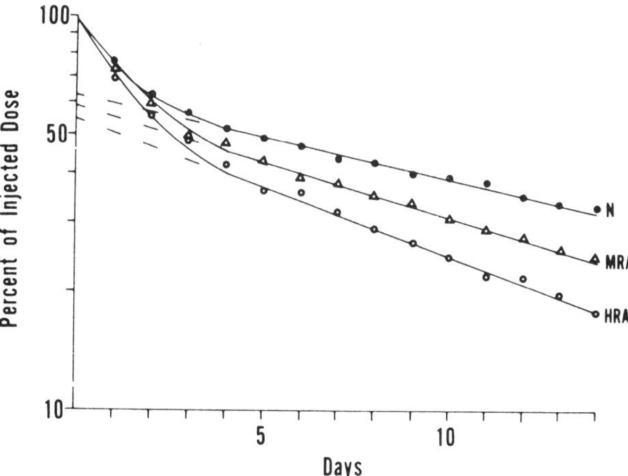

Figure 7-9   Mean curves of plasma decay for homo-IgG in normals (N, ●), MRA (△), and HRA (○). Derivation is by least squares analysis of mean data for days 4 to 14. The p values for slopes: N vs MRA, $p < 0.01$; N vs HRA, $<p\ 0.001$; and MRA vs HRA, $p < 0.01$. (Reproduced with permission, M. A. Catalano, E. H. Krick, D. H. De Heer et al., *J. Clin. Invest.* 60:313, 1977.)

flammatory response in the joints and synovial space.

Systemic Lupus Erythematosus

Perhaps no human disease has provided us with more in the way of direct information concerning the role of immune complexes than systemic lupus erythematosus (SLE). After the original LE cell phenomenon had been described (92, 93), additional serological abnormalities clearly implicated reactions between serum globulins and nuclear material (94–102). Thus, from the very outset in most of the modern clinical research involving SLE, attention has been directed to the importance of antibodies reacting with nuclear antigens. This focus was indeed fortunate; it has resulted in gradual evolution and refinement of our thinking in terms of the basic tissue lesions of SLE. To a great extent the current focus on DNA–anti-DNA antigen-antibody reactions as basic to the understanding of pathogenesis in SLE is a final result of the initial observation by Hargraves of the LE cell phenomenon (93) and the recognition by Klemperer and associates of material showing nuclear staining reactions within tissue lesions (92). By contrast the same type of parallel attention focused on the relation of gamma globulin to presence of rheumatoid factors in rheumatoid arthritis has not been as productive in terms of identification of basic pathogenetic mechanisms.

The Clinical Picture

An examination of the clinical picture of SLE emphasizes the diverse and widespread involvement in the disease. The extreme variety of presenting symptoms and clinical manifestations has been stressed in all of the current detailed assessments of this disorder (103). Presentation with fever, myalgia, muscle weakness, polyarthritis, serositis, pleurisy or pericarditis, predominant skin rash, thrombocytopenic purpura, acute hemolytic anemia, abdominal pain, pancytopenia, predominant personality or central nervous system changes, or intermittent psychosis all represent diffuse and integral manifestations of the disease.

It has always been clear that SLE is a gen-eralized disease. The multiplicity of tissue lesions ranging from the periarterial fibrosis in and around splenic vessels to the segmental arteriolar involvement and infarctions or vasculitis within the brain or other peripheral tissues are representative of a diffuse process often distributed in parallel with the vulnerable microvascular pathways. In this respect the central pattern of lesions is similar to that of rheumatoid arthritis, but much more extensive and necrotizing. In addition, the frequency of severe or progressive vascular involvement particularly in the kidney sets the disorder apart from the general course of rheumatoid disease. One is forced to admit that much of the chronicity and histological evolution of arterial lesions in SLE resemble those also seen during the course of an acute diffuse vasculitis as, for instance, in allergic vasculitis or even periarteritis nodosa. The difference, of course, is that antigen-antibody complexes (DNA–anti-DNA) have been identified in some of the basic lesions of SLE, whereas the same sort of identifiable basic immune derangement has not yet been directly proven in most cases of vasculitis of unknown cause.

Immune hyperresponsiveness to a wide variety of tissue antigens in SLE has now been documented. Antibodies or immune responses to a long list of such constitutents have been described. To date, immune complexes involving only a portion of these potential antigens have been identified as being directly involved with tissue lesions. The wide diversity of presumed autoantibodies recorded in SLE is a reflection of what is generally regarded as a generalized humoral hyperresponsiveness. Many patients show varying degrees of hypergammaglobulinemia along with what appears to be a relative decrease in effective cell-mediated responsiveness. This has been the subject of considerable study by a number of groups, and much parallel evidence for a decrease in cell-mediated immunity in SLE has been accumulated. As a general rule, one might say that B-cell–directed immune responses are amplified and that T-cell functions of cellular immunity are relatively impaired. Examples of these findings are summarized in Table 7-1. Generalized imbalance between humoral and cellu-

Table 7-1 Depression of cell-mediated immunity in systemic lupus erythematosus.

Observed effect	Possible relation to—	Clinical effect
Decrease in response to mitogens (phytohemagglutinin, concanavalin A, and pokeweed mitogen)	T-cell cytopenia(?) in vivo intracellular residence of virus	Possibly increased incidence of intracellular infections
Depressed reactivity in mixed leukocyte culture	Antilymphocyte antibody affecting T-responder cell population	Basic alteration in immune surveillance
Decrease in cellular response to specific antigens such as PPD and candida, as monitored by delayed hypersensitivity testing (paradoxical depression of MIF reactivity to measles antigen in face of elevated levels of humoral antibody)	T-cell cytopenia Suppression by immune complexes	General decline in effective cell-mediated immunity

lar immunity has also been extensively documented in the strikingly similar murine model for lupus as seen in the NZB/W mouse. This and other animal models of immune-complex disorders are discussed in detail in Chapter 13.

A popular explanation of humoral hyperresponsiveness and defective cellular reactivity has been that immunologic imbalance might result from lack of effective suppressor-cell function. While direct evidence to support such a concept is much more extensive in data accumulated from NZB mice studies, there are several human studies that provide evidence for defective suppressor-cell function (104–106). The lack of suppressor cells as a ready explanation for an increased, uncontrolled humoral response is an attractive hypothesis. It is important to point out that defective suppressor-cell activity cannot also directly explain impairment of cell-mediated immunity in the disease, unless one postulates that suppressor-cell mechanisms for cellular phenomena are somehow increased in reciprocal fashion.

Evidence for Immune-Complex Deposition and SLE

The first evidence that immune-complex deposition might be one of the fundamental changes occurring during the evolution of the clinical SLE disorder came from direct immunofluorescent studies of kidneys from patients in which extensive deposits of both IgG and C3 were recorded within glomerular capillaries and arteriolar vessels in multiple organs (106–108). Widespread distribution of immune-complex materials associated with tissue lesions was documented largely by immunofluorescent and subsequent electron microscopic studies. It was already known that patients with SLE showed marked heterogeneity of antinuclear antibodies in their sera, and a correlation had also been noted between the occurrence of anti-DNA antibodies and severe lupus nephritis (99, 101, 109). Serial studies of DNA and anti-DNA antibody activity among individuals with active SLE nephritis (110–115) further strengthened the argument for immune-complex activation in the ongoing disease process. An example of such serial determinations is shown in Figure 7-11. In parallel, it was known that exacerbations of lupus activity were often accompanied by marked reductions in total hemolytic complement in circulating plasma, suggesting in vivo complement activation (116, 117). Since antitissue antibodies of marked heterogeneity had been amply demonstrated in most lupus patients with a variety of techniques, initially it was unclear which were of most critical importance as participants in the actual immune deposits often noted in immunofluorescent studies of renal or skin deposits. Strong evidence was provided by a number of clinical studies that linked antibodies to native

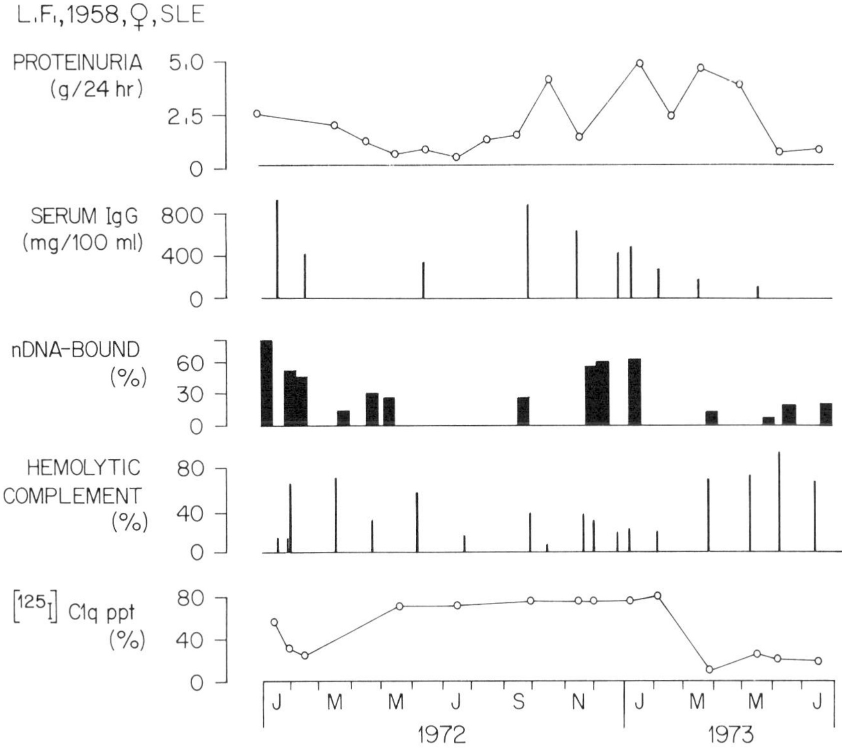

Figure 7-11 Comparison of the evolution of various parameters for SLE disease activity in the follow-up study of a fifteen-year-old girl. Periods with normal hemolytic complement activities are characterized by low [125I] C1q-binding activities. Low CH 50 activity, proteinuria, and high-titered anti-DNA antibodies further characterize periods associated with increased [125I] C1q binding. (Reproduced with permission, U. E. Nydegger, P. H. Lambert, H. Gerber et al., *J. Clin. Invest.* 54:297, 1974.)

double-stranded DNA (nDNA) more closely with the occurrence of nephritis. The most convincing evidence, however, implicating immune complexes and the basic lesions of lupus nephritis was provided by the direct elution studies of Krishnan and Kaplan (118) and Koffler and co-workers (108). These studies utilized preparations of renal glomeruli that could be made by simply finely mincing tissues and pushing tissue homogenates through a fine wire mesh. Tubular and interstitial elements passed through the filters, leaving relatively clean preparations of isolated glomeruli. These glomerular preparations were made from kidney tissues of patients dying of lupus nephritis and were subjected to elution procedures using buffers at acidic pH or other reagents capable of dissociating tissue-bound antigen-antibody complexes. Such glomerular eluates showed striking relative concentration of antinuclear antibody and in particular anti-DNA antibody. In addition, using sophisticated reagents with highly defined specificity such as rabbit or other lupus sera with known characteristic reactivity for DNA or nucleoprotein, actual tissue presence of DNA or other nuclear antigens was demonstrated by indirect immunofluorescence and appropriate blocking studies. When relative amounts of anti-DNA antibody activity were directly compared between whole serum and glomerular eluates, a marked relative glomerular enrichment for DNA-antibody was often recorded. Representative results of such experiments are shown in Table 7-2 from the report of Koffler and co-workers (108). Clinical detection of antinuclear or anti-DNA antibody showed a high degree of correlation with progression of severe lupus

Table 7-2 Comparison of the minimum gammaglobulin concentrations of serums and eluates giving antinuclear fluorescent reactions.

Case no.	Eluate	Eluate (μg γ-globulin/ml)	Serum (μg γ-globulin/ml)	Ratio of serum (γ-globulin/eluate γ-globulin)
1	A[a]	5	—	—
2	A	5	256	51
3	A	20	260	13
4	A	10	720	72
5[b]	A	60	2,400	40
6	A	200	660	3
7	A	90	3,600	40
	B[c]	9	3,600	400
8	A	32	200	6
	B	54	200	4
9	A	4	1,100	275
	B	12	1,100	92
10	A	9	[d]	—
	B	5	[d]	—
11	A	70	1,400	20
	B	50	1,400	28

Source: Reproduced with permission, D. Koffler, P. H. Schur, and H. G. Kunkel, *J. Exp. Med.* 126:607, 1967.

[a] Acid buffer eluate.

[b] Subacute glomerulonephritis.

[c] DNase eluate.

[d] Negative nuclear fluorescent reaction.

renal disease; low serum-complement activity often accompanied severe lupus activity. Immunoglobulin and complement could be demonstrated directly in the vascular, skin, and renal lesions of the disease, and most convincingly, eluates from actual affected lupus glomeruli showed a marked relative enrichment or concentration of anti-DNA and in some instances other antinuclear antibodies in comparison to serum or circulating plasma. These points established lupus nephritis as undoubtedly caused by immune deposits largely comprised of complexes containing DNA and anti-DNA antibodies. A typical example of these findings is shown in Figure 7-12, which illustrates the rather granular, lumpy-bumpy distribution of immunoglobulin and complement in renal tissue of a lupus patient with typical immune-complex glomerular involvement. In addition, when glomerular eluates such as those originally prepared by Koffler and co-workers (108) and Krishnan and Kaplan (118)

were applied to normal mouse liver sections, intense concentration of antinuclear antibody was demonstrated (Figure 7-13).

Several features of importance in the pathogenesis of SLE nephritis must also be mentioned. It is currently felt that within the category of antinuclear antibodies, anti-DNA antibodies can probably be classified into three distinct groups: those that show specificity for determinants only on nDNA, those that react with determinants on both nDNA and denatured or single-strand DNA (sDNA), and those with specificity only for antigenic configurations on sDNA (96, 99). The presence of high titers of antibodies to nDNA is unique to active SLE. However, antibodies to determinants on sDNA may also be present in other disorders such as chronic active liver disease, rheumatoid arthritis, mixed connective-tissue disorders, and a number of miscellaneous conditions (119, 120). Several technical improvements in the reliability and accuracy of measuring true

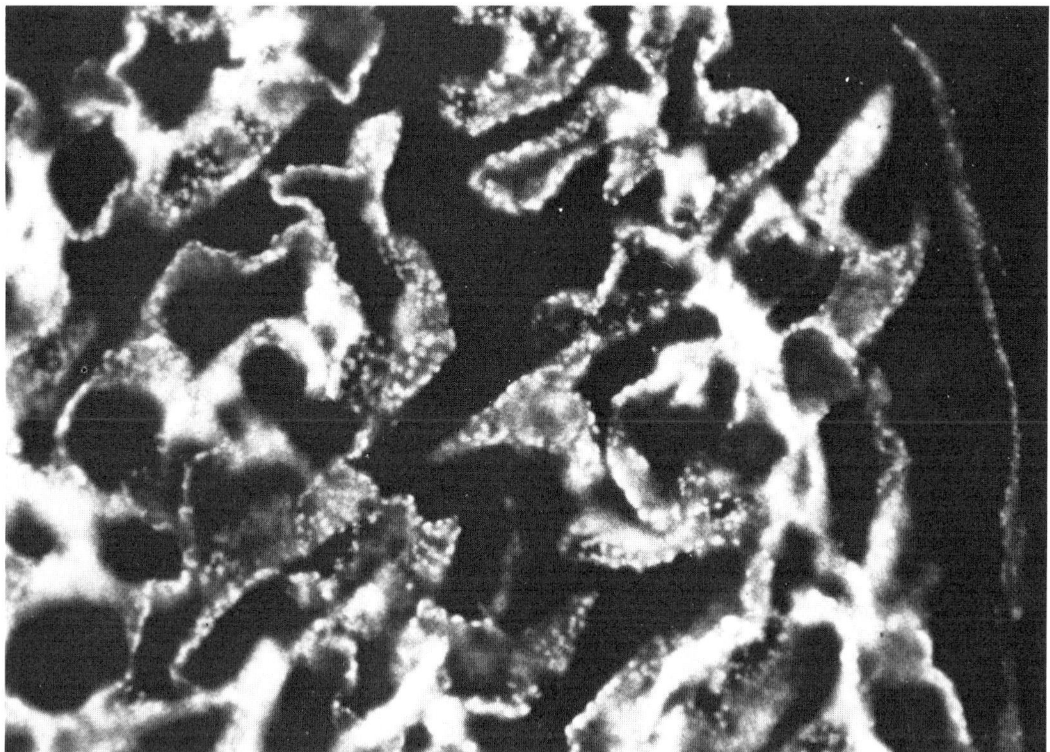

Figure 7-12 Granular lumpy-bumpy immune deposits within the glomeruli of C3 in a patient with diffuse lupus nephropathy. Magnification × 375.

anti-nDNA antibodies have recently been introduced—a useful advance in the technical reliability of clinical measurement. One ingenious method uses the circular native DNA of the parasite *Crithidia luciliae* as substrate for an immunofluorescent test (121, 122); the other method uses a synthetic DNA homologue of polynucleotides currently felt to be highly specific for antigenic determinants unique to nDNA (123). Application of these methods to diagnosis and clinical follow-up of individual patients should markedly improve perception of important disease sequelae.

Another feature of the immune-complex disease associated with SLE is that generation of high titers of anti-nDNA antibodies by these patients must represent a triggering mechanism for B-cell activation, which if clearly understood might be subject to effective therapeutic manipulation or control. Studies in our laboratory (124) have indicated that patients

with active SLE show relatively large numbers of cells capable of binding radiolabeled nDNA as putative antigen-binding cells and precursors of antibody-forming cells. Surprisingly, normal subjects also show a low but definite proportion of antigen-binding cells capable of binding radiolabeled nDNA as putative antigen-binding cells and precursors of antibody-forming cells. Data illustrating relative numbers of nDNA binding cells detected in both normal subjects and patients with active SLE are shown in Figure 7-14.

It is still unclear what triggers proliferation or relative increase of nDNA antigen-binding cells in SLE patients and what prevents such cells already present in normal subjects from proliferation and marked increased synthesis of anti-nDNA antibody. Our own studies of this problem indicate that most of the nDNA binding cells in patients with SLE and those present in much lower numbers in normal sub-

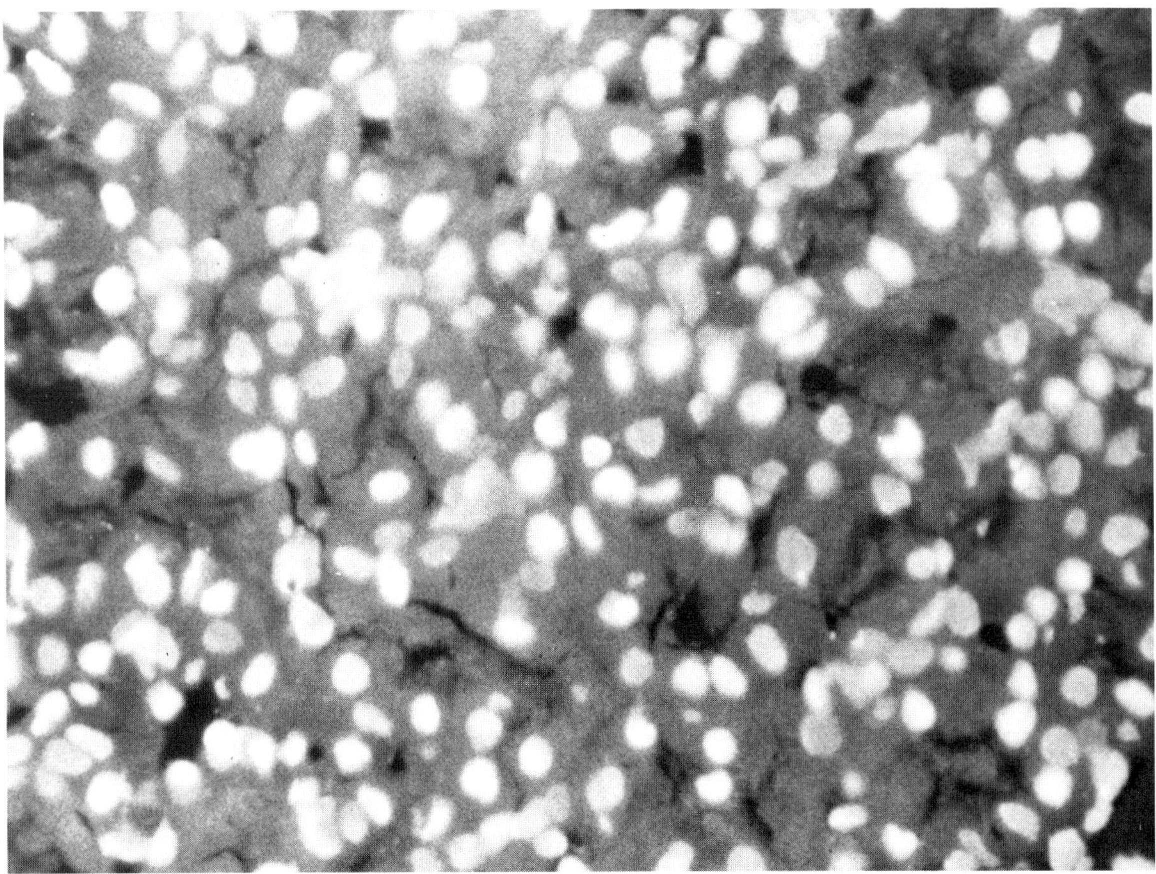

Figure 7-13 Antinuclear antibody reactivity of gamma-globulin eluate from isolated glomeruli of a patient with active SLE nephritis. Gamma globulin at 0.1 mg/ml produced this striking immunofluorescent reaction on normal mouse liver. Magnification × 350.

jects were B cells with membrane immunoglobulin. If a difference in ratios of proportions of nDNA antigen-binding B cells and T cells had been present, it might have been possible to suggest from such data that a disturbance in either helper or suppressor cells with specificity for nDNA was present. The fact that the cell profile of nDNA-binding cells in both normal and SLE patients was the same—mostly B cells—may mean that proliferation of nDNA-binding cells in SLE actually is not directly related to abnormalities in helper or suppressor mechanisms, but rather to a direct triggering or bypass phenomenon that occurs in active SLE.

A series of experiments conducted by several groups may be very important in the final interpretation of these phenomena. It was shown that administration of endotoxin, a known polyclonal B-cell activator, to mice not usually susceptible to the DNA–anti-DNA immune-complex disorders of other strains could markedly accelerate tissue deposition of such complexes in glomeruli (125). It is possible that the endotoxin acting as a polyclonal B-cell activator set off proliferation of nDNA antigen-binding cells normally present, and a marked increment in anti-DNA antibody with consequent immune-complex deposition ensued. The activation of anti-DNA antibody producing cells was not limited to only a few mouse strains but was noted when many different murine strains were challenged with lipopolysaccharides. Furthermore, subsequent studies

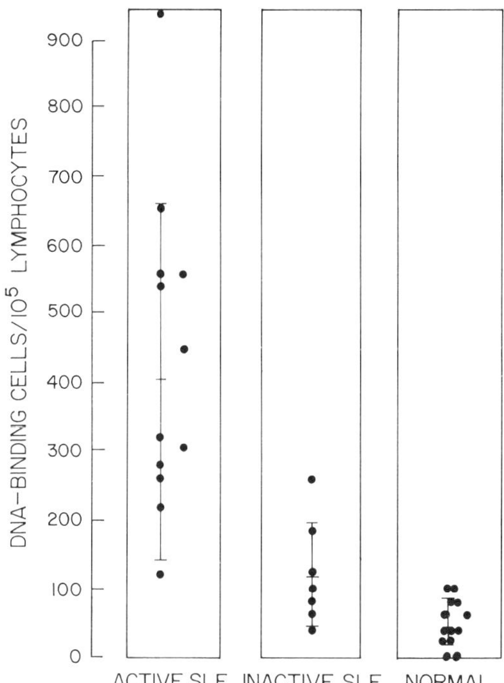

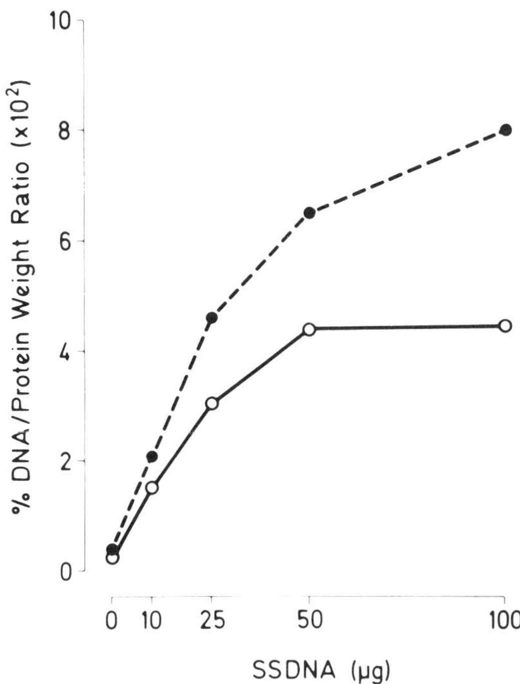

Figure 7-14 Relative numbers of antigen-binding cells (binding nDNA) among active and inactive SLE patients, and normal control subjects. (Reproduced with permission, A. D. Bankhurst and R. C. Williams, Jr., *J. Clin. Invest.* 56:1378, 1975.)

Figure 7-15 Binding curves of SSDNA to GBM (○). Increasing amounts of SSDNA were incubated with 100 µg of GBM or collagen. The DNA-binding capacity of these proteins is expressed on the vertical axis as weight ratio of DNA bound to GBM or collagen. (Reproduced with permission, S. Izui, P. H. Lambert, and P. A. Miescher, *J. Exp. Med.* 144:428, 1976.)

by Izui and colleagues (126) have shown that nDNA as an antigen itself may have an unusual predilection for collagen-like materials in the glomerular basement membrane (GBM). Examples of the striking binding that occurs in vitro between GBM collagen and DNA are shown in Figure 7-15 and may represent an extremely important feature amplifying any immune-complex nephritis in which nDNA functions as antigen. These findings may also apply to the deposition of immunoglobulin and complement in the dermal-epidermal junctional layers of the skin in patients with active systemic lupus (127–129). The phenomenon has been studied by a number of groups, who have tried with variable results to relate basal layer immunoglobulin and complement deposition directly to other parameters of lupus activity, particularly renal involvement (129, 130). It has never really been clear why immunoglobulin and complement components show deposition in these areas. Parallel conventional histo-

logical examination often does not reveal much in the way of vasculitis or tissue necrosis. It seems possible that collections of Ig and C3 in such skin deposits associated with SLE actually represent the phenomenon of DNA binding to collagen-like molecules within the integument, with subsequent deposition of anti-DNA antibody and complement locally in the same areas. Careful elution studies and search for local relative concentration of nDNA in such tissues will be necessary to confirm or refute this hypothesis.

Analyses of different histological and immunofluorescent distributions of Ig and complement in a certain proportion of renal lesions noted in SLE indicate that although GBM and subendothelial immune deposits are frequently present, there also is parallel histological change and immunoglobulin deposition within renal tubules and interstitial areas (131–133). These lesions appear to represent yet another example of renal immune-complex deposition related to SLE. Precisely what primary antigens may be involved is unknown. Demonstration of DNA or other nuclear antigens in these immune deposits has not been accomplished; it may well be that the primary antigens involved in these interstitial and tubular basement membrane localizations are related to those originally studied by several groups in conjunction with the so-called Heymann's nephritis model (134–136). Renal functional abnormalities often concerned with handling of acid and base, single amino acids, or calcium and phosphorus sometimes associated with a well-defined renal tubular acidosis in such patients may be related to similar overt or subclinical interstitial and tubular immune-complex disease.

Central Nervous System Involvement

Next to progressive and irreversible renal lesions, involvement of central nervous system (CNS) function is the most common serious complication recorded in any large series of patients with SLE followed over a number of years (137–140). Because many patients with overt arteritis or vague but progressive mental deficits or personality changes do poorly, attention has been focused on this particular problem and on an understanding of the basic pathological process involved. Central nervous system manifestations associated with SLE have also been the subject of several excellent clinical and pathological surveys (140, 141). Very little is really known concerning the genesis of either functional or anatomic lesions in CNS lupus involvement. A few patients can be shown at autopsy to have gross and microscopic changes of generalized cranial arteritis presumably from immune-complex deposition. Changes in the profile of cerebrospinal fluid complement components such as C3 or C4 or detectable immune complexes have been suggested as harbingers of serious clinical sequelae (115, 142). In addition, various types of noninvasive monitoring such as technetium or EMI scanning have proven useful in a few cases. Recently, we have been impressed with

the remarkable diversity of clearcut physiological abnormalities revealed by radioactive ^{15}O scanning as introduced by Pinching and associates for monitoring cerebral lupus involvement (143). This technique frequently shows large gaps in oxygen perfusion within multiple cerebral areas but requires proximity to a cyclotron or some other source capable of generating 15-labeled oxygen with the short half-life of several minutes. The obvious advantage of such a technique is its rapidity and the fact that it measures actual oxygen delivery to brain cells both in arterial oxygen and as labeled CO_2 in the venous phase. Examples of the remarkable changes shown in the cerebrum of an active SLE patient studied with this new technique are shown in Figure 7-16.

Several reports have provided evidence for involvement of immune complexes in CNS manifestations of SLE. Atkins and colleagues

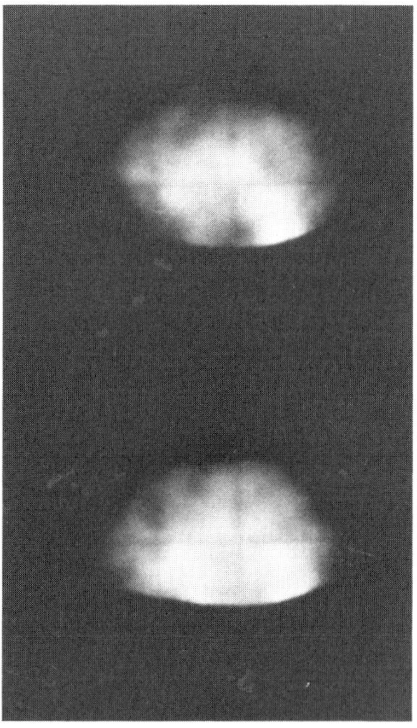

Figure 7-16   An example of the multiple cerebral defects noted using a ^{15}O brain scan in a patient with active SLE. The lower pattern was obtained with ^{15}O-labeled material, and the upper pattern shows the second phase where CO_2 is labeled with ^{15}O. (Photograph courtesy of Richard Seward and G. R. V. Hughes, Hammersmith Hospital, London.)

(144) demonstrated immunoglobulin, C3, and local vascular involvement of the choroid plexus in patients dying with cerebral lupus involvement. In addition, Lampert and Oldstone have shown similar choroid plexus involvement in animal models and in patients with SLE (145–147). These clinical and pathological findings are important, since they may reflect critical functional structural lesions in the choroid and microvascular bed very similar in its function of fluid and solute exchange to the renal glomerulus. Choroidal deposits of Ig and C3 conceivably could dramatically affect fluid exchange or solute concentrations within rapidly exchanging cerebrospinal fluid components. Whether such hypothetical shifts are capable of inducing the spectrum of neurophysiological changes seen in SLE is as yet undetermined. A diagrammatic representation emphasizing the similarities and differences between the topography within the renal glomerulus and the choroid plexus is shown in Figure 7-17. Of note is the thicker basement membrane present in the choroid compared to the same structure in the renal glomerulus and the scattered fibroblasts present in the choroid

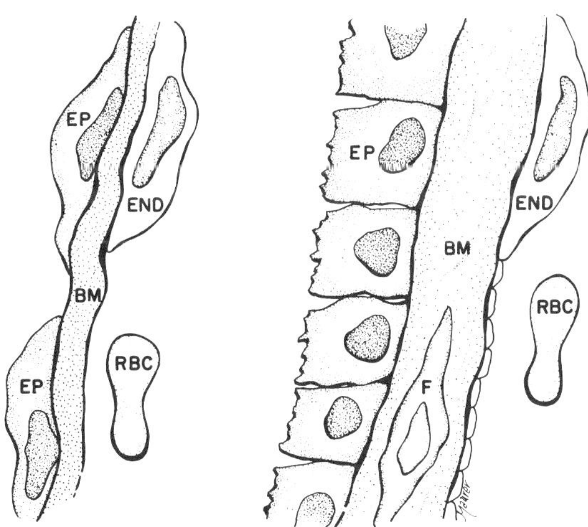

Figure 7-17 Structural differences between glomerular basement membrane in the kidney and in the choroid plexus. EP = epithelial cells; END = endothelial cells; BM = basement membrane; F = fibroblast; RBC = erythrocyte.

membrane. The finding of a receptor for activated complement components in the normal human glomerulus (148) and the demonstration of an Fc receptor within the human choroid (149) represent parallel findings supporting apparent endogenous receptors for immune complexes within these critical areas. In the past we have been impressed with the paucity of distinctly abnormal neuropathological findings in SLE patients dying with previous clinical manifestations of marked neurological dysfunction. It seems possible that other phenomena beside those directly mediated by immune complexes within the choroid or cerebral vessels may be involved. The fascinating results obtained with radiolabeled oxygen reported by Pinching and associates (143) suggest that changes in oxygen delivery to brain cells may vary transiently and may not correlate with patterns of cerebral blood flow as shown by parallel EMI scan or even angiography.

Immune Complexes and the Hematopoietic and Lymphoid Systems

Patients with SLE often show the presence of a wide variety of antibodies reactive with blood and lymphoid elements. Some patients may present with acute hemolytic anemia or the only initial disease manifestation may be idiopathic thrombocytopenic purpura or leukopenia and lymphopenia with fever and diffuse myalgias. In patients with acute hemolytic syndromes, antibodies with a wide spectrum of specificities have been implicated including anti–red-cell membrane antibodies restricted to the Rh complex (anti-e, anti-E) or other erythrocyte membrane antigens including IgM cold agglutinins capable of direct activation of the complement pathways. Although the occurrence of acute hemolytic anemia alone is probably rather rare as the only or primary manifestation of the disease, thrombocytopenia is more common as part of the presenting symptom complex. In many patients specific antiplatelet antibodies capable of complement consumption have been identified. Of great interest were a group of patients, studied by a number of workers (150–152), who presented with what initially appeared to be idiopathic or primary thrombocytopenia and responded appropriately to splenectomy only to show subsequent gradual evolution to a full-blown clinical picture of severe and often progressive SLE. These patients are particularly interesting in line with current thinking that since the spleen is known to contain a rich endowment of suppressor cells, splenectomy produces an acute depletion of suppressor cells and their precursors. Consequently, marked derangements in general immunologic control may supervene.

Similar to the situations encountered with erythrocytes or platelets, patients frequently show marked leukopenia and lymphopenia during acute SLE exacerbations. The lymphopenia in particular has been linked by several clinical studies to presence of antilymphocyte antibodies in the sera of such patients (153–157). This particular manifestation of cell-directed immune-complex disease may be of fundamental importance in somehow potentiating or amplifying many of the immunologic abnormalities of the disease. Antilymphocyte antibodies present in the sera of most patients with SLE show relative cold reactivity and are often found predominantly in the IgM subclass although they are also present in IgG fractions (156, 158). Such antibodies are capable of adsorption to lymphocyte membranes in vivo and may cause lysis of such cells on exposure to additional exogenous sources of complement (159). One of the most interesting aspects of antilymphocyte antibody is that some SLE sera show immunoglobulin components actually producing preferential reactivity for T cells or B cells of individual lymphocyte donors. This has now been demonstrated in various experimental systems where blocking of responder cells in mixed leukocyte cultures (160, 161) or binding to either T cells or B cells using radio-labeled protein A or direct cytotoxicity has been documented (158, 162).

One of the most puzzling features of antilymphocyte antibodies is indeed related to their primary specificity. The occurrence of these antibodies is not a phenomenon by any means limited to SLE, for they have now been described in a host of other disorders includ-

ing multiple sclerosis, pernicious anemia, inflammatory bowel disease, Hodgkin's disease, and viral disorders such as infectious mononucleosis (163–167). However, the broad reactivity against large panels of normal donor lymphocytes and their almost universal presence in association with SLE make them of considerable theoretical interest. It is possible that formation by lupus patients of antibodies to lymphocytes merely represents another example of the phenomenon of exaggerated hyperreactivity of the humoral immune system. Antilymphocyte antibodies with primary anti–B-cell specificity have recently been described in all normal subjects by Park and co-workers (168); this finding suggests that such antibodies could play a role in normal physiological immune homeostasis. On the other hand, the striking broad reactivity of antilymphocyte antibodies in SLE suggests that they may be important in some way in distorting or amplifying certain abnormal features of the immune response in systemic lupus. It is conceivable that some features of the depressed cell-mediated immune response in SLE are a direct result of coating or elimination of certain subpopulations of lymphocytes. Alternatively, if some antilymphocyte antibodies show preferential reactivity for suppressor T cells, such reactions might actually reduce functional suppressor T-cell effectiveness and accentuate potential autoimmune reactions. Some preliminary evidence for this has recently emerged and there are many indications (169) that similar antilymphocyte antibodies appear to preferentially inactivate or depress suppressor T-cell activity in NZB mice. These mice show high titers of lymphocytotoxic antibodies with relative specificity for thymocytes (170–172). The antibodies show preferential effects in influencing cell traffic or lymphocyte homing mechanisms within the intact animal. Now that the T_γ cells in human material have been identified as putative suppressor cells, this possibility must be directly examined using purified human T_γ and T_μ cells as targets for lymphocytotoxic antibodies in both cytotoxicity and functional assays (63, 173).

The striking potency of antilymphocyte antibodies in SLE also raises the possibility that they occur as an autologous response to antigens newly derived or hybridized with self-antigens already present on lymphocyte surfaces. Such an eventuality might occur if viral DNA segments had been intercalated into self-DNA to the extent that certain membrane antigens on lymphocyte surfaces were coded for by bits of "non-self" viral DNA hidden in the autologous host genetic material. Thus far, there is no direct evidence to support this sort of specificity in antilymphocyte antibodies present in SLE, but such approaches must be considered directly and experiments designed to ascertain whether antilymphocyte antibodies in lupus show some as yet undetermined specificity. Virtually all mouse strains thus far investigated possess DNA sequences that are homologous to the genomes of endogenous C-type particles (174). It has also been reported that normal mouse spleen cells activated by antigenic stimulation express murine leukemia virus GP71-like antigen on both T-cell and B-cell progeny (175). Thus human antilymphocyte antibodies such as are present in SLE reacting with virtually all normal human lymphocytes could theoretically show reactivity for some sort of "viral antigen" present on all normal lymphocytes.

Many sera from patients with SLE show varying degrees of cryoprecipitation at 4° C (176–178). Recently, studies of such cryoprecipitates have revealed relative concentration not only of antibodies to various polynucleotides (179) but of lymphocytotoxic antibodies as well (180). If antilymphocyte antibodies are present in large enough quantities to be represented in serum cryoprecipitates, they may participate directly in immune-complex–mediated tissue injury as insoluble immune complexes in various parts of the vascular system.

Studies conducted by Bluestein and Zvaifler (181) have indicated that antilymphocyte antibodies from some patients with SLE show distinct cross-reactivity with antigens present in normal human brain. The brain shares cross-reactive determinants with both hematopoietic stem cells and thymocytes particularly as studied in several mouse systems (182, 183). Studies of patients with clinical evidence of CNS involvement often show high titers of lymphocytotoxic antibodies, some of which can be absorbed out by preparations of human brain (181, 184). These findings raise the distinct possibility that initial antigenic stimulation toward their formation could arise by immunization through altered or damaged CNS tissues. These possible relationships now must be extended in longitudinal studies.

Another important feature related to the presence of lymphocytotoxic antibodies in patients with SLE has been pointed out in family studies presented by DeHoratius and co-workers (185, 186), which indicate a strikingly high prevalence of such antibodies in relatives of SLE patients—particularly those having close personal contact with the SLE proband. An example of the family distribution of antibodies from this study is shown in Table 7-3. Of particular significance is the finding that antilymphocyte antibodies were increased in non-blood-related relatives of SLE patients, again those having close personal association with SLE patients. In these studies a correlation was also noted between prevalence of antilymphocyte antibodies and antibodies to RNA as measured by radioactive binding techniques (186). Positive tests for lymphocytotoxic antibodies and anti-RNA antibodies apparently occurred together in many unaffected relatives. These data provide interesting material in terms of possible external agents being responsible for SLE. The initial family studies of the distribution of lymphocytotoxic antibodies have now been extended in several other population groups (187, 188). Similar clustering of positive family data as determined by Lowenstein and Rothfield (189) provides additional evidence for contact with patients and relatedness in the distribution of positive tests for dermal-epidermal junction skin immunofluorescence.

Other Remote Effects of Immune Complexes

A common clinical feature of SLE is the frequent presentation with polyserositis characterized by pleuritis, pericarditis, and even in some instances rapid accumulation of ascites. Little is known concerning mediation of serositis in such instances, but we have frequently been impressed with the rapidity of development of pleural or pericardial fluid

Table 7-3 Percentage of positive lymphocytotoxicity of sera from consanguineous relatives.

Relation to subject	Number of sera	Percentage of positive sera	
Control family members	60	3	
First-degree relatives	86	62	
Household contacts	68	72	} $p < 0.001$
Nonhousehold contacts	18	22	
Second-degree relatives	18	44[a]	
Household contacts	6	83	} $p < 0.02$
Nonhousehold contacts	12	25	

Source: Reproduced with permission, R. J. DeHoratius and R. P. Messner, *J. Clin. Invest.* 55:1254, 1975.
[a] Not significantly different than first-degree relatives.

and the findings of low complement levels and high gamma-globulin content in such fluids. Few clinical determinations are yet available in which quantitative levels of detectable immune complexes in serous effusions have been measured and compared to that present concurrently in blood. It seems highly likely that the polyserositis is an acute reaction to massive serosal surface stimulation by immune-complex deposition. There is possibly something about the clinical process in SLE that induces receptors for immune complexes in tissue locations where they are not ordinarily present in detectable form. If the intrinsic disease process were capable of such induction of Fc or C3b receptor differentiation on serous surfaces like the parietal pleura or pericardium, complex deposition understandably would ensue, and subsequent activation of chemotactic mechanisms with accumulation of PMN and mononuclear cells and later transudation of fluid effusions. Experimental models for polyserositis similar to that seen in SLE are discussed in Chapter 13.

Another clinical feature representing a unique complication frequently seen in patients with SLE is multiple areas of bony infarction or aseptic necrosis. The basic pathogenesis of this complication is poorly understood. It is usually seen in patients with peripheral evidence of active vasculitis, but is also noted in some patients with severe rheumatoid arthritis and in individuals undergoing prolonged immunosuppressive therapy after kidney transplantation. In each of these separate disease groups, increases in circulating immune complexes are often present. As has been mentioned earlier, there is extensive documentation for the presence of immune complexes in patients with rheumatoid arthritis (31–37, 79–81) and in subjects with SLE (106–109). A recent study of post–renal transplant patients (190) has documented the frequent occurrence of elevations of detectable immune complexes. A great deal of indirect evidence suggests that presence of aseptic necrosis in bone may be related to tissue deposition of immune complexes. The most obvious support for such a view relates to the fact that the bony lesions are essentially infarctions in which critical vascular supply to osseous tissues has been occluded. One of the most common lesions in SLE resembles central features of a diffuse vasculitis. It is therefore reasonable to assume that a similar pathogenetic mechanism may be involved in the problem of aseptic necrosis of bone. The demonstration of homing or fixation of antigens within dense connective tissue (60, 61) discussed in Chapter 5 lends additional support to this view.

In aseptic necrosis of bone associated with SLE, the tissue lesion is often that of a slowly evolving bony infarction. Typical x-ray findings of such lesions are shown in Figure 7-18. Few serial studies of such patients are available concerning changes in the osseous micro-

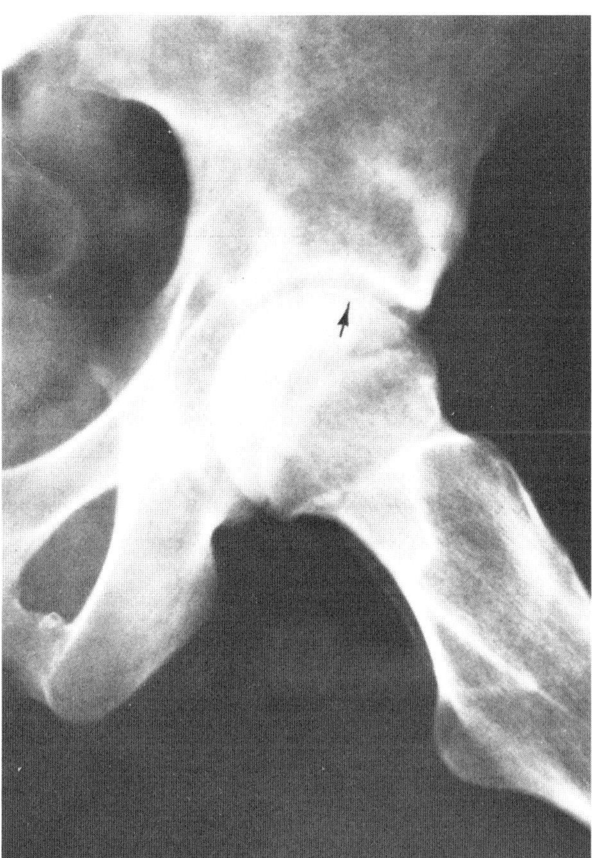

Figure 7-18 An example of early aseptic necrosis of the hip (*arrow*) in a patient with SLE and moderate previous corticosteroid therapy. (Photograph courtesy of J. S. Davis IV, Charlottesville, Virginia.)

vasculature during the early stages of necrosis. Certainly, the close association with long-term corticosteroid therapy in many patients is explainable by the experimental work of Haakenstad and co-workers (191), which indicates marked slowing and depression of immune-complex clearing in animals treated with corticosteroids. Further studies with an aim toward direct proof of immune-complex vasculitis as the initiating event in aseptic bony necrosis is difficult since biopsy, as in the kidney, is not feasible and may be fraught with severe complications such as superimposition of osteomyelitis or sinus formation. In this situation a noninvasive method of detecting immune-complex deposition is needed. Merely establishing obliteration of critical vascular supply by arteriography or bone scanning is not sufficient. Localization of labeled C3 or other isolated immune reactants to areas of aseptic necrosis would provide direct proof that such lesions are indeed associated with local immune-complex deposition. This particular clinical problem is an important one, particularly as newer features of therapy evolve, such as plasmapheresis or extracorporeal immune-complex removal. If elevations of detectable complexes were shown to be directly related to episodes of aseptic necrosis, some rational basis for direct complex removal as effective therapy might be established. All too often patients with this distressing and potentially crippling complication are managed passively and finally by resection and joint replacement when necrosis of osseous tissue is irreversible and complete.

Other Immune-Complex Systems

In the discussion thus far antigen-antibody systems have been stressed that have been most extensively studied and convincingly shown to be directly related to phenomena such as the nDNA–anti-nDNA reaction or possibly anti-lymphocyte antibodies. However, the remarkable heterogeneity of other autoantibodies in SLE suggests that other self-directed immune reactions are also present and may play as yet unidentified roles in direct pathogenesis. IgG, complement, and electron-dense deposits on renal tubular basement membranes and interstitial renal deposits represent reactions of this kind. Several other antigen-antibody systems studied in SLE may be of additional physiological interest, and much more is known about the antigens than at present is understood about the fate of immune complexes formed by their respective autoantibodies. A list of some of these antigen-antibody systems is presented in Table 7-4 along with specific disease associations and some of the most widely used methods of detection. Clear evidence implicating many of these systems in direct immune-complex–mediated tissue injury in SLE is not presently available, so that extended discussion is not warranted at this time. It is important, however, to stress that these immune reactions undoubtedly play an important part in the

Table 7-4   Antigen-antibody systems other than antilymphocyte antibody extensively studied in SLE.

Antigens (and references)	Method of detection and characterization	Disease association
Cytoplasmic antigens (192–195)	Immunofluorescence, precipitation, complement fixation [multiple antigens now described]	Low correlation with renal disease
Nucleoprotein (94, 95, 102, 196, 197)	Hemagglutination, precipitation, complement fixation	May be detected in renal eluates(?) associated with renal disease
Soluble nuclear antigens (198)	Precipitation, complement fixation, immunofluorescence, hemagglutination	Not directly related to renal disease
Histones or histone-binding proteins (199)		
RNA, RNP (200–204) and nucleolar antigens	Hemagglutination, complement fixation, radioimmunoassay, immunofluorescence	Mixed connective-tissue diseases; not usually associated with renal disease in MCTD
Sm antigens (100, 205)	Precipitation, complement fixation, hemagglutination	Often seen in patients with renal disease
Sjögren antigens (A and B) (206)	Precipitation, hemagglutination	Sjögren's syndrome
RA-related antigens (8, 9)	Precipitation, immunofluorescence	Rheumatoid arthritis, occasionally Sjögren's syndrome

genesis of various aspects possibly related to immune-complex injury. Formation of antibody to ENA (extractable nuclear antigen) has actually been shown in NZB/W hybrid mice to inhibit DNA–anti-DNA reactions (207). This may explain the relative rarity of progressive immune-complex renal disease in patients with mixed connective-tissue disease described initially by Sharp and co-workers (200, 201).

Selective Immune Deficiencies and SLE

One of the most fascinating paradoxical examples associated with SLE as a disorder of immune hyperreactivity or overresponse is the prevalence of SLE-like disease among patients with well-documented selective immunodeficiencies, particularly absence or marked decrease in isolated complement components. In many ways the situation is analogous to that of rheumatoid arthritis occurring in the face of agammaglobulinemia (208–210). An acute symmetrical polyarthritis resembling rheumatoid disease described in association with agammaglobulinemia is indeed puzzling. If one were to attempt to fit these clinical findings with the basic concept that immune complexes are fundamental to pathogenesis of rheumatoid arthritis, one might postulate that in an agammaglobulinemic individual it might take only infinitesimal quantities of antigen or complexes to initiate a disorder. Thus, any immune response whatsoever would put the patient immediately in antigen excess where tiny amounts of soluble complexes might be formed. This is an attractive argument, but one that has not to our knowledge been substantiated by experimental data.

The occurrence of SLE in patients with selective complement deficiencies is an analogous paradox, particularly if one invokes activation of the complement cascade and eventual tissue deposition of complexes as one of the basic pathological processes in the underlying disease. The clinical examples of SLE-like disease associated with complement deficiencies are convincing, and in many instances these patients have been studied in great detail. Several of the first patients described with selective complement component defects were subjects in whom the early reacting components such as C1 or C2 were either absent or markedly reduced (211–219). One of the subjects initially reported by Pickering and co-workers (218) as having glomerulonephritis on subsequent follow-up was found to have developed SLE (212). Further examples of SLE and several other autoimmune disorders including anaphylactoid purpura and dermatomyositis have also been reported where other later-acting complement deficiencies have been documented (220–227). Patients presenting with clinical evidence for SLE frequently showed striking skin rash, fevers, arthralgias, and most importantly clear evidence of immune-deposit disease on renal biopsy. An example of skin lesions recorded in the patient extensively studied by Moncada and co-workers (213) is shown in Figure 7-19. Expression of SLE in such patients with defective total complement activity was similar to that previously recorded in the usual patient without clear-cut complement deficiencies. The occurrence of immune-complex tissue deposition in patients with for instance C3 deficiency indicates that such deposits can form and probably activate the complement cascade directly through the alternate pathway. This recalls the animal studies discussed in Chapter 5 indicating that artificial decomplementation using cobra-venom factor or other procedures did not affect half-life or tissue disposition of passively infused immune complexes.

The occurrence of single-component complement deficiency may be considered from another aspect. A number of current studies indicate that small amounts of circulating immune complexes may be present transiently in normal subjects. Activation of complement and subsequently the C3b or Fc receptors in various portions of the reticuloendothelial system is effective in rapidly clearing circulating complexes, and normal homeostasis is usually

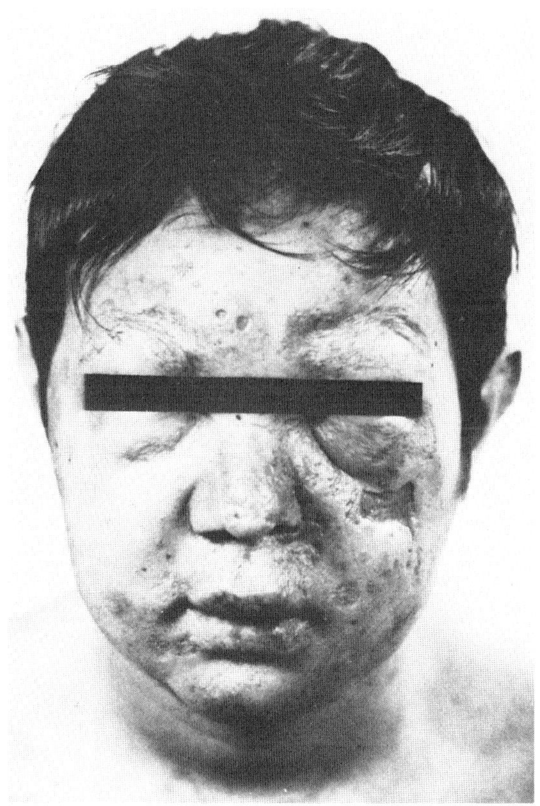

Figure 7-19 Striking skin lesions in a patient with SLE-like syndrome and complement deficiency. (Reproduced with permission, B. Moncada, N. K. B. Day, R. A. Good et al., *N. Engl. J. Med.* 286:689, 1972.)

maintained. In patients lacking any or all features of the natural clearing mechanism, prolongation or attenuation of effective clearing cycles will be present and immune-complex deposition is more likely to result. The presence of the second or alternative pathway in such subjects merely ensures that activation will eventually take place and immune-complex deposition occur. Several immunofluorescent and metabolic studies of SLE patients have demonstrated that the alternate complement pathway can function directly in immune-complex injury in patients with SLE (228, 229). If SLE were related to some type of persistent or slow virus infection, absence of individual complement components might also contribute to ineffective host inactivation of virus. Studies by Leddy and colleagues (230) using sera with selective complement deficiencies have shown marked impairment of neutralization using both DNA and RNA viruses. A number of experimental models have indicated that augmentation of either immune envelopment or killing of virus is often dependent on the presence of effective complement activity. If any single link in the chain is deficient, viral persistence or survival may well be amplified.

Clinical Application of Immune-Complex Assays

Any clinician is familiar with the most common clinical problem we face in SLE: how exactly is the patient doing? This particular question becomes vitally important in day-to-day or week-to-week follow-up of individual patients, particularly those on large doses of immunosuppressive drugs like corticosteroids, azathioprine, or cyclophosphamide. Accurate clinical assessment can be fraught with error or uncertainty with the usual parameters available to the clinician in an outpatient or even inpatient situation. Two types of serious complications are extremely difficult to follow and predict—that of the course of renal disease and that of CNS involvement. Recent studies of morbidity and mortality of patients with SLE (137–139) indicate that apart from the vasculitis affecting kidney or brain, immunodepletion and subsequent superimposed infection may be even more important in producing a fatal outcome. The physician attempting to suppress the disease with corticosteroids or cytostatic drugs frequently is rewarded by having to deal with unheralded overwhelming fungal, parasitic, or nosocomial bacterial infection.

In many instances renal biopsy serves as a reasonable basis for important judgments about therapeutic regimes, whether to utilize immunosuppressives, or even appropriate maintenance dosage of corticosteroid (231–235). It appears that focal, less extensive glomerular lesions detected either by light and electron microscopy or by immunofluorescent techniques have a considerably better overall prognosis than diffuse proliferative or membranous glomerular involvement. However, we have often observed the rapid change of the renal histological picture from a nonlesion or mild focal nephritis to a rampaging generalized proliferative lesion without much in the way of new therapy or without parallel clinical indication that the disease is undergoing a generalized intensification. What seems to be most urgently needed for rational therapy is an accurate predictive clinical assessment that can be correlated with other easily obtainable parameters such as urinalysis, blood urea nitrogen (BUN), creatinine clearance, level of complement activity, or renal histology.

One of the most vexing clinical problems is the fact that lupus nephropathy may be present or even progressive in the face of negative urine examinations or apparently normal renal function (236–238). This has recently been reemphasized in an interesting study by Mahajan and associates (237). Clinical findings and course were compared with renal biopsy pathology in 90 patients with SLE. Twenty-seven showed normal urinalysis and renal function in the face of biopsy-proven lupus nephropathy. Three patients with normal urine examinations and renal function showed focal glomerulonephritis that later progressed to diffuse glomerular involvement and eventual decrease in creatinine clearance. Twelve of the 27 patients with initial normal clinical findings showed diffuse glomerular changes on kidney biopsy. However, in the limited group examined, there did not appear to be any difference in overall course regardless of clinical findings of renal involvement at the time when histological evidence for a diffuse process was established.

The surprising finding of a significant proportion of patients without evidence of clinical renal disease who did have what might be considered silent diffuse nephropathy has been documented in other reports (238, 239). As the current sensitive assays for presence and amounts of detectable immune complexes are applied to the clinical assessment of patients, it will be of great interest to see whether such an additional parameter will indeed provide the clinician with a more meaningful assessment of the clinical status of individual patients. The general spectrum of what might be expected in any pathological study of a large group of patients with lupus nephritis has already been documented in several excellent reviews (240–246). The overall prognosis and the progression of disease in a considerable number of subjects with diffuse or membranous changes is still grim. With recently developed methods for immune-complex detection and more aggressive early attempts at newer therapeutic interventions (such as plasmapheresis or extracorporeal immunoabsorption), some real progress may be expected in patients with early or even moderate immune-complex renal disease.

Sensitive Tests for Detection of Complexes

Virtually all groups who have looked at patients with SLE via the newer methods for immune-complex detection have noted high proportions of positive tests. When Theofilopoulos and colleagues (76) applied the Raji-cell radioimmunoassay, all of 13 patients initially tested showed strongly positive tests ranging from 24 μg/ml to 800 or 1,000 μg/ml of aggregate-equivalent (76); data from this study are shown in Table 7-5. A negative correlation was seen between amount of com-

plexes and total hemolytic complement. A positive correlation, however, was noted between presence of immune complexes detectable in the Raji-cell radioimmunoassay and levels of anti-nDNA antibody. No correlation was recorded between amounts of complexes detected and parallel quantitative determination of serum IgG. Serial studies over a 12- to 24-month interval in 10 patients showed a definite relation between both depression of total hemolytic complement and elevation of complexes as measured in the Raji-cell assay and clinical exacerbations of disease (Figure 7-20). It can be seen that DNA binding was high in conjunction with depression of complement activity and marked elevation of levels of circulating complexes in the Raji-cell assay. Also significant in this study was the finding of marked interval decrease in detectable circulating complexes after initiation of prednisone treatment. No interference was recorded that could be attributed to binding of naturally occurring anti-lymphocyte antibodies to the indicator Raji cells. Since the actual binding of complexes to the Raji cell is a function of adherence of complexes to the cell through activated C3b, stud-

Table 7-5 Raji-cell radioimunoassay for immune complexes in patients with SLE.

Subject	AHG (μg eq/ml)	CH 50[a]	Anti-DNA[b]	Erythrocyte sedimentation rate	Proteinuria	Clinical activity	Serum IgG (mg/ml)
1	24	200	ND[c]	10	ND	0	14
2	98	85	43	39	ND	+	13.5
3	25	141	5	54	ND	0	15.7
4	400	114	55	92	0	+	18.5
5	24	125	34	69	±	±	14.9
6	65	147	ND	24	±	±	12.3
7	175	93	51	58	±	+	12.6
8	325	78	51	47	+	+	13.5
9	1,000	<30	62	15	0	+	11.8
10	164	<30	49	75	+	+	17.0
11	428	200	ND	89	0	0	11.0
12	52	121	ND	35	0	−	ND
13	800	74	57	26	0	+	14.7

Source: Reproduced with permission, A. Theofilopoulos, C. B. Wilson, and F. J. Dixon, *J. Clin. Invest.* 57:169, 1976.

[a] Normal values greater than 150.

[b] Determined by the Farr technique with [^{14}C]DNA. Upper limit for normals, 26 percent binding.

[c] ND = not determined.

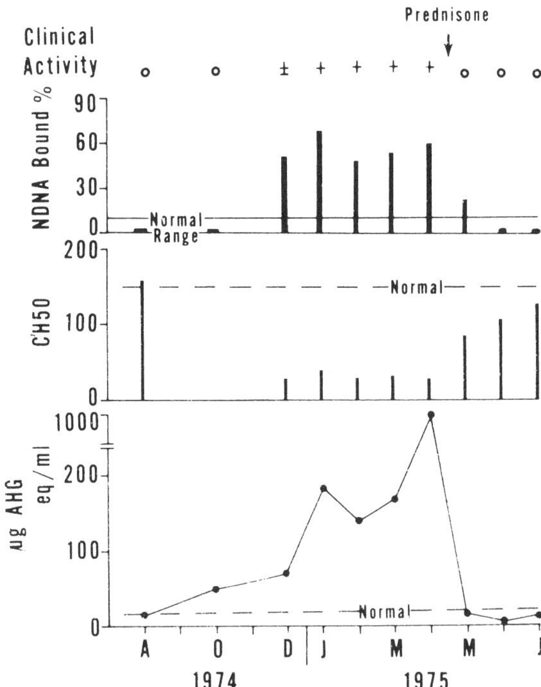

Figure 7-20 Serial study of a forty-seven-year-old woman with SLE showing the correlation among levels of immune complexes, C'H 50, antibodies to nDNA, and clinical activity. (Reproduced with permission, A. N. Theofilopoulos, C. B. Wilson, and F. Dixon, *J. Clin. Invest.* 57:169, 1976.)

ies were undertaken to ascertain whether in hypocomplementemic SLE sera addition of exogenous normal complement produced any enhancement of immune-complex binding to Raji cells. *No* enhancement was observed, indicating that even in markedly hypocomplementemic sera sufficient C3b activation had occurred to render the test uniformly positive.

Similar findings were also reported by Nydegger and co-workers (247), using precipitation with polyethylene glycol and the radiolabeled C1q-binding method. Sera from 22 SLE patients were analyzed and showed significant increases in C1q binding: 42 ± 27 percent versus 16 ± 16 percent in normal control sera. Again a definite negative correlation with total hemolytic complement activity was recorded. Sephadex G-200 gel filtration studies indicated that fractions reactive with C1q in the binding assay were generally found in the high-molecular-weight or exclusion fraction. From these

initial studies it appeared that high-molecular-weight complexes correlated with clinical flares in SLE renal activity. The relative importance of complexes of different sizes has recently been stressed by Levinsky and co-workers (248), who studied 29 patients with lupus nephritis using the sensitive latex agglutination method described in Chapter 6. Clinical disease appeared to closely parallel presence of detectable complexes. Size studies were performed in seven cases. An association was suggested between the presence of complexes of medium (>16S) molecular weight and renal disease. A variety of sizes of complexes was noted in these studies; it appeared that a spectrum of reactive materials constituting IgG dimers, 19 S materials containing IgG, and materials >19S was present in various patients. The circulating complexes detected in these patients are shown in Figure 7-21. A final conclusion cannot be drawn about the relative importance of size, since all patients studied did not have renal biopsies and the prevalence of lupus nephropathy without clinical evidence of renal disease is therefore unknown. Of interest, however, was the marked diminution of levels of detectable complexes after one-gram pulse therapy with methyl prednisone, a therapeutic approach that has gained recent support among some groups who follow substantial numbers of patients with SLE.

Using the Raji-cell radioimmunoassay and the solid-phase C1q test, we have found that most SLE patients serially studied show a marked degree of positive reactivity in these tests. One of the most important aspects of SLE is the fact that in our hands, the quantitative amounts of complexes (for instance, those estimated in the Raji-cell test) are sometimes enormous: 1,000 to 1,500 μg/ml, in comparison to mild elevation (50 to 100 μg/ml) recorded in other conditions. This is a very important point that perhaps has not been stressed heavily enough in the studies recorded to date. The actual microgram amounts of complexes in some SLE sera are extremely high in comparison to other disorders. We have also been impressed with the occurrence of complexes of both intermediate (11S) and relatively high molecular weight

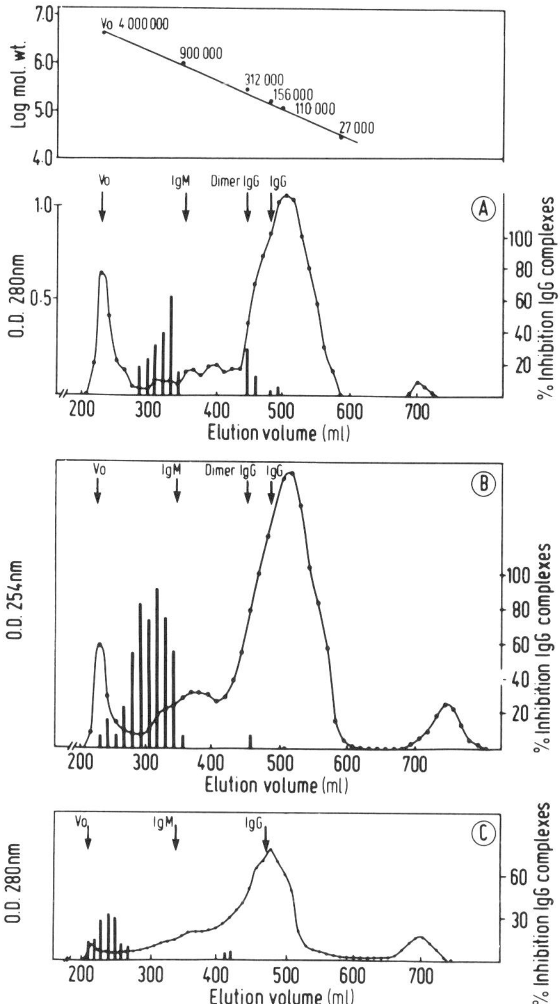

Figure 7-21 Sepharose CL 6B separation of proteins in sera of 3 patients with SLE. The column calibration is shown (*top*), with elution volume for proteins of different molecular weights: void volume (manufacturer's data), IgM (900,000), dimer IgG (312,000), IgG (156,000), F(ab')$_2$ (110,000), and pFc' (27,000). The void volume and elution peaks for IgM, dimer IgG, and monomer IgG are shown in the remaining graphs. Results of test for complexes using the anti-IgG reagent are shown; all fractions were tested and agglutination inhibition >3 percent plotted. The first trace, from a patient with SLE nephritis but no extrarenal manifestations, shows small and medium-sized complexes. The middle trace, from a patient with SLE nephritis with rash and vasculitis, shows small, medium-sized, and large complexes. The bottom trace, from a patient with active SLE but no clinical evidence of nephritis, shows small and large complexes, but none of medium size. (Reproduced with permission, R. J. Levinsky, J. S. Cameron, and J. F. Soothill, *Lancet* 1:564, 1977.)

(19 S or greater) in many patients with active lupus nephropathy.

The study recently recorded by Cano and colleagues (249) is also of interest. Twenty-one patients with SLE were studied using the C1q-deviation test. Only 11 showed elevations of immune complexes using this method, a figure and proportion much lower than that previously recorded in the studies by Theofilopoulos and associates (76) or by Nydegger and co-workers (247). Patients both with and without renal disease showed elevated C1q binding, but again there were no details indicating whether in fact all patients had undergone kidney biopsy. A definite positive correlation with anti-DNA antibodies and positivity in the C1q-binding test was also noted. As in the

findings of Levinsky and co-workers (248), density gradient ultracentrifugation of SLE sera positive for presence of complexes showed reactivity in intermediate (7 to 19 S) and 19 S and greater fractions within such separations. Of particular interest was the disappearance of C1q reactivity in several serum samples after DNase or RNase digestion, suggesting either that free DNA in some serum samples was responsible for positive reactivity or that antibodies to these various polynucleotides as complexes were involved in production of positive reactions. This particular line of approach must be extended; it is not at all clear just what antigens are present in the various types of complexes being detected during much of the research discussed. In the study by Cano and colleagues (249) RNase digestion was performed because RNA and particularly ribonucleoproteins constitute another important potential source of antigens in SLE. Surprisingly, little is known about their capacity to form or participate in immune-complex phenomena. Reichlin and Mattioli (194) have suggested that such antibodies against non-DNA nuclear constituents might even protect the kidney against immune-complex damage. It is also possible that antibodies against other antigens such as the Sm antigen (100) might be involved in the formation of some of the complexes detected in these experimental systems. The Sm antigen and the cytoplasmic antigens such as RO (194) are both less than 150,000 Daltons and might indeed account for some of the 7 to 19S complexes detected by various sensitive assay systems.

At present, no uniformity of opinion exists with regard to the weight or degree of importance to assign to serum DNA-binding or quantitative assessment of C3 or C4. In the studies by Cameron and co-workers (250) it was clear that C3 and C4 concentrations correlated poorly with nDNA binding. During serial studies in 32 individuals active nephritis was rarely found in patients showing a normal C4 or normal DNA binding; conversely, elevated DNA binding or depression of serum C4 did not always correlate with active renal disease. We too have been impressed that serial studies of C3 and C4 now readily available in most clinical laboratories as determined by radial diffusion Mancini technique are frequently not of much help in clinical assessment of the activity of lupus nephropathy. Patients currently being followed with episodes of severe CNS involvement often show no significant elevation of nDNA-binding and no depression of serum C3 or C4. Considerably more longitudinal study is needed with sensitive assays such as the Raji-cell radioimmunoassay, the C1q-binding tests, or the conglutinin-binding assay before the use of these tests will actually improve our clinical management of individual subjects. We must emphasize also that all of the current tests now in general use have blind spots—or at least there have been some moderate discrepancies when several tests are used in parallel on a similar panel of patients. The Raji-cell test and perhaps the conglutinin-binding test may show some preferential reactivity with immune complexes of relatively higher molecular weight. Serial studies in any group will, therefore, naturally be influenced by what test is being used to examine the samples involved.

Examples of the overlap and possible discrepancies of attempts to compare three different immune-complex assays in several groups of patients are illustrated in the report of Eisen-berg and colleagues (251). In SLE a much lower proportion were positive (21 percent) with the conglutinin-binding assay than were detected with the Raji-cell test (62 percent). Thus, parallel serial assessment with several test systems may prove helpful. Furthermore, there must be some reservation about whether circulating immune complexes detected in serum are in any way a complete solution to the question, in view of the fact that what is circulating and what has or will deposit in tissues may be two entirely different aspects of the problem. Detectable circulating immune complexes present in SLE may only be what is left over, the important complexes having already been deposited in various tissues after a transient pass through the circulation. What is really needed in these situations is a three-dimensional view of the kidney or other vulnerable microvascular beds, a thorough knowledge of the factors circulating in plasma as immune complexes or activated complement components, and an accurate appraisal of the degree of concurrent saturation of the reticuloendothelial system. A clear profile in all three directions would provide the basis for rational therapy in most cases. This is an important perspective, not only for disorders such as SLE but also for a broad spectrum of other immune-complex renal diseases, parasitic infections, and neoplastic states.

Some direct insight into the role of reticuloendothelial system (RES) function in SLE has been gained through recent research reported by Frank and colleagues (252). As noted in Chapter 5, studies in active lupus patients using ^{51}Cr-labeled erythrocytes sensitized with IgG indicated marked impairment of clearance attributed to defective splenic macrophage Fc-receptor function. Abnormal clearances correlated with immune-complex levels, as monitored by the C1q-binding assay, and appeared to correlate also with disease activity. These studies emphasize the importance of a three-dimensional view of complexes in the patient as a whole. In addition, they suggest that when RES clearance is saturated, immune complexes may be free to circulate unimpeded and induce tissue microvascular injury.

A parallel observation related to apparent

impairment of RES function in chronic liver disease has been recorded by Jaffe and colleagues (253). Clearance of isologous erythrocytes coated with IgM or IgG and C3b in patients with primary biliary cirrhosis (PBC), chronic hepatitis, or alcoholic cirrhosis was compared with that in normal controls. None of the patients showed a defect in clearance of aggregated serum albumin. None of 6 patients with PBC showed delayed clearance of IgG-coated erythrocytes; one of 6 individuals with chronic hepatitis showed delayed IgG-specific clearance. By contrast, all of the 6 patients with PBC had a defect in clearance mediated by RES C3b receptors. No similar defect was recorded in patients with chronic hepatitis or alcoholic cirrhosis. These studies emphasized what appeared to be a C3b-specific defect in RES function among patients with PBC. There is every reason to expect that continued functional assessment of receptor-specific clearance in such models will eventually clarify the physiological role of both tissue-fixed and circulating immune complexes in a number of disease states.

Juvenile Rheumatoid Arthritis

Juvenile rheumatoid arthritis (JRA) is a disorder thought to be related directly or indirectly to adult rheumatoid disease. However, the disease shows several distinct subclasses (254, 255). Systemic JRA often is accompanied by fever, skin rash, multiple joint involvement, and extra-articular manifestations such as pericarditis. A much milder form of the disease has been classified as the pauciarticular variety, with involvement of less than five joints and without signs of severe systemic disease. As yet, very little is known concerning the possible role of immune complexes in JRA. One study has indicated the presence of detectable complexes in 22 percent of 51 patients studied. Presence of detectable complexes appeared to be associated with the more severe or systemic manifestations of disease. Of interest was the relatively low incidence of anti-immunoglobulin rheumatoid factor in these sera and the fact that presence of antinuclear antibodies, often associated with a subgroup of children show-

ing iritis (256), did not correlate with presence of detectable complexes. In the JRA patient group studied by Rossen and colleagues (257) the quantitative elevations of complexes as monitored by C1q-binding activity, with the exception of 2 of 11 patients, were generally of a low order of magnitude. These findings reemphasize the difference between JRA and its adult equivalent and suggest that although immune complexes per se may be of great importance in rheumatoid disease, their handling or clearance in peripheral blood may be much more effective in JRA.

Mixed Connective-Tissue Disease

Mixed connective-tissue disease (MCTD) is an interesting disorder first described in 1972 by Sharp and co-workers (200, 201). Very little is known concerning its pathogenesis and development. It is probably fair to say that MCTD can actually be dissociated from other diseases with which it shares many clinical features by virtue of several abnormalities that set it slightly apart from its first cousins—SLE, rheumatoid arthritis, dermatomyositis, or even scleroderma. The most prominent clinical features are arthralgia or arthritis, Raynaud's phenomenon, a peculiar distal swelling of the phalanges, episodes of pleuritis or interstitial pulmonary fibrosis, disorders of esophageal motility, and presence of high titers of antinuclear antibody producing a characteristic speckled pattern of nuclear fluorescence (Figure 7-22). A number of serological and immunochemical studies have defined MCTD as being closely associated with speckled antinuclear antibody. The specific nuclear antigen involved has now been extensively characterized as a ribonucleoprotein (RNP) that is sensitive to RNase digestion. Thus, patients with MCTD may show titers of 1:100,000 in hemagglutination studies with cells coated with RNP antigens. However, when the antigen is treated with ribonuclease, the titers fall to 1:10, 1:20, or zero.

Definite presence of antibody to RNP fulfilling these serological criteria is currently considered crucial to a clear-cut diagnosis of MCTD. Rather than emerging as an example

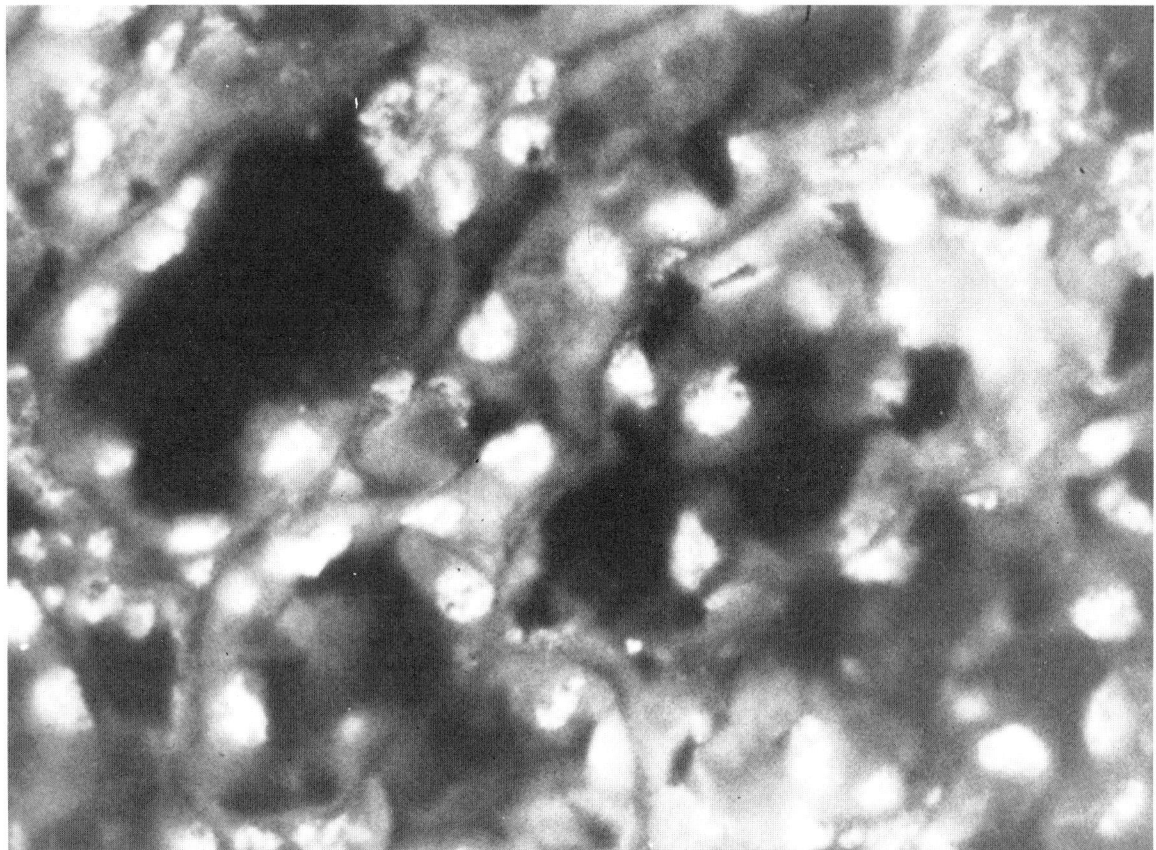

Figure 7-22 Speckled pattern of antinuclear antibody staining in serum from a patient with mixed
connective-tissue disease. Magnification × 450.

of distinct peripheral manifestation of immune-complex injury, somewhat the opposite
situation exists; in a way MCTD can be viewed
as a clinical foil to the broad general features of
SLE. Specifically, it appears unusual for immune-complex disease, particularly in the kidney, to be associated with MCTD. Although
several exceptions or convincing examples of
apparent immune-complex renal injury have
been reported in association with the disease
(258, 259), immune-complex renal involvement still appears to be uncommon. In many
ways the clinical course and precise manifestations of the disease should eventually be able to
tell us a great deal about both basic mechanisms and organ distribution of similar phenomena in comparable disorders such as
scleroderma, SLE, or rheumatoid arthritis.

Since many features of MCTD have been assumed in the past to be rather tacitly associated
with immune-complex phenomena, including
skin rash, arthritis, tenosynovitis, and pleuritis,
what is observed by the clinician may well be
generated by complexes, albeit of an entirely
different immunochemical type from those
generally encountered in the usual subject with
SLE. Thus, if nDNA–anti-DNA complexes are
the main offenders in SLE and by their particular physical and chemical nature show inor-
dinate affinity for skin or GBM collagen, complexes in MCTD may by virtue of their entirely
different physical qualities show organ and tissue distribution of a distinctive pattern caused
by the involvement of different fundamental
tissue antigens. As mentioned previously,
there is even some experimental work in ani-

mals suggesting that antibodies to RNA or RNP are capable of inhibiting reactions between nDNA and anti-DNA antibodies in experimental NZB/W hybrid mice (207). If this is clearly substantiated in clinical studies, it would explain the relative sparing of the kidney in most patients with this disorder. As more and more patients have been studied who fall into a difficult diagnostic category somewhere between SLE and MCTD, it is clear that one disease may at times evolve into the other. It is also obvious that if patients with high titers of anti-RNP antibodies and speckled nuclear antibody staining show high levels of antibody against the extractable nuclear Sm antigen originally characterized by Tan and Kunkel (100), the likelihood of eventual evolution into a typical SLE clinical syndrome with associated nephropathy is greatly enhanced.

The MCTD syndrome has now been described in children. Unlike the situation encountered in juvenile rheumatoid arthritis, it pursues a course more florid and sometimes equally as complicated and severe as that usually recorded in the adult counterpart (260).

Many clinical manifestations of SLE and MCTD overlap may eventually be enlightening in terms of actual perception of pathogenetic mechanisms, as for instance with respect to Raynaud's phenomenon, active skin lesions, frank arthritis, esophageal motility disturbances, or interstitial pulmonary infiltrates and fibrosis. To date there are few recorded observations of the presence of detectable immune complexes in such patients. Our own experience in a few patients studied to date, using both the Raji-cell radioimmunoassay and the solid-phase C1q tests, indicates that circulating complexes are present during active phases of the disease. The quantitative elevations of detectable complexes are, however, not nearly so impressive as those seen in SLE and have generally been in the neighborhood of 100 to 200 μg/ml.

A recent study by Halla and colleagues (261) reported assays of circulating immune complexes in sera from 20 patients with MCTD. Evidence for circulating complexes was found by at least one method in 94 percent of sera tested. This study utilized parallel immune-complex assays with Raji-cell radioimmunoassay, C1q-binding assay, and a monoclonal rheumatoid factor radioimmunoassay. The pattern of positive reactions in the three tests differed from that recorded with rheumatoid arthritis, where a much larger overlap was noted between positive tests in the monoclonal rheumatoid factor assay and C1q binding.

Patients with MCTD do not usually show presence of high levels of anti-nDNA antibody, although several exceptions have recently been encountered. It is possible that since only modest elevations of circulating complexes are present and no appreciable amounts of nDNA–anti-nDNA are found, clearance mechanisms for immune-complex removal in such patients are only moderately compromised and these patients fare better in eventual elimination or disposal of such materials than those with SLE who show high levels of detectable complexes (500 to 1,000 μg/ml) and a completely saturated clearance mechanism. Elution studies of gamma globulin from skin, synovial tissue, or other parenchymal lesions in the disease might serve as they have in SLE to point out those antigens involved in tissue deposition.

The clinical distinction being made between MCTD and SLE, rheumatoid arthritis, or scleroderma may be analogous to the designation of Felty's syndrome in rheumatoid arthritis as a separate or distinct phenomenon. This could be unfortunate, since recent evidence presented by Abdou and co-workers (262) now indicates that Felty's syndrome may show the characteristic leukopenia on the basis of an overactive suppressor T-cell phenomenon capable of directly affecting leukocyte maturation and proliferation in vivo and in vitro. To have segregated the patients with Felty's syndrome as a distinct clinical entity too early, merely on the basis of the presence of a low white-blood-cell count (as has been done in the patients with MCTD on the basis of the presence of high titers of anti-RNP antibody), would probably in retrospect have been incorrect. If, on the other hand, the designation of mixed connective-tissue disease as a separate clinical phenomenon will eventually clarify

important modulating influence in its pathogenesis, the distinction will have served a useful clinical purpose.

Ankylosing Spondylitis

Ankylosing spondylitis is generally regarded as a connective-tissue disorder of unknown etiology occurring principally in males and showing a remarkable linkage to HLA-B27 histocompatibility typing (263, 264). The clinical manifestations of the disease are often severe and progressive, with involvement of the axial skeleton and scattered peripheral joints. The striking relationship to B27 has focused attention on genetic and possible immunogenetic mechanisms involved in its pathogenesis. A recent report has also documented the occurrence of detectable circulating immune complexes in this disorder (265). Levels of complexes as detected by the C1q radioimmunoassay have not been as high as those in rheumatoid arthritis or SLE and have been found in a relatively low proportion of patients studied. The low levels of immune complexes in a few patients studied by Gabay and coworkers (265) do not suggest that they play a primary role in the disease.

Periarteritis Nodosa or Diffuse Vasculitis

Periarteritis nodosa or any of its clinical variants must be considered with the other connective-tissue diseases, for it has been classically regarded as one of the collagen vascular diseases. The necrotizing arterial lesions and the clinical presentation often intermingle with features of rheumatoid arthritis, SLE, polymyositis, or several of the other connective-tissue disorders. Again, little is known concerning basic pathogenesis, although histological examination of acute lesions is characteristic of an acute inflammatory arteritis with PMN cell, plasmacytic and lymphocytic infiltrations, and frequent areas of fibrinoid necrosis. In our experience, evidence that such a diffuse vasculitis process is the direct result of an antigen-antibody reaction is rarely documented in the individual case. Classification is

one of the problems relating to vasculitis. The original term *periarteritis nodosa* used by Kussmaul and Maier (266) has been criticized by Zeek and co-workers (267, 268) as a catchall for every type of inflammatory vascular lesion. Whether or not various histological classifications including hypersensitivity angiitis, eosinophilic granulomatous angiitis, vasculitis of connective-tissue diseases, and temporal arteritis have advanced our basic understanding of the pathogenesis of these disorders is a moot point. The morphological classifications suggested by Zeek were not based on immunologic proof of any distinct mechanisms involved. Establishment of temporal arteritis as a distinct clinical syndrome useful in classification and general perception of what may be expected in terms of eye complications or clinical course is certainly useful. However, in our opinion, dissection of multiple kinds of vasculitis on the basis of rather subjective clinical categories is bound to have a very short clinical usefulness. These classification problems have recently been reviewed by Alarçon-Segovia (269). Until direct proof is available of the precise pathological mechanisms involved, it is probably wise to regard these disorders as a heterogeneous group linked by common histopathological features, but not necessarily by similar basic etiologies.

Direct immunofluorescent studies of involved vessels may show traces of Ig or complement deposition but not nearly in the abundance documented with the similar vasculitic lesions of SLE. Exceptions have been the patients with hepatitis B immune-complex disease and a periarteritic-like presentation discussed at length in Chapter 3. Several patients with this symptom complex have been studied in detail by Fye and colleagues (270) using inhibition of antibody-dependent cell-mediated cytotoxicity (ADCC) and the Raji-cell radioimmunoassay, which demonstrated immune complexes in higher serum molecular weight fractions separated by gradient ultracentrifugation. However, quantitative amounts of complexes in the Raji-cell radioimmunoassay were 37 to 105 μg/ml, far below what is usually recorded in active SLE. It is problematic whether inhibition of ADCC can be relied upon to monitor complexes, since the assay may be affected by presence of antilymphocyte antibodies or rheumatoid factors.

Sensitive methods for immune-complex detection have been applied to other heterogeneous patients with vasculitis. In general, levels have been high and often associated with a variety of severe clinical manifestations. One patient studied recently by us presented with anuria, red-blood-cell casts, and diffuse purpuric lesions on the extremities. Levels of 1,000 to 1,200 μg/ml by Raji-cell radioimmunoassay were recorded during the first 10 days of his hospital course. Physical studies of the immune complexes revealed concentration of positive activity for complexes in high-molecular-weight (19 S or greater) serum fractions separated by gradient centrifugation. Levels of detectable complexes gradually fell, on institution of hemodialysis and high-dose corticosteroid. A clear picture of the findings in any large number of patients with polyarteritis is difficult to obtain from the current literature. Patients labeled as having vasculitis with quantitative determination of immune complexes are often categorically lumped with those having rheumatoid vasculitis or vasculitis associated with other primary diagnoses (76, 271). The few patients we have seen with true idiopathic periarteritis, in whom immune-complex elevations have been documented, have not shown very striking amounts of immunoglobulin or complement deposition in tissue biopsies or autopsy material. It may well be that minute amounts of complex deposition are sufficient to initiate the process, or that vascular-linked complexes are so toxic that they are rapidly cleared by invading phagocytic cells. Again, as in the clinical situation encountered in SLE with active nephropathy, a three-dimensional view of the patients is needed.

A priori one would expect that if diffuse vasculitis such as is seen in periarteritis were secondary to a phenomenon such as the Arthus reaction involving reaction between antigen and antibodies within the vascular wall, more direct evidence might be forthcoming in individual patients for presence of the immunological reactant—immunoglobulin, complement, and possibly antigen—within the adventitia or vascular tissues. Identification of putative antigens in such tissues, as in the case of the vasculitis associated with hepatitis B infection, makes the argument more convincing but there still appear to be other factors involved in the pathogenesis of many cases that remain relatively obscure.

A fascinating group of patients has been recognized, in whom chronic urticaria appears to accompany what may be an immune-complex–mediated vasculitis associated with necrotizing venulitis (272–276). The syndrome itself is characterized by recurrent episodes of urticaria and arthralgia or arthritis, abdominal pain, and diffuse glomerulonephritis. Soter has reported observations on 16 patients with this syndrome (275): some individuals showed normal complement levels, while others had low C1q, C4, and in some instances depressions of C3. Most of these subjects, the majority of whom were women, had elevations of sedimentation rate. Skin biopsies of urticarial-like lesions showed evidence of necrotizing venulitis, and renal biopsy in one patient with hematuria provided clear evidence for a diffuse glomerulitis and deposition of immunoglobulin and complement. Other patients with similar clinical features (274, 276) have been demonstrated to have actual immunoglobulin and complement deposits within cutaneous structures. In other subjects cellular infiltrates surrounding involved cutaneous vessels have suggested that more than one mechanism mediating vascular and perivascular inflammation may be involved (277). The observation that some persons with chronic urticaria may in effect show evidence for a low-grade vasculitis is important. In the past, many patients with this disorder may have been labeled as having simple chronic urticaria.

Acute Rheumatic Fever

The clinical presence of acute rheumatic fever is not as obvious now as it was several decades ago. However, its residual effects in the form of chronic disease and disability associated with rheumatic heart disease are still very much with us. In a way rheumatic fever stands apart from the other connective-tissue disorders; it is known to be clearly associated with antecedent streptococcal infection and thus (unlike SLE or rheumatoid arthritis) cannot be considered a disease of unknown etiology. The precise mechanisms involved in the development of the tissue lesions of rheumatic fever and subsequent rheumatic heart disease are still not understood. One of the most intriguing aspects of the rheumatic episode is the requirement for a certain interval of time between the onset of rheumatic fever and actual infection with the group A streptococcus. This interval was carefully studied during many of the early clinical and epidemiological investigations of acute rheumatic fever (278–280) and was found to average about 2.5 to 3 weeks. The precise interval from streptococcal exposure to onset of clinical disease may vary somewhat depending on the particular manifestations involved. For arthritis and carditis it appears to be 2 to 3 weeks, but for evolution of subcutaneous nodules or Sydenham's chorea, it may be considerably longer. Erythema marginatum tends to be manifest 3 to 4 weeks after streptococcal exposure.

Another fascinating aspect related to the latent interval between streptococcal infection and onset of clinical symptomatology is that in individual patients it has often been noted to be relatively constant in subsequent or repeated attacks. Once a clinical pattern of rheumatic involvement is established, it is frequently repeated many times (281). The interval between streptococcal infection and onset of the first clinical manifestations of the disease is actually slightly longer for acute rheumatic fever than it is for acute poststreptococcal glomerulonephritis, where 10 to 14 days is regarded as the most common intervening period between overt streptococcal infection and the onset of nephritic symptoms (282, 283). A great deal of epidemiological study has already been directed at attempts to decipher the meaning of these differences. Could it be that the development of arthritis or chorea after streptococcal exposure represents a primary immune response, whereas in acute poststreptococcal glomerulonephritis the immune reaction is accelerated after streptococcal exposure because it signals an anamnestic reac-

tion in a host previously sensitized to potential nephritogenic antigens? Many other modulating influences have been suggested, including the possibility that other nonimmunologic factors such as streptolysin S, one of the most potent of the bacterial toxins ever characterized, may modify actual expression of the disease. The strikingly different clinical manifestations of rheumatic fever and acute glomerulonephritis have been contrasted on a number of occasions. Identifiable differences between what are regarded as nephritogenic and rheumatic fever associated strains have been extensively studied and related to individual epidemics or outbreaks of the two diseases. It seems clear from the studies of Rammelkamp (282, 283) that certain strains or serotypes of group A streptococci are related to outbreaks of nephritis. A similar clear-cut definition of rheumatogenic strains is not currently available, although certain serotypes have been convincingly identified in several outbreaks. One feature that helped to solidify the clinical association between antecedent streptococcal infection and acute rheumatic fever was studies supporting an overreaction or high degree of humoral immune responsiveness in patients with acute rheumatic fever to streptococcal products such as streptococcal DNase B or streptolysin O (284–286). Titers were generally found to be much higher in rheumatic fever subjects than in similarly exposed controls without rheumatic fever ensuing as a complication.

Another puzzling feature of the disease is that it appears to affect a small proportion of the population at risk, or those clinically exposed to group A streptococcal infection. Studies conducted over several decades by Wilson and co-workers (287, 288) indicated that in certain families genetic factors might influence development or clinically detectable presence of the disease. Other studies, however, particularly those in identical twins, do not support the concept of strong genetic control (289, 290). Most attempts to relate HLA phenotypes to the occurrence of rheumatic fever, furthermore, have been inconclusive, failing to establish clear HLA linkage in patient groups studied to date. However, a striking association with one of the human Ia-like antigens and previous rheumatic fever has recently been reported (291).

The Clinical Picture

The clinical picture of acute rheumatic fever is an impressive and sometimes frightening generalized disorder. It may, of course, manifest itself initially in rather gradual or subclinical ways, as a slight behavior disorder or movement disturbance in the child with chorea. One of the most interesting features of Sydenham's chorea revolves around its predilection for females (292). In the patients studied in Cairo in conjunction with the group at the Free Rheumatic Heart Centre (293–295), our experience showed that the ratio of females to males with clearly defined chorea has been 2.5 or 3.0 to 1. A similar female preponderance has been noted in the children presenting with arthralgias and rapidly developing carditis. This lopsidedness may reflect the well-known female superiority in capacity to mount an immune response that has been documented in a number of experimental animal models (296–299). At the bedside one is struck by the frequent evanescence of joint or articular symptoms. True migratory arthritis is the general rule, often with an acute synovitis and periarticular inflammatory response present in a knee or ankle on one afternoon or morning, and almost complete subsidence and resolution by the next day, followed by similar clinical presentations in another one or two joints in rapid succession over a period of days or several weeks. Typical synovitis associated with rheumatic fever is shown in Figure 7-23.

There have been surprisingly few detailed studies of the changes in synovial fluid during such fleeting rheumatic symptoms. A recent report by Svartman and co-workers (300) noted mild synovitis characterized by modest cellular reactions and a profile of complement component changes entirely compatible with the presence of an arthritis mediated directly by immune-complex phenomena. If such episodes of synovitis and periarticular inflammation occurring during acute rheumatic fever are indeed related to activation of inflamma-

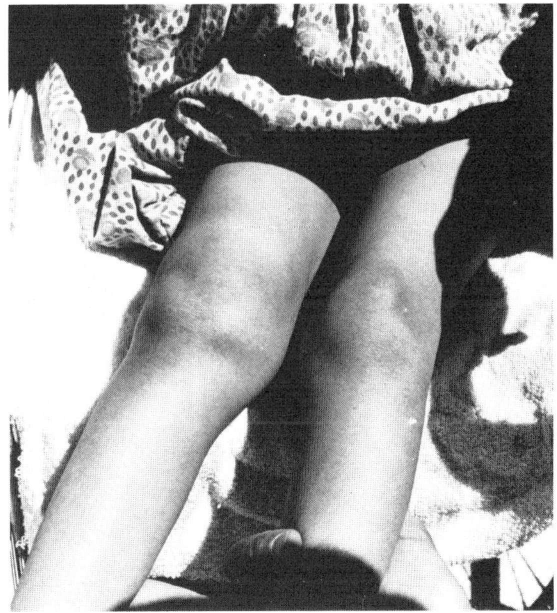

Figure 7-23 Acute synovitis of the right knee in a seven-year-old child with acute rheumatic fever. The knee contained a moderate effusion and was extremely tender to palpation.

tory cells and mechanisms set in motion by local trapping of immune complexes, the process must be very different from that encountered in rheumatoid arthritis, in which a slowly evolving and progressive reaction is initiated that often persists over a period of months or years. The physical nature or affinity of such complexes, therefore, if central to the etiology of acute rheumatic fever and its associated articular complaints, must be entirely different from that seen in rheumatoid synovitis.

No sophisticated histological or immunofluorescent studies such as have been performed in rheumatoid synovial inflammation are yet available in the case of rheumatic fever. It is not known, for instance, whether there are IgG or IgG-IgM complexes present in the synovium or synovial fluids of patients with rheumatic fever during transient episodes of arthritis. Obviously there are basic or fundamental differences involved in the synovitis of the two disorders. Persistence of inflammation, local generation of IgG and IgM rheumatoid factors within rheumatoid synovium, and clear evidence for both alternative and classical complement component activation suggest that the rheumatoid process may be involved in persistence and possible replication of causative antigens within the inflammatory focus. On the contrary, the clinical evanescence of inflammation and the rapid complete resolution of the synovitis in rheumatic fever suggest that if immune complexes are involved, they are not being generated de novo within the synovial space, but may be only temporarily trapped within such tissues long enough to create an inflammatory disturbance before being disposed of by normal phagocytic removal systems of the synovial lining cells and articular structures.

In like manner, skin lesions previously associated with rheumatic-fever involvement are extremely transitory and rapidly regressing. The characteristic appearance of erythema marginatum has often been useful in substantiating the diagnosis in individual patients. A typical skin lesion of this type is shown in Figure 7-24. To our knowledge there have been very few definitive immunopathological studies using either immunofluorescence or anti-streptococcal antibodies and immunoelectron-microscopy to identify localization of immune complexes in such tissues. In many ways the evanescent skin lesions suggest that activation of intrinsic vasoactive processes or vasoactive amine release within soft tissues may play a key role in such reactions.

Cardiac Involvement

The most important basic lesion in acute rheumatic fever involves the heart. Acute lesions are characterized by mononuclear cell infiltrations and changes in cardiac muscle cell fibers eventually evolving to the classic Aschoff lesion shown in Figure 7-25. Similar inflammatory lesions also involve the endocardium and heart valve structures. An extensive pancarditis with focal areas of inflammation within myocardium, endocardium, and pericardium is often present. Focal parts of such an inflammatory process are also seen with each individual recurrence of acute rheumatic fever and after many years gradual evolution of the repeated episodes or slow progress of more chronic processes produces the familiar scarring and de-

Figure 7-24 Erythema marginatum in a patient with acute rheumatic fever. (Photograph courtesy of Barbara Ansell, Northwick Park Clinical Research Centre, Harrow, England.)

formity characteristic of established rheumatic heart disease.

Surprisingly little is known concerning the mechanisms that occur to produce such a final end result. Rich suggested that delayed-type hypersensitivity was involved (301), whereas direct toxic reactions occurring between cellular components of group A streptococci and connective-tissue elements have also been suggested as potential mechanisms of tissue injury (302). The observations of myocardial and endocardial gamma globulin and complement deposition by Kaplan and co-workers (303) suggested that an immune process was active

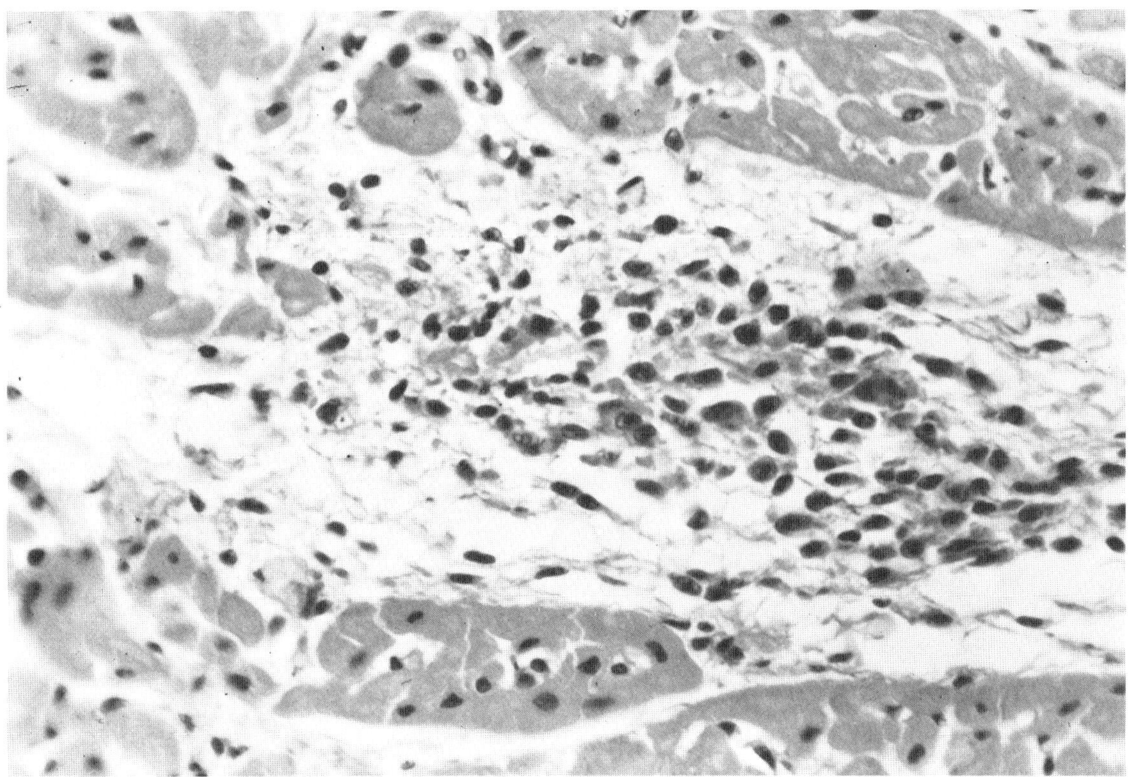

Figure 7-25   An early Aschoff lesion in the myocardium of a child dying of acute rheumatic fever. A collection of mononuclear cells with edema and some dissolution of tissue is noted. Magnification × 300. (Photograph courtesy of E. Ayoub, Gainesville, Florida.)

in the genesis of the acute and subacute lesions. Subsequently it was established that a strong degree of cross-reaction occurred between antigenic components of the group A hemolytic streptococcus and human myocardium, valvular glycoproteins, and human myocardial sarcolemmal membranes (304–315). From this work emerged the concept of molecular mimicry that has functioned as one of the leading theories in explaining the genesis of rheumatic heart disease (316).

The striking cross-reactions between group A streptococcal membranes and the antigens present in human myocardial membrane structures are shown in Figure 7-26. It has been suggested that an immune response originally produced by the host against group A streptococcal antigens also then reacts with vital host self-antigens distributed throughout many key cardiac structures and that combined humoral and cell-mediated host immune responses somehow result in the chronic inflammatory process and subsequent tissue damage present in the heart with chronic rheumatic involvement. Recent attempts to document other ancillary mechanisms possibly involved in such tissue damage have utilized cultured beating heart cells and the mechanisms of in vitro cell-mediated lymphocyte tissue destruction as reported by Yang and co-workers (317). Other studies of lymphocyte migration inhibition and cellular reactivity by Read and colleagues (318) have also demonstrated a cell-mediated immune response to streptococcal membrane-associated antigens in patients with acute rheumatic fever. Of interest in the Yang reports was the apparent absence in this particular experimental model of any evidence implicating antibody-mediated K-cell reactivity.

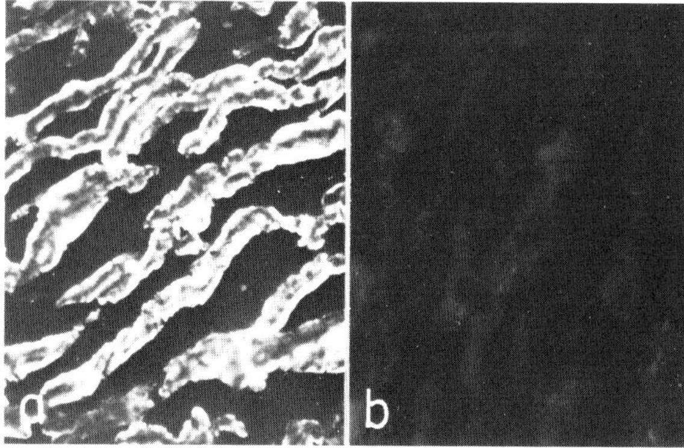

Figure 7-26 Immunofluorescent staining of human myocardium with purified heart-reactive antibody isolated from acute rheumatic fever patients. *A*, antibody bound to the sarcolemma or cardiac myofibers. *B*, absence of staining pattern when heart-reactive antibody was absorbed with purified group A streptococcal membrane antigen. Magnification × 450. (Reproduced with permission, I. van de Rijn, J. B. Zabriskie, and M. McCarty, *J. Exp. Med.* 146:579, 1977.)

Several other cross-reactions between streptococcal antigens and mammalian tissues have been recognized. A cross-reaction between the group A polysaccharide and thymic tissues was described by Lyampert and Danilova (319). In addition, Kingston and Glynn (320) have described cross-reactivity between group A streptococci and elements of CNS origin including astrocytes and glial tissues, and more recently elements of the bundle of His (321). We have also observed that sera from children afflicted with Sydenham's chorea show strong reactions with neuronal antigens present in unfixed frozen sections of normal human brain (293). Such antibodies could be completely removed after absorption of reactive sera with purified membranes of group A β-hemolytic streptococci. These findings indicated that antibodies with neuronal reactivity were actually directed at antigens common to the limiting membranes of group A streptococci. All of these examples of potentially important cross-reactions between human or mammalian tissues and various antigenic constituents of streptococci are of great interest and emphasize the extent to which streptococcal infection might initiate a self-directed process of injury.

Many of the immunopathological studies published to date regarding potential mechanisms of tissue injury in acute rheumatic fever have not satisfactorily explained the initiation and ongoing tissue destruction characteristic of the chronic cardiac lesions. We have recently attempted to reconcile the original observations of Kaplan and co-workers of immunoglobulin and complement myocardial tissue deposits during evolution of acute rheumatic pancarditis (303) to what may be reflected in serial serum studies during acute rheumatic pancarditis. A group of children with active rheumatic fever and either Sydenham's chorea or moderately severe rheumatic carditis has been studied during evolution of acute disease at the Free Rheumatic Heart Centre in Cairo. These patients were followed during acute clinical illness using quantitative determinations of immune complexes by the Raji-cell and solid-phase C1q assay. Of interest was the finding of marked elevations of immune complexes sometimes detected by both methods in parallel during disease evolution in virtually all patients studied. Elevations of immune complexes were usually present during the acute phases of disease and appeared to correlate directly with clinical fluctuations in both chorea and carditis (322). In some instances patients with apparent isolated episodes of rheumatic chorea had levels of circulating complexes equally as high as those studied during full-blown episodes of rheumatic pancarditis. Complexes present in the sera during acute rheumatic fever in both chorea and/or carditis were largely localized to 11 to 19S and larger molecular weight fractions.

As yet our studies have not yielded any evidence for clear-cut physical or immunochemical differences between the size or nature of complexes associated with chorea and those detected in association with rheumatic carditis. The apparent physical size similarity of immune complexes present in the sera of children with both kinds of rheumatic manifestations has not been explained. One might hypothesize that local tissue factors must somehow markedly influence the local pathological processes involved. It is conceivable that during the rheumatic fever episode extracellular streptococcal products (quite distinct from those already discussed with relation to the cross-reacting myocardial or brain antigens) are released and somehow modulate or govern the localization and tissue effects of circulating immune-complex materials. Thus, immune complexes detected in the circulation of patients with Sydenham's chorea may exert their effects on CNS function through deposition or localization within either the choroid plexus (as has been previously postulated for SLE) or the CNS vasculature. At present, no pathological confirmation of this concept has been obtained. Most subjects with Sydenham's chorea do not die but show gradual resolution of their movement disorder, and we have not had occasion to actually examine neuropathological material from this group of subjects. Furthermore, it is difficult to conceive of precisely how circulating complexes might traverse the blood-brain barrier in the acute state and thereby interfere with or influence CNS function. Finally, it is also possible that the elevations recently noted in circulating immune complexes during both carditis and chorea have nothing to do directly with the clinical manifestations of acute carditis or chorea itself. Their presence in serum at the time of either type of clinical syndrome may merely reflect a secondary event or materials circulating as complexes released during acute tissue injury but not directly related to the primary tissue damage. Considerably more in the way of clinical-pathological correlation is needed before the relationship between detectable circulating complexes and the underlying, often slowly progressive rheumatic process is clearly understood.

Early recognition of the correlation between initial group A streptococcal infection and acute rheumatic fever represents a clear advantage in any approach to its understanding. Although we now feel that nDNA–anti-nDNA antigen-antibody complexes are probably a fundamental mechanism in initiation of the immune complex nephritis in SLE, we have no precise insight into the exact relation of DNA to SLE. Is intrinsic or autologous DNA involved, or is the DNA material introduced into the body proper in the form of some extrinsic agent? The same might be said for all of the evidence implicating altered gamma globulin and autologous IgG complexes in the pathogenesis of rheumatoid arthritis. The reactants have been carefully and meticulously characterized but the raison d'être remains unclear. Actually, the reverse situation seems to obtain in the case of acute rheumatic fever. The etiology—namely, the streptococcus—has been identified and extensively characterized. The presence of large amounts of gamma globulin and complement in cardiac tissues in acute rheumatic fever has also been well documented. From the interval between the initial streptococcal infection and the first appearance of joint symptoms or acute carditis, we presume that some type of developing immune reaction has occurred. The presence of marked elevations of immune complexes, the clearly documented exhaustive catalogue of cross-reactivities between streptococcal products and streptococcal antigens, and the involved tissues are also well defined. What is needed are convincing demonstrations of how these potential mechanisms interrelate to produce the clinically recognized disease. Perhaps in no other connective-tissue disorder does the opportunity now seem so hopeful. Future studies must unfold the puzzle, and perhaps in so doing elucidate this fascinating but perplexing experiment of nature.

References

1. Williams, R. C., Jr. Brief historical review and clinical features of the disease. In *Rheumatoid Arthritis as a Systemic Disease*, p. 1. W. B. Saunders, Philadelphia, 1974.

2. Sokoloff, L., McCluskey, R. T., and Bunim, J. J. Vascularity of the early subcutaneous nodule of rheumatoid arthritis. *Arch. Pathol.* 55:475, 1953.

3. Sokoloff, L., Wilens, S. L., and Bunim, J. J. Arteritis of striated muscle in rheumatoid arthritis. *Am. J. Pathol.* 27:157, 1951.

4. Kulka, J. P., Bocking, D., Ropes, M. W., et al. Early joint lesions of rheumatoid arthritis. Report of eight cases, with knee biopsies of lesions of less than one year's duration. *Arch. Pathol.* 59:129, 1955.

5. Kulka, J. P. Vascular derangements in rheumatoid arthritis. In A. G. S. Hill, ed., *Modern Trends in Rheumatology,* p. 49. Butterworths, London, 1966.

6. Lindner, J. Der rheumatische Bindegewebs-Stoffwechsel und die pathologische Struktur der Bindegewebe bei rheumatoider Arthritis. *Verh. Dtsch. Ges. Inn. Med.* 74:1315, 1968.

7. Schumacher, H. R., and Kitridou, R. C. Synovitis of recent onset: a clinico-pathologic study during the first month of disease. *Arthritis Rheum.* 15:465, 1972.

8. Alspaugh, M. A., Talal, N., and Tan, E. M. Differentiation and characterization of autoantibodies and their antigens in Sjögren's syndrome. *Arthritis Rheum.* 19:216, 1976.

9. Alspaugh, M. A., and Tan, E. M. Serum antibody in rheumatoid arthritis reactive with a cell-associated antigen. Demonstration by precipitation and immunofluorescence. *Arthritis Rheum.* 19:711, 1976.

10. Alspaugh, M. A., Jensen, F. C., Robin, H., et al. Lymphocytes transformed by Epstein-Barr virus. Induction of nuclear antigen reactive with antibody in rheumatoid arthritis. *J. Exp. Med.* 147:1018, 1978.

11. Bevans, M., Nadell, J., De Martini, F. E., et al. The systemic lesions of malignant rheumatoid arthritis. *Am. J. Med.* 16:197, 1954.

12. Robinson, W. D., French, A. J., and Duff, I. F. Polyarteritis in rheumatoid arthritis. *Ann. Rheum. Dis.* 12:323, 1953.

13. Sokoloff, L., and Bunim, J. J. Vascular lesions in rheumatoid arthritis. *J. Chron. Dis.* 5:668, 1957.

14. Schmid, F. R., Cooper, N. S., Ziff, M., et al. Arteritis in rheumatoid arthritis. *Am. J. Med.* 30:56, 1961.

15. Cruickshank, B. The arteritis of rheumatoid arthritis. *Ann. Rheum. Dis.* 13:136, 1954.

16. Gruenwald, P. Visceral lesions in a case of rheumatoid arthritis. *Arch. Pathol.* 46:59, 1948.

17. Sinclair, R. J. G., and Cruickshank, B. A clinical and pathological study of sixteen cases of rheumatoid arthritis with extensive visceral involvement ('rheumatoid disease'). *Q. J. Med.* 25:313, 1956.

18. Adler, R. H., Norcross, B. M., and Lockie, L. M. Arteritis and infarction of the intestine in rheumatoid arthritis. *J.A.M.A.* 180:922, 1962.

19. Finkbiner, R. B., and Decker, J. P. Ulceration and perforation of the intestine due to necrotizing arteriolitis. *N. Engl. J. Med.* 268:14, 1963.

20. Torrigiani, G., and Roitt, I. M. Antiglobulin factors in sera from patients with rheumatoid arthritis and normal subjects. Quantitative estimation in different immunoglobulin classes. *Ann. Rheum. Dis.* 26:334, 1967.

21. Stage, D. E., and Mannik, M. 7SγM-globulin in rheumatoid arthritis. Evaluation of its clinical significance. *Arthritis Rheum.* 14:440, 1971.

22. Theofilopoulos, A. N., Burtonboy, G., Lo Spalluto, J. J., et al. IgM rheumatoid factor and low molecular weight IgM. An association with vasculitis. *Arthritis Rheum.* 17:272, 1974.

23. Zvaifler, N. J., and Schur, P. H. Reactions of aggregated mercaptoethanol treated gamma globulin with rheumatoid factor: precipitin and complement fixation studies. *Arthritis Rheum.* 11:523, 1968.

24. Schmid, F. R., Roitt, I. M., and Rocha, M. J. Complement fixation by a two-component antibody system: immunoglobulin G and immunoglobulin M antiglobulin (rheumatoid factor). Paradoxical effect related to immunoglobulin G concentration. *J. Exp. Med.* 132:673, 1970.

25. McCormick, J. N., Day, J., Morris, C. J., et al. The potentiating effect of rheumatoid arthritis serum in the immediate phase of nephrotoxic nephritis. *Clin. Exp. Immunol.* 4:17, 1969.

26. DeHoratius, R. J., and Williams, R. C., Jr. Rheumatoid factor accentuation of pulmonary lesions associated with experimental diffuse proliferative lung disease. *Arthritis Rheum.* 15:293, 1972.

27. Baum, J., Stastny, P., and Ziff, M. Effects of the rheumatoid factor and antigen-antibody complexes on the vessels of the rat mesentery. *J. Immunol.* 93:985, 1964.

28. Paulus, H. E., Machleder, H., Bangert, R., et al. A case report: thoracic duct lymphocyte drainage in rheumatoid arthritis. *Clin. Immunol. Immunopathol.* 1:173, 1973.

29. Paulus, H. E., Machleder, H. I., Levine, S., et al. Lymphocyte involvement in rheumatoid arthritis. Studies during thoracic duct drainage. *Arthritis Rheum.* 20:1249, 1977.

30. Andreis, M., Ziff, M., and Stastny, P. Experimental arthritis produced by injection of mediators of delayed hypersensitivity. *Fed. Proc.* 31:798, 1972.

31. Hannestad, K. Presence of aggregated γ-G-globulin in certain rheumatoid synovial effusions. *Clin. Exp. Immunol.* 2:511, 1967.

32. Winchester, R. J., Agnello, V., and Kunkel, H. G. An association between γG globulin complexes and complement depletion in joint fluids of patients with rheumatoid arthritis. *Arthritis Rheum.* 12:343, 1969.

33. Winchester, R. J., Agnello, V., and Kunkel, H. G. Gamma globulin complexes in synovial fluids

of patients with rheumatoid arthritis. Partial characterization and relationship to lowered complement levels. *Clin. Exp. Immunol.* 6:689, 1970.

34. Agnello, V., Winchester, R. J., and Kunkel, H. G. Precipitin reactions of the C1q component of complement with aggregated γ-globulin and immune complexes in gel diffusion. *Immunology* 19:909, 1970.

35. Winchester, R. J., Kunkel, H. G., and Agnello, V. Occurrence of γ-globulin complexes in serum and joint fluid of rheumatoid arthritis patients: use of monoclonal rheumatoid factors as reagents for their demonstration. *J. Exp. Med.* 134:286s, 1971.

36. Hurd, E. R., LoSpalluto, J., and Ziff, M. Formation of leukocyte inclusions in normal polymorphonuclear cells incubated with synovial fluid. *Arthritis Rheum.* 13:724, 1970.

37. Hurd, E. R., Kinsella, T. D., and Ziff, M. Immunohistologic studies of synoviocytes and synovial exudate cells. *J. Exp. Med.* 134:296s, 1971.

38. Mellors, R. C., Heimer, R., Corcos, J., et al. Cellular origin of rheumatoid factor. *J. Exp. Med.* 110:875, 1959.

39. Munthe, E., and Natvig, J. B. Immunoglobulin classes, subclasses, and complexes of IgG rheumatoid factor in rheumatoid plasma cells. *Clin. Exp. Immunol.* 12:55, 1972.

40. Munthe, E., and Natvig, J. B. Complement-fixing intracellular complexes of IgG rheumatoid factor in rheumatoid plasma cells. *Scand. J. Immunol.* 1:217, 1972.

41. Smiley, J. D., Sachs, C., and Ziff, M. *In vitro* synthesis of immunoglobulin by rheumatoid synovial membrane. *J. Clin. Invest.* 47:624, 1968.

42. Vaughan, J. H., Chihara, T., Moore, T. L., et al. Rheumatoid factor-producing cells detected by direct hemolytic plaque assay. *J. Clin. Invest.* 58:933, 1976.

43. Normansell, D. E., and Stanworth, D. R. Interactions between rheumatoid factor and native γ-G-globulins studied in the ultracentrifuge. *Immunology* 15:549, 1968.

44. Normansell, D. E. Anti-γ-globulins in rheumatoid arthritis sera. I. Studies on the 22S complex. *Immunochemistry* 7:787, 1970.

45. Stone, M. J., and Metzger, H. Binding properties of a Waldenström macroglobulin antibody. *J. Biol. Chem.* 243:5977, 1968.

46. Jerne, N. K. Theoretical considerations of the reaction mechanism, based on neutralization curves for individual sera under varying experimental conditions. In "A study of avidity based on rabbit skin responses to diphtheria toxin-antitoxin mixtures." *Acta Pathol. Microbiol. Scand.* 87:62, 1954 (suppl.).

47. Talmage, D. W. The kinetics of the reaction between antibody and bovine serum albumin using the Farr method. *J. Infect. Dis.* 107:115, 1960.

48. Michaelides, M. C., and Eisen, H. N. The strange cross-reaction of menadione (vitamin K_3) and 2,4-dinitrophenyl ligands with a myeloma protein and some conventional antibodies. *J. Exp. Med.* 140:687, 1974.

49. Richards, F. F., and Konigsberg, W. H. Speculations. How specific are antibodies? *Immunochemistry* 10:545, 1973.

50. Richards, F. F., Amzel, L. M., Konigsberg, W. H., et al. Polyfunctional antibody combining regions. In E. E. Sercarz, A. R. Williamson, and C. F. Fox, eds., *The Immune System: Genes, Receptors, Signals,* p. 53. Academic Press, New York, 1974.

51. Bokisch, V. A., Chiao, J. W., and Bernstein, D. Isolation and immunochemical characterization of rabbit 7S anti-IgG with restricted heterogeneity. *J. Exp. Med.* 137:1354, 1973.

52. Bokisch, V. A., Chiao, J. W., Bernstein, D., et al. Homogenous rabbit 7S anti-IgG with antibody specificity for peptidoglycan. *J. Exp. Med.* 138:1184, 1973.

53. Hannestad, K. Certain rheumatoid factors react with both IgG and an antigen associated with cell nuclei. *Scand. J. Immunol.* 7:127, 1978.

54. Hedberg, H. Studies on the depressed hemolytic complement activity of synovial fluid in adult rheumatoid arthritis. *Acta Rheum. Scand.* 9:165, 1963.

55. Hedberg, H. The depressed synovial complement activity in adult and juvenile rheumatoid arthritis. *Acta Rheum. Scand.* 10:109, 1964.

56. Pekin, T. J., Jr., and Zvaifler, N. J. Hemolytic complement in synovial fluid. *J. Clin. Invest.* 43:1372, 1964.

57. Ruddy, S., and Austen, K. F. The complement system in rheumatoid synovitis. I. An analysis of complement component activities in rheumatoid synovial fluids. *Arthritis Rheum.* 13:713, 1970.

58. Götze, O., Zvaifler, N. J., and Müller-Eberhard, H. J. Evidence for complement activation by the C3 activator system in rheumatoid arthritis. *Arthritis Rheum.* 15:111, 1972.

59. Ward, P. A., and Zvaifler, N. J. Complement-derived leukotactic factors in inflammatory synovial fluids of humans. *J. Clin. Invest.* 50:606, 1971.

60. Cooke, T. D., Hurd, E. R., Bienenstock, J., et al. The immunofluorescent identification of immunoglobulins and complement in rheumatoid ar-

ticular collagenous tissue. *Arthritis Rheum.* 15:433, 1972.

61. Cooke, T. D., Hurd, E. R., Ziff, M., et al. The pathogenesis of chronic inflammation in experimental antigen-induced arthritis. II. Preferential localization of antigen-antibody complexes to collagenous tissues. *J. Exp. Med.* 135:323, 1972.

62. King, R. A., Messner, R. P., and Williams, R. C., Jr. Human lymphocyte transformation induced by anti-gamma globulin factors. *Arthritis Rheum.* 12:597, 1969.

63. Moretta, L., Webb, S. R., Grossi, C. E., et al. Functional analysis of two human T-cell subpopulations: help and suppression of B-cell responses by T cells bearing receptors for IgM or IgG. *J. Exp. Med.* 146:184, 1977.

64. Kinsella, T. D. Induction of autologous lymphocyte transformation by synovial fluids from patients with rheumatoid arthritis. *Clin. Exp. Immunol.* 14:187, 1973.

65. Kinsella, T. D. Enhancement of human lymphocyte transformation by aggregated human gamma globulin. *J. Clin. Invest.* 53:1108, 1974.

66. DeHoratius, R. J., Abruzzo, J. L., and Williams, R. C., Jr. Immunofluorescent and immunologic studies of rheumatoid lung. *Arch. Intern. Med.* 129:441, 1972.

67. Rodman, W. S., Williams, R. C., Jr., Bilka, P. J., et al. Immunofluorescent localization of the third and fourth component of complement in synovial tissue from patients with rheumatoid arthritis. *J. Lab. Clin. Med.* 69:141, 1967.

68. Conn, D. L., McDuffie, F. C., and Dyck, P. J. Immunopathologic study of sural nerves in rheumatoid arthritis. *Arthritis Rheum.* 15:135, 1972.

69. Franklin, E. C., Holman, H. R., Müller-Eberhard, H. J., et al. An unusual protein component of high molecular weight in the serum of certain patients with rheumatoid arthritis. *J. Exp. Med.* 105:425, 1957.

70. Kunkel, H. G., Franklin, E. C., and Müller-Eberhard, H. J. Studies on the isolation and characterization of the "rheumatoid factor". *J. Clin. Invest.* 38:424, 1959.

71. Franklin, E. C., Kunkel, H. G., and Ward, J. R. Clinical studies of seven patients with rheumatoid arthritis and uniquely large amounts of rheumatoid factor. *Arthritis Rheum.* 1:400, 1958.

72. Mongan, E. S., Cass, R. M., Jacox, R. F., et al. A study of the relation of seronegative and seropositive rheumatoid arthritis to each other and to necrotizing vasculitis. *Am. J. Med.* 47:23, 1969.

73. Epstein, W. V., and Engleman, E. P. The relation of the rheumatoid factor content of serum to clinical neurovascular manifestations of rheumatoid arthritis. *Arthritis Rheum.* 2:250, 1959.

74. Kunkel, H. G., Müller-Eberhard, H. J., Fudenberg, H. H., et al. Gamma globulin complexes in rheumatoid arthritis and certain other conditions. *J. Clin. Invest.* 40:117, 1961.

75. Schrohenloher, R. E. Characterization of the γ-globulin complexes present in certain sera having high titers of anti-γ-globulin activity. *J. Clin. Invest.* 45:501, 1966.

76. Theofilopoulos, A. N., Wilson, C. B., and Dixon, F. J. The Raji cell radioimmune assay for detecting immune complexes in human sera. *J. Clin. Invest.* 57:169, 1976.

77. Tanimoto, K., Cooper, N. R., Johnson, J. S., et al. Complement fixation by rheumatoid factor. *J. Clin. Invest,* 55:437, 1975.

78. Tung, K. S. K., and Williams, R. C., Jr. Unpublished observations, 1977.

79. Luthra, H. S., McDuffie, F. C., Hunder, G. G., et al. Immune complexes in sera and synovial fluids of patients with rheumatoid arthritis. Radioimmunoassay with monoclonal rheumatoid factor. *J. Clin. Invest.* 56:458, 1975.

80. Zubler, R. H., Nydegger, U., Perrin, L. H., et al. Circulating and intra-articular immune complexes in patients with rheumatoid arthritis. Correlation of ^{125}I-C1q binding activity with clinical and biological features of the disease. *J. Clin. Invest.* 57:1308, 1976.

81. Nydegger, U. E., Zubler, R. H., Gabay, R., et al. Circulating complement breakdown products in patients with rheumatoid arthritis. Correlation between plasma C3d, circulating immune complexes, and clinical activity. *J. Clin. Invest.* 59:862, 1977.

82. Andersen, S. B., and Jensen, K. B. Metabolism of γG-globulin in collagen disease. *Clin. Sci.* 29:533, 1965.

83. Levy, J., Barnett, E. V., MacDonald, N. S., et al. Altered immunoglobulin metabolism in systemic lupus erythematosus and rheumatoid arthritis. *J. Clin. Invest.* 49:708, 1970.

84. Mills, J. A., Calkins, E., and Cohen, A. S. The plasma disappearance time and catabolic half-life of I-131-labeled normal human gamma globulin in amyloidosis and in rheumatoid arthritis. *J. Clin. Invest.* 40:1926, 1961.

85. Olhagen, B., Birke, G., Plantin, L. O., et al. Isotope studies of gamma-globulin catabolism in collagen disorders. *Acta Rheumatol. Scand.* 9:88, 1963.

86. Vaughan, J. H., Armato, A., Goldthwait, J. C. et al. A study of gamma globulin in rheumatoid arthritis. *J. Clin. Invest.* 34:75, 1955.

87. Wochner, R. D. Hypercatabolism of normal IgG; an unexplained immunoglobulin abnormality in the connective tissue diseases. *J. Clin. Invest.* 49:454, 1970.

88. Catalano, M. A., Krick, E. H., De Heer, D. H., et al. Metabolism of autologous and homologous IgG in rheumatoid arthritis. *J. Clin. Invest.* 60:313, 1977.

89. Johnson, P. M., Watkins, J., and Holborow, E. J. Antiglobulin production to altered IgG in rheumatoid arthritis. *Lancet* 1:611, 1975.

90. Johnson, P. M., Watkins, J., Scopes, P. M., et al. Differences in serum IgG structure in health and rheumatoid disease. Circular dichroism studies. *Ann. Rheum. Dis.* 33:366, 1974.

91. Mullinax, F., Hymes, A. J., and Mullinax, G. L. Molecular site and enzymatic origin of IgG galactose deficiency in rheumatoid arthritis and SLE. *Arthritis Rheum.* 19:813, 1976 (abstract).

92. Klemperer, P., Gueft, B., Lee, S. L., et al. Cytochemical changes of acute lupus erythematosus. *Arch. Pathol.* 49:503, 1950.

93. Hargraves, M. M., Richmond, H., and Morton, R. Presentation of two bone marrow elements: the "tart" cell and "L.E." cell. *Proc. Staff Meet. Mayo Clin.* 23:25, 1948.

94. Holman, H. R., and Kunkel, H. G. Affinity between the lupus erythematosus serum factor and cell nuclei and nucleoprotein. *Science* 126:162, 1957.

95. Robbins, W. C., Holman, H. R., Deicher, H., et al. Complement fixation with cell nuclei and DNA in lupus erythematosus. *Proc. Soc. Exp. Biol. Med.* 96:575, 1957.

96. Seligmann, M. Mise en évidence dans le sérum de malades atteints de lupus érythemateux disséminé d'une substance déterminant une réaction de précipitation avec l'acide desoxyribonucléique. *C. R. Acad. Sci. (D) (Paris)* 245:243, 1957.

97. Holman, H., and Deicher, H. R. The reaction of the lupus erythematosus (L.E.) cell factor with deoxyribonucleoprotein of the cell nucleus. *J. Clin. Invest.* 38:2059, 1959.

98. Stollar, D., Levine, L., Lehrer, H. I., et al. The antigenic determinants of denatured DNA reactive with lupus erythematosus serum. *Proc. Natl. Acad. Sci. USA* 48:874, 1962.

99. Arana, R., and Seligmann, M. Antibodies to native and denatured deoxyribonucleic acid in systemic lupus erythematosus. *J. Clin. Invest.* 46:1867, 1967.

100. Tan, E. M., and Kunkel, H. G. Characteristics of a soluble nuclear antigen precipitating with sera of patients with systemic lupus erythematosus. *J. Immunol.* 96:464, 1966.

101. Tan, E. M., Schur, P. H., Carr, R. I., et al. Deoxyribonucleic acid (DNA) and antibodies to DNA in the serum of patients with systemic lupus erythematosus. *J. Clin. Invest.* 45:1732, 1966.

102. Koffler, D., Carr, R. I., Agnello, V., et al. Antibodies to polynucleotides: distribution in human serum. *Science* 166:1648, 1969.

103. Dubois, E. L. The clinical picture of systemic lupus erythematosus. In E. L. Dubois, ed., *Lupus Erythematosus,* ed. 2, p. 232. University of Southern California Press, Los Angeles, 1974.

104. Abdou, N. I., Sagawa, A., Pascual, E., et al. Suppressor T-cell abnormality in idiopathic systemic lupus erythematosus. *Clin. Immunol. Immunopathol.* 6:192, 1976.

105. Bresnihan, B., and Jasin, H. E. Suppressor function of peripheral blood mononuclear cells in normal individuals and in patients with systemic lupus erythematosus. *J. Clin. Invest.* 59:106, 1977.

106. Vazquez, J. J., and Dixon, F. J. Immunohistochemical study of lesions in rheumatic fever, systemic lupus erythematosus, and rheumatoid arthritis. *Lab. Invest.* 6:205, 1957.

107. Paronetto, F., and Koffler, D. Immunofluorescent localization of immunoglobulins, complement and fibrinogen in human diseases. I. Systemic lupus erythematosus. *J. Clin. Invest.* 44:1657, 1965.

108. Koffler, D., Schur, P. H., and Kunkel, H. G. Immunological studies concerning the nephritis of systemic lupus erythematosus. *J. Exp. Med.* 126:607, 1967.

109. Schur, P. H., and Sandson, J. Immunologic factors and clinical activity in systemic lupus erythematosus. *N. Engl. J. Med.* 278:533, 1968.

110. Koffler, D., Agnello, V., Thoburn, R., et al. Systemic lupus erythematosus: prototype of immune complex nephritis in man. *J. Exp. Med.* 134:169s, 1971.

111. Pincus, T., Schur, P. H., Rose, J. A., et al. Measurement of serum DNA-binding activity in systemic lupus erythematosus. *N. Engl. J. Med.* 281:701, 1969.

112. Hughes, G. R. V., Cohen, S. A., and Christian, C. L. Anti-DNA activity in systemic lupus erythematosus. A diagnostic and therapeutic guide. *Ann. Rheum. Dis.* 30:259, 1971.

113. Lightfoot, R. W., Redecha, P. B., and Levesanos, N. Longitudinal studies of anti-DNA antibody levels in SLE. *Scand. J. Rheumatol.* 11:52, 1975 (suppl.).

114. Davis, P., Cumming, R. H., and Verrier-Jones, J. Relationship between anti-DNA antibodies, complement consumption and circulating immune

complexes in systemic lupus erythematosus. *Clin. Exp. Immunol.* 28:226, 1977.

115. Carr, R. I., Harbeck, R. J., Hoffman, A. A., et al. Clinical studies on the significance of DNA: anti-DNA complexes in the systemic circulation and cerebrospinal fluid (CSF) of patients with systemic lupus erythematosus. *J. Rheumatol.* 2:184, 1975.

116. Williams, R. C., Jr., and Law, D. H., IV. Serum complement in connective tissue disorders. *J. Lab. Clin. Med.* 52:273, 1958.

117. Kohler, P. F., and Ten Bensel, R. Serial complement component alterations in acute glomerulonephritis and systemic lupus erythematosus. *Clin. Exp. Immunol.* 4:191, 1969.

118. Krishnan, C., and Kaplan, M. H. Immunopathologic studies of systemic lupus erythematosus. II. Anti-nuclear reaction of γ-globulin eluted from homogenates and isolated glomeruli of kidneys from patients with lupus nephritis. *J. Clin. Invest.* 46:569, 1967.

119. Epstein, W. V., Tan, M., and Easterbrook, M. Serum antibody to double-stranded RNA and DNA in patients with idiopathic and secondary uveitis. *N. Engl. J. Med.* 285:1502, 1971.

120. Hahn, B. H., Sharp, G. C., Irvin, W. S., et al. Immune responses to hydralazine and nuclear antigens in hydralazine-induced lupus erythematosus. *Ann. Intern. Med.* 76:365, 1972.

121. Aarden, L. A., de Groot, E. R., and Feltkamp, T. E. W. Immunology of DNA. III. *Crithidia luciliae,* a simple substrate for the determination of anti-dsDNA with the immunofluorescence technique. *Ann. N.Y. Acad. Sci.* 254:505, 1975.

122. Crowe, W., and Kushner, I. An immunofluorescent method using *Crithidia luciliae* to detect antibodies to double-stranded DNA. *Arthritis Rheum.* 20:811, 1977.

123. Steinman, C. R., Deesomchok, U., and Spiera, H. Detection of anti-DNA antibody using synthetic antigens. Characterization and clinical significance of binding of poly (deoxyadenylate-deoxythymidylate) by serum. *J. Clin. Invest.* 57:1330, 1976.

124. Bankhurst, A. D., and Williams, R. C., Jr. Identification of DNA-binding lymphocytes in patients with systemic lupus erythematosus. *J. Clin. Invest.* 56:1378, 1975.

125. Fournié, G. J., Lambert, P. H., and Miescher, P. A. Release of DNA in circulating blood and induction of anti-DNA antibodies after injection of bacterial lipopolysaccharides. *J. Exp. Med.* 140:1189, 1974.

126. Izui, S., Lambert, P. H., and Miescher, P. A. *In vitro* demonstration of a particular affinity of glomerular basement membrane and collagen for DNA. A possible basis for a local formation of DNA-anti-DNA complexes in systemic lupus erythematosus. *J. Exp. Med.* 144:428, 1976.

127. Burnham, T. K., Neblett, T. R., and Fine, G. The application of the fluorescent antibody technique to the investigation of lupus erythematosus and various dermatoses. *J. Invest. Dermatol.* 41:451, 1963.

128. Tan, E. M., and Kunkel, H. G. An immunofluorescent study of the skin lesions in systemic lupus erythematosus. *Arthritis Rheum.* 9:37, 1966.

129. Gilliam, J. N., Cheatum, D. E., Hurd, E. R., et al. Immunoglobulin in clinically uninvolved skin in systemic lupus erythematosus: association with renal disease. *J. Clin. Invest.* 53:1434, 1974.

130. Caperton, E. M., Jr., Bean, S. F., and Dick, F. R. Immunofluorescent skin test in systemic lupus erythematosus. Lack of relationship with renal disease. *J.A.M.A.* 222:935, 1972.

131. McCluskey, R. T. The value of immunofluorescence in the study of human renal disease. *J. Exp. Med.* 134:242s, 1971.

132. Brentjens, J. R., Sepulveda, M., Baliah, T., et al. Interstitial immune complex nephritis in patients with systemic lupus erythematosus. *Kidney Int.* 7:342, 1975.

133. Unanue, E. R., and Dixon, F. J. Experimental allergic glomerulonephritis induced in the rabbit with heterologous renal antigens. *J. Exp. Med.* 125:149, 1967.

134. Klassen, J., McCluskey, R. T., and Milgrom, F. Nonglomerular renal disease produced in rabbits by immunization with homologous kidney. *Am. J. Pathol.* 63:333, 1971.

135. Andres, G. A., and McCluskey, R. T. Tubular and interstitial renal disease due to immunologic mechanisms. *Kidney Int.* 7:271, 1975.

136. Lehman, D. H., Wilson, C. B., and Dixon, F. J. Extraglomerular immunoglobulin deposits in human nephritis. *Am. J. Med.* 58:765, 1975.

137. Estes, D., and Christian, C. L. The natural history of systemic lupus erythematosus by prospective analysis. *Medicine* 50:85, 1971.

138. Sergent, J. S., and Lockshin, M. D. Editorial. Treatment of central nervous system lupus erythematosus. *Ann. Intern. Med.* 80:413, 1974.

139. Small, P., Mass, M. F., Kohler, P. F., et al. Central nervous system involvement in SLE. Diagnostic profile and clinical features. *Arthritis Rheum.* 20:869, 1977.

140. Bennett, R., Hughes, G. R. V., Bywaters, E. G. L., et al. Neuropsychiatric problems in systemic lupus erythematosus. *Br. Med. J.* 4:342, 1972.

141. Johnson, R. T., and Richardson, E. P. The neurological manifestations of systemic lupus erythematosus. A clinical-pathological study of 24 cases and review of the literature. *Medicine* 47:337, 1968.

142. Petz, L. D., Sharp, G. C., Cooper, N. R., et al. Serum and cerebral spinal fluid complement and serum auto-antibodies in systemic lupus erythematosus. *Medicine* 50:259, 1971.

143. Pinching, A. J., Travers, R., Hughes, G. R. V., et al. 15-oxygen brain scanning in systemic lupus erythematosus. Presented at annual meeting Heberden Society, November 18, 1977.

144. Atkins, C. J., Kondon, J. J., Quismorio, F. P., et al. The choroid plexus in systemic lupus erythematosus. *Ann. Intern. Med.* 76:65, 1972.

145. Lampert, P. W., and Oldstone, M. B. A. Host immunoglobulin G and complement deposits in the choroid plexus during spontaneous immune complex disease. *Science* 180:408, 1973.

146. Oldstone, M. B. A. Virus neutralization and virus-induced immune complex disease. Virus-antibody union resulting in immunoprotection or immunologic injury—two sides of the same coin. *Prog. Med. Virol.* 19:84, 1975.

147. Lampert, P. W., and Oldstone, M. B. A. Pathology of the choroid plexus in spontaneous immune complex disease and chronic viral infections. *Virchows Arch. (Pathol. Anat.)* 363:21, 1974.

148. Gelfand, M. C., Frank, M. M., and Green, I. A receptor for the third component of complement in the human renal glomerulus. *J. Exp. Med.* 142:1029, 1975.

149. Williams, R. C., Jr., Husby, G., Wedege, E., et al. Sydenham's chorea, anti-neuronal antibodies, circulating immune complexes and the choroid plexus Fc receptor. In B. Schwabe, ed., *Menarini Foundation and World Health Organization Conference on Autoimmunity of the Central and Peripheral Nervous System.* Basel, forthcoming.

150. Lee, S. L., Sanders, M., and Kahny, H. M. A disorder of blood coagulation in systemic lupus erythematosus. *J. Clin. Invest.* 34:1814, 1955.

151. Breckenridge, R. T., Moore, R. D., and Ratnoff, O. D. A study of thrombocytopenia: new histologic criteria for the differentiation of idiopathic thrombocytopenia and thrombocytopenia associated with disseminated lupus erythematosus. *Blood* 30:39, 1967.

152. Rabinowitz, Y., and Dameshek, W. Systemic lupus erythematosus after" idiopathic" thrombocytopenic purpura. *Ann. Intern. Med.* 52:1, 1960.

153. Mittal, K. K., Rossen, R. D., Sharp, J. T., et al. Lymphocyte cytotoxic antibodies in systemic lupus erythematosus. *Nature* 225:1255, 1970.

154. Terasaki, P. I., Mottironi, V. D., and Barnett, E. V. Cytotoxins in disease. Autocytotoxins in lupus. *N. Engl. J. Med.* 283:724, 1970.

155. Butler, W. T., Sharp, J. T., Rossen, R. D., et al. Relationship of the clinical course of systemic lupus erythematosus to the presence of circulating lymphocytotoxic antibodies. *Arthritis Rheum.* 15:231, 1972.

156. Winfield, J. B., Winchester, R. J., Wernet, P., et al. Nature of cold-reactive antibodies to lymphocyte surface determinants in systemic lupus erythematosus. *Arthritis Rheum.* 18:1, 1975.

157. Winfield, J. B., Winchester, R. J., and Kunkel, H. G. Association of cold-reactive antilymphocyte antibodies with lymphopenia in systemic lupus erythematosus. *Arthritis Rheum.* 18:587, 1975.

158. Williams, R. C., Jr., Bankhurst, A. D., and Montaño, J. D. IgG antilymphocyte antibodies in SLE detected by ^{125}I protein A. *Arthritis Rheum.* 19:1261, 1976.

159. Stastny, P., and Ziff, M. Antibodies against cell membrane constituents in systemic lupus erythematosus and related diseases. I. Cytotoxic effect of serum from patients with systemic lupus erythematosus (SLE) for allogeneic and for autologous lymphocytes. *Clin. Exp. Immunol.* 8:543, 1971.

160. Wernet, P., and Kunkel, H. G. Antibodies to a specific surface antigen of T-cells in human sera inhibiting mixed leukocyte culture reactions. *J. Exp. Med.* 138:1021, 1973.

161. Williams, R. C., Jr., Lies, R. B., and Messner, R. P. Inhibition of mixed leukocyte culture responses by serum and γ-globulin fractions from certain patients with connective tissue disorders. *Arthritis Rheum.* 16:597, 1973.

162. Lies, R. B., Messner, R. P., and Williams, R. C., Jr. Relative T-cell specificity of lymphocytotoxins from patients with systemic lupus erythematosus. *Arthritis Rheum.* 16:369, 1973.

163. Goldberg, L. S., Cunningham, J. E., and Terasaki, P. I. Lymphocytotoxins and pernicious anemia. *Blood* 39:862, 1972.

164. van den Noort, S., and Stjernholm, R. L. Lymphotoxic activity in multiple sclerosis serum. *Neurology* 21:783, 1971.

165. Mottironi, V. D., and Terasaki, P. I. Lymphocytotoxins in disease. I. Infectious mononucleosis, rubella, and measles. In P. I. Terasaki, ed., *Histocompatibility Testing*, p. 301. Munksgaard, Copenhagen, Williams & Wilkins Co., 1970.

166. Grifoni, V., Del Giacco, G. S., Tognella, S., et al. Lymphocytotoxins in Hodgkin's disease. *Ital. J. Immunol. Immunopathol.* 1:21, 1970.

167. Messner, R. P. Naturally occurring anti-

lymphocyte antibodies. In R. C. Williams, Jr., ed., *Lymphocytes and Their Interactions*, p. 169. Raven Press, New York, 1975.

168. Park, M. S., Terasaki, P. I., and Bernoco, P. Autoantibody against B lymphocytes. *Lancet* 2:465, 1977.

169. Klassen, L. W., Krakauer, R. S., and Steinberg, A. D. Selective loss of suppressor cell function in New Zealand mice induced by NTA. *J. Immunol.* 119:830, 1977.

170. Auer, I. O., Tomasi, T. B., Jr., and Milgrom, F. Natural thymocytolytic autoantibodies in NZB and other strains of mice. *Cell. Immunol.* 10:404, 1974.

171. Shirai, T., and Mellors, R. C. Natural cytotoxic autoantibody against thymocytes in NZB mice. *Clin. Exp. Immunol.* 12:133, 1972.

172. Gelfand, M. C., Parker, L. M., and Steinberg, A. D. Mechanism of allograft rejection in New Zealand mice. II. Role of a serum factor. *J. Immunol.* 113:1, 1974.

173. Oldstone, M. B. A., Tishon, A., and Moretta, L. Active thymus derived suppressor lymphocytes in human cord blood. *Nature* 269:333, 1977.

174. Callahan, R., Benveniste, R. E., and Lieber, M. M. Nucleic acid homology of murine type-C viral genes. *J. Virol.* 14:1394, 1974.

175. Wecker, E., Schimpl, A., and Hünig, T. Expression of MuLV GP71-like antigen in normal mouse spleen cells induced by antigenic stimulation. *Nature* 269:598, 1977.

176. Christian, C. L., Hatfield, W. B., and Chase, P. H. Systemic lupus erythematosus. Cryoprecipitation of sera. *J. Clin. Invest.* 42:823, 1963.

177. Hanauer, L. B., and Christian, C. L. Studies of cryoproteins in systemic lupus erythematosus. *J. Clin. Invest.* 46:400, 1967.

178. Stastny, P., and Ziff, M. Cold-insoluble complexes and complement levels in systemic lupus erythematosus. *N. Engl. J. Med.* 280:1376, 1969.

179. Winfield, J. B., Koffler, D., and Kunkel, H. G. Specific concentration of polynucleotide immune complexes in the cryoprecipitates of patients with systemic lupus erythematosus. *J. Clin. Invest.* 56:563, 1975.

180. Winfield, J. B., Winchester, R. J., Wernet, P., et al. Specific concentration of antilymphocyte antibodies in the serum cryoprecipitates of patients with systemic lupus erythematosus. *Clin. Exp. Immunol.* 19:399, 1975.

181. Bluestein, H. G., and Zvaifler, N. J. Brain-reactive lymphocytotoxic antibodies in the serum of patients with systemic lupus erythematosus. *J. Clin. Invest.* 57:509, 1976.

182. Golub, E. S. Brain-associated stem cell antigen: an antigen shared by brain and hemopoietic stem cells. *J. Exp. Med.* 136:369, 1972.

183. Reif, A. E., and Allen, J. M. V. The AKR thymic antigen and its distribution in leukemias and nervous tissues. *J. Exp. Med.* 120:413, 1964.

184. Bresnihan, B., and Hughes, G. R. V. Unpublished data, 1978.

185. DeHoratius, R. J., and Messner, R. P. Lymphocytotoxic antibodies in family members of patients with systemic lupus erythematosus. *J. Clin. Invest.* 55:1254, 1975.

186. DeHoratius, R. J., Pillarisetty, R., Messner, R. P., et al. Anti-nucleic acid antibodies in systemic lupus erythematosus patients and their families. Incidence and correlation with lymphocytotoxic antibodies. *J. Clin. Invest.* 56:1149, 1975.

187. Malavé, I., Papa, R., and Layrisse, Z. Lymphocytotoxic antibodies in SLE patients and their relatives. *Arthritis Rheum.* 19:700, 1976.

188. Folomeeva, O., Nassonova, V. A., Alekberova, A. S., et al. Comparative studies of antilymphocyte, antipolynucleotide, and antiviral antibodies among families of patients with systemic lupus erythematosus. *Arthritis Rheum.* 21:23, 1978.

189. Lowenstein, M. B., and Rothfield, N. F. Family study of systemic lupus erythematosus: analysis of the clinical history, skin immunofluorescence, and serologic parameters. *Arthritis Rheum.* 20:1293, 1977.

190. Ooi, Y. M., Ooi, B. S., Vallota, E. H., et al. Circulating immune complexes after renal transplantation. Correlation of increased ^{125}I-C1q-binding activity with acute rejection characterized by fibrin deposition in the kidney. *J. Clin. Invest.* 60:611, 1977.

191. Haakenstad, A. O., Case, J. B., and Mannik, M. Effect of cortisone on the disappearance kinetics and tissue localization of soluble immune complexes. *J. Immunol.* 114:1153, 1975.

192. Clark, G., Reichlin, M., and Tomasi, T. B., Jr. Characterization of a soluble cytoplasmic antigen reactive with sera from patients with systemic lupus erythematosus. *J. Immunol.* 102:117, 1969.

193. Mattioli, M., and Reichlin, M. Heterogeneity of RNA protein antigens reactive with sera of patients with systemic lupus erythematosus. Description of a cytoplasmic non-ribosomal antigen. *Arthritis Rheum.* 17:421, 1974.

194. Reichlin, M., and Mattioli, M. Correlation of a precipitin reaction to an RNA protein antigen and a low prevalence of nephritis in patients with systemic lupus erythematosus. *N. Engl. J. Med.* 286:908, 1972.

195. Provost, T. T., Ahmed, A. R., Maddison, P. J., et al. Antibodies to cytoplasmic antigens in lupus erythematosus: serologic marker for systemic disease. *Arthritis Rheum.* 20:1457, 1977.

196. Robitaille, P., and Tan, E. M. Relationship between deoxyribonucleoprotein and deoxyribonucleic acid antibodies in systemic lupus erythematosus. *J. Clin. Invest.* 52:316, 1973.

197. Tan, E. M. An immunologic precipitin system between soluble nucleoprotein and serum antibody in systemic lupus erythematosus. *J. Clin. Invest.* 46:735, 1967.

198. Akizuki, M., Powers, R., Jr., and Holman, H. R. Comparative study of immunologic methods for demonstration of antibodies to soluble nuclear antigens. Immunofluorescence, hemagglutination, complement fixation, and immunodiffusion. *Arthritis Rheum.* 20:693, 1977.

199. Stollar, B. D. Varying specificity of systemic lupus erythematosus sera for histone fractions and a periodate-sensitive antigen associated with histone. *J. Immunol.* 103:804, 1969.

200. Sharp, G. C., Irvin, W. S., Tan, E. M., et al. Mixed connective tissue disease. An apparently distinct rheumatic disease syndrome associated with a specific antibody to an extractable nuclear antigen (ENA). *Am. J. Med.* 52:148, 1972.

201. Sharp, G. C., Irvin, W. S., La Roque, R. L. et al. Association of autoantibodies to different nuclear antigens with clinical patterns of rheumatic disease and responsiveness to therapy. *J. Clin. Invest.* 50:350, 1971.

202. Parker, M. D. Ribonucleoprotein antibodies: frequency and clinical significance in systemic lupus erythematosus, scleroderma, and mixed connective tissue disease. *J. Lab. Clin. Med.* 82:769, 1973.

203. Talal, N., and Gallo, R. C. Antibodies to a DNA:RNA hybrid in systemic lupus erythematosus measured by a cellulose ester filter radioimmunoassay. *Nature (New Biol.)* 240:240, 1972.

204. Miyawaki, S., and Ritchie, R. F. Nucleolar antigen specific for antinucleolar antibody in the sera of patients with systemic rheumatic disease. *Arthritis Rheum.* 16:726, 1973.

205. Tan, E. M., Northway, J. D., Pinnas, J. L. The clinical significance of antinuclear antibodies. *Postgrad. Med.* 54:143, 1973.

206. Tan, E. M. Immunospecificities of antinuclear antibodies. *Arthritis Rheum.* 20:187s, 1977.

207. Morris, A. D., Littleton, C., Corman, L. C., et al. Extractable nuclear antigen effect on the DNA-anti-DNA reaction and NZB/NZW mouse nephritis. *J. Clin. Invest.* 55:903, 1975.

208. Good, R. A., Rötstein, J., and Mazzitello, W. F. The simultaneous occurrence of rheumatoid arthritis and agammaglobulinemia. *J. Lab. Clin. Med.* 49:343, 1957.

209. Peterson, R. D., Cooper, M. D., and Good, R. A. The pathogenesis of immunologic deficiency diseases. *Am. J. Med.* 38:579, 1965.

210. Janeway, C. A., Gitlin, D., Craig, J. M., et al. "Collagen disease" in patients with congenital agammaglobulinemia. *Trans. Assoc. Am. Physicians* 69:93, 1956.

211. Agnello, V., De Bracco, M. M. E., and Kunkel, H. G. Hereditary C2 deficiency with some manifestations of systemic lupus erythematosus. *J. Immunol.* 108:837, 1972.

212. Day, N. K., Geiger, H., McLean, R., et al. C2 deficiency. Development of lupus erythematosus. *J. Clin. Invest.* 52:1601, 1973.

213. Moncada, B., Day, N. K., Good, R. A., et al. Lupus-erythematosus-like syndrome with a familial defect of complement. *N. Engl. J. Med.* 286:689, 1972.

214. Douglass, M. C., Lamberg, S. I., Lorincz, A. L., et al. Lupus erythematosus-like syndrome with a familial deficiency of C2. *Arch. Dermatol.* 112:671, 1976.

215. Osterland, C. K., Espinoza, L., and Parker, L. P. Inherited C2 deficiency and systemic lupus erythematosus: studies on a family. *Ann. Intern. Med.* 82:323, 1975.

216. Stern, R., Fu, S. M., Fotino, M., et al. Hereditary C2 deficiency: association with skin lesions resembling the discoid lesion of systemic lupus erythematosus. *Arthritis Rheum.* 19:517, 1976.

217. Glass, D., Raum, D., Gibson, D., et al. Inherited deficiency of the second component of complement. Rheumatic disease associations. *J. Clin. Invest.* 58:853, 1976.

218. Pickering, R. J., Michael, A. F., Jr., Herdman, R. C., et al. The complement system in chronic glomerulonephritis: three newly associated aberrations. *J. Pediatr.* 78:30, 1971.

219. Wild, J., Zvaifler, N., Müller-Eberhard, H., et al. Deficiency of the second component of complement (C2) in a patient with discoid lupus erythematosus (DLE). *J. Clin. Invest.* 53:84, 1974 (abstract).

220. Rosenfeld, S. I., Kelly, M. E., and Leddy, J. P. Hereditary deficiency of the fifth component of complement in man. I. Clinical, immunochemical, and family studies. *J. Clin. Invest.* 57:1626, 1976.

221. Hauptmann, G., Grosshaus, E., and Heid, E. Lupus érythémateux aigus et deficits héréditaires en complement. Apropos d'un cas par déficit com-

plet en C4. *Ann. Dermatol. Syphiligr. (Paris)* 101:479, 1974.

222. Leddy, J. P., Griggs, R. C., Klemperer, M. R., et al. Hereditary complement (C2) deficiency with dermatomyositis. *Am. J. Med.* 58:83, 1975.

223. Boyer, J. T., Gall, E. P., Norman, M. E., et al. Hereditary deficiency of the seventh component of complement. *J. Clin. Invest.* 56:905, 1975.

224. Kohler, P. F., Percy, J., Campion, W. M., et al. Hereditary angioedema and" familial" lupus erythematosus in identical twin boys. *Am. J. Med.* 56:406, 1974.

225. Jasin, H. E. Absence of the eighth component of complement (C8) and SLE-like disease. *Arthritis Rheum.* 19:803, 1976.

226. Jasin, H. E. Absence of the eighth component of complement in association with systemic lupus erythematosus-like disease. *J. Clin. Invest.* 60:709, 1977.

227. Schaller, J. G., Gilliland, B. G., Ochs, H. D., et al. Severe systemic lupus erythematosus with nephritis in a boy with deficiency of the fourth component of complement. *Arthritis Rheum.* 20:1519, 1977.

228. Rothfield, N., Ross, H. A., Minta, J. O., et al. Glomerular and dermal deposition of properdin in systemic lupus erythematosus. *N. Engl. J. Med.* 287:681, 1972.

229. Ziegler, J. B., Rosen, F. S., Alper, C. A., et al. Metabolism of properdin in normal subjects and patients with renal disease. *J. Clin. Invest.* 56:761, 1975.

230. Leddy, J. P., Simons, R. L., and Douglas, R. G. Effect of selective complement deficiency on the rate of neutralization of enveloped viruses by human sera. *J. Immunol.* 118:28, 1977.

231. Ahmadian, Y. S., Given, G. Z., and Mendoza, S. A. Normal urine and positive immunofluorescence reaction in lupus nephritis. *Am. J. Dis. Child.* 123:121, 1972.

232. Bardana, E. J., Jr., Harbeck, R. J., Hoffman, A. A., et al. The prognostic and therapeutic implications of DNA: anti-DNA immune complexes in systemic lupus erythematosus (SLE). *Am. J. Med.* 59:515, 1975.

233. Dujovne, I., Pollak, V. E., Pirani, C. L., et al. The distribution and character of glomerular deposits in systemic lupus erythematosus. *Kidney Int.* 2:33, 1972.

234. Morel-Maroger, L., Méry, J. P., Delrieu, F., et al. Etude immunohistochemique de 29 biopsies rénales faites au cours du lupus érythémateux disséminé. *J. Urol. Nephrol. (Paris)* 77:367, 1971.

235. Soffer, L. J., Southren, A. L., Weiner, H. E., et al. Renal manifestations of systemic lupus erythematosus. A clinical and pathologic study of 90 cases. *Ann. Intern. Med.* 54:215, 1961.

236. Zweiman, B., Kornblum, J., Cornog, J., et al. The prognosis of lupus nephritis. Role of clinicopathologic correlations. *Ann. Intern. Med.* 69:441, 1968.

237. Mahajan, S. K., Ordóñez, N. G., Feitelson, P. J., et al. Lupus nephropathy without clinical renal involvement. *Medicine* 56:493, 1977.

238. Cruchaud, A., Chenais, F., Fournié, G. J., et al. Immune complex deposits in systemic lupus erythematosus kidney without histological or functional alterations. *Eur. J. Clin. Invest.* 5:297, 1975.

239. Bennett, W., Houghton, D., Bardana, E., et al. Staging of renal involvement in systemic lupus erythematosus (SLE) when clinical nephropathy is absent. *Clin. Res.* 24:161, 1976 (abstract).

240. Sinniah, R., and Feng, P. H. Lupus nephritis: correlation between light, electron microscopic and immunofluorescent findings and renal function. *Clin. Nephrol.* 6:340, 1976.

241. Rothfield, N. F., McCluskey, R. T., and Baldwin, D. S. Renal disease in systemic lupus erythematosus. *N. Engl. J. Med.* 269:537, 1963.

242. Pollak, V. E., Pirani, C. L., and Schwartz, F. D. The natural history of the renal manifestations of systemic lupus erythematosus. *J. Lab. Clin. Med.* 63:537, 1964.

243. Simenhoff, M. L., and Merrill, J. P. The spectrum of lupus nephritis. *Nephron* 1:348, 1964.

244. Baldwin, D. S., Lowenstein, J., Rothfield, N. F., et al. The clinical course of the proliferative and membranous forms of lupus nephritis. *Ann. Intern. Med.* 73:929, 1970.

245. Harvey, A. M., Shulman, L. E., Tumulty, P. A., et al. Systemic lupus erythematosus: review of the literature and clinical analysis of 138 cases. *Medicine* 33:291, 1954.

246. Dubois, E. L., and Tuffanelli, D. L. Clinical manifestations of systemic lupus erythematosus. Computer analysis of 520 cases. *J.A.M.A.* 190:104, 1964.

247. Nydegger, U. E., Lambert, P. H., Gerber, H., et al. Circulating immune complexes in the serum in systemic lupus erythematosus and in carriers of hepatitis B antigen. Quantitation by binding to radiolabeled C1q. *J. Clin. Invest.* 54:297, 1974.

248. Levinsky, R. J., Cameron, J. S., and Soothill, J. F. Serum immune complexes and diseases activity in lupus nephritis. *Lancet* 1:564, 1977.

249. Cano, P. O., Jerry, L. M., Sladowski, J. P., et al. Circulating immune complexes in systemic

lupus erythematosus. *Clin. Exp. Immunol.* 29:197, 1977.

250. Cameron, J. S., Lessof, M. H., Ogg, C. S., et al. Disease activity in the nephritis of systemic lupus erythematosus in relation to serum complement concentrations. DNA-binding capacity and precipitating anti-DNA antibody. *Clin. Exp. Immunol.* 25:418, 1976.

251. Eisenberg, R. A., Theofilopoulos, A. N., and Dixon, F. J. Use of bovine conglutinin for the assay of immune complexes. *J. Immunol.* 118:1428, 1977.

252. Frank, M. M., Hamburger, M. I., Lawley, T. J., et al. Defective reticuloendothelial system Fc-receptor function in systemic lupus erythematosus. *N. Engl. J. Med.* 300:518, 1979.

253. Jaffe, C. J., Vierling, J. M., Jones, E. A., et al. Receptor specific clearance by the reticuloendothelial system in chronic liver diseases. Demonstration of defective C3b-specific clearance in primary biliary cirrhosis. *J. Clin. Invest.* 62:1069, 1978.

254. Ansell, B. M., and Bywaters, E. G. L. Prognosis in Still's disease. *Bull. Rheum. Dis.* 9:189, 1959.

255. Brewer, E. J., Bass, J., Baum, J., et al. Current proposed revision of JRA criteria. JRA criteria subcommittee of the diagnostic and therapeutic criteria committee of the American Rheumatism Association section of the Arthritis Foundation. *Arthritis Rheum.* 20:195, 1977 (suppl.).

256. Schaller, J. G., Johnson, G. D., Holborow, E. J., et al. The association of antinuclear antibodies with the chronic iridocyclitis of juvenile rheumatoid arthritis (Still's disease). *Arthritis Rheum.* 17:409, 1974.

257. Rossen, R. D., Brewer, E. J., Person, D. A., et al. Circulating immune complexes and antinuclear antibodies in juvenile rheumatoid arthritis. *Arthritis Rheum.* 20:1485, 1977.

258. Venkateswara, R. K., Berkseth, R. O., Crosson, J. T., et al. Immune-complex nephritis in mixed connective tissue disease. (Letter.) *Ann. Intern. Med.* 84:174, 1976.

259. Fuller, T. J., Richman, A. V., Auerbach, D., et al. Immune-complex glomerulonephritis in a patient with mixed connective tissue disease. *Am. J. Med.* 62:761, 1977.

260. Sanders, D. Y., Huntley, C. C., and Sharp, G. C. Mixed connective tissue disease in a child. *J. Pediatr.* 83:642, 1973.

261. Halla, J. T., Volanakis, J. E., and Schrohenloher, R. E. Circulating immune complexes in mixed connective tissue disease. *Arthritis Rheum.* 22:484, 1979.

262. Abdou, N. I., Na Pombejara, C., Balentine, L., et al. Suppressor cell-mediated neutropenia in Felty's syndrome. *J. Clin. Invest.* 61:738, 1978.

263. Schlosstein, L., Terasaki, P. I., Bluestone, R., et al. High association of an HL-A antigen, W27, with ankylosing spondylitis. *N. Engl. J. Med.* 288:704, 1973.

264. Brewerton, D. A., Caffrey, M., Hart, F. D., et al. Ankylosing spondylitis and HL-A 27. *Lancet* 1:904, 1973.

265. Gabay, R., Zubler, R. H., Nydegger, U. E., et al. Immune complexes and complement catabolism in ankylosing spondylitis. *Arthritis Rheum.* 20:913, 1977.

266. Kussmaul, A., and Maier, R. Ueber eine bisher nicht beschriebene eigenthümliche Arterienerkrankung (Periarteritis nodosa), die mit Morbus Brightii und rapid fortschreitender allgemeiner Müskellähmung einhergeht. *Dtsch. Arch. Klin. Med.* 1:484, 1966.

267. Zeek, P. M. Periarteritis nodosa: a critical review. *Am. J. Clin. Pathol.* 22:777, 1952.

268. Zeek, P. M., Smith, C. C., and Weeter, J. C. Studies on periarteritis nodosa. Differentiation between vascular lesions of periarteritis nodosa and of hypersensitivity. *Am. J. Pathol.* 24:889, 1948.

269. Alarçon-Segovia, D. The necrotizing vasculitides. A new pathogenetic classification. *Med. Clin. North Am.* 61:241, 1977.

270. Fye, K. H., Becker, M. J., Theofilopoulos, A. N., et al. Immune complexes in hepatitis B antigen-associated periarteritis nodosa. Detection by antibody-dependent cell-mediated cytotoxicity and the Raji cell assay. *Am. J. Med.* 62:783, 1977.

271. Whitaker, J. N., and Engel, W. K. Vascular deposits of immunoglobulin and complement in idiopathic inflammatory myopathy *N. Engl. J. Med.* 286:333, 1972.

272. Soter, N. A., Austen, K. F., and Gigli, I. Urticaria and arthralgias as manifestations of necrotizing angiitis (vasculitis). *J. Invest. Dermatol.* 63:485, 1974.

273. Sissons, J. G. P., Williams, D. G., Peters, D. K., et al. Skin lesions, angio-oedema, and hypocomplementaemia. *Lancet* 2:1350, 1974.

274. McDuffie, F. C., Sams, W. M., Jr., Maldonado, J. E., et al. Hypocomplementemia with cutaneous vasculitis and arthritis. Possible immune complex syndrome. *Mayo Clin. Proc.* 48:340, 1973.

275. Soter, N. A. Chronic urticaria as a manifestation of necrotizing venulitis. *N. Engl. J. Med.* 296:1440, 1977.

276. Tuffanelli, D. L. Cutaneous immunopathology: recent observations. *J. Invest. Dermatol.* 65:143, 1975.

277. Soter, N. A., Mihm, M. C., Jr., Gigli, I., et al. Two distinct cellular patterns in cutaneous necrotizing angiitis. *J. Invest. Dermatol.* 66:344, 1976.

278. Rammelkamp, C. H., Jr., Denny, F. W., and Wannamaker, L. W. Studies on the epidemiology of rheumatic fever in the armed services. In L. Thomas, ed., *Rheumatic Fever: A Symposium,* p. 72. University of Minnesota Press, Minneapolis, 1952.

279. Stollerman, G. H. The epidemiology of primary and secondary rheumatic fever. In J. W. Uhr, ed., *The Streptococcus, Rheumatic Fever and Glomerulonephritis,* p. 311. Williams & Wilkins Co., Baltimore, 1964.

280. Taranta, A. Rheumatic fever: clinical aspects. In J. L. Hollander, ed., *Arthritis and Allied Conditions,* p. 694. Lea & Febiger, Philadelphia, 1966.

281. Feinstein, A. R., and Spagnuolo, M. Mimetic features of rheumatic-fever recurrences. *N. Engl. J. Med.* 262:533, 1960.

282. Rammelkamp, C. H., Jr. Epidemiology of streptococcal infections. *Harvey Lect.* 51:113, 1955–56.

283. Rammelkamp, C. H., Jr. Microbiologic aspects of glomerulonephritis. *J. Chronic Dis.* 5:28, 1957.

284. Wannamaker, L. W., and Ayoub, E. M. Antibody titers in acute rheumatic fever. *Circulation* 21:598, 1960.

285. Ayoub, E. M., and Wannamaker, L. W. Evaluation of the streptococcal desoxyribonuclease B and disphosphopyridine nucleotidase antibody tests in acute rheumatic fever and acute glomerulonephritis. *Pediatrics* 29:527, 1962.

286. Ayoub, E. M., and Wannamaker, L. W. Streptococcal antibody titers in Sydenham's chorea. *Pediatrics* 38:946, 1966.

287. Wilson, M. G., Schweitzer, M. D., and Lubschez, R. The familial epidemiology of rheumatic fever: genetic and epidemiologic studies: genetic studies. *J. Pediatr.* 22:468, 1943.

288. Wilson, M. G., and Schweitzer, M. D. Pattern of hereditary susceptibility in rheumatic fever. *Circulation* 10:699, 1954.

289. Taranta, A., Torosdag, S., Metrakos, J., et al. Rheumatic fever in monozygotic and dizygotic twins. *Atti X Congr. Lega Internaz. contro il Rheum.,* 2:96, 1961.

290. Spagnuolo, M., and Taranta, A. Rheumatic fever in siblings. Similarity of its clinical manifestations. *N. Engl. J. Med.* 278:183, 1968.

291. Patarroyo, M. E., Winchester, R. J., Vejerano, A., et al. Association of a B-cell alloantigen with susceptibility to rheumatic fever. *Nature* 278:173, 1979.

292. Stollerman, G. H. Clinical manifestations of acute rheumatic fever. In *Rheumatic Fever and Streptococcal Infection,* p. 169. Grune & Stratton, New York, 1975.

293. Husby, G., van de Rijn, I., Zabriskie, J. B., et al. Antibodies reacting with cytoplasm of subthalamic and caudate nuclei neurons in chorea and acute rheumatic fever. *J. Exp. Med.* 144:1094, 1976.

294. Lueker, R. D., Abdin, Z. H., and Williams, R. C., Jr. Peripheral blood T and B lymphocytes during acute rheumatic fever. *J. Clin. Invest.* 55:975, 1975.

295. Williams, R. C., Jr., Zabriskie, J. B., Mahros, F., et al. Lymphocyte surface markers in acute rheumatic fever and post-streptococcal acute glomerulonephritis. *Clin. Exp. Immunol.* 27:135, 1977.

296. Terres, G., Morrison, S. L., and Habicht, G. S. A quantitative difference in the immune response between male and female mice. *Proc. Soc. Exp. Biol. Med.* 127:664, 1968.

297. Butterworth, M., McClellan, B., and Allansmith, M. Influence of sex on immunoglobulin levels. *Nature* 214:1224, 1967.

298. Batchelor, J. R. Regulation of the antibody response. In B. Cinader, ed., *Hormonal Control of Antibody Formation,* p. 276. Charles C. Thomas, Springfield, Ill., 1968.

299. Kongshavn, P. A., and Bliss, J. Q. Sex differences in survival of H-2 incompatible skin grafts in mice treated with antithymocyte serum. *Nature* 226:451, 1970.

300. Svartman, M., Potter, E. V., Poon-King, T., et al. Immunoglobulins and complement components in synovial fluid of patients with acute rheumatic fever. *J. Clin. Invest.* 56:111, 1975.

301. Rich, A. R. Hypersensitivity in disease with especial reference to periarteritis nodosa, rheumatic fever, disseminated lupus erythematosus, and rheumatoid arthritis. *Harvey Lect.* 42:106, 1946–47.

302. Cromartie, W. J. Reactions of connective tissue to cellular components of group A streptococci. In J. W. Uhr, ed., *The Streptococcus, Rheumatic Fever and Glomerulonephritis,* p. 187. Williams & Wilkins Co., Baltimore, 1964.

303. Kaplan, M. H., Bolande, R., Rakita, L., et al. Presence of bound immunoglobulins and complement in the myocardium in acute rheumatic fever. Association with cardiac failure. *N. Engl. J. Med.* 271:637, 1964.

304. Kaplan, M. H., and Svec, K. H. Immunologic relation of streptococcal and tissue antigens. III. Presence in human sera of streptococcal antibody cross-reactive with heart tissue. Association

with streptococcal infection, rheumatic fever, and glomerulonephritis. *J. Exp. Med.* 119:651, 1964.

305. Kaplan, M. H. Localization of streptococcal antigens in tissues. I. Histologic distribution and persistence of M protein, types 1, 5, 12 and 19 in the tissues of the mouse. *J. Exp. Med.* 107:341, 1958.

306. Kaplan, M. H., and Meyeserian, M. An immunological cross-reaction between group-A streptococcal cells and human heart tissue. *Lancet* 1:706, 1962.

307. Kaplan, M. H. Immunologic relation of streptococcal and tissue antigens. I. Properties of an antigen in certain strains of group A streptococci exhibiting an immunologic cross-reaction with human heart tissue. *J. Immunol.* 90:595, 1963.

308. Zabriskie, J. B., and Freimer, E. H. An immunological relationship between the group A streptococcus and mammalian muscle. *J. Exp. Med.* 124:661, 1966.

309. Zabriskie, J. B., Hsu, K. C., and Seegal, B. C. Heart-reactive antibody associated with rheumatic fever: characterization and diagnostic significance. *Clin. Exp. Immunol.* 7:147, 1970.

310. Lyampert, I. M., Vvedenskaya, O. I., and Danilova, T. A. Study on streptococcus group A antigens common with heart tissue elements. *Immunology* 11:313, 1966.

311. Nakhla, L. S., and Glynn, L. E. Studies on the antigen in β haemolytic streptococci that cross-reacts with an antigen in human myocardium. *Immunology* 13:209, 1967.

312. Goldstein, I., Halpern, B., and Robert, L. Immunological relationship between streptococcus A polysaccharide and the structural glycoproteins of heart valve. *Nature* 213:44, 1967.

313. van de Rijn, I., Zabriskie, J. B., and McCarty, M. Group A streptococcal antigens cross-reactive with myocardium. Purification of heart-reactive antibody and isolation and characterization of the streptococcal antigen. *J. Exp. Med.* 146:579, 1977.

314. Kaplan, M. H. Multiple nature of the cross-reactive relationship between antigens of group A streptococci and mammalian tissue. In J. J. Trentin, ed., *Cross-Reacting Antigens and Neoantigens,* p. 48. Williams & Wilkins Co., Baltimore, 1967.

315. Kaplan, M. H. Cross-reaction of group A streptococci and heart tissue: varying serologic specificity of cross-reactive antisera and relation to carrier-hapten specificity. *Transplant. Proc.* 1:976, 1969.

316. Zabriskie, J. B. Mimetic relationships between group A streptococci and mammalian tissues. *Adv. Immunol.* 7:147, 1967.

317. Yang, L. C., Soprey, P. R., Wittner, M. K., et al. Streptococcal-induced cell-mediated-immune destruction of cardiac myofibers *in vitro. J. Exp. Med.* 146:344, 1977.

318. Read, S. E., Fischetti, V. A., Utermohlen, V., et al. Cellular reactivity studies to streptococcal antigens. Migration inhibition studies in patients with streptococcal infections and rheumatic fever. *J. Clin. Invest.* 54:439, 1974.

319. Lyampert, I. M., and Danilova, T. A. Immunological phenomena associated with cross-reactive antigens of micro-organisms and mammalian tissues. *Prog. Allergy* 18:423, 1975.

320. Kingston, D., and Glynn, L. E. A cross-reaction between *Str. pyogenes* and human fibroblasts, endothelial cells and astrocytes. *Immunology* 21:1003, 1971.

321. Kasp-Grouchowska, E., and Kingston, D. Streptococcal cross-reacting antigen and the bundle of His. *Clin. Exp. Immunol.* 27:63, 1977.

322. Williams, R. C., Jr., Walker, L., Kassaby, M., et al. Immune complexes in acute rheumatic fever. *J. Clin. Lab. Immunol.* 2:185, 1979.

CHAPTER 8

Neoplasia

No other area in clinical or experimental medicine has been examined more closely, during the last several decades, than that of tumor immunology. The availability of research funding has produced a recent tremendous flood of experimental data with some increment in knowledge of host reaction to tumors, but only a disappointing gain in insight into basic mechanisms. However, a number of important concepts have been established in many areas that point to practical use for patients with various tumors; these include knowledge of tumor antigens, mechanisms of tumor-cell destruction by the host, and the host immune response, which may actually aid tumor growth rather than impede it. One of the most interesting areas interrelating tumor progression or metastases with host protective mechanisms induced is the potential role of immune complexes. Many of the most carefully studied systems suggest that immune complexes may be deleterious as well as protective, depending on relative tumor antigenicity and host response. The presence of large amounts of circulating complexes does not augur well for the host and may correlate with metastasis and subsequent subversion of other potentially effective host defense mechanisms. A historical and possibly truncated introduction to the problem is presented in this chapter; practical implementation of the knowledge now accumulated must wait for future developments in this area.

Tumor Antigens

Cancers of many tissues show a variety of histological and physiological differences that identify them as distinct from their normal surrounding tissue. Perhaps the most important of these features is uncontrolled autonomous growth. For a number of years tumor tissues also were suspected to differ fundamentally from normal tissue in an immunological sense, that is, they possessed unique or distinctive antigens not usually expressed in their normal tissue counterparts. The existence of tumor-related or even tumor-specific antigens has now been demonstrated in a number of experimental animal systems and in a wide variety of human tumors. Thus, tumors induced in animals by chemical carcinogens, such as the methylcholanthrene-induced fibrosarcomas of mice extensively studied by a number of workers (1–4), show what appear to be unique surface antigens specific for these tumors. In addition, tumors induced by viruses or associated with viral infection clearly show tumor antigens distinct from normal tissue counterparts (5–10). Of interest is the fact that apparent virus-related antigens have now been identified on the surface of tumors produced by some of the most commonly used chemical agents for induction of tumors in experimental animals (11). Many naturally occurring animal and human tumors show unique surface antigens that have now been extensively characterized: mouse melanomas (12), human neuroblastomas (13), nephroblastomas (14), human melanomas (15–17), human carcinomas of the colon (18), human sarcomas (19–21), human and murine leukemias (22–26), and human carcinoma of the bladder (27, 28). In each of these systems, groups of antigens have been identified within malignant tissues that are not detectable with parallel normal tissues of similar origin. However, during the study of these apparent tumor-associated antigens, reservations have surfaced. These have usually related to what is and is not "self," and to whether there are any true tumor-specific antigens or only differentiation antigens unmasked by processes of rapid cell division and dedifferentiation inherent in the tumor process itself. This very important point is illustrated by close examination of several systems in which the original uniqueness or absolute tumor specificity of certain antigens has been explored in detail: the carcinoembryonic antigen initially related primarily to carcinoma of the colon; the α-fetoprotein, described most frequently with hepatoma or testicular teratoma; the antigens described in human acute leukemia; or those recently characterized in human melanoma.

After the initial description of the carcinoembryonic antigen (CEA) by Gold and Freedman (29) it appeared that these glycoproteins might be unique or true tumor-associated antigens specific for carcinomas of the lower digestive tract, specifically carcinomas of the colon. Recently test kits were prepared and marketed to physicians and clinics for use in cancer screening or detection and clinical follow-up of patients with previously established disease. Subsequent studies have indicated that CEA is also present in significant amounts in noncancerous conditions, including inflammatory bowel disease and an assortment of other gastrointestinal conditions, in heavy smokers, and in other tumors such as carcinoma of the breast, bronchus, or urinary tract (30–39). The appearance of CEA in other nontumor-related disease states immediately emphasized that this group of antigens were not only not tumor specific but were also released in a broad range of different inflammatory conditions. Moreover, a number of studies have shown that CEA antigens actually constitute a collection of similar, related glycoproteins (40–43), probably somehow involved in early events of cellular differentiation. It is still possible that various subfractions within the CEA group of related glycoproteins may indeed show true neoplastic specificity and better definition for colorectal malignancies. This possibility is being actively explored in several laboratories (41, 43).

The original work suggested that CEA, being present in fetal tissues, was actually an early or primitive material expressed in the initial stages of fetal organ differentiation (29, 44). Their presence in sera of heavy smokers or miscellaneous gastrointestinal inflammatory conditions has not precluded the usefulness of CEA determination, since the method adapted to sensitive techniques of radioimmunoassay and its many refinements is useful in the clinical follow-up of patients either at risk or known to have developed metastatic disease (45–47). The mass of data now accumulated relating to CEA has been of immense value, not only in establishing a perspective in which other potential tumor-specific antigens must be viewed, but also in setting the stage for clear definition and recognition of what are now generally regarded as oncofetal antigens. These antigens are expressed in tumors as a recall function of the original antigenic potential present since birth in the genome of some cells.

A second oncofetal antigen that has played an important role in the development of this concept is α-fetoprotein (AFP). This protein was originally described in 1963 by Abelev and co-workers (48). Later, it showed promise as a tumor-specific marker in relation to hepatoma and testicular teratomatas (49–52). Alpha-fetoprotein is very similar to normal human serum albumin, as emphasized by primary sequence analyses documented by Ruoslahti and Terry (53). The protein is produced by hepatic cells and in cases of nontumorous hepatic derangement, such as massive hepatic necrosis, it may also be elevated or detectable in serum (54–55). An example of cells showing cytoplasmic synthesis of AFP in a patient without tumor but with alcoholic hepatitis is shown in Figure 8-1. Its usefulness in the diagnosis and follow-up of tumor patients, however, again has not been entirely vitiated by the background occurrence in nonneoplastic states and it represents another interesting example of an oncofetal antigen expressed on dedifferentiated primitive cells, many times in association with tumor. Several other properties of AFP have made its study fascinating to those involved in problems related to cell differentiation or cellular interaction. Like CEA, a large

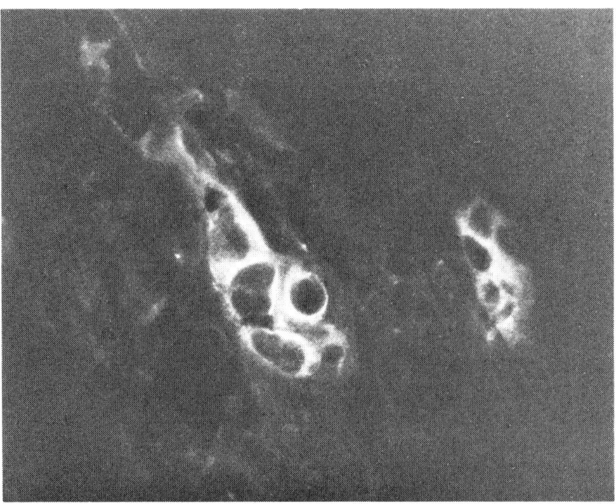

Figure 8-1 Immunofluorescent identification of a nest of hepatic cells producing AFP in liver biopsy sample from a patient with alcoholic hepatitis. Magnification × 450.

degree of microheterogeneity appears to be present within AFP (56–59). Using sensitive electrophoretic techniques combined with other fractionation procedures, AFP has been shown to consist of at least five major electrophoretically distinct fractions separated on the basis of differences in charge conferred by presence of varying numbers of sialic acid residues (60). Microheterogeneity has also been emphasized by the physical and functional assays of Lester and co-workers (59). Several initial reports support the concept that AFP possesses immunosuppressive capacity, since it is capable of diminishing mitogen-provoked in vitro lymphocyte response, in vivo primary and secondary response, and mixed leukocyte culture reactivity (61–63). Evidence is also present to suggest that AFP induces some of these phenomena through interaction with suppressor-cell systems (64). More recently, the general immunosuppressive effects of AFP have been questioned first on the basis of different functional behavior of subpopulations of AFP and second by examination of functional effects using a number of in vitro systems (65–67). Certainly, the final overall view of AFP, whether more generally immunosuppressive, sometimes immunostimulatory, or neutral, is as yet undecided. This work serves to emphasize the complexity of potential effects that may be attributed to certain oncofetal antigens.

With respect to the two oncofetal antigens CEA and AFP, only rarely have there been instances of host immune response per se to such antigens (68). Carcinoembryonic antigen has been identified by immunofluorescence in immune deposits of patients with renal involvement and primary carcinoma of the colon with metastases (69). An example of these findings is shown in Figure 8-2. However, a large or protracted host immune response with subsequent immune-complex formation to either CEA or AFP has not been identified as a common clinical phenomenon.

Still another example related to the reservations with which we must view the whole subject of specific tumor antigens is that recently described in association with acute lymphatic leukemia (ALL). Using antisera made in rabbits to human ALL cells, Greaves and co-workers (22, 23) described antigens that appear to be unique to these cells. After extensive absorption with normal thymus, bone marrow, B cells, and spleen, antisera that appeared to be specific for antigens on ALL cells were characterized. However, these same antigens also are present on a small fraction of normal stem cells in human fetal marrow (70, 71). Thus, the ALL antigen uniquely expressed on virtually all ALL (+) acute lymphatic leukemia cells may well be an antigen related to normal differentiation but not expressed on com-

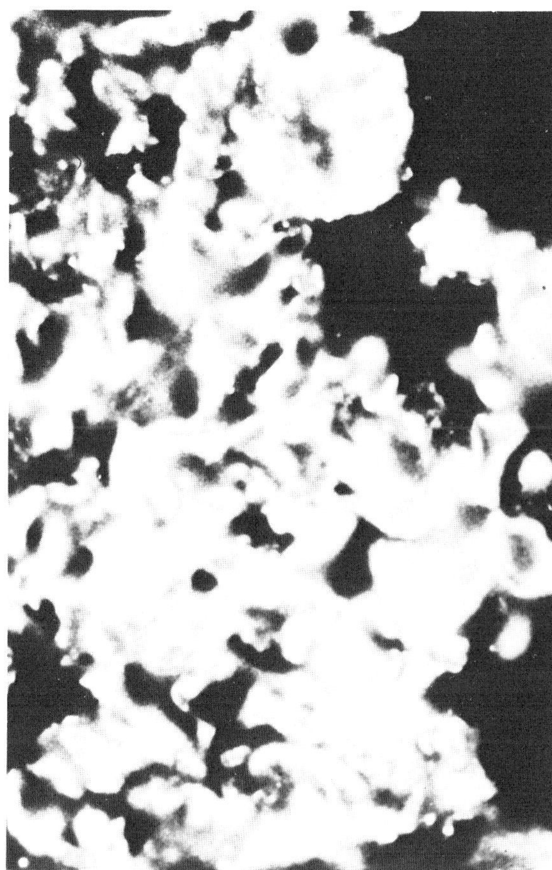

Figure 8-2 Photomicrograph of a glomerulus, showing immunofluorescent staining for CEA in a patient with carcinomatous nephropathy associated with colonic neoplasm. Similar distribution of immunofluorescence was noted with staining for IgG. Magnification × 400. (Reproduced with permission, M. E. Constanza, V. Pinn, R. S. Schwartz et al., *N. Engl. J. Med.* 289:520, 1973.)

pletely differentiated lymphocytes in normal human peripheral blood.

Acute lymphatic leukemia is divisible into several groups: T-cell leukemia, showing E-rosetting capacity; B-cell leukemia, showing readily detectable surface immunoglobulins; the so-called ALL (+) leukemia possessing the unique stem-cell related antigen of Greaves and co-workers and others (22, 23, 73); and a very small group of patients who have been for the moment classified as ALL null, that is, leukemic cells possessing no presently detectable T-cell or B-cell surface markers and no unique

or readily defined leukemia or differentiation antigens. This concept is illustrated in Table 8-1 taken from a recent report by Chessells and colleagues (72). The description and definition of antigens unique to or concentrated in various subsets of leukemic cells represents a finding of great practical usefulness since the ALL (+) group appears to bear a much more tractable prognosis and generally better record with chemotherapy than do patients in the T-cell, B-cell, or null-cell groups (72).

Finally, considerable evidence exists for tumor-specific antigens associated with human melanoma. Apart from evidence for humoral immunity, a number of studies have suggested cell-mediated immune reactions to what appear to be melanoma-specific antigens (15–17, 73–76). Recent studies by Carey and Shiku and their co-workers (77–79) have illustrated the remarkably narrow specificity of host antibodies reacting with the patient's own melanoma-tumor cell surface antigens, which in many ways appear to be individually specific. A second class of melanoma antigens was also recognized that showed shared reactions using sera from different patients, and was not expressed on other normal tissues. The remarkable diversity of these antibodies is a good example of the heterogeneous systems under current study. Shiku and associates found that melanoma-specific antibodies of one particular class, although not showing direct reactivity with other autologous or even xenogeneic cells, could be absorbed out by the latter (79). There are several other examples of autoantibodies of more broad general reactivity that are also associated in some instances with malignancies (80, 81), including those identified with anti–smooth muscle specificity.

The concept of an absolutely unique tumor-specific antigen must at present be viewed relatively. This view, or reservation, should probably also pertain to antigens associated with various virally induced tumors. As mentioned in Chapter 7, a considerable body of evidence now supports the concept that most normal murine cells show within their genome bits of information coding for antigens related to various C-type viruses (82–84). Here the precise definition of what is and what is not "self" fal-

Table 8-1 The presenting features and cell types of acute leukemia in childhood.

Type of ALL	Number of patients			Age (years)		White blood cell count ($\times 10^9/1$)			Mediastinal enlargement
	Male	Female	Total	Range	Median	<20	20–100	>100	
Common	39	32	71	0.5–15	4	45	18	8	1 (1%)
T cell	9	2	11	1.3–12.5	7	1	2	8	9 (82%)
B cell	1	1	2	3–5	—	1	1	0	0
Null cell	6	4	10	1.5–11	7	1	8	1	4 (40%)
Total	55	39	94	0.5–15		48	29	17	14 (15%)

Source: Reproduced with permission, J. M. Chessells, R. M. Hardisty, N. T. Rapson, et al., *Lancet* 2:1307, 1977.

ters considerably. Must one consider pieces of viral DNA intercalated into "autologous" DNA, which have perhaps been present in many generations, not self? As had been suggested by Moroni and colleagues, they may have been incorporated into the genomes of all living mammalian cells because they offer some survival advantage (84). At present, it seems best to take a broad utilitarian view of this subject. There is a great deal of evidence to suggest that *relatively* tumor-specific antigens do exist, and furthermore that the host invaded by tumor is capable of mounting an immune response to some of these antigens. We now proceed to an examination of what this immune response is and the specific role of immune complexes in the host response to neoplastic tissues. Some perplexing biological questions hang on this very point and relate to the actual tissue effects of tumor-directed immune response.

Tumor-Directed Immune Responses

Immune response by the host to a naturally occurring or implanted tumor is a central question toward which a number of experimental systems have provided useful data. One of the most fundamental questions concerns what really is important to host survival. Many experimental models employing cell-mediated destruction of isolated tumor cells have been studied both in vitro and in vivo in an attempt to establish guidelines for those basic mechanisms that are most crucial in allowing the host to overcome tumor encroachment. An interesting problem has inserted itself parenthetically into this question: the most effective intrinsic lines of defense against tumor cells may be very difficult to identify in the organism because effective obliteration of potential tumor cells may actually be occurring continuously in some normal subjects. Indeed this was one of the attractions in the original clonal selection theory of Burnet (85): namely that foreign or potentially inimical clones of malignant cells were immediately recognized as harmful and eliminated by the immune system. What becomes more complex is the problem of the way that the body deals with the tumor after such cells have surmounted the first barrier. In this situation secondary lines of defense are called into play. Obviously, from even a superficial examination of the clinical profile in many cancer patients, these ancillary lines of immunologic defense are not effective, since uncontrolled proliferation of tumor tissue results in eventual destruction of the host. Many features within the first, second, or subsequent reinforcing mechanisms present in the host immune response to various types of tumors are now reasonably well understood and, ironically, some seem to facilitate further tumor encroachment. One of the features involved in such mechanisms was first recognized by Kaliss in what he called immunologic enhancement (86–88). This particular phenomenon is especially important in any general consideration of immune complexes and cancer.

The Enhancement Phenomenon

Immunologic enhancement is a generalized biological phenomenon related to interaction between the host and any foreign tissue. The events of its initiation and perpetuation probably also relate to many clinical phenomena common to both tumor immune response and various homografts or allografts now so common in the burgeoning field of transplantation. Enhancement was first regarded as specific antibody-induced unresponsiveness to foreign tissues or foreign antigens carried by grafted tissues. Enhancement has also been regarded as a possible mechanism for specific immunosuppression and prolonged survival of kidney grafts. With respect to tumors, the experiments of Kaliss and co-workers (86, 87) showed that induction of a humoral immune response to certain tumors actually *facilitated* rather than *impeded* subsequent tumor growth. This phenomenon could be demonstrated by passive administration of serum or isolated antibody-containing fractions in animals while simultaneously challenged with viable grafts of tumor cells. Tumor administered with so-called enhancing antibody showed marked acceleration in growth and killing of the challenged animal. If the tumor alone were grafted in other controls, it proceeded to grow slowly or was eventually eliminated through other natural protective mechanisms.

During the evolution of thinking concerning the actual enhancement phenomenon, two general concepts were entertained and these are perhaps also applicable to the central problem surrounding immune complexes and cancer (88–93). First, enhancing antibody might actually facilitate tumor growth by masking all foreign determinants and evidence that the body might recognize and respond to as foreign. In simple terms, enhancing antibody directed at tumor-specific antigens occludes the effective afferent arm or recognition system of the immune response and allows the tumor time to become firmly established, unimpeded by any effective intrinsic immune response.

The second possibility is that enhancement also blocks the effector arm of the immune reaction (91, 92). Instead of merely masking the foreign tumor, it may effectively defuse the effector mechanism by a more intricate network of effects. Antigen-antibody complexes dissociated from tumor tissue that has already been saturated with large quantities of passively administered antibody might then be free to circulate and gradually cause obtundation and eventual complete saturation of Fc receptors on both natural defending killer cells and reticuloendothelial system cells that might normally remove such complexes. In addition, passive administration of antibody capable of combining directly with important immunodominant tumor antigens might very well work as an immunosuppressant for any primary humoral immune response of the host. It is well established that passive administration of antibody acts as a negative feedback in controlling the amounts of antibody an animal produces during either primary or secondary immune response (91, 93). Similarly, removal of antibody during the course of primary immune response will markedly boost the antibody secretion of primed antibody-forming cells. This reaction, moreover, shows a great deal of immunologic specificity, and in the case of passive infusion of quantities of antibody with primary reactivity for the most dominant tumor antigens present, it would effectively shut off intrinsic host immune response to this same group of antigens. Some of the processes possibly involved in the phenomenon of immunologic enhancement are illustrated in Figure 8-3.

Considerable work has been directed at an immunochemical understanding of the precise role of enhancing antibody, particularly in experimental animal systems. Early experiments established that enhancing immunoglobulins were largely IgG antibodies (94–96). Studies in mice have shown that the mouse IgG–2 subclass seems to be generally more effective in enhancement than IgG–1 (96–100). Clearly, IgM is not present in gamma-globulin fractions capable of producing effective enhancement. If the phenomenon of tumor enhancement were such as to abrogate lymphocyte-mediated destruction of either autochthonous or autologous tumor cells, one would at any given time, in fact, expect to find a substantial fraction of tumor cells coated with antibodies. The results presented by both E. and G. Klein and their colleagues (101, 102), and Ran and Witz (96, 98) suggest that this is indeed happening. Immunoglobulins eluted from membrane-rich subcellular fractions of

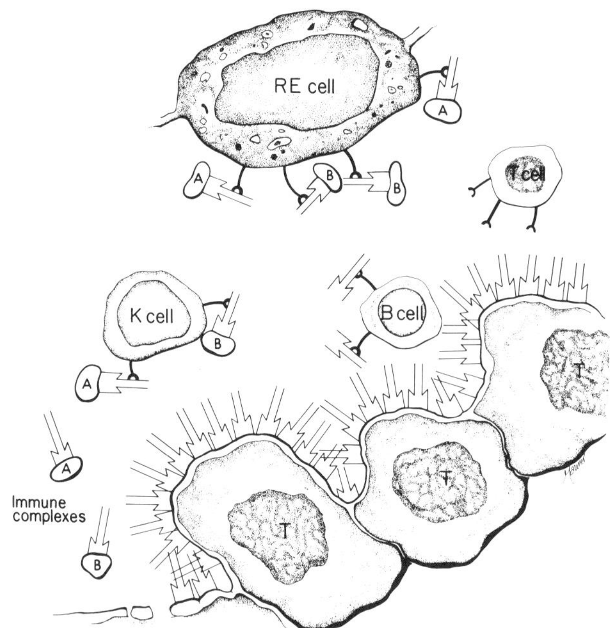

Figure 8-3 Potential mechanisms involved in the process of immunologic enhancement. Tumor cells are coated with antibody (*below*). Killer or K cells bearing Fc receptors may be blocked by antigen and antibody complexes. Similar complexes may obscure Fc receptors on fixed reticuloendothelial cells as shown in the B cells (*above*). T cells bearing Fc receptors may also adsorb enhancing antibody.

tumors showed enrichment or concentration of tumor enhancing capacity (98).

The phenomenon of immunologic enhancement illustrates a recurrent theme of work in many areas; that the immune response to neoplastic tissue may under certain circumstances actually be *harmful* and not protective to the host involved. Very little is known about the exact features of immunologic enhancement either at a basic level or in individual patients. In some animal models, little evidence for enhancing antibody can be detected so that it can by no means be regarded as a universal phenomenon. In addition, very little is understood about the genesis of naturally occurring enhancing antibody in human tumor patients. This is potentially a very important area, since manipulation of the antigenicity of tumor fractions to abrogate production of enhancing antibody and subsequently to favor production of other antibodies facilitating host destruction of tumors might possibly be used. This can best be illustrated by a theoretical model postulating three major immunodominant tumor-spe-

cific antigens (Figure 8-4). Two of these tumor antigens are potentially strong antigens, but are blocked by being spatially or sterically close on the cell surface to a third antigen, which is known to be capable of natural stimulation of enhancing antibody. As the tumor develops, considerable antigen A is released, stimulating B cells and subsequently, of course, IgG antibody possessing potent enhancing capabilities. If the clinical or experimental situation could be manipulated to allow deletion of tumor cell synthesis of antigen A, the other two tumor-specific antigens, B and C, would be given the opportunity to produce their own immune responses, which in turn would provide circulating humoral antibody lacking blocking or enhancing capability. Antibodies to determinants B and C might be of such physiochemical nature as to facilitate direct complement-mediated destruction of tumor tissue, or alternatively to provide natural effective access to killer cells bearing receptors for exposed Fc antibody portions. Killing of tumor cells might then ensue and resolution of the tumor follow.

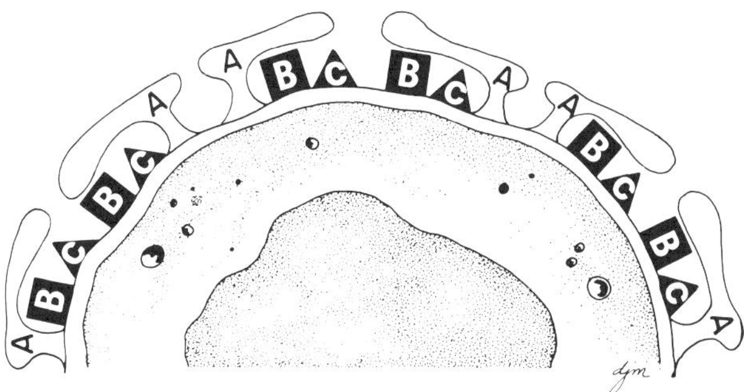

Figure 8-4 Diagram illustrating three closely spaced antigens on tumor cell surface. Antigens B and C are potentially strong tumor-associated antigens but are sterically blocked by antigen A, which is capable of inducing potent enhancing antibody.

Certain antitumor agents, particularly those initiating blockage of protein synthesis or DNA disruption within tumor cells, may be partially effective in inducing such a mechanism by deletion of the molecular machinery necessary for synthesis of, for instance, antigen A. A practical approach utilizing this sort of mechanism would first involve identification of the immunodominant antigens, such as those associated with leukemia. Next, an attempt might be made to determine which of these antigens were effective in producing enhancing antibody. Finally, drugs might be tested in vitro for their ability to block the assembly and cell-surface placement of the putative antigens, allowing the natural immune response to effective nonenhancement-producing antigens such as B and C in Figure 8-4. Similar mechanisms may conceivably be at work in the current impressive success with various chemotherapeutic regimens in childhood leukemia.

An alternative approach could also be taken in which heterologous antibody to the particular H-chain subclass of the enhancing antibody, or alternatively to the enhancing antigen itself, could be coupled to insoluble immunoabsorbents and the patients' circulating plasma pool exhaustively depleted of either antigen or antibody using an extracorporeal apparatus. A variation of this general approach has been initiated by Langvad and co-workers (103) using antibody isolated from patients with hypernephroma and subsequently coupled to insoluble surfaces of an immunoabsorbent apparatus. The keys to effective implementation of any such program are recognition of important immunodominant antigens for each tumor system, and establishment of proof that enhancing antibodies are actually of some clinical importance.

Recognition of the possible biological problems involved in immunologic enhancement is essential in any general program directed at immunotherapy. Current programs involving leukemia vaccines, immunostimulation by BCG, *Corynebacterium parvum*, or other immunopotentiating agents are being rather uncritically conducted in many parts of the world with the general hope that stimulation of the immune response in all sorts of cancers is a good thing. The original observations of Kaliss on enhancement (86–88), and all that has been learned subsequently concerning the mechanisms of tumor-host interaction, must be kept firmly in mind if rational immunotherapy is to succeed for cancer patients.

Cancer Immunity—Which Cells Are Really Important?

Central to any discussion of immune complexes and cancer is the question, as yet unsolved, of which host cell types are really important in eradication of tumors. A number of experimental systems have been devised in which it can be shown that lymphocytes actually participate in tumor killing (1–3, 5). The precise mechanisms involved when tumor killing is mediated by T cells have not been completely clarified, but in most systems studied some sort of physical contact between lymphocytes and target tumor cells appears to be involved. One of the general concepts postulated in such situations is that T cells, as final effectors of cell-mediated immunity, may bear recognition units or specific receptors for antigenic determinants on tumor cells and thus provide immunologic specificity in the homing to and eventual direct killing reactions that occur. Very little is yet understood about the immunologically specific receptors on sensitized or immune T cells. The current work of Taniguchi and co-workers (104), Tada and Takemori (105), Binz and Wigzell (106, 107), and Prange and co-workers (108) already discussed in some detail in Chapters 4 and 5 would indicate that the antigen-specific recognition unit on sensitized T cells shows the same degree of fine specificity as the antibody combining site and is also somehow linked to other constituents of the cell-surface marker and recognition system, including those defined by Ia antigens (104). Since the mechanism of specific killing by T cells somehow involves recognition and probable direct physical interaction with antigen, it follows that other materials containing alternative sites of antigen interaction, including either free circulating tumor antigen itself or antigen in the form of antigen-antibody complexes, could directly interfere with such killing mechanisms.

Two other forms of lymphocyte killing of target tumor cells have been extensively studied. One is the reaction of B cells bearing Fc receptors or K cells with cells sensitized with IgG antibody—the mechanism of antibody-dependent cell-mediated cytotoxicity (ADCC) (109–112); the other is that ascribed to natural killer or K cells, which may react without an antibody-coating intermediary (113). Finally, some direct effects on tumor cells by killer lymphocytes could conceivably also be mediated by short-distance release of small mediator molecules such as lymphotoxin or possibly interferon. It is important to point out that nearly all of the lymphocyte mechanisms of killing presented above involve Fc receptors on either killer cells or target cells, and with the possible exception of direct release of lymphokines all are inhibited by presence of antigen

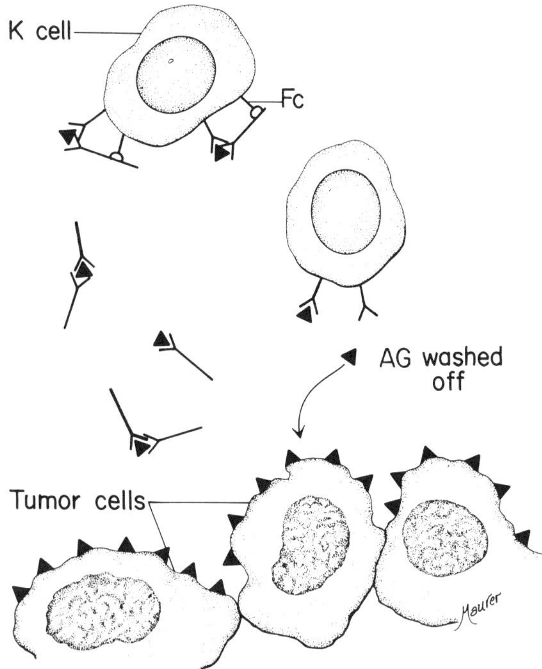

Figure 8-5   Killer or K cells with Fc receptors showing potential blocking of their reactivity with tumor cells by soluble complexes or by antigen released from tumor cell surface, subsequently forming complexes.

or antigen-antibody complexes (114–117). This is illustrated in Figure 8-5.

Suppressor Cells

An essential point in any general discussion of cellular immune response to tumors relates to the potential importance of suppressor cells in the modification of effective host response. There are numerous examples of tumors that by their very presence appear to be capable of inducing potent suppressor-cell activity on the part of the host (118–125). Virally induced tumors, tumors associated with chemical carcinogens, and naturally occurring transplantable tumor cell lines all share this insidious characteristic. In many instances the suppressor cells have been characterized as T cells, but in others they appear to be mononuclear cells or macrophage-like cells. Most suppressor-cell activities studied to date relate to their capacity to depress humoral immune response, but in other systems they also appear to be capable of effective suppression of T-cell–mediated phenomena such as delayed-type hypersensitivity. Recently, the suppressor cell involved with depression of cell-mediated immunity in patients with Hodgkin's disease has been characterized by our group as a prostaglandin-producing adherent cell (126). Suppressor cells may also be capable of directly shutting off T-cell–mediated killing of tumor cells. This is an important potential mechanism not yet well understood. The additional finding that certain human tumors known to be associated with intrinsic production of prostaglandin are often associated with relative ineffectiveness of tumor-directed immune response may be directly pertinent to this point. It is clear that tumors or their products can induce a marked relative immunosuppression in the host. Whether they do this by marked increments in local production of prostaglandins of the E series (PGE) or by other undefined mechanisms is not yet known. An example of marked increment in tumor tissue content of PGE in several human tumors as identified by indirect immunofluorescent techniques in our laboratory is shown in Figure 8-6 (127). The mechanisms by which a variety of human tumors actually induce suppressor-cell activity in the host is an important area. It is also probably important to the mechanisms of immunosuppression observed in widespread parasitic or bacterial infections, such as malaria, trypanosomiasis, schistosomiasis, or lepromatous leprosy. However, induction of suppressor cells has not yet been directly related to immune complexes, although a possible link may indeed be present.

A large body of experimental evidence has also focused on the importance of the macrophage in defense or natural protection against tumors. The concept of the activated macrophage was developed through the work of MacKaness (128, 129), Remington and colleagues (130, 131), and many other groups (132–135). When activated by a number of inflammatory stimuli, macrophages become angry, as it were, and potentially violent to bystanders in their particular environment. Angry or activated macrophages undergo sev-

eral interesting gross physical and metabolic changes. They spread out, appear to become more sticky, and show increased levels of energy consumption. When activated by intracellular infections in no way related to tumors themselves, such macrophages are capable of impressive destruction of tumor cells nearby. Recently, the potential importance of this mechanism in destruction of tumors has been of great interest (136). In this context it is again important to note that macrophages have an assortment of Fc receptors that are capable of interacting with components of immune complexes. It is not entirely clear from the experimental or clinical situations thus far examined whether immune complexes can, by saturating macrophage Fc receptors, actually defuse or attenuate their protective effects.

As mentioned earlier, clear definition of the single most important host cell mediating tumor destruction is not currently possible. For some tumors, it may well be the macrophage; for others, the natural K or other killer cells; and for still others, sensitized T cells. The host afflicted with a tumor often recognizes foreign antigens on the tumor and seems capable of mounting a humoral immune response, so that the natural consequence will be eventual formation of antigen-antibody complexes. In some situations the majority of these complexes remain affixed to tumor-cell membranes, but in many other instances they are released and circulate within extracellular sites and in the plasma of affected individuals. It is appropriate to examine what is known of their demonstrable effects in a variety of instances.

Immune Complexes in Experimental Tumor Models

During the early work exploring host immune response to a variety of tumors, it was repeatedly pointed out, particularly by the Hellströms, that serum from hosts affected by tumors was often capable of inhibiting an effective immune response (2, 3, 5). From these and other studies it was apparent that serum was capable of inhibiting lymphocyte-mediated destruction of tumors (94). Some of the blocking was probably correctly attributed to simple

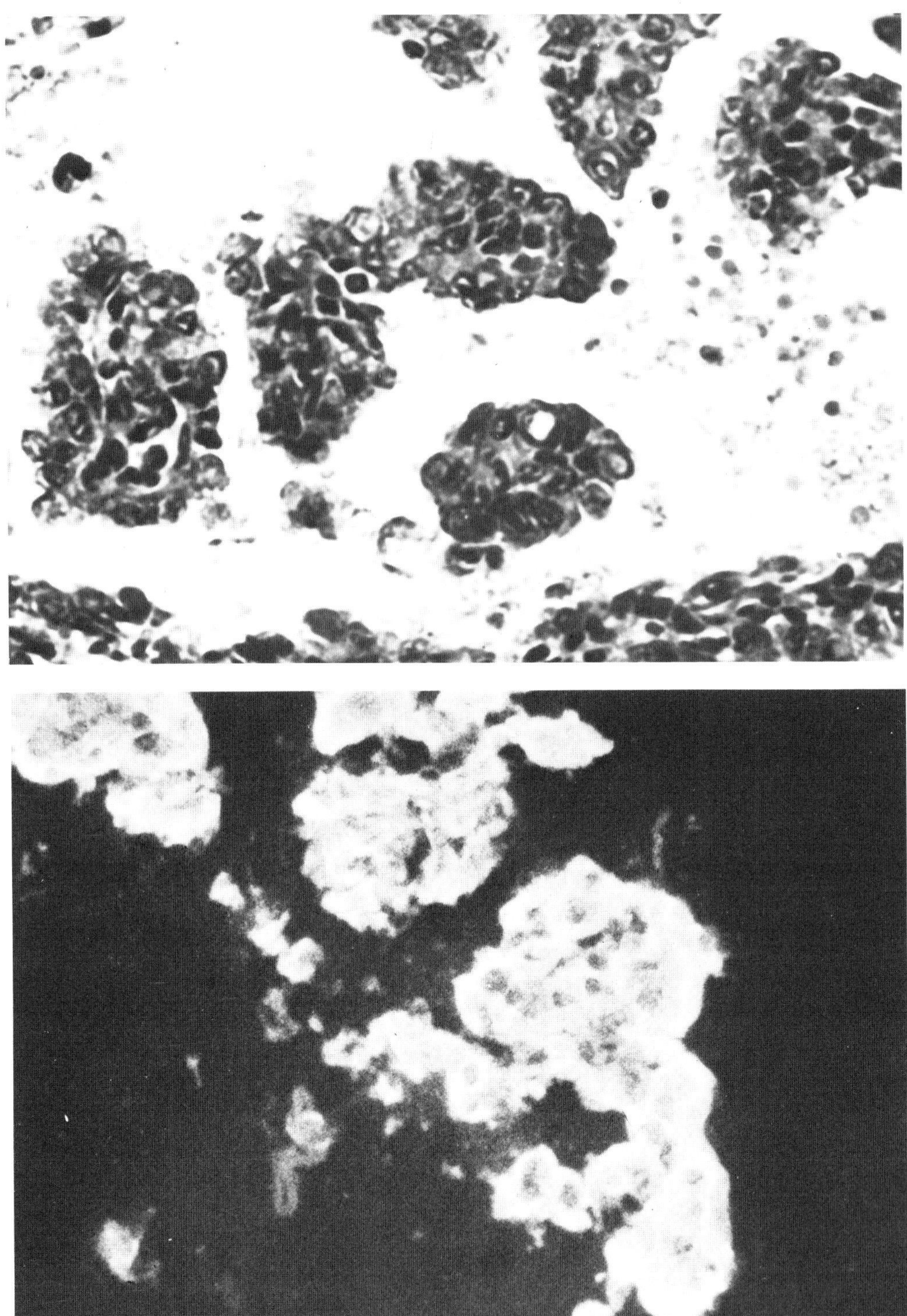

Figure 8-6 *Above,* gross appearance of carcinoma of lung showing clusters of tumor cells stained with H&E. Magnification × 400. *Below,* same tumor as above, stained with specific antiserum to PGE using immunofluorescent technique. (Reproduced with permission, G. Husby, R. G. Strickland, G. L. Rigler et al., *Cancer* 40:1629, 1977.)

masking or impedance of tumor-associated antigens (137, 138). The fact that antibody molecules were in some way involved in the blocking phenomena was established by showing immunologic specificity of autologous or cross-reacting serum for protection of autologous tumor cells from killing (138). In addition, it could be shown that serum-blocking activity in some experimental systems could be neutralized by addition of excess tumor antigen (139). In certain circumstances it was also possible to show that under proper conditions addition of small amounts of tumor membrane antigen to immune serum to form complexes resulted in blocking activity (139). In both experimental animals and in patients, blocking activity appeared to correlate with the clinical stage of the disease and to disappear from sera of patients who were tumor free after presumably curative therapy (140). Of great importance in this latter report was the observation that antibody-containing sera from tumor-free patients could abrogate the blocking effects of sera from patients containing progressive tumors of the same types (140). This "unblocking" phenomenon is one of high potential importance; initially it was attributed to masking of antigen in blocking sera that contained antigen bound as antigen-antibody complexes.

Another possible explanation for the unblocking phenomenon might be that cured cancer-patient or experimental-animal sera capable of unblocking sera with blocking immune complexes actually contained rheumatoid factor or anti-γ-globulin antibodies with particular specificity for tumor antigen-antibody complexes. If unblocking were indeed the result of the activity of either 7 S IgG or 19 S IgM anti-γ-globulins with specificity for autologous immune complexes, it is conceivable that such anti-γ-globulins might show reactivity only with complexes in which the antibodies were free and perhaps not bound to the cell surface. This might then explain why the same anti-γ-globulins would not subsequently block antibody-dependent lymphocyte or killer-cell phenomena directed against antibodies actually fixed to tumor cells. Of note in the report by Hellström and colleagues (140) was that unblocking sera obtained from tumor-free or

cured patients could unblock other sera from patients with progressive tumors of the same type. This sort of fine specificity is reminiscent of that attributed to rheumatoid factors. It also suggests that there may be something unique or idiotypic about blocking complexes for a particular tumor that unblocking antibodies must recognize. This concept of uniqueness or shared idiotypy has been significantly developed after the original observations relating to cold agglutinins and cross-reactive anti-idiotypic antibodies (141, 142). In the case of unblocking antibodies with apparent specificity for certain types of complexes, it seems unlikely that it would be antibody activity directed against combining sites of antitumor antibodies, as these would not be exposed in the blocking sera where antigen-antibody complexes would have already saturated most of the pertinent antibody combining sites. Specificity for a certain type of blocking complex would then perhaps depend on other conformational features of the complex beside that involved in its antibody-combining site (Figure 8-7). These arguments are all extensions of the hypothesis that the unblocking phenomenon is a function of some sort of anti-γ-globulin—to date a hypothesis that has not been established. Several alternative explanations of the unblocking phenomenon are shown diagrammatically in Figure 8-8.

Initial studies aimed at characterizing the blocking factors in animals carrying progressively growing sarcomas either induced by Moloney's virus or methylcholanthrene were carried out by Sjögren and colleagues (143). It was shown that the blocking effect could be absorbed out using the respective types of tumor cells and could then be eluted from cells with low pH buffers designed to dissociate antigen-antibody complexes. Blocking fractions were separated into low- and high-molecular-weight materials. Either fraction alone added to tumor cells did not show blocking activity; however, when added together, blocking occurred. These studies indicated that the blocking factors were indeed antigen-antibody complexes. It was not clear at this point that antigen alone as a blocking material was ruled out, since the low-molecular-weight materials

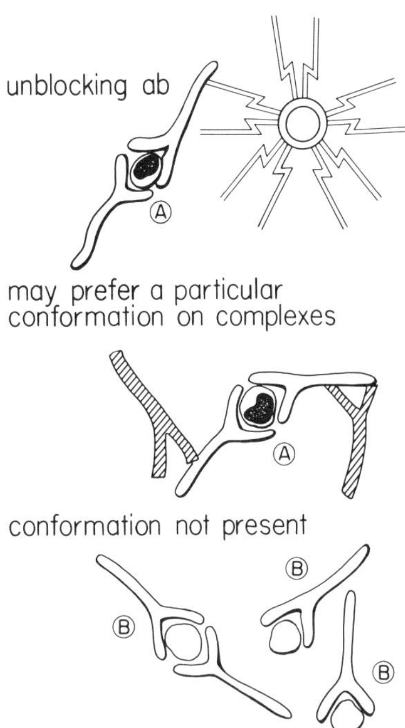

Figure 8-7 Several hypothetical ways in which unblocking antibodies might function. Unblocking 19S IgM (*upper panel*) or 7S (*middle panel*) might react with particular conformational antigenic determinants on blocking antibody A. In other complexes between antitumor antibody and tumor antigens (*lower panel*), no unblocking occurs because the blocking antibody is not of the proper shape or conformation.

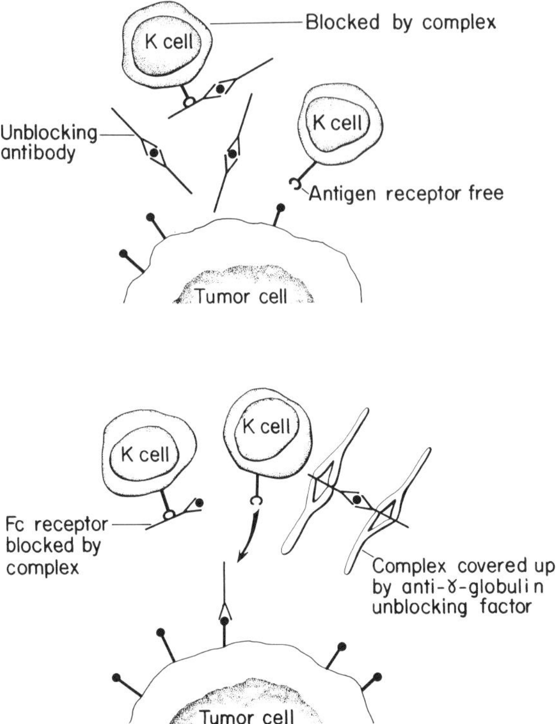

Figure 8-8 Other alternative ways in which unblocking antibodies might function. *Above,* two different types of killer-cell–mediated mechanisms are shown. On the left, the K cell has its Fc receptor blocked by soluble complexes. Unblocking antibody might react with free tumor antigen to produce a complex ineffectively adhering to K-cell Fc receptors, thus allowing antibody-mediated or direct tumor-cell killing. On the right, the primed killer cell shows a tumor-specific antigen receptor. Unblocking antibody has enveloped enough free antigen to allow direct T-cell killing. *Below,* the unblocking antibody is depicted as a type of anti-γ-globulin antibody that ties up Fc portions of immune complexes and allows killer cells with or without Fc receptors to function.

showed some blocking activity if added to tumor cells and allowed to incubate with tumor cells and killer lymphocytes over an extended 48-hour period (143). However, previous experiments using immunoabsorption with heterologous antibody to immunoglobulins had shown that removal of IgG antibody from blocking sera removed blocking activity (5).

These initial studies were extended by Jose and Skvaril using sera from children with malignant neuroblastoma (144). These sera could be shown specifically to block in vitro cytotoxicity of lymphocytes for cultured neuroblastoma cells; however, the blocking sera appeared to contain no detectable free tumor-specific antibody. Removal of IgG from blocking sera by repeated solid-phase immunoabsorbents removed blocking activity, and

blocking effect could also be recovered from eluates prepared from the solid-phase anti-IgG immunoabsorbent. The immunoglobulin H-chain subclasses of IgG antibodies involved in blocking phenomena were examined. Most of the blocking activity appeared to be present in IgG-1 and IgG-3 with some lesser activity in IgG-4, but virtually none associated with IgG-2 (144). These experiments utilized cell cultures of neuroblastoma tissues from the patients actually studied. Very little similar information concerning the relative efficiencies of the four major human IgG H-chain subgroups is available in terms of blocking activity for other tumors. More work is needed to extend information available through experiments such as those reported for the neuroblastoma model above. If certain tumors show marked restriction or unique patterns of H-chain IgG subgroup expression of antibodies participating in the blocking phenomena, advantage might be taken of this by various therapeutic manipulations of the host or his internal environment as discussed above.

The studies by Jose and Seshadri (145), using material from neuroblastoma, were further extended with elegant techniques including ^{125}I-labeling of surface antigens on isolated cultured tumor cells and a radiocounterimmunoelectrophoretic assay for both free antigen and immune complexes. No free antibody could be detected in sera from patients with progressively growing tumors; whereas when tests were performed in high-ionic-strength buffers capable of dissociating complexes, antitumor antibody titers of 1:64 to 1:5,000 were recorded. Of particular importance were serial studies conducted on patients with special emphasis on the importance of ratios of antigen

and antibody to the observed blocking phenomenon. It was found that maximum blocking of lymphocyte-mediated cytotoxicity was noted when antigen-antibody equivalence was present (Figure 8-9). Analysis of supernates showed that when either excess antigen or excess antibody was present, inhibition of cell-mediated tumor killing was not at a maximum.

These studies also provided some interesting data related to presence of detectable antigen in patients' remission or so-called progressor sera. Using the relatively sensitive radioelectrophoretic assay, serum samples from 5 patients with progressive tumors showed presence of detectable soluble antigens, suggesting either presence of excess free antigen or antigen bound by constantly dissociating low-affinity antibody. When the same sorts of experiments were performed in buffers designed for immune-complex dissociation, then increased detectable free antigens were noted. Of great importance was the finding that no free antigen or bound antigen was detected in any of the patients studied in established remission. Specificity controls showed no blocking of specific cytotoxicity using soluble tumor antigens or antigen-antibody complexes from children with Wilms' tumors or those with osteogenic sarcoma.

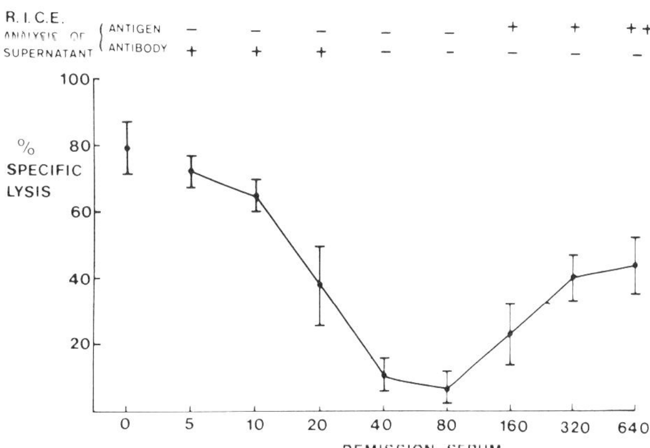

Figure 8-9 Effect of variation of ratio between Neuro V membrane-turnover antigen and remission serum antibody on an autochthonous cell-mediated cytotoxic assay. Maximum blocking found in microcultures where antigen-antibody equivalence was present in the supernatant. Data show mean cytotoxicity and SC of 6 microcultures per serum dilution in one typical experiment with Neuro V patient material. (Reproduced with permission, D. J. Jose and R. Seshadri, *Int. J. Cancer* 13:824, 1974.)

When progressor sera were examined during this study, maximum specific blocking of cytotoxic immunity was noted in patients where immune complexes of tumor antigen and antibody were present, but which did not appear to contain any detectable free tumor antigen. Less than 10 percent blocking occurred in the presence of antigen alone. This is particularly significant in view of the extended speculations and assessments of the relative importance of free tumor antigen as opposed to antigen-antibody complexes in such systems, a subject that will be addressed in more detail below. The results of this definitive study by Jose and Seshadri (145) are summarized in Table 8-2. The most important findings were that when antigen-antibody complexes were effective in blocking cell-mediated killing of test tumor cells, it was always in the zone of an equivalence ratio. The specificity of inhibition appeared to correspond to that of labeled antigenic material spontaneously shed from cell membrane of autochthonous tumor cells cultured in vitro. The blocking effects disappeared in antibody excess and were not present in significant amount when tumor antigen alone was present. It was therefore suggested that tumor antigens such as those studied in this particular system might be continuously released by many tumors during the spontaneous metabolic turnover of tumor cell membranes. In this study the 8 patients examined with progressive and ultimately fatal tumor showed persistent antigen excess. It might appear, therefore, that tumor membrane growth and turnover is eventually capable of outstripping the host's capacity to provide enough antibody to complex with it. These findings might also be extended to unblocking; it is possible that unblocking and subsequent tumor regression merely represent achievement of systemic antibody excess and thereby avoidance of the dangerous zone of equivalence in which cell-mediated immune reactions may be paralyzed. If the dose of antibody is insufficient to produce total-body antibody excess, and if equivalence instead is produced, progression rather than tumor regression may be the result (146). With respect to the observations reported by Jose and Seshadri (145), neuroblastoma of early childhood is one human tumor known to be associated with a relatively high rate of regression (147). Whether such natural regressions are associated with total body shifts from equivalence to antibody excess remains to be determined. The studies presented by these authors represent some of the most compelling arguments in favor of the critical immune balance in the host with tumor and also illustrate the importance of quantitative relationships between tumor antigen and amounts of antibody manufactured.

Extension of these general concepts was provided by the work of Mantovani and Spreafiaco (148), who studied an allogenic system of CBH mice transplanted with what was called the L_{1210} leukemia. This situation involved transplantation of a leukemia strain of cells with certain leukemia-specific antigens and other histocompatability antigens (known as H2 in the mouse) into recipients of a different histocompatibility type. The work of these investigators was important, for it showed that serum-blocking factors and antibodies sensitizing effector cells or their targets for killing target tumor cells acted on different effector cell populations. The proof for presence of immune complexes in these particular experiments was not as hard and fast as had been presented by Jose and Seshadri (145). However, the idea that perhaps different effector cell populations might be involved during various phases of the immune response may be important in interpreting complex waves of immune response during the evolution of several forms of human malignancy. In the usual forms of antibody-mediated cytotoxicity as a means of host killing of tumor cells, immune complexes would be capable of inhibition through direct interaction with K-cell Fc receptors. On the other hand, a different mechanism may have to be postulated for what occurs in modulating T-cell killing, where Fc receptors may or may not be involved.

Possible Role of Uncomplexed Circulating Antigen

Despite the convincing data presented by Jose and Seshadri (145) concerning the role of antigen-antibody complexes at equivalence in the

Table 8-2 The effect of specific antibody, antigen, or complexes in blocking autochthonous in vitro lymphocytotoxic assay.

| | Cytotoxic test | | | | | | | | |
| | Reaction mixture | | | | Result | | Supernatant analysis | | |
Target cells	Lymphoid cells	Serum	Soluble antigen	CPM ± SD[a]	Percent lysis[b]	Percent blocking[b]	Free antigen	Free antibody	Complexes
Neuro I	Normal	Normal	Nil	9564 ± 1032	5	0	Trace	Nil	Nil
Neuro I	Neuro I	Normal	Nil	3842 ± 722	62*	0	Trace	Nil	Nil
Neuro I Fibroblast	Osteo I	Normal	Nil	9286 ± 1381	7	0	Trace (0)	Nil	Nil
Neuro I Fibroblast	Normal	Normal	Nil	9862 ± 976	1	0	Nil	Nil	Nil
Neuro I	Neuro I	Normal	Nil	9694 ± 1324	4	0	Nil	Nil	Nil
Neuro I	Neuro I	Neuro I progressor	Nil	9642 ± 864	4	93*	Nil	Nil	++
Neuro I	Neuro I	Neuro I remission	Nil	3793 ± 646	62*	0	Nil	1/125	Nil
Neuro I	Neuro I	Normal	+	4025 ± 973	59*	—	+	Nil	Nil
Neuro I	Neuro I	Neuro I progressor	+	7721 ± 871	23*	63*	+	Nil	++
Neuro I	Neuro I	Neuro I remission	+	4684 ± 632	53*	14*	Nil	1/512	++
Neuro I	Normal	Neuro I progressor	Nil	9327 ± 763	7	0	Nil	Nil	++
Neuro I	Normal	Neuro I remission	Nil	9142 ± 1104	8	0	Nil	1/125	Nil

Source: Reproduced with permission, J. D. Jose and R. Seshadri, *Int. J. Cancer* 13:824, 1974.

[a] Radioactivity remaining in target cells after incubation and washing: mean and standard deviation of 6 microcultures after adjustment of total incorporated radioactivity to 10,000 CPM.

[b] Percent lysis and percent blocking as determined by release of radioactivity.

* Significantly different from normal control ($p < 0.01$).

blocking phenomena related to lymphocyte cytotoxicity in neuroblastoma patients, there is a good deal of attention given intermittently in the literature to the possible role of circulating antigen in modulating various blocking phenomena. Studies by Currie and Basham have been directed at this possibility (149). Using a microcytotoxicity assay, they tested lymphocytes from cancer patients on autologous and allogenic tumor cells in vitro. They found that extensive washing of the lymphocytes from many cases with particularly advanced disease greatly enhanced specific cytotoxic effects of individual lymphocyte populations. Although apparent immunologic specificity against autologous or similar tumors was retained, the cytotoxicity could be blocked once again by addition of patients' sera. Serum components capable of producing inhibition of lymphocyte-mediated killing had no detectable affinity for the target tumor cells, but rather appeared to interact with the effector killer-lymphocyte surface. These investigators suggested that they might be observing blockage of cytolytic effect through direct inactivation or interaction with surface antigen receptors on effector cells. The increase in lymphocyte cytotoxicity observed during this work occurred after repeated washing of the effector lymphocytes (up to six times). These results were obtained using material from patients with a wide variety of tumors including malignant melanoma, bladder carcinoma, hypernephroma, and fibrosarcomas. Of particular interest in the course of these studies and analogous to work later reported by Shiku and co-workers (78, 79) was that marked individual specificity of killing only by autologous cells was often noted in the experiments using melanoma patients' cells and tumors, although some degree of cross-reactivity within the melanoma system was recorded. Of note were results obtained in one patient after immunization with irradiated autologous melanoma cells: before such immunization, the lymphocytes from this subject required multiple washes before their intrinsic cytotoxicity could be demonstrated. However, after a course of immunization with irradiated autologous tumor cells, powerfully cytotoxic lymphocytes were obtained that needed no

washing to demonstrate their killing potential. Alternatively, addition of serum obtained before immunization to this latter system again effectively blocked autologous lymphocyte-mediated killing reactions.

Several interpretations of these interesting results are possible. First, the authors themselves thought that the fact that the apparent blocking factors had no demonstrable affinity for the target tumor cells, but rather appeared to show specific affinity for the effector cells made it more likely that the blockade was occurring somehow through primed specific antigen receptors on these effector cells. The effects noted after multiple washing procedures were also taken as evidence that blocking factors were adsorbed principally to the effector cells and not to the target tissues. It is also possible that the blockade itself involved interaction of specific antigen-antibody complexes with Fc receptors, or with Fc receptors in parallel with specific antigen receptors. Such a double attraction might explain why the blocking factors appeared to show greater affinity for effector than for target tumor cells.

Knowledge and insight into Fc receptors and their importance in many of the killing reactions of both natural killer cells and the variety of cells known to be potentially involved in direct killing of various sorts of target cells has increased considerably since these experiments were conducted. It is difficult to explain the results obtained after immunization with irradiated cells on this basis. After immunization it appeared that the serum contained very little in the way of blocking activity, and that instead it contained antitumor antibody activity, since parallel studies of binding specificities showed preferential binding of postimmunization serum to target cells instead of effector cells. These experiments reemphasized that binding ratios and perhaps intrinsic avidities of individual antibody populations are of critical importance in many of the tumor blocking phenomena or assays used by various workers. More importantly, they may play a critical role in the outcome of the tumor among individual patients.

Another possible interpretation of the results presented by Currie and Basham (149) is that the washing procedure itself partially damaged the effector lymphocyte membranes that were by this process rendered intrinsically more cytotoxic to their target cells. Contrary to such an explanation is that apparent immunologic specificity only against primary target cells was maintained after the washing procedures. There is, however, some recent evidence that exposure of certain activities of lymphocyte membranes may render them much more capable of background cytolytic or destructive effects (150).

The basic question relating load of tumor antigen to survival and to effects of local host immune response is a very important one in any consideration of the broad effects of antigen-antibody complexes in the host response to tumor. We are constantly reminded of this in the clinical setting when dealing with cancer patients. Patients with huge metastatic deposits at the time of initial tumor diagnosis are virtually always doomed. Patients with acute leukemia who present with a huge tumor load as manifested by extremely high total white-blood-cell counts usually show a poor prognosis (151).

The presence of antigenic load, whether it be neoantigen of the tumor or merely reexpression of the differentiation antigen, may also play a major role in the local immune response to the tumors themselves. Studies by Alexander and colleagues (152) of small limb tumors in the rat indicate that such tumors appear to be capable of inhibiting effective development of cell-mediated immune response in regional lymph nodes, presumably by antigen flooding of the local lymph nodes. Such effects may well be initiated by constant exposure to a low, but continuous, amount of tumor-specific antigens. As the tumor progresses and the trapping mechanisms inherent in the node are gradually overwhelmed, antigen may reach the general circulation, and central inhibition or even low-dose tolerance ensues.

The role of antigen as the mainstay of the blocking effect observed in some clinical or experimental immune tumor mechanisms has been further studied by Currie (153, 154) using material largely derived from clinical experience and attempts to monitor immunotherapy after surgical intervention. Patients studied after extensive surgical excision of melanoma showed rapid loss of blocking activity in in vitro assays. Moreover, immunizations with autologous irradiated tumor cells again produced rapid disappearance of serum inhibitory activity, and some correlation with continued stable clinical status was also noted. Serum inhibitory materials induced by the tumor and disappearing after immunization with autologous tumor showed separation of inhibitory activity in the 30,000 to 40,000 Dalton fraction of sera from patients with hypernephroma. This particular fractionation along with inhibition of the lymphocyte-mediated cytotoxic reactions against the autologous tumor are shown in Figure 8-10. A similar fall in serum-blocking activities was also reported by Sinkovics and co-workers (155) following chemotherapy. At present, it is difficult to generalize on the relative importance of free antigen and immune complexes as blocking factors. Realistically, it seems most likely that both are involved in specific clinical or experimental situa-

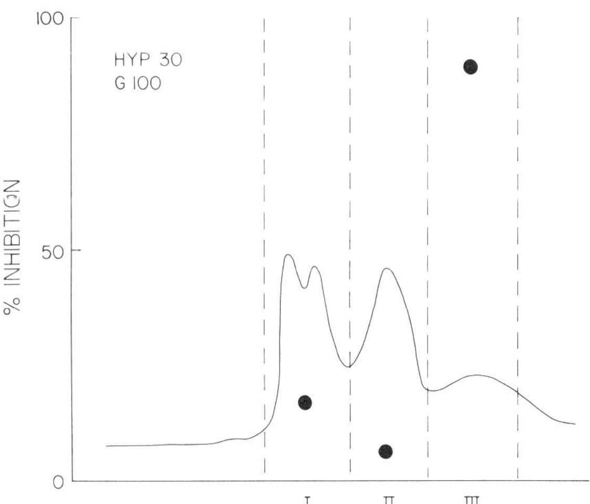

Figure 8-10 The effect of serum from a patient with disseminated hypernephroma (Hyp 30) on autologous lymphocyte cytotoxicity following fractionation on Sephadex G-100. The inhibitory activity is restricted to the fraction with a molecular weight range of 30,000 to 40,000 Daltons. (Reproduced with permission, G. A. Currie, *Br. J. Cancer* 28:153, 1973, suppl. 1.)

tions. If antibodies of high affinity are produced during the course of what may be a cyclic immune response of the host to tumor antigens, these antibodies may bind tightly to cell-fixed or fragmented antigens and be cleared by activation of the complement pathways and reticuloendothelial receptor mechanisms because of their particular immunochemical nature. Alternatively, in situations involving attenuation of humoral immunity and perhaps in a cycle of low-avidity antibody production, more free antigen may be available and the effects of dissociated uncomplexed antigens may predominate. Which circumstance is actually at work in any particular clinical situation requires precise physiochemical characterization of the putative antigen as well as the character and binding qualities of antibodies involved.

Immune Complexes and Blocking Factors

The preceding discussion has presented a summary of the evidence implicating antibodies and tumor-related antigens in blocking reactions in a variety of experimental systems. From the cumulative work in this area to date it is apparent that the various blocking factors thus far characterized are capable of abrogating both T-cell–mediated immunity to tumors (156) and non-T-cell or K-cell tumor killing. The most convincing recent demonstration that immune complexes per se participate in blocking phenomena is presented by Tamerius and colleagues (157). Columns for affinity chromatography were prepared by coupling tumor-immune antibodies to an insoluble porous matrix. These antibodies were specific for the particular tumors under study and were actually prepared from sera of animals who showed the capacity to unblock the blocking-serum phenomenon. Passage of blocking serum over such insolubilized antibodies removed all blocking activities. Subsequent elution of materials from these immunoabsorbent columns produced recovery of the blocking activities. This approach provided additional evidence for the presence of both 7 S IgG and lower-molecular-weight materials, presumably antigen, in the blocking materials

recovered. The direct blocking activity identified in chromatographed eluates from the affinity column occurred in fractions very close to 7 S and presumably consisting largely of IgG. It is possible that this 7 S eluate, active in blocking, still contained small antigenic fragments. The low-molecular-weight materials obtained in the same eluate did not contain blocking activity when tested individually.

These experiments provide further insight into the nature of unblocking activity previously frequently recorded in the sera of regressor animals (158). The data indicated that the unblocking activity was largely, if not entirely, IgG; furthermore, since it showed specific immune reactivity for the blocking activity of the various individual tumors tested, it must to some degree be related either to the original tumor antigens involved or to very selective idiotypic determinants as discussed above. These findings perhaps can be extended eventually to clinical usefulness. Serum samples from patients with unblocking antibodies might actually be utilized to clear plasma from patients with blocking activity by the use of extracorporeal apparatus such as has recently been suggested by Langvad and co-workers (103). Such procedures would have seemed like science fiction only a few years ago, but now may soon be open to direct clinical implementation. What is needed is a good reproducible assay for serum-blocking activity for the particular tumor to be studied, along with ample supplies of unblocking antibodies from patients in whom specific tumors have regressed. It might even be possible to manufacture heterologous unblocking antibody in another species by immunizations with blocking fractions from the patients involved. This approach seems much more rational and auspicious than the wholesale indiscriminate use of BCG, *C. parvum,* thymosin, levamisole, and other rather poorly understood current immunopotentiating agents.

Anti-Idiotypic Antibodies in Malignant Disease

Granted that antigen-antibody complexes per se and free antigen are two of the most important factors modulating the effectiveness of host immune responsiveness to many tumors, one other mechanism is also of practical relevance. The concept of idiotypy, already alluded to, purports that individual specific antibodies to isolated or very similar antigenic determinants often possess unique antigens themselves. An example of anti-idiotypic antibody related to tumor immunity is shown in Figure 8-11.

The whole process of immune regulation has been related by Jerne (159) to the idea that anti-idiotypic responses modulate or control all forms of immune interaction. This has generally been called the *network theory* and in simple terms states that for every specific antibody, there is in turn a second antibody directed at it or its combining site that serves to influence and regulate subsequent synthesis and secretion of the first antibody, and so perhaps ad infinitum. The same concept can be applied to every immunologically committed T cell: that one cell with individually specific commitment to another is in turn activated. The network theory of cellular interaction depends on the unique nature of each individual antibody or cellular response and is visualized as a system to dampen immune responses once set into action. It can be thought of as functioning as an endogenous "immunostat" for all types of humoral or cell-mediated immune responses.

Studies by Lewis and co-workers (160) probably relate directly to the general phenomenon of idiotypy. The formation of antibodies by the host directed at unique conformational or other individual determinants of antibody combining sites may represent an important, possibly harmful mechanism in the general problem of neoplasia. In their initial work Lewis and co-workers noted that autoimmunization of patients with their own irradiated melanoma tumor cells produced interesting and enigmatic reactions. Patients' sera taken prior to inducement of tumor-specific antibody through immunization procedures were capable of blocking detection of this antibody. Conversely, preimmunization sera that were supposedly negative for specific antitumor antibody did not block detection of the latter in immune sera if applied to tumor cells prior to addition of specific antitumor antibody. In addition, negative preself-immunization sera showed lines of precipitation in gels with immune sera, and the same negative preimmunization sera were capable of reduction of complement-dependent cytotoxicity of positive hyperimmune sera in the presence of target melanoma tumor cells. These findings suggested that the "negative" sera actually contained antibodies capable of combining with subsequently induced hyperimmune antimelanoma antibodies in such a way as to block their combination with tumor antigens. The simplest and most direct explanation of these findings is that the "negative" preimmunization sera were, in fact, not negative but actually contained anti-idiotypic antibody activity with unique specificity for the combining sites of antimelanoma specific antibodies. This is illustrated by the diagrammatic representation in Figure 8-11.

Later, Hartmann and Lewis (161) presented additional clinical data related to patients with malignant melanoma indicating that this sort of anti-idiotypic antibody might be related to clinical progression of tumor within individual patients. These studies showed an inverse relation between serum agglutinators—antibodies directed against Fab IgG determinants—and presence of antitumor antibodies as detected by membrane immunofluorescent reactions. An example of a serial clinical profile of the relationship taken from this work is shown in Figure 8-12. A number of patients were studied, including subjects with osteosarcoma, cancer of the colon, adenocarcinoma of the bowel,

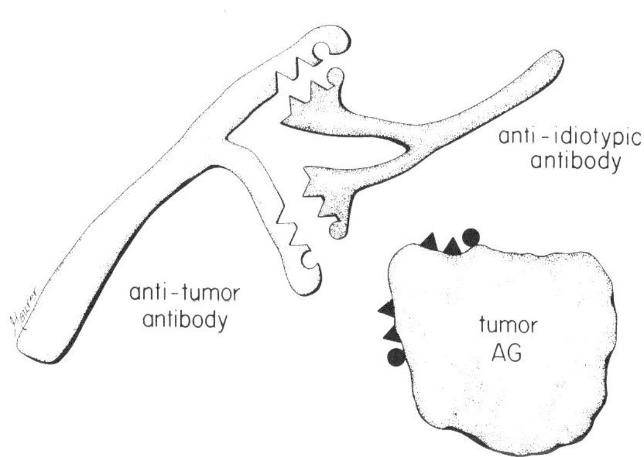

Figure 8-11 Anti-idiotypic antibody with specificity for antitumor-antibody combining site.

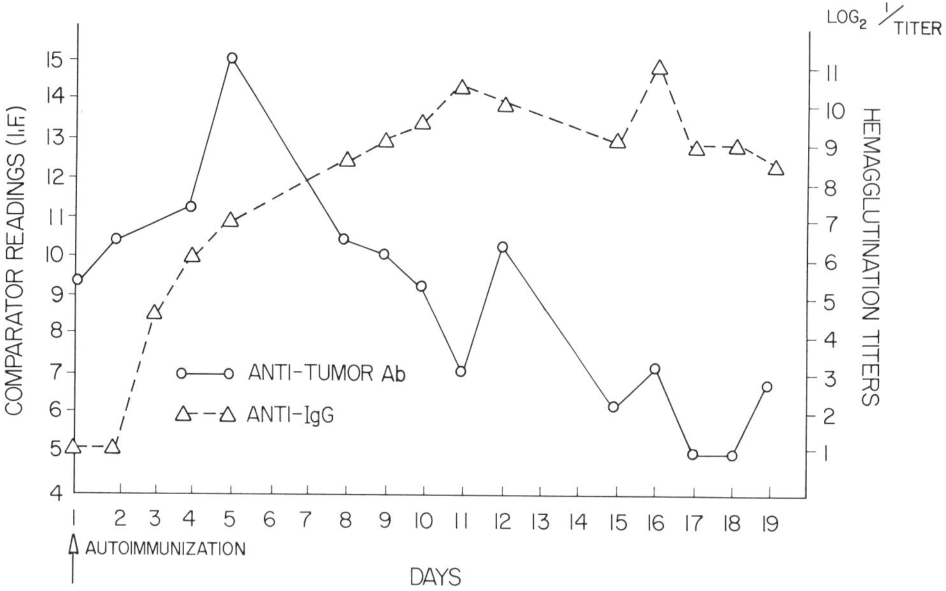

Figure 8-12 The relation between antitumor antibody and anti-IgG hemagglutinin titers in a patient with cutaneous malignant melanoma. (Reproduced with permission, D. Hartmann and M. G. Lewis, *Lancet* 1:1318, 1974.)

and malignant melanoma. A veritable spectrum of solid tumor malignancies was found to be associated with high titers of anti-Fab antibodies, particularly melanoma and carcinoma of the colon that had spread extensively beyond regional lymph node sites. In these same patients a consecutive serial fall in detectable antitumor antibodies was recorded. It was postulated that the patient's specific antitumor antibodies had gradually been blocked by autologous anti-idiotypic antibodies directed at the antitumor antibody combining sites. These studies have been amplified and extended in further work by several groups (162–164). Use of C1q-binding assays for immune complexes in patients studied with malignant melanoma showed presence of detectable complexes early in disease, with subsequent falls in complexes as the disease progressed (164, 165).

It is difficult to tell whether blocking of potential antibody combining sites on autologous antitumor antibodies by this sort of 7S IgG anti-idiotypic response is an important factor in other types of malignant disease. If it occurs as a universal phenomenon built into the immune system, it could participate to a consider-

able extent in the unimpeded progression of a number of tumors. Anti-idiotypic antibodies in general are somewhat difficult to detect. They may not exist in plasma actually complexed to their respective idiotype-bearing target antibody molecules, but only react when the idiotype antibody bends or unfolds through its hinge region in the process of combining with antigen. The usual anti-γ-globulin present in various human sera shows reactivity for determinants on H chains or, more specifically, portions of the Fc region of IgG. This certainly has been the case in most studies of the molecular mapping of specificity; for instance, with regard to 19S or 7S human rheumatoid factors. On the other hand, an interesting group of anti-γ-globulins has been described, theoretically with varying specificities for antigenic sites that might participate in antibody combining sites. These include anti-gamma-globulins with specificity for sites only exposed by combination of antigens with their respective antibodies (166), antibodies with reactivity for Fab or F(ab')$_2$ fragments of IgG (167, 168), and antibodies with specificity for determinants on L chains (169).

It is of particular interest that these antibodies appear to be present, albeit in relatively low titer, in most normal human sera. These reactions, particularly as related to the anti-idiotype concept of Lewis and associates (163–165), should be scrutinized in the sera of patients with cancer, to search for such reactions as an indication of possible anti-idiotype feedback control. A recent report by Pyrhonen and co-workers (170) showed presence of antigammaglobulins in 33 patients with bladder tumors that correlated with blocking of lymphocyte-mediated cytotoxicity against target bladder tumor cells.

Immune Complexes in Cancer Patients

With the recent availability of highly sensitive assays for detection of circulating immune complexes, a number of studies have appeared attempting to relate quantitative levels of complexes detected with clinical staging, survival, and various peripheral manifestations of cancer. Of the studies conducted to date, few have actually identified physical or immunochemical properties in putative antigens supposedly included in the complexes measured. However, some fascinating data have rapidly accumulated that emphasize the wide prevalence of detectable complexes in many neoplastic states.

An early study conducted by Ludwig and Cusumano (171) utilized ^{125}I labeled goat anti human monovalent F(ab') fragments and sucrose gradient centrifugation to detect 10 to 11 S immune-complex material in the sera of 5 cancer patients. The results provided some of the earliest evidence for the physical characteristics of IgG complexed to something else in plasma and correlating with apparent clinical load of tumor burden in individual patients. One patient studied in this small group showed presence of immune-complex glomerulonephritis in association with 10 to 11 S sedimenting IgG.

The strong implication of Epstein-Barr virus in Burkitt's lymphoma led to identification in 1974 of antigen-antibody complexes containing EB virus antigen in 2 patients with Burkitt's lymphoma by Oldstone and co-workers (172). In this study examination of renal glomeruli from 2 patients with African Burkitt's lymphoma revealed host IgG and C3 along the glomerular basement membrane (GBM) and renal mesangia in granular patterns characteristic of immune-complex disease. Elution of IgG bound to glomerular tissues indicated that eluted immunoglobulin contained specific antibody to viral capsid antigens and early viral antigens, but not to complement-fixing nuclear antigens, nor to membrane antigens of EB virus. In contrast, the serum samples showed antibodies to all of these component EB viral antigens. Studies of sera showed presence of circulating complexes using the Raji-cell radioimmunoassay in 9 of 15 patients examined. Marked quantitative elevation of complexes was recorded in the patients positive in the complex assay with ranges of 30 to 1,200 μg/ml and means of 256 μg/ml, compared with means of 29 μg/ml in appropriate controls. An immunofluorescent study of glomerular tissue examined during this work is shown in Figure 8-13, indicating the distribution of IgG in one of the Burkitt's patients studied. Calculations of quantitative relationships of IgG in glomerular eluates and demonstrable antibody activities in these eluates indicated that at least 26 percent of the IgG in the eluate could be accounted for as antibody to various EB viral antigens.

This study represents impressive documentation of the value of having specific heterologous reagents available by which glomerular or other tissue immune deposits and eluates can be precisely examined. So often in instances where immune complexes are suspected, no precise identification of the antigen portions of immune complexes is made and final proof of the true immune-complex nature of the basic lesion must be tacitly assumed from the pattern of tissue immunoglobulin and complement deposition.

The advantage afforded by availability of specific antiviral reagents related to the spectrum of antigens involved in the pathogenesis of EBV-related diseases was extended in subsequent work by Heimer and Klein (173), using sera from additional patients with Burkitt's lymphoma and subjects with nasopharyngeal

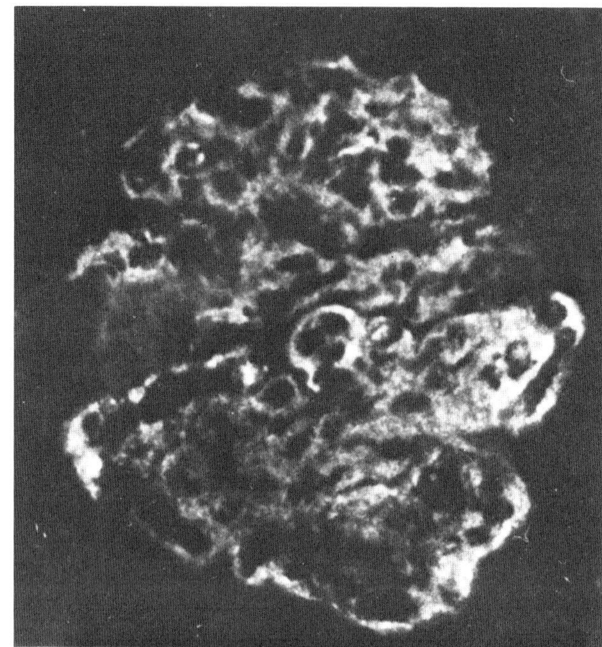

Figure 8-13 Immunofluorescent pattern in the glomerulus of a patient with African Burkitt's lymphoma, showing staining for host IgG. Sections were also positive for C3 and EB viral antigens. (Reproduced with permission, M. B. A. Oldstone, A. N. Theofilopoulos, P. Gurvén et al., *Intervirology* 4:292, 1974. Courtesy of S. Karger AG, Basel.)

carcinoma, a disorder also closely linked with Epstein-Barr virus infection (174). Hemolytic complement consumption was combined with molecular sizing via sucrose gradient centrifugation and reactivity with rheumatoid factors. Table 8-3, taken from this study, shows that 60 percent of Burkitt's subjects along with about half of the patients with nasopharyngeal carcinoma showed detectable complexes using the complement consumption method. Fractionation of positive sera showed that immune complex activity was present in intermediate molecular fractions between 7S and 19S. By means of insolubilized human rheumatoid factors, virtually all of the immune-complex activity could be removed, indicating that IgG antibody was the predominant immunoglobulin in these complexes. Adsorptions were also conducted using con-A Sepharose columns; immunoabsorbents removed the complexes, which could then be eluted specifically with the con-A dissociating ligand of α-methyl-D-mannoside and showed that the antigens involved in the immune complexes studied were glyco-

proteins. This approach is a valuable one and should be applied to other sera containing complexes of indeterminate nature. In the case of complexes in which reactive glycoproteins constitute part of the tumor antigen, the use of con-A Sepharose could even be contemplated in therapeutic maneuvers to remove complexes through extracorporeal means.

Tumor-Bound Immunoglobulins

Research has recently been directed at mechanisms involved in localization of immune complexes in tumor tissues. In one study by Irie and co-workers (175) a mixed hemadsorption technique utilized cells sensitized with whole immunoglobulins or activated C3. Tumors from a number of cancer patients showed presence of antibody and activated complement through use of these sensitive techniques; normal tissues obtained from control patients did not show this activity. Similar findings of immunoglobulin and complement binding to human tumors have been presented

Table 8-3 The complement consumption activity of sera from patients with Burkitt's lymphoma or nasopharyngeal carcinoma.

| | Number of patients | | | |
Condition	"Negative" (1:20 or <)	"Moderate" (1:40 to 1:160)	"Considerable" (1:320 or >)	Percent "positive"
Burkitt's lymphoma	10	6	9	60
Nasopharyngeal carcinoma	12	5	9	54
Healthy control	20	1	0	5

Source: Reproduced with permission, R. Heimer and G. Klein, *Int. J. Cancer* 18:310, 1976.

in the past using immunofluorescent and elution techniques (176–178). In addition, similar immune adherence techniques described were shown to detect antibody and complement affixed to surface antigens of human cancer cells studied immediately after surgical biopsy (179–180). Analysis of tumor cell membranes for the presence of immunoglobulins is merely the beginning of the puzzle. Whether the majority of such affixed immunoglobulins are indeed effective antitumor antibody, enhancing antibody, or immune complexes masked by additional piggyback anti-γ-globulins is not yet evident. This subject has been reviewed in detail with regard to enhancement by Witz (181).

The problem of immunoglobulins binding to tumor-cell membranes is further complicated by the presence of endogenous receptors for immune complexes (Fc receptors) on many different types of tumors. Studies by several groups using hemadsorption or rosetting of sensitized indicator erythrocytes to frozen tissue sections or suspensions of fresh tumor cells have indicated that a wide variety of human tumors express Fc receptors (182–184). Precise definition of which cells actually are expressing Fc receptors in sections or even suspensions of tumor tissues is often complicated by the presence of numbers of lymphoid and macrophage-type cells. However, much of the work in this area indicates that tumor cells often bear intrinsic membrane receptors for Fc portions of immunoglobulins. The problem has recently been explored using sensitized sheep erythrocytes labeled with technetium-99m (185). Indicator erythrocytes sensitized with F(ab′)$_2$ fragments of IgG antibody devoid of Fc determinants did not show adsorption to tumor tissues. It seems possible that one of the intrinsic self-protective mechanisms that the tumor may have at its disposal in protecting itself against the host is generation or expression of high concentrations of receptors for immune complexes. If strategically placed over the tumor-cell membrane, such receptors might be capable of adsorbing a variety of antigen-antibody complexes and thus providing a defensive shield against effective T-cell killing, direct antibody-mediated cytolysis of tumor membrane by the complement system, or by naturally occurring K cells. By reacting with the Fc portion of potentially harmful antitumor antibodies, the tumor cell might be circumventing what started out as an appropriate and effective host immune response. In summary, antibodies—and in many instances activated complement components—have been demonstrated on the membranes of a variety of tumor cells. What they actually are doing there and by what mechanisms they are bound to tumor cell membranes in many cases is unknown. It seems important to direct considerable attention to these particular questions, since accurate assessment of many individual tumors may be a key to implementation of rational and effective treatment. Several ways in which immunoglobulin G can react with tumor cell surface structures are presented in Figure 8-14.

A recent report (186) compares the presence of detectable immune complexes in sera of 90 patients with Hodgkin's disease to the binding of immunoglobulin and complement in these same samples to established monolayer tissue

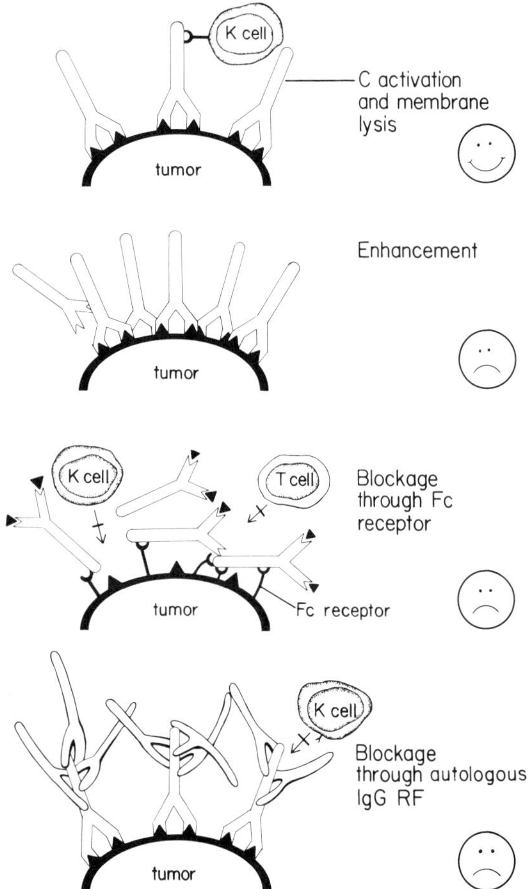

Figure 8-14   Several ways in which antitumor antibody molecules can react with tumor-cell membranes or various effector cells.

cultures of cells prepared from the patients' individual tumors. All 23 sera showing elevations of detectable complexes by the Raji-cell radioimmunoassay technique were bound to cultured Hodgkin's disease cells. Binding involved IgG heavy- and light-chain determinants and C3 complement component. Most importantly, adsorption of immune-complex–containing sera with cultured Hodgkin's disease cells removed detectable immune complexes and eliminated binding of any serum components by the tumor. Only 4 of 56 sera with immune complex levels of less than 10 μg/ml showed binding to tumor cells. Of interest was the absence of detectable Fc or conventional C3 receptors on the surfaces of cultured Hodgkin's disease cells. It was postulated that

free antibody combining sites in the immune complexes reacted with Hodgkin's disease specific antigens on the cultured cells, thus providing a ligand for specific absorption. This finding emphasizes not only the heterogeneity of ways in which immune complexes may bind to tumor cells but also the fact that free antibody combining sites still reactive against tumor-related antigens may actually be available in circulating complexes. Enhanced production of IgG immunoglobulin in vitro by splenic lymphocytes has been demonstrated in Hodgkin's disease by Longmire and co-workers (187), and abnormalities of complement components detected in patients with this disorder (188) suggest that an active immunologic process of complement activation often accompanies the disease in vivo.

Circulating Immune Complexes in Cancer

A number of reports have appeared documenting the prevalence and clinical implications of the presence of circulating immune complexes in various groups of cancer patients. The incidence of circulating complexes in melanoma was studied by Jerry and colleagues (189) using binding to polyclonal rheumatoid factors, C1q binding, and the C1q-deviation test. Sixty-four patients with malignant melanoma were studied; this included, in two instances, fresh tissue obtained from autopsy samples. Complexes were recorded in early and well-advanced stages of the disease; it was also noted that large amounts of complexes were frequently associated with progressive or advanced disease. C1q-reactive material was found in both intermediate 7S to 19S and greater than 19S high-molecular-weight fractions of 4 sera using sucrose density gradient techniques. Data acquired by careful serial measurements of antitumor antibodies in parallel with levels of circulating complexes in 51 patients were most informative in these studies. In many instances a slow cyclic fluctuation of levels of complexes over periods of 2 to 3 months was observed. These cycles are illustrated graphically in Figure 8-15. The most striking factor influencing detectable levels of

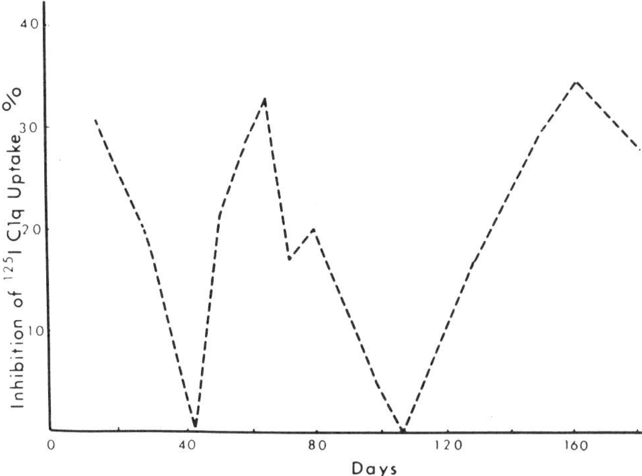

Figure 8-15   Cyclic variation with time in C1q-reactive material from a patient with stage II resected melanoma under treatment with oral BCG, 120 mg weekly. The C1q-reactive material in serum (measured by the C1q-deviation test) fluctuates in serial determinations over a 6-month period. (Reproduced with permission, L. M. Jerry, G. Rowden, P. O. Cano et al., *Scand. J. Immunol.* 5:845, 1976.)

circulating complexes appeared to be therapy with chemotherapeutic regimes. In 3 patients receiving chemotherapy, levels of detectable complexes dropped within 1 to 2 weeks following treatment only to reappear again in several weeks; BCG treatment was accompanied by continuous fluctuations in levels of complexes but not disappearance.

The most intriguing contribution of this study was the information derived from the serial studies of individual patients. The slow cyclic variation in levels of complexes and the rapid decline immediately after chemotherapy are of particular interest. A cyclical rise and fall in the immune response has been documented by numerous groups of workers and is felt to represent normal periodicity in the homeostatic control mechanisms within the immune system itself. A priori, one might have expected sudden rises in levels of detectable complexes after chemotherapy and destruction of tumor cells; instead, a fall was observed. This could be interpreted to mean that all available antibody to tumor antigens may already have been saturated at the time of initiation of chemotherapy or that antibodies complexed tightly to tumor antigens in cells killed by chemotherapy were quickly cleared and disposed of by the reticuloendothelial system,

thus never actually appearing as complexes within the circulating plasma. Considerably more experience with longitudinal studies of large numbers of patients similar to those conducted by Jerry and co-workers (189) is necessary before final insight into mechanisms of control of tumor growth is achieved.

Several other screening procedures for detection of immune complexes have been applied to large groups of cancer patients with a wide range of malignancies (190–192). In the study by Teshima and co-workers (190) from the Sloan Kettering Institute, ^{125}I-labeled C1q-deviation tests were performed on 459 sera from cancer patients. More than 50 percent of the sera tested showed strong inhibition of C1q binding, indicating significant levels of circulating immune complexes. Physical studies performed by density gradient centrifugations at low pH to allow dissociation of antigens from respective complexes showed that in general complexes were larger than 19S. In contrast to the studies previously reported by Jerry and colleagues (189), decreases in circulating immune complexes were noted after BCG treatment and after immunization with autologous nonviable melanoma tumor cells. A summary of the results of this screening study is given in Table 8-4. Useful data were also

Table 8-4 Immune complexes in sera of patients with various forms of malignancies.

Type of malignancy	Number of patients (n)	Mean AHG/ml (µg eq/ml)
Melanoma	128	15.0 (0–175.0)
Breast	91	13.0 (0–140.0)
Head and neck	50	16.0 (0–72.0)
Gynecological	48	14.0 (0–105.0)
Lung	41	15.5 (0–150.0)
Colon and rectal	37	12.0 (0–48.0)
CLL	19	8.4 (0–46.0)
Ovarian	16	5.8 (0–29.0)
Pancreas	4	26.0 (17.5–51.0)
Chronic myelocytic leukemia	4	14.0 (8.5–20.5)
Bone	4	23.0 (0–81.0)
Bile duct	2	17.3 (12.5–22.0)
Erythroleukemia	2	8.3 (0–16.5)
Hepatoma	2	5.5 (0–11.0)
Stomach	2	29.0 (0–58.0)
Sarcoma	2	9.5 (0–19.0)
Acute myoblastic leukemia	1	8.5
Acute lymphoblastic leukemia	1	0
Bladder	1	33.0
Gall bladder	1	7.8
Parotid	1	18.0
Reticulohistocytosis	1	0
Normal (healthy individuals)	50	4.5 (0–12.0)
SLE	10	60.0 (4.0–115.0)
Multiple sclerosis	17	7.0 (0–31.0)

Source: Reproduced with permission, H. Teshima, H. Wanebo, C. Pinsky et al., *J. Clin. Invest.* 59:1134, 1977.

provided by this same screening survey of Teshima and co-workers (190), in that 63 to 77 percent of sera from cancer patients showed reduced levels of total hemolytic complement or C3 and C1q in conjunction with elevated levels of detectable circulating complexes. Marked fluctuations of levels of complexes were noted within short periods of serial observations during this study, similar to the findings of Jerry and co-workers (189).

Of interest in the Teshima report were serial studies conducted on several patients receiving intensive autostimulation with irradiated melanoma cells mixed with BCG. In one such patient, a dramatic fall was noted in levels of detectable complexes 7 to 9 days after autostimulation (Figure 8-16). Subsequently, however, circulating complexes rose to previous elevated levels. It is important to mention in this context that very little hard data are actually available regarding what such fluctuations in levels of circulating complexes may mean in individual patients, such as the one whose course is outlined in Figure 8-16. It seems possible that brief or transient excessive stimulation of host immune responses results in relative saturation of circulating antigen binding sites by newly released antibody and temporary clearing of the circulating complexes from plasma. However, factors affecting the kinetics of dissociation and association of gamma globulins or complexes to and from the membranes of the tumor cell mass are ambiguous. One might presume that antitumor

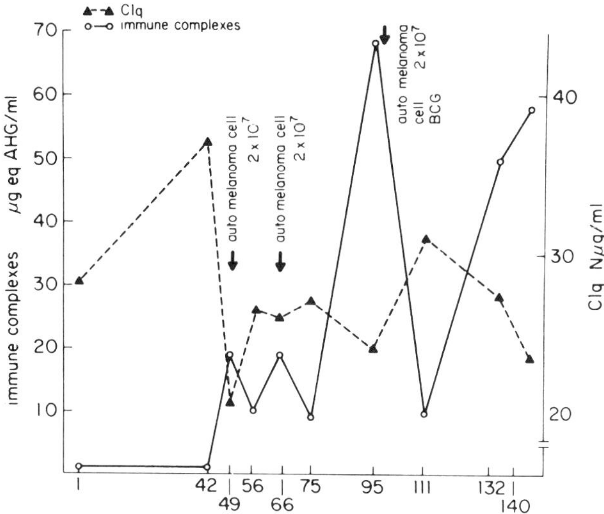

Figure 8-16 Levels of immune complexes and serum C1q of serial samples of a patient with melanoma after treatment with autologous tumor cells and BCG. (Reproduced with permission, H. Teshima, H. Wanebo, C. Pinsky et al., *J. Clin. Invest.* 59:1134, 1977.)

antibodies of high binding avidity might not dissociate or reassociate with tumor membranes in situ during such a procedure. What might be detected is analogous to an "iceberg effect": the fluctuations of easily dissociated complexes in plasma perhaps not truly reflecting the kinetics of immunoglobulin and immune-complex attachment to the tumor membranes. The serial assay of immune complexes both on fixed tumor surfaces and in plasma would be of great interest in patients where a large-scale attempt was made to physically remove such complexes either by plasmapheresis or extracorporeal immunoabsorption procedures. To our knowledge, data bearing on this latter point are not yet available.

A group of 134 cancer patients has been recently studied by Rossen and co-workers (191), using C1q binding as a primary screening procedure. Elevation of C1q binding was recorded in 83 percent of the patients studied. Unfortunately, in this particular report quantitative estimations of levels of complexes (referred to conventionally as μg equivalents, or μg/ml of human aggregated IgG) were not given. Serial follow-up studies of patients showing cancers of many different histological types were performed. From the data presented in this study, little prognostic value was noted when ultimate clinical course was related to initial determinations of immune complexes, with the exception of carcinoma of the lung where high levels of complexes were often related ($p = 0.04$) to disease progression. A small number of serum samples was also studied for size distribution of C1q-binding immune-complex materials. In general, reactivity was found in fractions of intermediate 7S to 19S size. A broad general survey of this particular variable is needed in a large number of cancer patients followed over a considerable period to determine whether physical size or other more subtle physicochemical characteristics of various immune complexes in cancer patient sera can be used to predict clinical course or long-term prognosis.

A survey conducted in 1976 by Samayoa and colleagues (192) at the Mayo Clinic included results obtained on sera from 146 cancer patients utilizing precipitin testing and radioimmunoassay with monoclonal rheumatoid factors. Unlike the results obtained in the two previously discussed large surveys, the Samayoa group found positive tests for complexes in only 29 percent of cancer sera. Thirty-five percent of patients with established metastatic disease showed positive tests—a slightly higher value. The particular monoclonal rheumatoid factor utilized in this work was said to show primary specificity for aggregated human IgG, although slight reactivity for uncomplexed native monomer IgG was also present. A summary of results recorded in this study is shown in Figure 8-17. It can be seen that very few patients showed extremely high values using the monoclonal rheumatoid-factor assay. Again, gradient centrifugal analysis was carried out and showed positive reactions in the 13 S to 32 S molecular-weight range.

At present the overall significance of the results of these three large-scale surveys of heterogeneous groups of cancer patients is difficult to assess. Using sensitive methodology such as the C1q-deviation or ^{125}I-labeled C1q-binding test, the prevalence of detectable complexes in large groups of serum samples from cancer patients varied from 50 to 83 percent. When a relatively specific but perhaps less sensitive assay such as binding to monoclonal rheumatoid factor was used, incidence of positive tests fell to 29 percent. The final usefulness of the various tests for detection of circulating complexes in cancer patients will require consider-

ably more in the way of longitudinal follow-up. Although helpful in evaluating the status of some patients with established malignancy who by other parameters appear to be faring well, the quantitative levels of detectable complexes must be related to other key features of each individual patient's illness. A multidimensional viewpoint is needed that takes into consideration the quantitative amounts of circulating complex, relative saturation of the reticulo-endothelial system clearing mechanisms, and, most importantly, the total tumor load along with the host capacity to continue to mount some sort of immune response.

In a study directed at patients with breast cancer, levels of circulating immune complexes were measured by radioimmunoprecipitation with ^{125}I-C1q (193). Before operation all 22 patients showed elevation of immune complexes significantly higher than that detected in normal controls. Twelve months following mastectomy, patients identified clinically as having a good prognosis showed almost normal levels of immune complexes; by contrast, patients who had not fared well and who demonstrated de-

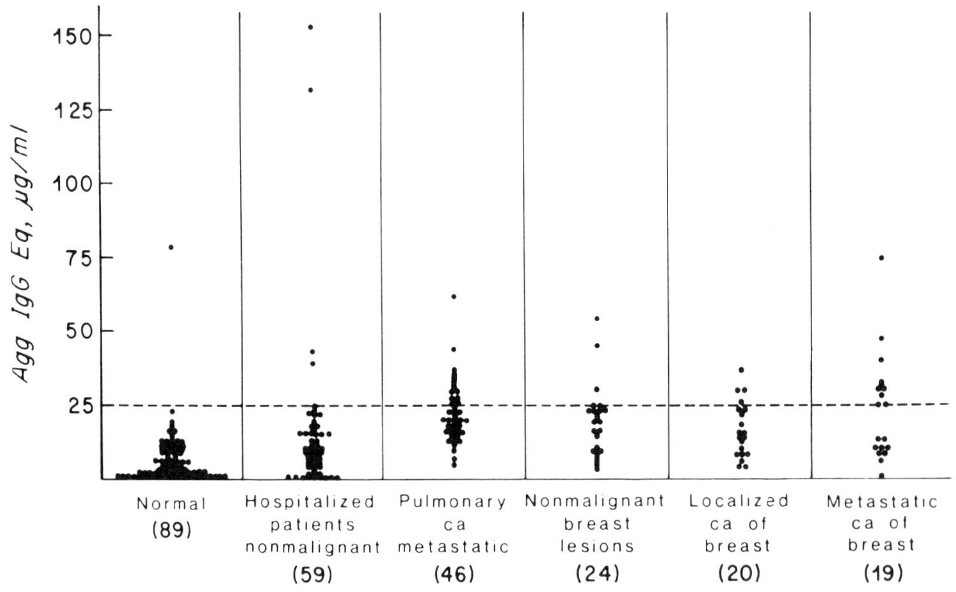

Figure 8-17 Immune-complex–like material in the sera of normal subjects, patients with nonmalignant diseases, and patients with tumors. Numbers in parentheses indicate the total number of individuals in each group. (Reproduced with permission, E. A. Samayoa, F. C. McDuffie, A. M. Nelson et al., *Int. J. Cancer* 19:12, 1977.)

tectable dissemination showed significantly elevated plasma levels of detectable complexes. These results are shown in Figure 8-18 taken from this study. Prior to surgery, many patients had high levels of detectable complexes but there was a wide scattering of values; levels of complexes remained high in patients who died or showed a poor prognosis. No precise identification of tumor antigens was given in this study; however, these results provide careful follow-up of patients with a single major type of cancer and emphasize the potential usefulness of serial determinations in such individuals.

Hodgkin's Disease

In the initial report by Theofilopoulos and co-workers describing standardization and clinical applications of the Raji-cell radioimmunoassay (194), a high proportion of patients with lymphoid tumors including Hodgkin's disease, lymphoma, and sarcomas showed detectable complexes. Using a slightly different approach, Amlot and colleagues (195) also studied the question of circulating complexes and symptoms in Hodgkin's disease. Increased quantities of the third component of complement (C3) were noted in high-molecular-weight plasma fractions from patients with untreated Hodgkin's disease. Certain clinical features such as night sweats, fever, and weight loss have been associated with a poor prognosis in patients with Hodgkin's disease (196, 197). Pruritus, which curiously is often also associated with Hodgkin's, does not, however, correlate with poor prognosis. Staging procedures such as laparotomy and splenectomy have shown that individuals with night sweats, fever, and weight loss who show the same apparent anatomical staging as those without these systemic symptoms actually fare much worse

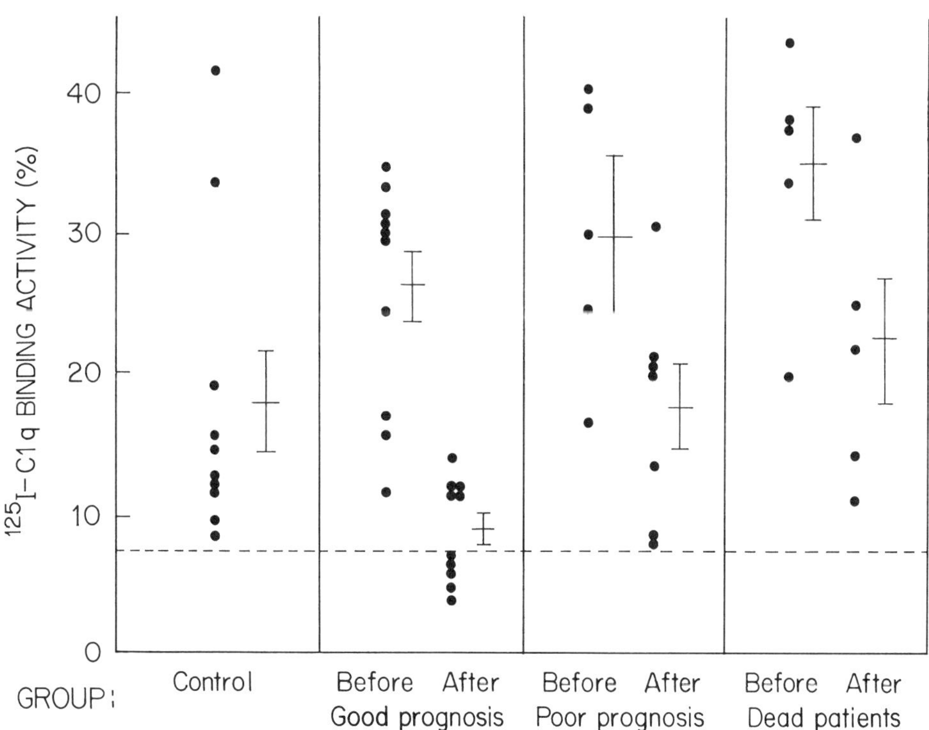

Figure 8-18 Mean ^{125}I-C1q-binding activities (±S.E.) in women with breast cancer before and 12 months after operation according to clinicopathological staging. The horizontal dotted line at 8 percent represents binding activity in normal sera. (Reproduced with permission, K. Hoffken, I. D. Meredith, R. A. Robins et al., *Br. Med. J.* 2:218, 1977.)

from the clinical standpoint. Considerable previous work has of course focused on mechanisms of fever induction and febrile response in humans. Several studies have indicated that immune complexes themselves may be pyrogenic and can induce the formation of endogenous pyrogen in vitro (198). Certain patterns of febrile response of intermittent variety have been given the eponym of Pel-Ebstein fever and often used to support a possible or anticipatory clinical diagnosis of occult Hodgkin's disease.

In the study by Amlot and co-workers (195) serum samples from normal controls and 18 patients with Hodgkin's disease were studied by Sephadex G-200 gel filtration. Appearance of C3 in macromolecular fractions rather than in its normal molecular-weight distribution corresponding to its molecular size of 185,000 Daltons was taken as evidence for immune complexes that had activated C3, thereby shifting its distribution to high-molecular-weight fractions. The representative Hodgkin's gel filtration pattern is shown in Figure 8-19 from this report.

There are a number of previous observations in the literature indicating that phagocytosis or cellular activation by immune com-

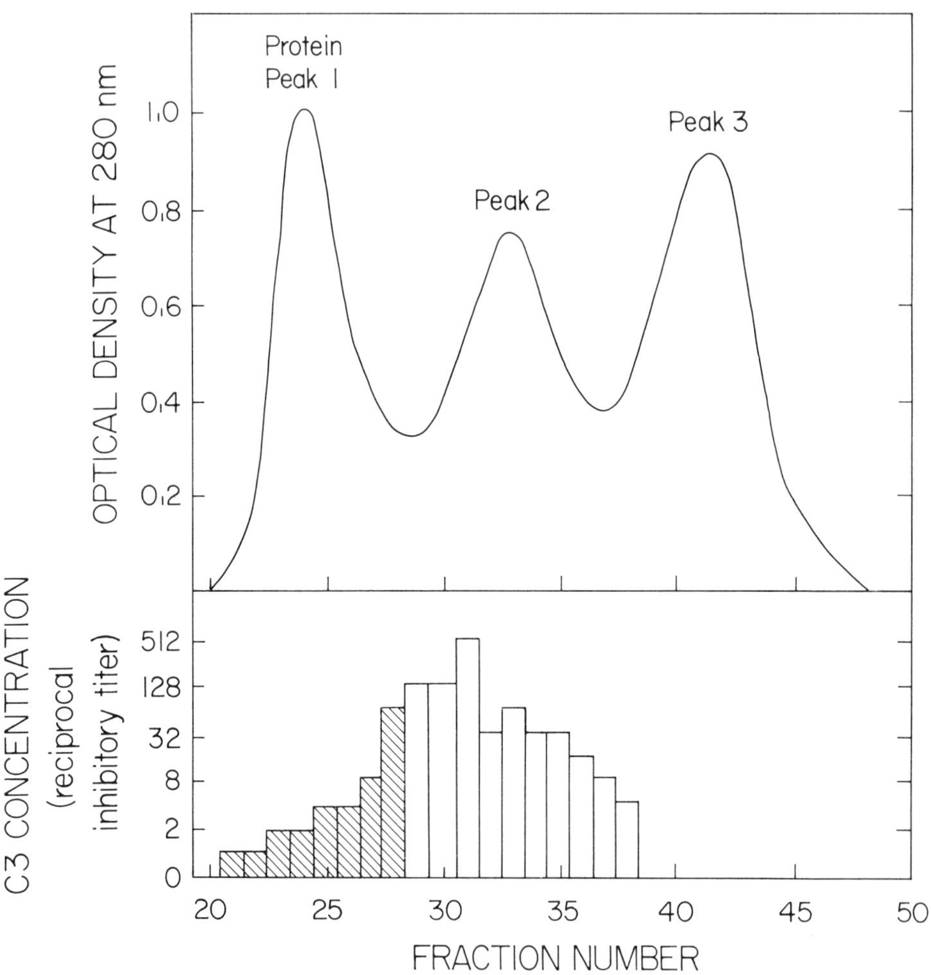

Figure 8-19 The distribution of C3 in plasma from a patient with stage IIIB Hodgkin's disease. The C3 present in the first protein peak is shown in the hatched areas. (Reproduced with permission, P. L. Amlot, J. M. Slaney, and B. D. Williams, *Lancet* 1:449, 1976.)

plexes may be occurring in Hodgkin's disease. Using aggregated albumin as a test for reticuloendothelial system function, clearance is more rapid in stages III and IVB of Hodgkin's disease than in milder cases or controls (199). In many ways this is not surprising, for the disease is often located in lymph nodes, spleen, and bone marrow—the principal locations of active reticuloendothelial elements, which presumably contain large numbers of activated macrophages. It has been noted that leukocyte alkaline phosphatase levels correlate with relative disease activity (200), and that leukocytosis in the absence of infection may be associated with a poor prognosis in this disease (201). These findings must be extended to assess whether the presence of detectable immune complexes is directly correlated with fever itself in a variety of patients with diverse forms of malignancy other than Hodgkin's disease and the lymphomas. In many such subjects onset of fever during clinical workup or subsequent therapy is assumed to be on the basis of infection. From a practical standpoint, patients who develop fever during or immediately after chemotherapy or radiation are often empirically placed on a panel of antibiotics. If certain immunochemical or molecular profiles of circulating immune complexes had been established for individual patients which were related to the basic disease, when these individuals became febrile because of superimposed nosocomial or other infections, sophisticated methods for detecting shifts in actual characteristics of complexes might be of great clinical usefulness.

The Amlot findings are convincing in assigning a probable relationship between presence of detectable complexes and the symptoms of fever, night sweats, and weight loss; however, it is not yet clear how these factors may be related. Does plasmapheresis or removal of complexes cause abatement of the accompanying symptoms? Are systemic symptoms always related to large complexes of 19 S or greater that activate the complement system? Are numerous intermediary mechanisms involving leukocyte synthesis of endogenous pyrogen and subsequent activation of other mediator molecules necessary for the apparent clinical link

between complexes and night sweats or between complexes and fever? It is exciting to think that perhaps at last some of these relatively vague but common clinical phenomena may be exposed to rational inspection. Now that something definite like immune complexes have been implicated, it will be important to look carefully at how such factors actually operate.

One of the corollaries to the study of fevers and night sweats related to generalized systemic disease is of course apparent in such poorly defined clinical syndromes as familial Mediterranean fever (FMF). Patients with this disorder have now been extensively examined for possible mechanisms inherent in the generation of their febrile episodes (202, 203). In many ways FMF resembles Hodgkin's disease with repeated hectic fevers, evidence of serositis, peritonitis, and many of the peripheral manifestations suggesting at least that mechanisms related to immune-complex activation may be involved. Like Hodgkin's, FMF is also frequently associated with the development of amyloidosis (204). Clinical and laboratory analyses of patients with FMF have not yet shown any one feature that convincingly explains the myriad peripheral manifestations. It seems possible that careful serial determinations of immune complexes in this group of disorders may provide direct insight into basic mechanisms related to the underlying disorder.

Leukemia and Myeloproliferative Disease

In contrast to the solid tumors such as melanoma, carcinoma of the lung, Hodgkin's disease, or carcinoma of the breast, in leukemia the clinical situation involves neoplastic transformation of cells circulating in both intravascular and extravascular spaces and the central tissues of the hematopoietic and reticuloendothelial system. Moreover, there is not a great deal of available evidence concerning the host's ability to mount an effective immune response to leukemia-specific antigens. Some of the early successes claimed concerning the efficacy of BCG and immunization procedures in acute leukemia were attributed to potentiation of autologous leukemic antigenicity (205–207); however, host immune responses to leukemia antigens have not been conclusively demonstrated.

Presence of immune complexes in patients with various forms of leukemia has been studied recently by Carpentier and colleagues (208) using ^{125}I-C1q-binding and the Raji-cell radioimmunoassay on 467 serum samples from 230 leukemia patients (208). Increased ^{125}I-C1q binding was recorded in 40 percent of subjects with acute myeloid leukemia, 23 percent with acute lymphatic, 46 percent during myeloid leukemia blast crisis, 12 percent with chronic lymphatic leukemia, and 13 percent with chronic myelogenous leukemia. Complexes were found to sediment as 14 to 28 S material on density gradient separation and contained IgG that could be dissociated at low or acidic pH. The C1q binding of complexes studied in the sera of acute leukemia patients was removed by anti-IgG immunoabsorbents and was lost after mild reduction and alkylation. Remission took place in 75.4 percent of patients with no detectable circulating complexes at time of clinical onset, whereas remission was achieved in only 32.7 percent of those who showed detectable complexes at time of initial clinical presentation. Good internal correlation was recorded in this work between results recorded in Raji-cell and C1q-binding assays. Physical characterization studies performed with these sera were carefully done and yielded additional information. Representative sucrose gradient analysis of serum from a patient with blastic crisis is shown in Figure 8-20. Acid dissociation of materials binding to C1q and analysis of distribution of relative amounts of 7 S and 19 S materials indicated a major 7 S component within immune complexes and a smaller amount of high-molecular-weight materials. Which of these fractions constituted antigen is unclear.

Since certain antigens related to acute lymphatic leukemia or acute myelogenous leukemia might contain determinants uniquely capable of producing host enhancing or blocking antibodies that would favor the leukemic process, such an analysis is of vital importance. It might well be that direct knowledge of such

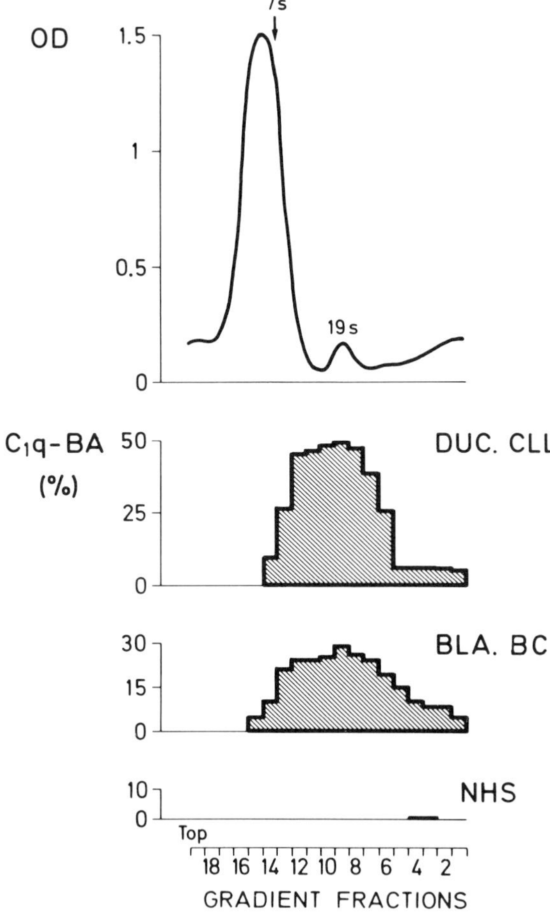

Figure 8-20 ^{125}I-C1q binding activity (C1q-BA) measured in each sucrose gradient fraction obtained by density fractionation of sera from a patient (DUC) with CLL, a patient (BLA) with blastic crisis, and a healthy blood donor (NHS). *Above,* the optical density pattern obtained with a 1:10 diluted serum is shown; the positions of the 7 S and 19 S markers are indicated. *Below,* C1q binding activity is represented by the shaded columns. (Reproduced with permission, N. A. Carpentier, G. T. Lange, D. M. Fiere et al., *J. Clin. Invest.* 60:874, 1977.)

features at the time of diagnosis would provide extremely useful guides in the design of therapy. If, for instance, it could be established that presence of enhancing antibody to the ALL-specific antigen of Greaves and co-workers (22, 23) were present in some cases, a concerted effort might be directed immediately after initial diagnosis toward plasmapheresis or extracorporeal immunoabsorption procedures that would eliminate any possible enhancing antibody. Such an approach seems clinically feasible at the present time. A similar attack on the possible participation of enhancing antibody in patients with acute myelogenous leukemia also seems justified. This may, however, have to await precise identification of myeloid-specific antigens related to the leukemia itself.

In the studies of leukemia, no apparent correlation existed between detection of sepsis in individual patients and circulating immune complexes. The latter were most often detected in leukemic patients during periods of rapid cell proliferation and turnover, as in the blast crisis stage. It is possible, therefore, that antibodies present in immune complexes occurring in such instances might be related to the leukemic cells, but directed specifically at unusual differentiation antigens actually expressed in the blastic state of the cells. Antigens possibly related to such differentiation or proliferative states have previously been described by several groups (209–211). During serial studies of patients with leukemia, no marked increase in levels of detectable complexes was noted after chemotherapy. This confirmed the earlier melanoma studies of Jerry and co-workers (189). More precise knowledge of the antigens present in immune complexes of leukemic patients is now needed.

A great deal of new information is available on the different types of leukemia-related or differentiation antigens present in the cells of such patients (212–217). The association of higher levels of detectable complexes at disease onset with bad prognosis, if confirmed, is a finding of great importance. It will be recalled that this particular relationship was not present in the group of patients with carcinoma of the breast studied by Hoffken and colleagues (193) where, instead, persistence of complexes after surgical excision and follow-up correlated with poor outcome. In many ways this difference may be related to the actual balance of host defenses and aggressiveness of the tumor in each particular clinical circumstance. In the case of acute lymphatic or myelogenous leukemia, the presence of complexes may represent the effect of intense immune enhancement in a rapidly progressive tumor that has at

one fell swoop gained entry to both the reticuloendothelial system, which is designed to eliminate it, and the peripheral blood and distant tissues. On the other hand, in carcinoma of the breast the balance of host defenses against the tumor may in many situations be much more favorable. This is obvious in the remarkable clinical results already achieved with estrogen therapy or with the newer combined modalities of chemotherapeutic agents. When complexes are detected late in patients with carcinoma of the breast, what we may be seeing is failure of other central clearing functions to hold the tumor in check. Thus, in each individual case the appearance of complexes in the peripheral blood must be interpreted in line with what is generally known about the normal clinical course and endogenous strength of natural host defenses. The presence of complexes in the cancer patient may be telling us something more than merely that the host has made some humoral response to the tumor. It is possible that their presence in the leukemia patient may be reflecting a general profile of the immune status of the host: namely, that of unbalanced production perhaps of antibody of low titer or even low avidity (218, 219). More work is certainly needed in the study of leukemia, particularly since the overall prognosis of acute myelogenous disease has not shown much in the way of convincing long-term beneficial results.

Nephrotic Syndrome and Neoplasia

One of the most convincing manifestations of the potential importance of immune-complex disease associated with neoplasia or cancer is the growing number of examples now amply documented in the literature of nephrotic syndrome or diffuse nephritis associated with specific tumors. The clinical association between cancer and nephrotic syndrome or between cancer and cryptic proteinuria and apparent glomerulonephritis was recognized long before the concept of immune-complex renal disease was postulated. As in many important areas linking immunology and clinical medicine, once the concept was established, a large number of examples of this particular clinical association appeared. An aphorism attributed to Louis Pasteur seems pertinent in this situation: "Observation favors the prepared mind." We often see clearly what we are specifically looking for. In the instance of renal disease associated with various forms of cancer, the evidence is indeed overwhelming.

One of the earliest studies relating then cryptogenic renal disease and cancer is that of Lee and co-workers (220), who in 1966 recorded the association of nephrotic syndrome in 11 adult patients with cancer studied over a ten-year period. At that time, much like today, the diagnosis of nephrotic syndrome was based on the presence of massive proteinura, urinary excretion of lipid materials, variable tendency toward edema, hypoalbuminemia, hyperlipidemia, and excretion of 3.5 gm or more of protein per 24 hours related to 1.73 square meters of body surface area. In addition, the patients studied by Lee showed negative or essentially minimal histological and ultrastructural changes on renal biopsy. Renal disease preceded discovery of malignancy in 7 of the 11 patients reported in this series.

As the possibility emerged that nephrotic syndrome or diffuse glomerular minimal-change nephritis might indeed be associated with some sort of immunologic reaction, subsequent analysis of various other patients began to fit data into the etiologic puzzle. Of the patients studied in some detail to date, Hodgkin's disease probably heads the list as the primary tumor associated with nephrotic syndrome. In the study by Sherman and colleagues (221), immunofluorescence and conventional microscopic examination showed little more than enlarged glomeruli, electron-microscopic fusion of foot processes, or GBM irregularities. The possibility of an acute toxic process related somehow to the disease was considered; however, the nephrotic syndrome responded to radiotherapy directed at Hodgkin's involvement quite distinct from the urinary system. In one patient being maintained on 100 mg of predisone per day, shortly after initiation of radiotherapy to mediastinal Hodgkin's involvement, a diuresis commenced and proteinuria diminished concomitant with rise in creatinine clearance. Several other groups of

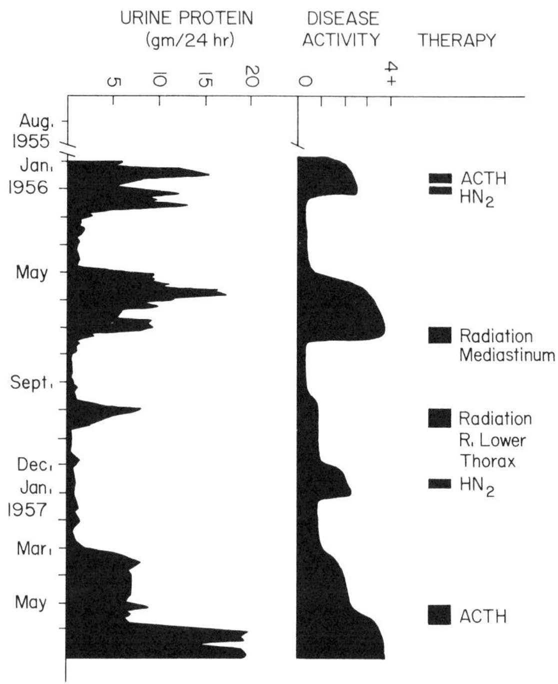

Figure 8-21   Correlation between Hodgkin's disease activity and proteinuria. Disease activity is illustrated on a 0 to 4+ scale, based on clinical and radiological evaluation. HN₂ represents a four-day course of nitrogen mustard therapy (0.4 mg/kg). (Reproduced with permission, J. Plager and L. Stutzman, *Am. J. Med.* 50:56, 1971.)

investigators have observed similar striking clinical improvements in nephrotic syndrome associated with Hodgkin's disease after therapy in the form of radiation or chemotherapy (221, 223, 225). A dramatic example of serial studies conducted on several patients with this disease association is shown in Figure 8-21, from the study of Plager and Stutzman (224).

A number of other studies have identified progressive structural changes and clear evidence for immunologic reactivity, documented by deposits of IgG or IgM and complement along with occasional massive glomerular subendothelial electron-dense deposits (226). In the 2 patients serially studied by Hyman and colleagues (226), the nephritis progressed from histological null lesions to clear-cut diffuse glomerulonephritis with focal proliferative changes, immune deposits, and electron-dense deposits largely in the subendothelial location. A second patient with Burkitt's lymphoma showed membranoproliferative changes accompanied by granular immune deposits and electron-dense subendothelial evidence of immune complexes.

One of the first demonstrations that immune reactivity to specific tumor-derived antigens might indeed be involved in such reactions was presented by Lewis and co-workers (227). A patient who presented with nephrotic syndrome associated with bronchial carcinoma was studied. Immunoglobulins eluted from glomeruli showed specific reaction with surface membranes of the bronchial tumor cells. In addition, a precipitin in agar gel was noted between tumor extract and the gamma globulins present in glomerular eluates and in serum. This report, demonstrating direct reactions between tumor extract and gamma globulins in the glomeruli, focused attention on the presumed immunologic mechanisms at work in such patients. Numerous other reports have documented the strong clinical association between a variety of malignant tumors and either nephrotic syndrome or diffuse nephritis. Patients studied by Cantrell (228) and by Revol and co-workers (229) showed resolution or temporary improvement of massive proteinuria following surgical removal of primary gastric carcinoma or bronchogenic carcinoma respectively.

Patients with the general association of carcinoma and nephropathy have also been studied by Ozawa and co-workers (230). These investigations represent some of the most convincing evidence for relating tumor membrane antigens and antigen-antibody complexes to the nephropathy associated with various tumors. In 3 patients with clear-cell renal carcinoma and 1 patient with intrarenal tumor associated with nephropathy, immunoglobulin and complement components were shown by immunofluorescent studies to be localized in the glomeruli and tumor membranes of all patients. Both sera and specific glomerular eluates showed fixation of immunoglobulin to antigens present in the *normal* brush border structures of proximal renal tubular cells and to similar structures of normal human jejunal mucosa. Tissue eluates also showed staining of glomeruli and autologous proximal tubular

structures of patients' tissues. A similarity was observed between tumor-associated antigens and antigens present in brush border materials of normal renal and intestinal mucosal structures. Positive reactions in immunofluorescence could be absorbed out by specific tumor extracts. The tumor antigens described within the immune complexes found in association with these patients with carcinoma localized to the kidney were apparently similar to the original renal tubular epithelial antigens described by Edgington and co-workers in association with Heymann's experimental nephritis (231). This latter work was of interest in that in such an experimental situation reactivity to the host's own similar material is somehow induced by injection of heterologous renal tubular antigens. The precise mechanisms involved in such self-potentiating immunologic reactivity have in the past been attributed to abrogation of tolerance to self-antigens through such immunization procedures. It also raises the important question, not yet satisfactorily answered, of whether immune complexes associated with a wide variety of immune reactions to autologous tumors may, in fact, be partially related to normal self-antigens. A similar problem in interpretation of underlying mechanisms is apparent in a careful consideration of the case reported by Constanza and colleagues (69), where CEA was identified in the diffuse granular deposits within glomeruli involved by a nephropathy associated with a primary carcinoma of the colon. Since information coding for the CEA is present in the fetal genome and has possibly been only temporarily derepressed in its expression within later occurring endogenous tumor, it is difficult to fathom why in some rare instances it is indeed recognized as foreign and followed by an immune response sufficient to induce immune-complex glomerulonephritis.

An alternative view related to other possible mechanisms of nephrotic syndrome, particularly in Hodgkin's disease, has been presented by Moorthy and co-workers (232), who pointed out that in a majority of instances thus far documented in the literature where Hodgkin's has been associated with nephrotic syndrome, examination of renal tissue by conventional and electron microscopic techniques has showed no specific abnormalities. A few reports do exist, however, in which findings at autopsy or biopsy do show apparent glomerular localization of complexes. In three-fourths of the patients reviewed by the Moorthy group the histological diagnosis in the Hodgkin's tumor tissues examined was of the mixed cellularity type. These researchers suggested that an alternative mechanism involving functional glomerular damage without much in the way of demonstrable tissue change could be attributable to lymphokines somehow released from lymphoid tissues involved in the mixed cellularity lesions of Hodgkin's tissue. The fact that the usual prevalence of mixed cellularity in Hodgkin's (35 percent) is much lower than the 75 percent incidence recorded in the 35 case reports of renal lesions associated with Hodgkin's suggested a relationship with this particular cellular lesion. It is an interesting point of view that must be studied in more detail. Very little current information is available to link glomerulonephritis or nephrotic syndrome to disorders of cell-mediated immunity. The suggestion that the two might be related has been made from time to time (233, 234), but direct experimental evidence in favor of such a hypothesis is lacking. Certainly this view must be further tested and evaluated in studies of additional patients. Several clinical features of the cases reviewed in detail by Moorthy may bear out other factors operative in the pathogenesis of proteinuria in these patients. One item is the documentation of rapid disappearance of proteinuria immediately after therapy, as in the patients studied by Plager and Stutzman (224). If immune-complex deposition were the only mechanism underlying proteinuria in all patients with Hodgkin's disease, one would not a priori expect such rapid reversal of proteinuria. Indeed, in the original models of immune-complex glomerulonephritis provided by experimental serum sickness, proteinuria was persistent many weeks after cessation of immune-complex deposition.

Finally, a case described by Higgins and co-workers (235) provides still another example of the complexity of the clinical problem surrounding nephropathy associated with malignant disease. In this patient, who had oat-cell carcinoma of the lung, antinuclear antibody was present in conjunction with immune-complex glomerulonephritis in renal glomeruli at autopsy. Examination of tissues with Feulgen stain showed masses of material with characteristics of DNA in the same distribution as that of the immune deposits. Moreover, renal eluates showed antinuclear activity. It was postulated that an immune-complex nephritis might have involved DNA–anti-DNA antigen-antibody complexes—the DNA having been released through necrosis and lysis in the tumor.

Studies of postmortem material obtained from large series of cancer patients suggest that minute and perhaps subclinical manifestations of immune-complex deposition may be much more common than is generally recognized. Studies by Sutherland and colleagues (236) of kidneys obtained at postmortem examination of a large group of 303 patients, 90 percent of whom had tumors, showed a surprisingly high frequency of immune complexes as detected by immunofluorescence. A summary of the findings in this particular study is given in Table 8-5. The highest prevalence of detectable immune complexes was recorded in renal tissues from patients with acute leukemia (14.3 percent) and lowest in individuals with solid tumors (1.6 percent). Many of the patients showed no clinical antemortem evidence for glomerulonephritis, and renal tissues appeared essentially normal by conventional light microscopy. Electron microscopic examinations in these same cases frequently showed dense subendothelial deposits (Figure 8-22.) The immunofluorescent distribution of immune complexes in this subclinical cancer material was most often capillary and, in only rare instances, mesangiocapillary in location.

A similar study focusing on Hodgkin's disease was recorded by this same group (237). Here, in contrast to the rather high proportions of subjects showing detectable complexes in the screening studies using sensitive assays such as the Raji-cell radioimmunoassay (194), only 2 of 23 postmortem kidneys and 5 of 22 patients (23 percent) who underwent renal biopsy during staging laparotomies showed clear

Table 8-5 Percentages of kidneys with immune complexes, by clinical groups.

Clinical group	Number of kidneys examined	Positive for both gamma globulin and complement		Positive for gamma globulin alone (number)
		Number	Percent	
Acute leukemia	83	12	14.3	2
Chronic leukemia	9	1	11	1
Lymphomas	54	2	3.5	1
Solid tumors	124	2	1.6	4
No tumor	33	4	11	5
Total	303	21	6.9	12

Source: Reproduced with permission, J. C. Sutherland, R. V. Markham, Jr., and M. R. Mardiney, Jr., *Am. J. Med.* 54:536, 1974.

immunofluorescent evidence for tissue immune-complex deposition. No obvious relationship between preterminal or terminal virus infections in the subjects and renal immune complexes was apparent, indicating that intercurrent viremia or other nosocomial infections were not responsible for the findings observed.

In many ways retrospective postmortem studies of this kind are difficult to interpret in terms of the real biologic relationship of immune complexes to the broad cancer problem. As with the observation of immune complexes in renal glomeruli during the acute phases of typhoid fever in patients without notable manifestation of renal disease (238), the real significance of these findings is not yet clear. Renal biopsy for immune-complex detection merely takes advantage of the fact that the human glomerulus and its capillary network are extremely sensitive histological indicators for the presence of immune complexes. Such an approach is hardly practical or safe in many acute or chronic clinical situations. Thus biopsy evaluation of the presence and significance of immune complexes will not be feasible or indeed indicated in many patients ill with cancer. On the other hand, studies of the precise composition of immune complexes using materials obtained by elution from renal biopsies may in some instances prove very instructive. The materials actually sticking within immune deposits may in some instances be entirely different from those identified as presumptive antigens

in circulating antigen-antibody complexes reacting with Raji-cell complement receptors or any of the various adaptations of the C1q-binding assay.

Elegant research directed at the problem of correlation between tumor-specific antibody response and the development of immune-complex renal disease has also been presented by Poskitt and co-workers (12) in the study of mice bearing a transplantable strain-specific melanoma tumor. During routine examination of tissues it was found that these animals developed a mild proliferative glomerulonephritis accompanied by moderate degrees of proteinuria. This histological change is shown in Figure 8-23. Immunofluorescent studies demonstrated striking immune deposits in these animals, as illustrated in Figure 8-24. Of interest were the findings of IgG, IgA, and IgM within these deposits in focal or granular distribution. Eluates of affected renal glomeruli showed strong reactivity for the respective autologous tumor cell membranes; this is illustrated in Figure 8-25. Additional data in this report showed that immune-complex deposition in this particular experimental model was actually correlated with progressive overcoming of host defense responses and subversion of cell-mediated immune reactivity. Thus an apparent inverse relationship was noted between presumably effective cell-mediated reactions, as exemplified by intense host mononuclear and inflammatory cell infiltrations

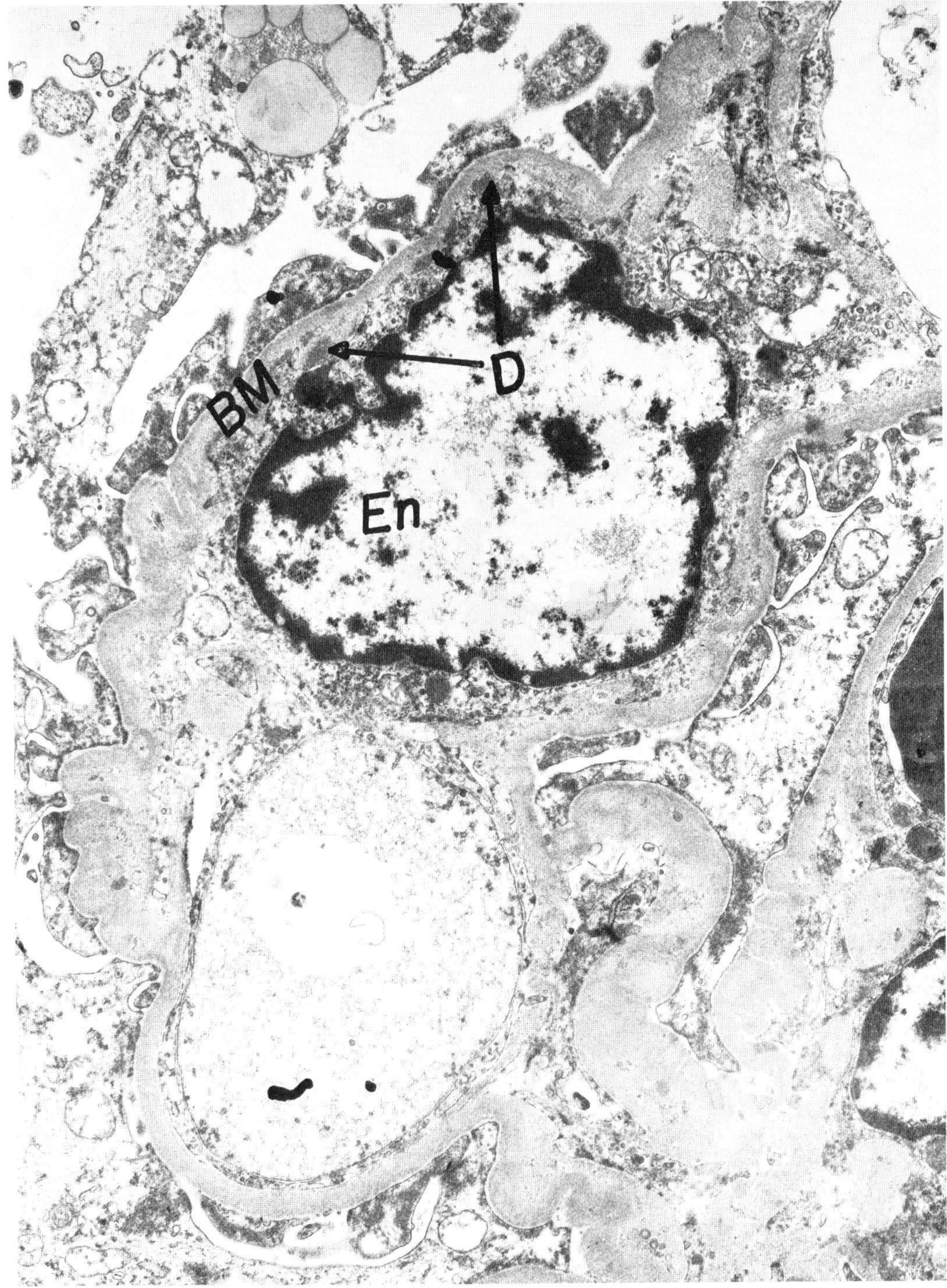

Figure 8-22   A portion of a capillary loop revealing irregularity and focal thickening of the basement membrane (BM) and the presence of dense subendothelial deposits (D); En = endothelial cell. Material is derived from a patient with acute myelocytic leukemia. Magnification × 7,900. (Reproduced with permission, J. C. Sutherland, R. V. Markham, Jr., and M. R. Mardiney, Jr., *Am. J. Med.* 57:536, 1974.)

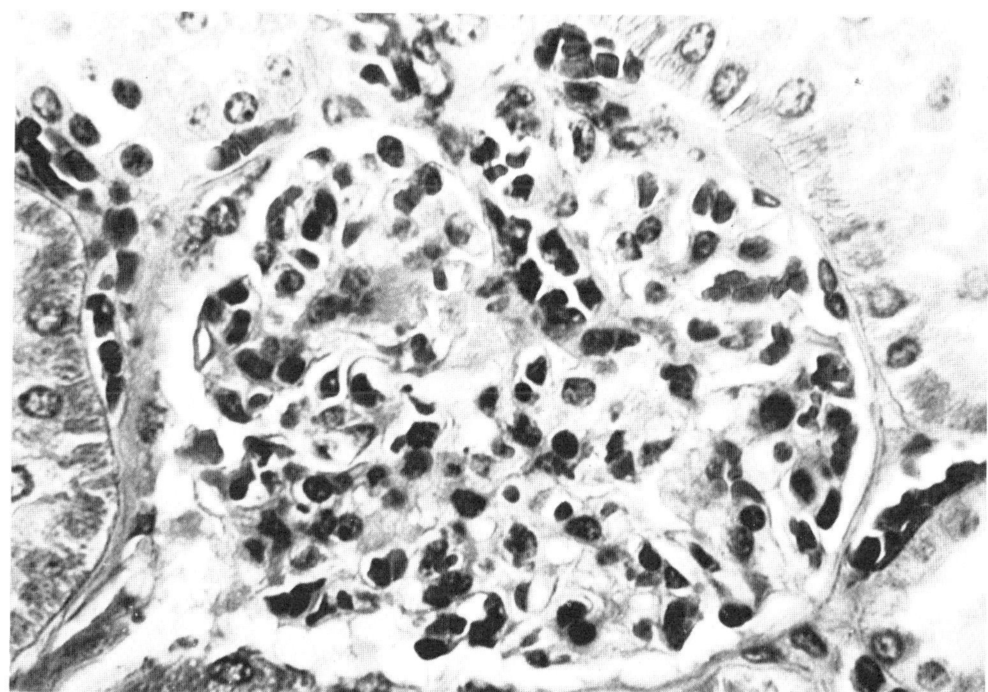

Figure 8-23 *A*, kidney from a normal 16-week-old C57BL/6J male mouse. *B*, kidney from a 16-week-old tumor-progressor male mouse of the same stain, showing prominent hypercellularity and increased mesangial matrix. Hematoxylin and eosin-stained 3 μ sections. Magnification × 324. (Reproduced with permission, P. K. F. Poskitt, T. R. Poskitt, and J. H. Wallace, *J. Exp. Med.* 140:410, 1974.)

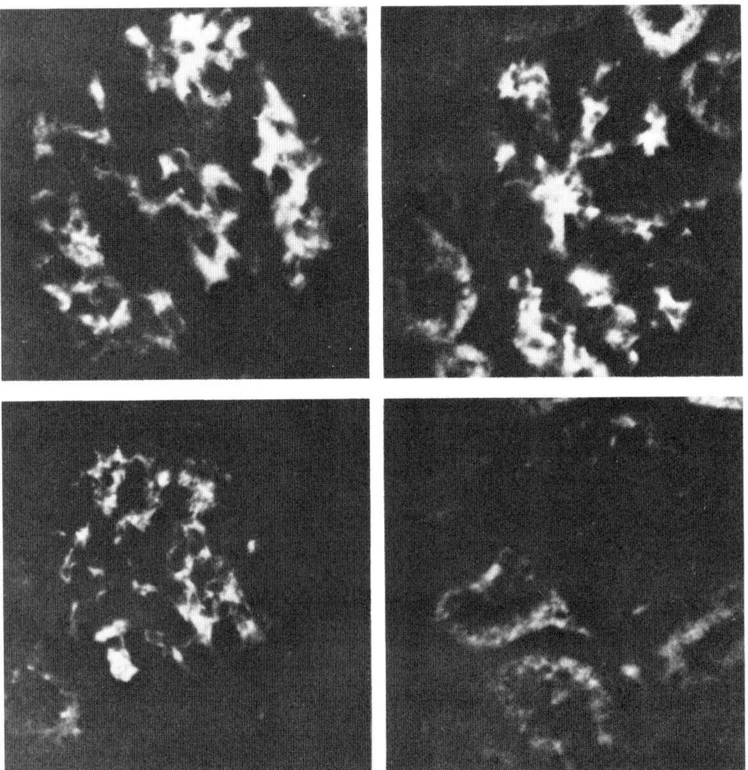

Figure 8-24 *Above left,* a tumor-progressor glomerulus stained with anti-IgG FITC, showing granular mesangial and GBM deposits. *Above right,* a tumor-progressor glomerulus stained with anti-IgM FITC. The deposits are primarily mesangial. *Below left,* a tumor-progressor glomerulus stained with anti-IgA FITC. The deposits are primarily mesangial. *Below right,* age-matched nontumor-bearing control stained with anti-IgM FITC. Magnification × 200. (Reproduced with permission, P. K. F. Poskitt, T. R. Poskitt, and J. H. Wallace, *J. Exp. Med.* 140:410, 1974.)

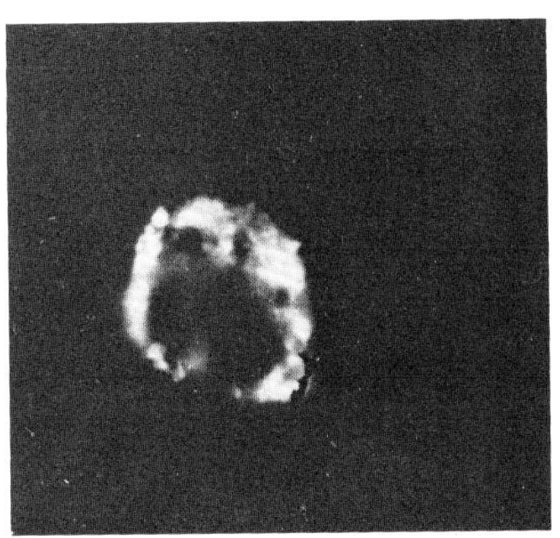
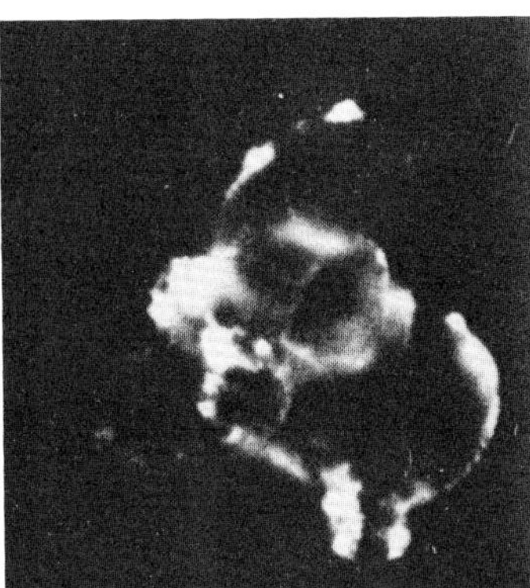

Figure 8-25 Indirect immunofluorescence for IgG antibody activity against B-16 cell membranes. *Left,* pooled (K1 and citrate) renal eluate from tumor-progressor mice. *Right,* pooled undiluted serum from tumor-progressor mice. (Reproduced with permission, P. K. F. Poskitt, T. R. Poskitt, and J. H. Wallace, *J. Exp. Med.* 140:410, 1974.)

around pulmonary or subcutaneous metastases, and presence of strong immunofluorescent renal deposits. This striking relationship is shown in Figure 8-26. Moreover, in vitro assays of serum or immune-complex–mediated blocking of lymphocyte-mediated killing of target tumor cells showed a direct correlation with presence of detectable immune complexes in renal glomeruli. These studies are of special significance in view of the possible role of anti-idiotypes and antigen-antibody complexes in affecting the course of human melanoma.

In summary, it is clear that immune complexes may function to modulate and alter the immune response of the host bearing a tumor. Deposition of immune complexes including normal tissue antigens or relatively unique

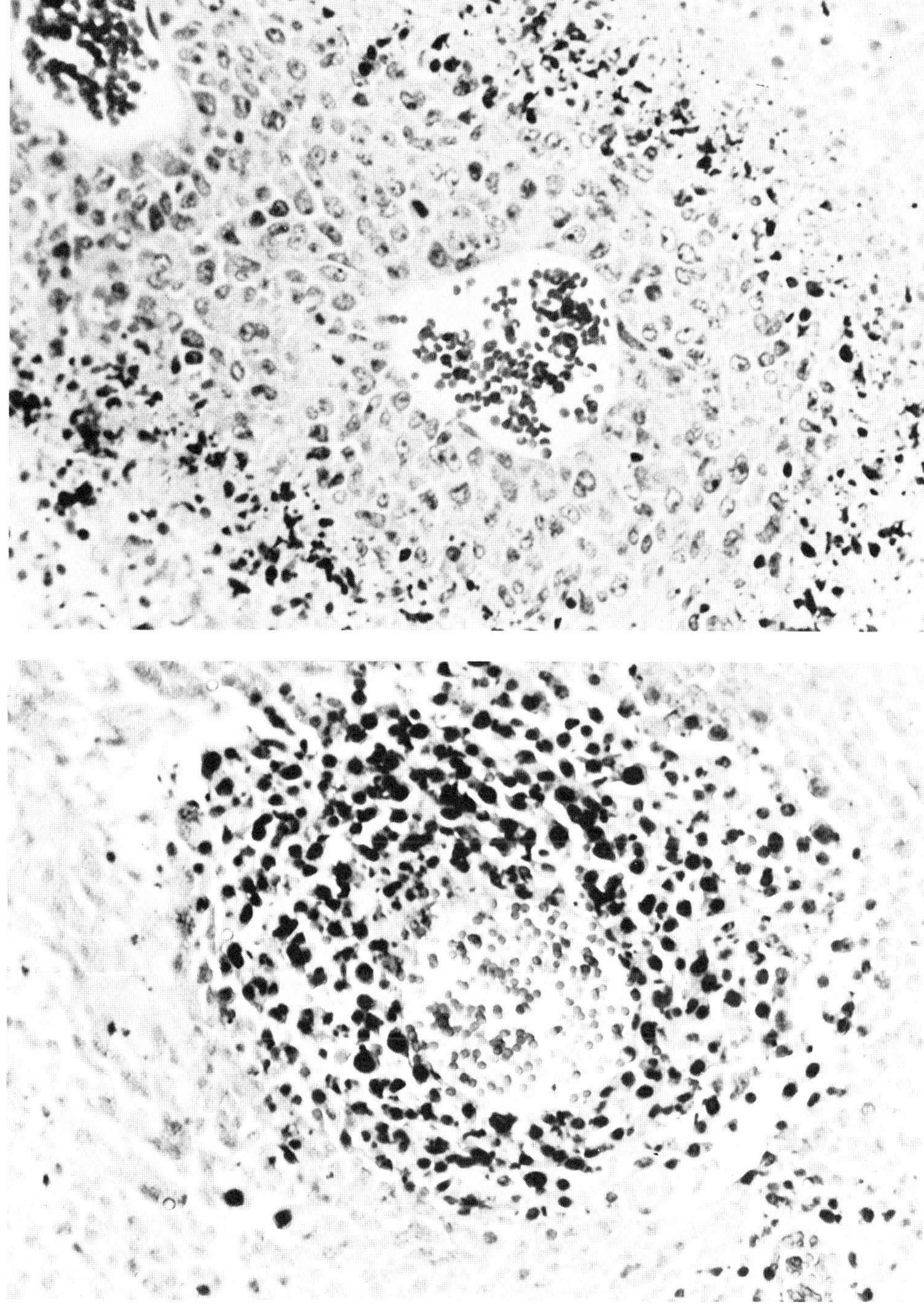

Figure 8-26 Hematoxylin and eosin-stained sections of subcutaneous B-16 melanoma. *Above,* sections from a representative animal with >2+ renal IgG, showing healthy tumor cells around the blood vessel with no MNL infiltrate. *Below,* sections from a representative animal with <1+ renal IgG, showing MNL infiltrate surrounding the blood vessel and dead or dying tumor cells in the vicinity of the infiltrate. Both photos, magnification × 160. (Reproduced with permission, P. K. F. Poskitt, T. R. Poskitt, and J. H. Wallace, *J. Exp. Med.* 140:410, 1974.)

tumor-related materials occur in the renal mesangium or GBM as a complication or direct result of excessive host response and subsequent manufacture of antibodies directed at tumor-related antigens. Much of the tumor-associated nephropathy seen with hypernephromas, carcinoma of the colon, or lung tumors may indeed involve antigen-antibody deposits related somehow to the original tumors. However, the findings in some patients with Hodgkin's disease and minimal-change nephrosis indicate that perhaps other mechanisms of massive proteinuria quite distinct from those mediated by local immune-complex deposition may also be involved.

One of the most critical areas in designing new and uncharted courses in the management of malignant disease is first to understand or identify precisely the level at which the presence of immune complexes is of most biological importance. Is it at the level of the actual tumor cell membrane, at the interface between natural killer cell or macrophage and tumor cell, or in the reticuloendothelial system that the primary effects are crucial? The answers to these questions may be forthcoming. Much of what we have learned about the immune reaction to tumors is unsettling; in some circumstances immune complexes actually may be self-defeating, as in the case of enhancement. However, there are other features of tumor immunity that appear to be eminently useful and potentially of great therapeutic benefit. An understanding of immune complex interaction with the defensive and effector immune systems of the host may eventually unravel some of the basic questions related to tumor metastasis and perhaps tumor autonomy itself.

References

1. Hellström, I., Hellström, K. E., and Pierce, G. E. *In vitro* studies of immune reactions against autochthonous and syngeneic mouse tumors induced by methylcholanthrene and plastic discs. *Int. J. Cancer* 3:467, 1968.

2. Hellström, I., Hellström, K. E., and Sjögren, H. O. Serum mediated inhibition of cellular immunity to methylcholanthrene-induced murine sarcomas. *Cell. Immunol.* 1:18, 1970.

3. Hellström, K. E., and Hellström, I. Immunological enhancement as studied by cell culture techniques. *Ann. Rev. Microbiol.* 24:373, 1970.

4. Möller, G. Effect on tumour growth in syngeneic recipients of antibodies against tumour-specific antigens in methylcholanthrene-induced mouse sarcomas. *Nature* 204:846, 1964.

5. Hellström, I., and Hellström, K. E. Studies on cellular immunity and its serum mediated inhibition in Moloney-virus-induced mouse sarcomas. *Int. J. Cancer* 4:587, 1969.

6. Klein, G., Clifford, P., Klein, E., et al. Search for tumor-specific immune reactions in Burkitt lymphoma patients by the membrane immunofluorescence reaction. *Proc. Natl. Acad. Sci. USA* 55:1628, 1966.

7. Lamon, E. W., Gatti, R. A., Kiessling, R., et al. Comparison of the allospecific and viral-specific immune responses to irradiated versus formaldehyde-fixed allogeneic Moloney lymphoma cells in CBA mice. *Cancer Res.* 35:962, 1975.

8. Nowinski, R. C., Kaehler, S. L., and Burgess, R. R. Immune response in the mouse to endogenous leukemia viruses. *Cold Spring Harbor Symp. Quant. Biol.* 39:1123, 1975.

9. Bolognesi, D. P., Luftig, R., and Shaper, J. H. Localization of RNA tumor virus polypeptides. I. Isolation of further virus substructures. *Virology* 56:549, 1973.

10. Hunsmann, G., Claviez, M., Moennig, V., et al. Properties of mouse leukemia viruses. X. Occurrence of viral structural antigens on the cell surface as revealed by a cytotoxicity test. *Virology* 69:157, 1976.

11. Grant, J. P., Bigner, D. D., Fischinger, P. J., et al. Expression of murine leukemia virus structural antigens on the surface of chemically induced murine sarcomas. *Proc. Natl. Acad. Sci. USA* 71:5037, 1974.

12. Poskitt, P. K. F., Poskitt, T. R., and Wallace, J. H. Renal deposition of soluble immune complexes in mice bearing B-16 melanoma. Characterization of complexes and relationship to tumor progress. *J. Exp. Med.* 140:410, 1974.

13. Hellström, I., Hellström, K. E., Pierce, G. E., et al. Demonstration of cell-bound and humoral immunity against neuroblastoma cells. *Proc. Natl. Acad. Sci. USA* 60:1231, 1968.

14. Diehl, V., Jereb, B., Stjernswärd, J., et al. Cellular immunity to nephroblastoma. *Int. J. Cancer* 7:277, 1971.

15. Lewis, M. G., Ikonopisov, R. L., Nairn, R. C., et al. Tumour-specific antibodies in human malignant melanoma and their relationship to the extent of the disease. *Br. Med. J.* 3:547, 1969.

16. Morton, D. L., Malmgren, R. A., Holmes, E. C., et al. Demonstration of antibodies against human malignant melanoma by immunofluorescence. *Surgery* 64:233, 1968.

17. Muna, N. M., Marcus, S., and Smart, C. Detection by immunofluorescence of antibodies specific for human malignant melanoma cells. *Cancer* 23:88, 1969.

18. Hellström, I., Hellström, K. E., Pierce, G. E., et al. Cellular immunity to colonic carcinomas in man. In W. J. Burdette, ed., *Carcinoma of the Colon and Antecedent Epithelium,* p. 176. Charles C Thomas, Springfield, Ill., 1970.

19. Eilber, F. R., and Morton, D. L. Sarcoma-specific antigens: detection by complement fixation with serum from sarcoma patients. *J. Natl. Cancer Inst.* 44:651, 1970.

20. Wood, W. C., and Morton, D. L. Host immune response to a common cell-surface antigen in human sarcomas. *N. Engl. J. Med.* 284:569, 1971.

21. Morton, D. L., Eilber, F. R., and Malmgren, R. A. Immune factors in human cancer: malignant melanomas, skeletal and soft tissue sarcomas. *Prog. Exp. Tumor Res.* 14:25, 1971.

22. Greaves, M. F., Brown, G., Rapson, N. T., et al. Antisera to acute lymphoblastic leukemia cells. *Clin. Immunol. Immunopathol.* 4:67, 1975.

23. Greaves, M. F., Janossy, G., Roberts, M., et al. Membrane phenotyping: diagnosis, monitoring and classification of acute lymphoid leukemias. In S. Therfelder, H. Rodt, and E. Thill, eds., *Immunological Diagnosis of Leukemias and Lymphomas,* p. 61. Springer-Verlag, Munich, 1976.

24. Liang, W., and Cohen, E. P. Activation of specific cellular immunity toward murine leukemia in mice rejecting syngeneic somatic hybrid cells. *J. Immunol.* 119:1054, 1977.

25. Yu, A., and Cohen, E. P. Studies on the effect of specific antisera on the metabolism of cellular antigens. I. Isolation of thymus leukemia antigens. *J. Immunol.* 112:1285, 1974.

26. Zighelboim, J., Bonavida, B., and Fahey, J. L. Antibody-mediated *in vivo* suppression of EL4 leukemia in a syngeneic host. *J. Natl. Cancer Inst.* 52:879, 1974.

27. O'Toole, C., Perlmann, P., Unsgaard, B., et al. Cellular immunity to human urinary bladder carcinoma. I. Correlation to clinical stage and radiotherapy. *Int. J. Cancer* 10:77, 1972.

28. O'Toole, C., Stejskal, V., Perlmann, P., et al. Lymphoid cells mediating tumor-specific cytotoxicity to carcinoma of the urinary bladder. Separation of the effector population using a surface marker. *J. Exp. Med.* 139:457, 1974.

29. Gold, P., and Freedman, S. O. Specific carcinoembryonic antigens of the human digestive system. *J. Exp. Med.* 122:467, 1965.

30. Moore, T. L., Kupchik, H. Z., Marcon, N., et al. Carcinoembryonic antigen assay in cancer of the colon and pancreas and other digestive tract disorders. *Am. J. Dig. Dis.* 16:1, 1971.

31. Stevens, D. P., and Mackay, I. R. Increased carcinoembryonic antigen in heavy cigarette smokers. *Lancet* 2:1238, 1973.

32. Rule, A. H., Straus, E., Vandevoorde, J., et al. Tumor-associated (CEA-reacting) antigen in patients with inflammatory bowel disease. *N. Engl. J. Med.* 287:24, 1972.

33. Munjal, D., Zamcheck, N., Kupchik, H. Z., et al. Correlation of carcinoembryonic antigen content with carboxylesterase activity in benign and malignant human tissues. *Cancer Res.* 34:2936, 1974.

34. Zamcheck, N., Moore, T. L., Dhar, P., et al. Immunologic diagnosis and prognosis of human digestive-tract cancer: carcinoembryonic antigens. *N. Engl. J. Med.* 286:83, 1972.

35. Zamcheck, N. The present status of CEA in diagnosis and therapy evaluation of colon cancer. *Cancer* 36:154, 1975.

36. Hall, R. R., Laurence, D. J., Darcy, D., et al. Carcinoembryonic antigen in the urine of patients with urothelial carcinoma. *Br. Med. J.* 3:609, 1972.

37. Chu, T. M., and Nemoto, T. Evaluation of carcinoembryonic antigen in human mammary carcinoma. *J. Natl. Cancer Inst.* 51:1119, 1973.

38. Concannon, J. P., Dalbow, M. H., Liebler, G. A., et al. The carcinoembryonic antigen assay in bronchogenic carcinoma. *Cancer* 34:184, 1974.

39. Martin, E. W., Jr., Kibbey, W. E., Di Vecchia, L., et al. Carcinoembryonic antigen: clinical and historical aspects. *Cancer* 37:62, 1976.

40. Coligan, J. E., Henkart, P. A., Todd, C. W., et al. Heterogeneity of the carcinoembryonic antigen. *Immunochemistry* 10:591, 1973.

41. Edgington, T. S., Astarita, R. W., and Plow, E. F. Association of an isomeric species of carcinoembryonic antigen with neoplasia of the gastrointestinal tract. *N. Engl. J. Med.* 293:103, 1975.

42. Hollinshead, A., McWright, C. G., Alford, T. C., et al. Separation of skin reactive intestinal cancer antigen from the carcinoembryonic antigen of Gold. *Science* 177:887, 1972.

43. Zamcheck, N., Kupchik, H. Z., and Pusztaszeri, G. CEA-S—a more specific CEA? *N. Engl. J. Med.* 293:145, 1975.

44. Gold, P., Gold, M., and Freedman, S. O.

Cellular location of carcinoembryonic antigens of the human digestive system. *Cancer Res.* 28:1331, 1968.

45. Martin, E. W., Skivolocki, W., Minton, J. P., et al. CEA as an adjunct in the diagnosis and prognosis of colorectal carcinoma. *Rev. Surg.* 32:214, 1975.

46. Livingstone, A. S., Hampson, L. G., Shuster, J., et al. Carcinoembryonic antigen in the diagnosis and management of colorectal carcinoma. Current status. *Arch. Surg.* 109:259, 1974.

47. Martin, E. W., Jr., James, K. K., Hurtubise, P. E., et al. The use of CEA as an early indicator for gastrointestinal tumor recurrence and second-look procedures. *Cancer* 39:440, 1977.

48. Abelev, G. I., Perova, S. D., Khramkova, N. I., et al. Production of embryonal α-globulin by transplantable mouse hepatomas. *Transplantation* 1:174, 1963.

49. Abelev, G. I. Alpha-fetoprotein in oncogenesis and its association with malignant tumors. *Adv. Cancer Res.* 14:295, 1971.

50. Sell, S., and Morris, H. P. Relationship of rat α_1-fetoprotein to rate and chromosome composition of Morris hepatomas. *Cancer Res.* 34:1413, 1974.

51. Waldmann, T. A., and McIntire, K. R. The use of a radioimmunoassay for alpha-fetoprotein in the diagnosis of malignancy. *Cancer* 34:1510, 1974.

52. McIntire, K. R., Waldmann, T. A., Moertel, C. G., et al. Serum alpha-fetoprotein in patients with neoplasms of the gastrointestinal tract. *Cancer Res.* 35:991, 1975.

53. Ruoslahti, E., and Terry, W. D. α-foetoprotein and serum albumin show sequence homology. *Nature* 260:804, 1976.

54. Murray-Lyon, I. M., Orr, A. H., Gazzard, B., et al. Prognostic value of serum alpha-fetoprotein in fulminant hepatic failure including patients treated by charcoal haemoperfusion. *Gut* 17:576, 1976.

55. Smuckler, E. A., Koplitz, M., and Sell, S. α-fetoprotein in toxic liver injury. *Cancer Res.* 36:4558, 1976.

56. Ruoslahti, E., and Seppälä, M. Studies of carcino-fetal proteins: physical and chemical properties of human α-fetoprotein. *Int. J. Cancer* 7:218, 1971.

57. Yachnin, S., and Lester, E. Inhibition of human lymphocyte transformation by human alpha-foetoprotein (HAFP); comparison of foetal and hepatoma HAFP and kinetic studies of *in vitro* immunosuppression. *Clin. Exp. Immunol.* 26:484, 1976.

58. Yachnin, S. Demonstration of the inhibitory effect of human alpha-fetoprotein on *in vitro* transformation of human lymphocytes. *Proc. Natl. Acad. Sci. USA* 73:2857, 1976.

59. Lester, E. P., Miller, J. B., and Yachnin, S. Human alpha-fetoprotein as a modulator of human lymphocyte transformation: correlation of biological potency with electrophoretic variants. *Proc. Natl. Acad. Sci. USA* 73:4645, 1976.

60. Zimmerman, E. F., Voorting-Hawking, M., and Michael, J. G. Immunosuppression by mouse sialylated α-foetoprotein. *Nature* 265:354, 1977.

61. Murgita, R. A., and Tomasi, T. B., Jr. Suppression of the immune response by α-fetoprotein. I. The effect of mouse α-fetoprotein on the primary and secondary antibody response. *J. Exp. Med.* 141:269, 1975.

62. Murgita, R. A., and Tomasi, T. B., Jr. Suppression of the immune response by α-fetoprotein. II. The effect of mouse α-fetoprotein on mixed lymphocyte reactivity and mitogen-induced lymphocyte transformation. *J. Exp. Med.* 141:440, 1975.

63. Dattwyler, R. J., and Tomasi, T. B. Inhibition of sensitization of T-cells by alpha-fetoprotein. *Int. J. Cancer* 16:942, 1975.

64. Murgita, R. A., Goidl, E. A., Kontiainen, S., et al. α-fetoprotein induces suppressor T cells *in vitro*. *Nature* 267:257, 1977.

65. Sheppard, H. W., Jr., Sell, S., Trefts, P., et al. Effects of α-fetoprotein on murine immune responses. I. Studies on mice. *J. Immunol.* 119:91, 1977.

66. Sell, S., Sheppard, H. W., Jr., and Poler, M. Effects of α-fetoprotein on murine immune responses. II. Studies on rats. *J. Immunol.* 119:98, 1977.

67. Fujinami, R. S., Paterson, P. Y., Parmely, M. J., et al. Lack of suppressive effect of α-foetoprotein on development of experimental allergic encephalomyelitis in rats. *Nature* 264:782, 1976.

68. Gold, P. Circulating antibodies against carcinoembryonic antigens of the human digestive system. *Cancer* 20:1663, 1967.

69. Costanza, M. E., Pinn, V., Schwartz, R. S., et al. Carcinoembryonic antigen-antibody complexes in a patient with colonic carcinoma and nephrotic syndrome. *N. Engl. J. Med.* 289:520, 1973.

70. Greaves, M. F. Recent progress in the immunological characterization of leukaemic cells. *Blut* 34:349, 1977.

71. Roberts, M., Greaves, M., Janossy, G., et al. Acute lymphoblastic leukaemia (ALL) associated antigen—I. Expression in different haematopoietic malignancies. *Leukemia Research* 2:105, 1978.

72. Chessells, J. M., Hardisty, R. M., Rapson, N.

T., et al. Acute lymphoblastic leukaemia in children: classification and prognosis. *Lancet* 2:1307, 1977.

73. Fass, L., Herberman, R. B., Ziegler, J. L., et al. Cutaneous hypersensitivity reactions to autologous extracts of malignant melanoma cells. *Lancet* 1:116, 1970.

74. Hellström, I., and Hellström, K. E. Some recent studies on cellular immunity to human melanomas. *Fed. Proc.* 32:156, 1973.

75. Lewis, M. G., Avis, P. J. G., Phillips, T. M., et al. Tumor-associated antigens in human malignant melanoma. *Yale J. Biol. Med.* 46:661, 1973.

76. Lewis, M. G., and Phillips, T. M. The specificity of surface membrane immunofluoresence in human malignant melanoma. *Int. J. Cancer* 10:105, 1972.

77. Carey, T. E., Takahashi, T., Resnick, L. A., et al. Cell surface antigens of human malignant melanoma. I. Mixed hemadsorption assays for humoral immunity to cultured autologous melanoma cells. *Proc. Natl. Acad. Sci. USA* 73:3278, 1976.

78. Shiku, H., Takahashi, T., Oettgen, H. F., et al. Cell surface antigens of human malignant melanoma. II. Serological typing with immune adherence assays and definition of two new surface antigens. *J. Exp. Med.* 144:873, 1976.

79. Shiku, H., Takahashi, T., Resnick, L. A., et al. Cell surface antigens of human malignant melanoma. III. Recognition of autoantibodies with unusual characteristics. *J. Exp. Med.* 145:784, 1977.

80. Whitehouse, J. M., and Holborow, E. J. Smooth muscle antibody in malignant disease. *Br. Med. J.* 4:511, 1971.

81. Yoshida, T. O. Autoantibodies in the sera of various cancer patients. *Gann Monogr.* 16:63, 1974.

82. McClintock, P. R., Ihle, J. N., and Joseph, D. R. Expression of AKR murine leukemia virus GP71-like and BALB (X) GP71-like antigens in normal mouse tissues in the absence of overt virus expression. *J. Exp. Med.* 146:422, 1977.

83. Wecker, E., Schimpl, A., and Hünig, T. Expression of MuLV GP71-like antigen in normal mouse spleen cells induced by antigenic stimulation. *Nature* 269:598, 1977.

84. Moroni, C., and Schumann, G. Are endogenous C-type viruses involved in the immune system? *Nature* 269:600, 1977.

85. Burnet, M. F. The history of immunological ideas. In *Self and Not Self: Cellular Immunology,* bk. 1, p. 12. Melbourne University Press and Cambridge University Press, Victoria and London, 1969.

86. Kaliss, N. Immunological enhancement of tumor homografts in mice: a review. *Cancer Res.* 18:992, 1958.

87. Kaliss, N. Immunological enhancement. *Int. Rev. Exp. Pathol.* 8:241, 1969.

88. Kaliss, N. Dynamics of immunologic enhancement. *Transplant. Proc.* 2:59, 1970.

89. Takasugi, M., and Hildemann, W. H. Regulation of immunity toward allogeneic tumors in mice. I. Effect of antiserum fractions on tumor growth. *J. Natl. Cancer Inst.* 43:843, 1969.

90. Billingham, R. E., Brent, L., and Medawar, P. B. "Enhancement" in normal homografts with a note on its possible mechanics. *Transplant. Bull.* 3:84, 1956.

91. Möller, G. Antibody-induced depression of the immune response. A study of the mechanism in various immunological systems. *Transplantation* 2:405, 1964.

92. Möller, E. Antagonistic effects of humoral isoantibodies on the *in vitro* cytotoxicity of immune lymphoid cells. *J. Exp. Med.* 122:11, 1965.

93. Feldmann, M., and Diener, E. Antibody-mediated suppression of the immune response *in vitro. J. Exp. Med.* 131:247, 1970.

94. Heppner, G. H. Studies on serum-mediated inhibition of cellular immunity to spontaneous mouse mammary tumors. *Int. J. Cancer* 4:608, 1969.

95. Bubeník, J., Iványi, J., and Koldovský, P. Participation of 7S and 19S antibodies in enhancement and resistance to methylcholanthrene-induced tumours. *Folia Biol. (Praha)* 11:426, 1965.

96. Ran, M., and Witz, I. P. Tumor-associated immunoglobulins. The elution of IgG2 from mouse tumors. *Int. J. Cancer* 6:361, 1970.

97. Witz, I. P., Yagi, Y., and Pressman, D. IgG associated with microsomes from autochthonous hepatomas and normal liver of rats. *Cancer Res.* 27:2295, 1967.

98. Ran, M., and Witz, I. P. Tumor-associated immunoglobulins. Enhancement of syngeneic tumors by IgG2-containing tumor eluates. *Int. J. Cancer* 9:242, 1972.

99. Irvin, G. L., III, Eustace, J. C., and Fahey, J. L. Enhancement activity of mouse immunoglobulin classes. *J. Immunol.* 99:1085, 1967.

100. Tokuda, S., and McEntee, F. Immunologic enhancement of sarcoma I by mouse gamma-globulin fractions. *Transplantation* 5:606, 1967.

101. Klein, E., Klein, G., Nadkarni, J. S., et al. Surface IgM-kappa specificity on a Burkitt lymphoma cell *in vivo* and derived cell lines. *Cancer Res.* 28:1300, 1968.

102. Klein, G., Clifford, P., Henle, G., et al. EBV-associated serological patterns in a Burkitt lymphoma patient during regression and recurrence. *Int. J. Cancer* 4:416, 1969.

103. Langvad, E., Hydén, H., Wolf, H., et al. Extracorporeal immunoadsorption of circulating specific serum factors in cancer patients. *Br. J. Cancer* 32:680, 1975.

104. Taniguchi, M., Hayakawa, K., and Tada, T. Properties of antigen-specific suppressive T cell factor in the regulation of antibody response of the mouse. II. *In vitro* activity and evidence for the I region gene product. *J. Immunol.* 116:542, 1976.

105. Tada, T., and Takemori, T. Selective roles of thymus-derived lymphocytes in the antibody response. I. Differential suppressive effect of carrier-primed T cells on hapten-specific IgM and IgG antibody responses. *J. Exp. Med.* 140:239, 1974.

106. Binz, H., and Wigzell, H. Shared idiotypic determinants on B and T lymphocytes reactive against the same antigenic determinants. I. Demonstration of similar or identical idiotypes on IgG molecules and T-cell receptors with specificity for the same alloantigens. *J. Exp. Med.* 142:197, 1975.

107. Binz, H., and Wigzell, H. Shared idiotypic determinants on B and T lymphocytes reactive against the same antigenic determinants. V. Biochemical and serological characteristics of naturally occurring, soluble antigen-binding T-lymphocyte-derived molecules. *Scand. J. Immunol.* 5:559, 1976.

108. Prange, C. A., Fiedler, J., Nitecki, D. E., et al. Inhibition of T-antigen-binding cells by idiotypic antisera. *J. Exp. Med.* 146:766, 1977.

109. Perlmann, P., and Holm, G. Cytotoxic effects of lymphoid cells *in vitro. Adv. Immunol.* 11:117, 1969.

110. Forman, J., and Möller, G. The effector cell in antibody-induced cell-mediated immunity. *Transplant. Rev.* 17:108, 1973.

111. Tracey, D. E., Pross, H. F., Jondal, M., et al. Antibody-dependent cell-mediated cytotoxic activity in syngeneic mouse ascites tumors. *Int. J. Cancer* 16:870, 1975.

112. Peters, C. J., and Theofilopoulos, A. N. Antibody-dependent cellular cytotoxicity against murine leukemia viral antigens: studies with human lymphoblastoid cell lines and human peripheral lymphocytes as effector cells comparing rabbit, goat, and mouse antisera. *J. Immunol.* 119:1089, 1977.

113. Nelson, D. L., Bundy, B. M., Pitchon, H. E., et al. The effector cells in human peripheral blood mediating mitogen-induced cellular cytotoxicity and antibody-dependent cellular cytotoxicity. *J. Immunol.* 117:1472, 1976.

114. Zighelboim, J., Bonavida, B., and Fahey, J. L. Evidence for several cell populations active in antibody dependent cellular cytotoxicity. *J. Immunol.* 111:1737, 1973.

115. Ramshaw, I. A., and Parish, C. R. Surface properties of cells involved in antibody-dependent cytotoxicity. *Cell. Immunol.* 21:226, 1976.

116. Greenberg, A. H. L., Hudson, L., Shen, L., et al. Antibody-dependent cell-mediated cytotoxicity due to a "null" lymphoid cell. *Nature (New Biol.)* 242:111, 1973.

117. Lamon, E. W., Whitten, H. D., Lidin, B., et al. IgM-induced tumor cell cytotoxicity mediated by normal thymocytes. *J. Exp. Med.* 142:542, 1975.

118. Kamo, I., Patel, C., Kateley, J., et al. Immunosuppression induced *in vitro* by mastocytoma tumor cells and cell-free extracts. *J. Immunol.* 114:1749, 1975.

119. DeLustro, F., and Argyris, B. F. Mechanism of mastocytoma-mediated suppression of lymphocyte reactivity. *J. Immunol.* 117:2073, 1976.

120. McCarthy, R. E. Modification of the immune response of mice to skin homografts and heterografts by Ehrlich ascites carcinoma. *Cancer Res.* 24:915, 1964.

121. Hrsak, I., and Marotti, T. Mechanism of the immunosuppressive effect of Ehrlich ascitic tumour. *Eur. J. Cancer* 11:181, 1975.

122. Frost, P., and Lance, E. M. Abrogation of lymphocyte trapping by ascitic tumours. *Nature* 246:101, 1973.

123. Gorczynski, R. M. Immunity to murine sarcoma virus-induced tumors. II. Suppression of T cell-mediated immunity by cells from progressor animals. *J. Immunol.* 112:1826, 1974.

124. Kirchner, H., Muchmore, A. V., Chused, T. M., et al. Inhibition of proliferation of lymphoma cells and T lymphocytes by suppressor cells from spleens of tumor-bearing mice. *J. Immunol.* 114:206, 1975.

125. Cerny, J., Grinwich, K. D., and Stiller, R. A. Immunosuppression by spleen cells from Moloney leukemia. III. Evidence for a suppressor cell that is not the leukemic, virus-producing cell. *J. Immunol.* 119:1097, 1977.

126. Goodwin, J. S., Messner, R. P., Bankhurst, A. D., et al. Prostaglandin producing suppressor cells in Hodgkin's disease. *N. Engl. J. Med.* 297:963, 1977.

127. Husby, G., Strickland, R. G., Rigler, G. L., et al. Direct immunochemical detection of prostaglandin-E and cyclic nucleotides in human malignant tumors. *Cancer* 40:1629, 1977.

128. Mackaness, G. B. Cellular resistance to infection. *J. Exp. Med.* 116:381, 1962.

129. Mackaness, G. B. The immunological basis of acquired cellular resistance. *J. Exp. Med.* 120:105, 1964.

130. Hibbs, J. B., Jr., Lambert, L. H., Jr., and Remington, J. S. Possible role of macrophage mediated nonspecific cytotoxicity in tumour resistance. *Nature (New Biol.)* 235:48, 1972.

131. Remington, J. S., Krahenbuhl, J. L., and Hibbs, J. B., Jr. A role for the macrophage in resistance to tumor development and tumor destruction. In R. van Furth, ed., *Mononuclear Phagocytes in Immunity, Infection and Pathology,* p. 869. Blackwell Scientific Publications, London, 1975.

132. Wing, E. J., Gardner, I. D., Ryning, F. W., et al. Dissociation of effector functions in populations of activated macrophages. *Nature* 268:642, 1977.

133. Evans, R., and Alexander, P. Mechanism of immunologically specific killing of tumour cells by macrophages. *Nature* 236:168, 1972.

134. Forman, J., and Britton, S. Heterogeneity of the effector cells in the cytotoxic reaction against allogeneic lymphoma cells. *J. Exp. Med.* 137:369, 1973.

135. Krahenbuhl, J. L., and Lambert, L. H., Jr. Cytokinetic studies of the effects of activated macrophages on tumor target cells. *J. Natl. Cancer Inst.* 54:1433, 1975.

136. Evans, R., and Alexander, P. Cooperation of immune lymphoid cells with macrophages in tumour immunity. *Nature* 228:620, 1970.

137. Takasugi, M., and Klein, E. The role of blocking antibodies in immunological enhancement. *Immunology* 21:675, 1971.

138. Jagarlamoody, S. M., Aust, J. C., Tew, R. H., et al. *In vitro* detection of cytotoxic cellular immunity against tumor-specific antigens by a radioisotopic technique. *Proc. Natl. Acad. Sci. USA* 68:1346, 1971.

139. Baldwin, R. W., Price, M. R., and Robins, R. A. Blocking of lymphocyte-mediated cytotoxicity for rat hepatoma cells by tumour-specific antigen-antibody complexes. *Nature (New Biol.)* 238:185, 1972.

140. Hellström, I., Hellström, K. E., Sjögren, H. O., et al. Serum factors in tumor-free patients cancelling the blocking of cell-mediated tumor immunity. *Int. J. Cancer* 8:185, 1971.

141. Kunkel, H. G., Mannik, M. D., and Williams, R. C., Jr. Individual antigenic specificity of isolated antibodies. *Science* 140:1218, 1963.

142. Williams, R. C., Jr., Kunkel, H. G., and Capra, J. D. Antigenic specificities related to the cold agglutinin activity of gamma M globulins. *Science* 161:379, 1968.

143. Sjögren, H. O., Hellström, I., Bansal, S. C., et al. Suggestive evidence that the "blocking antibodies" of tumor-bearing individuals may be antigen-antibody complexes. *Proc. Natl. Acad. Sci. USA* 68:1372, 1971.

144. Jose, D. G., and Skvaril, F. Serum inhibitors of cellular immunity in human neuroblastoma. IgG subclass of blocking activity. *Int. J. Cancer* 13:173, 1974.

145. Jose, D. G., and Seshadri, R. Circulating immune complexes in human neuroblastoma: direct assay and role in blocking specific cellular immunity. *Int. J. Cancer* 13:824, 1974.

146. Sjögren, H. O., and Bansal, S. C. Antigens in virally induced tumors. In B. Amon, ed., *Progress in Immunology,* p. 921. Academic Press, New York, 1971.

147. Fowler, G. A., and Nauts, H. C. The apparently beneficial effects of concurrent infections, inflammation or fever, and of bacterial toxin therapy on neuroblastoma. Monograph no. 11. New York Cancer Institute, New York, 1970.

148. Mantovani, A., and Spreafico, F. On the nature of blocking factors and their lymphoid target cells in an allogeneic tumor system. *Eur. J. Cancer* 11:451, 1975.

149. Currie, G. A., and Basham, C. Serum mediated inhibition of the immunological reactions of the patient to his own tumour: a possible role for circulating antigen. *Br. J. Cancer* 26:427, 1972.

150. Ferluga, J., Friou, G. J., and Allison, A. C. Cytotoxic activity of human lymphocyte plasma membranes. *Clin. Exp. Immunol.* 25:347, 1976.

151. Hersh, E. M., Whitecar, J. P., Jr., McCredie, K. B., et al. Chemotherapy, immunocompetence, immunosuppression and prognosis in acute leukemia. *N. Engl. J. Med.* 285:1211, 1971.

152. Alexander, P., Bensted, J., Delorme, E. J., et al. The cellular immune response to primary sarcomata in rats. II. Abnormal responses of nodes draining the tumour. *Proc. R. Soc. Lond. (Biol.)* 174:237, 1967.

153. Currie, G. A. Effect of active immunization with irradiated tumour cells on specific serum inhibitors of cell-mediated immunity in patients with disseminated cancer. *Br. J. Cancer* 28:25, 1973.

154. Currie, G. A. The role of circulating antigen as an inhibitor of tumour immunity in man. *Br. J. Cancer* 28:153, 1973 (suppl. 1).

155. Sinkovics, J. G., Cabiness, J. R., and Shullenberger, C. C. Disappearance after chemotherapy

of blocking serum factors as measured *in vitro* with lymphocytes cytotoxic to tumor cells. *Cancer* 30:1428, 1972.

156. Gorczynski, R., Kontiainen, S., Mitchison, N. A., et al. Antigen-antibody complexes as blocking factors on the T lymphocyte surface. In G. M. Edelman, ed., *Cellular Selection and Regulation in the Immune Response,* p. 143. Raven Press, New York, 1974.

157. Tamerius, J., Nepom, J., Hellström, I., et al. Tumor-associated blocking factors: isolation from sera of tumor-bearing mice. *J. Immunol.* 116:724, 1976.

158. Hellström, I., and Hellström, K. E. Colony inhibition studies on blocking and non-blocking serum effects on cellular immunity to Moloney sarcomas. *Int. J. Cancer* 5:195, 1970.

159. Jerne, N. K. Clonal selection in a lymphocyte network. In G. M. Edelman, ed., *Cellular Selection and Regulation in the Immune Response,* p. 39. Raven Press, New York, 1974.

160. Lewis, M. G., Phillips, T. M., Cook, K. B., et al. Possible explanation for loss of detectable antibody in patients with disseminated malignant melanoma. *Nature* 232:52, 1971.

161. Hartmann, D., and Lewis, M. G. Presence and possible role of anti-IgG antibodies in human malignancy. *Lancet* 1:1318, 1974.

162. Hartmann, D., Lewis, M. G., Proctor, J. W., et al. *In vitro* interactions between antitumour antibodies and anti-antibodies in malignancy. *Lancet* 2:1481, 1974.

163. Lewis, M. G. Immunology and the melanomas. *Curr. Top. Microbiol. Immunol.* 63:49, 1974.

164. Jerry, L. M., Lewis, M. G., and Cano, P. Anergy, anti-antibodies and immune complex disease: a syndrome of disordered immune regulation in human cancer. In M. Martin and L. Dionne, eds., *Immunocancerology in Solid Tumors,* p. 63. Stratton Intercontinental Medical Book Corp., New York, 1976.

165. Lewis, M. G., Hartmann, D. P., and Jerry, L. M. Antibodies and anti-antibodies in human malignancy. An expression of deranged immune regulation. *Ann. N.Y. Acad. Sci.* 276:316, 1976.

166. Milgrom, F., Dubiski, S., and Woźniczko, G. Human sera with "anti-antibody." *Vox Sang.* 1:172, 1956.

167. Osterland, C. K., Harboe, M., and Kunkel, H. G. Anti-γ-globulin factors in human sera revealed by enzymatic splitting of anti-Rh antibodies. *Vox Sang.* 8:133, 1963.

168. Waller, M., Curry, N., and Richard, A. Serological specificity of IgG and IgM antiglobulin antibodies in anti-Gm (a) antisera. *Clin. Exp. Immunol.* 3:631, 1968.

169. Williams, R. C., Jr. Heterogeneity of L-chain sites on Bence-Jones proteins reacting with anti-gamma-globulin factors. *Proc. Natl. Acad. Sci. USA* 52:60, 1964.

170. Pyrhonen, S., Timonen T., Heikkinen, A., et al. Rheumatoid factor as an indicator of serum blocking activity and tumour recurrences in bladder tumours. *Eur. J. Cancer* 12:87, 1976.

171. Ludwig, F. J., and Cusumano, C. L. Detection of immune complexes using ^{125}I goat anti (human IgG) monovalent F(ab'$_2$) antibody fragments. *J. Natl. Cancer Inst.* 52:1529, 1974.

172. Oldstone, M. B. A., Theofilopoulos, A. N., Gurvén, P., et al. Immune complexes associated with neoplasia: presence of Epstein-Barr virus antigen-antibody complexes in Burkitt's lymphoma. *Intervirology* 4:292, 1974.

173. Heimer, R., and Klein, G. Circulating immune complexes in sera of patients with Burkitt's lymphoma and nasopharyngeal carcinoma. *Int. J. Cancer* 18:310, 1976.

174. Wolf, H., Hausen, H. zur, and Becker, V. EB viral gemomes in epithelial nasopharyngeal carcinoma cells. *Nature (New Biol.)* 244:245, 1973.

175. Irie, K., Irie, R. F., and Morton, D. L. Detection of antibody and complement complexed *in vivo* on membranes of human cancer cells by mixed hemadsorption techniques. *Cancer Res.* 35:1244, 1975.

176. Gupta, R. K., and Morton, D. L. Suggestive evidence for *in vivo* binding of specific antitumor antibodies of human melanomas. *Cancer Res.* 35:58, 1975.

177. Phillips, T. M., and Lewis, M. G. A method for elution of immunoglobulin from the surface of living cells. *Rev. Eur. Etud. Clin. Biol.* 16:1052, 1971.

178. Thunold, S., Tönder, O., and Larsen, O. Immunoglobulins in eluates of malignant human tumors. *Acta Pathol. Microbiol. Scand. (A)* 236:97, 1973 (suppl.).

179. Irie, K. Detection of *in vivo* antigen/antibody/complement complexes on membranes of human cancer cells. *Proc. Am. Assoc. Cancer Res.* 15:88, 1974.

180. Irie, K., Irie, R. F., and Morton, D. L. Evidence for *in vivo* reaction of antibody and complement to surface antigens of human cancer cells. *Science* 186:454, 1974.

181. Witz, I. P. Tumor-associated immunoglobulins. *Isr. J. Med. Sci.* 7:230, 1971.

182. Cohen, D., Gurner, B. W., and Coombs, R. R. A. A phenomenon resembling opsonic adherence shown by disaggregated cells of the transmissible venereal tumour of the dog. *Br. J. Exp. Pathol.* 52:447, 1971.

183. Milgrom, F., Humphrey, L. J., Tönder, O., et al. Antibody-mediated hemadsorption by tumor tissues. *Int. Arch. Allergy Appl. Immunol.* 33:478, 1968.

184. Tønder, O., Morse, P. A., Jr., and Humphrey, L. J. Similarities of Fc receptors in human malignant tissue and normal lymphoid tissue. *J. Immunol.* 113:1162, 1974.

185. Wood, G. W., Gillespie, G. Y., and Barth, R. F. Receptor sites for antigen-antibody complexes on cells derived from solid tumors: detection by means of antibody sensitized sheep erythrocytes labeled with technetium-99m. *J. Immunol.* 114:950, 1975.

186. Long, J. C., Hall. C. L., Brown, C. A., et al. Binding of soluble immune complexes in serum of patients with Hodgkin's disease to tissue cultures derived from the tumor. *N. Engl. J. Med.* 297:295, 1977.

187. Longmire, R. L., McMillan, R., Yelenosky, B. S., et al. *In vitro* splenic IgG synthesis in Hodgkin's disease. *N. Engl. J. Med.* 289:763, 1973.

188. Lichtenfeld, J. L., Wiernik, P. H., Mardiney, M. R., Jr., et al. Abnormalities of complement and its components in patients with acute leukemia, Hodgkin's disease, and sarcoma. *Cancer Res.* 36:3678, 1976.

189. Jerry, L. M., Rowden, G., Cano, P. O., et al. Immune complexes in human melanoma: a consequence of deranged immune regulation. *Scand. J. Immunol.* 5:845, 1976.

190. Teshima, H., Wanebo, H., Pinsky, C., et al. Circulating immune complexes detected by ^{125}I-C1q deviation test in sera of cancer patients. *J. Clin. Invest.* 59:1134, 1977.

191. Rossen, R. D., Reisberg, M. A., Hersh, E. M., et al. The C1q binding test for soluble immune complexes: clinical correlations obtained in patients with cancer. *J. Natl. Cancer Inst.* 58:1205, 1977.

192. Samayoa, E. A., McDuffie, F. C., Nelson, A. M., et al. Immunoglobulin complexes in sera of patients with malignancy. *Int. J. Cancer* 19:12, 1977.

193. Hoffken, K., Meredith, I. D., Robins, R. A., et al. Circulating immune complexes in patients with breast cancer. *Br. Med. J.* 2:218, 1977.

194. Theofilopoulos, A. N., Wilson, C. B., and Dixon, F. J. The Raji cell radioimmune assay for detecting immune complexes in human sera. *J. Clin. Invest.* 57:169, 1976.

195. Amlot, P. L., Slaney, J. M., and Williams, B. D. Circulating immune complexes and symptoms in Hodgkin's disease. *Lancet* 1:449, 1976.

196. Carbone, P. P., Kaplan, H. S., Musshoff, K., et al. Report of the committee on Hodgkin's disease staging classification. *Cancer Res.* 31:1860, 1971.

197. Musshoff, K., Boutis, L., Laszlo, A. M., et al. Prognostische Krankheitssymptome und zeichen bei Morbus Hodgkin und ihre Bedeutung für die Therapie der Erkrankung. *Strahlentherapie* 131:482, 1966.

198. Root, R. K., and Wolff, S. M. Pathogenetic mechanisms in experimental immune fever. *J. Exp. Med.* 128:309, 1968.

199. Sheagren, J. N., Block, J. B., and Wolff, S. M. Reticuloendothelial system phagocytic function in patients with Hodgkin's disease. *J. Clin. Invest.* 46:855, 1967.

200. Bennett, J. M., Nathanson, L., and Rutenberg, A. M. Significance of leukocyte alkaline phosphatase in Hodgkin's disease. *Arch. Intern. Med.* 121:338, 1968.

201. Bethell, F. H., Andrews, G. A., Neligh, R. B., et al. Treatment of Hodgkin's disease with roentgen irradiation and nitrogen mustards. *Am. J. Roentgenol. Radium Ther. Nucl. Med.* 64:61, 1950.

202. Sohar, E., Gafni, J., Pras, M., et al. Familial Mediterranean fever: a survey of 470 cases and review of the literature. *Am. J. Med.* 43:227, 1967.

203. Ehrenfeld, E. N., Eliakim, M., and Rachmilewitz, M. Recurrent polyserositis (familial Mediterranean fever; periodic disease). A report of fifty-five cases. *Am. J. Med.* 31:107, 1961.

204. Gafni, J., Ravid, M. and Sohar, E. The role of amyloidosis in familial Mediterranean fever. A population study. *Isr. J. Med. Sci.* 4:995, 1968.

205. Mathé, G. Cancer active immunotherapy. Immunoprophylaxis and immunorestoration. An introduction. *Recent Results Cancer Res.* 55:1, 1976.

206. Mathé G., Amiel, J. L., Schwarzenberg, L., et al. Active immunotherapy for acute lymphoblastic leukemia *Lancet* 1:697, 1969

207. Mathé, G., Amiel, J. L., Schwarzenberg, L., et al. Follow-up of the first (1962) pilot study of active immunotherapy of acute lymphoid leukemia: a critical discussion. *Biomedicine* 26:29, 1977.

208. Carpentier, N. A., Lange, G. T., Fiere, D. M., et al. Clinical relevance of circulating immune complexes in human leukemia. Association in acute leukemia of the presence of immune complexes with unfavorable prognosis. *J. Clin. Invest.* 60:874, 1977.

209. Izui, S., Lambert, P. H., Carpentier, N., et al. The occurrence of antibodies against single-stranded DNA in the sera of patients with acute and chronic leukemia. *Clin. Exp. Immunol.* 24:379, 1976.

210. Klein, G., Steiner, M., Wiener, F., et al. Human leukemia-associated antinuclear reactivity. *Proc. Natl. Acad. Sci. USA* 71:685, 1974.

211. Steiner, M., Klein, E., and Klein, G. Antinuclear reactivity of sera in patients with leukemia

and other neoplastic diseases. *Clin. Immunol. Immunopathol.* 4:374, 1975.

212. Mann, D. L., Halterman, R., and Leventhal, B. Acute leukemia-associated antigens. *Cancer* 34:1446, 1974.

213. Baker, M. A., Ramachandar, K., and Taub, R. N. Specificity of heteroantisera to human acute leukemia-associated antigens. *J. Clin. Invest.* 54:1273, 1974.

214. Mohanakumar, T., Metzgar, R. S., and Miller, D. S. Human leukemia cell antigens: serologic characterization with zenoantisera. *J. Natl. Cancer Inst.* 52:1435, 1974.

215. Brown, G., Capellaro, D., and Greaves, M. Leukemia-associated antigens in man. *J. Natl. Cancer Inst.* 55:1281, 1975.

216. Harris, R. Leukemia antigens and immunity in man. *Nature* 241:95, 1973.

217. Greaves, M. F., Janossy, G., Roberts, M., et al. Membrane phenotyping: diagnosis, monitoring and classification of acute 'lymphoid' leukemias. *Haematol. Blood Transfus.* 20:61, 1977.

218. Soothill, J. F., and Steward, M. W. The immunopathological significance of the heterogeneity of antibody affinity. *Clin. Exp. Immunol.* 9:193, 1971.

219. MacLennan, I. C. M., Gale, D. G. L., and Wood, J. Resistance of certain leukaemic myeloblasts to immunological attack. *Int. J. Cancer* 15:995, 1975.

220. Lee, J. C., Yamauchi, H., and Hopper, J., Jr. The association of cancer and the nephrotic syndrome. *Ann. Intern. Med.* 64:41, 1966.

221. Sherman, R. L., Susin, M., Weksler, M. E., et al. Lipoid nephrosis in Hodgkin's disease. *Am. J. Med.* 52:699, 1972.

222. Kiely, J. M., Wagoner, R. D., and Holley, K. E. Renal complications of lymphoma. *Ann. Intern. Med.* 71:1159, 1969.

223. Ghosh, L., and Muehrcke, R. C. The nephrotic syndrome: a prodrome to lymphoma. *Ann. Intern. Med.* 72:379, 1970.

224. Plager, J., and Stutzman, L. Acute nephrotic syndrome as a manifestation of active Hodgkin's disease. Report of four cases and review of the literature. *Am. J. Med.* 50:56, 1971.

225. Kiy, Y. Síndrome nefrótica associada á doenca de Hodgkin. *Rev. Hosp. Clin. Fac. Med. Sao Paulo* 22:186, 1967.

226. Hyman, L. R., Burkholder, P. M., Joo, P. A., et al. Malignant lymphoma and nephrotic syndrome. A clinicopathologic analysis with light, immunofluorescence, and electron microscopy of the renal lesions. *J. Pediatr.* 82:207, 1973.

227. Lewis, M. G., Loughridge, L. W., and Phillips, T. M. Immunological studies in nephrotic syndrome associated with extrarenal malignant disease. *Lancet* 2:134, 1971.

228. Cantrell, E. G. Nephrotic syndrome cured by removal of gastric carcinoma. *Br. Med. J.* 1:739, 1969.

229. Revol, L., Viala, J. J., Revillard, J. P., et al. Protéinurie associée à des manifestations paranéoplasiques au cours d'un cancer bronchique. *Lyon Medicale* 212:907, 1964.

230. Ozawa, T., Pluss, R., Lacher, J., et al. Endogenous immune complex nephropathy associated with malignancy. I. Studies on the nature and immunopathogenic significance of glomerular bound antigen and antibody, isolation and characterization of tumor specific antigen and antibody and circulating immune complexes. *Q. J. Med.* 44:523, 1975.

231. Edgington, T. S., Glassock, R. J., and Dixon, F. J. Autologous immune complex nephritis induced with renal tubular antigen. I. Identification and isolation of the pathogenetic antigen. *J. Exp. Med.* 127:555, 1968.

232. Moorthy, A. V., Zimmerman, S. W., and Burkholder, P. M. Nephrotic syndrome in Hodgkin's disease. Evidence for pathogenesis alternative to immune complex deposition. *Am. J. Med.* 61:471, 1976.

233. Shalhoub, R. J. Pathogenesis of lipoid nephrosis: a disorder of T-cell function. *Lancet* 2:556, 1974.

234. Cohen, S., Fisher, B., Yoshida, T., et al. Serum migration-inhibitory activity in patients with lymphoproliferative diseases. *N. Engl. J. Med.* 290:882, 1974.

235. Higgins, M. R., Randall, R. E., Jr., and Still, W. J. S. Nephrotic syndrome with oat-cell carcinoma. *Br. Med. J.* 3:450, 1974.

236. Sutherland, J. C., Markham, R. V., Jr., and Mardiney, M. R., Jr. Subclinical immune complexes in the glomeruli of kidneys postmortem. *Am. J. Med.* 57:536, 1974.

237. Sutherland, J. C., Markham, R. V., Jr., Ramsey, H. E., et al. Subclinical immune complex nephritis in patients with Hodgkin's disease. *Cancer Res.* 34:1179, 1974.

238. Sitprija, V., Pipantanagul, V., Boonpucknavig, V., et al. Glomerulitis in typhoid fever. *Ann. Intern. Med.* 81:210, 1974.

CHAPTER 9

Allergic Disorders

For many years humoral factors of an unusual kind have often been associated with immediate-type hypersensitivity reactions. In spontaneous skin reactivity to pollens such as ragweed, the reactive effect was known to be transferred from sensitive to normally insensitive individuals by a heat-labile humoral factor inactivated at 56° C. If serum from an allergic patient is injected into a normal subject and the skin rechallenged with presumptive allergens, a definite immediate wheal and surrounding area of inflammation is noted. Passive transfer of immediate-type hypersensitivity by humoral factors in serum from allergic donors is known as the Prausnitz-Küstner (or P-K) reaction, after the clinicians who first used it to demonstrate passive transfer (1).

Reagin, IgE, and Immediate Hypersensitivity

During the early work on reagins (2–7), empirical clinical observations established that various desensitization procedures involving repeated small increments of rather crude preparations of antigens actually resulted in improvement in patients' symptoms. Despite uncertainties about how reagins worked, practical implementation of desensitization procedures was established and a great deal of useful clinical insight obtained long before precise knowledge of the immunochemical nature of either reagin or specific allergens evolved. Little relating to the actual molecular biology of this series of phenomena was understood until several highly unusual myeloma proteins

appeared on the scene. These myelomas did not react with any of the then available typing antisera with specificity for H-chain determinants on IgG, IgA, IgD, or IgM. Moreover, physical and immunochemical studies showed them to be slightly larger (8 S) than ordinary IgG antibody molecules and to possess unique H-chain antigens not shared by other immunoglobulins. The chemical structure of IgE is considerably different from IgG, IgA, IgM, or IgD (8–10). The molecule itself (shown schematically in Figure 9-1) appears to have more intrachain disulfide bonds, a higher methionine content, and an entirely different conformation than the other common immunoglobulins.

Studies by several groups indicated that skin injection of these isolated monoclonal IgE proteins was capable of inhibition of the Prausnitz-Küstner reaction (12) and was somehow directly linked to the immediate hypersensitivity reaction. IgE was present in much lower concentration than most of the other immunoglobulins in most normal sera. Methods of quantitation now used in most clinical laboratories involve radioimmunoassay inhibition techniques using specific anti-IgE antisera usually manufactured against several isolated IgE myeloma proteins (13–15). A comparison between quantitative amounts of IgE and other major classes of immunoglobulins in addition to other physical properties is shown in Table 9-1. Studies of patient groups afflicted with allergic disorders, such as extrinsic asthma and hay fever, have indicated quantitative elevations of IgE in the sera of many indi-

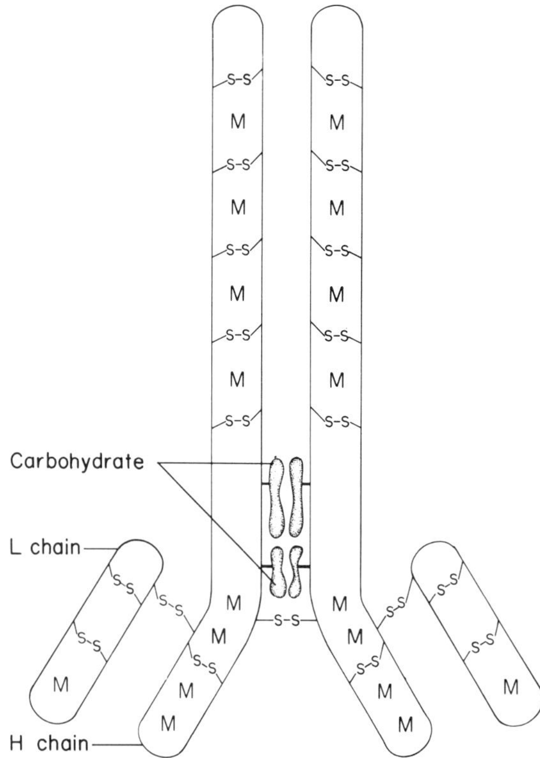

Figure 9-1 Probable structure of an immunoglobulin E or IgE molecule, indicating relatively high methionine content (M), large numbers of intra-H-chain disulfide bonds, and probable location of carbohydrate.

viduals (16, 17). It was also recognized that IgE elevations frequently were associated with a wide variety of parasitic infections—particularly with worms (18–21) where levels of 10,000 to 20,000 μg/ml have been recorded.

Clear association between reaginic antibody activity and IgE was established by the work of Ishizaka and Ishizaka (22, 23). With ^{131}I-labeled ragweed antigen E, only antibodies of the IgE class were shown to parallel demonstrable reaginic biologic activity measured by passive transfer into normal human skin. The subsequent explosion in knowledge and attempts to relate IgE-mediated mechanisms to a number of diverse human conditions represent remarkable progress relating basic immunology to clinical medicine.

When it was recognized that IgE had something to do with allergic reactions and particularly immediate hypersensitivity (24), studies directed at the exact mechanisms involved proceeded with great rapidity. It could be shown that IgE molecules exhibited preferential reactivity for a very small subpopulation of human or animal leukocytes—basophils and mast cells. When these target cells became sensitized or coated with even a few IgE molecules, the stage was set for triggering an abrupt immediate hypersensitivity reaction. It is now believed that basophils possessing specific Fc receptors for determinants present on IgE absorb such immunoglobulin molecules. When potential allergen is presented to sensitized cells, the antibody combining site of IgE antibody reacts with allergen and a rapid chain of reactions is set into motion, resulting in release of potent pharmacologic mediators of immediate hypersensitivity such as histamine, slow-reacting substance (SRS), and other small mediator molecules. This sequence of events, which is shown diagrammatically in Figure 9-2,

Table 9-1 Comparison of IgE and other main classes of immunoglobulins.

Immuno-globulin	Sedimentation coefficient	Carbo-hydrate (%)	Molecular weight (Daltons)	Mean serum level[a]	Half-life (days)
IgG	6.8–7.0 S	3	140,000	1200 mg%	23
IgA	7–8 S	10	160,000	400 mg%	6
	(9, 11, 13)[b]				
IgM	18.6–19 S	10	900,000	120 mg%	5
IgE	7.9–8.2 S	10–11	196,000	240 ng/ml	10
IgD	7.0 S	13	180,000	3 mg%	3

[a] In healthy adults.
[b] Possible polymeric forms in serum.

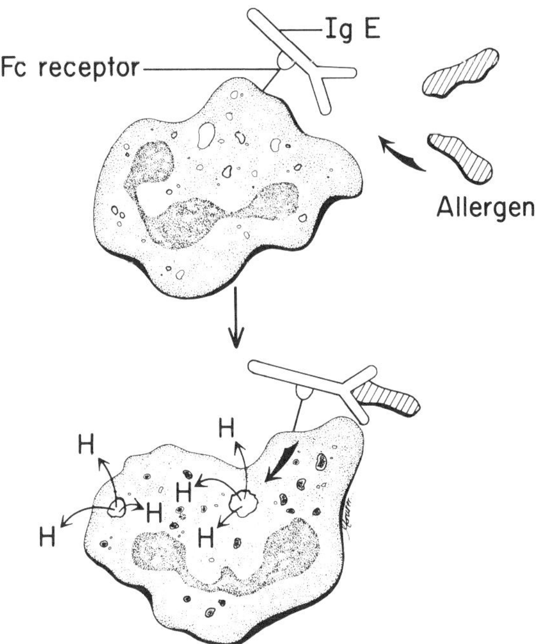

Figure 9-2 Sensitization by an IgE molecule of a basophil or mast cell through interaction with an IgE Fc receptor. When the sensitized basophil encounters allergen, reaction between the IgE antibody combining site and allergen triggers a number of intracellular events including release of histamine (H), slow-reacting substance, and other potent mediators of immediate hypersensitivity.

represents one of the most highly studied and incisive examples of the particularly selective physiological power of cell-localized immune complexes.

Potentially reactive cells such as tissue mast cells or basophils contain natural receptors for Fc portions of reaginic sensitizing antibodies. Histamine release from human blood cells had been studied by a number of investigators before recognition and definitive characterization of the IgE-mediated mechanisms were developed (25–29). More recently, the cellular model defining the actual release phenomena has been elegantly characterized using ragweed pollen antigens in the presence of various human leukocyte preparations (30–37). A representative quantitative histamine release experiment using various concentrations of antigen E obtained from ragweed is shown in Figure 9-3. Allergic histamine release in vitro

requires physiological conditions of pH, temperature, and salt concentration. Calcium and magnesium appear to be necessary for a maximum response, but no requirement for complement is present (30). Reaction of leukocytes sensitized with IgE antibody and histamine release can also be produced by application of heterologous rabbit anti-IgE antibody to human leukocytes (38).

Parallel investigations have shown that basophil-sensitizing IgE antibodies and indeed total quantitative levels of IgE are markedly elevated in certain groups of patients with allergic disorders, such as hay fever, seasonal rhinitis, eczema, and in some patients with asthma, rhinitis, and nasal polyposis. One of the most important features of the allergic patient therefore is his ability to manufacture sizable quantities of IgE antibody to potential allergens in his environment. Beneficial effects achieved when patients are subjected to desensitization procedures has in the past involved attempts to modify this particular response in individual patients. Acute allergic reactions appear to depend principally on rather minute

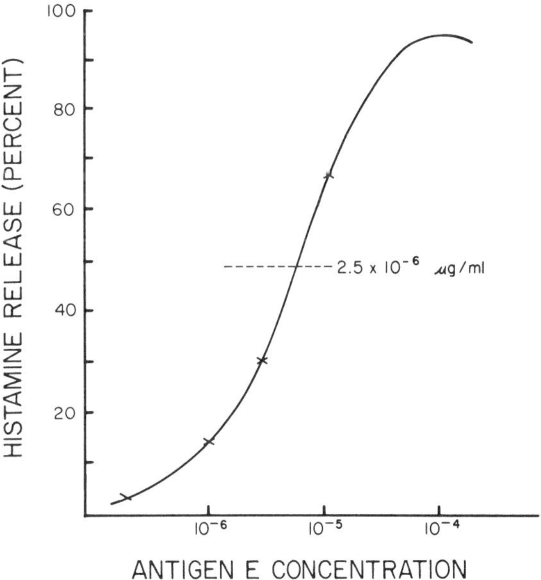

Figure 9-3 Representative curve of histamine release using increasing concentrations of ragweed antigen E. The area of 50-percent total release (2.5 × 10^{-6}) is shown.

amounts of cell-fixed antigen-antibody complexes. The important physiological responses of the patient in the nasal mucosa, bronchial tree, or skin depend upon the presence of sensitized basophils or similar cells such as mast cells with Fc receptors for IgE antibody. In many ways definition of this type of fixed-cell system dependent on minute amounts of an immunoglobulin usually present only in trace amounts in serum of normal subjects represents a completely unique system. Because of the knowledge that has been generated about the manner in which these microreactants interact, this area has been better defined and more carefully studied than many other disease states where both circulating complexes and those fixed to various tissue receptors may be of clinical importance.

The unique features of the IgE immediate hypersensitivity system have been used to develop various assays for measuring degrees of hypersensitivity in individual patients. When it was found that immediate hypersensitivity could be studied using peripheral blood leukocytes from patients, addition of test serum or IgE-containing fractions and potential allergens in vitro resulting in basophil degranulation and histamine release provided a quantitative assessment of the potential reactants in such a system and could be used to follow relative degrees of hypersensitivity in practical clinical situations. This particular technique can be sequentially studied and quantitative assessment made. During the course of ragweed desensitization procedures, the curve of in vitro histamine release on challenge of peripheral blood leukocytes with allergen (Figure 9-3) is often shifted far to the right. That is, it takes considerably more putative antigen added to the same number of leukocytes to effect a certain level of histamine release. Precisely what is happening in the patient as a whole is not yet completely understood.

Many of the earlier studies attempting to decipher events leading to obvious clinical improvement after desensitization procedures suggested what were called blocking antibodies. During the course of increasingly larger periodic injections of putative allergens, such as ragweed, the patient mounted an immune response that included production of a different *quality* of antibody reacting with antigen but that did not result in the release of vasoactive substances and mediator molecules capable of inciting an immediate allergic response. The concept of production of blocking antibody may in fact partially explain some of the beneficial effects of such desensitization procedures. Recent attempts to characterize the immunochemical nature of such blocking antibodies have provided considerable insight into their nature, turnover, and physiological effectiveness (39, 40).

Successful desensitization during immunotherapy for patients with ragweed hay fever is thought to involve production of nonbasophil- or mast-cell-binding IgG antibodies that are capable of combining with antigen without setting off the cycle of basophil or mast-cell degranulation and its unpleasant side reactions. Double-blind studies by several groups have now established that desensitized patients show less severe symptoms of ragweed allergy than those who had not undergone any type of immunotherapy or desensitization procedure (41–43). The beneficial effects of desensitization appear to depend on reduction in the abilities of peripheral blood leukocytes to release histamine with allergen challenge (34, 44). Benefits of desensitization also relate to increases in allergen-directed blocking IgG antibody and reduction in magnitude of seasonal rises of IgE antibodies (34, 37, 39, 40).

During studies conducted by Lichtenstein and colleagues (37) a relationship was recorded between the patient's serum level of IgE reactive with ragweed antigen and the amount of this antibody actually on the patient's basophils as judged by antigen-induced histamine release. The relationship is illustrated in Figure 9-4 using data from this study. In placebo-treated patients, ragweed antigen-specific IgE antibody usually declined gradually prior to ragweed season and was boosted by natural environmental exposure to ragweed pollens. In patients who had received desensitization therapy, IgE antibody specific for ragweed antigens rose at the beginning of a course of treatment but fell as the desensitization proceeded and had significantly decreased in 18 of

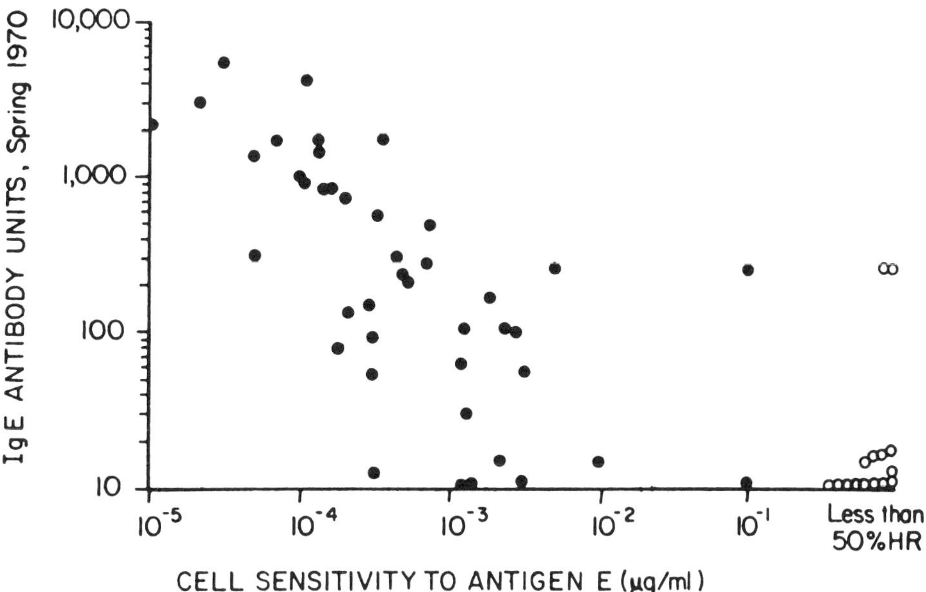

Figure 9-4 The relationship between the serum level of IgE-RaAg and the IgE-RaAg on the basophils of a patient, as judged by antigen-E–induced histamine release (HR). The Spearman-Rank correlation coefficient for the highly sensitive patients (*closed circles*) is 0.74, with $p < 0.01$. All but two of the relatively insensitive patients (*open circles*) have very low IgE-RaAg levels. (Reproduced with permission, L. M. Lichtenstein, K. Ishizaka, P. S. Norman et al., *J. Clin. Invest.* 52:472, 1973.)

19 patients by the end of the second year. Increase in blocking antibody during immunotherapy correlated significantly ($p < .05$) with the decrease in serum-IgE antibody specific for ragweed antigens. Seasonal changes in IgE antibodies were also studied by Yunginger and Gleich (39) who found that such antibodies were elevated in all allergic patients studied. Magnitude of ragweed-specific IgE antibody appeared to be a feature of the preseasonal ragweed IgE antibody level, since IgE antibody production was the same in the groups undergoing desensitization and immunotherapy as it was in the untreated groups when patients were matched on the basis of their preseasonal IgE antibody levels.

A relationship was noted between quantitative levels of IgE and IgG antiragweed antibody (anti-antigen E) in patients receiving high-dose perennial immunotherapy; this provides evidence that immunoglobulin levels are a feature of the basic makeup of certain patients and that IgG antibody rise is not specifically linked to IgE ragweed-specific fall in individual patients. An example of these findings is shown in Figure 9-5. These findings have recently been extended (40) analyzing immunotherapy results in 63 treated patients compared to 40 untreated patients with ragweed hay fever. Again it was found that changes in levels of ragweed-specific IgE were related to IgE levels before the onset of ragweed season, but that desensitization resulted in reduction of the seasonal decrease in IgE antibody from October to July in patients with low levels of IgE antibody. In many subjects undergoing immunotherapy both IgE and IgG-ragweed antibodies were low despite parenteral therapy reflecting the general lower levels of humoral immune response in these particular patients.

These studies have been greatly facilitated by use of the RAST or radioallergosorbent assay (45), an adaptation utilizing solid-phase ragweed antigen linked to cellulose particles. The allergen is allowed to combine with specific antibody in a test serum sample and, after washing, the specific IgE antibody combined with antigen is detected using addition of [131]I-

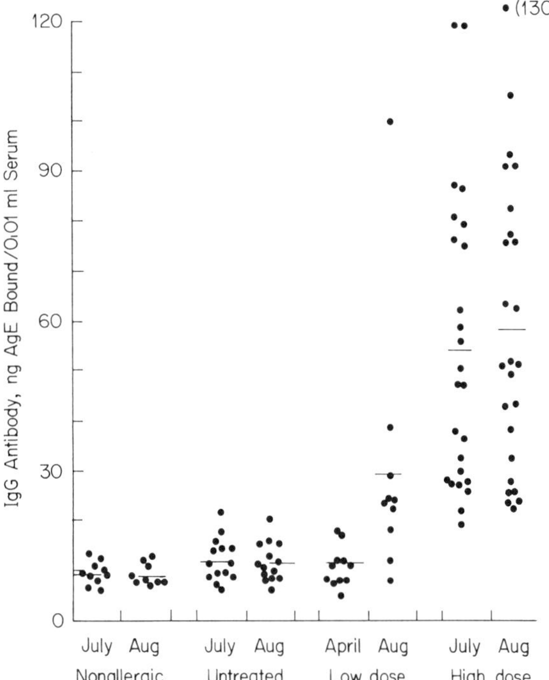

Figure 9-5 Changes in IgG antibodies to antigen E (AgE) in the study groups. Mean values are indicated by bars. (Reproduced with permission, J. W. Yunginger and G. J. Gleich, *J. Clin. Invest.* 52:1268, 1973.)

labeled specific anti-IgE. Diagrammatic representation of this particular assay is shown in Figure 9-6. In instances where some estimate is needed as to how much of the total serum IgE is actually comprised of antiragweed antibody, total serum IgE can be quantitated using the usual double-antibody radioimmunoassay (46) and the results compared with quantities identified as specific IgE ragweed-directed antibody in the RAST.

A variety of changes in the host proper appear to be present during effective clinical courses of desensitization. Studies by several investigators have shown that reactive leukocytes themselves become less liable to histamine release. Thus, regardless of IgE levels the leukocyte thermostatic setting, as it were, is turned far down by the actual desensitization procedure. Precise understanding of this particular aspect of the beneficial results of clinical desensitization is not yet available but is a cur-

rent area of intensive study in many laboratories (34, 37, 47). It may be that actual alteration of important second-messenger mediators such as cAMP or cGMP occurs during desensitization and this in turn produces a basic downshift in sensitivity of leukocytes or tissue mast cells regardless of their external IgE milieu.

Delayed-Type Hypersensitivity Reactions

In contrast to the immediate hypersensitivity reactions described above, the delayed-type reaction has a voluminous and classical history. Delayed-type hypersensitivity, developing in the skin and subcutaneous tissues 24 to 48 hours after cutaneous challenge with antigen, is a much more deliberate expression of host reactivity. Prominent cellular features of such reactions are infiltration by lymphocytes and mononuclear cells as well as edema, and a few polymorphonuclear leukocytes. Classically, de-

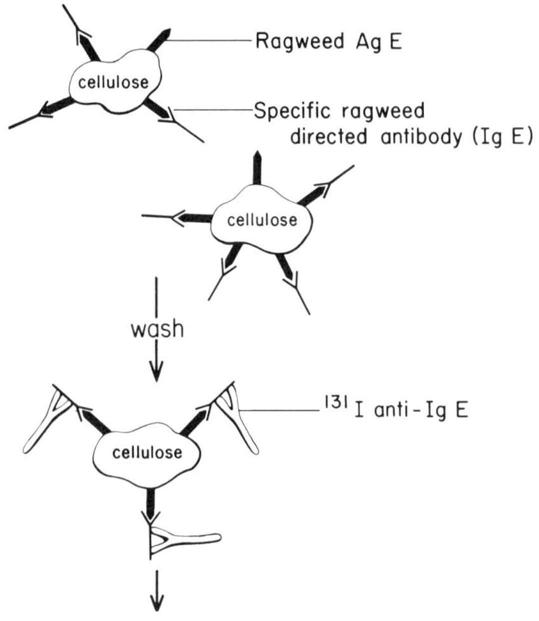

Figure 9-6 Diagrammatic representation of the commonly used RAST, or radioallergosorbent assay.

layed hypersensitivity has been equated with cell-mediated immunity and T-cell response. Monocytes or macrophages also appear to be essential for priming and development of a complete reaction. Many aspects of certain disorders grouped in the category of allergic disturbances may be related to activation of cellular immunity and prolonged rather chronic inflammatory reactions. Among these might be eczema, contact hypersensitivity, or perhaps even such diseases as celiac disease or gluten enteropathy. It is important to point out that macrophage processing and macrophage–T-cell interaction are essential for effective mediation of delayed-type hypersensitivity reactions. The influence of suppressor cells and helper cells in final expression of individual reactions is also of primary importance. The control mechanisms modulating final expression of delayed-type hypersensitivity are important in the regulation of immediate hypersensitivity responses. Thus, work using various experimental animal systems has shown that specific T-suppressor cells exist which control IgE-mediated immune reactions (48–52). Watanabe and co-workers (48) have characterized spleen cells capable of specific suppression of the IgE response in certain strains of mice as belonging to the Ly-1 subset of T cells. Moreover, helper cells apparently specific for IgE antibody production have also been characterized (49). Cell-free supernatants have been shown to contain specific suppressor activities that are not antigen specific and do not contain immunoglobulin determinants (50). A similar factor acting as an IgE-bearing cell facilitator has also been described by Urban and co-workers (51). It is important to point out the potential impact in complete understanding of the built-in regulatory controls for various aspects of IgE synthesis and secretion. These studies reinforce the importance of various normal control mechanisms for many aspects of the immune system and indicate that specific T suppressor cell systems exist that affect only IgE. Therefore, it seems likely that when IgE is elevated in the blood or tissues of certain individuals, the natural IgE-specific suppressor cell mechanism has either been turned off or

somehow attenuated in various clinical situations. Patients who develop IgE-mediated immediate hypersensitivity may in fact represent a subpopulation within the normal range of individuals who have less suppressor cell modulation of built-in IgE responses. It is also possible that activation of natural suppressor cells specific for IgE control and synthesis may occur in clinical situations where allergy to particular substances in the environment disappears normally or even during the course of successful desensitization procedures. Thus, if a pharmacologic way were found to induce IgE-specific suppressor cell activity, clinical control of various allergic reactions could be simplified and directly applied to the practical problem facing the clinician or patient with allergic disease.

IgE System—Independence of Control

The IgE system appears to be distinct from control feedback loops involved in regulation of other immunoglobulins such as IgA, IgG, or IgM. A good example of the basic independence of the IgE immune system is found in occasional patients with immune deficiency who show clear evidence for clinical immediate hypersensitivity and concurrently normal levels of IgE (53–55). In the patient with infantile x-linked agammaglobulinemia reported by Ganier and Lieberman (55), levels of 10 to 60 μg/ml IgE were recorded in serum. This subject showed an immediate hypersensitivity reaction to penicillin. A series of anti-immunoglobulin suppression experiments in mice have established that immunoglobulin-producing cells develop as IgM → IgG → IgA. This is suggested by the work of Kincade and colleagues (56), where administration of anti-μ chain antisera resulted in suppression of IgM, IgG, and IgA cell synthesis. On the other hand, administration of anti-γ-chain suppressed both IgG and IgA and administration of anti-α-chain suppressed only IgA cell synthesis. Dwyer and colleagues (57) showed that administration of anti-μ antisera had no effect on IgE production. These experiments, together with the experiments of nature in which patients with agammaglobulinemia show clear evidence for IgE-mediated immediate hypersensitivity reactions, emphasize the independence in the entire IgE control mechanism.

Cell-Surface Receptors for IgE

Several recent studies have aided in characterization of the mast-cell/basophil cell-surface receptor for IgE. Studies of the receptor in situ and after solubilization with detergent indicate that the effective valence of the IgE receptor is one (58, 59). Moreover, studies of the actual events leading to binding of IgE by mast cells or basophils indicate that some degree of cross-linking of cell-bound antibodies is necessary for final degranulation and histamine release. Cross-linking need not be antigen-mediated since, as noted above, antibody to IgE can also function in this way. This reaction has recently been studied using rat immunoglobulin E treated with a chemical cross-linking agent (60). Monomers produced no histamine release whereas dimers and higher polymers produced active positive responses. Previous observations indicated that mast-cell–basophil degranulation could be induced by bridging of IgE molecules by antigens or by other means. The experiments reported by Segal and colleagues (60) suggest that IgG antibody may bind reversibly but tightly to cell-surface receptors for IgE. These receptors are monovalent and move freely and independently in the plane of the membrane. When two or more receptors become cross-linked by receptor IgE complexes, the minimal signal for triggering is satisfied and cell degranulation occurs. Observations by Brostoff and co-workers (61) may be pertinent to these findings. Evidence of circulating high-molecular-weight forms of IgE appearing as 11 to 17 S material in density gradient analyses was obtained in serum samples from patients with hay fever or atopic eczema. Previous studies have also shown that some sera from patients with hay fever may contain antiglobulins capable of reacting with autologous IgE (62). The exact role played by the IgE complexes in hay fever or atopic eczema is still unclear. If dimers are necessary for cross-linking cell-surface receptors, the formation of

dimers may be somehow facilitated by the presence of these complexes.

Interaction of IgE Complexes and Other Cell Types

The most extensively studied interaction between IgE and cells involved basophils or tissue mast cells and sensitizing IgE antibody. Recently, however, a unique interaction between IgE complexes and macrophages has been described by Capron and colleagues (63), who showed that IgE antibodies complexed to schistosomal parasitic antigens were capable of adsorption to macrophages and induction of subsequent dramatic ultrastructural changes in these cells facilitating specific lytic activity for intermediate schistosomule forms. This IgE-specific arming of macrophages and enhancement of their lytic activity against parasite forms indicates that under certain circumstances IgE may function as a direct humoral mediator for one of the most important protective mechanisms of cell-mediated immunity. One of the striking manifestations of parasitic worm infections in both animals and humans is the production of large amounts of IgE (64, 65). The only well-identified function of IgE antibody itself in such clinical situations is in the induction of immediate hypersensitivity reactions. The almost universal IgE response to parasitic infections has been suggested as an important defense mechanism in its own right. It leads to localized anaphylaxis and a chain of events that eventually focuses the local host inflammatory reaction and provides ready access of other classes of immunoglobulin and immunocytes to the parasite, facilitating eventual worm expulsion. This has been termed the "self-cure" reaction described by Barth and co-workers (66) for rats infected with *Nippostrongylus brasiliensis*. Production of ovalbumin-induced anaphylaxis in rats passively immunized with antiserum to *N. brasiliensis* produced a significant reduction in transplanted populations of adult worms compared with rats that were passively immunized alone or with rats subjected to ovalbumin anaphylaxis alone. It had previously been observed that rats infected subcutaneously with a large worm burden of

500 or more *N. brasiliensis* larvae undergo a self-cure reaction toward the end of the second week of infection manifested by sudden drop in egg production followed over a few days by sudden expulsion of the worms from the intestine (67, 68). Moreover, a degree of immunity was thereby induced in the host to reinfection with either larvae or adult worms. If adult worms were subsequently reintroduced into the small intestine, they were rapidly reexpelled (68). This immunity could be passively transferred with serum. Later it was shown that rats having undergone self-cure could be shocked by an intravenous injection of *N. brasiliensis* antigen, but that the lesions of the shocking process were mainly intestinal in location and resembled changes present in the same rats at the time of self-cure (69).

In the work recorded by Barth and colleagues (66) rats were subjected to intestinal anaphylaxis induced by ovalbumin and *Haemophilus pertussis;* it was noted that the consequent physical alterations in the mucosa did *not* result in worm expulsion. However, if intestinal anaphylaxis was induced in passively immunized rats, significant worm expulsion resulted. These findings suggested that the physical changes associated with anaphylaxis had facilitated extravascular passage of antibody where its effect in this site was directed specifically against the worms leading to subsequent worm expulsion. Furthermore, the local edema and increased capillary permeability inherent in the anaphylaxis within the gut may have allowed immediate access of other immune reactants (such as immunocytes, macrophages, and polymorphs) to the worms, also facilitating expulsion. Evans blue dye studies done in conjunction with this work emphasized the marked degrees of capillary leakage that occurred at the time of successful worm expulsion. This is an attractive theory and one that may be partially involved in host defense against a number of worm parasitic forms.

A parallel has been noted between resistance to *Schistosoma mansoni* or *Schistosoma haematobium* infections and the ability of the host to produce reaginic IgE antibodies (70). More recently it was shown that interaction of IgG antibodies with neutrophils, eosinophils, or macrophages may also be effective in mediating various kinds of direct killing of parasites (71, 72). In the studies recorded by Capron and co-workers (63) in vitro killing of schistosomules by normal macrophages proceeded with remarkable effectiveness in the presence of specific IgE antibody activity. Anti–*S. mansoni* antibody was determined using *S. mansoni* immunoabsorbent and radioimmunoassay. The killing of schistosomules by macrophages was assayed by ^{51}Cr release in the presence of serum containing specific antischistosomal IgE antibody. Of particular interest was that whereas specific antischistosomal antibody was capable of arming macrophages for killing, aggregated rat myeloma IgE protein had no effect. Ultrastructural studies of macrophages incubated with immune IgE-containing serum showed close contact between macrophage membranes and the schistosome and perforation of the parasitic surface by macrophage microvillae—along with phagocytosis of schistosome materials. These findings are shown in Figure 9-7. Studies of IgE binding to macrophages indicated that the numbers of binding sites for IgE appeared to be about the same order of magnitude as those for aggregated IgG. These experiments suggest that in addition to interacting with mast cells or basophils, IgE and antigen complexes are capable of arming killer macrophages and mediating macrophage activation themselves. This amplification of the possible role for IgE in parasite-directed immune reactions represents an important new extension of biologic activity of such complexes and a new class of effector cells. It may be that similar interactions between IgE-antigen complexes play an important role in other more familiar lesions mediated by IgE.

Distribution of IgE-Forming Cells

Since IgE represents a rather unique system implicated as the main immunoglobulin mediator in a variety of immediate hypersensitivity reactions and since, as previously noted, the immune-complex reactions in which immediate-type IgE antibodies participate are largely the result of those fixed to a rather specialized

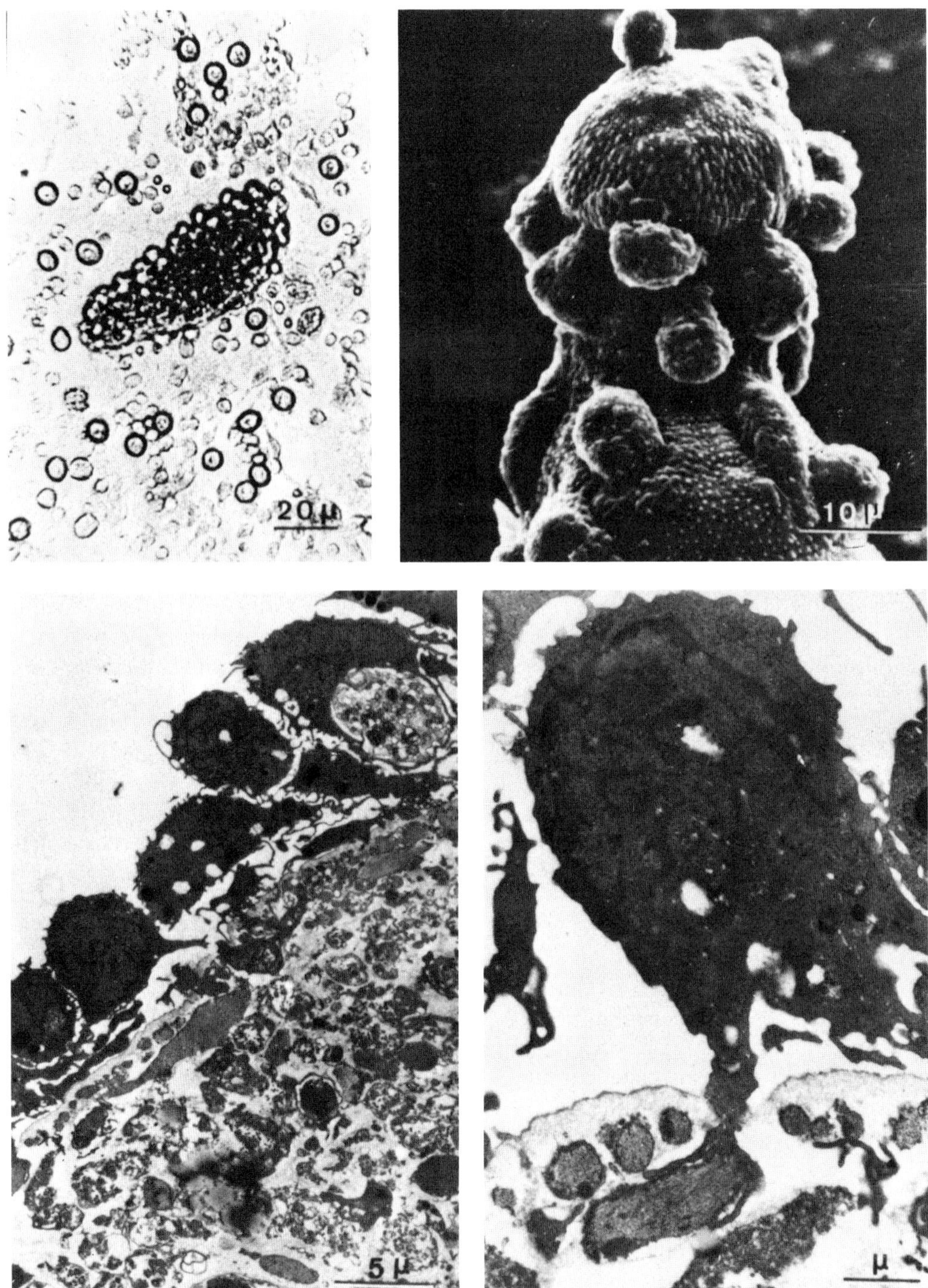

Figure 9-7 The interaction of macrophages incubated with immune rat serum and *S. mansoni* schistosomules. *Top left,* photograph of schistosomule covered with adherent peritoneal exudate cells; *top right,* scanning EM of the same preparation showing close contact between macrophages and the target schistosome; *bottom frame,* ultrastructural studies of macrophage-schistosomule interface showing the perforation of the membrane (*left*) and phagocytosis of the parasitic materials (*right*) by macrophages. (Reproduced with permission, A. Capron, J -P. Dessaint, M. Joseph et al., *Europ. J. Immunol.* 7:315, 1977.)

assortment of tissue mast cells or basophils, it is important to review what is currently known about local sites of synthesis and secretion of IgE itself. Early in the development of basic knowledge in this area, general distribution of IgE-forming cells was studied by immunofluorescence in various tissues of the monkey and human by Tada and Ishizaka (73). Frozen sections were treated with guinea pig anti-IgE and stained with fluorescent antibody against guinea pig immunoglobulins. Frequently present in the respiratory tract and gastrointestinal mucosa and in regional lymph nodes were IgE-forming plasma cells. Some areas within tonsils, adenoids, bronchial, or mesenteric lymph nodes showed germinal centers stained by anti-IgE reagents. By contrast, cells staining for IgE were relatively scarce in the spleen and subcutaneous lymph node system. The numbers of IgE plasma cells detected in lymphoid tissues appeared to be higher than one would expect from the relative serum IgE concentrations. Thus, normal serum levels of IgE average about 0.3 μg/ml, which is approximately 0.001 percent that of IgG and 0.6 to 0.7 percent of IgA. An extreme example of the difference or discrepancy between serum levels and apparent IgE-producing cells was found in the lamina propria of the gastrointestinal mucosa where more IgE than IgG-containing cells were noted in some areas. Nasal polyps from atopic patients were also found to contain many IgE-producing plasma cells. The finding of prominent IgE-containing plasma cells within lamina propria and in other sites within the gastrointestinal tract is a surprising phenomenon and one that we have recently confirmed in our own laboratory. Of interest in this regard is the detection of marked relative elevations of IgE among a large group of miscellaneous patients with chronic liver disease (74). This may represent nonspecific recruitment of IgE helper cells during chronic active liver disease or it may be related in part to basic immune imbalance in such patients with hyperactive B-cell responses and relative T-cell insufficiency represented by lack of an effective suppressor T-cell system.

The detection of concentrations of IgE-containing plasma cells within portions of the respiratory tract was not surprising in view of the common nasal and bronchopulmonary manifestations of acute allergic disorders such as hay fever and asthma. It will be important eventually to map local concentrations of IgE-specific or antigen-specific helper and suppressor cells in tissues of allergic patients. At present reliable reagents capable of identifying tissue localization of human suppressor or helper cells participating perhaps in the vital area of local modulation and control of IgE-mediated hypersensitivity are not yet generally available.

Genetic Control of the Allergic Immune Response

Familial predisposition toward allergic manifestations has been known to occur in some kindreds. This has been documented in each of several major clinical manifestations of allergic disease: hay fever, asthma, and atopic eczema (75–77). The development of HLA typing systems and the recognition that many levels within the immune response are under the control of specific immune-response genes have greatly facilitated this type of analysis. Examples of these associations have been recorded in reports linking ragweed allergen Ra5 and HLA–B7 cross-reacting groups (77–79). Similar associations have been recorded between IgE-mediated sensitivity to the rye group I antigen and HLA–B8 (80), and between sensitivity to ragweed allergen Ra3 and HLA–A2 and B12 (81). A recent study by Bruce and co-workers (82) examined 41 ragweed allergic nonasthmatics on the basis of similar total IgE levels. No significant differences were observed in their sensitivity to ragweed antigen E as monitored by histamine release or in their skin reactivity to ragweed antigens E, Ra3, and Ra5. In this study an increased frequency of HLA–B5 was observed in nonasthmatics as compared to asthmatics. Although frequencies of HLA–A1 and B8 were also elevated in nonasthmatics and HLA–B40 in asthmatics, the differences were not significant. This study is representative of much of the work undertaken to date in attempts to define significant HLA associations with various allergic states. The entire problem is complicated by what probably relates to multiple levels of control related to a number of different genes—all of which can profoundly influence the immediate hypersensitivity immune response. This is illustrated by the fact that several groups have now recorded distinct differences between asthmatics and nonasthmatics in basal cAMP levels within peripheral blood leukocytes; such differences become even more marked following catecholamine stimulation (83–85). No evidence has been produced that basal leukocyte cAMP levels are linked to IR genes. However, these fascinating findings illustrate part of the problem involved with precise identification of genetic factors involved in allergic states. The relative confusion or discrepancies recorded between different groups now working directly on this problem at present probably relate to difficulties in classifying particular clinical groups of patients examined. Thus, in the study cited above by Bruce and co-workers (82) ragweed-sensitive asthmatics were matched with ragweed-sensitive nonasthmatics on the basis of similar IgE levels. Such a comparison makes the tacit assumption that the same or similar genes in both such groups control or ultimately govern total IgE levels. The assumption may be erroneous, since IgE levels in the two groups may actually reflect genetic control at entirely different levels by separate regulatory mechanisms that in some way have a great deal to do with whether or not a ragweed-sensitive individual will develop asthma. The basic difficulty with such analyses is illustrated by the slightly different findings of Thorsby and co-workers (86), who reported increased incidence of haplotypes HLA–A1, B8 and HLA–A2, Bw40 relative to nonasthmatic subjects. The basic difficulties inherent in such analyses were illustrated in the work of Bruce and colleagues (82), which showed the actual similarities in 50-percent leukocyte histamine released in a group of ragweed-sensitive seasonal asthmatics and ragweed-sensitive nonasthmatics. Again it will be noted that patients were paired in this study on the basis of similar total IgE levels. From the data accumulated it would appear that perhaps separate genetic mechanisms are at work in producing: (1) setting of the IgE production apparatus; (2) capacity or inclination for development of ragweed sensitivity; and (3) final susceptibility to intrinsic mechanisms actually resulting in asthma itself. This sort of analysis was predicted perhaps by Rackemann in 1918, when he felt that asthma per se was a separate entity from allergic rhinitis (87). The genetic control of both IgE response and possible susceptibility to ragweed hay fever has also been studied by Levine and colleagues (88). Linkage to HLA–A1, B8 appeared to be involved not only with IgE elevation but with ragweed sensitivity. Considerably more work in larger numbers of patients will be necessary before precise understanding of the linkage of various HLA cell-surface antigens to the variety of clinical manifestations of allergic diathesis is finally reconciled.

Chemical Properties of Allergens

All of us are exposed constantly to a variety of external antigens in our environment through inhalation, ingestion, or surface contact. Fortunately, only a certain proportion of genetically predisposed individuals—estimated at about 10 percent of the population at risk—become sensitized to these antigens during the course of natural exposure (89). The environmental sources of atopic allergens include pollens of grasses, trees, weeds, animal danders, fungi, insects, foods, drugs, chemicals, and laundry detergents including additives such as bacterial enzymes (90). Much progress has been made in the actual characterization and purification of atopic allergenic compounds from various sources (91, 92).

Perhaps the most extensively characterized allergen is that related to late summer hay fever in the eastern United States and Canada, or ragweed pollen. Five antigens derived from ragweed have now been purified. The two most important—antigens E and K—are acidic proteins with molecular weights of 38,000 Daltons. These two materials, which represent 6 and 3 percent respectively of pollen proteins, have been extensively characterized by King and co-workers (93–95). The three other allergens of ragweed pollen have been designated as antigens Ra3, Ra5, and Ra4. They are all basic proteins with lower molecular weights of 11,000, 4,970, and 23,000 Daltons respectively and represent 0.4, 0.4, and 0.9 percent of actual ragweed pollen proteins. The complete amino acid sequence of Ra5 has now been determined (96). Ragweed antigen E is the most active component in producing leukocyte histamine release (93). Antigen K showed about half the histamine-releasing activity of antigen E (94) and its activity appeared to be closely related to antigen E, probably because these materials share common reactive determinants. In ragweed-sensitive patients antigen-E–specific IgE appears to account for an average of 45 percent of all IgE antibodies reacting with ragweed pollen antigens (97, 98). Purification and analysis of ragweed antigen E indicated that the protein consisted of two nonidentical polypeptide chains bound together in the native molecule by noncovalent forces (95, 99, 100).

Studies with various portions of ragweed antigen E have provided insight into what appear to be major antigenic determinants of the molecule, particularly as regards T-cell–B-cell interaction. B-cell stimulating antigens of antigen E depend on the shape of the whole native molecule. However, antigens capable of stimulating helper T-cell function were still preserved in urea-denatured antigen E and its isolated α and β chains (101, 102).

Many other important allergens have recently received extensive study. These include grass pollen allergens, rye grass antigens, and tree pollen allergens—all capable of stimulation of specific reaginic IgE antibody (103). Most of the allergens thus far characterized have been proteins of low molecular weight (10,000 to 30,000 Daltons). Patients who are sensitive to animal danders often are also sensitive to animal serum proteins. Thus, in a survey of cat-sensitive patients by the radioallergosorbent test, 66 percent of serum samples showed positive reactions only with dander extracts, 27 percent were positive with both dander and cat serum, and 7 percent were positive with cat-serum proteins alone (104). Active antigenic fractions in both animal danders and house dust appear also to be in 10,000 to 20,000 molecular weight fractions.

Allergy to insect stings such as bees, yellow jackets, wasps, and hornets of the Hymenoptera order represents an important medical problem. Each year in the United States it is estimated that more patients die after anaphylactic reactions to insect bites than die of poisonous snake envenomation. Bee venom has been extensively characterized and contains several major antigenic components: phospholipase, hyaluronidase, hemolytic peptide, and neurotoxic peptide (103). The hyaluronidase and the phospholipase appear to represent the most important potential allergens of this group. Various induced chemical modifications of bee venom phospholipase have been prepared by King and colleagues (105). However, marked variability was noted in actual physiological activity when tested in a range of sensitive patients. Thus, relative activity of the succinylated enzyme compared to the native protein ranged from 0.003 to 0.7 in 5 allergic patients tested. This is a good example of the wide variety of different antigenic determinants recognized by different allergic subjects on the same small protein. If a range of antigenic determinants is involved in the production of specific reagin IgE, attempts at chemical modifications of the original material in the hopes of producing an effective but less toxic substance to be used for desensitization procedures appear to be less feasible. This is illustrated diagrammatically in Figure 9-8. Chemical modifications of many allergens have been prepared with the hope of producing less toxic but effective biologic products that could be used in various desensitization procedures.

Most allergens are absorbed on inhalation or ingestion and require absorption through the respiratory tract, gastrointestinal mucosa, or skin. As noted above, these areas are common sites of distribution of IgE-reactive plasma cells in the normal subject. Since there must undoubtedly be an upper size limit to the molecules that can pass freely through these surfaces (perhaps 65,000 Daltons), the fact that most potent allergens thus far described are of relatively small size becomes understandable. An exception to this general rule seems to be the situation with keyhole limpet hemocyanin (molecular weight 1×10^6). Salvaggio and co-

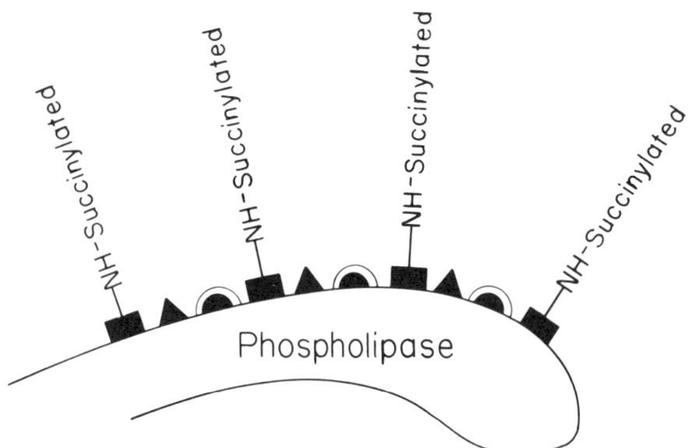

Figure 9-8 Enzyme phospholipase bearing three major allergenic determinants. Succinylation of one of these groups may markedly reduce antigenicity and effectiveness for use in, for instance, desensitization procedures in some sensitive individuals.

workers (106) have shown that intranasal immunization of normal subjects or atopic patients leads to the production of specific IgE antibody. However, hemocyanins are known to comprise subunits of 30,000 Daltons and it is possible that specific IgE was generated to determinants present on dissociated subunits rather than the giant molecule itself. Studies comparing permeability of nasal mucosa in normal subjects and atopic patients have generally shown no significant difference (107).

Many attempts have been made to modify well-known allergens in the hope that materials useful for desensitization might result. The most widely used resulting materials have probably been modified preparations of ragweed antigen E treated with the cross-linking preparation glutaraldehyde. Patterson and coworkers (108, 109) prepared cross-linked antigen E which could be separated into high- and low-molecular-weight fractions with molecular weight ranges of 0.2 to 4 $\times$ 10^6 and 4 to 20 $\times$ 10^6 Daltons. In rabbits, both fractions were as effective as the native unaltered materials in inducing specific IgG antibody production. Native antigen produced a transient IgE response. Low-molecular-weight cross-linked material produced a weaker IgE response than native material, whereas the high-molecular-weight substances showed a stronger and longer-lasting IgE response than was recorded with the native antigen (110). Subsequent clini-

cal trials with polymerized antigen E have now been reported (111, 112). It appears that this material may be capable of rapid induction of blocking IgG antibody and of reducing allergenicity, thereby decreasing the incidence of unpleasant side reactions during initiation and maintenance of desensitization procedures. Another advantage noted during these initial trials of polymerized antigens was that it took less than one-third the usual time to reach the standard full maintenance dose for continued desensitization.

A rather novel, potentially exciting approach to the practical problem of desensitization has been presented by Lee and Sehon (113). Their method was to attempt to abrogate reaginic antibody formation using conjugates of haptens with nonimmunogenic carriers. The method employed coupling of allergens tested to the nonimmunogenic hydrophilic polymer, polyethylene glycol. This work was prompted by a previous report indicating that coupling of good antigens such as catalase or bovine serum albumin to polyethylene glycol resulted in loss of immunogenicity of these two proteins (114). Intravenous administration of antigen-polyethylene glycol conjugates immediately before challenge of sensitized mice primed for antigen-specific IgE production completely eliminated reaginic antibody response both of primary and secondary type. These remarkable results are shown in Figure 9-9. Injection of conjugates into presensitized mice that were making specific IgE reaginic antibody led to suppression of the specific IgE responses as well. Finally, the polyethylene glycol conjugates themselves did not combine directly with preformed antibody and did not possess any intrinsic allergenicity themselves. Clear understanding of the mechanisms involved in these reactions is not yet available. Lee and Sehon (113) have suggested that abrogation of specific IgE and other humoral responses in this system may be related to interference with T-cell–B-cell interaction and perhaps activation of antigen-specific and immunoglobulin-E–specific suppressor cells. It has also been demonstrated that partly denatured antigen E is capable of stimulating T-suppressor cells (115), and it is conceivable that

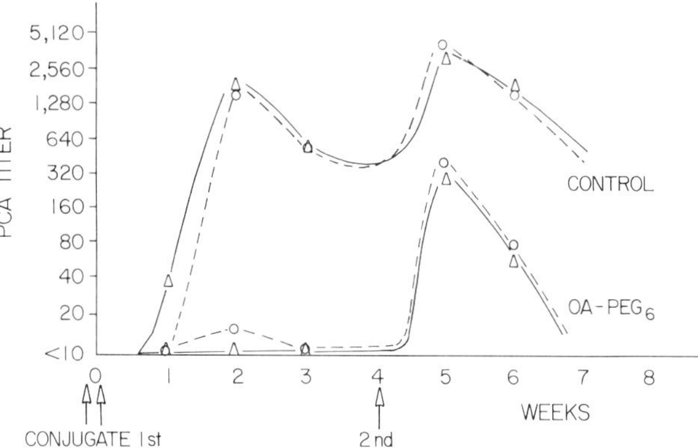

Figure 9-9 Suppression of the reaginic antibody response with ovalbumin-PEG₆. Test mice were injected intravenously with 1 mg of ovalbumin-PEG 4 hours before receiving the first sensitizing dose of DNP-ovalbumin on day 0. The mice received intraperitoneally a second sensitizing dose of antigen on day 28 without further administration of the conjugate. $\triangle$--$\triangle$, anti-ovalbumin IgE response; $\bigcirc$--$\bigcirc$, anti-DNP Ig response. (Reproduced with permission, W. Y. Lee and A. H. Sehon, *Nature* 267:618, 1977.)

when certain antigens are presented to the immune system in nonimmunogenic form, they may in turn activate suppressor-cell mechanisms. If the basic cellular mechanisms involved in the results presented by Lee and Sehon (113) can be safely adapted to a human model, it seems likely that a rational basis for further precise and perhaps more clinically successful methods of specific immunotherapy will become available.

Basophils

From the inception of studies of immediate hypersensitivity, it has been recognized that the key cell mediating much of the reaction in skin, bronchial subepithelium, or nasal mucosa is the tissue mast cell or basophil. A rough correlation was recorded between amounts of IgE in serum and actual quantitative amounts bound to individual basophils (116). This has been explored using electron microscopic observations by several groups; such observations indicate that amounts of IgE per basophil might vary from 10,000 to 500,000 IgE molecules per cell

(117). Cell-bound IgE has also been studied by van Elven and colleagues (118) comparing quantitative estimation of basophil IgE binding using immunofluorescent techniques in conjunction with horseradish peroxidase-labeled anti-IgE. Cell-bound IgE demonstrated on basophilic leukocytes using immunoelectron microscopy appeared to correlate with results obtained by semiquantitative immunofluorescent procedures. Representative appearance of cells visualized in this work is shown in Figure 9-10.

Antigen-induced degranulation of basophils from atopic subjects was also studied by electron microscopy (119). Incubation of basophils with antigen to which the leukocyte donor was sensitive caused histamine release and exocytic degranulation as expected. Degranulated basophils showed an irregular surface to which platelets and other leukocytes were often adherent. Residual granular material was noted both in exocytic cavities and at the cell surface and coated vesicles as well as cisternae of smooth endoplasmic reticulum often related directly to the plasma membrane at sites of exocytosis. These findings refute the concept that histamine release might be accomplished by destruction of the basophil. No support was obtained for the notion that microtubules play a role in response to antigen in these studies. It is important to note that the exocytic degranulation observed during this in vitro study has not as yet been observed in vivo. An alternative, more gradual degranulation process termed "piecemeal degranulation" has been suggested by Dvorak and co-workers (120, 121). From these and many other studies, it is evident that there is still much to learn about the precise functions of this class of cells.

Asthma

Asthma, or reversible episodic obstructive airway disease, is the most serious common allergic disorder with which physicians must deal. Asthma afflicts an estimated 9 million individuals in the United States and is responsible for about 2,000 to 3,000 deaths annually (122). The disorder is familiar to most practicing physicians and is characterized by episodic

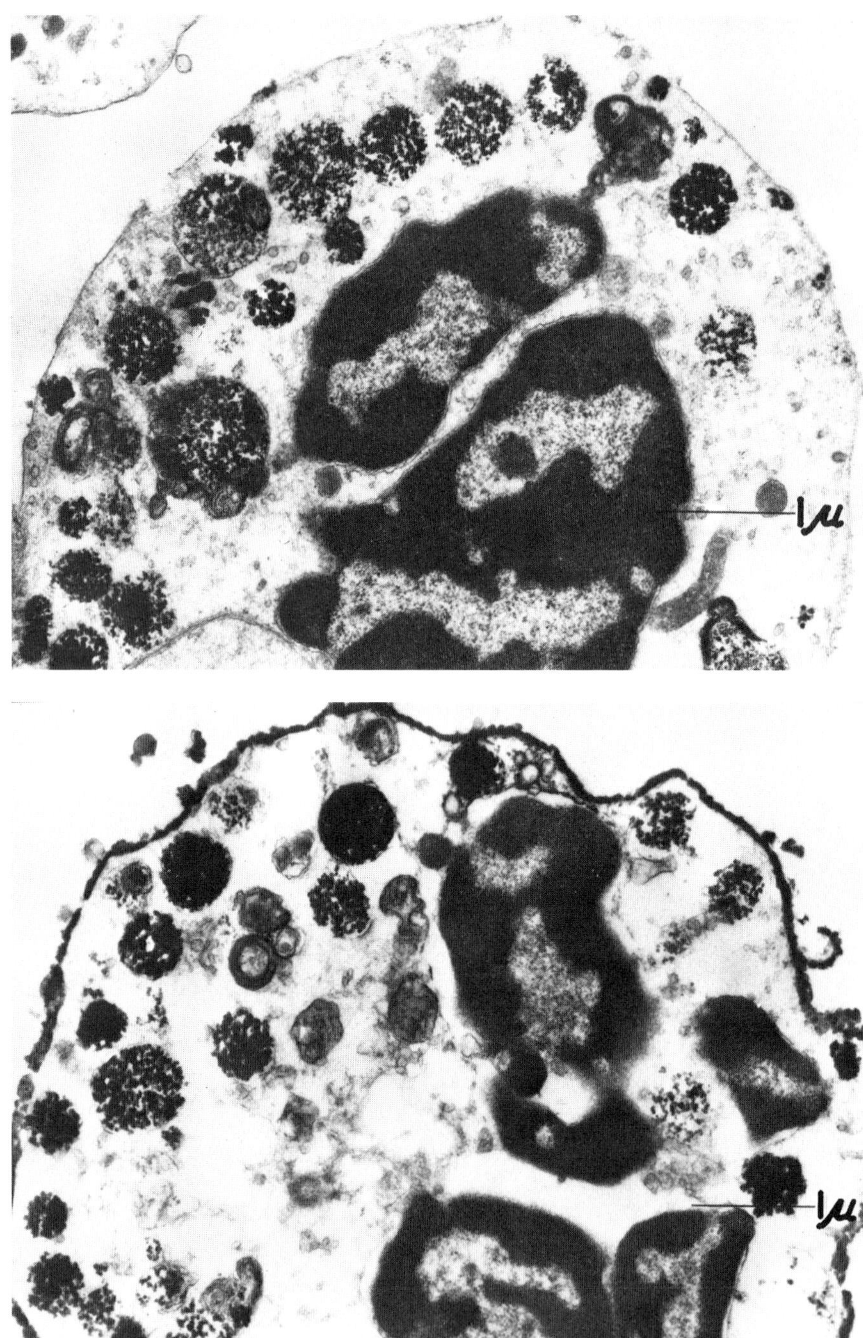

Figure 9-10 *Above,* a basophilic granulocyte fixed in 1-percent paraformaldehyde and incubated with antihuman IgE is conjugated with horseradish peroxidase showing weakly positive staining. *Below,* a basophilic granulocyte from another atopic patient showing strongly positive membrane staining for surface IgE. (Reproduced with permission, E. H. van Elven, P. J. Stallman, and P. H. C. Brühl, *Int. Arch. Allergy Appl. Immunol.* 54:560, 1977. Courtesy of S. Karger AG, Basel.)

bronchial obstructive phenomena related to bronchial mucosal edema, viscous plugs of mucus in both bronchi and bronchioles, and bronchial smooth-muscle contraction. Histological features include peripheral blood eosinophilia, infiltration of eosinophils into bronchial walls, and shedding of superficial columnar epithelial cells as well as eosinophils into the bronchial lumen. Also occurring are frequent dilation of submucosal capillaries, mast-cell degranulation, and thickening of bronchial mucosal membrane. Essentially, similar features are found in extrinsic asthma, for which a provoking allergen can be identified, and intrinsic asthma, the cause of which is poorly understood. Although increased serum IgE levels are found in many patients with extrinsic asthma, not all such individuals are shown to exhibit consistently elevated levels of this immunoglobulin. Many of the features of immunologically mediated tissue injury interact in production of the asthmatic episode. However, a broad variety of diverse events or agents can trigger an asthmatic attack. These include cold air, dust, chemical fumes, exercise, infection, and certainly emotional stress. These various stimuli can produce irritation or stimulation of the respiratory tract to such an extent that excessive reflex stimulation of efferent parasympathetic nerves innervating smooth muscle components, glands, mucous membranes, and blood vessels culminates in sudden or gradual narrowing of airways (123, 124).

The actual chemical sequences triggering the immediate-type inflammatory reaction in the genesis of the asthmatic attack include histamine, slow-reacting substance of anaphylaxis (SRS–A), eosinophil chemotactic factor (ECF–A), basophil kallikrein, platelet-activating factor, and possibly kinins and prostaglandins of the F series. These substances are released from mast cells and basophils subsequent to allergen combining with IgE molecules affixed to their surfaces. This series of reactions is shown schematically in Figure 9-11. Activity of the many mediators involved in this intricate series of reactions can be controlled at three different levels: (1) regulation of generation and release; (2) alteration of target-cell response by modification of actual receptor binding or cell activation; and (3) inactivation by biodegradation. Of the six primary mediators shown in the rectangles within Figure 9-11, only histamine is known to inhibit its own release and that of other mediators by way of action on H_2 receptors with subsequent elevation of intracellular levels of cAMP. Tripeptides inhibit chemotaxis by interaction and blocking of the eosinophil receptors for ECF–A, the primary eosinophil chemotactic factor. The chemotactic activities of eosinophils are actually enhanced by histamine and suppressed by the presence of SRS–A. Finally, eosinophils mod-

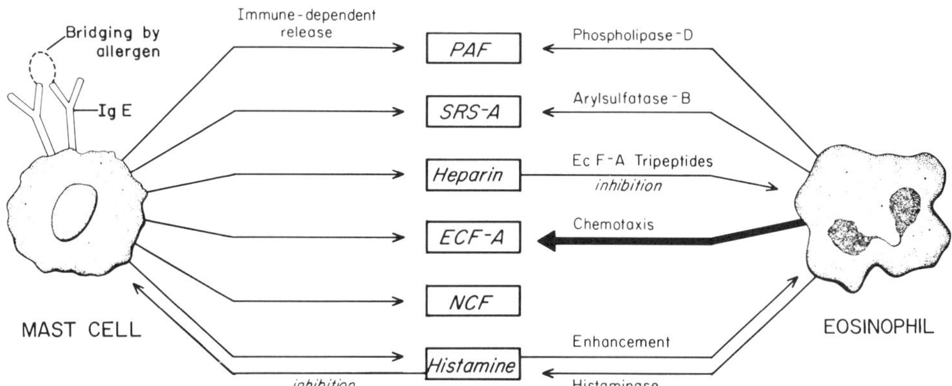

Figure 9-11 Interrelation of chemical mediators and intracellular processes involved in mast-cell–IgE interaction as well as induction of eosinophil response.

ulate mediator activities through biodegradation of histamine through histaminase. They also influence or exert mediator control by release of two other enzymes, phospholipase-D and arylsulfatase-B, which modulate platelet activating factor (PAF) and SRS–A, respectively. The concept of eosinophilic participation and modulation of many of the intermediate messages and molecules directly involved in this sequence of reactions is an important one that helps to explain local eosinophilic infiltration and presence in bronchial mucosal and secretions during acute asthmatic episodes. This schema of interactions has been discussed in detail by Goetzl and Austen (124).

A great explosion of knowledge has recently been prompted by definitive understanding of how various mediator substances actually influence cellular functions through changes effected by cAMP and cGMP. Many hormones that do not directly stimulate adenylate cyclase have been shown to induce the formation of cGMP from GTP by an analogous reaction through guanylate cyclase, an enzyme present in both plasma membranes and the cytosol of cells. Hormones and other agents important in

modulating the actual clinical process involved in the asthmatic attack and capable of stimulating accumulation of cAMP or cGMP in lymphocytes, mast cells, lung, or smooth-muscle-containing structures such as bronchioles are shown in Table 9-2 and Figure 9-12.

Cyclic AMP mediates hormonal signals by an increment in the enzymatic activity of intracellular protein kinases (125). Mechanisms by which cAMP inhibits a variety of immunologic responses have been the subject of study by many groups (126–128). Inhibition of these responses, such as mediator release from mast cells or basophils, is important in the induction of an acute asthmatic attack. In every instance thus far examined, an effect opposing that of cAMP has been demonstrated for cGMP or for agents that increase intracellular cGMP levels. Cells possess several mechanisms by which drugs or hormones used in the treatment of clinical asthma influence special functions. Cyclic AMP has a retarding or negative influence on allergic or inflammatory responses, whereas cGMP together with calcium ions exert opposing actions. In relation to asthma itself, an

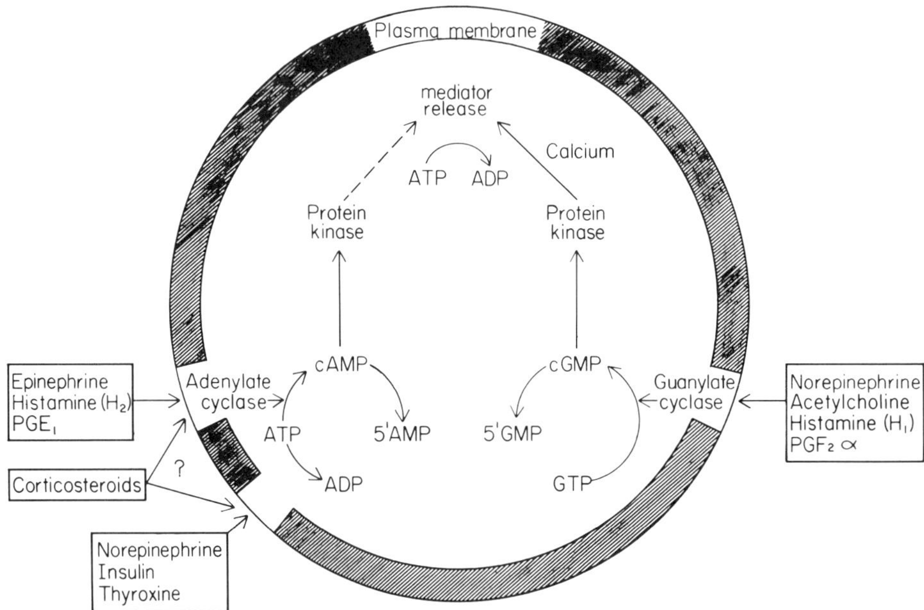

Figure 9-12 Hormonal and intracellular processes thought to be involved in some of the basic processes of mediator regulation and homeostasis pertinent to asthma.

Table 9-2 Agents altering cyclic nucleotide levels that influence clinical asthma.

Agent	Mast cell		Lung		Smooth muscle	
	cGMP	cAMP	cGMP	cAMP	cGMP	cAMP
α-Adrenergic		↓		↓	↑	0
β-Adrenergic		↑	↓	↑	↓	↑
Cholinergic			↑	0	↑	0
Corticosteroids		↑	↓			
Histamine H–1			↑	0	↑	
Histamine H–2				↑		
PGF$_{2\alpha}$				0 or ↑	↑	0
PGE				↑	↓	↑

increase in cAMP relaxes tracheobronchial smooth muscle, produces vasodilatation of bronchial and pulmonary vasculature, stimulates corticosteroid synthesis by adrenal cortex, inhibits mediator release by basophils and mast cells, and decreases eosinophil release and eosinophil leukotaxis.

One general theory applied to an understanding of the asthmatic condition is that asthma, once established, actually represents an imbalance in both α- and β-adrenergic receptor responsiveness and subsequent cholinergic hyperresponsiveness. Virtually all agents used in the immediate treatment of allergic disorders like asthma are associated with increased cAMP or decreased cGMP levels. The origin of the controlling mechanisms actually inducing cell receptor imbalance are presently unknown. Definitive understanding will only be achieved through studies in which the specific receptors and their modulating mediators are isolated and studied directly. There is no histological or immunofluorescent evidence for extensive tissue immune-complex deposition in asthma. This in itself emphasizes the tremendous biologic amplification system involved after IgE on sensitized mast cells or basophils interacts with antigen in a critical anatomic position: namely, in the bronchial or respiratory mucosa. Unlike the other more dramatic histological examples, lesions of asthma do not contain intense deposits of immunoglobulins nor complement.

The interrelationship of the clinical phenomenon of asthma with both direct immediate hypersensitivity phenomena related to mast cells and the IgE system as well as to the complicated pathophysiology of the autonomic control of airway obstruction represents one of the most important and challenging areas in clinical medicine. In general, physicians do not like to take care of asthmatics. In our own experience asthmatics, much like alcoholics, are often regarded with scorn or indulgence by many attending physicians since they continually return, unable to break the cycles of external and internal influences that produce repeated and often discouraging attacks. With all that is known of the intricate mechanisms involved in IgE-mediated release of various noxious components, the patient with repeated severe attacks of asthma still represents one of the most difficult and challenging problems for the practicing physician.

Hypersensitivity Pneumonitis

In 1713 Ramazini first noted that cough, shortness of breath, and cachexia resulted from the inhalation of improperly dried cereal-grain dust. As indicated by Pepys, this was perhaps the first clinical description of pulmonary hypersensitivity disease (129). During the past 25 years an increasing awareness of hypersensitivity pneumonitis or what Pepys called "extrinsic allergic alveolitis" (130) has been demonstrated by numerous descriptions of acute or chronic interstitial pneumonitis secondary to an ever increasing number of organic dust inhalants. Most of the materials implicated in the production of this syndrome are related to particulate allergenic or antigenic materials present in molds, insect, plant, or animal matter. By a large margin the two clinical examples most extensively studied to date are farmer's lung caused by antigens derived from various actinomycetes fungi, which are present in moldy hay, and pigeon breeder's (fancier's) disease, related to multiple antigens present in pigeon droppings and pigeon serum. Hypersensitivity pneumonitis seems to be initiated by immune complexes in the alveoli and alveolar septal areas induced by direct inhalation of antigen. The process is later amplified by secondary cellular mechanisms including delayed-type hypersensitivity phenomena, ensuing after the initial inflammatory response has been initiated. This pattern of inflammatory reaction serves as a model for a clinical inflammatory disorder initiated by immune complexes. It initially features some of the characteristics of an Arthus reaction, followed by a more chronic inflammatory component of cellular immunity. At a superficial level, a parallel might be drawn between hypersensitivity pneumonitis and diseases such as rheumatoid arthritis: both occur either as diseases of acute onset or in subacute or chronic form. Initial inflammatory stimuli presumably triggered by immune complexes are present in both disorders and evidence has accumulated for presence of immune complexes discernible by direct immunofluorescence in tissues or tissue fluids in both diseases. Finally, as the inflammatory process becomes more chronic, cellular infiltrates of lymphocytes and plasma cells accumulate bearing many of the histological features of a delayed-type hypersensitivity or graft versus host phenomenon.

Farmer's Lung

Farmer's lung was first described in detail by Dickie and Rankin (131). It was found in upper middle western agricultural workers who had been repeatedly exposed to moldy fodder or hay. The disease is manifested either as an acute, rather dramatic, and sometimes fatal pulmonary syndrome characterized by chills, fever, rapidly progressive dyspnea, acute pulmonary insufficiency, and occasion-

ally death, or as a more chronic persistent tracheobronchitis, interstitial pneumonitis-dyspnea syndrome (132–136). Chest x-rays often show a prominent but patchy interstitial infiltrate (Figure 9-13). Shortly after farmer's lung was recognized, many patients were found to show a range of antibodies to antigenic components present in the thermophilic actinomycetes fungi, *Micropolyspora faeni* and *Thermoactinomyces vulgaris*. These antibodies frequently produced precipitins in agar gel media with antigens prepared from the strain of fungi isolated from moldy hay or silage in the patient's own environment. Biopsy during various stages of clinical evolution of the disease has shown an interstitial pneumonitis characterized by thickening of alveolar septae, lymphocytic and plasma cell infiltration, interstitial pulmonary fibrosis, and scarring of lung tissue in areas where the disease has progressed over a period of months or years. Typical changes seen on lung biopsy in this disorder are shown in Figure 9-14. It became apparent that administration of corticosteroids was often helpful in aborting a long and distressing convalescence particularly if the disease was recognized early or in its acute exudative stages. However,

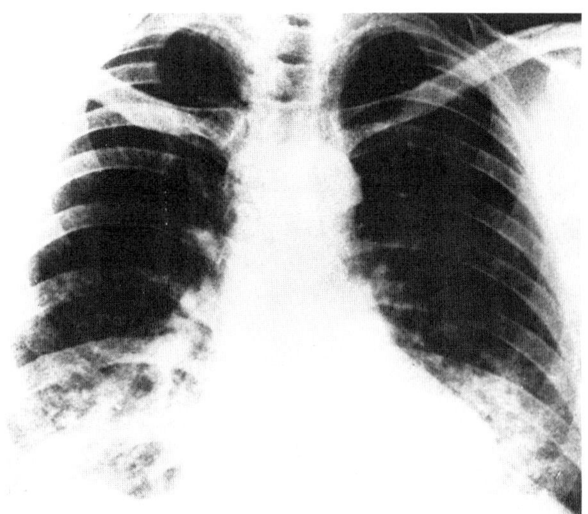

Figure 9-13 Chest x-ray of patient with farmer's lung showing bilateral basilar interstitial infiltrates. (Photograph courtesy of Helen Dickie, Madison, Wisconsin.)

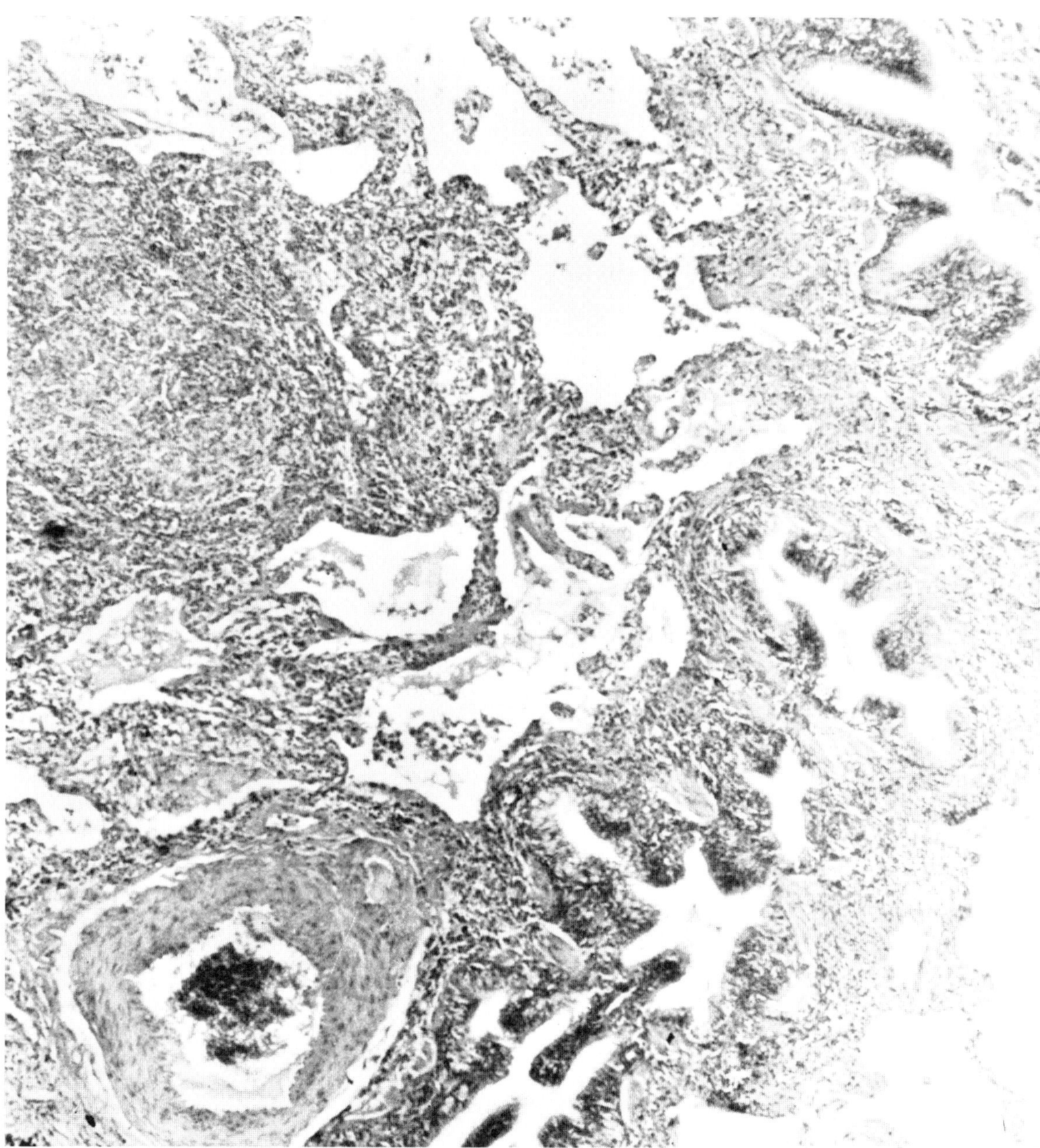

Figure 9-14 Severe interstitial pneumonitis associated with farmer's lung marked by alveolar wall thickening, massive infiltrates characterized by lymphocytes, mononuclear cells, and interstitial edema. H&E × 150. (Photomicrograph courtesy of Helen Dickie, Madison, Wisconsin.)

avoidance of the inciting antigens implicated seemed the only sure method of preventing recurrence and further progression of symptoms. Since the molds involved in the genesis of farmer's lung are indigenous to the work environment of many patients potentially at risk to develop the disorder, it represents a serious potential health risk to many such personnel. When the actual clinical histories of these patients are examined in detail, it is apparent that onset of the disease often follows intense exposure within an enclosed space as, for instance, filling a silo or standing for hours with moldy hay while breathing in antigens of the thermophilic actinomycetes.

Pigeon Breeder's (Bird Fancier's) Disease

At about the same time that the clinical picture of farmer's lung was evolving, it was recognized that bird fanciers also were subject to an acute or chronic hypersensitivity pneumonitis much like that of farmer's lung (137–139). Clinical features showed a remarkable similarity to those present in farmer's lung. Patients presented with an acute, subacute, or chronic respiratory disorder, interstitial pulmonary infiltrates, and restrictive-obstructive or diffusion defect by conventional pulmonary function testing (140). The granulomatous interstitial histological process noted on open lung biopsy in such patients is very similar to that of farmer's lung shown in Figure 9-14. Again, as with farmer's lung, precipitating antibodies to antigens present in pigeon droppings or pigeon serum were recorded in many of these subjects. Interpreting the presence of these precipitating antibodies to pigeon-related antigens has been difficult because such antibody is also found in a considerable proportion of bird fanciers who do *not* show clinically apparent hypersensitivity pneumonitis. Serological surveys of populations of bird fanciers show as many as 50 percent with antibody to pigeon serum or material in droppings (130, 141, 142). Early studies indicated that the precipitating antibody to these inhaled antigens was mainly IgG (143), although further serological studies have shown detectable IgM or IgA antibodies in lower titers using indirect immunofluorescent techniques (144–146) in

the case of farmer's lung antigens. An example of the heterogeneity of the precipitating antibodies present in a single serum from a patient with pigeon breeder's disease is shown in Figure 9-15. Distinct antibodies were demonstrated against antigens present in droppings, egg white, pigeon serum, and extract of pigeon feathers. Absorption of serum with extract of pigeon droppings removed precipitin lines against extract of feathers in these studies (147). Complement-fixing activities of the antibodies involved in pigeon breeder's hypersensitivity pneumonitis have been studied (148) in an attempt to differentiate symptomatic patients who have the clinically recognizable disease from subjects at risk who show no clinical symptoms but do show detectable precipitating antibodies. Quantitative amounts of precipitating IgG antibody were higher in the serum of pigeon breeders who were ill, and complement-fixing activities were greater than in asymptomatic pigeon breeders. However, the latter showed IgG antibodies also capable of activating the complement system. These data are shown in Table 9-3, taken from this particular report (148). Similar findings were also reported by a separate group of investigators who noted that pigeon breeder serum was capable of activating C4 (149). These data indicate that pigeon antigen and host antibody probably interact with the complement system through the classic pathway. When studies of asymptomatic pigeon breeders were performed using inhalation challenge with pigeon serum (150), depression in serum complement levels after inhalation exposure was recorded. No depression in complement levels was noted in symptomatic breeders after similar aerosol challenges. These data are paradoxical and may indicate differences in relative permeability of challenged airways to the antigen aerosols in the two groups—the ill patients having already mobilized sufficient inflammatory exudates and thickened alveolar walls to the extent that direct in vivo activation of complement did not occur to a detectable amount within the circulating plasma.

This area is still under active investigation and is complicated somewhat by the heterogeneity of precipitating and perhaps other

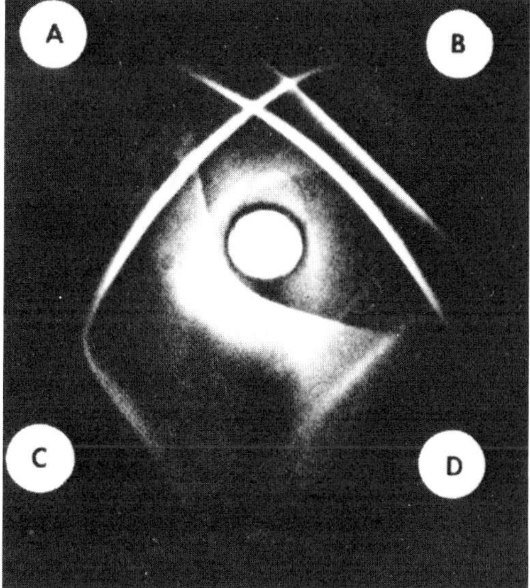

Figure 9-15 *Left,* immunodiffusion pattern of the patient's serum against pigeon antigens. *Center well,* patient's serum; *A*, extract of pigeon droppings; *B*, pigeon's serum; *C*, pigeon egg white; *D*, extract of pigeon feathers. *Right,* immunodiffusion pattern of the patient's serum absorbed with pigeon serum (location of antigens as indicated in left-hand figure). (Reproduced with permission, J. Barboriak, A. J. Sosman, and C. E. Reed, *J. Lab. Clin. Med.* 65:600, 1965.)

Table 9-3 Quantitative precipitation and complement fixation in symptomatic and asymptomatic pigeon breeders.

Subject	μg Ab protein precipitated/ ml serum	Ab/Ag at equivalence	CH 50 units fixed/ml serum	CH 50 units fixed/μg Ab precipitate
Symptomatic breeders				
1	826	7.9	299	0.36
2	959	9.0	160	0.18
3	1,256	6.3	735	0.58
4	1,890	17.2	214	0.11
5	538	8.7	169	0.31
6	2,358	11.1	1,062	0.45
	1,304[a]		440[a]	
	(519; 2,090)		(48; 832)	
Asymptomatic breeders				
1	1,581	14.9	313	0.20
2	598	9.5	117	0.20
3	497	10.6	115	0.23
4	416	12.2	103	0.24
	773[a]		162[a]	
	(−92; 1,638)		(2; 323)	

Source: Reproduced with permission, V. L. Moore and J. N. Fink, *J. Lab. Clin. Med.* 85:540, 1975.

[a] Mean and 95-percent confidence limits.

nonprecipitating systems present in individual patients. Berrens and Guikers (151) reported that pigeon-dropping antigens depleted C3 in the serum of ill pigeon breeders but did not fix complement by the classic pathway in combination with antiserum. Since IgG is the most prominent immunoglobulin involved in the detectable immune response to pigeon-related antigens, it would be of considerable interest to study relative IgG H-chain subgroup composition of antibodies involved in the various reactions. Since complement fixation can be relatively easily demonstrated in many sera, it would appear that IgG-1 and IgG-3 and perhaps less IgG-2 and IgG-4 are directly involved in initiation of the pathophysiological events. It is of great theoretical interest that symptomatic as well as some asymptomatic breeders develop an Arthus-like reaction after intracutaneous challenge with pigeon serum (150).

In clinical situations the detection of precipitating antibody against offending animal or mold antigens is often used to confirm a tentative diagnosis in individual patients. Three methods were studied in parallel double-blind fashion by several laboratories and it was determined that the gel template and microscope slide micro-Ouchterlony methods were comparable in reproducibility and sensitivity to the counterimmunoelectrophoresis technique (152). Precise diagnostic tests utilizing highly purified and immunochemically distinct antigens with such techniques as radioimmunoassay must await the type of characterizations that have been performed for materials like ragweed antigen E. Preliminary studies have been directed at chemical characterization of antigens responsible for hypersensitivity pneumonitis (153), but final definition of the range of offending antigens is not yet complete.

The clinical importance of the phenomena exemplified by farmer's lung or bird fancier's disease is the astonishing and ever growing number of clinical syndromes that seem to be related to the same general phenomena. A summary of some of these conditions appears in Table 9-4. The antigens involved are largely of mold or plant origin with the exception of pituitary snuff and bird fancier's disease.

An interesting variant of hypersensitivity pneumonitis has also been described in association with air-conditioning units or humidifiers contaminated with thermophilic actinomycetes (154–156). Implication of the organism in the production of the syndrome was confirmed by positive Arthus reactions in some cases and by development of positive serum precipitins against antigen extracts prepared from the strain of thermophilic actinomycetes isolated from the units in question. Inhalation chal-

Table 9-4 Diversity of clinical syndromes of hypersensitivity pneumonitis.

Disease	Source	Antigen
Farmer's lung	Moldy hay	*Micropolyspora faeni*
Mushroom worker's lung	Mushroom compost	*Thermoactinomyces vulgaris*
Bagassosis	Moldy sugar cane	*Thermoactinomyces vulgaris*
Malt-worker's lung	Germinating barley	*Aspergillus clavatus*
Maple-bark disease	Dry moldy bark	*Cryptosporium corticale*
Suberosis	Moldy cork dust	?
Sequoiosis	Moldy sawdust	*Graphium pullularia*
Mill worker's lung	Mill dust	*Sitophilus granularises*
Coffee worker's lung	Coffee bean dust	Fungal antigens
Byssinosis	Cotton	Cotton antigens
Bird breeder's lung	Feathers, droppings, egg whites, serum	Multiple
Pituitary snuff	Powdered pituitary extracts	Bovine and porcine sera and pituitary tissue
Hypersensitivity pneumonitis	Contamination of air conditioners	Thermophilic actinomycetes

lenge produced symptoms in patients afflicted with this sensitivity. It is clear then that the clinical entity of hypersensitivity pneumonitis is present in a wide variety of forms. The presence of precipitating IgG antibody and a high degree of association with various fungal antigens make it unique and in many ways distinct from the inflammatory processes invoked by IgE and the immediate hypersensitivity reaction.

Animal Models of Hypersensitivity Pneumonitis

Several animal models for hypersensitivity pneumonitis have been studied by different groups. Experimental pneumonitis produced in the guinea pig by Richerson (157) was induced in various ways favoring either humoral antibody production or cell-mediated delayed-type hypersensitivity. These studies utilized several diverse antigens including ovalbumin, tuberculin, and an azobenzenearsonate hapten. Guinea pigs immunized with or without Freund's adjuvant developed PCA or γ-1 antibody with or without γ-2 hemolytic antibody. The azo-hapten used produced pure delayed-type hypersensitivity. After initial immunization, animals were challenged with aerosol inhalation and killed at intervals to follow the sequence of histological changes. Presence of γ-1-type IgG antibody was associated with acute anaphylaxis and peribronchial eosinophilia, whereas induction of γ-2 complement-fixing antibody was later associated with severe hemorrhagic pneumonitis and extensive leukocytic infiltrations of delayed-type hypersensitivity with focal areas of alveolitis. Small or large mononuclear cells were the predominant cell type in these latter lesions. These experiments indicated that the pattern of lung pathology in the guinea pig depended on the initial type of immune responses induced. Unfortunately, this experimental animal is a relatively poor producer of precipitating antibody compared with other species. These findings may bear on related mechanisms of delayed type hypersensitivity involved in such reactions (158) where the guinea pig has proved extremely helpful in elucidating basic pathological processes.

A closer and perhaps more pertinent model for human hypersensitivity pneumonitis has been studied in the monkey by Hensley and co-workers (159). In this work the presence of circulating precipitating antibody to pigeon serum was associated with a hemorrhagic alveolitis within 6 hours after inhalation challenge with antigen. Passive transfer of lymphoid cells from immunized monkeys showed arrest of lymphocytes within pulmonary capillaries and mild alveolar septal infiltration at 6 hours after challenge. The lymphocyte transfer experiments were not, however, associated with a hemorrhagic pneumonia or an extensive polymorphonuclear leukocytic component. These findings emphasize that, in a primate closely related to humans, the presence of precipitating antibody in the serum of the challenged animals played a dominant role in the production of the initial acute alveolitis and hemorrhagic pneumonia. This implies that an acute intraalveolar immune-complex–type reaction is important in initiating the basic process involved in hypersensitivity pneumonitis to antigens present in pigeon serum. However, the human lesion has much more in the way of features of a delayed-type hypersensitivity reaction. Subsequent development of a more chronic progressive cell-mediated inflammatory process in the disease may be the result of a second wave of immune reactivity.

Of interest in this regard is a report by Pirie and co-workers (160) of what seemed to be spontaneously occurring farmer's lung appearing appropriately enough in a cow. This animal had precipitating antibodies to the thermophilic actinomycete *M. faeni* and experienced an exacerbation of disease on inhalation challenge with this antigen. Twenty-four hours after challenge the cow was killed, and advanced interstitial pneumonia with intraalveolar hemorrhage and granulocytic exudates were noted.

The cellular phase of delayed-type hypersensitivity possibly involved in this disease in humans was also studied in rabbits by Moore and colleagues (161). Animals exposed by aerosol to large quantities of pigeon antigens developed a humoral but not a cellular immune response and their lungs showed essentially normal histology. However, a single intravenous injection of BCG in oil permitted the induction of cell-mediated immunity to the inhaled antigens and induced pulmonary lesions more pronounced than those associated with intravenous BCG administration alone. These findings again support the idea that an initial humoral antibody-mediated acute alveolitis gradually evolves into a more indolent chronic response during continued antigenic exposure. During this study animals with normal pulmonary histology and circulating complement-fixing antibodies showed falls in serum complement after an aerosol challenge with pigeon antigens. However, in similar rabbits with BCG-induced lesions and lungs already inflamed, no complement depression after aerosol challenge was recorded. This work confirmed similar changes found in symptomatic and asymptomatic pigeon breeders (148), suggesting that a prior inflammatory process in

the alveoli profoundly affected distribution of antigen inhaled, effectively shunting it away from uptake by the circulating plasma.

Figure 9-16 shows serial changes in total hemolytic serum complement noted in aerosol challenge experiments. These experiments indicate that something other than continued inhalation is indeed necessary for the development of the chronic sort of interstitial pneumonitis dominated by lymphocytes, plasma cells, and foam cells commonly noted in the usual subacute or chronic human case. In this regard, some experiments using bentonite particles coated with schistosoma antigen are of interest (162, 163). Addition of inert particles markedly increased the size of schistosomal pulmonary granulomata. A similar mechanism might well be at work in the instance of hypersensitivity pneumonitis. Since the pigeon antigens or fungal materials are

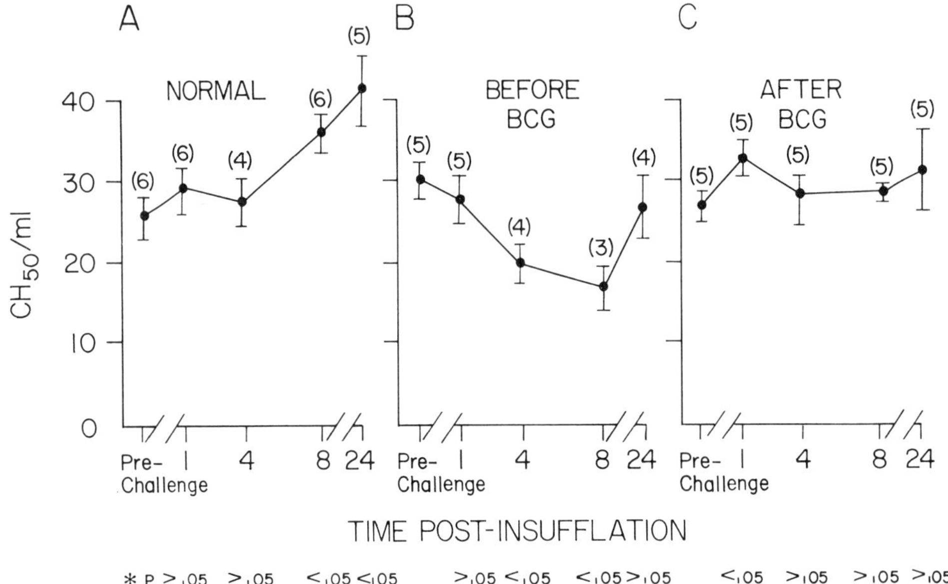

Figure 9-16 Serum-complement (CH 50) changes in rabbits after an aerosol challenge with pigeon dropping extract (PDE). *A*, normal rabbits. *B*, before BCG, rabbits were insufflated 5 days/week with PDE for 3 months (group I); 3 days later the changes in serum CH 50 values were noted after an aerosol challenge with PDE. *C*, after BCG, rabbits were insufflated 5 days/week with PDE for 3 months, given 100 μg of killed BCG in oil intravenously, and again insufflated 5 days/week with PDE for 3 weeks; 3 days after the last insufflation the changes in serum CH 50 values were noted following aerosol challenge with PDE. Values are mean ± SEM. The number of determinations appears in parentheses. * = prechallenge vs postchallenge, Student's *t* test. (Reproduced with permission, V. Moore, G. T. Hensley, and J. N. Fink, *J. Clin. Invest.* 56:937, 1975.)

usually inhaled along with other particulate matter, some of the latter may be capable of an adjuvant effect merely by particle size or particulate nature. In the haste to identify specific and crucial antigens important in actual induction of the immune response, insufficient attention might have been directed toward the potential importance of inert particulate material bearing the antigens. Such materials might be critical in the transition from acute immune-complex–mediated lesion to chronic cell-mediated lesion.

Several published clinical observations are useful longitudinal views of the actual pathological process in hypersensitivity pneumonitis. Caldwell and colleagues (149) studied 5 patients with pigeon breeder's disease using intradermal challenge with pigeon antigen and measurements of cell-mediated immunity including assay of MIF in the presence of pigeon-derived antigen. Skin challenge produced an immediate wheal and flare reaction within 15 minutes and an Arthus-type reaction within 4 to 8 hours. Immunofluorescent study of the secondary Arthus-type reaction showed IgG, C3, and C4 deposits. Precipitating IgG antipigeon antibody isolated from sera of patients formed immune complexes capable of in vitro complement activation. However, peripheral blood lymphocytes from 4 of 5 patients produced MIF when challenged with dilute pigeon serum, providing evidence for cell-mediated immunity in some phase of the ongoing disease process.

The studies recorded by Wenzel and co-workers (164) and van Toorn (165) provide evidence for acute deposition of immunoglobulin in the lung during the early course of hypersensitivity pneumonitis. Van Toorn studied a patient with extrinsic allergic alveolitis secondary to inhalation of coffee dust and noted what appeared to be protein deposits along alveolar capillary basement membranes. No definite proof that this represented an antigen-antibody complex was presented, however. More convincing were the reports of Wenzel and co-workers (164), who noted high concentrations of antibody to *M. faeni* in the lung tissues of patients with farmer's lung. Similar studies of more chronic cases failed to reveal immuno-

fluorescent evidence for antibodies. In acute patients Wenzel and co-workers (164) noted great numbers of histiocytic cells that contained large quantities of C3, suggesting immune complexes. However, there are few published studies specifically using acute material and documenting relative concentration of antigen, antibody, and complement in such individuals. Elution studies and demonstration of marked relative concentration of such reactants within the actual tissue lesions are needed.

Immunologic Reactions Involving Immune Complexes and Chronic Fibrotic Lung Disease

Many clinical conditions have as their final common pathway the establishment of an interstitial fibrotic pulmonary parenchymal lesion leading eventually to various degrees of obstructive and restrictive lung disease. Among the conditions are sarcoidosis, scleroderma, idiopathic pulmonary fibrosis, emphysema, and fibrosis related to smoking, histoplasmosis, chronic interstitial pneumonitis, and a host of other conditions including chronic hypersensitivity pneumonitis. Analysis of cellular and protein content of bronchopulmonary lavage fluids from such patients (166) has revealed an inflammatory and eosinophilic cellular response with significant elevation of IgG in lung fluids from patients with idiopathic pulmonary fibrosis. However, in patients with chronic hypersensitivity pneumonitis, relative increments in IgM and lymphocytes, and some elevation in lung fluid IgG was found. In patients with chronic hypersensitivity pneumonitis a significant proportion of T lymphocytes was also recorded. The presence of T lymphocytes in lung fluids from these patients showed some correlation with prior histological studies of the same individuals on lung biopsy. The importance of T lymphocytes in the final induction of pulmonary fibrosis has also been emphasized by the recent studies of Kravis and co-workers (167), who have shown that T cells from patients with various forms of pulmonary fibrosis take part in processes where recognition of collagen results in immunologically specific migration inhibition. These data indicate that T cells may participate directly in an autoimmune cell-directed process aimed at autologous collagen determinants. In these studies specific T-lymphocyte–mediated MIF reactions were blocked by anti–T-cell antiserum. Thus, the final common result of a host of human disease processes, some of which are associated with intrapulmonary immune-complex deposition and some of which are still of obscure etiology, may be linked to activated T cells and autosensitization to autologous collagen determinants.

The clinical and experimental data now available regarding hypersensitivity pneumonitis are interesting, for they combine problems relating to the evolution of chronic disease and lesions characterized by all the hallmarks of a delayed-type or cell-mediated immune phenomenon with those recognizable at the onset as being associated with acute in situ deposition of immune complexes. Thus, they differ from those commonly recognized as initiated by acute immune-complex injury in sites such as the choroid plexus or renal glomerulus. In these instances no clear evolution to a process strictly mediated by cellular immunity has been convincingly demonstrated. Hypersensitivity pneumonitis is also an interesting example of an allergic or immune-complex disease unlike so many other allergic disorders intimately linked to IgE. It is important now to consider other clinical examples of allergic disorders in an attempt to understand their pathogenesis vis-à-vis immune complexes.

Systemic Anaphylaxis

The term anaphylaxis was introduced in 1902 by Poitier and Richet (168) to describe the shock and subsequent death induced in dogs after injection of sea anemone poison. A fatal profound shock state occurred after a repeat injection rather than prophylaxis or protection to the foreign material previously injected. Acute anaphylactic reactions represent critical medical emergencies and are a dramatic example of the potency of immune complexes including the series of reactions that they are sometimes capable of initiating (169). The clin-

ical manifestations are the result of release of diverse chemical mediators previously discussed in the section on IgE and asthma. They include chemical mediators such as histamine, slow-reacting substance of anaphylaxis (SRS–A) and eosinophil chemotactic factor, all of which interact to increase vascular permeability, contract smooth muscle, and attract inflammatory cells.

Patients who experience anaphylaxis show a variety of clinical symptoms including severe respiratory distress. These are rapidly followed by hypoxia and secondary vascular collapse. In some individuals progressive respiratory insufficiency, wheezing, or stridor are not clinically apparent and primary vascular collapse predominates. It is in this latter clinical presentation that a fatal outcome may occur, since there is little external warning: syncope, collapse, and hypotension may be followed rapidly by low perfusion state, ventricular arrhythmia, and death. Bronchial and bronchiolar constrictions are noted by the patient as a feeling of increasing tightness in the chest. Audible wheezing and laryngeal edema appear as hoarseness, stridor, and tightening in the throat and hypopharynx. Gastrointestinal features include nausea, vomiting, crampy abdominal pain, and occasional bloody diarrhea. One of the most characteristic features of almost all anaphylactic reactions is an eruption of well-circumscribed, erythematous wheals with serpiginous borders and pale or blanched centers. These urticarial wheals are often intensely pruritic and diffusely distributed or localized in one particular area and may coalesce to form giant hives, which seldom persist longer than 48 hours. In addition, the skin may show a more deep-seated edema (angioedema) that generates a deep burning or stinging sensation.

Patients who die of anaphylactic shock associated with bronchial obstruction show marked hyperinflation of lungs; however, microscopic findings are surprisingly localized and sparse and are limited largely to bronchi and bronchioles. Large amounts of bronchial secretions, peribronchial congestion, submucosal edema, and moderate eosinophilic infiltration are found. Angioedema in deeper tissues may actually contribute to mechanical obstruction in the epiglottis, larynx, and hypopharynx, where submucosal eosinophilic infiltration is often evident. In patients who die rapidly of vascular collapse without prominent bronchial obstruction, visceral pooling of blood is often present; such individuals may exhibit electrocardiographic changes of acute myocardial infarction (170) probably the result of hypoxia, poor venous return, and acute coronary insufficiency. A sudden reduction in central blood volume may also explain such changes (171).

Constitutional predisposition may facilitate anaphylaxis. Atopic patients may be more prone to develop anaphylactic reactions with a previous history of symptoms on exposure to a particular allergen, an immediate family history of a similar event, and positive intradermal skin tests. In one study, 5 of 17 patients dying of anaphylaxis after penicillin were asthmatic (172); in another 12 of 15 atopic subjects showed skin-sensitizing IgE antibody after penicillin treatment as compared with 31 of 110 persons with no prior atopy (173).

Materials capable of eliciting systemic anaphylactic reactions in humans include heterologous foreign proteins such as antiserum, hormones, enzymes, bee venom, pollen extracts, foods, diagnostic agents such as iodinated organic contrast materials, BSP dye, and a growing list of drugs including even vitamins. Under certain circumstances, low-molecular-weight compounds like drugs may act as haptens forming covalent or looser associations with autologous body proteins. In some instances both the parent compounds and their conjugated products are capable of forming bonds with host protein to produce an immunogenic substance. As the numbers of new drugs used in clinical practice grows, the potential for systemic anaphylaxis expands accordingly. Unsuspected circumstances play a curious role in systemic anaphylaxis: recently, antigens introduced in seminal plasma during sexual intercourse have been implicated in rare instances of anaphylaxis (174). In addition, systemic anaphylaxis following transfusion of blood from an atopic donor containing high titers of reaginic antibody to components recently ingested by the blood transfusion re-

cipient have also been documented (175). In this instance, the blood transfusion recipient ingested beans and peas; the donor plasma contained high titers of reaginic antibody to leguminous foods. Such severe reactions are rare since known atopic individuals are excluded as blood donors. The classic reaction of this type was reported in a much celebrated case described by Ramirez (176), in which the recipient of a blood transfusion developed asthma during a carriage ride 2 weeks following the transfusion from a donor sensitive to horse dander.

The mechanisms involved in the sudden development of anaphylactic shock have been reviewed previously in early sections. Heat-labile reagin IgE has been conclusively demonstrated from heart blood of a patient dying of systemic anaphylaxis by passive transfer (P-K) reaction into the skin of a normal donor followed by wheal and flare reaction on intracutaneous challenge with suspected antigen (177). Subsequent release from tissue mast cells and basophils of SRS-A, histamine, eosinophil chemotactic factor, and other potent mediators is all that is required for an intense generalized reaction to occur.

In a practical clinical situation the attending physician has several problems to contend with. If the patient has severe stridor or upper airway obstruction caused by laryngeal edema, an airway must be provided either by direct intubation, or if infeasible, by extension of the neck to gain maximum tracheal expansion. The treatment of choice is appropriately diluted intravenous epinephrine: 0.2 to 0.5 ml of a 1:1,000 solution given intravenously in a central vein followed by bolus therapy with a water-soluble preparation of corticosteroid such as dexamethasone or betamethasone (80 mg) intravenously. Glucocorticoids are unlikely to alter the anaphylactic reaction, but a reasonably high dose may alter capillary permeability sufficiently to sustain blood pressure. Epinephrine—combining effects of α and β sympathetic stimulation—will help to sustain blood pressure while at the same time counteracting the intracellular consequences of anaphylaxis. If hypotension improves but bronchial constriction persists, it is reasonable to give intravenous aminophylline which potentiates the intracellular β-adrenergic effects of epinephrine. Intravenous epinephrine must be appropriately diluted to avoid possible ventricular arrhythmias in the shocked patient. The sequence of what to give and how much has recently been debated in a series of letters (178–180) following recommendations for anaphylaxis made by Davies and co-workers (181). In most patients prompt administration of the agents suggested above will be beneficial.

Urticaria

Estimates of the prevalence of urticaria differ widely, influenced perhaps by the perspectives of the various observers; nonetheless, this manifestation of immune-complex disease is quite common. Exhaustive analysis of patients with chronic urticaria often fails to establish an allergic cause. In one series, 100 patients with chronic idiopathic urticaria were actually admitted to hospital for detailed workup and in only one could food allergy be reasonably advanced as the causative factor (182). Many patients exhibiting this unpleasant and vexing symptom may possibly show a basic abnormality in regulating their intrinsic system of pharmacologic mediators placing the lesion beyond that form of urticaria classically associated with IgE-mediated histamine release. The observation that aspirin releases histamine in patients with urticaria pigmentosa (183) has led to a practical and useful approach to this general problem that may be used in screening common agents for possible identification of drugs or additives and materials in foodstuffs that should be eliminated (184–186). Substances suspected of inducing urticaria directly include various azo dyes used in food and drug coloring; sodium benzoate and 4-hydroxybenzoic acid used as preservatives in pickles, sauces, instant coffee and other beverages; and indomethacin and penicillin. Sequential testing of individual patients with numbered capsules and patients' careful recording of any exacerbation of symptoms may be very helpful in the practical management of such patients. A report by Warin and Smith (187) using this procedure defined one or more test substances as being implicated in exacerbations of urticarial episodes. Materials tested in numbered capsules included: tartrazine, sodium benzoate, 4-hydroxybenzoic acid, tyrosine, penicillin, aspirin, brewer's yeast, candida, and lactose (as a control). Some of these substances are now so extensively used by the food industry that complete elimination is far from simple. Avoidance of tartrazine or sodium benzoate, therefore, is extremely difficult to follow.

Since something other than the rather vague concept of autonomic imbalance or receptor defects must be at fault in patients with chronic idiopathic urticaria, an attempt has been made to study these patients directly to arrive at an understanding of their problems. Studies by Kern and Lichtenstein (188) utilized histamine release by peripheral blood leukocytes in 20 patients with chronic urticaria in parallel with controls. Since the offending allergen was unknown, histamine release was produced by challenge with antihuman IgE antibody. Histamine response to a broad range of antibody concentrations was significantly *lower* in chronic urticaria patients than in controls. Although total serum-IgE levels were higher in patients than controls, total histamine content of 10^7 pooled leukocytes showed no differences between patients and controls. Autoradiographic studies with ^{125}I-anti-IgE showed no obvious quantitative abnormality in the distribution of basophil-bound IgE in patients with chronic idiopathic urticaria. Ionophore stimulation of leukocytes of patients demonstrated that normal amounts of histamine were released, in contrast to the results obtained using anti-IgE challenge. Such ionophores bypass usual histamine release-mechanism sequences. Furthermore, unlike asthmatic patients, there was no significant difference in basal or isoproterenol-stimulated leukocyte cAMP levels. It therefore appeared that patients with chronic urticaria have a defect in leukocyte histamine release which occurs in a step subsequent to IgE–anti-IgE reaction, but before the actual releasing process. This sort of physiological setting by the patient is similar to that acquired during the process of desensitization. Representative data from these studies are shown in Figure 9-17.

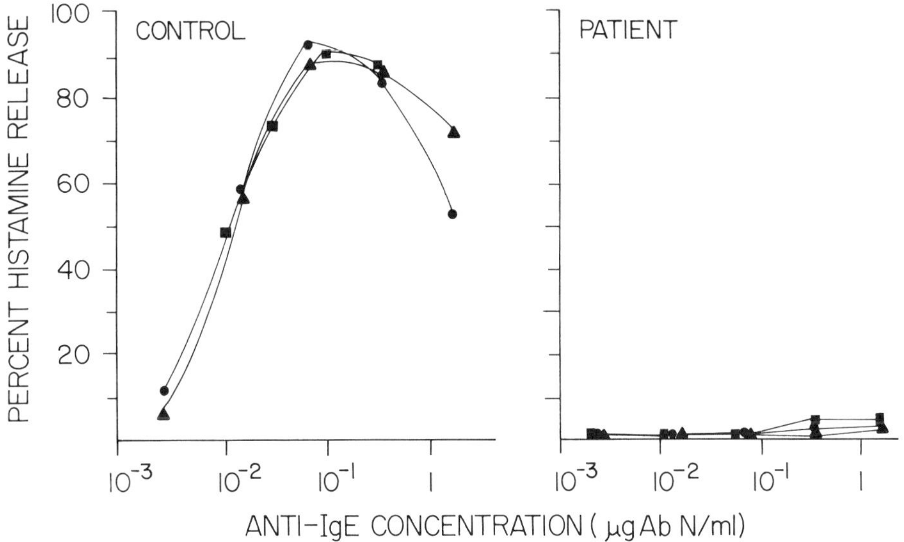

Figure 9-17 Leukocyte histamine release curves of a control subject and a patient with chronic urticaria. The three determinations for each subject were performed over a 10-week period and indicate the highly reproducible nature of the histamine release assay. Ab = antibody. (Reproduced with permission, F. Kern and L. M. Lichtenstein, *J. Clin. Invest.* 57:1369, 1976.)

Similar results have been reported by Greaves and colleagues (189). These enigmatic findings complicate the problem of chronic urticaria even more than simply calling it idiopathic; no evidence was uncovered during these studies of low basophil numbers or an abnormal IgE. Since urticaral patients showed increased IgE levels in comparison to controls, simple explanations on the basis of these findings seemed untenable. No abnormalities related to defective basophil receptors for IgE were noted during the autoradiographic studies cited above. Since the physiological basophil setting in these chronic urticaria patients resembles that previously encountered during immunotherapy for allergic rhinitis (190), chronic urticaria, and diminished histamine release on anti-IgE challenge with which it is associated, may be linked with a chronic natural process of desensitization that is ineffective in alleviating symptoms but that produces relative deactivation of the release mechanism (191). If some mechanism were available to isolate IgE-bound unknown antigen in such patients, perhaps effective desensitization could be eventually induced using such a procedure. These observations relating to the continued enigma surrounding aspects of the problem of urticaria emphasize the tremendous advances in fundamental understanding of basic control mechanisms actually involved in mediating the immediate hypersensitivity phenomenon.

Cold Urticaria

Cold-induced urticaria is a fascinating clinical phenomenon in which patients develop urticarial eruptions after exposure to lowered temperatures. The urticaria may then progress to a more generalized and subacute angioedema. The disorder is associated with the presence of cryoglobulins, cryoprecipitable fibrinogens, or cold-reactive hemolysins in some patients, but the etiology is unknown in about two-thirds of patients afflicted with this disorder. In this major idiopathic group a serum factor is present that can, if transferred to normal recipient skin, induce urticaria after challenge with cold (192). Passive-transfer experiments suggest that the actual process must involve IgE or reaginic antibody (193). Also, if an extremity is immersed in a cold environment, histamine release occurs (194–197). Studies of the mechanisms of cold-induced urticarial reactions (198, 199) indicate that both histamine and eosinophil chemotactic factor levels rise in the arm of an experimental subject where cold immersion had been induced for three minutes. No changes in the same parameters were noted in the control nonimmersed arm, and no discernible changes were found in either classic or alternate complement pathways. These studies suggest that histamine release through tissue mast cells plays a significant role in the cold urticarial process. Representative data from these experiments are shown in Figures 9-18 and 9-19. Erythema, urticaria, and angioedema persist for hours after the histamine level in the extremity returns to normal preimmersion levels, which is considerably longer than the effects of intravenous histamine— generally persisting only 45 to 60 minutes (200). Administration of antihistamines has limited effectiveness in either preventing or controlling attacks of cold-induced urticaria or persistent subsequent angioedema. The experiments of Soter and colleagues (198) may explain the relative ineffectiveness of antihistamines alone; other potent mediators, such as SRS–A, eosinophil chemotactic factor–A, and platelet-activating factor, may be intimately involved in perpetuating the inflammatory process.

Cold urticaria itself is an unpleasant and sometimes disabling disorder. The clear association with histamine release and other mediators of immediate-type hypersensitivity has also been confirmed by demonstration of degranulation of skin mast cells during induction of the lesions (201). Studies by Bentley-Phillips and co-workers (199) attempted to desensitize patients to severe cold-related attacks by inducing cold tolerance through exposure in limited repetitive fashion. These studies also confirmed cold-associated histamine release in venous blood draining urticated skin lesions and documented that no detectable changes either in prostaglandins or kinins occurred. Repeated cold exposure resulted in depletion of skin histamine reserves and temporary tolerance.

These studies have established that cold urticaria is indeed secondary to histamine and other mediator release, but they have not yet satisfactorily explained the occurrence of this syndrome in patients with idiopathic cold urti-

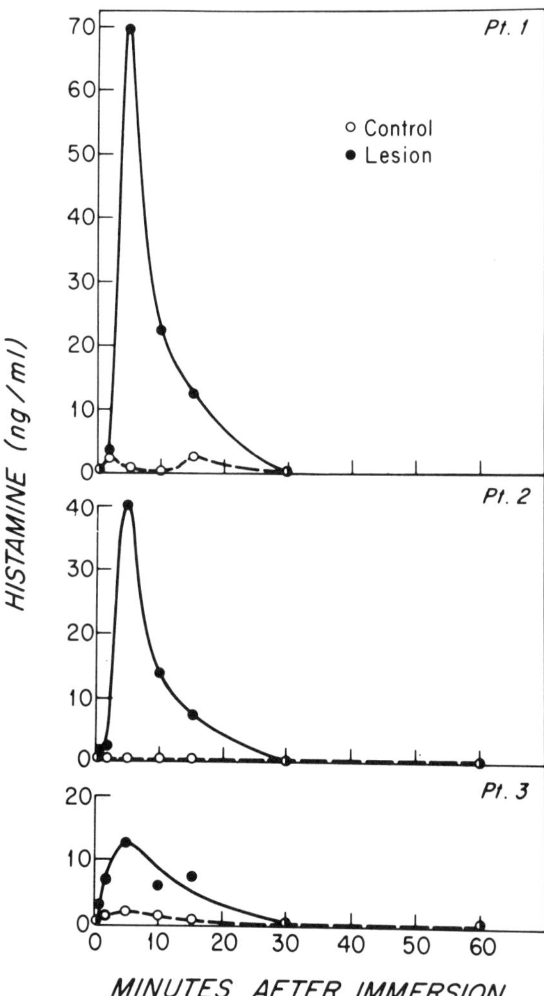

Figure 9-18   Time course of histamine release in each of 3 patients with cold urticaria in an extremity immersed in ice water at time 0 for 3 minutes (●). Histamine levels in serum of the contralateral arm (○) are shown. The histamine value plotted for time 0 was obtained just before immersion. (Reproduced with permission, N. A. Soter, S. I. Wasserman, and K. F. Austen, *N. Engl. J. Med.* 294:687, 1976.)

caria. In patients with a cold-precipitable immunoglobulin or fibrinogen, it is conceivable that local deposition near and around tissue mast cells in the skin is sufficient to initiate urticaria. This in itself is difficult to explain on the basis of classic IgE-mediated histamine release. Many of the cryoglobulins associated with cold-induced urticaria contain both IgG and IgM; such cryoglobulins often have been demon-

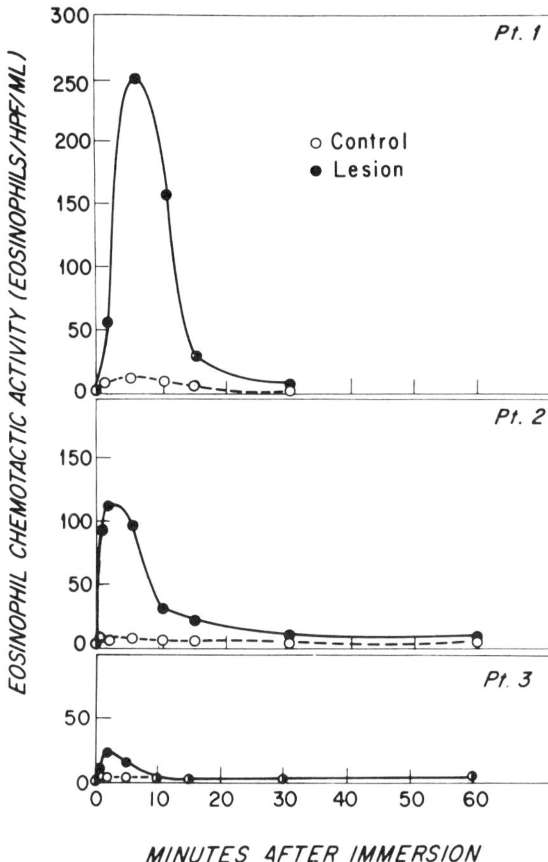

Figure 9-19 Time course of eosinophil chemotactic activity release in the 3 patients of Figure 9-18 in the immersed extremity (●) and the contralateral arm (○). (Reproduced with permission, N. A. Soter, S. I. Wasserman, and K. F. Austen, *N. Engl. J. Med.* 294:687, 1976.)

strated to harbor anti-γ-globulin or rheumatoid factor activity. It seems possible, therefore, that activation of IgE fixation to tissue mast cells may involve cold-precipitable anti-immunoglobulins that bear primary or cross-reacting specificities for determinants present on IgE. Such naturally occurring anti-γ-globulins with apparent anti-IgE specificity have been described in normal sera and in sera from patients with allergic disorders (61, 62). Such a mechanism may conceivably be involved in the production or precipitation of cold urticaria in skin exposed to low temperatures. The hypothesis would conveniently explain most of the current data attributed to this curious clinical phenomenon. The natural availability of small amounts of both antigen (IgE) and antibody to autologous IgE would be present in the skin at all times and only cold exposure would be needed to precipitate mast-cell or basophil fixation and subsequent release of potent mediators. Experimental testing of this hypothesis only awaits availability of patients with such a syndrome.

Gluten Enteropathy

The problem of what was formerly called non-tropical sprue or coeliac disease was revolutionized by the finding that materials in certain grain foods, particularly gluten or gliadin, might play an important part in the pathogenesis of the disease (202, 203). Subsequently, a significant number of experimental and clinical studies have implicated an immune response to various fractions of gluten and related substances as being directly involved in the production of at least some of the lesions in this disorder. Whether gluten itself causes the disorders of both childhood and adult coeliac disease is still unsettled; however, there is now little doubt that gluten is fundamentally involved in potentiation of the basic lesions of villous intestinal atrophy and of cell-mediated and humoral immune reactivity to its various constituents. Whether the basic disorder is related to secondary effects of the immune response (204) or to lack of intestinal enzymes which allow gliadin or its degradation products to accumulate and produce direct cellular damage (202) is still unknown. In patients with gluten-sensitive enteropathy, gluten challenge produces an increase in the local production of immunoglobulins within the involved gastrointestinal mucosa (205). A major portion of these locally stimulated immunoglobulins can be accounted for by antigliadin antibody (206). Moreover, the striking effects of gluten on intestinal epithelial cells is also demonstrated using an in vitro organ culture system and jejunal biopsy specimens from patients with gluten-sensitive enteropathy (207). In vitro evidence for exacerbation of the enteropathy was only observed in biopsy tissues from patients in exacerbation but not in remission. The effects, demonstrated in these latter studies by striking changes in intestinal enzyme content and villous morphology, could result from local immune mechanisms set into action during disease exacerbation.

For many years various models of intestinal anaphylaxis have been studied as a possible mechanism in food allergy. However, the precise events mediating what appear to be food allergies have at times been ascribed to a number of diverse etiologies including immediate hypersensitivity mediated by IgE, delayed-type hypersensitivity, or nonimmunologic processes such as enzymatic defects (208–210).

Early work in the immunologic reactions present in the disease indicated that coeliac patients frequently showed presence of antibodies to various dietary proteins, including wheat and gluten extracts (210, 211). Later this same group of patients showed antibodies to a broad variety of other heterogeneous dietary antigens, including milk, oats, sheep, bovine, and egg proteins (212–214). Most investigators have attributed these heterogeneous antibody responses to the basic inflammatory process occurring in a diffuse area of the gut absorptive surface and consequent increased permeability to a variety of macromolecules or potential antigens. When serum and intestinal secretions were studied in parallel in coeliac and control children (215), serum precipitins were noted in 27 of 33 coeliacs to antigens in wheat flour, gluten, oatmeal, rice flour, milk, bovine calf serum, sheep serum, and egg—and in only a small fraction of the controls.

Many patients with dermatitis herpetiformis (DH) showed the presence of an enteropathy similar to that found in adult coeliac disease; this enteropathy frequently showed dramatic improvement on gluten withdrawal (216–220). In addition, tissue antibodies were described in both DH and adult coeliac disease that appeared to react with reticulin (221). (DH is discussed in detail in Chapter 11.)

Present evidence for a generalized immune-complex etiology in the gluten-sensitive enteropathies is at best only fragmentary. All investigators who have examined this question directly are not in complete agreement. In one highly quoted study, Shiner and Ballard (222) performed immunofluorescence on unfixed sections of 13 children with coeliac disease before and after gluten challenge. Positive staining was reported in areas of basement membranes of villous and crypt epithelium in 10 of 13 patients. The predominant immunoglobulin that was found was IgA; fixation or tissue deposition of C3 was recorded only in one subject. Concurrent conventional histological examination showed intense infiltration of polymorphonuclear leukocytes resembling certain features of a possible local Arthus reaction. IgA staining was most intense 15 to 98 hours after gluten challenge. Prewashing of unfixed frozen sections with acidic buffers at pH 2.5 abolished staining. This was presented as evidence that immune complexes actually comprised the immunoglobulin staining. Tissue fixation of C3 in this study is difficult to explain as participating in IgA immune-complex formation; this particular Ig class does not usually fix complement, except by the alternate pathway and only then as IgA aggregates.

Further evidence for immune-complex formation was presented by Doe and co-workers (223). They challenged 3 adult patients who had been previously maintained on a gluten-free diet for at least 2 years and whose jejunal morphology was normal. Sequential studies immediately after 30 gm of intraduodenal gluten showed significant decrease in serum CH 50 and C3 in all three patients. Histological changes showed marked hyperemia, cellular infiltration, and swelling of endothelial cells within lamina propria. Again, the total picture was suggestive of an immune reaction of the Arthus type. Unfortunately, no direct immunofluorescence data were presented.

Other studies utilizing gluten challenge have suggested local immune mechanisms at work. Marked increases in lamina propria plasma cells, lymphocytes, eosinophils, and intraepithelial lymphocytic infiltrates have been recorded by a number of examiners (224–226). Basement membrane jejunal staining with anti-IgA serum occurred in coeliacs and was most intense in untreated patients. Moreover, jejunal mucosal immunoglobulin-containing cells, presumably plasma cells concerned with local Ig synthesis, were increased in coeliac children on diets containing gluten (226). Cells making all three major immunoglobulins (IgG, IgA, and IgM) were increased whereas on gluten-free diets only IgM-containing cells were noted to be elevated. Similar findings have also been recorded by others (227–229).

Since the cellular infiltrates within gluten enteropathy have suggested participation of both humoral and cellular immunity, a number of attempts have been made to demonstrate cell-mediated immunity. Documentation for the latter was recently provided by Ferguson and colleagues (230), who demonstrated specific MIF activity generated by jejunal biopsy specimens cultured in the presence of lymphocytes and α-gliadin. Clear-cut evidence for lymphocyte transformation has been presented using Frazer's fraction III from gluten representing a portion of the pepsin-trypsin digest of gluten which does not precipitate at pH 4.5 (231). Positive skin tests denoting definite cutaneous reactivity to subfractions of gluten antigens have now been recorded in a number of patients (232, 233). In the study by Baker and Read (233) skin tests showed induration and erythema appearing 2 to 3 hours after introduction of antigen and concurrent immunofluorescent studies showed local deposition of IgG and C3 in tissues with polymorphonuclear infiltration suggesting an Arthus reaction rather than delayed-type hypersensitivity. A direct correlation was noted between presence of antibody to gluten and positive skin tests which were recorded in half of the untreated patients studied. Similar Arthus-type reactions were also recorded subsequently by Arnand and co-workers (232).

In the case of gluten enteropathy, direct linkage to genetic factors may be present. HLA-8, as well as HLA-Dw3, has been recorded by several groups (234, 235); however, the primary association seems to be with HLA-Dw3 and probably only secondarily with HLA-8 by linkage disequilibrium with the Dw3 determinant (235). In the latter study a strong association with Dw3 was noted in patients with dermatitis herpetiformis as well.

The clinical examples of asthma, hypersensitivity pneumonitis, acute anaphylaxis, urticaria, and finally gluten enteropathy have been included in the discussion of immune-complex diseases related to allergy in the broad sense. They illustrate how immune complexes, as in asthma or hypersensitivity pneumonitis, play the initial and sometimes dominating role in triggering events that lead to an acute or later chronic disease state. On the other hand, allergic diseases such as hypersensitivity pneumonitis or gluten enteropathy probably involve immune-complex deposition as a transient but not predominant feature of basic pathogenesis. The diverse syndromes and disorders discussed here have been chosen as illustrative examples of the ways in which immune-complex–mediated phenomena of many types can cause tissue injury and important clinical disorders in a number of organ systems.

References

1. Prausnitz, C., and Küstner, H. Studien ueber die Ueberempfindlichkeit. *Zentralbl. Bakter.* 86:160, 1921.

2. Miller, H., and Campbell, D. H. Reagins: preliminary report on experimental evidence in support of a new theory of their nature. *Ann. Allergy* 5:236, 1947.

3. Loveless, M. H., and Cann, J. R. Distribution of "blocking" antibody in human serum proteins fractionated by electrophoresis-convection. *J. Immunol.* 74:329, 1955.

4. Loveless, M. H. Immunological studies of pollinosis: IV. The relationship between thermostable antibody in the circulation and clinical immunity. *J. Immunol.* 47:165, 1943.

5. Perelmutter, L., Rose, B., and Goodfriend, L. The relationship between the skin-sensitizing antibody and γA protein in the sera of ragweed-allergic individuals. *J. Allergy* 37:236, 1966.

6. Porter, R. R. The reagin content of human gamma-globulin fractions. *Int. Arch. Allergy Appl. Immunol.* 11:61, 1957.

7. Osler, A. G., Lichtenstein, L. M., and Levy, D. A. *In vitro* studies of human reaginic allergy. *Adv. Immunol.* 8:183, 1968.

8. Johansson, S. G. O., Bennich, H., and Wide, L. A new class of immunoglobulin in human serum. *Immunology* 14:265, 1968.

9. Johansson, S. G. O., and Bennich, H. Studies on a new class of human immunoglobulins. In J.

Killander, ed., *Gamma Globulins: Third Nobel Symposium,* P. 193. Almquist & Wiksell, Stockholm, 1968.

10. Johannson, S. G. O., and Bennich, H. Immunological studies of an atypical (myeloma) immunoglobulin. *Immunology* 13:381, 1967.

11. Ogawa, M., Kochwa, S., Smith, C., et al. Clinical aspects of IgE myeloma. *N. Engl. J. Med.* 281:1217, 1969.

12. Stanworth, D. R., Humphrey, J. H., Bennich, H., et al. Specific inhibition of the Prausnitz-Küstner reaction by an atypical human myeloma protein. *Lancet* 2:330, 1967.

13. Bennich, H., and Johansson, S. G. O. Structure and function of human immunoglobulin E. *Adv. Immunol.* 13:1, 1971.

14. Salmon, S. E., Mackey, G., and Fudenberg, H. H. "Sandwich" solid phase radioimmunoassay for the quantitative determination of human immunoglobulins. *J. Immunol.* 103:129, 1969.

15. Gleich, G. J., Averbeck, A. K., and Swedlund, H. A. Measurement of IgE in normal and allergic serum by radioimmunoassay. *J. Lab. Clin. Med.* 77:690, 1971.

16. Berg, T., and Johannson, S. G. O. IgE concentrations in children with atopic diseases. A clinical study. *Int. Arch. Allergy Appl. Immunol.* 36:219, 1969.

17. Juhlin, L., Johansson, S. G. O., Bennich, H., et al. Immunoglobulin E in dermatoses. Levels in atopic dermatitis and urticaria. *Arch. Dermatol.* 100:12, 1969.

18. Johansson, S. G. O., Mellbin, T., and Vahlquist, B. Immunoglobulin levels in Ethiopian preschool children with special reference to high concentrations of immunoglobulin E. (IgND). *Lancet* 1:1118, 1968.

19. Hogarth-Scott, R. S., Johansson, S. G. O., and Bennich, H. Antibodies to toxocara in the sera of visceral larva migrans patients: the significance of raised levels of IgE. *Clin. Exp. Immunol.* 5:619, 1969.

20. Rosenberg, E. B., Whalen, G. E., Bennich, H., et al. Increased circulating IgE in a new parasitic disease—human intestinal capillariasis. *N. Engl. J. Med.* 283:1148, 1970.

21. Ball, P. A. J., and Bartlett, A. Serological reactions to infection with *Necator americanus. Trans. R. Soc. Trop. Med. Hyg.* 63:362, 1969.

22. Ishizaka, K., and Ishizaka, T. Human reaginic antibodies and immunoglobulin E. *J. Allergy* 42:330, 1968.

23. Ishizaka, K., and Ishizaka, T. Biological function of γE antibodies and mechanisms of reaginic hypersensitivity. *Clin. Exp. Immunol.* 6:25, 1970.

24. Stanworth, D. R., Humphrey, J. H., Bennich, H. H., et al. Inhibition of Prausnitz-Küstner reaction by proteolytic-cleavage fragments of a human myeloma protein of immunoglobulin class E. *Lancet* 2:17, 1968.

25. Katz, G., and Cohen, S. Experimental evidence for histamine release in allergy. *J.A.M.A.* 117:1782, 1941.

26. Noah, J. W., and Brand, A. Release of histamine in the blood of ragweed-sensitive individuals. *J. Allergy* 25:210, 1954.

27. Noah, J. W., and Brand, A. Histamine release with differing antigen-antibody reactions. *J. Allergy* 34:203, 1963.

28. Middleton, E., Jr., Sherman, W. B., Fleming, W., et al. Some biochemical characteristics of allergic histamine release from leukocytes of ragweed-sensitive subjects *J. Allergy* 31:448, 1960.

29. Van Arsdel, P. P., Jr., Middleton, E., Jr., Sherman, W. B., et al. A quantitative study on the *in vitro* release of histamine from leukocytes of atopic persons. *J. Allergy* 29:429, 1958.

30. Lichtenstein, L. M., and Osler, A. G. Studies on the mechanisms of hypersensitivity phenomena: IX. Histamine release from human leukocytes by ragweed pollen antigen. *J. Exp. Med.* 120:507, 1964.

31. Lichtenstein, L. M., and Osler, A. G. Studies on the mechanisms of hypersensitivity phenomena: XI. The effect of normal human serum on the release of histamine from human leukocytes by ragweed pollen antigen. *J. Immunol.* 96:159, 1966.

32. Lichtenstein, L. M., and Margolis, S. Histamine release *in vitro:* inhibition by catecholamines and methylxanthines. *Science* 161:902, 1968.

33. Lichtenstein, L. M., Norman, P. S., and Winkenwerder, W. L. Clinical and *in vitro* studies on the role of immunotherapy in ragweed hay fever. *Am. J. Med.* 44:514, 1968.

34. Levy, D. A., Lichtenstein, L. M., Goldstein, E. O., et al. Immunologic and cellular changes accompanying the therapy of pollen allergy. *J. Clin. Invest.* 50:360, 1971.

35. Ishizaka, K., Tomioka, H., and Ishizaka, T. Mechanisms of passive sensitization: I. Presence of IgE and IgG molecules on human leukocytes. *J. Immunol.* 105:1459, 1970.

36. May, C. D., Lyman, M., Alberto, R., et al. Procedures for immunochemical study of histamine release from leukocytes with small volume of blood. *J. Allergy* 46:12, 1970.

37. Lichtenstein, L. M., Ishizaka, K., Norman, P. S., et al. IgE antibody measurements in ragweed hay fever. Relationship to clinical severity and the re-

sults of immunotherapy. *J. Clin. Invest.* 52:472, 1973.

38. Ishizaka, T., Tomioka, H., and Ishizaka, K. Degranulation of human basophil leukocytes by anti-γE antibody. *J. Immunol.* 106:705, 1971.

39. Yunginger, Y. W., and Gleich, G. J. Seasonal changes in IgG antibodies and their relationship to IgG antibodies during immunotherapy for ragweed hay fever. *J. Clin. Invest.* 52:1268, 1973.

40. Gleich, G. J., Jacob, G. L., Yunginger, J. W., et al. Measurement of the absolute levels of IgE antibodies in patients with ragweed hay fever. Effect of immunotherapy on seasonal changes and relationship to IgG antibodies. *J. Allergy Clin. Immunol.* 60:188, 1977.

41. Lowell, F. C., and Franklin, W. A double-blind study of the effectiveness and specificity of injection therapy in ragweed hay fever. *N. Engl. J. Med.* 273:675, 1965.

42. Norman, P. S., Winkenwerder, W. L., and Lichtenstein, L. M. Immunotherapy of hay fever with ragweed antigen E: comparisons with whole pollen extract and placebos. *J. Allergy* 42:93, 1968.

43. Norman, P. S. A rational approach to desensitization. *J. Allergy* 44:129, 1969.

44. Sadan, N., Rhyne, M. B., Mellits, E. D, et al. Immunotherapy of pollinosis in children: investigation of the immunologic basis of clinical improvement. *N. Engl. J. Med.* 280:623, 1969.

45. Gleich, G. J., and Jones, R. T. Measurement of IgE antibodies by the radioallergosorbent test. I. Technical considerations in the performance of the test. *J. Allergy Clin. Immunol.* 55:334, 1975.

46. Gleich, G. J., Auerbeck, A. K., and Swedlund, H. A. Measurement of IgE in normal and allergic serum by radioimmunoassay. *J. Lab. Clin. Med.* 77:690, 1971.

47. Evans, R., Pence, H., Kaplan, H., et al. The effect of immunotherapy on humoral and cellular responses in ragweed hay fever. *J. Clin. Invest.* 57:1378, 1976.

48. Watanabe, N., Kojima, S., Shen, F. W., et al. Suppression of IgE antibody production in SJL mice. II. Expression of Ly-1 antigen on helper and nonspecific suppressor T cells. *J. Immunol.* 118:485, 1977.

49. Kimoto, M., Kishimoto, T., Noguchi, S., et al. Regulation of antibody response in different immunoglobulin classes. II. Induction of *in vitro* IgE antibody response in murine spleen cells and demonstration of a possible involvement of distinct T-helper cells in IgE and IgG antibody responses. *J. Immunol.* 118:840, 1977.

50. Suemura, M., Kishimoto, T., Hirai, Y., et al. Regulation of antibody response in different immunoglobulin classes. III. *In vitro* demonstration of "IgE class-specific" suppressor functions of DNP-mycobacterium-primed T cells and the soluble factor released from these cells. *J. Immunol.* 119:149, 1977.

51. Urban, J. F., Jr., Ishizaka, T., and Ishizaka, K.: IgE formation in the rat following infection with *Nippostrongylus brasiliensis*. III. Soluble factor for the generation of IgE-bearing lymphocytes. *J. Immunol.* 119:583, 1977.

52. Watanabe, N., and Ovary, Z. Suppression of IgE antibody production in SJL mice. III. Characterization of a suppressor substance extracted from normal SJL spleen cells. *J. Exp. Med.* 145:1501, 1977.

53. Polmar, S. H., Waldmann, T. A., and Terry, W. D. IgE in immunodeficiency. *Am. J. Pathol.* 69:499, 1972.

54. Polmar, S. H., Lischner, H. W., Huang, N. N., et al. IgE levels in immunological deficiency states. *Clin. Res.* 18:431, 1970.

55. Ganier, M., and Lieberman, P. Infantile agammaglobulinemia and immediate hypersensitivity to penicillin G. *J.A.M.A.* 237:1852, 1977.

56. Kincade, P. W., Lawton, A. R., Bockman, D. E., et al. Suppression of immunoglobulin G synthesis as a result of antibody-mediated suppression of immunoglobulin M synthesis in chickens. *Proc. Natl. Acad. Sci. USA* 67:1918, 1970.

57. Dwyer, J. M., Rosenbaum, J. T., and Lewis, S. The effect of anti-mu suppression of γM and γG on the production of γE. *J. Exp. Med.* 143:781, 1976.

58. Mendoza, G., and Metzger, H. Distribution and valency of receptor for IgE on rodent mast cells and related tumour cells. *Nature* 264:548, 1976.

59. Newman, S. A., Rossi, G., and Metzger, H. Molecular weight and valence of the cell-surface receptor for immunoglobulin E. *Proc. Natl. Acad. Sci. USA* 74:869, 1977.

60. Segal, D. M., Taurog, J. D., and Metzger, H. Dimeric immunoglobulin E serves as a unit signal for mast cell degranulation. *Proc. Natl. Acad. Sci. USA* 74:2993, 1977.

61. Brostoff, J., Johns, P., and Stanworth, D. R. Complexed IgE in atopy. *Lancet* 2:741, 1977.

62. Williams, R. C., Jr., Griffiths, R. W., Emmons, J. D., et al. Naturally occurring human antiglobulins with specificity for γE. *J. Clin. Invest.* 51:955, 1972.

63. Capron, A., Dessaint, J-P., Joseph, M., et al. Interaction between IgE complexes and macrophages in the rat: a new mechanism of macrophage activation. *Eur. J. Immunol.* 7:315, 1977.

64. Johansson, S. G. O., Bennich, H. H., and

Berg, T. The clinical significance of IgE. *Prog. Clin. Immunol.* 1:157, 1972.

65. Dessaint, J-P., Capron, M., Bout, D., et al. Quantitative determination of specific IgE antibodies to schistosome antigens and serum IgE levels in patients with schistosomiasis (*S. mansoni* or *S. haematobium*). *Clin. Exp. Immunol.* 20:427, 1975.

66. Barth, W. F. H., Jarrett, E. E. E., and Urquhart, G. M. Studies on the mechanism of the self-cure reaction in rats infected with *Nippostrongylus brasiliensis. Immunology* 10:459, 1966.

67. Africa, C. M. Studies on the host relations of *Nippostrongylus muris,* with special reference to age resistance and acquired immunity. *J. Parasitol.* 18:1, 1931.

68. Mulligan, W., Urquhart, G. M., Jennings, F. W., et al. Immunological studies on *Nippostrongylus brasiliensis* infection in the rat: the "self-cure" phenomenon. *Exp. Parsitol.* 16:341, 1965.

69. Urquhart, G. M., Mulligan, W., Eadie, R. M., et al. Immunological studies on *Nippostrongylus brasiliensis* in the rat: the role of local anaphylaxis. *Exp. Parasitol.* 16:210, 1965.

70. Sadun, E. H., and Gore, R. W. *Schistosoma mansoni* and *S. haematobium:* Homocytotropic reagin-like antibodies in infections of man and experimental animals. *Exp. Parasitol.* 28:435, 1970.

71. Dean, D. A., Wistar, R., Murrell, K. D. Combined *in vitro* effects of rat antibody and neutrophilic leukocytes on schistosomula of *Schistosoma mansoni. Am. J. Trop. Med. Hyg.* 23:420, 1974.

72. Butterworth, A. E., Sturrock, R. F., Houba, V., et al. Eosinophils as mediators of antibody-dependent damage to schistosomula. *Nature* 256:727, 1975.

73. Tada, T., and Ishizaka, K. Distribution of γE-forming cells in lymphoid tissues of the human and monkey. *J. Immunol.* 104:377, 1970.

74. Van Epps, D. E., Husby, G., Williams, R. C., Jr., et al. Liver disease—a prominent cause of serum IgE elevation. *Clin. Exp. Immunol.* 23:444, 1976.

75. Bias, W. B. The genetic basis of asthma. In F. Austen and L. Lichtenstein, eds., *Asthma,* p. 39. Academic Press, New York, 1973.

76. Black, P. L., and Marsh, D. G.: The genetic basis for atopic allergy in man. In M. S. Segal and E. B. Weiss, eds., *Bronchial Asthma: Mechanisms and Therapeutics,* p. 53. Little, Brown and Co., Boston, 1978.

77. Marsh, D. G. Allergens and the genetics of allergy. In M. Sela, ed., *The Antigens,* vol. 3, p. 271. Academic Press, New York, 1975.

78. Marsh, D. G. Purification of pollen allergens: use in genetic studies of immune responsiveness in man. In Y. Yamamura, O. L. Frick, Y. Horuchi et al., eds., *Proceedings of the Eighth International Congress of Allergology,* p. 381. American Elsevier Publishing Co., New York, 1974.

79. Santilli, J., Marsh, D., Bias, W., et al. Puncture skin testing with purified pollen antigens: a useful tool for genetic studies in atopic man. *J. Allergy Clin. Immunol.* 55:108, 1975.

80. Marsh, D. G., and Bias, W. B. Control of specific allergic response in man: HL-A associated and IgE-regulating genes. *Fed. Proc.* 33:774, 1974.

81. Marsh, D. G., Chase, G. A., and Bias, W. B. An immune response gene for ragweed Ra3: most probable location within the HL-A2, 12 haplotype. *Fed. Proc.* 34:980, 1975.

82. Bruce, C. A., Bias, W. B., Norman, P. S., et al. Studies of HL-A antigen frequencies, IgE levels, and specific allergic sensitivities in patients having ragweed hayfever, with and without asthma. *Clin. Exp. Immunol.* 25:67, 1976.

83. Logsdon, P. J., Middleton, E., Jr., and Coffey, R. G. Stimulation of leukocyte adenyl cyclase by hydrocortisone and isoproterenol in asthmatic and non asthmatic subjects. *J. Allergy Clin. Immunol.* 50:45, 1972.

84. Parker, C. W., and Smith. J. W. Alterations in cyclic adenosine monophosphate metabolism in human bronchial asthma. Leukocyte responsiveness to β-adrenergic agents. *J. Clin. Invest.* 52:48, 1973.

85. Gillespie, E., Valentine, M. D., and Lichtenstein, L. M. Cyclic AMP metabolism in asthma: studies with leukocytes and lymphocytes. *J. Allergy Clin. Immunol.* 53:27, 1974.

86. Thorsby, E., Engeset, A., and Lie, S. O. HL-A antigens and susceptibility to diseases. The study of patients with acute lymphoblastic leukaemia, Hodgkin's disease, and childhood asthma. *Tissue Antigens* 1:147, 1971.

87. Rackemann, F. M. A clinical study of 150 cases of bronchial asthma. *Arch. Intern. Med.* 22:517, 1918.

88. Levine, B. B., Stember, R. H., and Fotino, M. Ragweed hayfever: genetic control and linkage to HL-A haplotypes. *Science* 178:1201, 1972.

89. Cooke, R. A. In *Allergy in Theory and Practice.* W. B. Saunders Co., Philadelphia, 1974.

90. Norman, P. S. Antigens that cause atopic disease. In M. Samter, ed., *Immunological Diseases,* ed. 2, p. 775. Little, Brown and Co., Boston, 1971.

91. Marsh, D. G. Allergens and the genetics of allergy. In M. Sela, ed., *The Antigens,* p. 271. Academic Press, New York, 1975.

92. Stanworth, D. R. In *Immediate Hypersensitiv-*

ity. North-Holland Publishing Co., Amsterdam, 1973.

93. King, T. P., Norman, P. S., and Connell, J. T. Isolation and characterization of allergens from ragweed pollen. II. *Biochemistry* 3:458, 1964.

94. King, T. P., Norman, P. S., and Lichtenstein, L. M. Isolation and characterization of allergens from ragweed pollen. IV. *Biochemistry* 6:1992, 1967.

95. King, T. P., Norman, P. S., and Tao, N. Chemical modifications of the major allergen of ragweed pollen, antigen E. *Immunochemistry* 11:83, 1974.

96. Mole, L. E., Goodfriend, L., Lapkoff, C. B., et al. The amino acid sequence of ragweed pollen allergen Ra5. *Biochemistry* 14:1216, 1975.

97. Gleich, G. J., and Jacob, G. L. Immunoglobulin E antibodies to pollen allergens account for high percentages of total immunoglobulin E protein. *Science* 190:1106, 1975.

98. Zeiss, C. R., Pruzansky, J. J., Patterson, R., et al. A solid phase radioimmunoassay for the quantitation of human reaginic antibody against ragweed antigen E. *J. Immunol.* 110:414, 1973.

99. Griffiths, B. W. The subunits of antigens of ragweed pollen. *J. Chromatogr.* 69:391, 1972.

100. Griffiths, B. W. Structural studies on antigen E of ragweed pollen. *Can. J. Biochem.* 51:1275, 1973.

101. Ishizaka, K., Kishimoto, T., Delespesse, G., et al. Immunogenic properties of modified antigen E. I. Presence of specific determinants for T cells in denatured antigen and polypeptide chains. *J. Immunol.* 113:70, 1974.

102. Ishizaka, K., Okudaira, H., and King, T. P. Immunogenic properties of modified antigen E. II. Ability of urea-denatured antigen and α-polypeptide chain to prime T cells specific for antigen E. *J. Immunol.* 114:110, 1975.

103. King, T. P. Chemical and biological properties of some atopic allergens. *Adv. Immunol.* 23:77, 1976.

104. Brandt, R., Ponterius, G., and Yman, L. The allergens of cat epithelia and cat serum. Comparative studies based on the radioallergosorbent technique (RAST). *Int. Arch. Allergy Appl. Immunol.* 45:447, 1973.

105. King, T. P., Sobotka, A. K., Kochoumian, L., et al. Allergens of honey bee venom. *Arch. Biochem. Biophys.* 172:661, 1976.

106. Salvaggio, J., Castro-Murillo, E., and Kundur, V. Immunologic response of atopic and normal individuals to keyhole limpet hemocyanin. *J. Allergy* 44:344, 1969.

107. Kontou-Karakitsos, K., Salvaggio, J. E., and Matthews, K. P. Comparative nasal absorption of allergens in atopic and nonatopic subjects. *J. Allergy Clin. Immunol.* 55:241, 1975.

108. Patterson, R., Suszko, I. M., and McIntire, F. C. Polymerized ragweed antigen E. I. Preparation and immunologic studies. *J. Immunol.* 110:1402, 1973.

109. Patterson, R., Suszko, I. M., Pruzansky, J. J., et al. Polymerized ragweed antigen E. II. *In vivo* elimination studies and reactivity with IgE antibody systems. *J. Immunol.* 110:1413, 1973.

110. Patterson, R., and Suszko, I. M. Polymerized ragweed antigen E. III. Differences in immune response to three molecular weight ranges of monomer and polymer. *J. Immunol.* 112:1855, 1974.

111. Metzger, W. J., Patterson, R., Zeiss, C. R., et al. Comparison of polymerized and unpolymerized antigen E for immunotherapy of ragweed allergy. *N. Engl. J. Med.* 295:1160, 1976.

112. Cockcroft, D. W., Cuff, M. T., Tarlo, S. M., et al. Allergen injection therapy with glutaraldehyde-modified-ragweed pollen-tyrosine adsorbate. *J. Allergy Clin. Immunol.* 60:56, 1977.

113. Lee, W. Y., and Sehon, A. H. Abrogation of reaginic antibodies with modified allergens. *Nature* 267:618, 1977.

114. Abuchowski, A. The effects of covalent attachment of polyethylene glycol on bovine serum albumin and bovine liver catalase. Doctoral dissertation, Rutgers University, 1975.

115. Takatsu, K., and Ishizaka, K. Reaginic antibody formation in the mouse. VII. Induction of suppressor T cells for IgE and IgG antibody responses. *J. Immunol.* 116:1257, 1976.

116. Conroy, M. C., and Lichtenstein, L. M. Measurement of IgE binding to human leukocytes. *Fed. Proc.* 35:809, 1976.

117. Stallman, P. J., and Aalberse, R. C. Quantitation of basophil-bound IgE in atopic and nonatopic subjects. *Int. Arch. Allergy Appl. Immunol.* 54:114, 1977.

118. van Elven, E. H., Stallman, P. J., and Brühl, P. H. C. Electron microscopic studies on human basophils from atopic and nonatopic subjects, using horse radish peroxidase labelled anti-IgE. *Int. Arch. Allergy Appl. Immunol.* 54:560, 1977.

119. Hastie, R., Chir, B., Levy, D., et al. The antigen-induced degranulation of basophil leukocytes from atopic subjects studied by electron microscopy. *Lab. Invest.* 36:173, 1977.

120. Dvorak, A. M., Dickersin, G. R., Connell, A., et al. Degranulation mechanisms in human leukemic basophils. *Clin. Immunol. Immunopathol.* 5:235, 1976.

121. Dvorak, A. M., Mihm, M. C., Jr., and

Dvorak, H. F. Degranulation of basophilic leukocytes in allergic contact dermatitis reactions in man. *J. Immunol.* 116:687, 1976.

122. Nadel, J. A. Neurophysiologic aspects of asthma. In K. F. Austen and L. M. Lichtenstein, eds., *Asthma: Physiology, Immunopharmacology and Treatment*, p. 29. Academic Press, New York, 1973.

123. Levinson, H., Collins-Williams, C., Bryan, A. C., et al. Asthma: current concepts. *Pediatr. Clin. North Am.* 21:951, 1974.

124. Goetzl, E. J., and Austen, K. F. Generation, function, and disposition of chemical mediators of the mast cell in immediate hypersensitivity. In J. Hadden, R. G. Coffey, and F. Spreafico, eds., *Comprehensive Immunology Immunopharmacology,* p. 113. Plenum Medical Book Co., New York and London, 1977.

125. Langan, T. A. Protein kinases and protein kinase substrates. *Adv. Cyclic Nucleotide Res.* 3:99, 1973.

126. Assem, E. S. K. Inhibition of allergic reactions by beta-adrenergic stimulants. *Postgrad. Med. J.* 47:31, 1971 (suppl.).

127. Kaliner, M., Orange, R. P., and Austen, K. F. Immunological release of histamine and slow reacting substance of anaphylaxis from human lung. IV. Enhancement by cholinergic and alpha adrenergic stimulation. *J. Exp. Med.* 136:556, 1972.

128. Lichtenstein, L. M. The control of IgE-mediated histamine release: implications for the study of asthma. In K. F. Austen and L. M. Lichtenstein, eds., *Asthma: Physiology, Immunopharmacology, and Treatment,* p. 91. Academic Press, New York, 1973.

129. Pepys, J. Pulmonary hypersensitivity disease due to inhaled organic antigens. *Ann. Intern. Med.* 64:943, 1966.

130. Pepys, J. Hypersensitivity diseases of the lungs due to fungi and organic dusts. In P. Kallós, M. Hasak, and T. M. Inderbitzen, eds., *Monographs in Allergy,* vol. 4, p. 1. S. Karger, Basel, 1969.

131. Dickie, H. A., and Rankin, J. Farmer's lung—an acute granulomatous interstitial pneumonitis occurring in agricultural workers. *J.A.M.A.* 167:1069, 1958.

132. Emanuel, D. A., Wenzel, F. J., Bowerman, C. I., et al. Farmer's lung: clinical, pathologic and immunologic study of twenty-four patients. *Am. J. Med.* 37:392, 1964.

133. Seal, R. M., Hapke, E. J., Thomas, G. O., et al. The pathology of the acute and chronic stages of farmer's lung. *Thorax* 23:469, 1968.

134. Edwards, J. H. The isolation of antigens associated with farmer's lung. *Clin. Exp. Immunol.* 11:341, 1972.

135. Reed, C. E. Hypersensitivity pneumonitis. *Postgrad. Med.* 51:120, 1972.

136. Feldman, G., and Gordon, V. H. Hypersensitivity pneumonitis. *South. Med. J.* 68:952, 1975.

137. Reed, C. E., Sosman, A., and Barbee, R. A. Pigeon-breeder's lung. A newly observed interstitial pulmonary disease. *J.A.M.A.* 193:81, 1965.

138. Hargreave, C. E., Pepys, J., Longbotton, J. L., et al. Bird breeder's (fancier's) lung. *Lancet* 1:446, 1966.

139. Boyd, G., Dick, H. W., Lorimer, A. R., et al. Bird breeder's lung. *Scott. Med. J.* 12:69, 1967.

140. Fink, J. N., Sosman, A. J., Barboriak, J. J., et al. Pigeon breeder's disease. A clinical study of a hypersensitivity pneumonitis. *Ann. Intern. Med.* 68:1205, 1968.

141. Fink, J. N., Sosman, A. J., Salvaggio, J. E., et al. Precipitins and the diagnosis of a hypersensitivity pneumonitis. *J. Allergy Clin. Immunol.* 48:179, 1971.

142. Fink, J. N., Schlueter, D. P., Sosman, A. J., et al. Clinical survey of pigeon breeders. *Chest* 62:277, 1972.

143. Fink, J. N., Tebo, T., and Barboriak, J. Characterization of human precipitating antibody to inhaled antigens. *J. Immunol.* 103:244, 1969.

144. Boyd, G., and Parratt, D. Improved diagnosis of farmer's lung using the fluorescent antibody technique. *Thorax* 29:417, 1974.

145. Parratt, D., and Peel, J. A. A fluorescent antibody test in the diagnosis of farmer's lung. *J. Clin. Pathol.* 25:846, 1972.

146. Kurup, V. P., Barboriak, J. J., and Fink, J. N. Indirect immunofluorescent detection of antibodies against thermophilic actinomycetes in patients with hypersensitivity pneumonitis. *J. Lab. Clin. Med.* 89:533, 1977.

147. Barboriak, J. J., Sosman, A. J., and Reed, C. E. Serological studies in pigeon breeder's disease. *J. Lab. Clin. Med.* 65:600, 1965.

148. Moore, V. L., and Fink, J. N. Immunologic studies in hypersensitivity pneumonitis—quantitative precipitins and complement-fixing antibodies in symptomatic and asymptomatic pigeon breeders. *J. Lab. Clin. Med.* 85:540, 1975.

149. Caldwell, J. R., Pearce, D. E., Spencer, C., et al. Immunologic mechanisms in hypersensitivity pneumonitis. I. Evidence for cell-mediated immunity and complement fixation in pigeon breeder's disease. *J. Allergy Clin. Immunol.* 52:225, 1973.

150. Moore, V. L., Fink, J. N., Barboriak, J. J., et al. Immunologic events in pigeon breeder's disease. *J. Allergy Clin. Immunol.* 53:319, 1974.

151. Berrens, L., and Guikers, C. L. H. An immunochemical study of pigeon-breeder's disease.

IV. A highly selective *in vitro* test for pigeon fancier's lung based on complement (C3) inactivation. *Int. Arch. Allergy Appl. Immunol.* 43:347, 1972.

152. Flaherty, D. K., Barboriak, J., Emanuel, D., et al. Multilaboratory comparison of three immunodiffusion methods used for the detection of precipitating antibodies in hypersensitivity pneumonitis. *J. Lab. Clin. Med.* 84:298, 1974.

153. Roberts, R. C. Fractionation and chemical characterization studies on *Micropolyspora faeni* antigens. *Ann. N.Y. Acad. Sci.* 221:199, 1974.

154. Banaszak, E. F., Thiede, W. H., and Fink, J. N. Hypersensitivity pneumonitis due to contamination of an air conditioner. *N. Engl. J. Med.* 283:271, 1970.

155. Tourville, D. R., Weiss, W. I., Wertlake, P. T., et al. Hypersensitivity pneumonitis due to contamination of home humidifier. *J. Allergy Clin. Immunol.* 49:245, 1972.

156. Sweet, L. C., Anderson, J. A., Callies, Q. C., et al. Hypersensitivity pneumonitis related to a home furnace humidifier. *J. Allergy Clin. Immunol.* 48:171, 1971.

157. Richerson, H. B. Acute experimental hypersensitivity pneumonitis in the guinea pig. *J. Lab. Clin. Med.* 79:745, 1972.

158. Gell, P. G. H., and Benacerraf, B. Delayed hypersensitivity to simple protein antigens. *Adv. Immunol.* 1:319, 1961.

159. Hensley, G. T., Fink, J. N., and Barboriak, J. J. Hypersensitivity pneumonitis in the monkey. *Arch. Pathol.* 97:33, 1974.

160. Pirie, H. M., Dawson, C. O., Breeze, R. G., et al. A bovine disease similar to farmer's lung: extrinsic allergic alveolitis. *Vet. Rec.* 88:346, 1971.

161. Moore, V. L., Hensley, G. T., and Fink, J. N. An animal model of hypersensitivity pneumonitis in the rabbit. *J. Clin. Invest.* 56:937, 1975.

162. von Lichtenberg, F., Smith, T. M., Lucia, H. L., et al. New model for schistosome granuloma formation using a soluble egg antigen and bentonite particles. *Nature* 229:199, 1971.

163. Boros, D. L., and Warren, K. S. Specific granulomatous hypersensitivity elicited by bentonite particles coated with soluble antigens from schistosome eggs and tubercle bacilli. *Nature* 229:200, 1971.

164. Wenzel, F. J., Emanuel, D. A., and Gray, R. L. Immunofluorescent studies in patients with farmer's lung. *J. Allergy* 48:224, 1971.

165. van Toorn, D. W. Coffee worker's lung. A new example of extrinsic allergic alveolitis. *Thorax* 25:399, 1970.

166. Reynolds, H. Y., Fulmer, J. D., Kazmierowski, J. A., et al. Analysis of cellular and protein content of broncho-alveolar lavage fluid from patients with idiopathic pulmonary fibrosis and chronic hypersensitivity pneumonitis. *J. Clin. Invest.* 59:163, 1977.

167. Kravis, T. C., Ahmed, A., Brown, T. E., et al. Pathogenic mechanisms in pulmonary fibrosis: collagen-induced migration inhibition factor production and cytotoxicity mediated by lymphocytes. *J. Clin. Invest.* 58:1223, 1976.

168. Poitier, P., and Richet, C. De l'action anaphylactique de certains venins. *C.R. Soc. Biol. (Paris)* 54:170, 1902.

169. James, L. P., Jr., and Austen, K. F. Fatal systemic anaphylaxis in man. *N. Engl. J. Med.* 270:597, 1964.

170. Petsas, A. A., and Kotler, M. N. Electrocardiographic changes associated with penicillin anaphylaxis. *Chest* 64:66, 1973.

171. Hanashiro, P. K., and Weil, M. H. Anaphylactic shock in man: report of two cases with detailed hemodynamic and metabolic studies. *Arch. Intern. Med.* 119:129, 1967.

172. Kern, R. A., and Wimberley, N. A., Jr. Penicillin reactions: their nature, growing importance, recognition, management and prevention. *Am. J. Med. Sci.* 226:357, 1953.

173. Levine, B. B. Immunologic mechanisms of penicillin allergy: a haptenic model system for the study of allergic diseases of man. *N. Engl. J. Med.* 275:1115, 1966.

174. Levine, B. B., Siraganian, R. P., and Schenkein, I. Allergy to human seminal plasma. *N. Engl. J. Med.* 288:894, 1973.

175. Routledge, R. C., De Kretser, D. M. H., and Wadsworth, L. D. Severe anaphylaxis due to passive sensitization by donor blood. *Br. Med. J.* 1:434, 1976.

176. Ramirez, M. A. Horse asthma following blood transfusion: report of a case. *J.A.M.A.* 73:984, 1919.

177. Hunt, E. L. Death from allergic shock. *N. Engl. J. Med.* 228:502, 1943.

178. McEwen, L. M. Corticosteroids in treatment of anaphylaxis. *Br. Med. J.* 3:649, 1975.

179. Frankland, A. W., and Addel-Maguid, R. Adrenalin in the treatment of anaphylaxis. *Br. Med. J.* 4:162, 1975.

180. McEwen, L. M. Adrenalin in treatment of anaphylaxis. *Br. Med. J.* 4:519, 1975.

181. Davies, P., Roberts, M. B., and Roylance, J. Acute reactions to urographic contrast media. *Br. Med. J.* 2:434, 1975.

182. Thompson, J. S. Urticaria and angioedema. *Ann. Intern. Med.* 69:361, 1968.

183. Calnan, C. D. Release of histamine in urticaria pigmentosa. *Lancet* 1:996, 1957.

184. Moore-Robinson, M., and Warin, R. P. Effect of salicylates in urticaria. *Br. Med. J.* 4:262, 1967.

185. Michaëlsson, G., and Juhlin, L. Urticaria induced by preservatives and dye additives in food and drugs. *Br. J. Dermatol.* 88:525, 1973.

186. Doeglas, H. M. G. Reactions to aspirin and food additives in patients with chronic urticaria, including the physical urticarias. *Br. J. Dermatol.* 93:135, 1975.

187. Warin, R. P., and Smith, R. J. Challenge test battery in chronic urticaria. *Br. J. Dermatol.* 94:401, 1976.

188. Kern, F., and Lichtenstein, L. M. Defective histamine release in chronic urticaria. *J. Clin. Invest.* 57:1369, 1976.

189. Greaves, M. W., Plummer, V. M., McLaughlan, P., et al. Serum and cell bound IgE in chronic urticaria. *Clin. Allergy* 4:265, 1974.

190. Lichtenstein, L. M., and Levy, D. A. Is "desensitization" for ragweed hayfever immunologically specific? *Int. Arch. Allergy Appl. Immunol.* 42:615, 1972.

191. Baxter, J. H., and Adamik, R. Control of histamine release: effects of various conditions on rate of release and rate of cell desensitization. *J. Immunol.* 114:1034, 1975.

192. Sherman, W. B., and Seebohm, P. M. Passive transfer of cold urticaria. *J. Allergy* 21:414, 1950.

193. Houser, D. D., Arbesman, C. E., Ito, K., et al. Cold urticaria: immunologic studies. *Am. J. Med.* 49:23, 1970.

194. Rose, B. Histamine, hormones, and hypersensitivity. *J. Allergy* 25:168, 1954.

195. Henderson, L. L., Code, C. F., and Roth, G. M. Increased blood histamine in thermal intolerance: report of a patient with cryoglobulinemia. *J. Allergy* 29:122, 1958.

196. Beall, G. N. Plasma histamine concentrations in allergic diseases. *J. Allergy* 34:8, 1963.

197. Kaplan, A. P., Gray, L., Schaff, R. E., et al. *In vivo* studies of mediator release in cold urticaria and cholinergic urticaria. *J. Allergy Clin. Immunol.* 55:394, 1975.

198. Soter, N. A., Wasserman, S. I., and Austen, K. F. Cold urticaria: release into the circulation of histamine and eosinophil chemotactic factor of anaphylaxis during cold challenge. *N. Engl. J. Med.* 294:687, 1976.

199. Bentley-Phillips, C. B., Black, A. K., and Greaves, M. W. Induced tolerance in cold urticaria caused by cold-evoked histamine release. *Lancet* 2:63, 1976.

200. Weiss, S., Robb, G. P., and Ellis, L. B. The systemic effects of histamine in man, with special reference to the responses of the cardiovascular system. *Arch. Intern. Med.* 49:360, 1932.

201. Juhlin, L., and Shelley, W. B. Role of mast cell and basophil in cold urticaria with associated systemic reactions. *J.A.M.A.* 177:371, 1961.

202. Frazer, A. C. Discussion on some problems of steatorrhea and reduced stature. *Proc. Ry. Soc. Med.* 49:1009, 1956.

203. Frazer, A. C., Fletcher, R. F., Ross, C. A. C., et al. Gluten-induced enteropathy: the effect of partially digested gluten. *Lancet* 2:252, 1959.

204. Booth, C. C. The enterocyte in coeliac disease. *Br. Med. J.* 4:14, 1970.

205. Loeb, P. M., Strober, W., Falchuk, Z. M., et al. Incorporation of L-leucine-^{14}C into immunoglobulins by jejunal biopsies of patients with celiac sprue and other gastrointestinal diseases. *J. Clin. Invest.* 50:559, 1971.

206. Falchuk, Z. M., Laster, L., and Strober, W. Gluten sensitive enteropathy: intestinal synthesis of antigluten antibody *in vitro*. *Clin. Res.* 19:390, 1971.

207. Falchuk, Z. M., Gebhard, R. L., Sessoms, C., et al. An *in vitro* model of gluten-sensitive enteropathy. Effect of gliadin on intestinal epithelial cells of patients with gluten-sensitive enteropathy in organ culture. *J. Clin. Invest.* 53:487, 1974.

208. Bleumink, E. Food allergy. The chemical nature of the substances eliciting symptoms. *World Rev. Nutr. Diet.* 12:505, 1970.

209. Goldstein, G. B., and Heiner, D. C. Clinical and immunological perspectives in food sensitivity. *J. Allergy* 46:270, 1970.

210. Taylor, K. B., Thompson, D. L., Truelove, S. C., et al. An immunological study of coeliac disease and idiopathic steatorrhea. Serological reactions to gluten and milk proteins. *Br. Med. J.* 2:1727, 1961.

211. Heiner, D. C., Lahey, M. E., Wilson, J. F., et al. Precipitins to antigens of wheat and cow's milk in coeliac disease. *J. Pediatr.* 61:813, 1962.

212. Alarçon-Segovia, D., Herskovic, T., Wakim, K. G., et al. Presence of circulating antibodies to gluten and milk fractions in patients with nontropical sprue. *Am. J. Med.* 36:485, 1964.

213. Kenrick, K. G., and Walker-Smith, J. A. Immunoglobulins and dietary protein antibodies in childhood coeliac disease. *Gut* 11:635, 1970.

214. Rossipal, E. Precipitins to aqueous extracts of flour in coeliac disease. *Lancet* 1:251, 1970.

215. Ferguson, A., and Carswell, F. Precipitins to dietary proteins in serum and upper intestinal secretions of coeliac children. *Br. Med. J.* 1:75, 1972.

216. Marks, J., Shuster, S., and Watson, A. J. Small-bowel changes in dermatitis herpetiformis. *Lancet* 2:1280, 1966.

217. Fraser, N. G., Murray, D., and Alexander, J. O. D. Structure and function of the small intestine in dermatitis herpetiformis. *Br. J. Dermatol.* 79:509, 1967.

218. Fry, L., Keir, P., McMinn, R. M. H., et al. Small-intestinal structure and function and haematological changes in dermatitis herpetiformis. *Lancet* 2:729, 1967.

219. Fry, L., McMinn, R. M. H., Cowan, J. D., et al. Gluten-free diet and re-introduction of gluten in dermatitis herpetiformis. *Arch. Dermatol.* 100:129, 1969.

220. Shuster, S., Watson, A. J., and Marks, J. Coeliac syndrome in dermatitis herpetiformis. *Lancet* 1:1101, 1968.

221. Seah, P. P., Fry, L., Hoffbrand, A. V., et al. Tissue antibodies in dermatitis herpetiformis and adult coeliac disease. *Lancet* 1:834, 1971.

222. Shiner, M., and Ballard, J. Antigen-antibody reaction in jejunal mucosa in childhood coeliac disease after gluten challenge. *Lancet* 1:1202, 1972.

223. Doe, W., Henry, K., Holt, L., et al. An immunological study of adult coeliac disease. *Gut* 13:324, 1972.

224. Lancaster-Smith, M., Kumar, P. J., and Dawson, A. M. The cellular infiltrate of the jejunum in adult coeliac disease and dermatitis herpetiformis following the reintroduction of dietary gluten. *Gut* 16:683, 1975.

225. Lancaster-Smith, M., Packer, S., Kumar, P. J., et al. Cellular infiltrate of the jejunum after reintroduction of dietary gluten in children with treated coeliac disease. *J. Clin. Pathol.* 29:587, 1976.

226. Lancaster-Smith, M., Packer, S., Kumar, P. J., et al. Immunological phenomena in the jejunum and serum after reintroduction of dietary gluten in children with treated coeliac disease. *J. Clin. Pathol.* 29:592, 1976.

227. Douglas, A. P., Crabbé, P. A., and Hobbs, J. R. Immunochemical studies of the serum, intestinal secretions and intestinal mucosa in patients with adult celiac disease and other forms of the celiac syndrome. *Gastroenterology* 59:414, 1970.

228. Soltoft, J. Immunoglobulin-containing cells in non-tropical sprue. *Clin. Exp. Immunol.* 6:413, 1970.

229. Pettingale, K. W. Immunoglobulin-containing cells in the coeliac syndrome. *Gut* 12:291, 1971.

230. Ferguson, A., MacDonald, T. T., McClure, J. P., et al. Cell-mediated immunity to gliadin within the small-intestinal mucosa in coeliac disease. *Lancet* 1:895, 1975.

231. Sikora, K., Anand, B. S., Truelove, S. C., et al. Stimulation of lymphocytes from patients with coeliac disease by a subfraction of gluten. *Lancet* 2:389, 1976.

232. Anand, B. S., Truelove, S. C., and Offord, R. E. Skin test for coeliac disease using a subfraction of gluten. *Lancet* 1:118, 1977.

233. Baker, P. G., and Read, A. E. Positive skin reactions to gluten in coeliac disease. *Q. J. Med.* 45:603, 1976.

234. Falchuk, Z. M., Rogentine, G. N., and Strober, W. Predominance of histocompatibility antigen HL-A8 in patients with gluten-sensitive enteropathy. *J. Clin. Invest.* 51:1602, 1972.

235. Keuning, J. J., Peña, A. S., van Leeuwen, A., et al. HLA DW3 associated with coeliac disease. *Lancet* 1:506, 1976.

CHAPTER 10

Miscellaneous Disease States

Application of immune-complex assays to a large number of diverse disease states has emphasized that immune complexes are indeed a feature of an incredibly broad range of human conditions. Since their occurrence is not limited to such well-defined entities as systemic lupus erythematosus or even acute glomerulonephritis, but is now apparent in an increasingly wide spectrum of human diseases, one of the problems that emerges is what indeed is their actual relevance to pathogenesis of the disease states themselves? Like the erythrocyte sedimentation rate or zeta-potential, immune-complex elevations appear in a broad variety of circumstances. Their presence may of course merely reflect an epiphenomenon generated by the primary disease process. Conversely, elevations of circulating immune complexes represent a phenomenon about which a great deal more is now known than the physiological consequences of an elevation in sedimentation rate or blood viscosity, and considerable information is currently available about the composition and handling of such materials. Most important of all, we understand that tissue deposition and transient circulation of immune complexes are central phenomena to certain well-ordered mechanisms of the host immune response. Thus, rather than emphasizing the finding of immune-complex elevations in diseases where they were not thought to belong or where no clear immediate connection exists to their presence and our understanding of the disease, it seems more prudent to regard their presence in such disorders as an example of how various immune mechanisms can either accentuate or dampen underlying pathological processes. No major brief will be made in this chapter for the ultimate importance of immune complexes in many of the conditions or disorders discussed; rather, at this stage, it seems more appropriate to catalogue and describe their presence.

Pregnancy

In addition to their ability to initiate tissue injury as in the serum sickness animal model, immune complexes can interfere with various features of cellular immunity. This has already been discussed in relationship to cancer, where circulating antigen-antibody complexes or so-called blocking factors are capable of abrogating several vital cell-mediated host functions (1, 2). A number of factors directed against placental or fetal antigens have now been described in pregnancy serum which seem capable of interfering with cellular immunity (3–5). Moreover, data have been presented to support the role of immune complexes as blocking factors during pregnancy itself (6). In this latter report sera from pregnant mice were shown to inhibit killing of syngeneic tumor cells by lymph-node cells in a microcytotoxicity assay. Passage of pregnancy sera through immunoabsorbents of anti-mouse IgG_{2a} or anti-IgG_{2b} removed blocking activity. Moreover, passage of blocking sera through an immunoabsorbent column charged with antibody to whole mouse embryo also removed blocking activity. These experiments indicated that blocking factors in pregnant mouse serum were capable of directly interfering with K-cell activity against syngeneic tumors and, furthermore, that blocking factors contained mouse antibody and fetal antigens, presumably in the form of immune complexes. Such data did not exclude the possibility that free antigen or antibodies might participate independently in some blocking phenomena observed with pregnancy sera in various assay systems. A similar situation also pertains to cancer.

A recent report provides interesting data with respect to human pregnancy (7): using a test that employed isolated rabbit IgM rheumatoid-factor agglutination of IgG-coated latex particles (8), 84 sera collected from 55 women during various stages of pregnancy showed elevated titers of inhibition of this agglutination reaction (Figure 10-1). Pregnancy sera showing presumed immune complexes with this sensitive assay were studied by gel filtration and in all instances high-molecular-weight complexes ($>10^6$) were detected. Fixation of C3 was detected in a significantly increased number of pregnancy sera in association with high molecular weight IgG (500,000 Daltons or over). High-molecular-weight materials in inhibiting pregnancy sera (presumably complexes) were concentrated and adjusted to low pH by dialysis to dissociate complexes. When repassed through gels at the same acidic pH, this dissociated material lost inhibitory activity. These experiments provided evidence for the presence of immune complexes in the sera of normal healthy women during the course of their pregnancies. Precisely what antigens are involved, whether placental or fetal, was not determined. The antigens appear to be capable of C3 activation and were approximately 400,000 Daltons in size.

If confirmed by other studies, the presence of significant amounts of immune complexes in the sera of pregnant women represents a phenomenon of considerable interest. It is conceivable that mechanisms initiated by or at least involving complement-activating complexes could be involved in the pathogenesis of some forms of preeclampsia. In this regard, deposits of both IgG and C3 have been detected in the renal glomeruli of normal pregnant guinea pigs and mice (9). No similar extensive immunofluorescent data are currently available in the case of kidney biopsies from human patients during pregnancy, but when various samples have been examined for complex deposition, generally none has been found (10). Immune-complex deposits in pregnant guinea pigs and mice mentioned

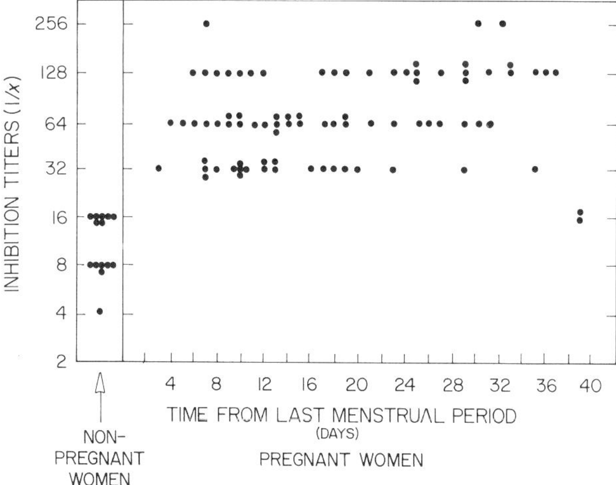

Figure 10-1 Inhibitory activity of sera from pregnant and nonpregnant women toward rabbit rheumatoid factor. (Reproduced with permission, P. L. Masson, M. Delire, and C. L. Cambiaso, *Nature* 265:542, 1977.)

above are comprised of granular deposits in capillary loops and mesangial matrix. An example of these findings from the work of Tung (9) is shown in Figure 10-2.

For years one of the most intriguing of immunologic puzzles has revolved around maternal and fetal factors contributing to the notion of pregnancy as a privileged, rather unique immunologic phenomenon. Many aspects of the maternal-fetal relationship have been suggested as being important in protecting the fetus from immunologic rejection by the maternal host. Some of these aspects may be related to humoral mechanisms. Serum factors with immunosuppressive properties have been demonstrated in pregnancy serum by a number of laboratories (11–13). In some instances these have been associated with alpha-globulin fractions (11), but in others the factors as yet are undefined. Small amounts of circulating complexes may contribute to the preservation and balance of opposing forces during normal human pregnancy. This concept is unique; most of the other discussions in this book have centered upon the pathogenetic role of complexes in a wide variety of disease states. The physiological setting in pregnancy is of course quite different. It represents a natural condition and cannot in any way be considered a disorder, but rather a reordering of intrinsic bodily functions. On one side of the placenta is the fetus, growing rapidly and differentiating its embryonic buds of tissue into full-fledged organs. Half of its histocompatibility phenotype is derived from the paternal genome and thus represents foreign tissue insofar as the immune recognition of the mother is concerned. Between the mother and the half-foreign fetus are interposed placental tissues arranged to allow vital oxygen and nutrient exchange but to exclude close mixing of most circulating cellular elements. Since the fetus represents an organism in close circulatory connection to the mother but with the potential for generation of an immune rejection by the mother, it can be considered a special sort of allograft.

Protection of the fetus from potentially adverse maternal immunologic rejection has been ascribed to the barrier imposed by the trophoblast (14) either by covering up of transplantation antigens or by the presence in this tissue of an extracellular masking layer. The precise immunologic function of the human trophoblast may have a great deal to do with protection of the fetus from immunologic rejection by the mother, but definition of mechanisms involved with such protection is not yet available. It seems possible that immune complexes present in maternal plasma have a great deal to do with initiating this protection. In 1967 Currie (15) showed that maternal lymphocytes are capable of directly lysing human trophoblastic cells in vitro. This indicated that such maternal cells actually recognized foreign antigenic groups on trophoblast. There is still disagreement on whether immunologic recognition in such instances involves perception of HLA antigens or other types of cell-surface recognition structures. It has been found that trypsinized trophoblastic cells react strongly with multispecific anti-HLA serum (16); however, actual physical expression of trophoblast antigens may be masked by dense layers of acidic mucoprotein.

An alternative antigen-masking mechanism in pregnancy could indeed be secondary to immunologic enhancement, as originally suggested by Kaliss and Dagg (17). Depression of mixed leukocyte culture reactions by primigravida pregnancy sera (18) or by IgG eluted from human placentas (19) has been reported. Studies described by Taylor and Hancock (4) utilized cultured human trophoblastic cells and maternal lymphocytes. Direct cytotoxic effects were seen in trophoblastic monolayers after 72 hours of incubation and depended on the presence of nonlymphoid cell types in addition to lymphoid elements. Lysis of target trophoblastic cells was preceded by cell division and blast-cell formation and involved close contact between maternal K cells and trophoblast targets. The changes from this particular study are illustrated in Figure 10-3. Cytotoxic effects of maternal lymphocytes on trophoblast were completely prevented by presence of maternal serum; the protective effect of the latter was markedly reduced after removal of IgG from maternal serum. Preincubation studies with target trophoblast and killer maternal lympho-

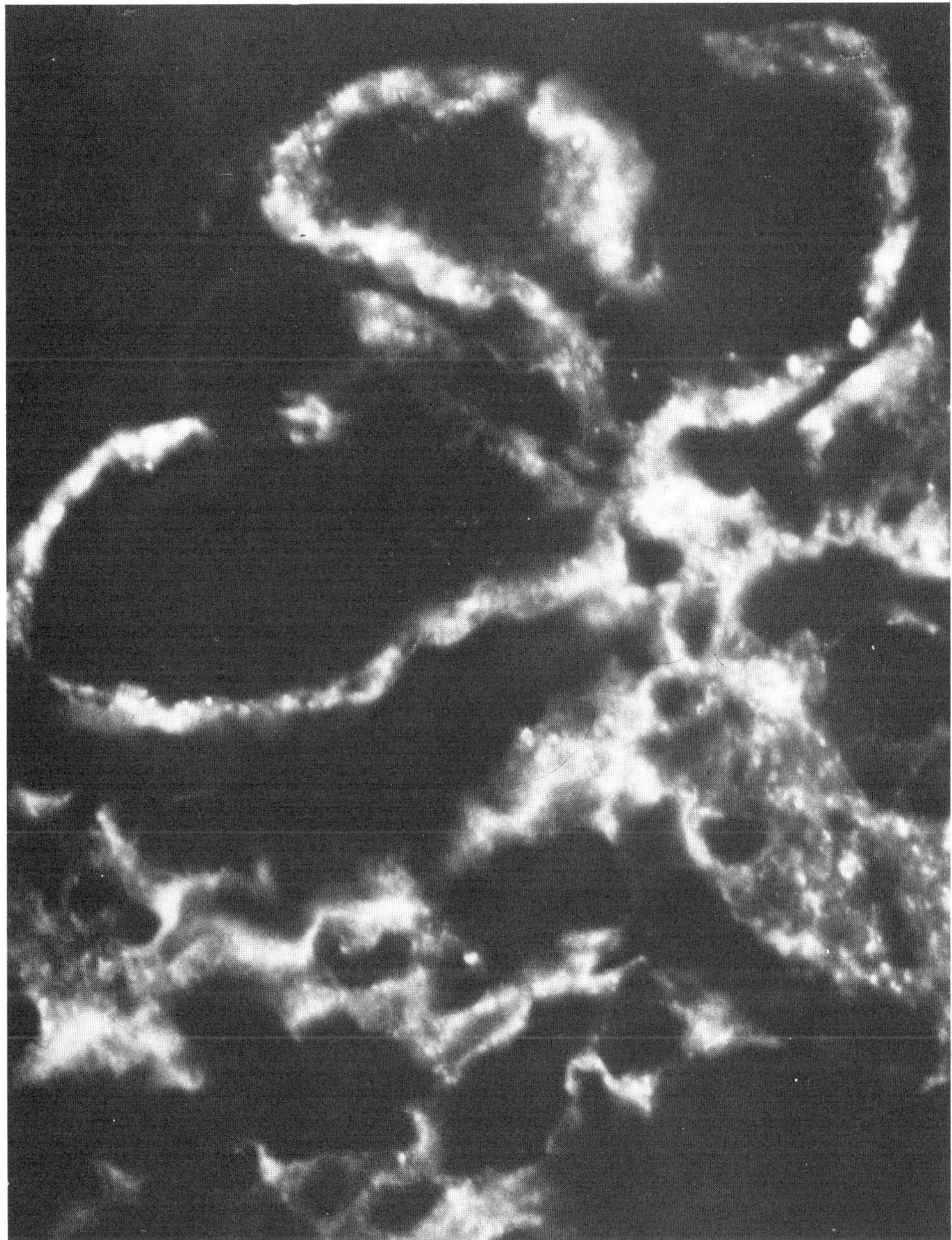

Figure 10-2 Immunofluorescence photomicrograph of the renal glomerulus of a pregnant guinea pig, to demonstrate the granular nature of IgG deposition in the capillary loops and in the mesangial matrix. Magnification × 1,280. (Reproduced with permission, K. S. K. Tung, *J. Immunol.* 112:186, 1974.)

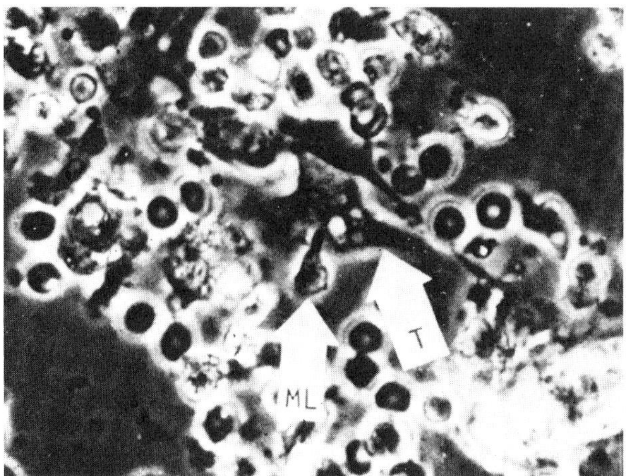

Figure 10-3 Frame from a time-lapse cinematographic study showing attachment of maternal lymphocyte (ML) to trophoblast cell (T). Magnification × 640. (Reproduced with permission, P. V. Taylor and K. W. Hancock, *Immunology* 28:973, 1975.)

cytes suggested that these effects were mediated through interaction of maternal antibody with trophoblast rather than with killer lymphoid cells. These studies are of particular interest, as they parallel much of what is known concerning blocking phenomena in tumors. In exactly opposite fashion to the instance of blocking or enhancing with respect to tumors, so-called blocking factors of pregnancy serum preserve integrity of the fetus. Thus in many ways the same sort of reactants may be working in antithetical fashion in pregnancy as opposed to neoplasia. Antigen-antibody complexes in maternal circulation and on the trophoblast protect the fetus from maternal immunologic rejection, whereas in the instance of tumors they allow the normal defense process to be subverted.

Several recent extensions of these concepts have been presented by a number of groups. Pence and co-workers (5) showed that autologous plasma from multigravida women specifically blocked MIF production by maternal lymphocytes using cells from their husbands as antigenic stimuli. Blocking activity could be absorbed out using paternal cells. Gel filtration studies showed that this blocking activity was present in 7S IgG fractions. An extension of these interesting findings indicated that patients with habitual abortion lacked this blocking factor (20). Since the factor lacked anti-

HLA, B, or C specificity in these studies, such antibodies might indeed be directed against products of the D locus possibly related to the human Ia system. No direct evidence, however, was noted for the presence of high-molecular-weight immune complexes as blocking factors.

Activation of a suppressor-cell mechanism could be important in further defusing or turning off potential immunologic rejection of the fetus by the maternal host. This possibility is suggested by the recent work of Olding (21–23) and Oldstone and their co-workers (24), whose reports indicate that human cord blood contains increased suppressor T-cell reactivity, which may be capable of protecting the fetus from immunologic attack by the mother. The experiments supporting this fascinating concept involved nonblocked mixed leukocyte cultures using cord-blood lymphocytes from male babies and maternal lymphocytes. The only lymphocytes that proliferated in this circumstance were those from the male babies, identified through use of male chromosome markers. Later it was shown that cord blood contained an increased proportion and physiological activity of Tγ or T suppressor cells (24). Of particular interest in this regard is a report by Murgita and colleagues (25) indicating that fetal cord-blood suppressor cells may be activated through mechanisms involving α-fetoprotein. Thus, activation of fetal suppressor T cells by the pregnant state may provide a built-in modulator for potential maternal lymphocyte host-versus-allograft responses. From the data accumulated to date, a number of immunologic mechanisms have been implicated in protecting the fetal allograft from maternal rejection. The relative importance of circulating immune complexes in this picture remains to be determined.

Gastrointestinal Disorders

The gastrointestinal tract is a unique area of the body where the primary immune reactivity appears to be vested in the secretory IgA system. One of the principal functions of IgA in this regard is to form complexes with various foreign materials and by so doing to exclude them from absorption or penetration of mucosal defenses, thereby abrogating their potential immunogenicity. Occasionally miscellaneous disease states affecting portions of the gastrointestinal tract itself such as the liver, small bowel, or biliary tree have been implicated as participating in immune-complex–mediated tissue injury. The following section focuses on several examples of such phenomena, although it is by no means clear that immune complexes per se represent a major mechanism in pathogenesis.

Chronic Liver Disease

A few reports ascribe various degrees of glomerular injury to chronic liver disease associated with cirrhosis (26–29). The designation of "cirrhotic glomerulosclerosis" was proposed by Bloodworth and Sommers (30), who felt that glomerular lesions in such patients represented a characteristic picture; immunofluorescent studies have occasionally demonstrated presence of gamma globulin within glomeruli of cirrhotic patients (31–33). Studies by Callard and co-workers (34) have amplified these earlier findings, indicating glomerular lesions in 9 of 10 patients with cirrhosis; the lesions were characterized by thickening of basement membranes, electron-dense deposits in capillary walls and mesangial areas, and presence of IgA with IgG and/or IgM and C3 in such deposits. Patients included in this study comprised mainly those with alcoholic cirrhosis (8 of 10) who underwent surgical biopsies of liver and kidneys during portacaval shunt procedures. The predominant immunoglobulin detected within glomerular deposits in these patients was mesangial IgA. IgG, IgM, and C3 localization were also observed but were much less prominent. None of the patients in this study had manifest renal failure or proteinuria; low serum C3 levels in several patients were attributed to presence of chronic active liver disease. In view of the absence of parallel clinical findings of renal functional impairment or proteinuria, these findings probably represent another example of the sensitivity of careful immunofluorescence studies of renal glomeruli as an assay for subclinical deposition of immune complexes in yet another human disease state. All patients studied by Callard and co-workers (34) had severe liver disease, as exemplified by the fact that all were undergoing portosystemic shunts for esophageal varices. Predominance of IgA in the glomerular deposits noted in this study is of interest, since marked elevations of this immunoglobulin are known to be frequently associated with chronic liver disease (35). The antigens responsible for the production of IgA-containing immune complexes in patients with cirrhosis and chronic active liver disease are not known. It seems likely that they are derived from bacterial, viral, or dietary sources within the gastrointestinal tract. Experimental cirrhosis in rats induced with carbon tetrachloride produces a marked IgA increase in response to oral immunization (36). It is well established that an increase in humoral antibody levels to a number of dietary materials and bacterial antigens occurs in association with chronic liver disease (37, 38). The hypergammaglobulinemia associated with cirrhosis may predispose to ready formation of small amounts of complexes composed at least in part by antigens derived from the gastrointestinal tract which are shunted more readily into the circulation because of inefficient Kupffer-cell function in the cirrhotic liver.

Certain types of chronic liver disease may fit more closely with immune-complex etiology than with what is attributed to the basic pathological process in cirrhosis or liver-cell damage caused primarily by alcohol. This may be the case in primary biliary cirrhosis as suggested by Thomas and colleagues (39). Patients with primary biliary cirrhosis usually are middle-aged women who develop insidious onset of cholestasis, which progresses to deep jaundice and ultimately to liver-cell failure. The characteristic lesion within the liver shows small bile-duct destruction and associated small granulomata (Figure 10-4). The clinical picture is often associated with features of rheumatoid arthritis, arteritis, glomerulitis, and sicca syndrome (40–44). One of the principal serological features of this disease is the occurrence of serum anti-mitochondrial antibody in over 90 percent of patients (45). Studies by Thomas and colleagues (46) have demonstrated the presence of circulating immune complexes in the sera of most patients with primary biliary cirrhosis irrespective of the histological stage of the lesion. Complexes were both small and large showing sedimentation coefficients of 8S to 11S as well as >20S. Larger complexes ap-

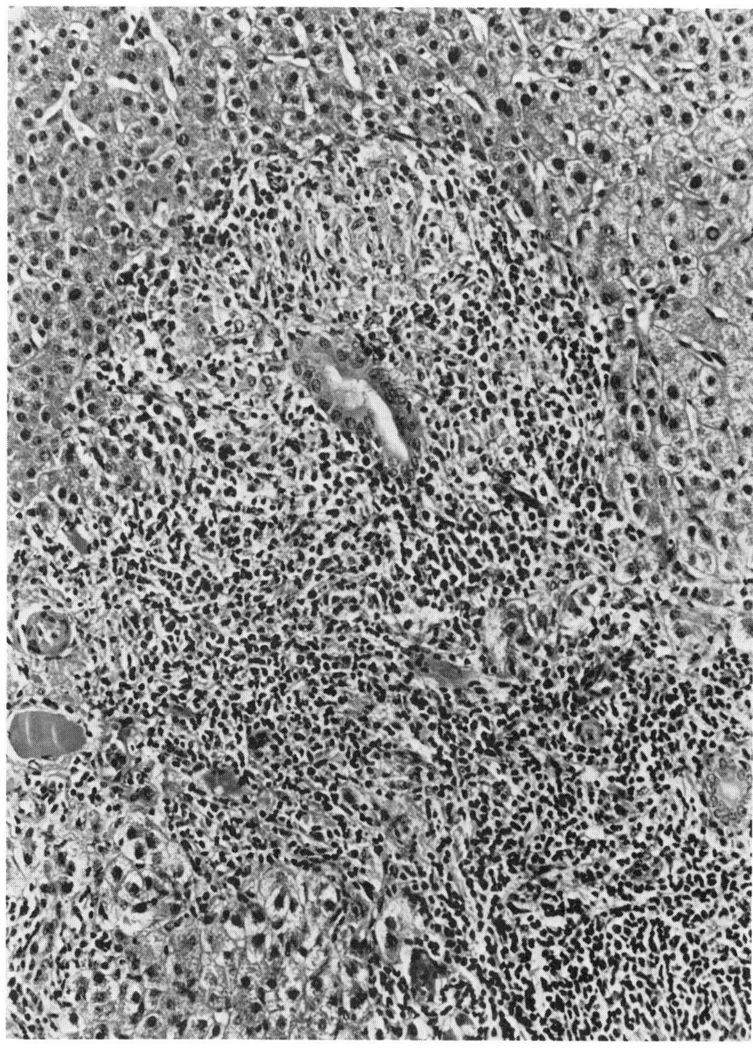

Figure 10-4   Photomicrograph of the early lesion in primary biliary cirrhosis; a bile duct surrounded by inflammatory cells with beginning granuloma formation is visible in the lower right-hand corner of the photograph. H&E × 167. (Photograph courtesy of P. J. Scheuer, Royal Free Hospital, London.)

peared to be characteristic of biliary cirrhosis, whereas smaller 8S to 11S complex-like materials were also detected in both hepatitis B-positive and negative chronic hepatitis.

The relation between detectable immune complexes and liver-cell injury as well as the foci of hepatic granulomata near biliary radicles is not yet clear. Paronetto and co-workers (47) noted extracellular aggregates of immunoglobulin and complement in the lesions of primary biliary cirrhosis. Moreover, such patients show an increased catabolism of C3, suggesting complement activation (48). Cleavage products of C3—C3b (49)—and the occurrence of antibodies to activated C3b in the form of immunoconglutinins (50) also suggest an active process of complement consumption, particularly since hepatitis B-positive and negative hepatitis or alcohol-induced liver disease show only slightly increased C3 catabolism. What the primary antigens are which are responsible for the presence of high-molecular-weight immune complexes in patients with biliary cirrhosis and precisely how they could initiate tissue damage has not yet been clarified.

Additional evidence for the importance of circulating immune complexes and complement activation in primary biliary cirrhosis was provided recently by studies reported by Wands and colleagues (51). Immune complexes were detected in 95 percent of 20 patients. Extremely high concentrations (474 μg/ml mean with range from 16.2 to 2,192) were recorded by the Raji-cell radioimmunoassay. Cryoproteins were also present in high concentration in 90 percent of the individuals studied. The cryoprecipitates were composed of IgM (60 percent); IgG-IgM (25 percent); and IgA-IgM (5 percent); these materials showed the capacity to activate the complement system directly in vitro. Evidence for alternate complement pathway activation was noted in 8 of 20 subjects. Serum C3 and C4 levels were normal in most patients, although clear evidence for alternate complement activation was present in EDTA plasma. The composition of cryoproteins among the patients with primary biliary cirrhosis differed from that seen with chronic hepatitis B; cryoprecipitates in primary biliary cirrhosis contained pre-

dominantly IgM instead of IgG. Antimitochondrial antibody in these same sera was not cryoprecipitable and was not concentrated in any of the cryoprecipitates examined.

Tissue localization of lesions of granulomatous type principally within portal tracts, and how such lesions are related to bile duct antigens, is not well understood. Although when preformed immune complexes were injected into the systemic circulation, a mononuclear infiltration of portal tracts occurred, no granuloma formation was recorded (52). On the contrary, if immune complexes were injected into the biliary tree, epithelial cell damage was noted along with an acute exudative inflammatory lesion (53). Thomas and co-workers (39) suggest that if this process were prolonged, it could produce tissue changes similar to those present in biliary cirrhosis. Such a circumstance whereby immune complexes themselves would be formed in the bile seems unlikely. Thomas has suggested that complexes are produced in the walls of bile ductules or in the surrounding tissues—analogous to lesions developing in an Arthus phenomenon. Thus, antigens absorbed from the bile could combine with antibody circulating in the portal circulation to produce complexes within the bile ductular walls or interstitial portal spaces. Chronic or repetitive deposition of complexes could presumably result in chronic granuloma formation and eventual tissue injury. Furthermore, the presence of the spleen as a major lymphoid organ and potential source of antibody production might also favor the continued local generation of immune complexes. Various aspects of this hypothesis are diagrammed in Figure 10-5. Many aspects of primary biliary cirrhosis are compatible with this hypothesis, including spillover of excess complexes from inflamed tissues and more distant peripheral effects such as arthritis or occasional glomerulitis. There are, however, obvious vacant areas or unknowns associated with such a scheme. For one thing, no primary antigen specific for or unique to biliary cirrhosis has been identified. Also, there is scanty evidence for immunoglobulin and complement deposition within biliary ductular walls during the early stages of disease evolution. On the other hand, the im-

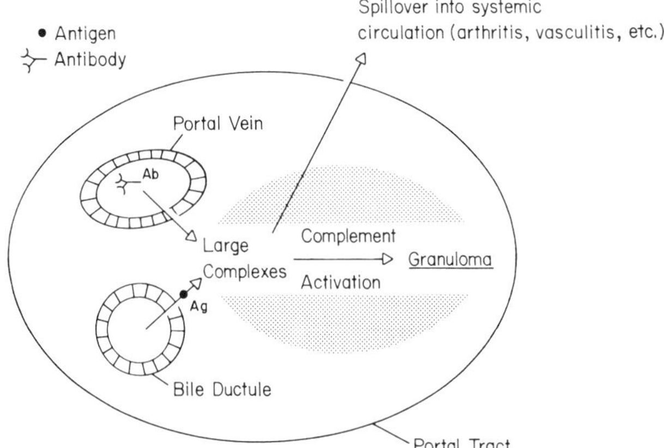

Figure 10-5 Possible mechanism of bile-ductular injury in primary biliary cirrhosis. (Reproduced with permission, H. C. Thomas, B. J. Potter, and S. Sherlock, *Lancet* 2:126, 1977.)

munologic abnormalities known to be associated with the disease including the presence of antimitochondrial antibody and hypergammaglobulin M suggest that a defect in immunologic control may be a basic feature of the disease. Many of the mechanisms relevant to chronic active hepatitis associated with hepatitis B (discussed at length in Chapter 3) are possibly applicable to the situation with primary biliary cirrhosis. It also seems likely that there may be important local factors influencing initial interactions of circulating complexes and their ultimate tissue distribution. Whether this relates to activation of Fc receptors or C3 receptors within the biliary canaliculi or Kupffer cells adjacent to portal tracts or to tissue-localizing features of the antigens involved is not yet clear. Studies of the local tissue distribution of circulating systemic or portal blood complexes might reveal whether certain physical or chemical properties of the antigens involved are indeed of more importance than the actual size of the complexes.

Cystic Fibrosis

Cystic fibrosis is a disorder characterized by chronic viscid mucoid bronchopulmonary secretions and frequent superimposition of severe purulent bacterial pulmonary infections. Organisms such as *Pseudomonas aeruginosa, Staphylococcus aureus, Hemophilus influenzae,* and *Diplococcus pneumoniae* are often responsible for recurrent purulent infections. Necropsy samples from patients with cystic fibrosis have provided immunofluorescent evidence for deposition of immune complexes in spleen, thymus, liver, stomach, duodenum, pancreas, lung, and trachea (54). Formation of immune complexes may act as a secondary or amplifying mechanism in producing injury to delicate and particularly vulnerable tissues within the lungs and respiratory tracts, although the basic lesion relates to the abnormal secretions in this disorder. In many ways patients with cystic fibrosis are similar to those with infective endocarditis or leprosy in that they develop tremendous humoral hypergammaglobulinemic responses in parallel with repeated bronchopulmonary infections. This is amply illustrated in the studies by Høiby and colleagues identifying a wide spectrum of precipitating antibodies against various pseudomonas antigens in serum from such patients (55–57). Examples of the strikingly diverse serum precipitins against pseudomonas components are shown in Figure 10-6.

A study recently published by Schiøtz and co-workers (58) showed immune complexes in the serum of 6 of 11 patients with cystic fibrosis, using a complement consumption assay. Of particular interest was the finding of granular deposits of IgM in the skin of 10 patients chronically infected with *P. aeruginosa* and in 7 patients without *P. aeruginosa* infections. A few

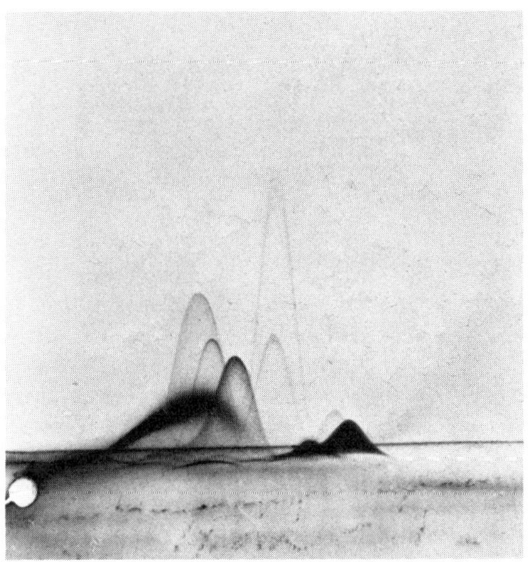

Figure 10-6 Typical findings in serum from a cystic fibrosis patient who had been chronically colonized in the respiratory tract with *Pseudomonas aeruginosa* for 5.3 years. Crossed immunoelectrophoresis of *P. aeruginosa* antigens (polyspecific antigen extract composed of water-soluble antigens from 40 groups of *P. aeruginosa* obtained by sonication) against patient serum is depicted. First-dimension electrophoresis: right anode; second-dimension electrophoresis: top anode; staining: Coomassie brilliant blue. Twenty-six precipitates were seen, whereas sera from normal persons contain less than one precipitin against *P. aeruginosa*. (Reproduced with permission, N. Høiby, E. W. Flensborg, B. Beck et al., *Scand. J. Resp. Dis.* 58:65, 1977.)

patients in both groups also showed C1q, C3, and fibrinogen skin deposition. An example of these findings is given in Figure 10-7, showing that the immunofluorescence was concentrated at the dermal-epidermal junction. Many of these same patients showed nonorgan-specific antinuclear factors but no specific anti-DNA antibodies were reported. The investigators were unable to detect pseudomonas antigens directly in the same immunofluorescent deposits. It is possible that such dermal-epidermal localization of complexes is unrelated to antigen-antibody complexes comprised of pseudomonas-derived antigens but rather represent the same unique localizing properties of DNA–anti-DNA complexes noted by others in the case of SLE.

These findings are a good example of the uncertainty of interpretation in the finding of localized tissue distribution of apparent immune-complex reactants such as immunoglobulin and complement when the antigen responsible for such complexes is unknown. Direct identification of antigen within immunofluorescent deposits has proved extremely difficult in the hands of many workers even when there is already a reasonable idea of the source of primary antigens. This has been true, for instance, in many studies of poststreptococcal glomerulonephritis where granular deposits of immunoglobulins and complement are frequently present but actual streptococcal antigen has been difficult to demonstrate. In the studies of cutaneous deposits in patients with cystic fibrosis, failure to show pseudomonas-related antigens may well be the result of masking or entrapment of such materials by blanketing antibodies. This important point may relate to the known tendency for skin lesions, occurring during pseudomonas sepsis, to localize deeply within the dermis and perivascular areas.

Augmentation of the basic chronic inflammatory pulmonary lesions in cystic fibrosis by local deposition of immune complexes seems highly likely. Experimental models in animals have demonstrated that localized pulmonary hypersensitivity reactions may be produced by tissue-complex deposition (59–61). The presence of high titers of multiple precipitating antibodies to various pseudomonas antigens would provide an ideal milieu for direct immune-complex–mediated injury in alveoli and small respiratory passages analogous in many ways to an Arthus reaction. The findings related to cystic fibrosis may be extrapolated to other more common clinical situations such as the debilitated patient with pseudomonas bronchiolitis or purulent pneumonia. This particular organism is notorious for production of rapid tissue necrosis and intense inflammatory response within infected pulmonary tissues. Many patients with chronic obstructive lung disease and the need for ancillary ventilatory support may show patterns of repeated pseudomonas pulmonary infection that elicit precipitating antipseudomonas anti-

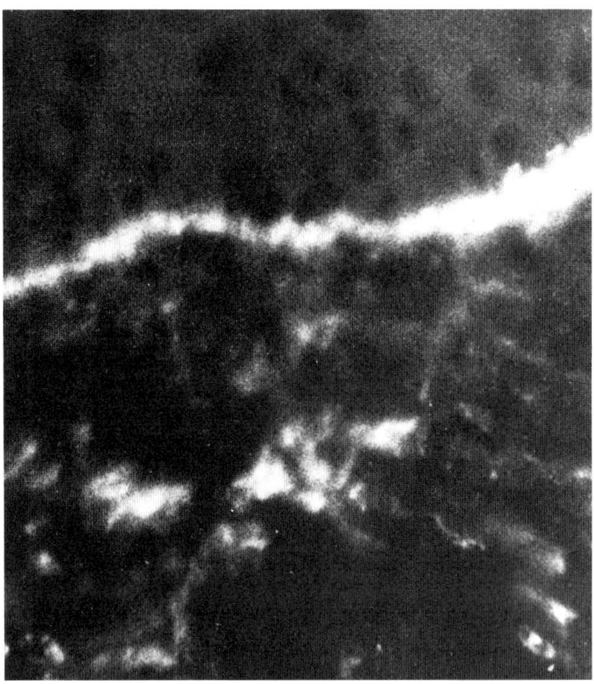

Figure 10-7 Deposits of IgM in a granular pattern at the dermal-epidermal junction. (Reproduced with permission, P. O. Schiøtz, N. Høiby, F. Juhl et al., *Acta Path. Microbiol. Scand.* 85(C):57, 1977.)

body. Similar mechanisms may be occurring in a number of patients without cystic fibrosis but with chronic or intermittent colonization of portions of their respiratory tract by pseudomonas organisms.

Inflammatory Bowel Disease

Patients with chronic inflammatory bowel disease often represent a difficult and vexing therapeutic problem for the practicing physician. Frequently, when acute or in severe exacerbation, the disease manifests itself with various presentations completely outside the gastrointestinal tract. Examples of such distant manifestations associated with ulcerative colitis or chronic regional ileitis are pyoderma gangrenosum, arthritis, and occasionally iritis. An example of pyoderma gangrenosum is shown in Figure 10-8. Many investigators have suggested that such peripheral manifestations could indeed be directly caused by local deposition and activation of inflammatory processes through immune complexes. Chronic cystic fibrosis and chronic inflammatory bowel disease, localized to the colon, terminal ileum, or exten-

sive areas of the gastrointestinal tract, provide a clinical situation in which a great surface area within the body proper is irritated, inflamed, and constantly undergoing either destructive or reparative processes. Since many of the mucosal and submucosal lesions occur within the fecal stream, these diseases provide a potential constant source of gut-derived bacterial antigens and dietary antigens with ready access to immunologic reactivity normally efficiently shut off by the intact mucosal barrier and the secretory IgA system. Having bypassed the usual natural barriers, such antigens may be processed by the local mesenteric lymphoid system and spleen or they may pass directly to the liver and beyond, perhaps to participate in a general immune response. The frequency with which a variety of nonspecific or moderately severe infiltrative liver lesions are associated with regional ileitis or ulcerative colitis suggests that concurrent inflammation in the liver may compromise normal hepatic clearing mechanisms and allow some antigens from the gut direct access to the general circulation.

A number of investigators have reported the

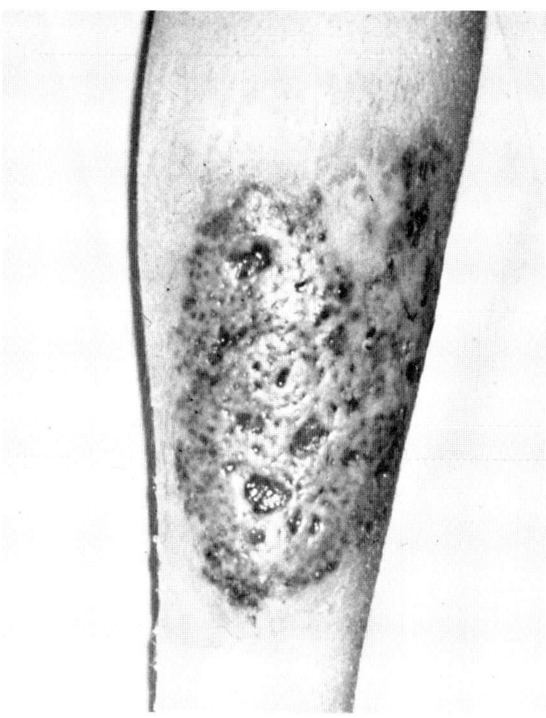

Figure 10-8 Typical pretibial localization and appearance of pyoderma gangrenosum skin lesions associated with ulcerative colitis. (Photograph courtesy of Derek Jewell, Royal Free Hospital, London.)

presence of immune complexes in sera from patients with ulcerative colitis and Crohn's disease (62–64). A recent study by Hodgson and co-workers (65) included determinations on 156 patients with ulcerative colitis or Crohn's disease using anticomplementary activity as one assay and precipitation of ^{125}I-labeled C1q as a parallel method. The anticomplementary test appeared to be most sensitive to complexes of 11 S in size, whereas C1q precipitation was most useful in detecting complexes of 20 S or greater. Complexes were commonly found in patients with active bowel inflammation, particularly in those with acute arthritis, associated spondylitis, or liver disease. Large complexes ($>10^6$) were most frequently seen in patients with liver disease. Levels of anticomplementary activity among the disease and control groups from this study are shown in Figure 10-9. No distinct relationship was noted between elevated anticomplementary activity in sera and age, sex, length of disease, or corti-

costeroid therapy. Furthermore, levels of anticomplementary activity generally fell as patients were studied before and after clinical remission. Four patients were studied who showed acutely inflamed joints; all of these individuals showed extremely high levels of anticomplementary activity. One of these subjects showed erythema nodosum and conjunctivitis. A single patient with pyoderma gangrenosum and two with iritis showed no elevations of anticomplementary activity. Gel filtration studies of sera showing high levels of complexes by the anticomplementary test indicated presence of apparent high molecular weight IgG in association with positive activity. Unfortunately, no molecular or immunochemical characterization of the presumed antigens involved is currently available.

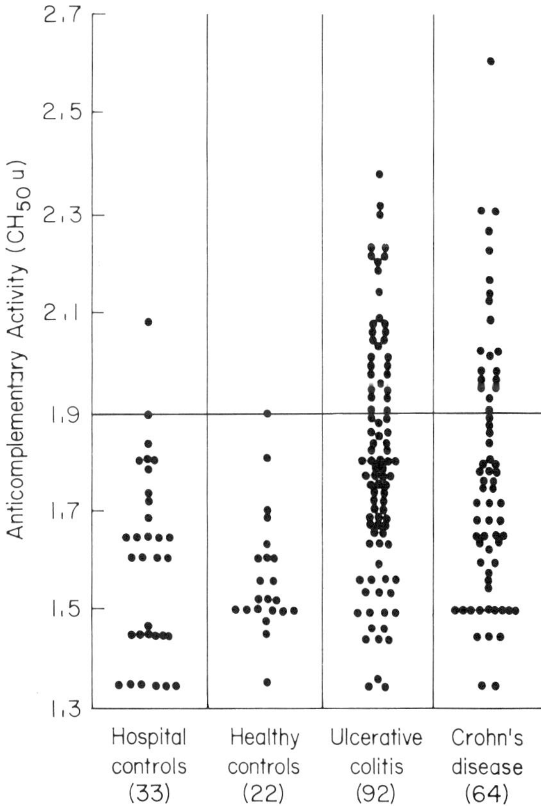

Figure 10-9 Levels of anticomplementary activity in sera from patients with inflammatory bowel disease and in control subjects. (Reproduced with permission, H. J. F. Hodgson, B. J. Potter, and D. P. Jewell, *Clin. Exp. Immunol.* 29:187, 1977.)

The extensive mucosal damage that occurs during the course of bowel disease allows access of gut or possibly bacterial antigens and subsequent production of immune complexes. The inflamed intestinal mucosa of Crohn's disease or ulcerative colitis often contains a marked increase in immunoglobulin-producing cells (66), and some of the immunoglobulin produced locally shows combining specificity for colonic or enteric bacteria (67). If complexes were formed between Gram-negative bacterial antigens and their respective antibodies, they might be capable of potent local inflammatory effects because of the direct complement activation by certain lipopolysaccharide components. During these studies no direct evidence was obtained for local gut-associated inflammatory reaction by complexes. Mechanisms underlying the basic lesion in the bowel wall itself have been the subject of extensive study by many groups over the past 30 years. Participation of cell-mediated immunity and other as yet poorly defined mechanisms may also play a considerable role in pathogenesis. The presence of detectable circulating complexes in the course of inflammatory bowel disease is probably an epiphenomenon; however, continued study of these relationships may do much to clarify understanding of many of the peripheral disease manifestations of these disorders.

Intestinal Bypass Surgery

Some patients who undergo intestinal jejunoileal bypass procedures as treatment for their morbid obesity develop recurrent tenosynovitis or chronic polyarthritis (68). There are now considerable published data supporting an immune-complex–mediated mechanism in the pathogenesis of the polyarthritis occasionally noted postoperatively. Wands and co-workers (69) studied 5 patients after such intestinal bypass operations. Sera from 3 of these individuals contained cryoprotein complexes, composed of IgG, IgM, IgA, complement components C3, C4, C5, and IgG antibody against *Escherichia coli* and *Bacillus fragilis*. Moreover, the C3-activator component of the properdin complex was identified in fresh serum samples from several of the patients with circulating cryoprotein complexes and arthritis. It was therefore suggested that circulating complexes were capable of activating both classic and alternate complement pathways and might be important in the pathogenesis of the arthritis associated with intestinal bypass procedures.

The clinical picture of these patients is of some interest. They may present with a monoarticular or polyarticular acute arthritis with redness, swelling, and extreme joint pain on motion of involved joints. Tests for rheumatoid factor or antinuclear antibodies are negative, and serum uric acid and synovial fluid analysis gives no direct support for gout. Serum C3 and C4 may be reduced during acute arthritic episodes (69); x-rays are generally unremarkable. The episodes of acute synovitis are painful but apparently self-limited. No documented progression to joint destruction or deforming arthritis has been presented as yet. Sedimentation rate may be markedly elevated during acute attacks and white-blood-cell counts are generally normal.

In the patients studied by Wands and co-workers (69), circulating cryoprotein complexes were identified only in patients with arthritis and disappeared with resolution of attacks of acute synovitis. The demonstration of IgG antibody against coliform or *B. fragilis* organisms—bacteria commonly present in gut flora—together with evidence for complement activation suggested that the source of the complexes was the gastrointestinal tract. Moreover, a relative concentration of these antibacterial antibodies compared to their presence in serum provided indirect evidence for the source of the complexes themselves. Since the initial report by Shagrin and colleagues (68) indicated that 25 percent of patients undergoing jejunocolostomy showed episodes of polyarthritis, this unique complication appears to be relatively common. The involvement of tendons and wrists in acute episodes of tenosynovitis is also of interest, for it suggests that these structures may contain certain poorly defined localizing factors that accentuate immune-complex–mediated inflammation in these areas. Also, one patient with severe, disabling bouts of arthritis had cessation of attacks following intestinal reanastomosis; this particular individual also experienced remission of arthritis during tetracycline therapy for a urinary tract infection, further supporting a gut-related source for primary antigens in this syndrome. Bacteriological studies of intestinal flora in patients undergoing jejunoileal bypass surgery have indicated that the blind loop resulting from the bypass procedure often is heavily colonized with *E. coli* or *Bacteroides* species (70).

Studies presented by Wands and co-workers (69) indicated that circulating cryoprotein complexes were capable of activating both classic and alternate complement pathways since C4, an early component of the conventional complement sequence, was present in the complexes and serum C4 levels were reduced. Furthermore, reduction in serum C3 activator during acute arthritis episodes implicated participation of the alternate pathway as well. The isolated cryoprotein obtained from one patient was shown to activate the alternate complement pathway in vitro with conversion of C3PA to C3A.

Subsequent studies of complications after jejunoileal bypass procedures have also been recorded by Moake and colleagues (71) and indicate that intravascular destruction of blood elements might also occur on the basis of immune complexes. A patient was studied who developed intravascular hemolysis, thrombocytopenia, and neutropenia two years after jejunoileal bypass for massive obesity. Studies revealed that the erythrocytes of the patient were coated with C4/C3 complement components, and serum induced direct lysis of chromium-51–labeled platelets. Circulating immune-complex assays using binding to labeled C1q showed increased amounts of complexes, and serum C3 and C4 were depressed. It appeared that immune-complex activation and adsorption to circulating blood elements had occurred in this patient.

From a superficial standpoint the problems attributed to immune complexes in patients with intestinal bypass procedures are different from those associated with inflammatory bowel disease, which raises some fascinating theoretical questions. In the situation of inflammatory bowel disease it is postulated that multiple inflamed regions on the gut surface represent the portal of entry of antigens and complexes into the circulation. The physical setting present in the bypass patients is exactly the opposite in that their gut absorptive surface, instead of being opened up or further exposed, has been markedly curtailed. Despite this latter restriction, circulating immune complexes appear to be present and are probably responsible for some of the complications including repeated bouts of acute arthritis or, rarely, blood element destruction. The contrast in the two clinical settings involved in the gut as a potential source of antigens participating in immune-complex manifestations is of interest, since it affords additional insight into other mechanisms operative in these situations. The source for bacterial antigen-antibody complexes in the case of the patients with bypass procedures apparently resides in the blind loop that becomes colonized by enteric bacteria. Certain features common to problems of immune-complex formation in such situations, and more importantly, their means of access to the general circulation may be important in the pathogenesis of many diseases of unknown etiology. In particular, this relates to possible access of gut-sequestered antigens to the general immune system. This point has been refocused recently in reports that measles antigen is apparently detectable in intestinal biopsies from a substantial proportion of patients with multiple sclerosis (72, 73). Although there is continuing controversy about the potential significance of this finding (74), it has served to alert us to the possible importance of the gastrointestinal tract as a source for antigens participating in immune-complex–mediated tissue injury in diverse and distant peripheral sites. There is, of course, very little direct evidence that multiple sclerosis or lesions of demyelinization within the central nervous system are caused by immune-complex injury. However, the transient episodes of synovitis occurring in the ileal bypass patients emphasize the potential contribution of the gastrointestinal tract to diseases such as rheumatoid arthritis, sarcoidosis, or even SLE as a portal of entry for antigens that could participate directly in pathogenesis. Much is still to be learned about specific aspects that regulate and control immune responses generated from antigens absorbed by or sequestered in the gut.

Arthritis occurring in patients with morbid obesity and probably secondary to episodic release of immune complexes from blind gut loops colonized by enteric bacteria is a rare condition. The fact that it occurs in episodes and not on a continuous basis is not well understood. No major diversion of portal venous or mesenteric arterial supply is involved when bypass procedures are performed. Changes in arterial and consequently venous blood supply are a familiar feature of other well-studied circulatory conditions such as the subclavian steal syndrome, which involves the carotid and other major vessels arising directly or indirectly from the aortic arch (75). It is possible that similar but intermittent arterial or venous steal phenomena somehow induced by the change in local bowel physiology after intestinal bypass are conducive to blood flow allowing immune complexes from the gut to enter the systemic circulation. Similar phenomena may be operative in the case of chronic inflammatory bowel disease or possibly in the arthritis that sometimes accompanies rare causes of inflammatory bowel disease such as Whipple's disease. Perhaps more important than these speculations concerning alterations in visceral blood supply is the fact that the gastrointestinal tract per se has been neglected as a possible source of antigens for a number of disorders of unknown etiology. Interest in this phenomenon has suddenly been reawakened by the reports of gut-sequestered viral measles antigens in multiple sclerosis. Perhaps these indications are sufficient to realert investigators to the potential importance of the gastrointestinal tract in such disorders.

Wegener's Granulomatosis

Wegener's granulomatosis is a disease of unknown etiology that has been variously grouped in the connective-tissue disorders or classified as a vasculitis of unknown cause. Pathological findings include necrotizing granulomatous lesions of the upper and lower respiratory tract, generalized focal necrotizing vas-

culitis, and glomerulitis. Their basic etiology is obscure; however, many manifestations of the disease, particularly the close juxtaposition of granulomatous lesions within the respiratory tract, suggest that some type of hypersensitivity lesion is present (76–78). An example of an orbital granulomatous lesion associated with this disease is shown in Figure 10-10. Important features of the disease that have evolved during the last several decades are the impressive responses achieved in many patients with cyclophosphamide and other potent immunosuppressive agents. Although chronic granulomatous inflammatory foci dominate

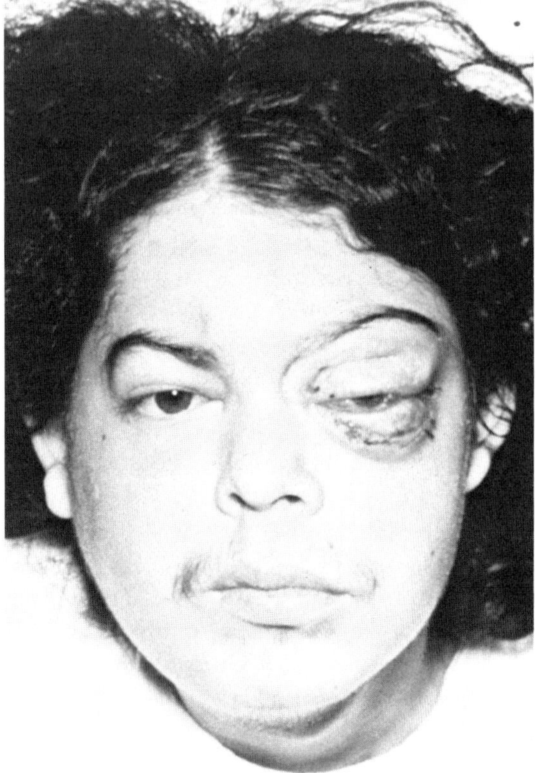

Figure 10-10 Orbital lesion in a patient with probable Wegener's granulomatosis. The patient subsequently expired, and pathological examination could not distinguish whether the granulomatous orbital involvement was that typical for Wegener's or a lymphoma with similar changes. (Photograph courtesy of Rodanthi Kitridou, University of Southern California Medical Center, Los Angeles.)

the pathological picture, some evidence has accumulated for the deposition of immunoglobulins and complement in glomeruli and subepithelial dense deposits detected by electron microscopy (76–81).

Howell and Epstein (82) have reported observations on circulating immune complexes in two patients with Wegener's granulomatosis. Complexes were detected using the C1q precipitin reaction and correlation made during serial studies that included renal biopsy. Both patients studied showed C1q-reactive materials during initial acute clinical illness. Complexes tended to diminish and disappear rather rapidly after initiation of azathioprine or cyclophosphamide and corticosteroid in these subjects. Of particular interest with respect to their true pathogenetic significance was that in these patients renal biopsy failed to show evidence for immunoglobulin or immune-complex deposition, though marked fibrin deposition was noted. Cryoglobulins were not present in the serum of these patients and no general complement profile supporting extensive intravascular complement activation was present.

Criteria for Clinical Importance

These studies emphasize the caution that must be exercised with respect to any final interpretations of the finding of circulating immune complexes in various human disease states. With increasingly sophisticated and sensitive methods for immune-complex detection, circulating complexes in small or moderate quantitative amounts are turning up in an amazing variety of human disease states. In many disorders their presence may reflect epiphenomena secondary to primary tissue injury through other primary inflammatory mechanisms. This certainly would appear to be the case in a chronic granulomatous condition such as Wegener's granulomatosis. In order to satisfy basic criteria for primary pathogenesis of disease states, it must be directly shown that immune complexes themselves participate at the action site and that they can be identified as principal agents in any ongoing inflammatory process. Such criteria certainly are not satisfied in the case of Wegener's granulomatosis. Studies of this condition and perhaps many others

must be viewed in clear perspective before complexes are assigned any major priority in initiating basic disease processes. Furthermore, strict attention must be given to the precise nature of the immune complexes and to studies aimed at characterization of the antigens implicated in the formation of such complexes. This is an especially hazy area in much of the discussion in the literature alluding to the role of immune complexes in miscellaneous disease states. In the disorders already discussed, for example, no clear immunochemical identification has been made of the putative antigens involved in the complexes present in human pregnancy, biliary cirrhosis, jejunoileal shunt procedures, or Wegener's granulomatosis. In some cases definition of the antigens may not be essential for proof of a pathological role in the specific disease states. Thus, the cryoproteins noted in the case of jejunoileal shunt patients show relative concentration of anti–Gram-negative gut-derived antibacterial antibody and appear to be temporally related to episodes of acute arthritis.

Complete or formal proof of the relative importance of immune complexes in the pathogenesis of disease states in which they occur should ideally include demonstration of such complexes in the sites of presumed immune-complex–mediated tissue injury; identification of the physical parameters, size, Ig content, and complement-activating properties of such complexes; characterization of the precise nature of the antigens involved; and demonstration that removal or disappearance of complexes in tissues or in the circulation results in improvement of the clinical condition with which they appear to be associated. As mentioned in previous chapters, most of these rigid criteria have only been satisfactorily met in a few human disease states such as SLE or hepatitis B-virus immune-complex disease. Since the occurrence of complexes is probably part of the normal immune response, mere detection of their presence in various disease states cannot be taken as proof of their importance in fundamental disease mechanisms. Ideal (or perhaps nearly ideal) justification for implicating immune complexes in the basic pathogenesis of disease states, and reasonable satisfaction of rigid criteria for their importance, are summarized in Table 10-1 in which data now accumulated with respect to SLE or hepatitis B-virus immune-complex vasculitis are provided.

Sickle Cell Anemia

Sickle cell disease and the anemia associated with this disorder result from genetically determined structural abnormalities of hemoglobin occurring in the red blood cells of affected homozygous patients. Various renal abnormalities have been reported in association with sickle cell (SS) disease (83–85); hematuria, tubular defects, and even nephrotic syndrome have been noted in conjunction with sickle cell trait (SA) (86, 87). Some individuals with sickle cell anemia show glomerular lesions that present as a membranoproliferative glomerulonephritis.

This clinical picture is not a common feature recognized overtly in most individuals, but several recent observations on the possible pathogenesis of renal lesions in such patients may be pertinent. The studies of Strauss and colleagues (88) focused on the nature of glomerular-bound antibody in a patient with sickle cell disease and membranoproliferative glomerulonephritis with immune-complex deposits de-

monstrable by immunofluorescence. Renal proximal tubular antigen (RTE) and IgG, IgM, C1q, and C3 were noted in granular patterns along the glomerular basement membrane of kidneys studied at autopsy. IgG and IgM eluted from the glomeruli were capable of directly fixing to antigen present in proximal tubules of normal human kidney. Examples of these findings are shown in Figure 10-11. The immunofluorescent localization of these glomerular eluates was abolished by absorption of immunoglobulins using RTE antigen. Moreover, glomerular eluates blocked localization of rabbit IgG antibody to human RTE on normal proximal renal tubules. These studies suggested that an immune-complex nephritis may occur in some patients with sickle cell disease because of deposition of immune complexes composed of autologous renal tubular antigens and antibodies to them. Of interest in this same vein was a later report (89) documenting similar RTE–immune-complex nephropathy in a child with sickle cell trait (SA) and asymptomatic proteinuria associated with cryoprecipitable complexes of RTE–anti-RTE. Structural studies in this patient showed sickled cells in renal glomeruli, immunoglobulin, and complement deposits in glomerular tissues and interstitial tubular infiltrates.

These findings emphasize how broadly the

Table 10-1   Criteria for classification of immune complexes of fundamental importance in the pathogenesis of disease.

Criterion	SLE	Hepatitis B vasculitis
1. Demonstration of complexes in actual sites of tissue injury	Immunofluorescence, electron microscopy, direct tissue elution	Immunofluorescence, electron microscopy, elution from tissues
2. Identification of physical nature, Ig content, and complement-activating properties of complexes	High-molecular-weight 19S or greater; IgG-containing, activates classic and alternate complement pathways	Broad range of molecular sizes —many 19S or greater; fix complement and contain IgG, IgM
3. Direct identification and characterization of antigens involved	nDNA, possibly nucleoprotein and SM antigen	Hepatitis B virus and related antigens
4. Documentation that removal or disappearance results in amelioration of basic inflammatory process	Plasmapheresis or spontaneous disappearance results in clinical improvement	Resolution of presence of complexes produces clinical improvement

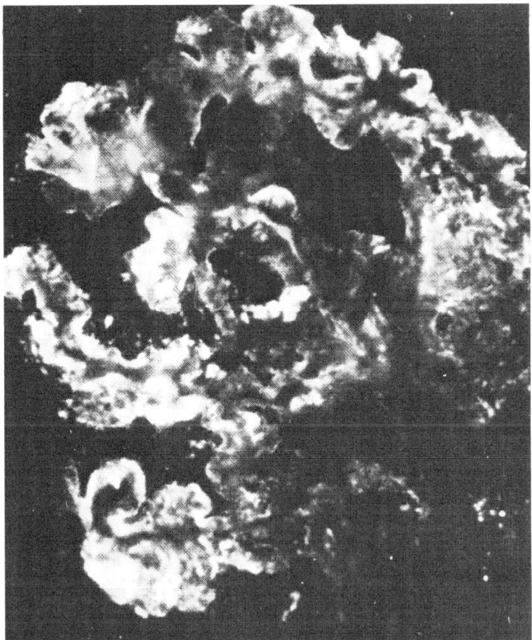 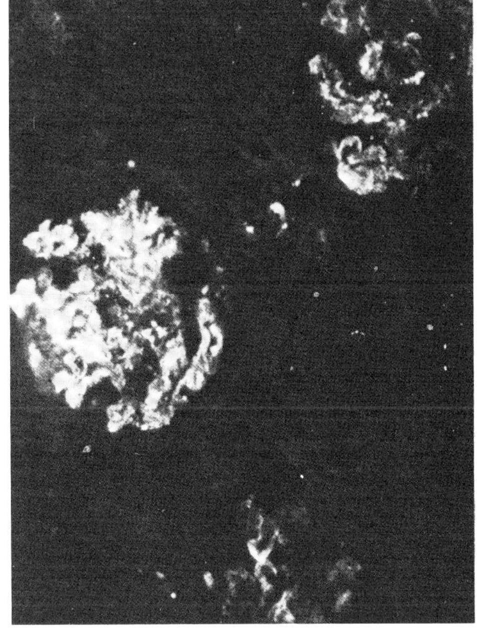

Figure 10-11 *Left,* a representative glomerulus from a patient with sickle cell disease, stained with fluorescein-conjugated rabbit antiserum to human IgG, showing granular deposits along the glomerular basement membrane. Magnification × 320. *Right,* a representative glomerulus from the same patient stained with anti-RTE antigen, showing granular deposits along the glomerular capillary wall. Magnification × 180. (Reproduced with permission, J. Strauss, V. Pardo, M. N. Koss et al., *Am. J. Med.* 58:382, 1975.)

possibilities of immune-complex–mediated mechanisms of tissue injury apply to a wide variety of human disease states. Sickle cell crises may be associated with drinking, acidosis, intercurrent infections, hypoxemia, exercise, high altitude, or inadvertent exposure to reducing agents. The renal lesions in the patients studied thus far have not been clinically linked to overt crisis related to the hemoglobinopathy. Several potential mechanisms may be involved in the pathogenesis of sickle cell nephropathy. Patients with sickle cell disease may undergo autosensitization to a number of partially altered autologous erythrocyte antigens during the course of repeated hemolytic episodes associated with crisis. Furthermore, since they are often treated with transfusion, sensitization to foreign antigens through transfused blood becomes another distinct possibility, which increases as the patient lives longer and longer. Many subjects with sickle cell disease are unusually susceptible to intercurrent infections. It is difficult to relate any of these possibilities directly to the autologous immune-complex nephritis involving renal tubular antigens as part of the glomerular immune deposits. With the chronic anemia and possibly during repeated crises, it is conceivable that renal ischemia leading to necrosis of proximal renal tubules occurs repeatedly in subclinical form. Also, alteration of proximal renal tubules may occur as various drugs or metabolites are handled by the excretory mechanism. There appears to be something unique with respect to sickle cell disease or even sickle cell trait that predisposes to tubular injury and production of autologous antigen-antibody complexes composed of renal tubular antigens or materials that cross-react with the latter. Experimental models of glomerular injury initiated by immunization with autologous renal tubular antigen have been extensively studied by several groups of investigators (90, 91). In this latter work, immunization with heterologous RTE was shown to induce an immune-complex glomerulonephritis that was somehow self-sustaining and associated finally with antibody and immune-complex deposition involving autologous renal tubular antigens. Breaking of self-tolerance to the renal tubular antigen involved has been postulated as one way in which such a sequence of events might occur. The broader implications of this general problem have been emphasized by the report of Naruse and co-workers (92), indicating presence of RTE within the immune-complex deposits of a certain proportion of patients with conventional membranous glomerulonephritis of unknown etiology. Further careful studies of diseases associated with other types of cryptic immune deposits in the kidney may eventually reveal a common mechanism involved in pathogenesis.

Immune-complex deposition involving renal tubular antigens or other antigens possibly related to intercurrent infections occurring in sickle cell patients cannot account for all of the nephropathy seen in many patients with this hemoglobinopathy. A number of reports have documented the occurrence of nephrotic syndrome in subjects with sickle cell disease (83, 85, 93–100). In addition, renal cortical changes reported in sickle cell patients *without* nephrotic syndrome include small cortical infarcts (101), hemosiderin deposits in epithelial cells of proximal convoluted tubules, glomerular congestion, hypertrophy of juxtamedullary glomeruli (102), and eventual glomerulosclerosis. One of the most interesting, rather unique changes occurring during the course of sickle cell nephropathy relates to focal reduplication of glomerular basement membranes associated with mesangial proliferation (103, 104). Patients with both sickle cell disease and nephrotic syndrome show reduplication of glomerular basement membranes, mesangial proliferation, iron-containing deposits in glomerular epithelial cells, and some degree of glomerular sclerosis. There is still considerable controversy about the relationship of all or any of these changes to the pathogenesis of the nephrotic syndrome in such patients. A careful

reappraisal of the spectrum of renal changes occurring in sickle cell disease has been published by Elfenbein and co-workers (87). In this study 5 of 6 patients with sickle cell disease and nephrotic syndrome showed extensive reduplication of glomerular basement membranes along with mild mesangial proliferation; similar but less extensive changes occurred in sickle cell disease without nephrosis, but not in sickle cell trait or controls. It was also found that significant glomerular hypertrophy occurred in association with sickle cell disease when contrasted with patients having sickle trait or controls. A plot of mean glomerular size versus age from this study is shown in Figure 10-12. While glomerular size in the sickle cell group increased with age, it was not strictly age-dependent. No clear correlation between glomerular size and blood pressure, blood urea nitrogen, presence of heart failure, or heart and kidney weight was recorded.

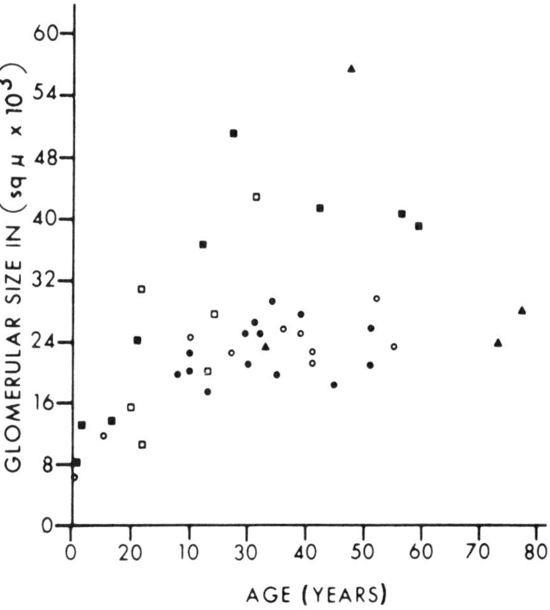

Figure 10-12 Glomerular size vs age in hemoglobinopathies and controls. (■ = SS hemoglobulin; □ = SS + nephrosis; ○ = AS + nephrosis + AS hemoglobin; ▲ = other hemoglobins; ● = controls. Magnification × 450. (Reproduced with permission, B. Elfenbein, A. Patchefsky, W. Schwartz et al., *Am. J. Pathol.* 77:357, 1974.)

Many suggestions have been made concerning the etiology of nephrotic syndrome seen in some patients with sickle cell disease. It is worthwhile briefly to review this material, particularly with an eye toward keeping the relative importance of possible immune-complex–mediated nephropathy in perspective. McCoy felt that the nephrotic syndrome might result from iron overload (83). It was suggested that the process might in some way be analogous to the iron overloading experiments of Ellis (105, 106) where administration of large boluses of saccharated iron oxide precipitated in glomerular capillaries, massively occluded them and eventually led to a proliferative and fibrotic process. No reduplication of glomerular basement membranes was recorded in Ellis' experiments. The mechanism of pure iron overload seems unlikely in humans, since no Prussian-blue–stainable iron is generally noted in glomeruli. The patients studied by Elfenbein and co-workers (87) showed no significant amounts of immunofluorescent deposits in glomerular tissues;

thus, it seems likely that although immune-complex mechanisms play a role in occasional patients with sickle cell anemia and nephropathy, such mechanisms are probably not primarily operative in the majority of patients. Intracapillary red-cell fragmentation and phagocytosis of erythrocytes may possibly play a direct role in the pathogenesis of nephrotic syndrome associated with sickle cell disease. These mechanisms also may pertain directly to the reduplication of glomerular basement membranes often recorded in renal tissues as a relatively early process. Examples of this unique change are shown in Figure 10-13.

Cryoglobulins and Immune-Complex Disease

Some of the most striking phenomena in clinical medicine are noted in association with the occurrence of cryoglobulins accompanying many disease states. Serum cryoglobulins appear to arise de novo within the organism without obvious association to the particular

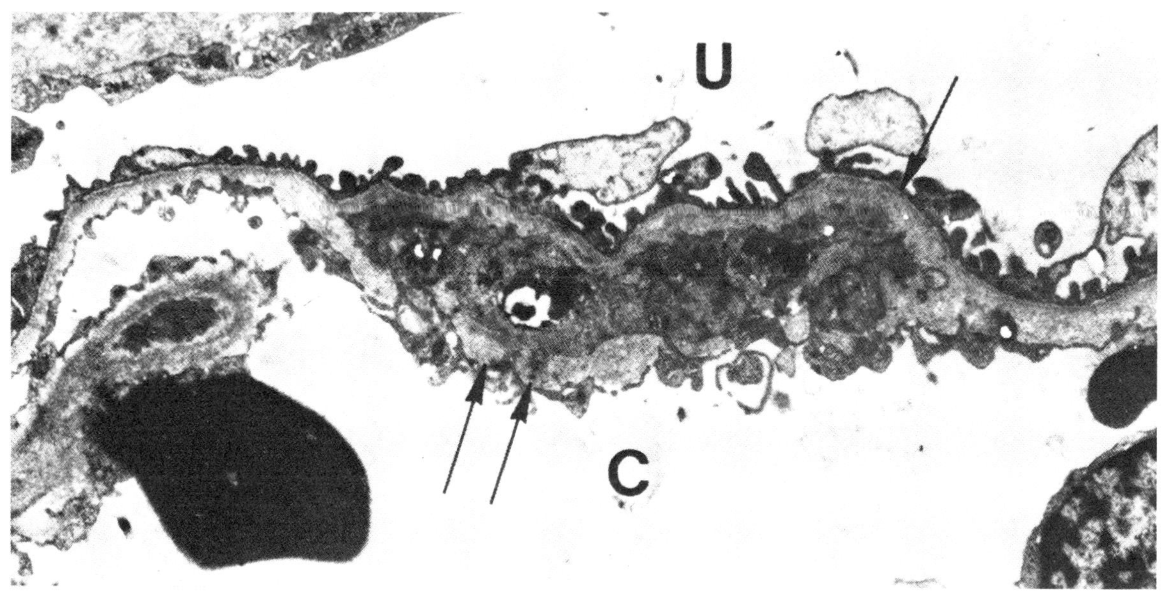

Figure 10-13 Peripheral capillary loop from a patient with sickle cell disease and nephrotic syndrome showing only focal reduplication of the glomerular basement membrane (*single arrow*) by mesangial cell cytoplasm. Neither dense deposits nor fibrin were seen in these regions. Magnification × 4,500. (Reproduced with permission, B. Elfenbein, A. Patchefsky, W. Schwartz et al., *Am. J. Pathol.* 77:357, 1974.)

disorders involved. Tissue lesions and clinical presentation in patients have provided insight into many of the important clinical manifestations of immune-complex disease associated with a wide variety of disorders (107). Patients may show a diffuse vasculitis, progressive glomerular and small blood vessel inflammatory changes, or only mild episodes of synovitis and skin lesions. As noted in Chapter 5, the physical behavior and characterization of such cryoproteins has revealed much of fundamental importance in the understanding of immune-complex phenomena. Moreover, the studies of Levo and co-workers (108) indicated that in some instances the antigens involved in generating these unique cryoglobulin proteins may actually be related to the hepatitis B virus.

The clinical picture of circulating cryoglobulins has been reviewed in detail by Meltzer and colleagues (109, 110). Patients may show homogeneous monoclonal proteins of IgG, IgA, or IgM type or cryoglobulins may occur as complexes of monoclonal IgM rheumatoid factor with nonhomogeneous autologous gamma globulins. A classification can be made on the basis of the immunoglobulin composition of the actual cryoprecipitates. Three main types can be described on the basis of immunoglobulin content and composition: (1) a single homogeneous monoclonal immunoglobulin may be present; (2) two or more immunoglobulins are present, one of which is homogeneous and monoclonal (mixed type); and (3) one or more immunoglobulins are found, none of which appear to be homogeneous or monoclonal (polyclonal type). Any of the major immunoglobulins can participate in this phenomenon and even cryo–Bence Jones proteins have been observed in some instances.

Very little is understood about the physical or chemical features that may predispose some of these circulating cryoproteins to deposit in vascular beds such as skin capillaries or renal glomeruli. Behavior of monoclonal cryoglobulins has served as a useful comparative model in the study of clinical conditions of diverse presumed etiology. Cryoglobulins, probably representing immune complexes, have focused attention on the composition of such reactants in many diseases, including systemic lupus erythematosus, hepatitis B prodromal syndromes, poststreptococcal glomerulonephritis, various parasitic diseases, and relatively rare syndromes such as immune-complex nephropathy associated with sickle cell disease or jejunoileal shunt bypass arthritis.

The primary antibody specificities of the various immunoglobulin components participating in cryoglobulin formation are often unknown. A number of clinical syndromes associated with the so-called idiopathic mixed cryoglobulinemias have been recognized for some time since the original analyses by Meltzer and co-workers (109, 110). Some patients show a rapidly progressive vasculitis and glomerulonephritis; serum complement values are frequently low in patients with "essential" or even secondary mixed cryoglobulinemias associated with a diverse variety of disease states ranging from infectious mononucleosis (111–113) and the postperfusion syndrome associated with cytomegalovirus infection (113, 114) to secondary syphilis, lymphogranuloma venereum, leprosy, and kala azar (115–118).

In some patients direct identification of cryoglobulin components can be made by immunofluorescence or ultrastructural analysis of material from kidney biopsies or areas of cutaneous vasculitis (110, 119, 120). Recent studies in our laboratory (121) have also utilized anti-idiotypic antisera specific for certain monoclonal immunoglobulins to detect these monoclonal cryoglobulins by immunofluorescence in renal tissues and biopsy samples from patients with monoclonal cryoglobulin M components clinically related to progressive glomerular injury. In one of our patients who was studied intensively over a period of several years, progressive renal failure was associated with deposition of the monoclonal cryoglobulin M component in glomeruli. The patient was treated with prednisone and potent cytotoxic agents in an attempt to abolish any clones of cells involved in production of the aberrant M component. Eventually, she underwent renal transplantation with a compatible allograft donor and, to our dismay, once again developed deposition of residual traces of the original and persisting IgG M-component cryoprotein in the transplanted kidney. This emphasizes that apparently certain physical or immunochemical features of such monoclonal M components, particularly those with cryoglobulin properties, predispose to their deposition with eventual microvascular glomerular damage in certain patients. The mechanisms involved in such renal injury have been difficult to define. No antiglomerular basement membrane activity or other specific renal localizing properties of such M components have been conclusively demonstrated as yet. Nor have specific receptors for various immunochemical determinants or molecular conformations on such monoclonal cryoproteins been identified. It is important to extend primary knowledge about basic mechanisms of microvascular or glomerular injury in such individuals, since these patients occur as an experiment of nature eventually providing considerable insight into underlying mechanisms involved in tissue injury in a number of heterogeneous conditions.

In view of our experience with a number of patients showing the clinical association of monoclonal paraprotein cryoglobulinemia and renal disease with participation of the M component in the microvascular renal injury, we favor repeated plasmapheresis as the primary treatment of choice early in the course, if possible. Removal of 1,000 ml of plasma at a time coupled with cytotoxic therapy can dramatically diminish detectable levels of cryoglobulin M component in some patients. Although recommended by others (107), we have had no satisfactory or lasting results with the use of ACTH or corticosteroids in such patients. Since thiol compounds are known to dissociate 19S IgM into 7 S subunits by reduction of disulfide bonds in vitro and also inhibit formation of actual cryogelling phenomena, penicillamine has been proposed in clinical situations where monoclonal IgM cryoglobulins are present (111, 122). One of the difficulties involved with the use of this drug is that at least several months are required before full effect is induced in vivo; also, the untoward side effects of loss of taste, occasional leukopenia or depression of platelets, and the complication of nephrotic syndrome or heavy proteinuria in some patients detract from its full therapeutic

usefulness. Despite intensive work related to this particular aspect of the disorder, surprisingly little is known about the features of such proteins favoring tissue deposition.

Tissue Injury Associated with External Toxic Injury and Immune-Complex Formation

Gold Nephropathy

Gold salts have been used in the treatment of rheumatoid arthritis for four decades (123). More recently, they have been introduced in the therapy of pemphigus (124). Besides occasional leukopenia, thrombocytopenia, and the occurrence of skin rashes, the most important side effect of gold therapy is related to induction of an immune-complex–type glomerulonephritis (125, 126). In many cases, the pathological picture is indistinguishable from the findings noted in idiopathic membranous nephropathy (125, 127, 128). Very little is understood concerning the sequence of events involved in the pathogenesis of renal injury in these patients. Recent observations by Palosuo and colleagues (129) indicate that endogenous generation of immune complexes may be involved in production of tissue lesions in this disorder. A patient with pemphigus vulgaris was studied who was receiving 30 to 50 mg per week of intramuscular gold/sodium thiomalate (129). This was given in addition to 40 mg of prednisone and 150 mg of azathioprine per day. After having received 665 mg of gold, proteinuria developed, and therapy was discontinued. Presence of detectable circulating immune complexes was assayed using the platelet aggregation technique. Various human tissue antigens were tested in several sensitive assay systems. Because serum samples were available on this particular subject prior to the development of proteinuria secondary to gold, it was possible to show presence of circulating immune complexes that coincided directly with the onset of proteinuria. Sucrose gradient analysis of serum samples obtained coincident with onset of gold nephropathy showed presence of high-molecular-weight (> 19S) and intermediate-sized (7 to 19S) complexes. Pemphigus antibody titers previously elevated before initiation of gold therapy fell to much lower levels following gold treatment.

Previous studies have indicated that deposition of immunoglobulins and complement may frequently occur in glomerular capillary walls in patients developing gold nephropathy (125, 126). Studies of serum samples from the patient of Palosuo and co-workers (129) showed the presence of circulating tissue antigens prior to the development of gold nephropathy. In addition, precipitation of patient's serum with preparations of human kidney containing renal tubular antigen (RTE) was also observed. It seems possible therefore that part of the nephropathy after chronic parenteral gold administration in patients with rheumatoid arthritis or other connective tissue diseases may be related to deposition of gold in renal tubules and subsequent release of tissue antigens such as RTE or other tubular components which then serve as primary antigens for immune-complex formation and eventual glomerular deposition leading to proteinuria and gold nephropathy. No renal biopsy nor tissue elution studies were performed in the patient studied by Palosuo and colleagues (129); further work along these lines is needed to confirm or amplify these possibilities.

Very little is understood regarding the positive or beneficial effects observed in patients with rheumatoid arthritis or pemphigus who receive gold treatment. Recent studies by Lipsky and Ziff (130) indicate that administration of gold seems to interfere specifically with macrophage phagocytic and processing functions. These effects were related to a basic diminution of the quantitative intensity of the underlying inflammatory process in the rheumatoid process itself. Thus, if gold halted or subdued the host antigen-processing functions, it could theoretically attenuate initiation of the entire inflammatory cascade involving immune complexes, complement activation, and phagocytosis of such materials by mononuclear cells and other cells important in continuation of the inflammatory process. Gold modulation of macrophage activity might also play a key role in some patients by allowing longer persistence in circulation of other immune

complexes formed, for instance, in situ as renal tubular antigens are released from renal tubules damaged or perturbed by deposition of gold salts. Such a postulated chain of events is shown schematically in Figure 10-14. Direct proof of such an hypothesis is unavailable. For instance, no extensive series of observations has yet been published on patients treated with gold, documenting the presence of circulating immune complexes in such patients before and after onset of gold nephropathy; the patient reported by Palosuo and co-workers (129) represents only a single case. Also, nothing is known concerning the actual source of immune complexes in gold toxicity or in fact whether all of the renal toxicity can be explained on this basis. If a certain size or molecular class of

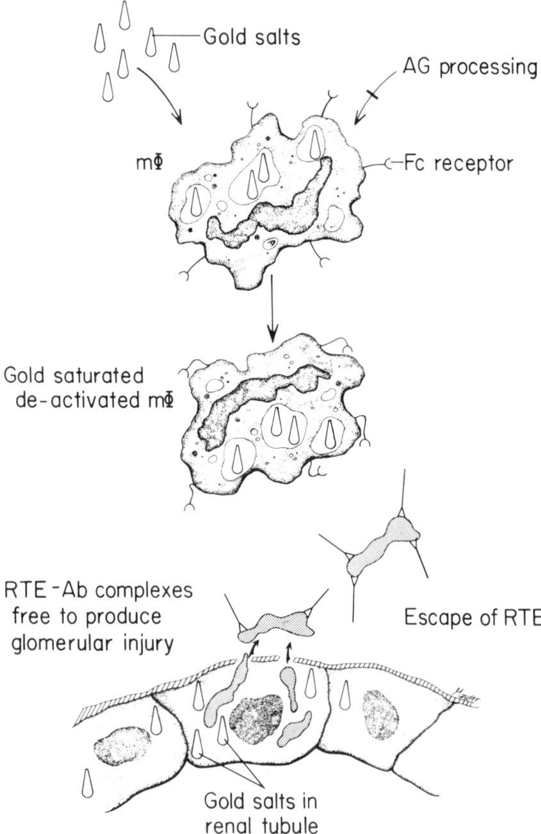

Figure 10-14   Possible mechanisms involved in immunosuppression by gold treatment or gold-induced membranous nephropathy. RTE = renal tubular antigen; MΦ = macrophage.

immune complex is associated with gold nephropathy in a predictable way, the newly developed quantitative assays may be of considerable help in the practical follow-up and management of patients during the initiation of therapy and long-term follow-up. In the absence of extensive data it must be emphasized that these possibilities still fall into the realm of speculation. However, they point up how a toxic reaction to a widely used therapeutic agent might involve direct mediation by immune-complex injury.

Vinyl Chloride Toxicity

Exposure to vinyl chloride compounds during industrial processes employing this material results in a spectrum of serious medical sequelae. Hepatic angiosarcoma in vinyl chloride workers (131, 132) may not actually be the most serious of its potential medical hazards. Acro-osteolysis was first recognized in 1966 in workers employed in the polymerization of vinyl chloride to produce various plastic products (133); numerous other cases have subsequently been described (134, 135). In all of the early reports, affected vinyl chloride workers helped in cleaning the autoclaves after the polymerization process. Later the disorder was also recognized in a worker who had never been involved at this stage of the industrial process (136). More widespread manifestations of tissue injury than acro-osteolysis alone have subsequently been recognized, and the term *vinyl chloride disease* is now given to the general toxic disorder, which includes sclerotic changes in skin, osteolysis, circulatory diseases such as Raynaud's phenomenon, thrombocytopenia, portal fibrosis, and impaired hepatic and pulmonary function.

A great deal of investigation has recently been directed at the pathogenesis of the entire disease complex, and several fascinating lines of evidence suggest that it may be linked with immune-complex formation. The striking clinical similarity of the peripheral manifestations of vinyl chloride disease to progressive scleroderma emphasizes the potential importance of the epidemiologic findings in this industrial disorder. Studies by Ward and colleagues (137, 138) have emphasized the multisystemic nature of the disease and, more importantly, the occurrence of circulating immune complexes in 19 of 28 patients with the disease and in 2 of 30 workers exposed to vinyl chloride. Among the subjects studied, mean exposure to vinyl chloride was 39 months; actual degree of exposure varied with the phase of the industrial process, so patients were divided into high- and low-exposure groups. High-exposure subjects generally worked within the reactor buildings where vinyl chloride polymerization was performed, or in the drying plant. Low-exposure workers included maintenance fitters and warehousemen. However, in the group studied, half had at some time worked in the reactor building or dry-bagging plant operation. A high proportion of the workers examined admitted to what is termed *vinyl chloride narcosis*, or toxic inhalation of vinyl chloride fumes, on at least one occasion.

In the studies reported by Ward and co-workers (137), the major abnormalities observed were a polyclonal increase of immunoglobulin (usually IgG), frequent presence of mixed cryoglobulins composed of IgG, C3, and fibrinogen, and evidence for in vivo conversion of C4 and C3. Using these criteria, evidence for circulating immune complexes was noted in 19 of 28 patients with vinyl chloride disease. Moreover, apparent immune complex activation closely paralleled the degree of vinyl chloride exposure experienced by the workers. Direct immunofluorescent studies of biopsy samples of skin (10 cases), muscle (1 case), and lung (1 case) showed aggregates of IgG, C4, C3, and fibrogen in the lumens of vessels, adherent to vascular endothelium. In addition, IgG, C4, C3, and fibrin were also detected in the media and subintimal regions of small and medium-sized arterioles. The immunofluorescent studies of biopsy material are particularly impressive, since an immune complex or cryoglobulinemic vasculitis would be consistent with previous findings by Markowitz and co-workers (135) of prominent perivascular infiltrates in dermal vessels in this condition. One weakness in the hypothesis offered by Ward and co-workers (137) that immune complexes might be involved in tissue injury in generalized vinyl chloride disease is the failure directly to document the occurrence and molecular characteristics of immune complexes in the disorder by sensitive assays such as the C1q or Raji-cell techniques. Also, if immune complexes are indeed involved, it would be of interest to know what precisely characterizes the antigen in such a disorder. Is it a normal tissue constituent like RTE or some other cellular constituent released by repeated exposure to the vinyl chloride reagent; or is it indeed vinyl chloride–tissue complex? During the study by Ward and colleagues (137) tests for autoantibodies showed a high proportion of positive antinuclear reactivity in subjects with high-exposure risk. However, more direct examination of the actual immune complexes and the physicochemical characteristics of the putative antigens involved will be necessary to relate their presence directly to the clinical phenomena observed. Other workers who have studied the evolution and pathogenesis of generalized vinyl chloride disease have failed to obtain documentation of any autoaggressive process (139, 140), although it was noted that thrombocytopenia often persisted in individual patients long after they were removed from continued exposure.

The metabolism of vinyl chloride in humans is not yet completely understood. Studies in rats by Hefner and colleagues (141) indicated that metabolism involved an alcohol dehydrogenase pathway at low concentration and production of an intermediate chloroethylene oxide at higher tissue levels. Furthermore, it was proposed by Williamson (142) that an intermediate metabolic product was more likely to be a cyclic dioxide. Both the oxide and dioxide would, if present, be highly reactive molecules capable of binding to free tissue sulfhydryl and amino groups. If such materials included free amino acids incorporated into various body structural proteins such as collagen, reticulin, or elastin, the inclusion of such additional groups might well produce autologous proteins that could function as potential autoantigens.

A more likely mechanism possibly involved in the genesis of vinyl chloride disease has been proposed by Ward and co-workers (137). Metabolic products of vinyl chloride, presumably

as the reactive dioxide, bind to plasma protein producing either a haptenic group or subtle conformational change within the protein molecule. This combination would then escape tolerance and stimulate autologous B-cell proliferation and subsequent immunoglobulin production. Circulating antibody complexed with antigen might interact to produce immune-complex injury presumably mediated by activation of the complement system. Predilection for immune-complex deposition in capillaries and endothelial cells near the extremities might then initiate fibrinogen-fibrin conversion and a prolonged low-grade thrombocytopenic process analogous in some respects to chronic defibrination. This sequence of events is sufficient to explain the vascular occlusions, skin, skeletal, and pulmonary changes noted in generalized vinyl chloride disease. Whether or not subsequent findings will bear out this interesting hypothesis remains to be seen. The whole story of vinyl chloride and the remarkable clinical syndrome associated with chronic exposure reemphasizes the potential importance of external reactive materials in the pathogenesis of various human disease states.

Halothane Anesthesia and Hypersensitivity

A condition that is somewhat analogous to gold nephrotoxicity, vinyl chloride toxicity, or other toxic hypersensitivity reactions is halothane toxicity. Although the incidence of jaundice after halothane anesthesia is still believed to be low (143), a continuing controversy exists about whether a direct association is present between repeated anesthetic exposure and predictable development of postoperative hepatic necrosis (144). Mechanisms involved in the production of the liver injury are not clearly understood, but several features of the clinical picture including the frequent history of repeated halothane exposure, eosinophilic infiltrates of hepatic lesions, and the time course of the illness suggest that a delayed hypersensitivity response to halothane or one of its metabolic products could be directly involved in production of liver-cell injury. In most cases very little evidence exists to suggest a pathogenesis involving circulating immune complexes. However, an interesting case report and detailed study by Williams and colleagues (145) provide insight into one aspect of the disorder that may be clinically operative in some patients with halothane toxicity.

The patient studied by the Williams group developed hepatitis after receiving three halothane anesthesias in a period of 22 days. Of particular interest was the development 24 hours after onset of jaundice of an acute serum sickness syndrome with polyarthralgia, proteinuria, and transient decrease in renal function. Serum concentrations of C1q, C4, and C3 showed marked reduction, and immune complexes capable of directly activating the complement system via the classical pathway were demonstrated both in serum and synovial fluid. A definite metabolite of halothane was associated with these immune complexes. Later, after clinical recovery, it was shown that exposure of the patient's lymphocytes to halothane produced lymphocyte stimulation but only in the presence of 7 S fractions of autologous serum. These results were interpreted as evidence that halothane or its metabolic products may in some individuals be immunogenic and that the immunogenicity was related to binding of one of the metabolic products of halothane to autologous plasma proteins. In this case immune-complex determinations on serum samples utilizing direct precipitation with C1q showed concentration of active materials in Sephadex G-200 gel fractions of high molecular weight (19 S). These same fractions were most efficient in producing C3 activation in fresh normal human serum. Gas-liquid chromatography identified the presence of halothane metabolite within immune complexes from both serum and synovial fluid during the acute serum-sickness episode associated with the reaction.

Multiple exposures to halothane, particularly within a four-week interval, appear to increase the probability of developing halothane-related hepatitis and shorten the interval between exposure and the development of jaundice and hepatic necrosis. The pattern of high-molecular-weight materials containing a halothane metabolic product in patient serum and synovial fluid capable of activating the complement pathway in vitro appears to be direct evidence for immune-complex involvement in the serum sickness phenomena observed. Although jaundice, severe hepatic necrosis, and prolonged convalescence or progression to liver failure often characterize the clinical picture of halothane liver injury, rashes, fever, and arthralgias have been noted, although uncommonly, after exposure to halothane (146, 147). Alternatively, other mechanisms involving direct metabolic injury or perhaps delayed hypersensitivity may be much more important in the actual liver-cell necrosis.

Recently many attempts have been made to study possible cell-mediated immune responses to halothane or its metabolites in patients with presumed halothane hypersensitivity (148–150) and occasional documentation of lymphocyte reactivity to drug has been presented (148). In the patient studied by Williams and colleagues (145) lymphocyte transformation only occurred in the presence of autologous 7 S serum fractions, suggesting that immune complexes rather than drug or drug metabolite alone were responsible for lymphocyte reactivity in this instance. No evidence is available on whether immune-complex–mediated tissue injury plays a direct role in the central and most important aspect of posthalothane toxicity—namely, hepatocyte necrosis. If metabolic products of drugs in some instances bind directly to glycoproteins of hepatic cells, then several specific mechanisms could be envisaged whereby liver-cell damage might be produced. Binding of antibody to drug or drug-protein complex could sensitize hepatocytes to destruction via antibody-mediated lysis of cells occurring through local activation of the intrinsic complement system. Thus far no evidence has been produced to support the involvement of such mechanisms in halothane-related hepatic necrosis.

Thrombocytopenic Purpura

Idiopathic thrombocytopenic purpura (ITP) is a disorder of unknown etiology characterized by marked diminution of circulating platelets, and peripheral as well as systemic bleeding. Some patients show a positive response to therapeutic splenectomy and in many individuals this appears to correlate with an improvement in the degree of thrombocytopenia on prior high-dose corticosteroid therapy. Therapy with corticosteroids, splenectomy, and in a small proportion of patients immunosuppressive therapy or even plasmapheresis may be effective in controlling the major manifestations and evolution of the disorder. The basic pathogenesis of the disease is not completely understood, but a number of experiments have related the destruction of platelets in ITP to the occurrence of a serum factor containing IgG (151–153). This factor might be antiplatelet autoantibody (153, 154) or it might also represent immune complexes that can be readily adsorbed onto platelets and cause their agglutination and consumption (155, 156). This latter possibility is suggested in the demonstration by Israels and co-workers (156) of an Fc receptor on platelets capable of adsorbing immune complexes. In order to differentiate antiplatelet antibody-mediated platelet reactivity and lysis from that produced by antigen-antibody complexes adsorbed to platelet Fc receptors, it would be necessary to demonstrate that the IgG molecules involved react with platelets via their Fab fragments. There is no substantial evidence in the current literature relating directly to this point. In fact, the studies published by Karpatkin and co-workers (157), who fractionated ITP sera by gel filtration, showed that the antiplatelet factor was found in a region of 330,000 M.W. and not actually in the 7 S or 150,000 M.W. region, which would have been expected with isolated IgG antibodies. Also of interest in this regard was that subsequent studies by Karpatkin and co-workers (157) indicated that antiplatelet factors contained IgG antibodies, mainly of the IgG-3 subclass known to be capable of substantial polymeric formation. Additional studies (158) have indicated that the Fc fragment of IgG-3 has a high affinity for platelet membranes.

A recent report by Lurhuma and colleagues (159) is pertinent to this problem. Sera from 72 patients with ITP were studied for inhibitory activity in the agglutination of IgG-coated particles by human rheumatoid factor or C1q. Eighty-three percent of serum samples showed inhibitory activity against both agglutinating materials, whereas only 17 percent showed presence of endogenous rheumatoid factor. A negative correlation was noted between titers of inhibition and platelet counts in individual patients. Gel filtration studies showed inhibitory factors in high-molecular-weight fractions eluting before 7 S IgG. IgG was found in high-molecular-weight serum fractions and appeared to be present as part of an immune complex since it was dissociable at acid pH. DNA was detected in high-molecular-weight complexes or serum fractions in all ITP sera examined by gel filtration and was thought to represent potential antigen in immune complexes. Counterelectrophoresis was utilized for detection of viral antigens in all sera, and hepatitis B antigen was found in 20 sera, EB virus antigen in 5 sera, and adenovirus antigen in 6 sera. Representative gel filtration experiments performed using these two sensitive assays for presumed immune complexes are shown in Figure 10-15. Inhibition of C1q or RF agglutination reactions by high-molecular-weight serum fractions was present. One of the most remarkable aspects of this report is the statement that 48 percent of the serum samples from ITP contained hepatitis B antigen—a claim that requires confirmation in other laboratories using radioimmunoassay or other sensitive assay techniques.

Other forms of thrombocytopenia appear to be more closely related to immune complexes than specifically to antiplatelet antibody. Thus, acute postinfectious thrombocytopenia (160) or drug-induced thrombocytopenic purpura (161, 162) appear to be more closely related to immune-complex adsorption by platelets than to the direct action of antiplatelet antibody on platelet antigens alone. These observations together with the findings of Lurhuma and colleagues (159) raise an important question related to the effects of circulating immune complexes in various disease states. In Chapter 5 the importance of the relative balance between load of circulating complexes, physicochemical qualities of these complexes, and saturation of tissue or cellular receptors for complexes was discussed in detail. In the case of a disorder such as immune thrombocytopenic purpura, yet another factor is intro-

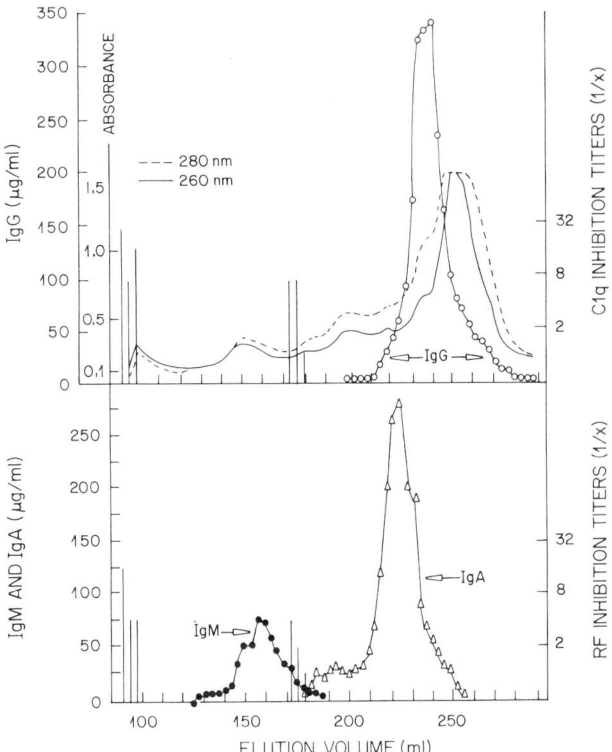

Figure 10-15 Chromatography on Ultrogel AcA22 of the serum (3 ml) of a patient with ITP. The elution (fractions of 3 ml) was monitored by absorbances at 260 and 280 mm; immunoassays of IgG, IgM, and IgA; and inhibition of the agglutination of IgG-coated latex by RF or C1q (*vertical bars*). (Reproduced with permission, A. Z. Lurhuma, H. Riccomi, and P. L. Masson, *Clin. Exp. Immunol.* 28:49, 1977.)

duced: that of intrinsic receptors for complexes on platelets themselves. Since ITP is a relatively rare disorder, and transient appearance of detectable immune complexes is a common feature of many human conditions (including human pregnancy, pneumococcal pneumonia, and other bacterial or viral infections), other factors than presence of circulating complexes must feature in induction of the pathological thrombocytopenic state. It may well require relative saturation of tissue Fc receptors or certain as yet poorly defined physical or immunochemical qualities of immune complexes to make platelets particularly vulnerable to adsorption and subsequent injury or lysis. In ITP, characteristically there is often proliferation or marked relative increase in megakaryocytes but absence of effective platelet release. This picture suggests the interesting features related to some of the rare

aregenerative hematologic syndromes recently studied in detail by several groups. For instance in Blackfan-Diamond syndrome characterized by an aregenerative anemia, it has recently been shown that erythropoiesis and effective maturation of normal red-cell processes may in some patients be directly inhibited by suppressor T cells (163, 164). Thus, normal marrow cocultured with T lymphocytes from affected patients is inhibited from normal erythroid maturation by what might be broadly termed suppressor T cells. Still another example of possible cell-mediated immune effects in Felty's syndrome, an analogous hematopoietic disorder, has been presented by Abdou and co-workers (165); they showed that the leukopenia and marked granulocytopenia in this interesting complication of rheumatoid arthritis is mediated by suppressor T cells capable of direct inhibition of granulocyte maturation and proliferation in an in vitro assay marrow-culture system. Therefore, similar mechanisms could be operative in the case of ITP, apart from the platelet lysis or sequestration induced either directly by antiplatelet antibodies or by adsorbed antigen-antibody complexes. The classic picture of marked relative increase in precursor mega-karyocytes might be easier to explain; that is, that full maturation and release of platelets is being shut off not by antiplatelet antibody, but by suppressor T-cell factors.

Retinal Vasculitis

Retinal vasculitis is a common accompaniment of several connective-tissue diseases such as systemic lupus erythematosus, periarteritis, or occasionally in mixed connective-tissue syndromes. In other instances, vasculitis of the retina is an inflammatory process predominantly involving the retinal venous system although occasionally extending to the arterial vessels. Several varieties have been reported. The peripheral type was first described by Eales in 1880 (166); this particular disorder is most often noted in young adult males and is frequently associated with repeated intraocular hemorrhage and severe loss of vision. Central retinal vasculitis, a clinical entity first described by Lyle and Wybar in 1961 (167), is generally regarded as a benign, unilateral disorder occurring predominantly in males, which occasionally produces permanent or severe visual impairment. To some workers the central form of subacute or chronic retinal vasculitis is the result of central venous occlusion in an otherwise normal retinal vascular network (168); however, the occasional occurrence first in one eye and then in the other (167) suggests an inflammatory or more generalized etiology. Examples of the appearance of the fundus and retinal angiograms in this condition are shown in Figures 10-16 and 10-17. Experimental evidence suggests that an immunologic reaction is involved in the mediation of central retinal vasculitis. Thus, antigens injected directly into the vitreous humor of sensitized animals produce an Arthus-type reaction in some ways resembling retinal vasculitis (169, 170) since the reactions are often accompanied by retinal vascular thrombosis within the venous system.

A group of 17 patients with central or peripheral retinal vasculitis have recently been studied by Andrews and co-workers (171). Evidence for the presence of circulating immune complexes was obtained using reactivity with C1q, monoclonal rheumatoid factor, anticomplementary activity of serum, and presence of complement activation. Two or more parameters judged to be presumptive evidence for circulating complexes were positive in 13 of 17 patients. The primary importance of these findings is beclouded by the fact that two of the patients showed Behçet's syndrome, two also showed glomerulonephritis confirmed by renal biopsy, and one had associated rheumatoid arthritis. Thus, it is difficult to ascertain which disorder was indeed related to the occurrence of detectable complexes in some patients included in this series.

More direct assessment of the local effects of immune complexes in the eye itself has been presented by Howles and McKay (172), who studied changes in local vascular permeability produced in rabbit eyes by intravenous injection of large quantities of immune complexes into previously immunized animals. In these studies soluble complexes were prepared in 20 to 25 times antigen excess, and local alterations in permeability monitored by the ocular accumulation of ^{125}I-labeled serum albumin. The local effects of immune complexes in ocular structures were most pronounced in vessels supplying iridial portions of the ciliary processes. Edema and transudation of fluid were the earliest findings described. This distribution of ocular injury is similar to that previously noted after endotoxin; however, with the latter, much more extreme and irreversible capillary changes were noted with platelet plugging, endothelial injury, and deposition of intravascular fibrin strands. These animal experiments are of importance; the uveal tract and structures immediately contiguous with the ciliary processes may be the most sensitive ocular structure to immune-complex injury.

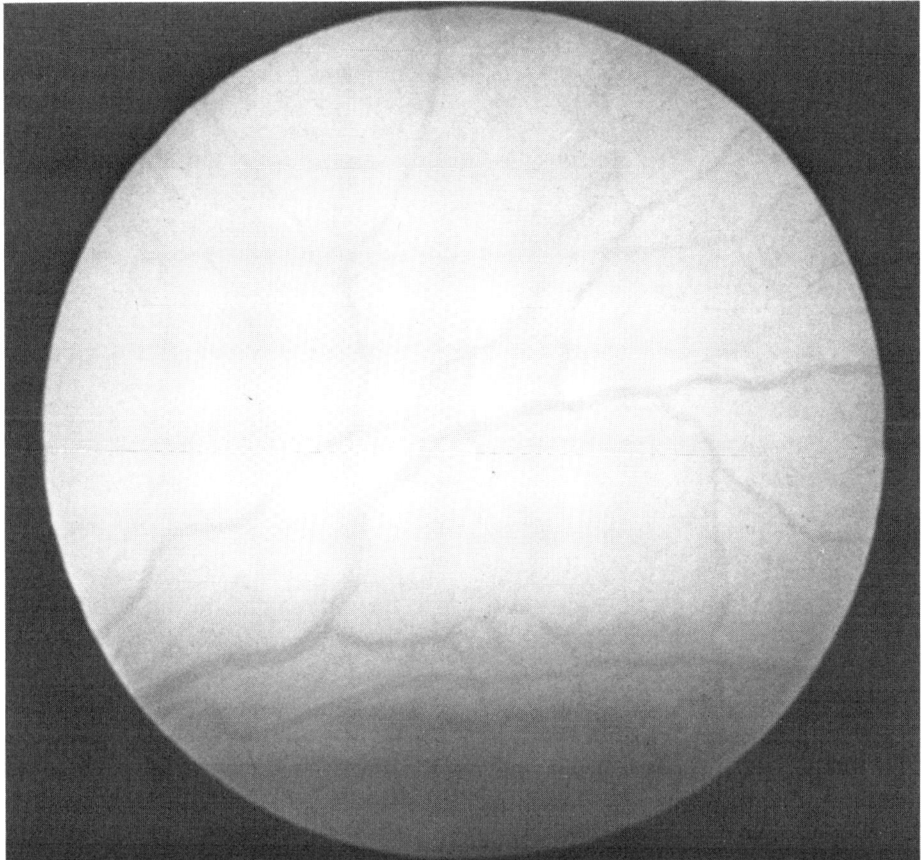

Figure 10-16   Retinal vasculitis as visualized by fundoscopy. Attenuation, primarily in the venous system, is apparent. (Photograph courtesy of Douglas Coster, London.)

Such localization might be significant, for instance, in the iridocyclitis associated with a wide variety of diseases in which immune complexes have at least been implicated, such as the peripheral manifestations of inflammatory bowel disease, ankylosing spondylitis, sarcoidosis, and juvenile pauciarticular rheumatoid arthritis. Further studies are needed in an attempt to define whether ciliary tissues or other discrete ocular structures show a relative concentration of receptors for immune complexes or whether, alternatively, there is something about the immunochemical or physical nature of some complexes that makes them unusually attracted to ocular structures.

Sarcoidosis

Human sarcoidosis has frequently been presumed to involve portions of the immune system. Several aspects of the primary disease suggest that formation of immune complexes may be associated with basic tissue lesions. Frequent elevation of immunoglobulin levels, coupled with relative depression of cell-mediated or delayed-type hypersensitivity, further emphasizes an apparent imbalance in the immune setting or regulation in the basic disease process (173, 174). Indirect evidence for possible clinical importance of immune complexes in this disease can be found in the fact that rheu-

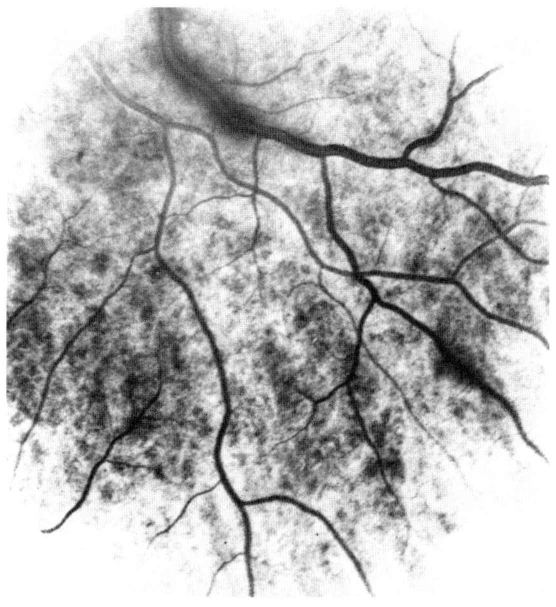

Figure 10-17   Retinal angiogram in a patient with retinal vasculitis, showing segmental venous leakage of contrast material in areas affected by acute inflammation. (Photograph courtesy of Douglas Coster, London.)

matoid factor present in the serum of many patients with the disease appears to correlate to a certain extent with activity of the disease (175).

Many of the clinical presentations of sarcoidosis, including erythema nodosum, polyarticular synovitis, repeated inflammation of the uveal tract or iritis, pulmonary infiltrates and interstitial fibrosis, skin lesions, and episodic flare-ups of the disease are manifestations possibly mediated by immune complexes. In contrast to this are the frequent histological findings of noncaseating granulomata in many tissue sites. From one standpoint, sarcoid seems to be an immune disease in search of an antigen or basic unifying concept of pathogenesis. Much like systemic lupus, the disease is correlated with hyperreactivity of the humoral immune system and relative depression of cell-mediated immune responses.

Deposition of immunoglobulins and complement has been noted in or surrounding the granulomatous lesions of sarcoidosis in lymph nodes (176, 177), and in sarcoid lesions studied

from lung biopsy samples (178). Hedfors and Norberg (179) recorded circulating immune complexes using the platelet aggregation assay in about 25 percent of 26 patients with sarcoid and in 4 of 5 patients with erythema nodosum and bilateral hilar adenopathy. Studies by Verrier-Jones and co-workers (180) in 22 patients with erythema nodosum and presumed sarcoid showed evidence for C1q precipitating materials in only 2 of 13 patients tested, whereas 6 of 10 patients were positive for complexes using the platelet aggregation test. Anticomplementary activity was present in 8 of 16 patients tested but CH 50 was reduced in only 4 of 18 patients. Activation products of C3 were recorded in 14 of these 18 patients.

The precise role of immune complexes in the general clinical picture of sarcoidosis is presently difficult to define. The occurrence of positive reactions in some patients early in their course is not surprising and the technical difficulties introduced in the interpretation of features such as anticomplementary activity or platelet aggregation in the presence of hypergammaglobulinemia make evaluation of positive tests nebulous. It is not surprising that a generalized granulomatous disorder such as sarcoidosis might be associated with presence of immune complexes during certain features of its clinical evolution. Similarly one might expect other diseases in which the agent is well known and characterized as in the case of disseminated tuberculosis or histoplasmosis producing multiple granulomata in numerous tissue sites also to be associated with presence of detectable circulating complexes at intervals during active disease. The presence of immune complexes in the circulation may well reflect multiple foci of tissue reaction and injury along with relative saturation of fixed and circulating cells bearing Fc receptors. One cannot conclude from any of the data available thus far that immune-complex deposition per se is the driving force in a disease such as sarcoidosis. This is particularly pertinent in view of the absence of any well-defined agent or primary antigen in the disease process. Thus the presence of detectable circulating complexes in sarcoidosis may have little pathological significance, and until proven otherwise they may be regarded as little more than an elevation of the sedimentation rate or C-reactive protein in this disorder. On the contrary, if immune complexes and their primary tissue deposition are found to represent the initial event in initiation of the many parenchymal tissue granulomatous lesions, more significance can be attached to their relation to the basic underlying disease process.

Transplantation

The most widely practiced transplantation procedure today is represented by renal allografts from either living related or cadaveric donors. The major related problem, of course, is recipient rejection of the allograft. Similar graft-recipient problems are encountered with transplantation of widely differing types, including heart, pancreas, skin, testicle, and many other tissues. Renal allografts have been extensively studied and currently represent the most common clinical transplant situation encountered by practicing physicians. The interrelated mechanisms influencing rejection are complex and represent both cell-mediated and humoral effects (181). Direct evidence for the importance of deposition of antibodies or soluble antigen-antibody complexes in grafts comes from the demonstration of granular deposits of immunoglobulins and complement in glomeruli during the process of graft rejection (182–184). Although immune-complex deposition in the allograft may be of importance in the logistical development of allograft injury, it is also clear that cell-mediated phenomena play a major role.

The role of circulating complexes in rejection and in the critical periods before and after renal transplantation has recently been studied by Ooi and co-workers (185). Sera from 45 normal subjects, 24 allografted patients undergoing acute rejection, and 11 allografted patients in the quiescent phase were tested using C1q binding radioimmunoassay. A marked increase in C1q binding activity was noted in 14 patients with acute rejection. In 9 subjects concurrent renal biopsies showed fibrin deposition in renal vasculature with tubulointerstitial cellular infiltrates. Ten other patients with acute

rejection, whose biopsies also showed cellular infiltrates characteristic of the rejection process, showed no increased levels of immune complexes by C1q binding assay. In the patients with acute rejection and elevated complexes a clinical correlation between levels of complexes and gradual resolution of rejection with therapy was recorded. A summary of representative sequential data accumulated during this study is shown in Figure 10-18. Physical studies of immune complexes were performed using sucrose density gradient ultracentrifugation techniques. Fractions showing positive reactions for C1q sedimented between 15 and 18.4 S, and after dissociation in acidic buffers were shown to contain IgG. Immunofluorescence studies on renal biopsy ma-

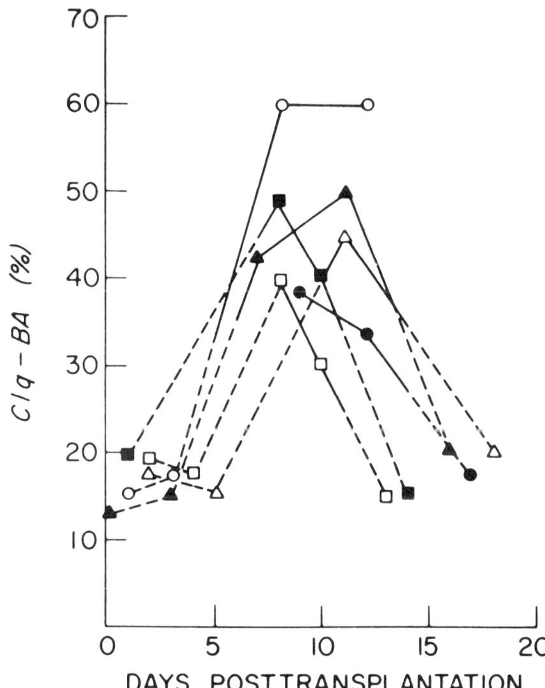

Figure 10-18 Sequential studies of serum C1q binding activity of 6 patients after renal allografting. Normal values of C1q binding were 16 ± 7.2 (mean, 2 S.D.). Increased serum C1q binding was recorded during rejection episodes as compared with levels during prerejection and postrejection periods. (*Dashed lines,* periods before or after treated rejection.) (Reproduced with permission, Y. M. Ooi, B. S. Ooi, E. H. Vallota et al., *J. Clin. Invest.* 60:611, 1977.)

terial revealed granular deposits of Ig or, less frequently, complement in glomeruli or tubular basement membranes of kidneys undergoing acute rejection. Deposition of immune complexes therefore may be an important part of the rejection process; furthermore these events seem in some cases to be correlated with intrarenal fibrin deposition. In a study of this type intrinsic immune complexes antedating the transplant and participating in the chronic progressive renal injury are of potential importance. Ten of the patients undergoing apparent humoral rejection were derived from patient groups not thought clinically to be involved with renal pathology primarily initiated by immune mechanisms (polycystic kidney disease, hereditary nephritis, hypertensive nephrosclerosis, reflux pyelonephritis, and diabetic glomerulosclerosis). In addition, although a distinct possibility in some patients, the role of administered antilymphocyte globulin (ALG) was excluded in the humoral immune-complex–mediated pathogenesis of 4 humoral-rejection patients, since two did not receive ALG and two showed humoral rejection at times unrelated to ALG administration.

Allograft rejection may take the form of predominantly cell-mediated phenomena characterized by lymphocytic and mononuclear cellular infiltration of the tubulointerstitial structures (186). However, in rejection dominated by humoral events, the major histological characteristic is often fibrin and microthrombi formation in renal microvasculature. The studies reported by Ooi and co-workers (185) provide evidence that microvascular changes of fibrin plugging and deposition may be related directly to local immune-complex–mediated effects in the renal vasculature. Several laboratory and experimental animal models have explored the relationship between activation of the complement system by antigen-antibody complexes and the coagulation process (187). In hyperimmunized animals infusion of small amounts of antigens may under certain circumstances be followed by acute cortical necrosis with marked fibrin deposition (188).

The experimental and clinical data presented by Ooi suggest that there may be a correlation between humoral rejection and development of fibrin microthrombi in renal vessels. Whether this is directly mediated by immune complexes or by other local tissue factors produced during allograft rejection remains to be established. It is conceivable that the detection of circulating immune complexes in the patients with transplantation rejection and a general picture of humoral mediation were secondary to basic underlying tissue injury and were present as a reflection of the process rather than its basic cause. Certainly characterization of the antigens involved in the production of such complexes and serial disappearance or homing studies of the latter would be helpful in assigning them a primary or secondary role. Renal transplant patients represent a complex mixture of simultaneous and dramatic processes. They are often heavily immunosuppressed and receive quantities of potent agents such as corticosteroids, ALG, or cytotoxic agents that may produce major shifts in immune balance. On the other hand, the features of allograft rejection represent a fascinating arena where immune-complex formation may play a critical role.

References

1. Baldwin, R. W., Price, M. R., and Robins, R. A. Blocking of lymphocyte-mediated cytotoxicity for rat hepatoma cells by tumour-specific antigen-antibody complexes. *Nature (New Biol.)* 238:185, 1972.

2. Sjögren, H. O., Hellström, I., Bansal, S. C., et al. Suggestive evidence that the "blocking antibodies" of tumor-bearing individuals may be antigen-antibody complexes. *Proc. Natl. Acad. Sci. USA* 68:1372, 1971.

3. Youtananukorn, V., and Mantangkasombut, P. Specific plasma factors blocking human maternal cell-mediated immune reaction to placental antigens. *Nature (New Biol.)* 242:110, 1973.

4. Taylor, P. V., and Hancock, K. W. Antigenicity of trophoblast and possible antigen-masking effects during pregnancy. *Immunology* 28:973, 1975.

5. Pence, H., Petty, W. M., and Rocklin, R. E. Suppression of maternal responsiveness to paternal antigen by maternal plasma. *J. Immunol.* 114:525, 1975.

6. Tamerius, J., Hellström, I., and Hellström, K. E. Evidence that blocking factors in the sera of multiparous mice are associated with immunoglobulins. *Int. J. Cancer* 16:456, 1975.

7. Masson, P. L., Delire, M., and Cambiaso, C. L. Circulating immune complexes in normal human pregnancy. *Nature* 266:542, 1977.

8. Lurhuma, A. Z., Cambiaso, C. L., Masson, P. L., et al. Detection of circulating antigen-antibody complexes by their inhibitory effect on the agglutination of IgG-coated particles by rheumatoid factor or C1q. *Clin. Exp. Immunol.* 25:212, 1976.

9. Tung, K. S. K. Immune complex in the renal glomerulus during normal pregnancy. A study in the guinea pig and the mouse. *J. Immunol.* 112:186, 1974.

10. Morris, R. H., Vassalli, P., and McCluskey, R. T. Immunofluorescent studies on renal biopsies in pregnancy. *Clin. Obstet. Gynecol.* 11:522, 1968.

11. Stimson, W. H. Studies on the immunosuppressive properties of a pregnancy-associated α-macroglobulin. *Clin. Exp. Immunol.* 25:199, 1976.

12. Hill, C. A., Finn, R., and Denye, V. Depression of cellular immunity in pregnancy due to a serum factor. *Br. Med. J.* 3:513, 1973.

13. Jha, P., Talwar, G. P., and Hingorani, V. Depression of blast transformation of peripheral leukocytes by plasma from pregnant women. *Am. J. Obstet. Gynecol.* 122:965, 1975.

14. Billingham, R. E. The transplantation biology of mammalian gestation. *Am. J. Obstet. Gynecol.* 111:469, 1971.

15. Currie, G. A. Immunological studies of trophoblast *in vitro*. *J. Obstet. Gynaecol. Br. Commonw.* 74:841, 1967.

16. Loke, Y. W., Joysey, V. C., and Borland, R. HL-A antigens on human trophoblast cells. *Nature* 232:403, 1971.

17. Kaliss, N., and Dagg, M. K. Immune response engendered in mice by multiparity. *Transplantation* 2:416, 1964.

18. Kasakura, S. A factor in maternal plasma during pregnancy that suppresses the reactivity of mixed leukocyte cultures. *J. Immunol.* 107:1296, 1971.

19. Faulk, W. P. Biological activity of placental immunoglobulins. 1st International Congress on Immunology in Obstetrics and Gynecology. *Excerpta Medica* 281:18, 1973.

20. Rocklin, R. E., Kitzmiller, J. L., Carpenter, C. B., et al. Maternal-fetal relation. Absence of an immunologic blocking factor from the serum of women with chronic abortions. *N. Engl. J. Med.* 295:1209, 1976.

21. Olding, L. B., and Oldstone, M. B. A. Lymphocytes from human newborns abrogate mitosis of their mother's lymphocytes. *Nature* 249:161, 1974.

22. Olding, L. B., Benirschke, K., and Oldstone, M. B. A. Inhibition of mitosis of lymphocytes from human adults by lymphocytes from human newborns. *Clin. Immunol. Immunopathol.* 3:79, 1974.

23. Olding, L. B., and Oldstone, M. B. A. Thymus-derived peripheral lymphocytes from human newborns inhibit division of their mother's lymphocytes. *J. Immunol.* 116:682, 1976.

24. Oldstone, M. B. A., Tishon, A., and Moretta, L. Active thymus derived suppressor lymphocytes in human cord blood. *Nature* 269:333, 1977.

25. Murgita, R. A., Goidl, E. A., Kontiainen, S., et al. α-fetoprotein induces suppressor T cells *in vitro*. *Nature* 267:257, 1977.

26. Horn, R. C., Jr., and Smetana, H. Intercapillary glomerulosclerosis. *Am. J. Pathol.* 18:93, 1942.

27. Raphael, S. S., and Lynch, M. J. G. Kimmelstiel-Wilson glomerulonephropathy: its occurrence in diseases other than diabetes mellitus. *Arch. Pathol.* 65:420, 1958.

28. Baxter, J. H., and Ashworth, C. T. Renal lesions in portal cirrhosis. *Arch. Pathol.* 41:476, 1946.

29. Patek, A. J., Jr., Seegal, D., and Bevans, M. The coexistence of cirrhosis of the liver and glomerulonephritis: report of 14 cases. *Am. J. Med. Sci.* 221:77, 1951.

30. Bloodworth, J. M. B., Jr., and Sommers, S. C. "Cirrhotic glomerulosclerosis", a renal lesion associated with hepatic cirrhosis. *Lab. Invest.* 8:962, 1959.

31. Sakaguchi, H., Dachs, S., Grishman, E., et al. Hepatic glomerulosclerosis. An electron microscopic study of renal biopsies in liver diseases. *Lab. Invest.* 14:533, 1965.

32. Salomon, M. I., Sakaguchi, H., Churg, J., et al. Renal lesions in hepatic disease: a study based on kidney biopsies. *Arch. Intern. Med.* 115:704, 1965.

33. Fisher, E. R., and Perez-Stable, E. Cirrhotic (hepatic) lobular glomerulonephritis. Correlation of ultrastructural and clinical features. *Am. J. Pathol.* 52:869, 1968.

34. Callard, P., Feldmann, G., Prandi, D., et al. Immune complex type glomerulonephritis in cirrhosis of the liver. *Am. J. Pathol.* 80:329, 1975.

35. Tomasi, T. B., Jr., and Tisdale, W. A. Serum gamma-globulins in acute and chronic liver diseases. *Nature* 201:834, 1964.

36. Triger, D. R., and Wright, R. Studies on hepatic uptake of antigen. II. The effect of hepato-

toxins on the immune response. *Immunology* 25:951, 1973.

37. Bjørneboe, M., Prytz, H., and Ørskov, F. Antibodies to intestinal microbes in serum of patients with cirrhosis of the liver. *Lancet* 1:58, 1972.

38. Triger, D. R., Alp, M. H., and Wright, R. Bacterial and dietary antibodies in liver disease. *Lancet* 1:60, 1972.

39. Thomas, H. C., Potter, B. J., and Sherlock, S. Is primary biliary cirrhosis an immune complex disease? *Lancet* 2:1261, 1977.

40. Rubin, E., Schaffner, F., and Popper, H. Primary biliary cirrhosis. Chronic non-suppurative destructive cholangitis. *Am. J. Pathol.* 46:387, 1965.

41. Golding, P. L., Smith, M., and Williams, R. Multisystem involvement in chronic liver disease. Studies on the incidence and pathogenesis. *Am. J. Med.* 55:772, 1973.

42. Alarçon-Segovia, D., Díaz-Jouanen, E., and Fishbein, E. Features of Sjögren's syndrome in primary biliary cirrhosis. *Ann. Intern. Med.* 79:31, 1973.

43. Sherlock, S., and Scheuer, P. J. The presentation and diagnosis of 100 patients with primary biliary cirrhosis. *N. Engl. J. Med.* 289:674, 1973.

44. Child, D. L., Mathews, J. A., and Thompson, R. P. Arthritis and primary biliary cirrhosis. *Br. Med. J.* 2:557, 1977.

45. Doniach, D., and Walker, G. Mitochondrial antibodies (AMA). *Gut* 15:664, 1974.

46. Thomas, H. C., De Villiers, D., Potter, B., et al. Immune complexes in acute and chronic liver disease. *Clin. Exp. Immunol.* 31:150, 1978.

47. Paronetto, F., Schaffner, F., and Popper, H. Antibodies to cytoplasmic antigens in primary biliary cirrhosis and chronic active hepatitis. *J. Lab. Clin. Med.* 69:979, 1967.

48. Potter, B. J., Elias, E., and Jones, E. A. Hypercatabolism of the third component of complement in patients with primary biliary cirrhosis. *J. Lab. Clin. Med.* 88:427, 1976.

49. Teisberg, P., and Gjone, E. Circulating conversion products of C3 in liver disease. Evidence for *in vivo* activation of the complement system. *Clin. Exp. Immunol.* 14:509, 1973.

50. Thomas, H. C., De Villiers, D., and Sherlock, S. Unpublished data, 1977.

51. Wands, J. R., Dienstag, J. L., Bhan, A. K., et al. Circulating immune complexes and complement activation in primary biliary cirrhosis. *N. Engl. J. Med.* 298:233, 1978.

52. Paronetto, F., and Popper, H. Chronic liver injury induced by immunologic reactions. Cirrhosis following immunization with heterologous sera. *Am. J. Pathol.* 49:1087, 1966.

53. Paronetto, F., Woolf, N., Koffler, D., et al. Response of the liver to soluble antigen-antibody complexes. *Gastroenterology* 43:539, 1962.

54. McFarlane, H., Holzel, A., Brenchley, P., et al. Immune complexes in cystic fibrosis. *Br. Med. J.* 1:423, 1975.

55. Høiby, N. *Pseudomonas aeruginosa* infection in cystic fibrosis. Relationship between mucoid strains of *Pseudomonas aeruginosa* and the humoral immune response. *Acta Pathol. Microbiol. Scand. (B)* 82:551, 1974.

56. Høiby, N., Jacobsen, L., Jørgensen, B. A., et al. *Pseudomonas aeruginosa* infection in cystic fibrosis. Occurrence of precipitating antibodies against *Pseudomonas aeruginosa* in relation to the concentration of sixteen serum proteins and the clinical and radiographical status of the lungs. *Acta Paediatr. Scand.* 63:843, 1974.

57. Høiby, N., and Wiik, A. Antibacterial precipitins and autoantibodies in serum of patients with cystic fibrosis. *Scand. J. Respir. Dis.* 56:38, 1975.

58. Schiøtz, P. O., Høiby, N., Juhl, F., et al. Immune complexes in cystic fibrosis. *Acta Pathol. Microbiol. Scand. (C)* 85:57, 1977.

59. Gordon, D. S., Hunter, R. G., O'Reilly, R. J., et al. *Pseudomonas aeruginosa* allergy and humoral antibody-mediated hypersensitivity pneumonia. *Am. Rev. Respir. Dis.* 108:127, 1973.

60. Johnson, K. J., and Ward, P. A. Acute immunologic pulmonary alveolitis. *J. Clin. Invest.* 54:349, 1974.

61. Mass, B., Ikeda, T., Meranze, D. R., et al. Induction of experimental emphysema. Cellular and species specificity. *Am. Rev. Respir. Dis.* 106:384, 1972.

62. Jewell, D. P., and MacLennan, I. C. M. Circulating immune complexes in inflammatory bowel disease. *Clin. Exp. Immunol.* 14:219, 1973.

63. Doe, W. F., Booth, C. C., and Brown, D. L. Evidence for complement-binding immune complexes in adult coeliac disease, Crohn's disease, and ulcerative colitis. *Lancet* 1:402, 1973.

64. Ezer, G., and Hayward, A. R. Inhibition of complement-dependent lymphocyte rosette formation: a possible test for activated complement products. *Eur. J. Immunol.* 4:148, 1974.

65. Hodgson, H. J. F., Potter, B. J., and Jewell, D. P. Immune complexes in ulcerative colitis and Crohn's disease. *Clin. Exp. Immunol.* 29:187, 1977.

66. Baklien, K., and Brandtzaeg, P. Comparative mapping of the local distribution of immunoglobulin-containing cells in ulcerative colitis and Crohn's disease of the colon. *Clin. Exp. Immunol.* 22:197, 1975.

67. Monteiro, E., Fossey, J., Shiner, M., et al. Antibacterial antibodies in rectal and colonic mucosa in ulcerative colitis. *Lancet* 1:249, 1971.

68. Shagrin, J. W., Frame, B., and Duncan, H. Polyarthritis in obese patients with intestinal bypass. *Ann. Intern. Med.* 75:377, 1971.

69. Wands, J. R., LaMont, J. T., Mann, E., et al. Arthritis associated with intestinal-bypass procedure for morbid obesity. Complement activation and characterization of circulating cryoproteins. *N. Engl. J. Med.* 294:121, 1976.

70. Mezey, E., Potter, J. J., Rent, K., et al. Is endogenous ethanol production responsible for hepatic dysfunction following jejuno-ileal anastomosis for morbid obesity? *Clin. Res.* 22:694A, 1974.

71. Moake, J. L., Kageler, W. V., Cimo, P. L., et al. Intravascular hemolysis, thrombocytopenia, leukopenia, and circulating immune complexes after jejunal-ileal bypass surgery. *Ann. Intern. Med.* 86:576, 1977.

72. Pertschuk, L. P., Cook, A. W., Gupta, J. K., et al. Jejunal immunopathology in amyotrophic lateral sclerosis and multiple sclerosis. Identification of viral antigens by immunofluorescence. *Lancet* 1:1119, 1977.

73. Prasad, I., Broome, J. D., Pertschuk, L. P., et al. Recovery of Paramyxovirus from the jejunum of patients with multiple sclerosis. *Lancet* 1:1117, 1977.

74. Woyciechowska, J. L., Madden, D. L., and Sever, J. L. Absence of measles-virus antigen in jejunum of multiple-sclerosis patients. *Lancet* 2:1046, 1977.

75. Snider, R. L., Porter, J. M., and Eidemiller, L. R. Axillary-axillary artery bypass for the correction of subclavian artery occlusive disease. *Ann. Surg.* 180:888, 1974.

76. Fauci, A. S., and Wolff, S. M. Wegener's granulomatosis: studies in eighteen patients and a review of the literature. *Medicine (Baltimore)* 52:535, 1973.

77. Godman, G. C., and Churg, J. Wegener's granulomatosis: pathology and review of the literature. *Arch. Pathol.* 58:533, 1954.

78. Wolff, S. M., Fauci, A. S., Horn, R. G., et al. Wegener's granulomatosis. *Ann. Intern. Med.* 81:513, 1974.

79. Roback, S. A., Herdman, R. C., Hoyer, J., et al. Wegener's granulomatosis in a child. Observations on pathogenesis and treatment. *Am. J. Dis. Child.* 118:608, 1969.

80. Horn, R. G., Fauci, A. S., Rosenthal, A. S., et al. Renal biopsy pathology in Wegener's granulomatosis. *Am. J. Pathol.* 74:423, 1974.

81. Aldo, M. A., Benson, M. D., Comerford, F. R., et al. Treatment of Wegener's granulomatosis with immunosuppressive agents. Description of renal ultrastructure. *Arch. Intern. Med.* 126:298, 1970.

82. Howell, S. B., and Epstein, W. V. Circulating immunoglobulin complexes in Wegener's granulomatosis. *Am. J. Med.* 60:259, 1976.

83. McCoy, R. C. Ultrastructural alterations in the kidney of patients with sickle cell disease and the nephrotic syndrome. *Lab. Invest.* 21:85, 1969.

84. Schlitt, L. E., and Keitel, H. G. Renal manifestations of sickle cell disease: a review. *Am. J. Med. Sci.* 239:773, 1960.

85. Sweeney, M. J., Dobbins, W. T., and Etteldorf, J. N. Renal disease with elements of the nephrotic syndrome associated with sickle cell anemia. A report of 2 cases. *J. Pediatr.* 60:42, 1962.

86. Bennett, M. A., Heslop, R. W., and Meynell, M. J. Massive haematuria associated with sickle-cell trait. *Br. Med. J.* 1:677, 1967.

87. Elfenbein, I. B., Patchefsky, A., Schwartz, W., et al. Pathology of the glomerulus in sickle cell anemia with and without nephrotic syndrome. *Am. J. Pathol.* 77:357, 1974.

88. Strauss, J., Pardo, V., Koss, M. N., et al. Nephropathy associated with sickle cell anemia: an autologous immune complex nephritis. I. Studies on nature of glomerular-bound antibody and antigen identification in a patient with sickle cell disease and immune deposit glomerulonephritis. *Am. J. Med.* 58:382, 1975.

89. Ozawa, T., Mass, M. F., Guggenheim, S., et al. Autologous immune complex nephritis associated with sickle cell trait: diagnosis of the haemoglobinopathy after renal structural and immunological studies. *Br. Med. J.* 1:369, 1976.

90. Glassock, R. J., Edgington, T. S., Watson, J. I., et al. Autologous immune complex nephritis induced with renal tubular antigen. II. The pathogenetic mechanisms. *J. Exp. Med.* 127:573, 1968.

91. Edgington, T. S., Glassock, R. J., and Dixon, F. J. Autologous immune complex nephritis induced with renal tubular antigen. I. Identification and isolation of the pathogenetic antigen. *J. Exp. Med.* 127:555, 1968.

92. Naruse, T., Kitamura, K., Miyakawa, Y., et al. Deposition of renal tubular epithelial antigen along the glomerular capillary walls of patients with membranous glomerulonephritis. *J. Immunol.* 110:1163, 1973.

93. Sweeney, M. H., Dobbins, W. T., and Etteldorf, J. N. Renal disease with elements of the

nephrotic syndrome associated with sickle cell anemia. *J. Pediatr.* 60:42, 1962.

94. Barnett, H. L., and Bernstein, J. Clinical pathological conference. *J. Pediatr.* 73:936, 1968.

95. Berman, L. B., and Schreiner, G. E. Clinical and histologic spectrum of the nephrotic syndrome. *Am. J. Med.* 24:249, 1958.

96. Berman, L. B., and Tublin, I. The nephropathies of sickle-cell disease. *Arch. Intern. Med.* 103:602, 1959.

97. Miller, R. E., Hartley, M. W., Clark, E. C., et al. Sickle cell nephropathy. *Ala. J. Med. Sci.* 1:233, 1964.

98. Strom, T., Muehrcke, R. C., and Smith, R. D. Sickle cell anemia with the nephrotic syndrome and renal vein obstruction. *Arch. Intern. Med.* 129:104, 1972.

99. Tellem, M., Rubenstone, A. I., and Frumin, A. M. Renal failure and other unusual manifestations in sickle-cell trait. *Arch. Pathol.* 63:508, 1957.

100. Walker, B. R., Alexander, F., Birdsall, T. R., et al. Glomerular lesions in sickle cell nephropathy. *J.A.M.A.* 215:437, 1971.

101. Kimmelstiel, P. Vascular occlusion and ischemic infarction in sickle cell disease. *Am. J. Med. Sci.* 216:11, 1948.

102. Bernstein, J., and Whitten, C. F. A histologic appraisal of the kidney in sickle cell anemia. *Arch. Pathol.* 70:407, 1960.

103. Pitcock, J. A., Muirhead, E. E., Hatch, F. E., et al. Early renal changes in sickle cell anemia. *Arch. Pathol.* 90:403, 1970.

104. Arakawa, M., and Kimmelstiel, P. Circumferential mesangial interposition. *Lab. Invest.* 21:276, 1969.

105. Ellis, J. T. Glomerular lesions and the nephrotic syndrome in rabbits given saccharated iron oxide intravenously, with special reference to part played by intercapillary precipitates in pathogenesis of lesions. *J. Exp. Med.* 103:127, 1956.

106. Ellis, J. T. Glomerular lesions in rabbits with experimentally induced proteinuria as disclosed by electron microscopy. *Am. J. Pathol.* 34:559, 1958.

107. Grey, H. M., and Kohler, P. F. Cryoimmunoglobulins. *Semin. Hematol.* 10:87, 1973.

108. Levo, Y., Gorevic, P. D., Kassab, H. J., et al. Association between hepatitis B virus and essential mixed cryoglobulinemia. *N. Engl. J. Med.* 296:1501, 1977.

109. Meltzer, M., and Franklin, E. C. Cryoglobulinemia—a study of twenty-nine patients. I. IgG and IgM cryoglobulins and factors affecting cryoprecipitability. *Am. J. Med.* 40:828, 1966.

110. Meltzer, M., Franklin, E. C., Elias, K., et al. Cryoglobulinemia—a clinical and laboratory study. II. Cryoglobulins with rheumatoid factor activity. *Am. J. Med.* 40:837, 1966.

111. Barnett, E. V., Bluestone, R., Cracchiolo, A., III., et al. Cryoglobulinemia and disease. *Ann. Intern. Med.* 73:95, 1970.

112. Capra, J. D., Winchester, R. J., and Kunkel, H. G. Cold-reactive rheumatoid factors in infectious mononucleosis and other diseases. *Arthritis Rheum.* 12:67, 1969.

113. Wager, O., Räsänen, J. A., Hagman, A., et al. Mixed cryoimmunoglobulinaemia in infectious mononucleosis and cytomegalovirus mononucleosis. *Int. Arch. Allergy Appl. Immunol.* 34:345, 1968.

114. Kantor, G. L., Goldberg, L. S., Johnson, B. L., et al. Immunologic abnormalities induced by post-perfusion cytomegalovirus infection. *Ann. Intern. Med.* 73:553, 1970.

115. Bonomo, L., and Dammacco, F. Immune complex cryoglobulinemia in lepromatous leprosy—a pathogenetic approach to some clinical features of leprosy. *Clin. Exp. Immunol.* 9:175, 1971.

116. Lassus, A. Development of rheumatoid factor activity and cryoglobulins in primary and secondary syphilis. *Int. Arch. Allergy Appl. Immunol.* 36:515, 1969.

117. Lassus, A., Mustakallio, K. K., and Wager, O. Autoimmune serum factors and IgA elevation in lymphogranuloma venereum. *Ann. Clin. Res.* 2:51, 1970.

118. Lerner, A. B., Barnum, C. P., and Watson, C. J. Studies of cryoglobulins. II. The spontaneous precipitation of protein from serum at 5° C in various disease states. *Am. J. Med. Sci.* 214:416, 1947.

119. Feizi, T., and Gitlin, N. Immune-complex disease in the kidney associated with chronic hepatitis and cryoglobulinaemia. *Lancet* 2:873, 1969.

120. Golde, D., and Epstein, W. Mixed cryoglobulins and glomerulonephritis. *Ann. Intern. Med.* 69:1221, 1968.

121. Avasthi, P. S., Erickson, D. G., Williams, R. C., Jr., et al. Benign monoclonal gammaglobulinemia and glomerulonephritis. *Am. J. Med.* 62:324, 1977.

122. Goldberg, L. S., and Barnett, E. V. Essential cryoglobulinemia. Immunologic studies before and after penicillamine therapy. *Arch. Intern. Med.* 125:145, 1970.

123. The Research Sub-committee of the Empire Rheumatism Council. Gold therapy in rheumatoid arthritis: report of a multi-centre controlled trial. *Ann. Rheum. Dis.* 19:95, 1960.

124. Penneys, N. S., Eaglstein, W. H., Indgin,

S., et al. Gold sodium thiomalate treatment of pemphigus. *Arch. Dermatol.* 108:56, 1973.

125. Silverberg, D. S., Kidd, E. G., Shnitka, T. K., et al. Gold nephropathy: a clinical and pathologic study. *Arthritis Rheum.* 13:812, 1970.

126. Williams, R. C. Jr. Treatment. In *Rheumatoid Arthritis as a Systemic Disease,* p. 242 W. B. Saunders Co., Philadelphia, 1974.

127. Ehrenreich, T., and Churg, J. Pathology of membranous nephropathy. In S. C. Sommers, ed., *Pathology Annual,* p. 145. Appleton-Century-Crofts, New York, 1968.

128. Törnroth, T., and Skrifvars, B. Gold nephropathy: prototype of membranous glomerulonephritis. *Am. J. Pathol.* 75:573, 1974.

129. Palosuo, T., Provost, T. T., and Milgrom, F. Gold nephropathy: serologic data suggesting an immune complex disease. *Clin. Exp. Immunol.* 25:311, 1976.

130. Lipsky, P. E., and Ziff, M. Inhibition of antigen-and mitogen-induced human lymphocyte proliferation by gold compounds. *J. Clin. Invest.* 59:455, 1977.

131. Editorial. Vinyl chloride, P.V.C., and cancer. *Lancet* 1:1323, 1974.

132. Editorial. Vinyl chloride and cancer. *Br. Med. J.* 1:590, 1974.

133. Cordier, J. M., Fievez, C., Lefèvre, M. J., et al. Acroostéolyse et lésions cutanées associés deux ouvriers affectés au nettoyage d'autoclaves. *Cah. Med. Travail* 4:3, 1966.

134. Harris, D. K., and Adams, W. G. F. Acro-osteolysis occurring in men engaged in the polymerization of vinyl chloride. *Br. Med. J.* 3:712, 1967.

135. Markowitz, S. S., McDonald, C. J., Fethiere, W., et al. Occupational acro-osteolysis *Arch Dermatol.* 106:219, 1972.

136. Stewart, J. D., Williams, D. M. J., and McLachlan, M. S. F. Acro-osteolysis in a poly-vinyl chloride worker with atypical industrial history. *J. Soc. Occup. Med.* 25:103, 1975.

137. Ward, A. M., Udnoon, S., Watkins, J., et al. Immunological mechanisms in the pathogenesis of vinyl chloride disease. *Br. Med. J.* 1:936, 1976.

138. Ward, A. M. Immune complex disease in vinyl chloride workers. *J. Clin. Pathol.* 29:83, 1976.

139. Lange, C. E., Jühe, S., Stein, G., et al. Die sogenannte Vinylchlorid-Krankheiteine berufsbedingte Systemsklerose. *Int. Arch. Arbeitsmed.* p. 32, 1974.

140. Veltman, G., Lange, C. E., Jühe, S., et al. Clinical manifestations and course of vinyl chloride disease. *Ann. N.Y. Acad. Sci.* 246:6, 1975.

141. Hefner, R. E., Jr., Watanabe, P. G., and Gehring, P. J. Preliminary studies of the fate of inhaled vinyl chloride monomer in rats. *Ann. N.Y. Acad. Sci.* 246:135, 1975.

142. Williamson, K. S. Vinyl chloride: review of animal studies. *Proc. R. Soc. Med.* 69:281, 1976.

143. Subcommittee on the National Halothane Study of the Committee on Anesthesia, National Academy of Sciences, National Research Council. Summary of the national halothane study: possible association between halothane anesthesia and postoperative hepatic necrosis. *J.A.M.A.* 197:775, 1966.

144. Inman, W. H. W., and Mushin, W. M. Jaundice after repeated exposure to halothane: an analysis of Reports to the Committee on Safety of Medicines. *Br. Med. J.* 1:5, 1974.

145. Williams, B. D., White, N., Amlot, P. L., et al. Circulating immune complexes after repeated halothane anaesthesia. *Br. Med. J.* 2:159, 1977.

146. Walton, B., Simpson, B. R., Strunin, L., et al. Unexplained hepatitis following halothane. *Br. Med. J.* 1:1171, 1976.

147. Böttiger, L. E., Dalén, H., and Hallén, B. Halothane-induced liver damage: an analysis of the material reported to the Swedish Adverse Drug Reaction Committee, 1966–1973. *Acta Anaesthesiol. Scand.* 20:40, 1976.

148. Paronetto, F., and Popper, H. Lymphocyte stimulation induced by halothane in patients with hepatitis following exposure to halothane. *N. Engl. J. Med.* 283:277, 1970.

149. Walton, B., Dumonde, D. C., Williams, C., et al. Lymphocyte transformation. Absence of increased responses in alleged halothane jaundice. *J.A.M.A.* 225:494, 1973.

150. Moult, P. J. A., Adjukiewicz, A. B., Gaylarde, P. M., et al. Lymphocyte transformation in halothane-related hepatitis. *Br. Med. J.* 2:69, 1975.

151. Harrington, W. J., Minnich, V., Hollingsworth, J. W., et al. Demonstration of a thrombocytopenic factor in the blood of patients with thrombocytopenic purpura. *J. Lab. Clin. Med.* 38:1, 1951.

152. Shulman, N. R., Marder, V. J., and Weinrach, R. S. Similarities between known anti-platelet antibodies and the factor responsible for thrombocytopenia in idiopathic purpura. Physiologic, serologic, and isotopic studies. *Ann. N.Y. Acad. Sci.* 124:499, 1965.

153. Karpatkin, S., and Siskind, G. W. *In vitro* detection of platelet antibody in patients with idiopathic thrombocytopenic purpura and systemic lupus erythematosus. *Blood* 33:795, 1969.

154. Dixon, R. H., and Rosse, W. F. Platelet antibody in autoimmune thrombocytopenia. *Br. J. Haematol.* 31:129, 1975.

155. Osler, A. G., and Siraganian, R. P. Immunologic mechanisms of platelet damage. *Prog. Allergy* 16:450, 1972.

156. Israels, E. D., Nisli, G., Paraskevas, F., et al. Platelet Fc receptor as a mechanism for Ag-Ab complex-induced platelet injury. *Thromb. Diath. Haemorrh.* 29:434, 1973.

157. Karpatkin, S., Schur, P. H., Strick, N., et al. Heavy chain subclass of human anti-platelet antibodies. *Clin. Immunol. Immunopathol.* 2:1, 1973.

158. Palosuo, T., and Leikola, J. Platelet aggregation by isolated and aggregated human IgG. *Clin. Exp. Immunol.* 20:371, 1975.

159. Lurhuma, A. Z., Riccomi, H., and Masson, P. L. The occurrence of circulating immune complexes and viral antigens in idiopathic thrombocytopenic purpura. *Clin. Exp. Immunol.* 28:49, 1977.

160. Myllylä, G., Vaheri, A., Vesikari, T., et al. Interaction between human blood platelets, viruses and antibodies. IV. Post-rubella thrombocytopenic purpura and platelet aggregation by rubella antigen-antibody interaction. *Clin. Exp. Immunol.* 4:323, 1969.

161. Miescher, P., and Miescher, A. Die Sedormid-Anaphylaxie. *Schweiz. Med. Wochenschr.* 82:1279, 1952.

162. Shulman, N. R. A mechanism of cell destruction in individuals sensitized to foreign antigens and its implications in autoimmunity. *Ann. Intern. Med.* 60:506, 1964.

163. Hoffman, R., Zanjani, E. D., Vila, J., et al. Diamond-Blackfan syndrome: lymphocyte-mediated suppression of erythropoiesis. *Science* 193:899, 1976.

164. Kagan, W. A., Ascensão, J.A., Pahwa, R. N., et al. Aplastic anemia: presence in human bone marrow of cells that suppress myelopoiesis. *Proc. Natl. Acad. Sci. USA* 73:2890, 1976.

165. Abdou, N. I., NaPombejara, C., Balentine, L., et al. Suppressor cell-mediated neutropenia in Felty's syndrome. *J. Clin. Invest.* 61:738, 1978.

166. Eales, H. Primary retinal haemorrhage in young men. *Birmingham Med. Rev.* 3:262, 1880.

167. Lyle, T. K., and Wybar, K. Retinal vasculitis. *Br. J. Ophthalmol.* 45:778, 1961.

168. Hart, C. D., Sanders, M. D., and Miller, S. J. H. Benign retinal vasculitis. Clinical and fluorescein angiographic study. *Br. J. Ophthalmol.* 55:721, 1971.

169. deMuro, P., and Focosi, M. Vascular allergy: experimental studies on allergic thrombosis of the retinal veins. *J. Allergy* 22:114, 1951.

170. Levine, R. A., and Ward, P. A. Experimental acute immunologic ocular vasculitis. *Am. J. Ophthalmol.* 69:1023, 1970.

171. Andrews, B. S., McIntosh, J., Petts, V., et al. Circulating immune complexes in retinal vasculitis. *Clin. Exp. Immunol.* 29:23, 1977.

172. Howes, E. L., Jr., and McKay, D. G. Circulating immune complexes. Effects on ocular vascular permeability in the rabbit. *Arch. Ophthalmol.* 93:365, 1975.

173. Buckley, C. E., III., and Dorsey, F. C. A comparison of serum immunoglobulin concentrations in sarcoidosis and tuberculosis. *Ann. Intern. Med.* 72:37, 1970.

174. Jones, J. V. Development of sensitivity to dinitrochlorobenzene in patients with sarcoidosis. *Clin. Exp. Immunol.* 2:477, 1967.

175. Oreskes, I., and Siltzbach, L. E. Changes in rheumatoid factor activity during the course of sarcoidosis. *Am. J. Med.* 44:60, 1968.

176. Mellors, R. C., Ortega, L. G., Noyes, W. F., et al. Further pathogenetic studies of diseases of unknown etiology, with particular reference to disseminated lupus erythematosus and Boeck's sarcoid. *Am. J. Pathol.* 33:613, 1957.

177. Wanstrup, J., and Elling, P. Immunohistochemistry of sarcoidosis. *Acta Pathol. Microbiol. Scand.* 73:37, 1968.

178. Ghose, T., Landrigan, P., and Asif, A. Localization of immunoglobulin and complement in pulmonary sarcoid granulomas. *Chest* 66:264, 1974.

179. Hedfors, E., and Norberg, R. Evidence for circulating immune complexes in sarcoidosis. *Clin. Exp. Immunol.* 16:493, 1974.

180. Verrier-Jones, J., Cumming, R. H., Asplin, C. M., et al. Circulating immune complexes in erythema nodosum and early sarcoidosis. *Lancet* 1:153, 1976.

181. Najarian, J. S., and Foker, J. E. The expression of immunity: the efferent arc. In J. S. Najarian and R. L. Simmons, eds., *Transplantation*, p. 94. Lea & Febiger, Philadelphia, 1972.

182. Porter, K. A., Andres, G. A., Calder, M. W., et al. Human renal transplants. II. Immunofluorescent and immunoferritin studies. *Lab. Invest.* 18:159, 1968.

183. McKenzie, I. F. C., and Whittingham, S. Deposits of immunoglobulin and fibrin in human allografted kidneys. *Lancet* 2:1313, 1968.

184. Rosenau, W., Lee, J. C., and Najarian, J. S. A light, fluorescence, and electron microscopic study of functioning human renal transplants. *Surg. Gynec. Obstet.* 128:62, 1969.

185. Ooi, Y. M., Ooi, B. S., Vallota, E. H., et al. Circulating immune complexes after renal transplantation. Correlation of increased ^{125}I-C1q binding activity with acute rejection characterized by fi-

brin deposition in the kidney. *J. Clin. Invest.* 60:611, 1977.

186. Porter, K. A. Renal transplantation. In R. H. Heptinstall, ed., *Pathology of the Kidney,* ed. 2, p. 977. Little, Brown and Co., Boston, 1974.

187. Ratnoff, O. D. Some relationships among hemostasis, fibrinolytic phenomena, immunity, and the inflammatory response. *Adv. Immunol.* 10:145, 1969.

188. Lee, L. Antigen-antibody reaction in the pathogenesis of bilateral renal cortical necrosis. *J. Exp. Med.* 117:365, 1963.

CHAPTER 11

Immune Complexes and the Skin

In no other major organ system are the obvious physical effects of immune-complex injury more apparent to the attending physician than in the skin. Skin disorders have been alluded to in previous sections of this book, including the vasculitic lesions of disseminated gonococcal infection or the erythema nodosum lesions associated with lepromatous leprosy or active inflammatory bowel disease. In some conditions such as hepatitis B associated vasculitis or disseminated lupus erythematosus, the nature of the immune-complex–related phenomena are well established. However in other disease states such as erythema nodosum or erythema multiforme, considerable information is lacking about why complexes localize to skin and how they are directly involved in basic pathogenesis.

The skin-irritating effects of immune complexes were first noted in 1924 by Opie (1), who studied the inflammatory reactions of immune animals to cutaneous antigen challenge. In 1958 Ishizaka and Campbell (2) showed that antigen-antibody complexes injected into skin produced a marked local increase in capillary permeability. These reactions were attributed to effects of soluble antigen-antibody complexes formed at equivalence and in antigen excess using rabbit antibodies and guinea pigs as experimental animals. Later work by Spector and Heesom (3) showed that injections of immune complexes formed at equivalence were also capable of producing granuloma formation. In clinical medicine there are many striking examples of antigen diffusing across microcapillary walls and meeting reactive antibody. This was recognized 40 years ago in a report by Kohn and co-workers (4) of what was termed "anaphylactic gangrene" following administration of horse serum to children. Arthus reactions are occasionally observed in modern clinical practice when patients with precipitating antibody are skin-tested with various antigens (5). Thus, there is abundant experimental and clinical evidence to suggest that the skin may be an organ which by its very physical properties and distribution of blood supply is unusually susceptible to microvascular immune-complex injury.

Cutaneous lesions have been recognized periodically as reflecting a variety of complex and sometimes inscrutable internal metabolic derangements. Thus the presence of acanthosis nigricans or sudden onset of heliotrope dermatomyositis may represent harbingers of occult carcinomas of the bowel, lung, breast, or ovary (6–8). In a somewhat different vein, many skin disorders considered diseases of unknown etiology for years may involve phenomena mediated by immune-complex deposition. The recent availability of precise immunofluorescent and electron microscopic techniques has proven very informative. However, initial experience with these techniques indicates that in some skin disorders it is very difficult to discern what results from primary immune-complex deposition as an initial event and what represent epiphenomena of immunoglobulin and/or complement component adherence occurring in conjunction with the natural inflammatory response to a completely distinct and nonimmune-complex–related mechanism. One of the technical problems in many studies involving analysis of the significance of apparent immune deposits within the skin relates to the presence in a variety of lesions of what may or may not be "background" immunofluorescence for Ig and/or complement components. It is possible that like the normally occurring C3b receptor located in the renal glomerulus, cutaneous structures show similar receptors for activated C3 or Fc portions of immunoglobulins. Very few data are currently available regarding this point and considerably more direct experimental work is needed.

Erythema Multiforme

Erythema multiforme represents a syndrome of widespread erythema and irritation that may be precipitated by a broad variety of inciting agents including drugs, external allergens, and frequently viral infections. The skin lesions themselves are characteristic and may become extremely widespread in severe cases. This condition has long been viewed by dermatologists as a probable allergic or immunologically mediated phenomenon. Recent studies by Kazmierowski and Wuepper (9) have shown that prospective study of 597 skin-biopsy specimens for immunofluorescent localization of Ig or C3 in microvasculature of cutaneous structures included a significant proportion (16 percent) with erythema multiforme. Specific findings in 17 erythema multiforme lesions indicated deposition of C3 alone or in conjunction with IgM in the small vessels of the papillary dermis. Representative findings are shown in Figure 11-1A. *Herpesvirus hominis* (HSV) was commonly implicated among the patients included in this series, while the remainder showed no readily definable inciting agent. These findings suggest that the primary disorder may be mediated by deposition of immune reactants in cutaneous microvasculature. Identification of presence of specific herpes anti-gens within such deposits will provide proof of a direct cause-and-effect relationship.

One of the earliest descriptions of the clinical picture of the disorder is attributed to Osler who recorded the findings observed in 11 patients in 1895 (10). However, as later pointed out by Baer (11), many of Osler's cases probably would not fit the usual clinical definition of the disease today, as he included patients with Henoch-Schönlein purpura and possibly subjects with gonococcal sepsis. The skin manifestations of erythema multiforme themselves may show a number of forms including "target" or "iris"-shaped eruptions presenting in papular, vesiculobullous, or bullous distribution (Figure 11-1B). Histological changes include necrosis of keratinocytes and vacuolar alteration with lymphocytic and histiocytic infiltrates at dermal-epidermal junctions and around blood vessels of the superficial dermal plexus (12–14). The actual skin changes, including toxic killing of epidermal cells, edema, and lymphoid inflammatory infiltrates, are compatible with local immune-complex–mediated injury. Participation of cell-mediated reactivity is suggested in an interesting report by Krueger and co-workers (15), who found macrophage aggregating factor in serum from a group of patients with erythema multiforme along with the presence of a serum factor that produced rapid appearance of erythema when injected in guinea pig skin. These findings raised the question of whether local skin inflammatory reactions might somehow also be associated with a significant outpouring of products of activated lymphocytes augmenting the inflammatory process.

Erythema multiforme may also be associated with extensive mucous membrane lesions accompanied by hemorrhagic bullae and involvement of mouth, eyes, genitalia, and anal mucous surfaces. When such lesions are present, they are grouped together as the Stevens-Johnson syndrome. This clinical picture is often accompanied by extreme toxicity, prostration, or high fever; it was associated with significant mortality (16, 17), particularly before treatment with systemic corticosteroid became widely available.

Various precipitating causes and types of

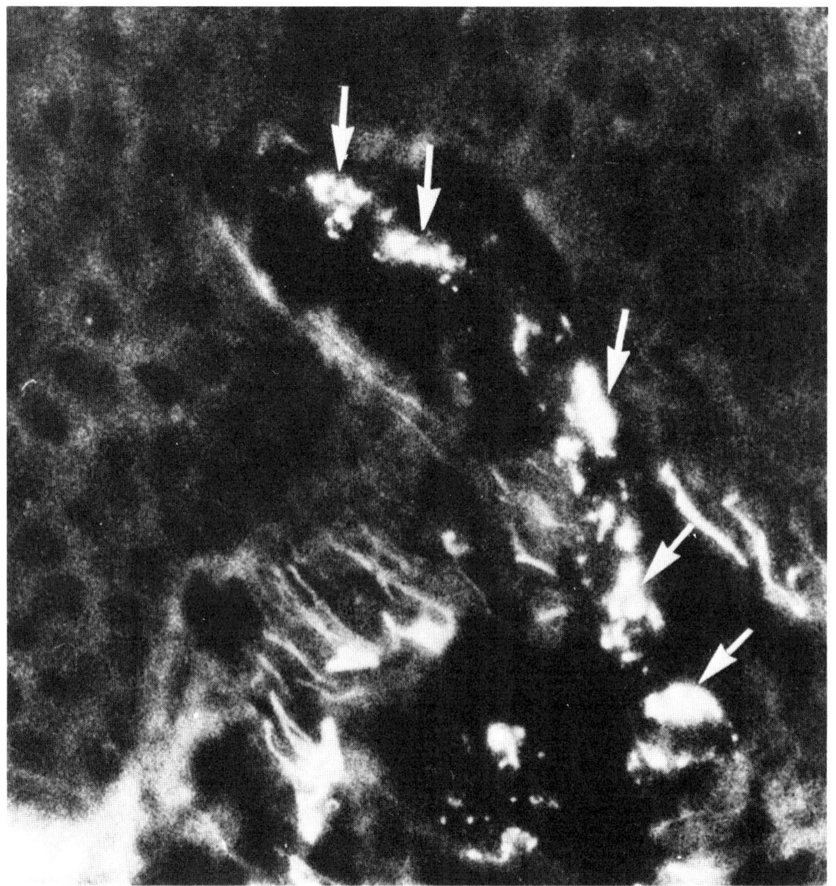

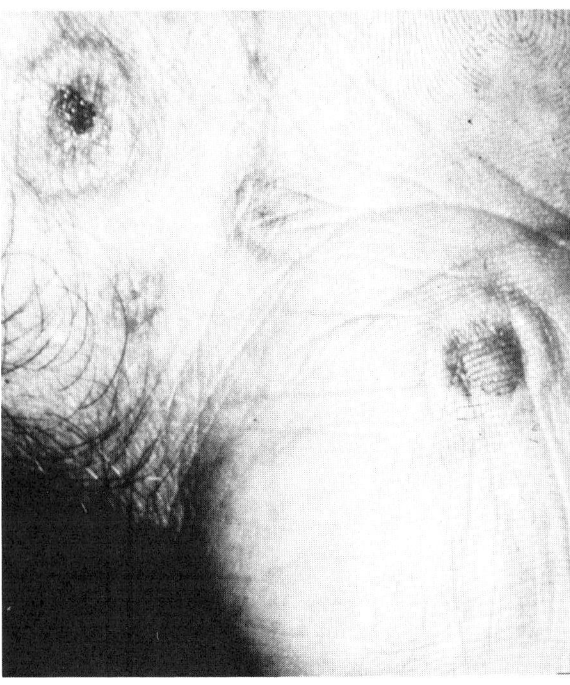

Figure 11-1 *A*, deposits of IgM in dermal vessels associated with erythema multiforme. *B*, typical iris-like lesions in the skin associated with erythema multiforme. (Photographs courtesy of John Kazmierowski, University of Oregon Medical Center, Portland.)

drug or chemical exposure associated with erythema multiforme (18) are shown in Table 11-1. In addition, erythema multiforme has been noted in conjunction with the connective-tissue diseases, malignancy, pregnancy, various foods, Wegener's granulomatosis, or after exposure to physical stimuli such as radiation therapy or sun exposure. Whether these latter conditions are primary or merely serve to trigger latent infections such as herpes has not been clarified. A growing awareness of the possible relation of erythema multiforme to herpetic infections is reflected in several recent studies (9, 14, 19, 20). Since dormant herpes infection appears to persist for extremely long periods of time in many patients, it may possibly be involved in the generation of erythema multiforme lesions in a number of instances where some other acute event such as meningitis, a streptococcal infection, or severe sunburn suddenly alters the host immune balance.

The findings of Kazmierowski and Wuepper (9) of immunofluorescent evidence of a microvascular injury involving some type of immune complex are the first direct indication that such a process may be involved in the evolution of the generalized syndrome. In this context it is important to mention a recent study by Braverman and Yen (21) directed at sequential events involved in cutaneous immune-complex deposition in a group of patients with cutaneous vasculitis. Histamine-induced wheals were produced in uninvolved skin of patients known to have concurrent active angiitis. Electron microscopic and immunofluorescent studies of biopsies taken from induced wheal tissues showed evidence of immune complexes in vessel walls. Neutrophils were recorded in various stages of disintegration and lysosomal enzyme release. Thus, induction of histamine-modulated local inflammation in uninvolved skin was capable of simulating histological and immunofluorescent findings present in naturally occurring angiitis. Electron microscopic and immunofluorescent studies of normal nonmanipulated or histamine-injected skin also revealed electron-dense deposits and IgG deposition, indicating that vascular immune-complex deposition was occurring *before* any local cellular inflammatory infiltrate was mobilized. If a similar process is taking place in the initial stages of erythema multiforme, examination of other possible local modulating factors is certainly indicated.

Table 11-1 Infections and compounds implicated in the cause of erythema multiforme.

Viral	Herpes simplex, herpes zoster, influenza A, lymphogranuloma venereum, psittacosis, ornithosis, variola vaccinia, milkers' nodules, orf, mumps, poliomyelitis, ECHO virus, Coxsackie virus, adenoviruses, infectious mononucleosis
Fungal	Histoplasmosis, coccidioidomycosis
Bacterial	Hemolytic streptococcus, diphtheria, typhoid, syphilis, meningococcus, pseudomonas, tuberculosis, tularemia, BCG vaccine, glanders, brucellosis, erysipeloid, *Vibrio parahemolyticus*
Mycoplasmal	Mycoplasma pneumonia
Parasitic	Malaria, *Trichomonas*, ankylostomiasis
Drugs, chemicals, and allergens	Penicillins, tetracyclines, sulfonamides, phenylbutazone, chlorpropamide, tolbutamide, acetylsalicylic acid, nitrogen mustard, phenolphthalein, barbiturates, arsenic, bromides, iodides, antipyrine, dilantin, gold, hydralazine, mercurials, 9-bromofluorene, poison ivy, primula allergen

Mucocutaneous Lymph-Node Syndrome

During the past few years observers in Japan have recorded the clinical picture of a fascinating newly recognized disease called mucocutaneous lymph-node syndrome (22). Generally the illness is seen in infants and young children and is characterized by initial cervical lymph-node swelling followed by a localized or extensive erythematous rash that frequently closely resembles erythema multiforme. However, several clinical features serve to distinguish this disorder from erythema multiforme. The entire clinical picture suggests an infectious etiology; a substantial proportion of patients show cardiac involvement with evidence of focal myocarditis or in some instances a clinical picture resembling infantile periarteritis nodosa (23). As yet, no extensive information is available concerning immunofluorescent findings in the skin or other vessels involved in this disease.

Immune-Complex Mechanisms in Erythema Multiforme

Two patients studied by Safai and co-workers (24) have provided additional insight into mechanisms related to the pathogenesis of erythema multiforme. Determination of complement components C1q, C2, C3, and C4 in blister fluid showed marked reduction. Moreover, cleavage of more than 90 percent of C3, C4, and properdin factor B was observed. Using a concurrent ^{125}I-labeled C1q deviation test, elevated levels of immune complexes were detected in erythema multiforme blister fluids, but not in simultaneously studied serum. Quantitative levels of IgG were markedly elevated both in serum and blister fluid. No evidence for in vivo fixation of C3 or IgG to skin vessels was found by immunofluorescence. Precise timing of such biopsies may, however, be critical if immune deposits are to be recognized by this technique. These results support the concept of an important role for immune complexes in the pathogenesis of erythema multiforme. The direct immunofluorescent studies presented by Kazmierowski and Wuepper (9) together with the demonstration of detectable immune complexes within actual blister fluid from involved lesions and a complement profile consistent with conventional pathway activation represent strong support for immune-complex involvement in genesis of the primary skin lesions.

There are several other observations implicating the importance of immune mechanisms in erythema multiforme. As noted above, the disorder is seen occasionally in subjects with connective-tissue disease. Two patients have now been reported who showed erythema multiforme in association with both hypocomplementemia and a lupus-like syndrome (25, 26). Marked diminution of serum complement activity was associated with C1q precipitins of low-molecular-weight type. These latter findings are difficult to fit with immune-complex deposition, since C1q-reacting materials representing soluble immune complexes should presumably be of intermediate or high molecular weight. However, it is possible that profound hypocomplementemia may in some way also predispose to other immune-complex–mediated syndromes—for example, erythema multiforme.

Erythema Nodosum

Erythema nodosum, like erythema multiforme, represents a clinical syndrome associated with a wide variety of different infectious and poorly understood conditions, most of which are suspected of arising on the basis of immunologic derangements. Erythema nodosum can be described as an immunologically reactive inflammatory syndrome involving the small blood vessels of subcutaneous tissue and dermis and producing crops of red nodules of relatively short duration. The clinical diagnosis is based mainly on the sudden appearance of the typical nodular lesions. Characteristic lesions are shown in Figure 11-2. A partial listing of presumed causes or associations noted with this condition is given in Table 11-2. Previous studies of large series of these patients have implicated tuberculosis as a cause in Europe and streptococcal infection or drug exposure as most common causes in the eastern United States (27–30). More recently *Yersinia enterocolitica* has been increasingly noted in association with the disorder in Scandinavia and Europe

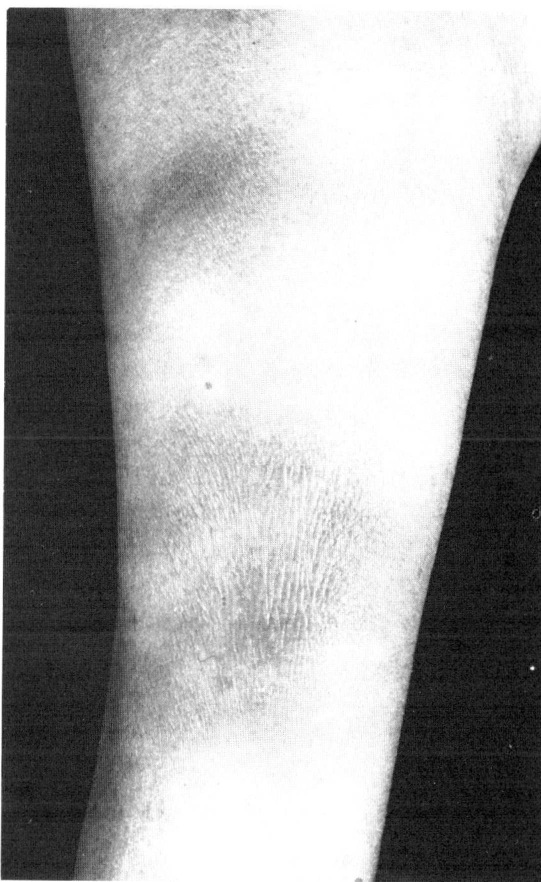

Figure 11-2 Typical erythema nodosum lesions located on pretibial regions. The lesions often resemble bruises at later stages. (Photograph courtesy of St. John's Hospital for Diseases of the Skin, London.)

(31); contraceptive medications have also been recognized as significant precipitating agents. In certain endemic areas of the southwestern United States, coccidioidomycosis probably bears the most common association (32). Although erythema nodosum is recognized as a complication occurring in association with inflammatory bowel disease, its prevalence in this latter condition is rare (33). It also occurs occasionally in conjunction with malignant states such as leukemia (34); however, the latter association may be difficult to differentiate from primary leukemic skin involvement.

Histological Picture

The major histological features of erythema nodosum include a major vasculitis usually involving veins with phlebitis characterized by lymphocytic and neutrophilic infiltrates and local hemorrhage (35). Later the perivenular areas of inflammation may progress to subacute or chronic granuloma formation. The predominant venous reaction in this condition was stressed by Löfgren and Wahlgren (36) in early descriptions of the disease. Other histological features are septal inflammation in connective tissue dividing subcutaneous fat lobules and both an acute and a later chronic panniculitis in these areas. The lymphocytic infiltrates and the persistence of histological changes for weeks or months in the more chronic lesions suggest a process more in keeping with cell-mediated than with humoral immunity.

Currently controversy exists on whether erythema nodosum lesions per se represent tissue-directed effects of immune complexes. Much of this controversy centers around the attention focused on leprosy and the active le-

Table 11-2 Presumptive causes or associated conditions noted in erythema nodosum.

Infections	Tuberculosis, leprosy, coccidioidomycosis, histoplasmosis, streptococci, lymphogranuloma venereum, *Yersinia enterocolitica*, psittacosis, toxoplasmosis, leptospirosis, brucellosis
Diseases of unknown cause	Sarcoidosis, ulcerative colitis, regional ileitis
Drugs	Penicillins, sulfonamides, broad spectrum antibiotics, contraceptive drugs
Malignancy	Leukemia

sions of the clinical phenomenon termed erythema nodosum leprosum (ENL). As can be seen from an examination of Table 11-2, there are a number of clinical conditions beside leprosy that might be examined in parallel for evidence of immune-complex phenomena. For various reasons, immunologic studies of erythema nodosum during the last 10 years have focused on the lesions and clinical association of erythema nodosum in active lepromatous leprosy. This is unfortunate, since the choice of this clinical condition is fraught with other complex and complicated factors making basic underlying mechanisms difficult to ascertain. Thus the clinical phenomena of ENL suggest that a generalized systemic reaction is occurring concurrently with manifestations of the pretibial nodose lesions. Patients with ENL often show impressive signs of generalized systemic toxicity such as chills, fever, malaise, arthralgias, pain over involved nerves, and a pronounced leukocytosis together with fall in hematocrit. Often the nodose skin lesions are extremely tender and, as pointed out by Rea and Levan (37), patients may show joint swelling or tenderness and testicular and nerve trunk tenderness. Examination of ENL biopsy material shows an impressive infiltrate of polymorphonuclear granuloma formation mixed with masses of activated foamy histiocytes or fixed tissue macrophages. Clinical testing of such patients during these systemic reactions fails to show a consistent diminution in cell-mediated immune functions (37). Participation of immune complexes in tissue lesions of ENL was first reported by Waters and colleagues (38) who described deposits of Ig and complement in vessel walls from biopsy material of acute lesions. Later material detectable in serum by precipitating reactions with C1q was reported by several groups (39–41). Whether or not these precipitin reactions were not caused by bacterial polysaccharides or free-DNA released during cellular injury was explored by several of these groups. DNase digestion of serum failed to abolish C1q reactivity in one study (41). Our own studies failed to show a high correlation between positive findings in C1q or Raji-cell tests and presence of ENL in a group of patients from Ethiopia

with various clinical forms of leprosy (42). Other groups (37) have failed to confirm fixation of IgG and C3 in vessels during ENL episodes, and a recent report (43) indicates immunofluorescence localization of C3 without evidence of concurrent IgG or other immunoglobulin in a series of patients studied for IgG H-chain subclass fixation of immune reactants. Some of these discrepancies may relate to the stages at which tissues or sera are examined. At present it would seem best to reserve final judgment on the basic pathological process occurring in ENL. Other forms of disease associated with erythema nodosum such as coccidioidomycosis, histoplasmosis, or drug sensitization may indeed provide a more definitive answer to some of these questions. In ENL the clinical situation itself is complicated by the presence of extreme hypergammaglobulinemia in some cases and presence of many serum autoantibodies including anti-DNA, rheumatoid factors, and anti–smooth-muscle antibodies (44).

Reichlin and co-workers (45) examined concentration and molecular profile of euglobulins present in sera of patients with ENL reactions. Elevation of euglobulin IgG was often noted in these sera, but analytic ultracentrifuge examination failed to show any evidence for polymeric IgG or IgG-IgG complexes in the same samples; euglobulin IgG appeared to sediment primarily in 7S fractions in this study. These findings in themselves do not support the occurrence of large quantities of intermediate IgG-IgG (11 to 17S) complexes in the serum of such patients.

It seems likely that local tissue fixation of immune complexes plays some role in the pathogenesis of the ENL lesions. Some evidence has been presented that appears to support the concept that ENL reactions as a clinical phenomenon may not become frequent until almost all leprosy bacilli are nonviable, as judged by the morphological index (46). This has recently been questioned by Rea and Levan (37) and further direct observations may be necessary to settle the question. Direct examination of ENL lesions often reveals histological elements denoting Arthus reactions and neutrophilic infiltration of degenerating dermis (47).

If leprosy bacteria are mostly nonviable at the time of ENL reactions, the immune complexes directly involved may be represented by autologous cytoplasmic antigens concurrently released from damaged or dying cells.

Erythema nodosum occurs in association with sarcoidosis; like lepromatous leprosy sarcoid is a disorder characterized by a number of features suggesting hyperreactivity of the immune response. Many patients show moderate or extreme levels of hypergammaglobulinemia. In addition, serum from a considerable proportion of these patients shows presence of rheumatoid factors particularly during active phases of the disease (48, 49). Deposits of immunoglobulin and complement have been noted by immunofluorescence in granulomatous lesions of lymph nodes (50, 51) or sarcoid lung-biopsy samples (52). Several reports have appeared that support the presence of circulating immune complexes during active sarcoidosis and erythema nodosum. A study by Hedfors and Norberg (53) showed presence of complexes detected by the sensitive platelet agglutination technique in 4 of 5 patients with erythema nodosum and bilateral hilar adenopathy. Furthermore, a prospective study by Verrier-Jones and co-workers (54) showed presumed evidence of circulating complexes during acute episodes of erythema nodosum in 8 of 16 cases by assay of serum anticomplementary activity. Parallel studies of total hemolytic complement showed low CH 50 in half of the 8 patients positive in the anticomplementary activity test. Of interest were the findings of detectable breakdown products of C3 in 14 of 18 instances and positive platelet aggregation in 6 of 10 tested. Also of note was the finding of C1q precipitins in only 2 cases in this study. The finding of C3 activation products in the face of normal total hemolytic complement in some of these patients is difficult to interpret without precise complement-component turnover data. Molecular size estimates of the immune complexes indicated that as a rule they were larger than 19S. No direct analysis of concurrent histological immunofluorescent events were presented. It is particularly unclear why the lesions of erythema nodosum develop in the specific sites in which they are found. As yet no evidence has demonstrated that pretibial or ulnar sites are endowed with local properties that make them unduly susceptible to immune-complex trapping. Extensor surfaces of arms and elbows seem unusually predisposed as sites for the development of rheumatoid nodules. This sort of anatomical localization has been attributed to the minor trauma that such sites generally experience in the course of normal daily activities. The local factors predisposing to distribution and actual occurrence of erythema nodosum lesions require further study.

Immune Complexes in the Skin in Systemic Lupus Erythematosus

Systemic lupus erythematosus (SLE) was discussed in detail in Chapter 7, which dealt with the connective-tissue disorders. Evolution of knowledge concerning the relationships between clinical skin lesions and the patient's general physical condition provides direct insight into possible important factors that influence skin localization of immune complexes in various other disease states. The association between SLE and important clinical manifestations mediated by immune-complex deposition is long recognized. The most intensively studied area in this regard has been SLE nephropathy where strong evidence was obtained that immune complexes containing DNA and anti-DNA represent one of the most important factors in the production of renal damage. While clinicians were studying renal tissue, other groups began examining skin activity. Typical cutaneous SLE involvement is shown in Figure 11-3. A number of studies provided evidence for immunoglobulin and complement deposition at the basement membrane area of the skin in a characteristic linear or band-like pattern (55–58). The exact significance of these findings was not initially apparent; it seemed possible at the time that the antibody fixing in the basal membranes of the skin might indeed represent reaction with specific local cutaneous material. The well-known tendency for SLE dermatitis to flare in some patients after sun exposure was attributed to intrinsic alterations of local antigens by ultra-

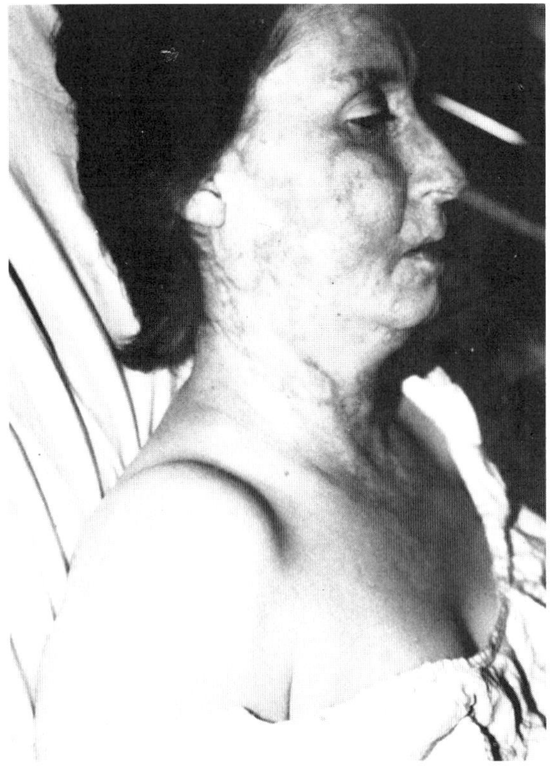

Figure 11-3 Cutaneous lesions of disseminated SLE, showing both skin atrophy and concomitant erythema.

violet light exposure. Initially the significance of binding of immunoglobulins and complement to the area of the dermal-epidermal junction was felt by some workers to represent specific antibody to the cutaneous basement membrane, since binding could be blocked by prior incubation with bullous pemphigoid antibody (59). Localization of properdin and IgG, IgM, C3, and C4 was reported by Rothfield and co-workers (60) in skin biopsies obtained from SLE lesions, and a clinical association between renal and dermal deposits was suggested. Subsequent studies by Landry and Sams (61) included immunofluorescence and elution of both skin lesions and apparently normal skin. Acid eluates from both involved and normal-appearing SLE skin biopsies contained antinuclear antibody fixing complement. The immunofluorescent appearance of SLE skin again showed immunoglobulin and complement along the basement membrane zone sep-

arating dermis from epidermis (Figure 11-4). Skin eluates contained antibody showing strong affinity for the basement membrane areas of epithelial tissue (Figure 11-5). The immunofluorescent antinuclear antibody pattern of skin eluates varied from peripheral to speckled and persisted after treatment of substrate tissues with RNase. Although pemphigoid antibody appeared to block basement membrane staining by serum or skin eluates, slightly different specificity was suggested by parallel titration and blocking studies. Similar results were presented by others (62). The data indicating blocking after prior incubation with pemphigoid sera are difficult to interpret; the sera may have masked other structures, such as receptors for immune complexes, thereby blocking dermal-epidermal staining by a slightly different mechanism than merely occupying the same antigens within these same tissues.

As these studies were extended by a number of different groups (55), a correlation appeared between presence of dermal-epidermal junction immunoglobulin deposits and activity of the underlying SLE process as assessed by serum complement activity and presence of renal disease. In one study immunoglobulins of the class found in skin were detected in glomeruli of the same patients examined concurrently by renal biopsy (63). This relationship, however, was not confirmed in other studies examining the same question (64, 65). It became apparent that a natural variation in the degree of immunoglobulin localized to the basement membrane was noted in normal uninvolved skin depending on whether light-exposed or protected skin was sampled (66, 67). Light-protected sites tended to show a lower incidence of positive results (68). Ultrastructural studies of dermal lesions in SLE showed electron-dense deposits suggesting presence of immune complexes (69). Since in some studies the renal lesions in SLE and in the skin appeared to parallel one another, it was suggested that the skin deposits might in fact represent focal collections of DNA–anti-DNA complexes. Moreover, in discoid LE where renal disease is not present, immunoglobulin deposits were recorded only in areas of active

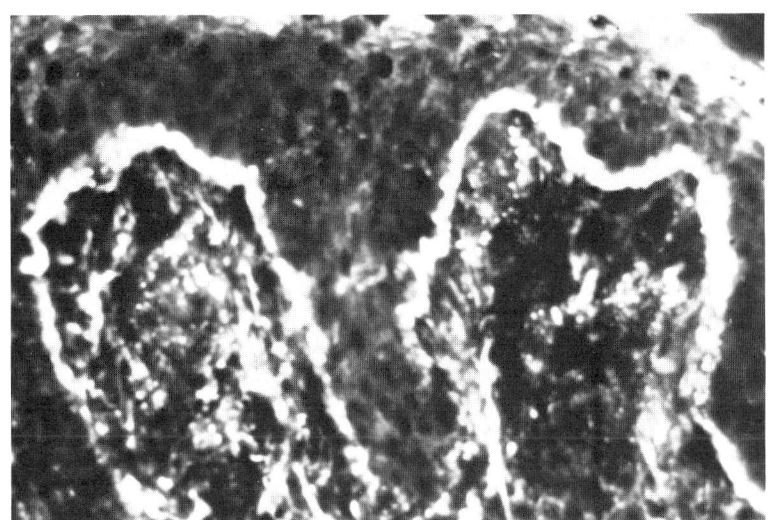

Figure 11-4 Granular deposits of IgG along the basement membrane zone separating epidermis from dermis (fluorescein-conjugated anti-human IgG.) Magnification × 250. (Reproduced with permission, M. Landry and W. M. Sams, Jr., *J. Clin. Invest.* 52:1871, 1973.)

skin involvement rather than in normal skin (68). The pattern of immunoglobulin and complement deposition in normal and involved skin in systemic lupus was examined by Jordon and co-workers (70). Their studies confirmed the frequent presence of IgG and IgM, and C1q and C3 in dermal-epidermal zones. C3PA and properdin deposits, though present in some biopsies, did not appear as prominent as elements related to the conventional complement pathway. However, a larger group of 61 patients studied by Schrager and Rothfield (65) showed presence of properdin in 50 percent of normal and lesion samples. An example of dermal-epidermal junctional properdin deposition from the latter study is shown in Figure 11-6.

Recently an interesting group of patients with glomerulonephritis but without extrarenal manifestations of SLE showing positive skin immunofluorescence were studied by Lief and co-workers (71). The only serological abnormality suggestive of SLE was a positive antinuclear antibody test; complement studies and anti-DNA antibody tests were repeatedly normal. The clinical course of these patients appeared to be more benign than that of the usual patient with severe lupus nephropathy and apparent favorable responses to prednisone and/or azathioprine were present. This group of patients presents an interesting enigma: one might on purely theoretical grounds question the diagnosis of SLE in the absence of definite anti-DNA antibody. Also, if these patients do indeed represent some kind of *forme fruste* of SLE, they raise additional questions concerning the specificity of reactions showing dermal-junctional zone immunofluorescence (72). Direct elution studies of skin and renal tissues would have been of interest, for it seems possible that anti-DNA might have been concentrated in these areas without being detectable in the serum.

Herpes Gestationis

Recent studies related to herpes gestationis (73, 74) are fascinating extensions of knowledge in this general area. Herpes gestationis (HG) is a rare recurrent disorder of pregnancy or the postpartum period, associated with intensely pruritic subepidermal blistering (Figure 11-7). It is generally considered to be a variant of erythema multiforme or dermatitis herpetiformis. Provost and Tomasi (75) were among the first to demonstrate skin basement membrane deposition of C3, properdin, and C5 in patients with this disorder. These findings were later confirmed in separate studies by other groups (76–78). One of the most puzzling features of the distribution of immune reactants in the skin basement membrane zone noted during these early studies was that despite the finding of C3, properdin, and other complement components, initially no clear evidence for immunoglobulin deposition in the skin was detected. A humoral factor

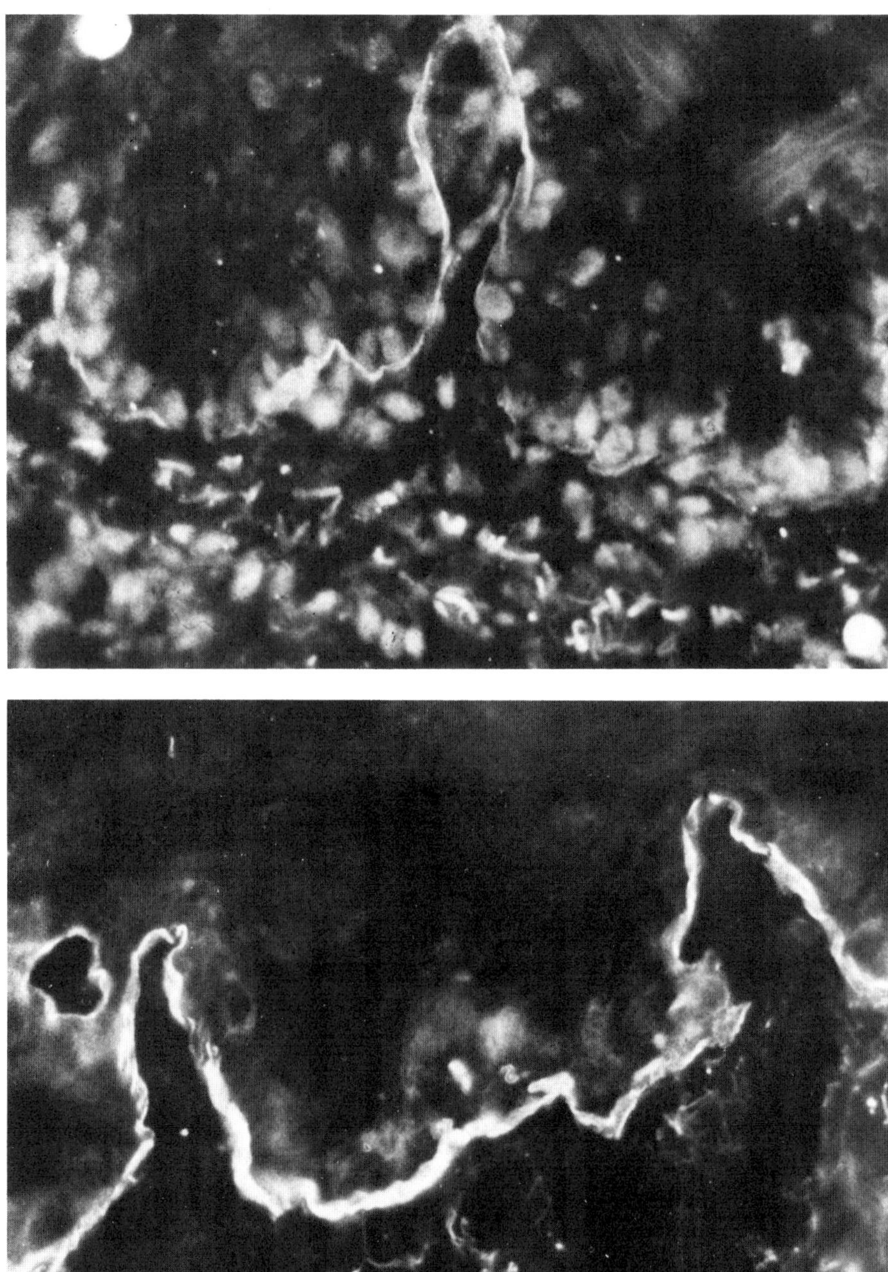

Figure 11-5 *Above,* skin eluate after application to guinea pig esophagus, showing both antinuclear and antibasement membrane zone antibodies (fluorescein-conjugated antihuman IgG). *Below,* skin eluate after application to rabbit esophagus, showing very strong antibasement membrane zone antibody that displays a tubular, folded appearance. Although this tissue gave a better demonstration of antibasement membrane antibody than did guinea pig esophagus, it did not demonstrate antinuclear antibody (fluorescein-conjugated antihuman IgG). Magnification × 332 above, × 340 below. (Reproduced with permission, M. Landry and W. M. Sams, Jr., *J. Clin. Invest.* 52:1871, 1973.)

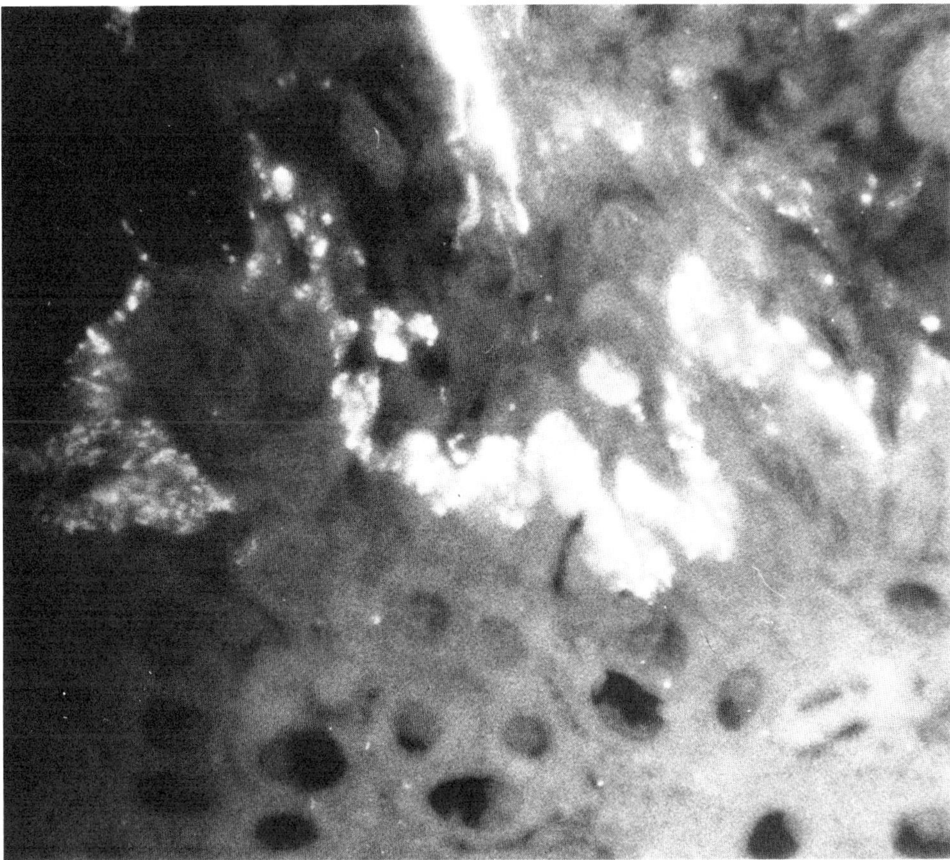

Figure 11-6 Immunofluorescence of the dermal-epidermal junctional zone of normal skin at the deltoid region, from a patient with active SLE stained for properdin. An intense staining band of granular fluorescence is present. Magnification × 216. (Reproduced with permission, M. A. Schrager and N. F. Rothfield, *J. Clin. Invest.* 57:212, 1976.)

initially thought to be heat labile was detected in serum samples from patients with HG. A number of studies indicated that this HG factor was capable of activation of C3 via the alternative complement pathway. Later Bushkell and co-workers (79) reported a patient with HG whose skin lesions showed IgG, C1q, C3, and properdin on direct immunofluorescence at the basement membrane zone. Moreover, serum from this patient contained antibody with a titer against basement membrane structures of 1:320. Subsequent studies by two additional groups (73, 74) have indicated that HG factor is indeed an IgG immunoglobulin which often, for reasons as yet unresolved, is not detected in immunofluorescent studies of active cutaneous lesions. Examples of the impressive amounts of complement (C3) deposition seen in basement membranes within affected skin in this disease are shown in Figure 11-8 from the study by Jordon and colleagues (73). The presence of antibody in this disease with apparent specificity for determinants within the basement membrane zone of skin raises some fascinating theoretical questions that bear directly on SLE and bullous pemphigoid. First, since antibodies that show apparent basement membrane localizing ability are generated during the course of HG, self-antigens present in this anatomic distribution may in fact undergo some sort of alteration sufficient for induction of autoimmune reactivity and production of such antibody by the host. Whether changes are actually induced by

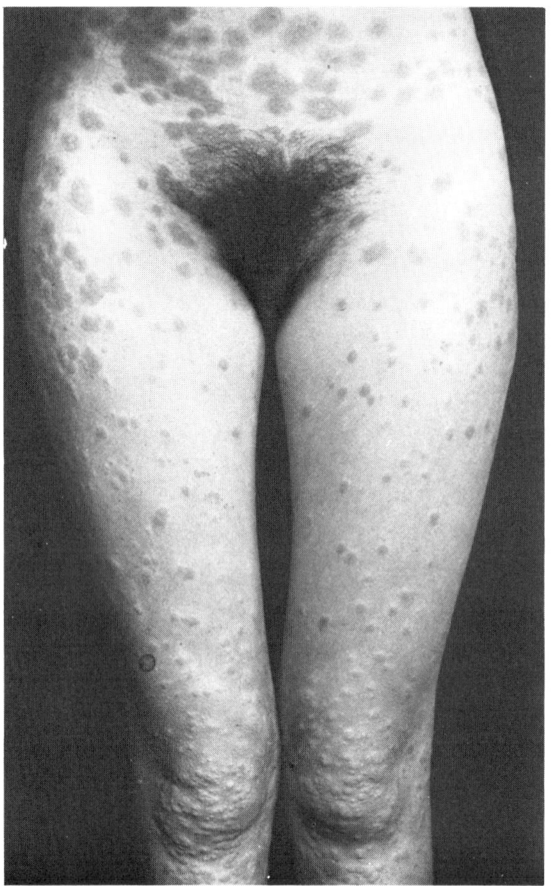

Figure 11-7 Characteristic eruption seen in herpes gestationis. (Photograph courtesy of St. John's Hospital for Diseases of the Skin, London.)

virus itself or by a combination of effects resulting from occult long-standing virus infection together with changes in immune reactivity induced by pregnancy is as yet undetermined. Furthermore, herpes infection itself may alter the structures within cutaneous basement membrane allowing them to express latent receptors for activated C3 or possibly Fc that were absent prior to activation of the disease. This obviously could also apply to SLE or bullous pemphigoid without the necessity to ascribe such changes to intrinsic herpes virus infection per se but rather to some other latent viral agent. Alternatively the turnover of cells within the epidermis, and local release of DNA encountering anti-DNA antibody near the basement membrane zones of skin might

account for the focal collection of immune deposits in these areas (80–82). The process is shown schematically in Figure 11-9. Further amplification of local mechanisms in the subepidermal zone might also be influenced by the direct reactivity of collagen fibrils with released DNA itself, since there appears to be a strong binding between collagen-like molecules and DNA, demonstrated by Izui and co-workers (83). If tissue injury or the lupus process itself were capable of activating local Fc or C3b receptors not ordinarily expressed in such tis-

Figure 11-8 *Above,* in vitro complement (C3) staining of normal human skin with herpes gestationis serum. A DEAE-Sephadex-purified HG factor has been used. Positive BMZ staining (*arrows*) is evident. *Below,* substitution of C2-deficient serum for normal human serum, since the complement source has inhibited positive in vitro C3 staining (*arrows*) with HG factor. Both photographs, magnification × 250. (Reproduced with permission, R. E. Jordon, K. G. Heine, G. Tappeiner et al., *J. Clin. Invest.* 57:1426, 1976.)

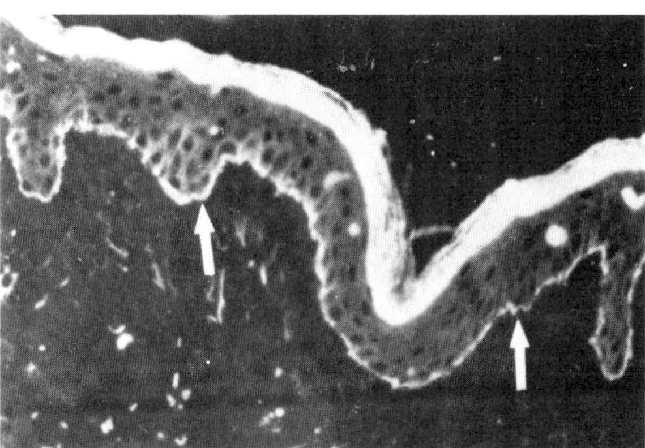

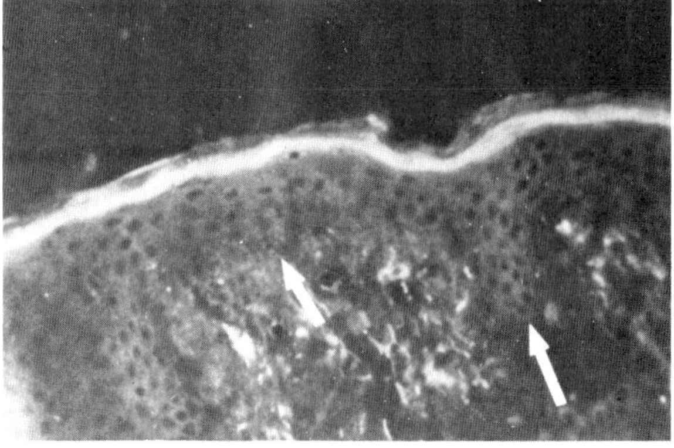

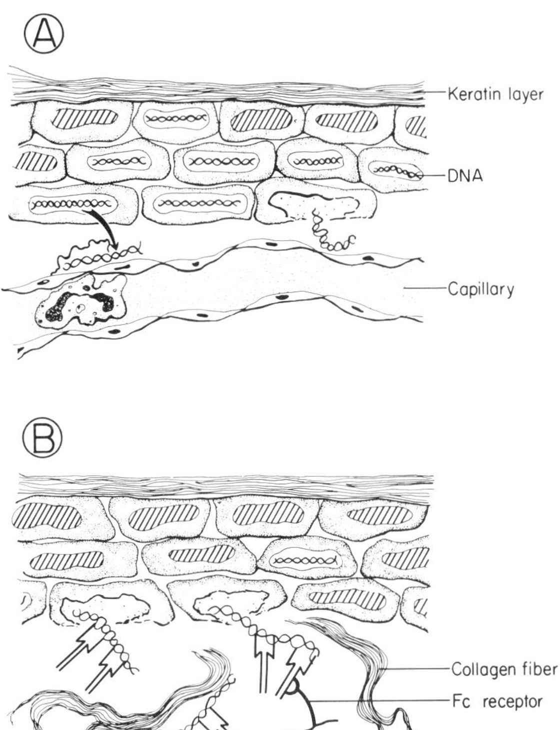

Figure 11-9 Proposed mechanism of subepidermal Ig accumulation. *A*, liberation of epidermal nuclear material during the process of normal keratinization may result in back-diffusion of nDNA into the dermis. Under normal circumstances this nDNA would pass through the subepidermal zone and be removed by the blood and lymphatic vessels. *B*, when anti-nDNA is present, the epidermal nDNA and the anti-nDNA precipitate in the subepidermal zone. Thus the formation of this subepidermal precipitate of nDNA–anti-nDNA is influenced by both local and systemic factors. (Adapted from J. N. Gilliam, *J. Invest. Dermatol.* 65:154, 1975.)

sues, a third mechanism for immune-complex sticking in this particular region might be postulated. It is clear that precise definition of all of these factors in the localization of immune reactants within the skin basement membrane will require more data before the relative importance of each becomes apparent.

An interesting study has appeared that documents an increased prevalence of dermal-epidermal membrane fixation of immune reac-

tants within the skin of unaffected relatives of patients with SLE (84). These findings provide additional evidence for a familial predisposition toward derangement in basic immune mechanisms involved in the genesis of the disease. Similar family studies by other groups, documenting what appears to be a marked increment in lymphocytotoxic antibodies among relatives of patients with SLE (85, 86), also provide evidence that either genetic or environmental factors may be of importance in the expression of the disease. In the case of dermal-junctional immune deposits in nonaffected relatives, one would have to postulate that the same underlying process must be at work in this anatomical site as in the patient with fully developed disease, but that full expression of SLE does not occur owing to the absence of full-blown immune dysfunction in otherwise apparently healthy family members. The relative importance of anti-DNA antibody is also brought into question by these family studies. If presence of true anti-DNA antibody is necessary for the formation of immune deposits at the basement membrane zones of skin, slightly increased local amounts of anti-DNA must be present in family members showing positive dermal tests for immunoglobulin deposition. That potential autoantibody formation occurs, albeit at low subclinical levels, in normal individuals has been amply documented in previous studies. The finding of marked increases in antibody to RNA in a number of unaffected relatives of SLE patients during a previous study is pertinent here (86). Also implicating an environmental or transmissible factor were the findings in two separate studies of lymphocytotoxic antibody and immune deposits in skin in spouses of SLE probands (84, 85). Most of the work on incidence of abnormalities in relatives of SLE probands indicates genetic and possible environmental factors influencing the various parameters tested.

Cutaneous Vasculitis in Systemic Diseases

Necrotizing vasculitis, originally termed hypersensitivity angiitis by Zeek (87), has been described in a number of systemic diseases including the connective-tissue diseases, drug reactions, bacterial infections or their sequelae, and even in association with malignancies such as lymphoma. The actual histological lesions of necrotizing or hypersensitivity angiitis contain features of both the Shwartzman and Arthus reactions. The Arthus reaction is induced by fixation of antigen within the walls of small vessels, where diffusion and direct contact with circulating antibody can induce complement activation, rapid ingress of polymorphonuclear leukocytes and other inflammatory cells, intense local reaction, and adjacent tissue necrosis. In 1967, using immunofluorescent techniques, Parish and Rhodes demonstrated aggregates of gamma globulin and group A streptococcal polysaccharide in lesions from a patient with nodular vasculitis following a streptococcal infection (88). IgG was noted in all areas of lesions containing streptococcal antigens. These workers also demonstrated that soluble complexes prepared from the patient's own gamma globulins containing antistreptococcal antibody, and group A polysaccharide could produce a local vasculitis when injected into baboons. Subsequently, lesions associated with cutaneous vasculitis have been investigated using immunofluorescence by a number of groups (88–92).

One of the problems in analysis of necrotizing angiitis involving the skin is that a number of heterogeneous conditions often have been included in the patient material studied. In some instances undoubtedly this resulted in inclusion of widely disparate clinical groups in the natural effort to amass "a series" of patients with apparently similar histological findings. Thus, in a group of 26 cases studied by Schroeter and colleagues (92), patients with necrotizing vasculitis associated with such diverse clinical conditions as facial granuloma, livedo vasculitis, systemic lupus erythematosus, carcinoma, lymphoma, periarteritis nodosa, Sjögren's syndrome, Coombs' positive hemolytic anemia, and thyroiditis with elevated antithyroid antibodies were included. Certainly, in many of these primary disease conditions ample possibility for the generation of immune complexes would have been afforded by the primary disease process. Many of the early studies related to cutaneous vasculitis presented clear evidence principally on the basis of immunofluorescent data of immune deposits within the dermal microvasculature. A representative summary of such data from the heterogeneous group studied by Schroeter is shown in Table 11-3. Of special interest was the observation of dense basement membrane, IgG, IgM, IgA, and C3 staining in three subjects with facial granuloma in this group. (Figure 11-10 shows an example.) Moreover, the finding of immunoglobulin in perivascular spaces indicates that vessel-wall damage was extensive enough to allow rather wide diffusion of immune reactants outside the vessels themselves. Striking histological changes of acute infiltration of dermal capillaries in paral-

Table 11-3 Vascular immunofluorescence in 33 patients with vasculitis.

Lesions	IgG	IgA	IgM	Of cell granules	β_1C and β_1A With vessels IgG	IgM	Fibrin
Necrotizing angiitis (diffuse perivascular)	15/26	0.18	8/18	9/15	6/7	6/7	11/18
Livedo vasculitis (medial)	3/4	0/3	3/3	0/3	3/3	3/3	3/3
Facial granulomata (reticulate periadventitial)	3/3	3/3	3/3	3/3	3/3	3/3	3/3

Source: Reproduced with permission, A. L. Schroeter, P. W. M. Copeman, R. E. Jordon et al., *Arch. Dermatol.* 104:254, 1971. Copyright 1971, American Medical Association.

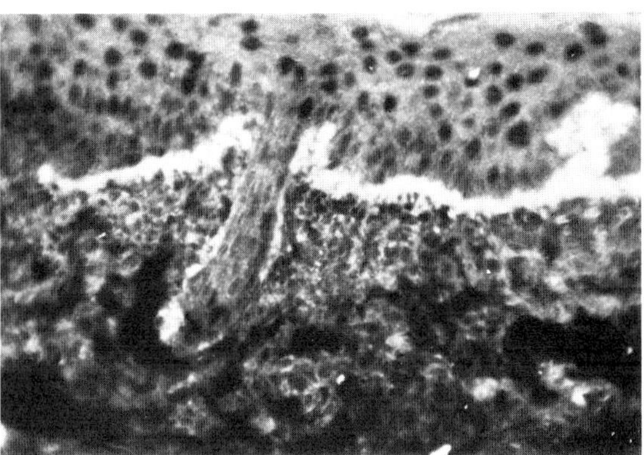

Figure 11-10 Facial granuloma, where direct immunofluorescence has demonstrated IgG in the thick basement membrane zone. Similar patterns for IgM, IgA, and $\beta_1 C/1-A$ globulin also were demonstrated by direct immunofluorescence. Magnification × 250. (Reproduced with permission, A. L. Schroeter, P. W. M. Copeman, R. E. Jordon et al., *Arch. Dermatol.* 104:254, 1971. Copyright 1971, American Medical Association.)

lel with immunofluorescent localization of immune reactants is illustrated in Figure 11-11 from the report by Stringa and co-workers (89). The obvious parallel with experimental studies of the Arthus reaction in animals is clear (93). Quite early in the clinical and experimental approaches to this general problem it was recognized that the principal weakness in studies documenting intense immunoglobulin and complement dermal vessel immune deposits was the failure to demonstrate the nature of the particular antigens involved.

Hypocomplementemia and Anticomplementary Activity

In 1973 McDuffie and co-workers (94) described a group of 4 patients with recurrent attacks of erythematous, urticarial, and hemorrhagic skin lesions associated with clinical evidence of synovitis and occasionally with abdominal distress. Skin biopsies in these patients showed necrotizing vasculitis with deposition of immunoglobulins and complement. Special features of these patients included marked hypocomplementemia with low levels of both early- and late-acting complement components during attacks and precipitins for C1q in sev-

eral sera suggesting presence of circulating immune complexes. Two of these patients showed lumpy deposits on renal glomerular basement membranes with histological evidence of mild glomerulonephritis. Examples of the cutaneous eruptions noted in this syndrome are shown in Figure 11-12. Both SLE and mixed cryoglobulinemia have also frequently been associated with hypocomplementemia but no clear evidence for either of these conditions was established in the patients studied by McDuffie and co-workers (94). Thus LE cells and anti-DNA antibody were not present and skin biopsies themselves showed no basement membrane immunofluorescence. Several features of the clinical illness in these patients suggested a parallel to those accompanying hereditary angioneurotic edema, in that recurrent severe episodes of abdominal pain were present in one patient and a second subject showed an attack of facial and laryngeal edema. No ready explanation is apparent for the urticarial skin lesions in these patients, and it is conceivable that the factors precipitating local areas of cutaneous vasculitis were in some way also associated with release of skin-reactive vasopeptides or other mediator molecules. Mild renal involvement, particularly in association with marked hypocomplementemia during vasculitis attacks, further supports an immune-complex etiology; however, the general profile of the disease appears separate from that associated with membranous glomerulonephritis and C3NeF, since no profound or persistent hypocomplementemia was documented *between* attacks and C3NeF was not present.

Similar patients with necrotizing angiitis of the skin were reported by Soter and colleagues (95), who studied patients with concomitant rheumatoid arthritis, Sjögren's syndrome, or SLE. The clinical evidence for cutaneous vasculitis included macules, papules, nodules, infarcts, and even skin ulcerations. Different complement profiles were noted depending on the underlying disease state and the nature of associated serum cryoproteins present. Thus in patients with either rheumatoid arthritis or Sjögren's syndrome the early complement components—C1, C4, and C2—were depressed. When cryoproteins containing mainly

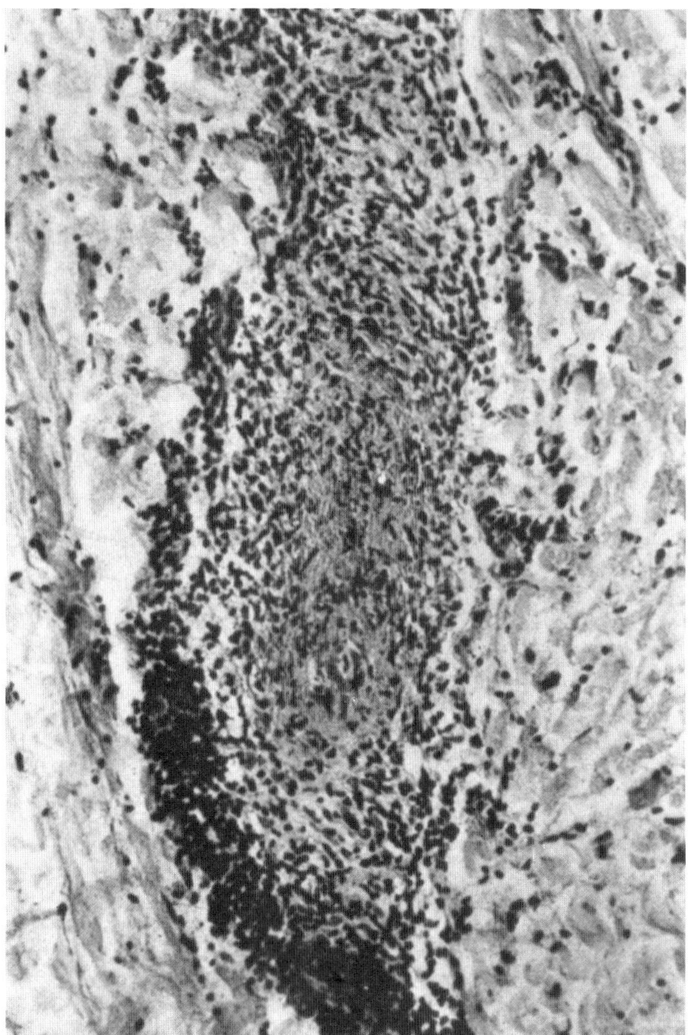

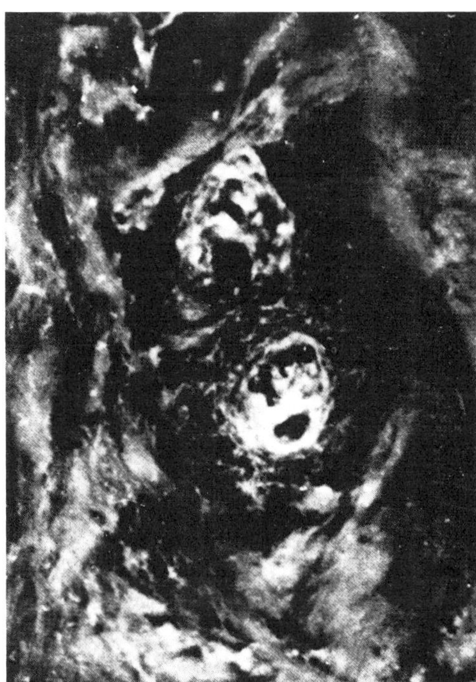

Figure 11-11 *Left,* thrombosis of a dermal capillary, showing pronounced fibrinoid necrosis in the vascular wall and inflammatory infiltrates with marked nuclear destruction. H&E × 100. *Right,* dermal vessels showing bright fluorescence after incubation with anti-IgG conjugated with fluorescein isothiocyanate. Magnification × 20 obtained with a monocular Zeiss 6 microscope, and ocular magnification × 12 and × 5 with an Exacta Varex camera with microscope adapter and extension tube. (Reproduced with permission, S. G. Stringa, C. Bianchi, A. M. Casala et al., *Arch. Dermatol.* 95:23, 1967. Copyright 1967, American Medical Association.)

IgG and IgM were present, there was evidence of further preferential reduction in serum C4 and C2. One interesting patient with Sjögren's syndrome and a cryoprotein containing large amounts of IgA showed serum C3 depression without demonstrable effects on the early complement components—suggesting predominant alternate complement pathway activation. By contrast, patients with active necrotizing cutaneous vasculitis and SLE showed marked depressions of both early and late complement component activities with striking C1q depression. One salient problem in the evaluation of patients with connective-tissue diseases and necrotizing vasculitis is that it may be wrong to classify them together under a cate-

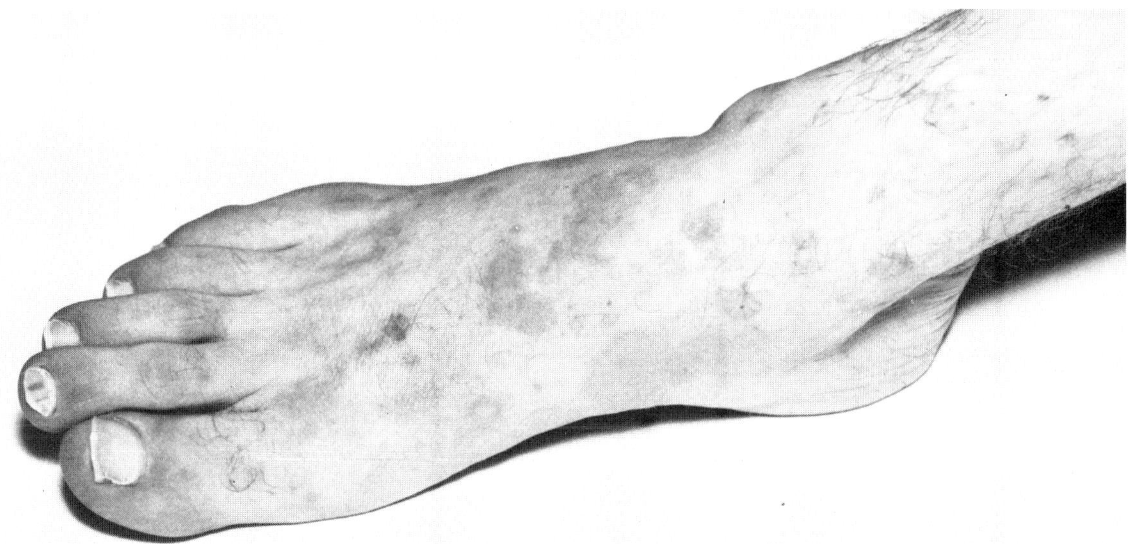

Figure 11-12 Cutaneous eruption of slightly elevated, erythematous lesions with a tendency toward central clearing. Note the purpuric area above the base of the second toe. (Reproduced with permission, F. C. McDuffie, W. M. Sams, J. E. Maldonado et al., *Mayo Clin. Proc.* 48:340, 1973.)

gory of cutaneous vasculitis rather than on the basis of their underlying disease state. This has been amply illustrated in a prospective analysis by Conn and colleagues (96), dealing with cutaneous vessel deposits in rheumatoid arthritis. Normal skin was biopsied in 39 patients with rheumatoid arthritis; immune deposits in dermal vessels were found in 20 of 32 patients with seropositive rheumatoid disease. Of importance was the fact that frequency of such deposits was only slightly higher in patients with clinical evidence of rheumatoid vasculitis than in those without. In patients with clinical vasculitis it appeared that there was an association between cutaneous vessel immune deposits and presence in serum of antinuclear antibody or elevation of IgM and IgA. The major immunoglobulin detected in cutaneous vessels was IgM associated with C3 deposits. Such findings support the concept that in a disease such as rheumatoid arthritis there is widespread immune-complex deposition, regardless of its clinical recognition as an associated necrotizing angiitis. However, when vasculitis manifests itself clinically, it may be the harbinger of acceleration of a basic disease process present apparently from the beginning. Clini-

cally recognizable vasculitis in rheumatoid arthritis may be associated with elevations in rheumatoid factor (97), serum hypocomplementemia (98), and peripheral manifestations of moderate or severe neuropathy (99). Vascular lesions probably related to immune-complex deposition represent one of the earliest basic pathological changes in the synovitis of rheumatoid disease (100) and in the generation of the rheumatoid nodule (101)

Previous studies of the prevalence of cutaneous immune deposits in patients with rheumatoid arthritis have varied in their findings. Two reports indicated no evidence of such immune deposits in forearm skin biopsies of patients with rheumatoid arthritis (102, 103). However, samples taken from less dependent areas may not be representative of the most advanced changes in this disease, since it is well known that peripheral vasculitic lesions are most often apparent in the lower extremities. The studies of Larsson (104) and our own observations (105) have confirmed the dermal deposits of Ig in skin capillaries from a wide range of subjects with rheumatoid arthritis irrespective of clinical evidence of overt vascular involvement. It therefore seems artificial to select out patients with different connective-tissue diseases and to lump them together as a clinical entity merely on the basis of a common manifestation of cutaneous vasculitis. Perhaps much more relevant and productive would be a careful analysis of the actual deposits by elution studies and more recently available methods of analysis such as gel electrophoresis for the nature of the antigens involved in such deposits. The tendency of investigators to lump heterogeneous mixtures of such patients together persists, as witnessed by a recent report claiming increased frequency of HLA-A11, Bw35 in patients with cutaneous necrotizing vasculitis which included patients with SLE, rheumatoid arthritis, Sjögren's syndrome, lymphoma, and arthritis with lymphoma (106). It is conceivable that such an HLA phenotype, when associated with a connective-tissue disease, predisposes to the development of cutaneous necrotizing vasculitis.

The possibility that circulating immune complexes might be related to the skin lesions in cutaneous vasculitis was examined in 1973 by Cream (107), who studied anticomplementary activity in serum from 32 patients. The patients studied included 21 with crops of purpura of the variety seen in Henoch-Schönlein purpura. Two patients showed additional clinical features supporting a diagnosis of systemic polyarteritis nodosa and one patient showed plaques typical of erythema elevatum diutinum. Patients with skin diseases of miscellaneous types not thought to be caused by circulating immune complexes were studied in parallel as controls. Anticomplementary activity in serum was demonstrated to be present in 11 of 32 patients with cutaneous vasculitis. Five of these anticomplementary sera were derived from samples containing mixed IgG-IgM cryoglobulins. This is one of the first studies to attempt quantitative estimation of levels of materials resembling immune complexes in the sera of patients with necrotizing cutaneous vasculitis. One of the major problems in the use of anticomplementary activities of serum samples as a measure of circulating complexes is that the test may be positive on the basis of IgG aggregates actually formed in vitro after blood samples are collected. Thus aggregates of IgG

particularly in hypergammaglobulinemic sera are known to fix complement (108) and may indeed account for the anticomplementary activity appearing in vitro in serum samples after storage (109, 110).

Further immunofluorescent findings in patients with cutaneous vasculitis have been reported by Weidner (111), who studied distribution of IgD and fibrin in such lesions. It was noted that IgD appeared in close apposition to the neutrophilic infiltrates in many lesions. Occasional homogeneous deposits of IgD within the walls of cutaneous blood vessels were recorded. These data are of interest, since IgD itself is present in extremely low concentrations within normal sera (112). There is very little clear insight into the actual physiological significance of IgD and its presence in lesions associated with necrotizing vasculitis requires further examination. Several studies have indicated that this particular immunoglobulin class can be shown to participate in specific antigen-binding activity (113) and autoantibody formation (114). Recently studies of IgD on cell surface membranes have suggested that it may function as an important receptor in lymphocyte differentiation (115). Particularly interesting with respect to its possible role in the pathogenesis of cutaneous vasculitis are recent reports that IgD may be important in protection versus tolerance (116, 117). It has been shown that removal of IgD lymphocyte receptors markedly increases cell susceptibility to tolerance induction. Since part of the process of necrotizing vasculitis may represent loss of tolerance to autologous antigens, it is possible that the local deposits of IgD in such lesions might result from the body's own response toward restoration of tolerance against an antigen that has for unknown reasons escaped the usual tolerance generating mechanisms. Since many of the currently utilized assays employ C1q binding as a primary method for detection of immune complexes, it is difficult to ascertain whether such assays would show reactivity with immune complexes containing IgD as the principal immunoglobulin; a portion of such complexes might be noncomplement fixing, at least via the C1q-driven conventional pathway.

Livedo Vasculitis

Atrophie blanche en plaque was first described by Milian in 1929 (118) as a skin disorder associated with smooth, ivory-white plaque-like lesions surrounded by hyperpigmented borders and telangiectatic blood vessels occurring on the legs and ankles. Typical lesions associated with this disorder are shown in Figure 11-13. In his original descriptions Milian believed that the skin lesions resulted from syphilis. This presumption may have been the hyperbole of a French imagination: many of the lesions were observed in their end stages accompanied by atrophic, porcelain-white stellate scars. About 30 years later Feldaker and co-workers (119) studied 12 patients with ulcerations that recurred during winter and summer. These ulcers were associated with livedo reticularis of the legs and ulcerations on the ankles and feet. Histological examination of the ulcers showed hyalinization of vessels in the dermis, panniculus, middermis, and in some instances papillary dermis. New vessel formation with perivascular lymphocytic or neutrophilic infiltration was also noted. Subsequently a number of histological studies of the basic process in the skin lesions (120–124) established segmental hyalinization of dermal vessels with apparent relative absence of associated dense neutrophilic or lymphocytic infiltrates. In retrospect it seems fair to say that the lesions of atrophie blanche are most probably the result of infarctive changes of skin in legs, ankles, and dorsum of the feet—a process that seems to result from a progressive segmental vasculitis of vessels supplying the dermis in these areas. A histological and immunopathological study of 15 patients was conducted by Schroeter and co-workers (125). IgM was the predominant immunoglobulin found, along with IgG deposition in 6 of 15 subjects studied. Concurrent

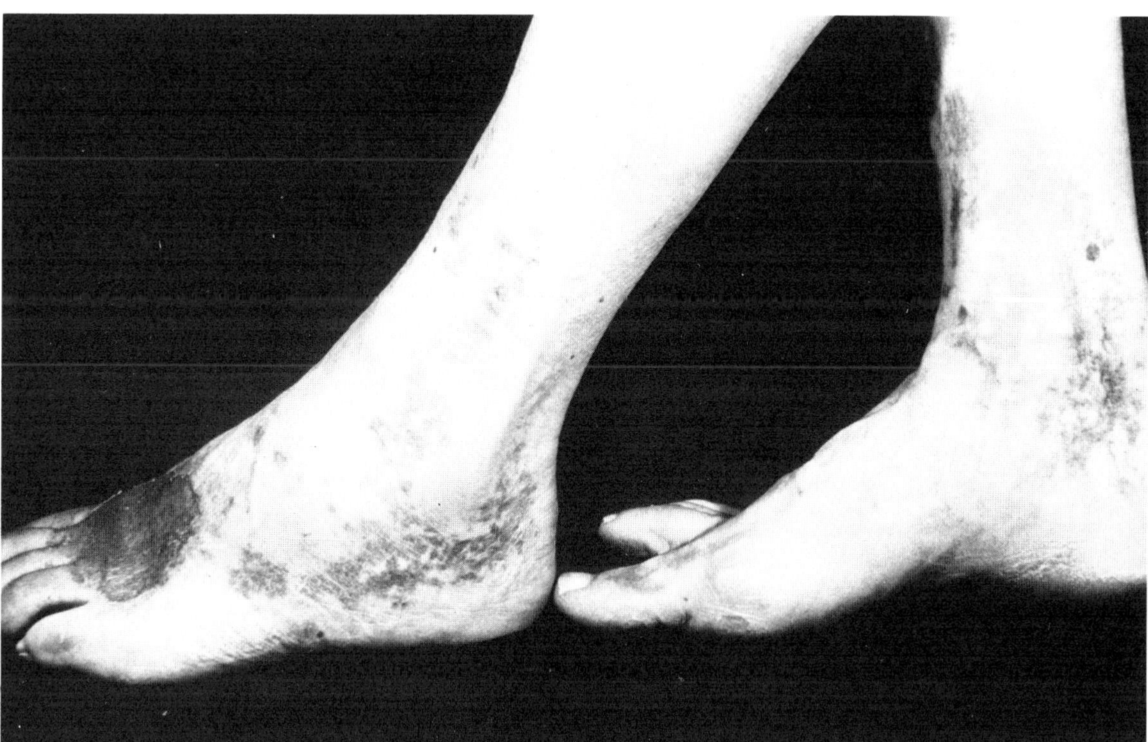

Figure 11-13 Skin lesions of *atrophie blanche en plaque*. (Photograph courtesy of St. John's Hospital for Diseases of the Skin, London.)

studies using antisera to C3 and C3PA provided evidence for parallel complement tissue deposits. Control skin biopsies from leg samples of patients without known systemic or cutaneous disease were negative. Comparison with conventional histology showed that Ig and complement deposition was localized to vessels found to be hyalinized, as demonstrated by PAS staining. Thus it appears that the vascular lesions associated with livedo reticularis represent another example of immune-complex vasculitis involving vessels supplying several layers of the skin itself.

Graft Versus Host Disease

In cases of leukemia or aplastic anemia, graft versus host disease represents one of the principal complications of human bone-marrow transplantation. The immunologic events transpiring in bone-marrow graft recipients are a complex mixture of rejection phenomena mounted by the recipient and agressive reactions against the host produced by grafted cells themselves. Often a clinical distinction between the assault of donor lymphoid cells on host tissues and the consequences of this process —deranged organ function, or even superimposed nosocomial infection—proves extremely difficult. However, the major target organs showing involvement in graft versus host disease are the skin, gastrointestinal tract, and the liver (126). The precise reasons for this distribution are still unknown. Changes in skin graft versus host reaction range from mild involvement with basal vacuolar degeneration of necrosis to focal and microscopic epidermal separation and frank epidermal loss with more severe involvement. In most cases the first organ system involved is the skin. Biopsy evaluation in such cases is often mandatory, as the patients are usually receiving a variety of immunosuppressive and antibiotic regimes. It seems likely that graft versus host lesions probably involve cell-mediated immune reactions; however, humoral antibody-mediated responses may also be of importance (127). Skin biopsies from both early and late graft versus host reactions were recently examined by Ullman and co-workers (128). C3 deposits in a dif-

fuse granular pattern were present at the dermal-epidermal junction in a patient with acute reaction, with concomitant staining of vessel walls for IgG, IgM, and C3. A patient with more chronic graft versus host disease showed deposits of IgM at the dermal-epidermal junction with IgM, IgA, and C3 in dermal vessel walls. These findings suggest that immune complexes of unknown type are participating at some level in the generation of the skin lesions seen in these patients. Whether they occur as a result of other, more primary disease processes involving graft versus host assault on host tissues is still unknown. Again, the finding of apparent immune-complex deposits within the basement membrane zones of skin in these patients underscores the potential central role of this particular anatomic location for saturation by or adsorption to immune-complex reactants. In the case of these particular deposits, it should eventually be possible to use eluates of skin in microcytotoxicity inhibition to ascertain whether HLA antigens of donor or recipient represent the prominent antigens found in such deposits.

Erythema Elevatum Diutinum

Erythema elevatum diutinum (EED) is a rare chronic skin disease associated with persistent red, purple, and yellow papules, plaques, and nodules distributed over fingers and extensor surfaces (129, 130). The histopathological findings usually show a leukocytoclastic angiitis associated with dense dermal infiltrates of neutrophils and mononuclear cells (131, 132). As the disease progresses, late lesions show fibrous replacement of the normal dermis. At present, the basic cause of the disease is unknown.

Studies of 5 patients with EED by Katz and colleagues (133) implicate involvement of cutaneous immune-complex deposition in the pathogenesis of the disease. A rather dramatic response to dapsone therapy was noted in 4 subjects. Representative skin involvement in one of the patients from this study is shown in Figure 11-14. Three of the 5 patients studied by Katz and colleagues (133) gave long histories of repeated bacterial infections most

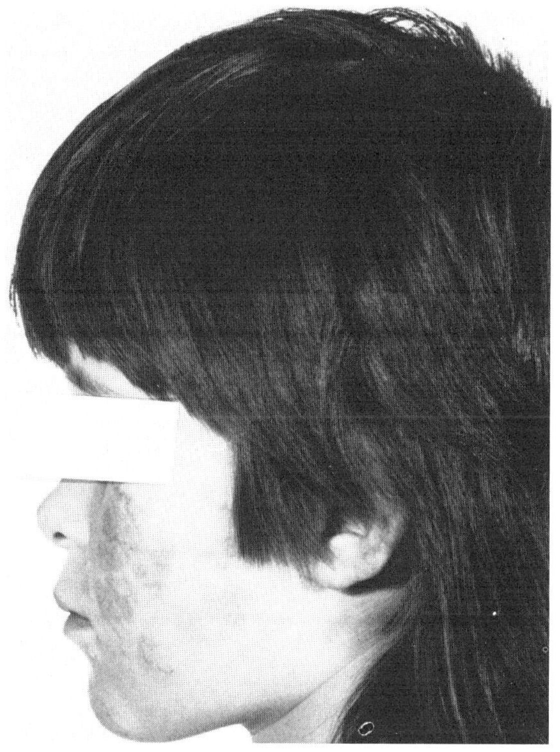

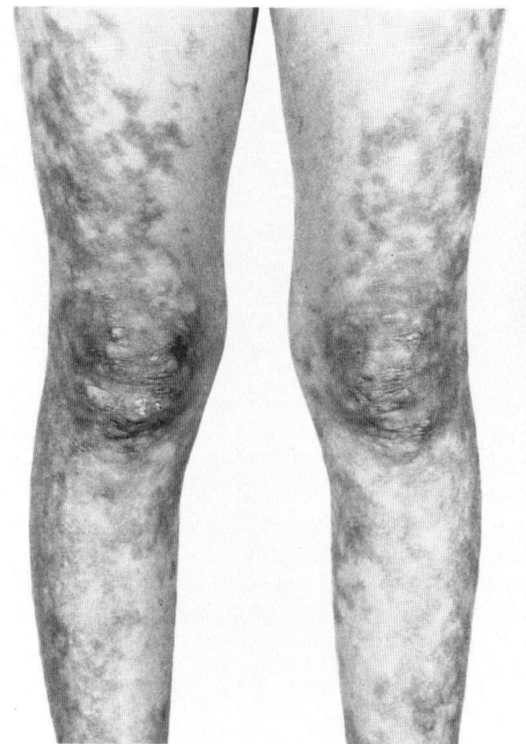

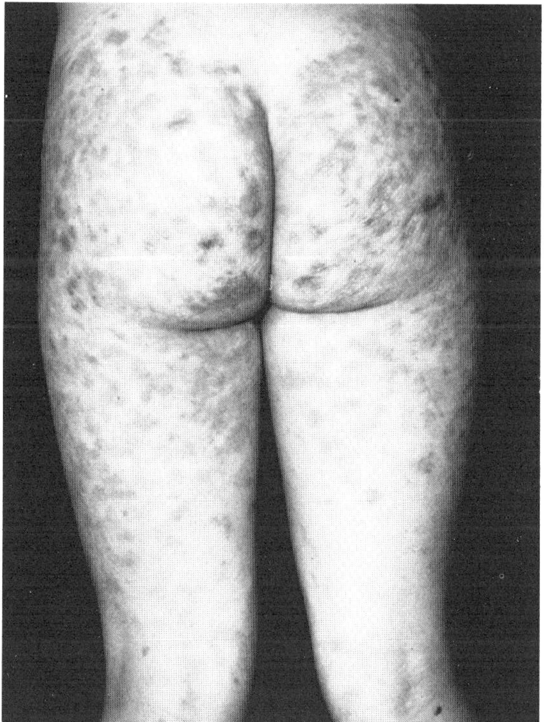

Figure 11-14 Patient with erythema elevatum diutinum before treatment showing papules, nodules, and plaques on face, legs, and buttocks. (Reproduced with permission, S. I. Katz, J. I. Gallin, K. C. Hertz et al., *Medicine* 56:443, 1977.)

prominently streptococcal; 4 of 5 subjects showed strongly positive skin tests to streptokinase-streptodornase, an extracellular product of Lancefield group C streptococci. Biopsy of the actual skin test sites showed most of the histological changes of the spontaneously occurring leukocytoclastic angiitis. In the small group studied no clear association was noted between occurrence of the disease and HLA type. Contrary to previous reports, it was found that systemic symptoms in these patients were sometimes severe, including malaise and generalized arthralgias. The dramatic response of skin lesions and systemic manifestations to dapsone was followed by prompt reappearance of symptoms and lesions on withdrawal of the drug. Various possible mechanisms of action of dapsone in the treatment have been postulated, including interference with activation of the alternate complement pathway (134); however, later work has not supported this view (135).

Extensive studies have been performed in an attempt to identify immunoglobulin and complement within the skin lesions of patients with EED (135). A mixture of eosinophils in the infiltrates was thought to obviate critical analysis of this approach, since these cells themselves were fluorophilic and granules appeared to take up fluoresceinated antibody and free fluorescein. Furthermore, ultrastructural evidence for electron-dense deposits in vessels of involved tissues was absent. Several lines of evidence, however, appeared to support an immune-complex etiology in the genesis of EED lesions. C1q binding activity was present in the sera of 3 patients. Moreover, when streptokinase-streptodornase skin testing was applied, particularly in subjects with history of repeated streptococcal throat infections, rapid development of Arthus-like lesions and striking acute inflammatory changes within the skin test sites suggested immune-complex activation. It may be that other indirect mechanisms are at work in this disorder. Thus immune complexes may activate neutrophils within the circulating blood without actually depositing within vessel walls. From the data at hand, it is still not entirely clear that EED can be classified as a disorder of primary immune-complex etiology. The

finding of C1q binding within patients' sera cannot be equilibrated with primary immune-complex etiology in a number of other clinical disorders. Many serum factors including Gram-negative lipopolysaccharides, other bacterial products, or even release of free DNA itself from damaged cells can produce C1q binding. Moreover, the relatively dramatic response to dapsone in this condition remains rather mysterious and poorly understood. It is possible that the drug inhibits a series of intermediary mechanisms that are important in the potentiation of local dermal vascular inflammation. Certainly the cautious use of the drug might be warranted in other nonrelated forms of necrotizing vasculitis. An isolated report by Thompson and Souhami (136) indicates that the Arthus reaction may be suppressed in guinea pig tissues by prior treatment with dapsone. Since that reaction is strongly dependent on both complement activation and rapid ingress of polymorphonuclear leukocytes, it seems probable that the primary modulating effect of the drug may affect function of one or both of these mechanisms. Many useful agents have been discovered long before their underlying means of action have been sorted out. Dapsone may well prove to be beneficial in other widely divergent types of immune-complex phenomena.

Necrobiosis Lipoidica and Diabetes

Necrobiosis lipoidica is an unusual skin condition characterized by asymptomatic, slightly depressed plaques often occurring along the lower anterior tibial surfaces. Typical lesions are shown in Figure 11-15. The disease is associated with diabetes mellitus in about half of the cases studied. Examination of skin biopsies of involved areas shows a zone of thickened and hyalinized collagen (necrobiosis) surrounded by histiocytes, lymphocytes, epithelial cells, and occasional giant cells. Blood vessels frequently show thickened walls, occlusions, and swelling of endothelial cells (137, 138). These changes show histological similarity to rheumatoid arthritis nodules or the lesions of erythema annulare. Recent studies of this condition by Ullman and Dahl (139) included im-

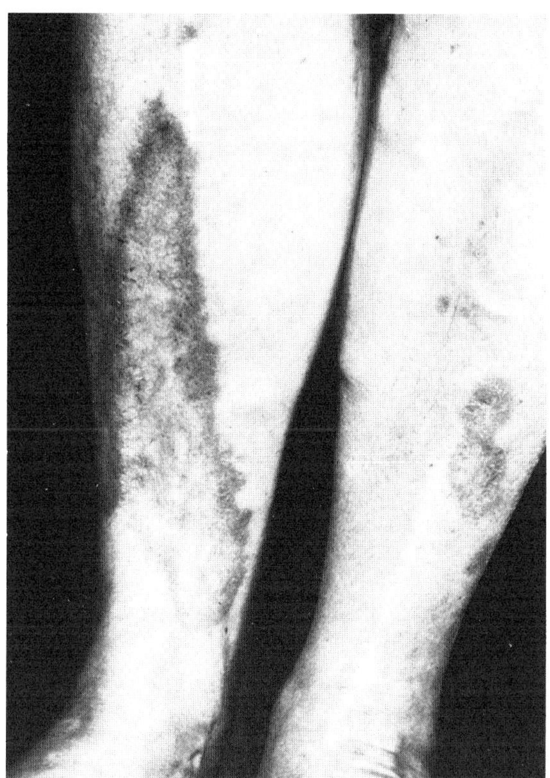

Figure 11-15 Typical skin lesions of necrobiosis lipoidica. (Photograph courtesy of St. John's Hospital for Diseases of the Skin, London.)

munofluorescence of skin biopsies in 12 subjects. IgM deposition was noted in vessel walls of involved skin in 6 patients and C3 fixation in 7 patients. A few subjects showed IgA within vessel walls. IgM, C3, and fibrinogen were also recorded at the dermal-epidermal junction of involved skin in 7 patients.

Immune complexes have been detected in the sera of patients with diabetes (140, 141). In a study by Irvine and co-workers (141) soluble immune complexes were found by the Raji-cell assay in 7 of 13 newly diagnosed insulin-dependent diabetics, 6 of whom also had islet-cell serum antibodies. No clear correlation was noted between various antiviral antibodies and recent onset of diabetes and none of these newly diagnosed diabetics showed serum antibodies to insulin. There is now a strong body of evidence implicating the importance of immune processes in the pathogenesis of what

has been termed type I diabetes which eventually results in insulin dependency (142). In the newly diagnosed patients studied by Irvine actual levels of complexes ranged from 32 to 64 μg/ml. In comparative studies significant elevations of immune complexes were recorded in 53 percent of 32 insulin-treated diabetics of longer standing, but in only 10 percent of 21 patients treated with diet alone. There appeared to be a general relationship between occurrence of insulin antibodies in insulin-treated diabetics and quantitative estimations of immune complexes in simultaneously studied serum samples. Of the 32 insulin-treated diabetics, 16 had various complications of diabetes including diabetic retinopathy, retinal hemorrhages, exudates, retinal or vitreous new blood-vessel formation, or diabetic nephropathy. Twelve of these 16 patients showed presence of soluble immune complexes in sera, while only 5 of the remaining 16 uncomplicated insulin-treated diabetics showed positive tests.

Several additional observations also suggest that immune complexes may be related to diabetic complications. Fine, granular deposits on the renal glomerular basement membrane have been described by Bloodworth (143) in patients with diabetic nephropathy. In addition such glomeruli are shown to contain insulin-binding capacity and also to exhibit insulin detectable by immunologic techniques (144). These same features are also present in ocular vessels of the diabetic eye (145). Direct immunofluorescent studies of the renal involvement of diabetic glomerulosclerosis, however, show not only insulin, IgG, IgM, and complement components, but also other nonimmune plasma protein deposits (146). Similar studies must be directed at the skin lesions of necrobiosis lipoidica in an effort to resolve these problems. One of the most difficult differential aspects of such investigations resides in the fact that the diabetic process itself is involved in generation of a diffuse microangiopathy, part of which may result from intrinsic abnormalities in glucose and lipid metabolism. Isolating those features of the angiopathy associated with diabetes mediated by immune-complex deposition may prove to be problematical. One obvious approach lies in the initiation of long-range prospective studies in which levels of detectable circulating immune complexes are assessed over a period of time in association with other essential parameters. Distribution of microvascular lesions associated with diabetes in the eye, skin, peripheral nerves, and kidneys has long intrigued many groups of investigators. In particular the changes occurring in retinal and vitreous vessels seem worthy of special study; if immune complexes are indeed of importance, it would seem worthwhile to examine such tissues directly for the presence of receptors for immune complexes interacting with C3b or the Fc portions of gamma globulin.

Granuloma Annulare

Granuloma annulare is a benign chronic skin disease of unknown cause characterized clinically by dermal papules and nodules usually arranged in annular fashion. Microscopic examination shows foci of necrobiotic collagen and mucinous change surrounded by mononuclear cells often arranged in a palisade fashion (147). In most cases histological study of the lesions shows infiltration of dermal collagen by mononuclear cells with occasional instances of granulomatous reaction showing giant cells and epithelioid elements. These latter changes may resemble some features of cutaneous sarcoidosis. The etiology of granuloma annulare is unknown. A variety of possible causes has been suggested by various workers including insect bites (148), sunlight (149–151), diabetes mellitus (152, 153), and reaction to tuberculin testing (154).

Direct immunofluorescent studies were first carried out by Umbert and Winkelmann (155). These studies showed presence of fibrin masses in all 11 specimens studied. Fibrin was localized in extravascular portions of the dermis corresponding to granulomatous and necrobiotic areas. No distinct localization of fibrin was recorded in blood vessels. IgM and C3 deposits were noted in the vessels of 1 patient and basement membrane immunofluorescence consisting of IgM or C3 staining was present in 3 subjects. These findings did not provide strong evidence for a primary immune-complex etiology in the pathogenesis of the lesions. However, Umbert and Winkelmann interpreted the extensive fibrin deposits as an indication that delayed-type hypersensitivity was a prominent feature of the basic reaction. Presence of extensive extravascular deposits of fibrin has been recognized as a distinctive feature of delayed-type hypersensitivity skin reaction in humans (156). Studies of fibrin deposition using radiolabeled reagents and immunofluorescence have been used to quantitate the delayed-type hypersensitivity reaction in experimental animals (156). Retention and progressive accumulation of fibrinogen in delayed-type skin reactions appeared to be related to local activation of the coagulation process.

Different findings have been reported by Dahl and co-workers (157), also based on immunofluorescent and histological studies of biopsy samples from 38 patients. In 6 of 20 subjects IgM was recorded in vessels of involved skin. In addition IgM, C3, or fibrinogen were noted at the dermal-epidermal junctions in 8 patients. Examination of biopsy material from 38 patients with granuloma annulare showed vessel wall necrosis, fibrinoid changes, or thickening and vascular occlusion in most samples. In confirmation of the previous study (156), fibrin was frequently present within necrobiotic areas. The vascular changes and depositions of IgM and C3 are shown in Figures 11-16 and 11-17 from this study. If indeed the lesions of granuloma annulare are produced on the basis of immune-complex deposition, they must occur on a different basis from those seen in the classic Arthus reaction, since they tend to remain and persist for weeks, months, or years. On the other hand lesions of typical allergic vasculitis usually disappear within a period of days or weeks. These differences suggest that the process involved in granuloma annulare is much more indolent and chronic than the usual Arthus reactions, where Ig and complement can be demonstrated in vessels only during the first 24 hours after induction (158). It is noteworthy that in certain patients lesions of necrobiosis lipoidica and granuloma annulare occur together. Again, as in the nu-

Figure 11-16 IgM at dermal-epidermal junction (*arrow*) of involved skin in patient with granuloma annulare (antihuman IgM). Magnification × 192. (Reproduced with permission, M. V. Dahl, S. Ullman, and R. W. Goltz, *Arch. Dermatol.* 113:463, 1977. Copyright 1977, American Medical Association.)

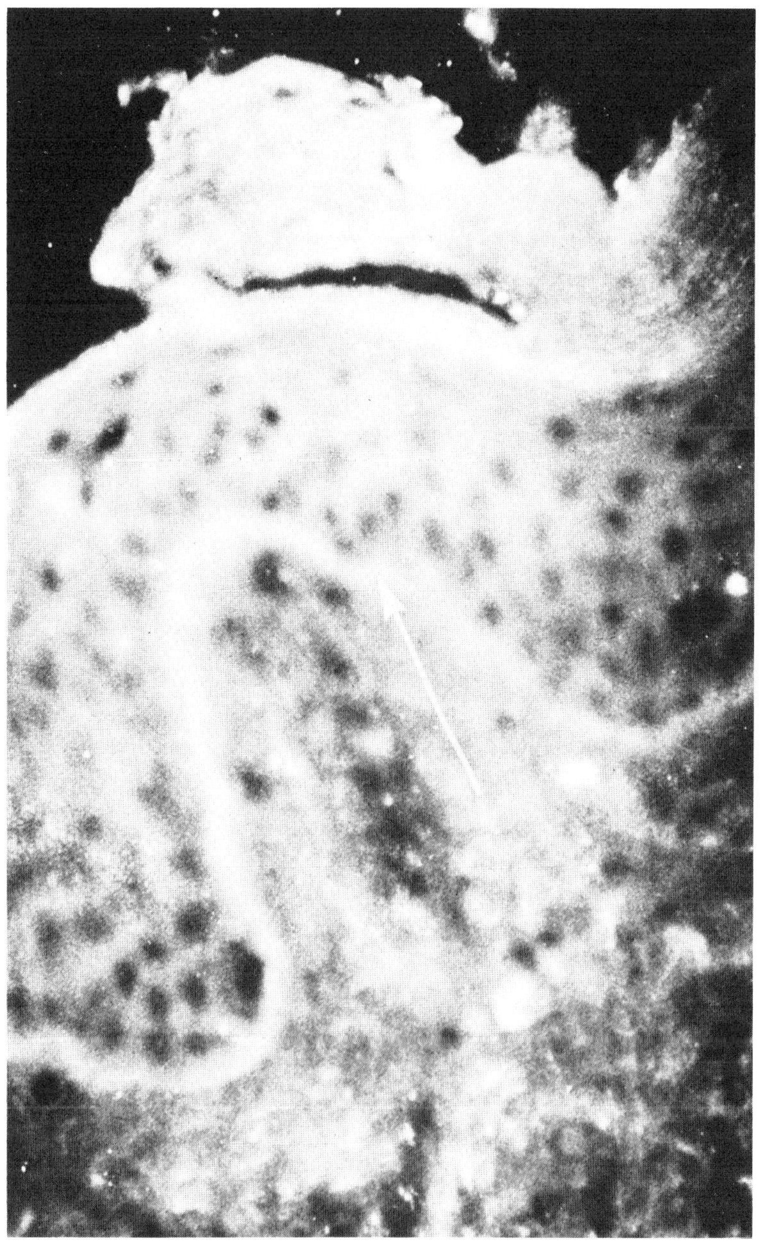

merous observations related to immunofluorescence of skin in necrotizing cutaneous vasculitis, many studies are hampered by lack of direct information about what antigens may be involved. Also the precise physiological significance of dermal-epidermal junctional deposits of immunoglobulin and complement remains an ill-defined area that now includes positive findings in a large number of unrelated primary conditions.

Dermatitis Herpetiformis

Dermatitis herpetiformis (DH) is a blistering skin condition that appears to be related to gluten-sensitive enteropathy and coeliac disease.

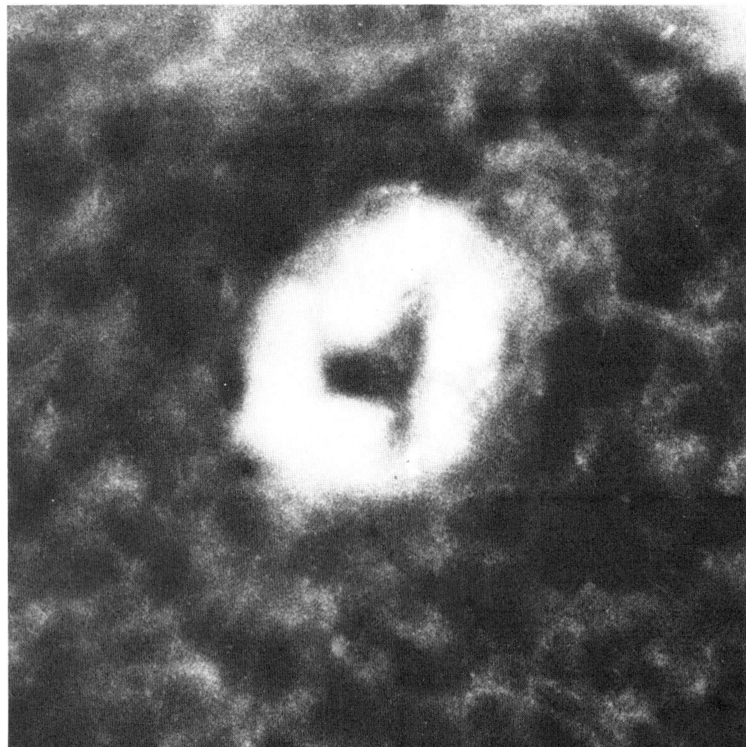

Figure 11-17 C3 in blood vessel of involved skin from a patient with granuloma annulare (antihuman C3). Magnification × 192. (Reproduced with permission, M. V. Dahl, S. Ullman, and R. W. Goltz, *Arch. Dermatol.* 113:463, 1977. Copyright 1977, American Medical Association.

DH is characterized by a symmetric pleomorphic eruption of urticarial plaques, papules, and groups of vesicles often occurring on extensor surfaces such as elbows, knees, shoulders, sacrum, or buttocks, and on the face and scalp. Presently the disease is considered one of unknown etiology; however, a prompt response often follows empirical therapy with sulfone or sulfapyridine. The skin lesions show characteristic histopathology including papillary edema, neutrophilic papillary microabscesses, and subepidermal blisters. Typical skin lesions seen in association with this disease are shown in Figure 11-18.

Dermatitis herpetiformis has been one of the most exhaustively studied disorders with respect to understanding of basic immune phenomena and actual mechanisms of pathogenesis (159). In DH, perhaps more than in any other skin disorder with the exception of SLE, modern techniques of immunofluorescence and interest in genetic control of the immune response have been rewarded with striking data supporting an immune-complex mecha-

nism in the genesis of skin lesions. There is also some support for possible IR gene control in the expression of the disease itself. One of the best criteria for a definite diagnosis of DH is immunofluorescent demonstration of IgA deposits at tips of dermal papillae or in a continuous band at the dermal-epidermal junction. A number of studies have been instrumental in establishing IgA skin deposits as one of the most reliable primary criteria for diagnosis of the disease and have also provided considerable insight into possible mechanisms relating DH directly to gluten-sensitive enteropathy or coeliac disease. In fact data bearing on the two disorders are so closely interwoven and related that both conditions may represent clinical expressions of the same underlying immunologic derangement.

Several early studies emphasized the importance of cutaneous immune deposits of immunoglobulins in DH (160, 161). It has become clear that dermal papillary and basement membrane IgA deposits represent an almost universal feature of active skin lesions or unin-

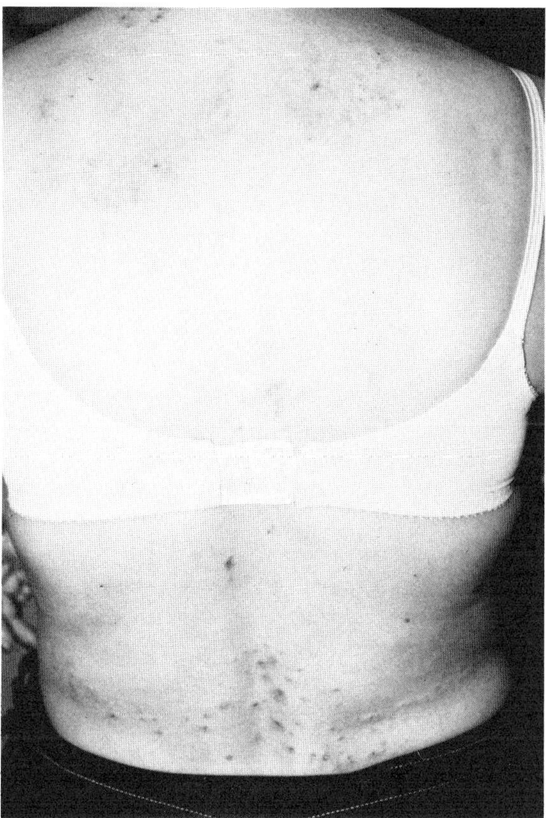

Figure 11-18 Skin lesions in dermatitis herpetiformis. (Photograph courtesy of Lawrence Becker, University of New Mexico School of Medicine, Albuquerque.)

volved normal-appearing skin in this condition. In the summary study involving 80 biopsies from 50 patients by Seah and Fry (162), IgA deposition was found in two basic patterns: the more common one involved IgA staining in dermal papillae and was recorded as the only pattern in 67 of 78 biopsies; the less common pattern was that of continuous band-like staining of IgA deposits at the dermal-epidermal junction. This was seen as the only pattern in 7 of 78 biopsies. In only 2 biopsies included in this study combined patterns showing papillary and basement membrane staining were noted. IgM and occasionally IgG were present in similar distribution. Several reports have extended these original observations, principally using electron microscopic examination and immunologic techniques

(163–165). In the studies by Stingl and colleagues (165) IgA was found in the upper papillary dermis in association with microfibrillar bundles and the microfibrillar components of elastic tissues. In this particular study there was apparent sparing of IgA physically fixed to the basal lamina. It was suggested by these authors that binding to microfibrils in skin might be related to gluten-antigluten IgA-bearing complexes present in such patients. Several reports had previously shown that patients with DH and coeliac disease demonstrated serum antireticulin antibodies (166, 167). In addition, previous studies by Seah and co-workers (161) had indicated that antireticulin antibodies in sera from patients with DH or coeliac disease could be removed by absorption with gluten or purified gluten fraction III. In view of the binding of IgA to fibrillar structures in dermal papillae in immunoelectron microscopic studies, it is possible that adherence was occurring on the basis of cross-reactions between antigluten antibodies and reticulin fibrils localized to these segments. Against such an interpretation, however, was that antireticulin antibodies had previously been demonstrated to be mainly of IgG class (166, 167).

The strong clinical and immunologic overlap between DH and gluten-sensitive enteropathy has been apparent from the beginning in many of the clinical and laboratory studies of these disorders. Since immune reactivity to gluten and antigluten antibodies had been extensively studied with respect to coeliac disease, it seemed possible that IgA skin fixation of immunoglobulin that occurred in DH alone, or DH in combination with gluten-sensitive enteropathy, might represent antibodies against gluten manufactured or stimulated by a primary immune response in the gut and localizing for unknown reasons to dermal structures. A test of this hypothesis would necessarily involve direct elution of IgA from DH-immune skin deposits and measurement of specific antibody activities against gluten and a variety of other antigens. To our knowledge such data are not yet available. Several studies have indicated that maintenance of DH patients on gluten-free diets for periods of 6 to 36 months is often associated with striking improvement in their skin lesions and/or requirement for maintenance suppressive dapsone or sulfone medication (168, 169). In one study (169) complete remissions were only observed in patients who maintained a gluten-free program.

In similar fashion a large proportion of patients with DH show morphological changes on intestinal biopsy compatible with gluten-sensitive enteropathy (170, 171). Furthermore, when patients with DH showing normal intestinal microvilli were challenged with gluten, subsequent morphological changes of flattened intestinal microvilli were noted (172). From these and numerous other clinical observations, it seems clear that sensitivity to gluten and clinical or subclinical sprue are directly related to the pathogenesis of DH.

The finding of predominant IgA deposits in the skin in this condition stands out as an exception to most of the other cutaneous disorders associated with immune-complex formation. If IgA-containing complexes are associated in any primary way with the genesis of the skin lesions, their presence in substantial amounts within the dermis must be explained. A problem in any theoretical consideration of this kind is the practical steps by which IgA deposits might be inciting or amplifying an inflammatory response. In the early report by Seah and co-workers (161), several patients with apparent C3 binding in addition to IgA were noted. It was suggested that aggregated IgA could perforce activate the alternate complement pathway thereby inducing chemotaxis and other parameters of the inflammatory process. This particular aspect of the clinical problem, at this juncture, needs more detailed sequential study. A search for secretory or 11 S IgA of gut origin would be in order with respect to DH, since if the deposits contained mainly secretory IgA instead of IgA derived from serum it would be a strong argument for primary derivation of sensitization through secretory surfaces of the gastrointestinal tract. Cutaneous IgA deposits in DH are characteristically found in normal-appearing uninvolved skin, so it seems to us most likely that they represent an epiphenomenon, which may be related to the nature or immunochemical qualities of the primary sensitizing antigen. Thus it

is possible that features of the primary antigenic stimulus, whether it be gluten or some other component related to gluten, are particularly efficient in calling forth an IgA immune response. Certain physical properties of the putative antigens involved may make them predisposed to stick to or lodge in the dermal papillae and basement membranes. After this sort of fixation IgA antibodies become trapped when antigen is fixed, and cutaneous deposits may be formed often without gross association to the papular or vesicular lesions. Until the identity and physical characteristics of the precise antigens participating in the skin deposits can be ascertained, this question will not be clarified. The theoretical problem of the presence of IgA in cutaneous structures associated with DH is similar to that posed by patients with IgA nephropathy, since the responsible antigens in both conditions are still unknown.

Dermatitis Herpetiformis and HLA

Dermatitis herpetiformis appears to be closely linked to HLA-B8. The association is particularly strong and has now been confirmed by a number of independent laboratories (173–177). The HLA-B8 antigen is present in approximately three to four times the prevalence in patients with DH as compared with controls. This association implies that predisposition to develop the disorder may be directly related to HLA-phenotype or more importantly IR genes linked to such a phenotype. Since IR genes in humans are most closely associated with the HLA-D or B-cell typing systems, it is apparent that HLA-D typing may further amplify or refine this particular relationship.

Circulating Immune Complexes in DH

The specific association between actual circulating immune complexes and the skin lesions of DH is still not completely understood. Examination of complement component profiles including C1q, C4, C2, C3, C3PA, and total hemolytic complement by Berrens and colleagues (178) showed no evidence of consumption of complement or activation of either the conventional or alternate complement pathways in serum from DH patients. Local activation of the alternate complement pathway by the action of polymeric or aggregated IgA as suggested by the studies of Seah and co-workers (179) might conceivably still take place without manifesting itself by detectable gross alterations of C3 or C3PA in whole serum. Research on catabolism and synthesis of isolated complement components in patients with DH will be necessary before this question can be resolved.

Several other observations suggest that elevations of circulating immune complexes are present in serum samples of patients with DH. Using an anticomplementary method, an initial report (180) indicated apparent complexes in 80 percent of 15 patients taking a normal diet, whereas only 36 percent of 11 subjects on a gluten-free regime showed anticomplementary activity. Sephadex gel filtration showed that anticomplementary activity in serum coincided with fractions of intermediate (8 to 10 S) size. No absorptions or tests for the immunoglobulin composition of these complexes were presented in this paper. A subsequent report (181) employing three parallel methods for immune-complex assay revealed complexes in all of 59 patients with DH studied. In contrast to the previous work of Berrens and co-workers (178), low serum C3 was detected in approximately half the DH patients examined. The three methods used for immune-complex assay in this study included polyethylene glycol precipitation, the guinea pig macrophage radioimmunoassay technique, and C1q binding. Analysis of immunoglobulin content of polyethylene glycol precipitates from sera showing positive tests for immune complexes revealed IgG and IgM but no evidence of IgA. The variety of different immunoglobulins in these precipitates was interpreted as evidence for presence of different types of complexes in the DH sera. Absence of IgA within the complexes studied was thought to be strong evidence against their direct correlation with tissue deposition in skin where IgA predominates. Thus although circulating serum immune complexes were detected in a majority of the large number of patients studied by Mohammed and colleagues (181), their direct implication in the pathogenesis of skin lesions was not established. These studies reemphasize the importance of exercising restraint in equilibrating presence of detectable immune complexes in any disease state with the pathology involved in a discrete location. This is highlighted by the work of Cooney and co-workers (182), who studied skin biopsies and small bowel tissue from a group of 18 patients with DH. No correlation was found between the histological severity of the skin and small bowel lesions, emphasizing that the degree of disease activity discernible by microscopic examination in the two areas most commonly affected by the disorder may not be the same in individual patients.

Pemphigus and Bullous Pemphigoid

Pemphigus and bullous pemphigoid involvement of the skin are vesiculobullous disorders analogous to renal diseases such as Goodpasture's syndrome and are characterized by specific antibody to various basement membrane structures. The basic lesion in pemphigus is clinically associated with flaccid weeping bullous lesions and denuded areas of skin, and microscopically associated with intraepidermal bulla formation and loss of cohesion between epidermal cells termed acantholysis. Typical clinical appearance of such lesions is shown in Figure 11-19. Bullous pemphigoid, which chiefly affects elderly subjects, is characterized by large tense blisters often involving intertriginous areas and formation of subepidermal bullae. These two conditions may be compared to Goodpasture's syndrome, since they correlate with circulating autoantibodies apparently directed at epidermal and mucosal antigens associated with the disease. In pemphigus the antigens have been localized to intercellular sites and in the case of bullous pemphigoid to basement membrane zones (183–186). Tissue-directed antibodies are capable of fixing complement in vivo; components of both classical and alternative pathways have been identified in skin lesions from both diseases in association with immunoglobulins (187–189). Bullous pemphigoid antibodies in serum, but not pemphigus antibodies, can be shown to fix complement in vitro using an immunofluorescent system (190, 191). Comple-

whereas in others the level of C1q binding and antibody to skin increased and decreased in parallel. It was presumed that C1q binding in this large series was unaffected by reactivity with free DNA in serum, because DNAse digestion of positive samples did not substantially reduce C1q binding values. It is unclear from cumulative data to date that the finding of circulating immune complexes in such patients occurs as a secondary phenomenon or whether, alternatively, immune complexes as such participate in generation or augmentation of the characteristic skin lesions. The previous studies documenting low complement levels in blister fluid with concomitant normal serum complement activities (192, 193) suggest that local activation of complement may occur largely in bullous and other skin sites rather than in the circulation as a whole. However, strong support for an immune-complex–mediated mechanism is apparent from the study of immunoglobulin and complement deposits within skin lesions of these two disorders.

Anaphylactoid Purpura

Generally the syndrome of anaphylactoid purpura is associated with purpuric skin lesions, synovial swelling, and arthralgias; occasionally with frank arthritis, glomerulonephritis, and hemorrhagic gastrointestinal lesions. Much like systemic lupus, the basic disease process seems to be accompanied by a generalized vasculitis (196, 197). Particularly when it occurs in late childhood and among adults, this disorder has been associated with a severe and progressive degree of glomerular injury. Direct examination of skin biopsy material in small groups of individuals has provided evidence for an immune-complex etiology. In a study published in 1973 by Faille-Kuyper and colleagues (198) IgA deposits were noted within cutaneous vessel walls. A subsequent study of skin lesions (199) revealed IgM, IgA, and C3 at the dermal-epidermal junction and in vessel walls of clinically involved and apparently normal skin. These findings are similar to those previously documented in SLE and in the numerous other examples of presumed immune-complex cutaneous injury previously

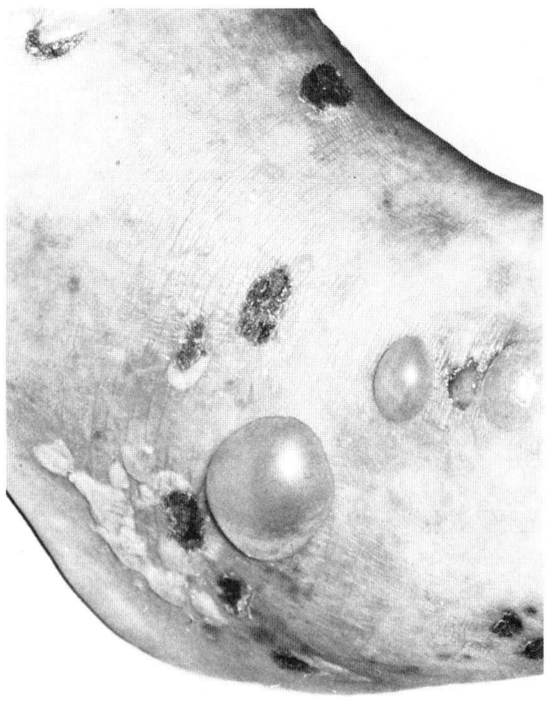

Figure 11-19 Skin lesions seen in pemphigus. (Photograph courtesy of St. John's Hospital for Diseases of the Skin, London.)

ment component profile studies of blister fluids from patients with both of these diseases reflect predominant classical complement pathway activation (192, 193). Studies of serum samples from these patients have also shown anticomplementary activity in high-molecular-weight fractions from pemphigus and pemphigoid blister fluids (192, 194).

A recent study (195) has extended these findings using the C1q radioimmunoassay and precipitation of serum samples with 1.5 percent polyethylene glycol. Detectable immune complexes were found in 40 percent of sera from 71 patients with pemphigus and 20 percent of 142 patients with bullous pemphigoid. A relationship between C1q binding and disease activity was apparent. In some patients an increase of C1q binding followed a detectable increment in antibody to cutaneous antigens,

discussed in this chapter. Parallel renal biopsy frequently shows immune deposits of immunoglobulins, properdin (200), other complement components, and fibrinogen within glomeruli. High titers of antinuclear antibody or DNA binding are not present. As yet, a clear explanation of the process involved cannot be given since the actual antigens are unidentified.

Mechanisms of Cutaneous Immune-Complex Deposition

It is apparent from the many observations noted here that immune complexes in the vessels and at the dermal-epidermal junction of the skin have been recorded in an increasingly wide variety of localized and systemic diseases involving the skin. Rapid expansion of the list of disorders showing such findings is to be expected, particularly with the ever broader application of immunofluorescent and electron microscopic techniques.

One of the principal unanswered questions in various examples of immune-complex–mediated phenomena within the skin, beside the identity and immunochemical characterization of the antigens involved, relates to the time sequence of events that occur during the development of lesions. Sams and colleagues (201) studied events in clinically normal skin from 13 patients with necrotizing vasculitis; 9 of the 13 showed C3, and 6 showed IgM or IgA in biopsies of vasculitis lesions. In adjacent apparently normal skin, 7 patients showed either IgM or IgA immune deposits. These findings, together with the previous study that utilized histamine wheal formation in similar patients (21), emphasize that immune-complex deposition occurs before ingress of polymorphonuclear leukocytes and subsequent active fibrinoid necrosis of vessels. It is evident that the timing of biopsies in relation to the actual histological evolution of tissue damage may be important in accurate documentation of immune reactants in the same locations.

The experiments in animal models by Cochrane and Weigle (202) also stress the fact that polymorphonuclear leukocytes will ingest and catabolize immune complexes and similar reactants within 24 to 28 hours of actual deposition. The precise mechanisms at work in localization of immune complexes in some vascular areas and not others are still poorly understood and must relate to the influence of other, as yet undefined, local factors. One of the puzzling features is the frequent finding of C3 or even properdin component fixation in blood vessels without concurrent convincing parallel demonstration of reacting immunoglobulin. Several theoretical possibilities may explain such findings: it is conceivable that antigens implicated in the vasculitis are capable of direct complement activation without intermediary immunoglobulin of any type. This mechanism has now been convincingly demonstrated for Gram-negative bacterial lipopolysaccharides and may possibly relate to a number of other classes of still undefined common materials. More likely is the possibility that the complement components visible by immunofluorescence represent an amplification system whereby small numbers of Ig-antigen complexes are capable of activation of much larger numbers of complement molecules.

Immune-Complex Materials

Few definitive studies have been published bearing directly on the exact nature of circulating or skin-fixing complexes associated with immune-complex–mediated phenomena in the skin. This probably represents the single most glaring omission in the work done on this subject to date. One observation of interest suggesting phlogistic properties somehow intrinsic to certain cryoproteins was emphasized in the studies of Whitsed and Penny (203). Both whole plasma and isolated cryoglobulin protein from a patient with mixed cryoglobulinemia and necrotizing vasculitis produced skin lesions similar to those that occurred spontaneously when injected intradermally in the same patient. Similar results have been reported by Verrier-Jones and colleagues (204), who also studied a patient with acute necrotizing vasculitis. In this instance negative tests for circulating immune complexes were present in serum as monitored by anticomplementary activity, reaction with monoclonal rheumatoid factor, and precipitin formation with C1q. However, when the patient's whole serum was injected intradermally, lesions were produced that again closely approximated the spontaneous lesions associated with the disorder itself. Fractionation of serum indicated that the skin-reactive components were associated with IgG of higher molecular weight than normal IgG, suggesting intrinsic complex formation. Immunofluorescent studies showed that cutaneous lesions induced by the higher-molecular-weight IgG contained both IgG and complement deposited in the epidermal basement membrane zone and within the dermal vessels. Subsequent plasmapheresis induced some clinical improvement. From the physical separation data involving Sephadex G–200 gel filtration of serum given in this report, the active fraction appeared somewhere between the 19 S and 7 S peaks. A peculiar finding was that the isolated skin-reactive IgG fractions were negative in the anticomplementary test for presumed immune complexes. This could have occurred as a result of adsorption to the complex materials of complement components that had already undergone spontaneous activation in vivo, thus blocking reactive sites necessary for activity in the anticomplementary assay. Of particular note was the finding of localization of injected presumed complex material to the dermal basement membrane zones.

These data suggest that this constantly recurring theme—dermal-epidermal junctional localization—must be telling us something about the local topography or absorbent properties for immune complexes in the skin. In addition, dermal junctional deposits are seen in miscellaneous vasculitis associated with facial granuloma or cutaneous vasculitis. We have already suggested two possible mechanisms for immune-complex trapping in this area related to induction or exposure of receptors for activated C3, Fc, or immunoglobulins; or in the case of SLE local release of DNA from normal cell turnover. It is possible that the physical density of the various layers of the skin acts as a gel-filtering mechanism whereby immune complexes of a particular size and associated with a number of heterogeneous conditions are filtered out and trapped at the junctional or basement membrane zone. Direct physical testing with a range of labeled molecules of differing sizes or physical properties might be used to test this hypothesis. In the case of SLE, the natural affinity between DNA and collagen fibrils might reinforce or accentuate a natural built-in mechanism for trapping complexes that are either locally produced or enter the area through lymphatics and circulating blood supply. Dermal-epidermal junctional trapping of high-molecular-weight or intermediate-sized immune complexes might even be looked on as a built-in protective mechanism whereby the largest organ by wet weight in the body—namely, the skin—can trap complexes and therefore splint or protect more vulnerable capillary networks, as in the glomeruli or choroid plexus. A diagrammatic representation of this hypothesis is shown in Figure 11-20. It should be recognized that this schema at present merely represents an hypothesis and must still be tested directly for degree of validity. The importance of the dermal-epidermal junctional layer in immune-complex localization within the skin is emphasized by Table 11-4, which shows the wide variety of conditions that have been recorded with this type of finding.

One of the most important aspects affecting insight into skin diseases of presumed immune-complex etiology is lucid definition of the putative antigens involved. Finding immunoglobulins and complement in dermal capillaries of normal or affected skin in various diverse conditions is only half the battle. The real problem lies in understanding how various antigens or external agents precipitate the lesions in many of the diseases in question. From the state of the art at present, considerable attention must be directed at animal models or in vivo assays in affected patients to ascertain why immune-complex reactants keep turning up at the dermal-epidermal junction. Moreover, experimental approaches aimed at an understanding of the physical or immunochemical changes that may occur in the porosity or adhesiveness of this structure during various disease states is also in order. Such

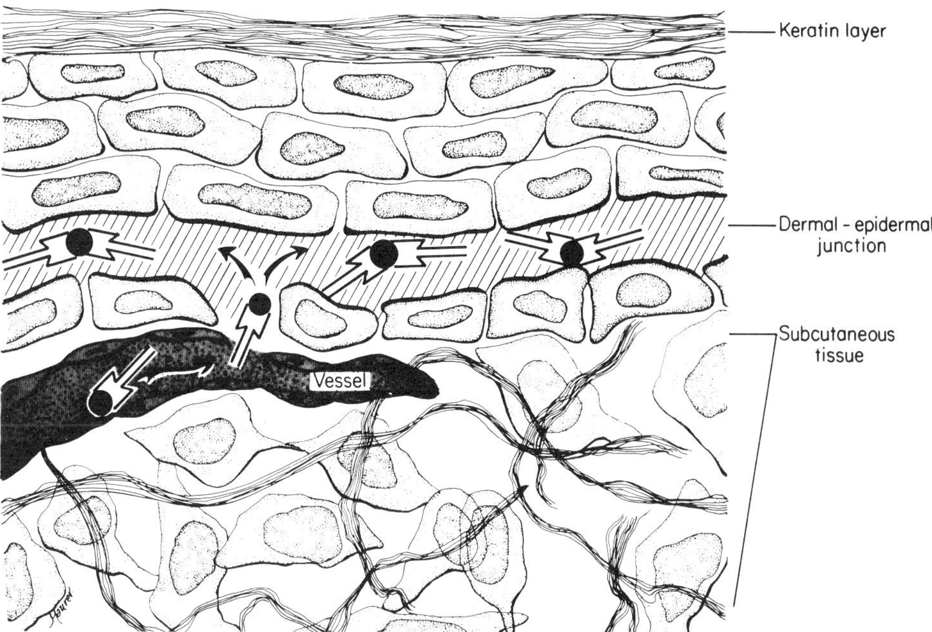

Figure 11-20   Possible schema for physical or immunochemical properties of the dermal-epidermal junction zone that attract or localize immune complexes reaching the area through dermal capillaries.

parallel changes occurring independently of actual immune-complex deposition might be much more important than the adherence of immune complexes themselves. The skin and its vascular supply afford a large and accessible arena for the study of these various phenomena. Future work must clarify the broad spectrum of changes now attributed to cutaneous immune-complex phenomena.

Table 11-4   Primary conditions in which immunoglobulins and/or complement have been observed at dermal-epidermal junctions.

Disease state (reference)	Most common immune deposits observed
Systemic lupus erythematosus (55–70)	IgG, IgM, C3, C4, properdin, C3A
Porphyria (205)	IgG, IgM
Leprosy (206)	IgG, IgM, C3
Graft vs host reactions (128)	IgM, C3
Facial granuloma (92)	IgG, IgM, IgA, C3
Necrotizing vasculitis (90–92, 111)	IgG, IgM, C3, IgD
Anaphylactoid purpura (207)	IgM, IgA, C3
Necrobiosis lipoidica (139)	IgM, C3
Granuloma annulare (157)	IgM, C3
Dermatitis herpetiformis (161, 162)	IgA, IgM
Herpes gestationis (73–75, 79)	C3, properdin, C5, IgG, C1q

References

1. Opie, E. L. Inflammatory reaction of the immune animal to antigen (Arthus phenomenon) and its relation to antibodies. *J. Immunol.* 9:231, 1924.

2. Ishizaka, K., and Campbell, D. H. Biological activity of soluble antigen-antibody complexes. I. Skin reactive properties. *Proc. Soc. Exp. Biol. Med.* 97:635, 1958.

3. Spector, W. G., and Heesom, N. The production of granulomata by antigen-antibody complexes. *J. Pathol.* 98:31, 1969.

4. Kohn, J. L., McCabe, E. J., and Brem, J. Anaphylactic gangrene following administration of horse serum. *Am. J. Dis. Child.* 55:1018, 1938.

5. Pepys, J. Hypersensitivity diseases of the lungs due to fungi and organic dusts. In *Monographs in Allergy,* No. 4. Karger, Basel, 1969.

6. Osment, L. S. Acanthosis nigricans due to gastric adenocarcinoma. *Int. J. Dermatol.* 15:450, 1976.

7. Liddell, K., and Jensen, N. E. Malignant acanthosis nigricans and its unusual association with carcinoma of the colon and carcinoma of the cervix. *Br. J. Surg.* 63:248, 1976.

8. Williams, R. C., Jr. Dermatomyositis and malignancy: a review of the literature. *Ann. Intern. Med.* 50:1174, 1959.

9. Kazmierowski, J. A., and Wuepper, K. W. Immune complex vasculitis of the superficial cutaneous microvasculature. *Clin. Res.* 25:282A, 1977.

10. Osler, W. On the visceral complications of erythema exudativum multiforme. *Am. J. Med. Sci.* 110:629, 1895.

11. Baer, R. L. Perspective erythema multiforme—1976. *Am. J. Med. Sci.* 271:119, 1976.

12. Ackerman, A. B., Penneys, N. S., and Clark, W. H. Erythema multiforme exudativum: distinctive pathological process. *Br. J. Dermatol.* 84:554, 1971.

13. Lever, W. F., and Schaumburg-Lever, G. Erythema multiforme. In *Histopathology of the Skin,* ed. 5, p. 122. J. B. Lippincott Co., Philadelphia, 1975.

14. Bedi, T. R., and Pinkus, H. Histopathological spectrum of erythema multiforme. *Br. J. Dermatol.* 95:243, 1976.

15. Krueger, G. G., Weston, W. L., Thorne, E. G., et al. A phenomenon of macrophage aggregation activity in sera of patients with exfoliative erythroderma, erythema multiforme and erythema nodosum. *J. Invest. Dermatol.* 60:282, 1973.

16. Ashby, D., and Lazar, T. Erythema multiforme exudativum major (Stevens-Johnson syndrome). *Lancet* 1:1091, 1951.

17. Costello, M. Erythema multiforme exudativum (erythema bullosum malignans-pluriorificial type). Personal observations of cases in Willard Parker Hospital for Contagious Diseases (1932–1946). *J. Invest. Dermatol.* 8:127, 1947.

18. Champion, R. H. Disorders affecting small blood vessels—erythema and telangiectasia. In A. J. Rook, D. S. Wilkinson, and F. J. G. Ebling, eds., *Textbook of Dermatology,* ed. 2, p. 891. Blackwell Scientific Publications, Oxford, 1972.

19. MacDonald, A., and Feiwel, M. Isolation of herpes virus from erythema multiforme. *Br. Med. J.* 2:570, 1972.

20. Britz, M., and Sibulkin, D. Recurrent erythema multiforme and Herpes genitalis (type 2). *J.A.M.A.* 233:812, 1975.

21. Braverman, I. M., and Yen, A. Demonstration of immune complexes in spontaneous and histamine-induced lesions and in normal skin of patients with leukocytoblastic angitis. *J. Invest. Dermatol.* 64:105, 1975.

22. Kawasaki, T., Kosaki, F., Okawa, S., et al. A new infantile acute febrile mucocutaneous lymph node syndrome (MLNS) prevailing in Japan. *Pediatrics* 54:271, 1974.

23. Yanagisawa, M., Kobayashi, N., and Matsuya, S. Myocardial infarction due to coronary thromboarteritis, following acute febrile mucocutaneous lymph node syndrome (MLNS) in an infant. *Pediatrics* 54:277, 1974.

24. Safai, B., Good, R. A., and Day, N. K. Erythema multiforme: report of two cases and speculation on immune mechanisms involved in the pathogenesis. *Clin. Immunol. Immunopathol.* 7:379, 1977.

25. Agnello, V., Ruddy, S., Winchester, R., et al. Hereditary C2 deficiency in systemic lupus erythematosus and acquired complement abnormalities in unusual SLE-related syndromes. In D. Bergsma, R. A. Good, and J. Finstad, eds., *Immunodeficiency in Man and Animals,* p. 312. Birth Defects Original Article Series, vol. 11. Krieger, New York, 1975.

26. Oishi, M., Takano, M., Miyachi, K., et al. A case of unusual SLE related syndrome characterized by erythema multiforme, angioneurotic edema, marked hypocomplementemia, and C1q precipitins of the low molecular weight type. *Int. Arch. Allergy Appl. Immunol.* 50:463, 1976.

27. Gordon, H. Erythema nodosum: a review of one hundred and fifteen cases. *Br. J. Dermatol.* 73:393, 1961.

28. Löfgren, S. Erythema nodosum: studies on

etiology and pathogenesis in 185 adult cases. *Acta Med. Scand.* 24:1, 1946 (suppl. 174).

29. Wallgren, A. Erythema nodosum and pulmonary tuberculosis. *Lancet* 1:359, 1938.

30. Doxiadis, S. A. Erythema nodosum in children: a review. *Medicine* 30:283, 1951.

31. Mygind, N., and Thulin, H. Yersinia enterocolitica: a new cause of erythema nodosum. *Br. J. Dermatol.* 82:351, 1970.

32. Schwarz, J., and Muth, J. Coccidiomycocis: a review. *Am. J. Med. Sci.* 221:89, 1951.

33. Jacobs, W. H. Erythema nodosum in inflammatory diseases of the bowel. *Gastroenterology* 37:286, 1959.

34. Sumaya, C. V., Babu, S., and Reed, R. J. Erythema nodosum-like lesions of leukemia. *Arch. Dermatol.* 110:415, 1974.

35. Winkelmann, R. K., and Förström, L. New observations in the histopathology of erythema nodosum. *J. Invest. Dermatol.* 65:441, 1975.

36. Löfgren, S., and Wahlgren, F. On the histopathology of erythema nodosum. *Acta Derm. Venereol. (Stockh.)* 29:1, 1949.

37. Rea, T. H., and Levan, N. E. Erythema nodosum leprosum in a general hospital. *Arch. Dermatol.* 3:1575, 1975.

38. Waters, M. F., Turk, J. L., and Wemambu, S. N. Mechanisms of reactions in leprosy. *Int. J. Lepr.* 39:417, 1971.

39. Moran, C. J., Ryder, G., Turk, J. L., et al. Evidence for circulating immune complexes in lepromatous leprosy. *Lancet* 2:572, 1972.

40. Rojas-Espinosa, O., Mendez-Navarrete, I., and Estrada-Parra, S. Presence of C1q-reactive immune complexes in patients with leprosy. *Clin. Exp. Immunol.* 12:215, 1972.

41. Gelber, R. H., Drutz, D. J., Epstein, W. V., et al. Clinical correlates of C1q-precipitating substances in the sera of patients with leprosy. *Am. J. Trop. Med. Hyg.* 23:471, 1974.

42. Tung, K. S. K., Kim, B., Bjorvatn, B., et al. Discrepancy between C1q deviation and Raji cell tests in the detection of circulating immune complexes in leprosy. *J. Infect. Dis.* 136:216, 1977.

43. Londono, F., Patarroyo, M. E., Duran de Rueda, M. M., et al. Erythema nodosum leprosum. *Arch. Dermatol.* 113:234, 1977.

44. Williams, R. C., Jr., Tung, K. S. K., and Montano, J. D. Unpublished observations.

45. Reichlin, M., Pranis, R. A., Gelber, R. H., et al. Correlation of euglobulin immunoglobulin G levels with erythema nodosum leprosum in lepromatous leprosy. *Clin. Immunol. Immunopathol.* 8:335, 1977.

46. Pettit, J. H. S., and Waters, M. F. R. The etiology of erythema nodosum leprosum. *Int. J. Lepr.* 35:1, 1967.

47. Ridley, D. S. Reactions in leprosy. *Lepr. Rev.* 40:77, 1969.

48. Kunkel, H. G., Simon, H. J., and Fudenberg, H. H. Observations concerning positive serologic reactions for rheumatoid factor in certain patients with sarcoidosis and other hyperglobulinemic states. *Arthritis Rheum.* 1:289, 1958.

49. Oreskes, I., and Siltzbach, L. E. Changes in rheumatoid factor activity during the course of sarcoidosis. *Am. J. Med.* 44:60, 1968.

50. Mellors, R. C., Ortega, L. G., Noyes, W. F., et al. Further pathogenetic studies of diseases of unknown etiology, with particular reference to disseminated lupus erythematosus and Boeck's sarcoid. *Am. J. Pathol.* 33:613, 1957.

51. Wanstrup, J., and Elling, P. Immunohistochemistry of sarcoidosis. *Acta Pathol. Microbiol. Scand.* 73:37, 1968.

52. Ghose, T., Landrigan, P., and Asif, A. Localization of immunoglobulin and complement in pulmonary sarcoid granulomas. *Chest* 66:264, 1974.

53. Hedfors, E., and Norberg, R. Evidence for circulating immune complexes in sarcoidosis. *Clin. Exp. Immunol.* 16:493, 1974.

54. Verrier-Jones, J., Cumming, R. H., Asplin, C. M., et al. Evidence for circulating immune complexes in erythema nodosum and early sarcoidosis. *Ann. N.Y. Acad. Sci.* 278:212, 1976.

55. Burnham, T. K., Neblett, T. R., and Fine, G. The application of fluorescent antibody technique to the investigation of lupus erythematosus and various dermatoses. *J. Invest. Dermatol.* 41:451, 1963.

56. Cormane, R. H. "Bound" globulin in skin of patients with chronic discoid lupus erythematosus and systemic lupus erythematosus. *Lancet* 1:534, 1964.

57. Tan, E. M., and Kunkel, H. G. An immunofluorescent study of the skin lesions in systemic lupus erythematosus. *Arthritis Rheum.* 9:37, 1966.

58. Pohle, E. L., and Tuffanelli, D. L. Study of cutaneous lupus erythematosus by immunohistochemical methods. *Arch. Dermatol.* 97:520, 1968.

59. Landry, M., and Sams, W. M., Jr. Basement-membrane antibodies in two patients with systemic lupus erythematosus. *Lancet* 1:821, 1972.

60. Rothfield, N., Ross, H. A., Minta, J. O., et al. Glomerular and dermal deposition of properdin in systemic lupus erythematosus. *N. Engl. J. Med.* 287:681, 1972.

61. Landry, M., and Sams, W. M., Jr. Systemic

lupus erythematosus. Studies of the antibodies bound to skin. *J. Clin. Invest.* 52:1871, 1973.

62. Thivolet, J., Beyvin, A. J., and Le Mot, J. Elution des anticorps fixes *in vivo* au niveau de la peau au cours du pemphigus, de la pemphigoide bulleuse et du lupus érythémateux. *Lyon Medicale* 227:241, 1972.

63. Gilliam, J. N., Cheatum, D. E., Hurd, E. R., et al. Immunoglobulin in clinically uninvolved skin in systemic lupus erythematosus. Association with renal disease. *J. Clin. Invest.* 53:1434, 1974.

64. Caperton, E. M., Jr., Bean, S. F., and Dick, F. R. Immunofluorescent skin test in systemic lupus erythematosus. Lack of relationship with renal disease. *J.A.M.A.* 222:935, 1972.

65. Schrager, M. A., and Rothfield, N. F. Clinical significance of serum properdin levels and properdin deposition in the dermal-epidermal junction in systemic lupus erythematosus. *J. Clin. Invest.* 57:212, 1976.

66. Burnham, T. K., and Fine, G. The immunofluorescent "Band" test for lupus erythematosus. III. Employing clinically normal skin. *Arch. Dermatol.* 103:24, 1971.

67. Burnham, T. K. Immunofluorescent test for lupus erythematosus: relation to renal disease. *J.A.M.A.* 223:798, 1973.

68. Grishman, E., and Churg, J. Ultrastructure of dermal lesions in systemic lupus erythematosus. *Lab. Invest.* 22:189, 1970.

69. Tuffanelli, D. L. Lupus erythematosus. *Arch. Dermatol.* 106:553, 1972.

70. Jordon, R. E., Schroeter, A. L., and Winkelmann, R. K. Dermal-epidermal deposition of complement components and properdin in systemic lupus erythematosus. *Br. J. Dermatol.* 92:263, 1975.

71. Lief, P. D., Barland, P., and Bank, N. Diagnosis of lupus nephritis by skin immunofluorescence, in the absence of extrarenal manifestations of systemic lupus erythematosus. *Am. J. Med.* 63:441, 1977.

72. Levitin, P. M., Weary, P. E., and Giuliano, V. J. The immunofluorescent "band" test in mixed connective tissue disease. *Ann. Intern. Med.* 83:53, 1975.

73. Jordon, R. E., Heine, K. G., Tappeiner, G., et al. The immunopathology of herpes gestationis. Immunofluorescence studies and characterization of 'HG factor'. *J. Clin. Invest.* 57:1426, 1976.

74. Katz, S. I., Hertz, K. C., and Yaoita, H. Herpes gestationis. Immunopathology and characterization of the HG factor. *J. Clin. Invest.* 57:1434, 1976.

75. Provost, T. T., and Tomasi, T. B., Jr. Evidence for complement activation via the alternate pathway in skin diseases. I. Herpes gestationis, systemic lupus erythematosus, and bullous pemphigoid. *J. Clin. Invest.* 52:1779, 1973.

76. Jablonska, S., Chorzelski, T. P., Beutner, E. H., et al. Immunologic phenomena in herpes gestationis. *Arch. Dermatol. Forsch.* 252:267, 1975.

77. Kocsis, M., Eeg, T. L., Husby, G., et al. Immunofluorescence studies in herpes gestationis. *Acta Derm. Venereol. (Stockh.)* 55:25, 1975.

78. Carruthers, J. A., and Black, M. M. Immunopathological findings in herpes gestationis. *Br. J. Dermatol.* 93:17 (abstract), 1975 (suppl. 11).

79. Bushkell, L. L., Jordon, R. E., and Goltz, R. W. Herpes gestationis. New immunologic findings. *Arch. Dermatol.* 110:65, 1974.

80. Sommer, V. M., Rudofsky, U. H., and Gabrielsen, A. E. Immune complexes in skin of NZB/NZW mice. *Clin. Exp. Immunol.* 22:461, 1975.

81. Gilliam, J. N. The significance of cutaneous immunoglobulin deposits in lupus erythematosus and NZB/NZW F_1 hybrid mice. *J. Invest. Dermatol.* 65:154, 1975.

82. Natali, P. G., and Tan, E. M. Experimental skin lesions in mice resembling systemic lupus erythematosus. *Arithritis Rheum.* 16:579, 1973.

83. Izui, S., Lambert, P. H., and Miescher, P. A. *In vitro* demonstration of a particular affinity of glomerular basement membrane and collagen for DNA. A possible basis for a local formation of DNA-anti-DNA complexes in systemic lupus erythematosus. *J. Exp. Med.* 144:428, 1976.

84. Lowenstein, M. B., and Rothfield, N. F. Family study of systemic lupus erythematosus. Analysis of the clinical history, skin immunofluorescence, and serologic parameters. *Arthritis Rheum.* 20:1293, 1977.

85. DeHoratius, R. J., and Messner, R. P. Lymphocytotoxic antibodies in family members of patients with systemic lupus erythematosus. *J. Clin. Invest.* 55:1254, 1975.

86. DeHoratius, R. J., Pillarisetty, R., Messner, R. P., et al. Anti-nucleic acid antibodies in systemic lupus erythematosus patients and their families. Incidence and correlation with lymphocytotoxic antibodies. *J. Clin. Invest.* 56:1149, 1975.

87. Zeek, P. M. Periarteritis nodosa and other forms of necrotizing angiitis. *N. Engl. J. Med.* 248:764, 1953.

88. Parish, W. E., and Rhodes, E. L. Bacterial antigens and aggregated gamma globulin in the lesions of nodular vasculitis. *Br. J. Dermatol.* 79:131, 1967.

89. Stringa, S. G., Bianchi, C., Casala, A. M., et

al. Allergic vasculitis. Gougerot-Ruiter syndrome: immunofluorescent study. *Arch. Dermatol.* 95:23, 1967.

90. Miescher, P. A., Paronetto, F., and Koffler, D. Immunofluorescent studies in human vasculitis. In P. Grabar and P. Miescher, eds., *4th International Symposium on Immunopathology, Monte Carlo,* p. 446. Grune & Stratton, New York, 1965.

91. Scott, D. G., and Rowell, N. R. Preliminary investigations of arteritic lesions using fluorescent antibody techniques. *Br. J. Dermatol.* 77:211, 1965.

92. Schroeter, A. L., Copeman, P. W. M., Jordon, R. E., et al. Immunofluorescence of cutaneous vasculitis associated with systemic disease. *Arch. Dermatol.* 104:254, 1971.

93. Levenson, H., and Cochrane, C. G. Nonprecipitating antibody and the Arthus vasculitis. *J. Immunol.* 92:118, 1964.

94. McDuffie, F. C., Sams, W. M., Jr., Maldonado, J. E., et al. Hypocomplementemia with cutaneous vasculitis and arthritis. Possible immune complex syndrome. *Mayo Clin. Proc.* 48:340, 1973.

95. Soter, N. A., Austen, K. F., and Gigli, I. The complement system in necrotizing angiitis of the skin. Analysis of complement component activities in serum of patients with concomitant collagen-vascular diseases. *J. Invest. Dermatol.* 63:219, 1974.

96. Conn, D. L., Schroeter, A. L., and McDuffie, F. C. Cutaneous vessel immune deposits in rheumatoid arthritis. *Arthritis Rheum.* 19:15, 1976.

97. Epstein, W. V., and Engleman, E. P. The relation of the rheumatoid factor content of serum to clinical neurovascular manifestations of rheumatoid arthritis. *Arthritis Rheum.* 2:250, 1959.

98. Hunder, G. G., and McDuffie, F. C. Hypocomplementemia in rheumatoid arthritis. *Am. J. Med.* 54:461, 1973.

99. Conn, D. L., McDuffie, F. C., and Dyck, P. J. Immunopathologic study of sural nerves in rheumatoid arthritis. *Arthritis Rheum.* 15:135, 1972.

100. Kulka, J. P., Bocking, D., Ropes, M. W., et al. Early joint lesions of rheumatoid arthritis: report of eight cases, with knee biopsies of lesions of less than one year's duration. *Arch. Pathol.* 59:129, 1955.

101. Sokoloff, L., McCluskey, R. T., and Bunim, J. J. Vascularity of the early subcutaneous nodule of rheumatoid arthritis. *Arch. Pathol.* 55:475, 1953.

102. Muijs van de Moer, W. W., and Cats, A. Immunofluorescence of the skin in patients with rheumatoid arthritis: a preliminary report. *Dermatologica* 134:351, 1967.

103. Huber, O., and Higmans, W. Immuno-

fluorescence on skin biopsies from patients with rheumatoid arthritis. In W. Müller, H.-G. Harwerth, and K. Fehr, eds., *Rheumatoid Arthritis: Pathogenetic Mechanisms and Consequences in Therapeutics,* p. 429. Academic Press, New York, 1971.

104. Larsson, O. Studies of small vessels in patients with diabetes: a clinical, histological and immunohistochemical study of diabetic and non-diabetic subjects with special reference to the occurrence of various plasma proteins in the dermal vessel walls. *Acta Med. Scand. (Suppl.)* 480:1, 1967.

105. Williams, R. C., Jr., and Montaño, J. D. Unpublished observations, 1976.

106. Glass, D., Soter, N. A., Gibson, D., et al. Association between HLA and cutaneous necrotizing venulitis. *Arthritis Rheum.* 19:945, 1976.

107. Cream, J. J. Anticomplementary sera in cutaneous vasculitis. *Br. J. Dermatol.* 89:555, 1973.

108. Ishizaka, T., Ishizaka, K., and Borsos, T. Biological activity of aggregated γ-globulin. IV. Mechanism of complement fixation. *J. Immunol.* 87:433, 1961.

109. Castañedo, J. P., and Williams, R. C., Jr. Anticomplementary activity of sera from patients with connective tissue disease and normal subjects. *J. Lab. Clin. Med.* 69:217, 1967.

110. Polley, M. J., and Mollison, P. L. The role of complement in the detection of blood group antibodies: special reference to the antiglobulin test. *Transfusion* 1:9, 1961.

111. Weidner, F. Immunofluorescent investigations in cutaneous vasculitis. II. Histotopical demonstration of IgD and fibrin. *Arch. Dermatol. Res.,* 254:215, 1975.

112. Rowe, D. S., and Fahey, J. L. A new class of human immunoglobulins. I. A unique myeloma protein. *J. Exp. Med.* 121:171, 1965.

113. Gleich, G. J., Bieger, R. C., and Stankievic, R. Antigen combining activity associated with immunoglobulin D. *Science* 165:606, 1969.

114. Kantor, G. L., Van Herle, A. J., and Barnett, E. V. Auto-antibodies of the IgD class. *Clin. Exp. Immunol.* 6:951, 1970.

115. Vitetta, E. S., and Uhr, J. W. Immunoglobulin-receptors revisited. A model for the differentiation of bone-marrow derived lymphocytes is described. *Science* 189:964, 1975.

116. Scott, D. W., Layton, J. E., and Nossal, G. J. V. Role of IgD in the immune response and tolerance. I. Anti-δ pretreatment facilitates tolerance induction in adult B cells *in vitro. J. Exp. Med.* 146:1473, 1977.

117. Vitetta, E. S., Cambier, J. C., Ligler, F. S., et al. B-cell tolerance. IV. Differential role of surface

IgM and IgD in determining tolerance susceptibility of murine B cells. *J. Exp. Med.* 146:1804, 1977.

118. Milian, G. Les atrophies cutanées syphilitiques. *Bull. Soc. Fr. Dermatol. Syphiligr.* 36:865, 1929.

119. Feldaker, M., Hines, E. A., Jr., Kierland, R. R. Livedo reticularis with ulcerations. *Circulation* 13:196, 1956.

120. Nelson, L. M. Atrophie blanche en plaque. *Arch. Dermatol.* 72:242, 1955.

121. Gray, H. R., Graham, J. H., Johnson, W., et al. Atrophie blanche: periodic painful ulcers of lower extremities: a clinical and histopathological entity. *Arch. Dermatol.* 93:187, 1966.

122. Bard, J. W., and Winkelmann, R. K. Livedo vasculitis: segmental hyalinizing vasculitis of the dermis. *Arch. Dermatol.* 96:489, 1967.

123. Winkelmann, R. K. Lividoid vasculitis (segmental hyalinizing vasculitis). *Jap. J. Dermatol. (B)* 82:84, 1972.

124. Pierard, J., and Geerts, M. L. Vascularité hyalinisante segmentaire (livedo vasculitis). *Arch. Belg. Dermatol. Syphiligr.* 27:103, 1971.

125. Schroeter, A. L., Diaz-Perez, J. L., Winkelmann, R. K., et al. Livedo vasculitis (the vasculitis of atrophie blanche). Immunohistopathologic study. *Arch. Dermatol.* 11:188, 1975.

126. Thomas, E. D., Storb, R., Cliff, R. A., et al. Bone-marrow transplantation. *N. Engl. J. Med.* 292:895, 1975.

127. Merritt, C. B., Mann, D. L., and Rogentine, G. N., Jr. Cytotoxic antibody for epithelial cells in human graft versus host disease. *Nature* 232:638, 1971.

128. Ullman, S., Spielvogel, R. L., Kersey, J. H., et al. Immunoglobulins and complement in skin in graft-versus-host disease. *Ann. Intern. Med.* 85:205, 1976.

129. Goltz, R. W. Erythema elevatum diutinum. In T. B. Fitzpatrick et al., eds., *Dermatology in General Medicine,* p. 750. McGraw Hill Co., New York, 1971.

130. Radcliffe-Crocker, H., and Williams, C. Erythema elevatum diutinum. *Br. J. Dermatol.* 6:1, 1894.

131. Haber, H. Erythema elevatum diutinum. *Br. J. Dermatol.* 67:121, 1955.

132. Ketron, L. W. Erythema elevatum diutinum. *Arch. Dermatol. Syphilogr.* 50:363, 1944.

133. Katz, S. I., Gallin, J. I., Hertz, K. C., et al. Erythema elevatum diutinum: skin and systemic manifestations, immunologic studies, and successful treatment with dapsone. *Medicine* 56:443, 1977.

134. Millikan, L. E., and Conway, F. R. Effect of drugs on the Pillemer pathway—Dapsone. *J. Invest. Dermatol.* 62:541, 1974.

135. Katz, S. I., Hertz, K. C., Crawford, P. S., et al. Effect of sulfones on complement deposition in dermatitis herpetiformis and on complement-mediated guinea-pig reactions. *J. Invest. Dermatol.* 67:688, 1976.

136. Thompson, D. M., and Souhami, R. Suppression of the Arthus reaction in the guinea-pig by dapsone. *Proc. R. Soc. Med.* 68:273, 1975 (abstract).

137. Rollins, T. G., and Winkelmann, R. K. Necrobiosis lipoidica granulomatosis. Necrobiosis lipoidica diabeticorum in the non-diabetic. *Arch. Dermatol.* 82:537, 1960.

138. Bauer, M., and Levan, N. E. Diabetic dermangiopathy. A spectrum including pigmented pretibial patches and necrobiosis lipoidica diabeticorum. *Br. J. Dermatol.* 83:528, 1970.

139. Ullman, S., and Dahl, M. Necrobiosis lipoidica. An immunofluorescence study. *Arch. Dermatol.* 113:1671, 1977.

140. Jayarao, K. S., Faulk, W. P., Karam, J. H., et al. Measurement of immune complexes in insulin-treated diabetics. *J. Immunol. Methods* 3:337, 1973.

141. Irvine, W. J., Al-Khateeb, S. F., DiMario, U., et al. Soluble immune complexes in the sera of newly diagnosed insulin-dependent diabetics and in treated diabetics. *Clin. Exp. Immunol.* 30:16, 1977.

142. Irvine, W. J. Classification of idiopathic diabetes. *Lancet* 1:638, 1977.

143. Bloodworth, J. M. B. Diabetic microangiopathy. In J. M. B. Bloodworth, ed., *Endocrine Pathology,* p. 389. Williams & Wilkins Co., Baltimore, 1968.

144. Berns, A. W., Owens, C. T., Hirata, Y., et al. The pathogenesis of diabetic glomerulosclerosis. II. A demonstration of insulin-binding capacity of the various histopathological components of the disease by fluorescence microscopy. *Diabetes* 11:308, 1962.

145. Coleman, S. L., Becker, B., Canan, S., et al. Fluorescent insulin staining of the diabetic eye. *Diabetes* 11:375, 1962.

146. Westberg, N. G., and Michael, A. F. Immunohistopathology of diabetic glomerulosclerosis. *Diabetes* 21:163, 1972.

147. Civatte, J. *Histopathologie cutanée.* Flammarion, Paris, 1967.

148. Moyer, D. G. Papular granuloma annulare. *Arch. Dermatol.* 89:41, 1964.

149. Tolmach, J. A. Case 5: disseminated granuloma annulare (atypical). *Arch. Dermatol.* 84:167, 1961.

150. Dicken, C. H., Carrington, S. G., and Winkelmann, R. K. Generalized granuloma annulare. *Arch. Dermatol.* 99:556, 1969.

151. Leppard, B., and Black, M. M. Dissemi-

nated granuloma annulare: a variant in which the lesions involve the sun-exposed areas. *Trans. St. John's Hosp. Dermatol. Soc.* 58:186, 1972.

152. Hammond, R., Dyess, K., and Castro, A. Insulin production and glucose tolerance in patients with granuloma annulare. *Br. J. Dermatol.* 87:540, 1972.

153. Haim, S., Friedman-Birnbaum, R., Haim, N., et al. Carbohydrate tolerance in patients with granuloma annulare: study of fifty-two cases. *Br. J. Dermatol.* 88:447, 1973.

154. Beer, W. E., and Wilson Jones, E. Granuloma annulare following tuberculin Heaf tests. *Trans. St. John's Hosp. Dermatol. Soc.* 52:68, 1966.

155. Umbert, P., and Winkelmann, R. K. Granuloma annulare: direct immunofluorescence study. *Br. J. Dermatol.* 95:487, 1976.

156. Colvin, R. B., and Dvorak, H. F. Role of the clotting system in cell-mediated hypersensitivity. II. Kinetics of fibrinogen/fibrin accumulation and vascular permeability changes in tuberculin and cutaneous basophil hypersensitivity reactions. *J. Immunol.* 114:377, 1975.

157. Dahl, M. V., Ullman, S., and Goltz, R. W. Vasculitis in granuloma annulare: histopathology and direct immunofluorescence. *Arch. Dermatol.* 113:463, 1977.

158. Cream, J. J., Bryceson, A. D. M., and Ryder, G. Disappearance of immunoglobulin and complement from the Arthus reaction and its relevance to studies of vasculitis in man. *Br. J. Dermatol.* 84:106, 1971.

159. Marks, J. M. Dogma and dermatitis herpetiformis. *Clin. Exp. Dermatol.* 2:189, 1977.

160. van der Meer, J. B. Granular deposits of immunoglobulins in the skin of patients with dermatitis herpetiformis: an immunofluorescent study. *Br. J. Dermatol.* 81:493, 1969.

161. Seah, P. P., Fry, L., Stewart, J. S., et al. Immunoglobulins in the skin in dermatitis herpetiformis and coeliac disease. *Lancet* 1:611, 1972.

162. Seah, P. P., and Fry, L. Immunoglobulins in the skin in dermatitis herpetiformis and their relevance in diagnosis. *Br. J. Dermatol.* 92:157, 1975.

163. Dabrowski, J., Jablónska, S., Chorzelski, T. P. et al. Electron microscopic studies in dermatitis herpetiformis in relation to the pattern of immune deposits in the skin. *Arch. Dermatol. Res.* 259:213, 1977.

164. Yaoita, H., and Katz, S. I. Immunoelectron-microscopic localization of IgA in skin of patients with dermatitis herpetiformis. *J. Invest. Dermatol.* 67:502, 1976.

165. Stingl, G., Hönigsmann, H., Holubar, K., et al. Ultrastructural localization of immunoglobulins in skin of patients with dermatitis herpetiformis. *J. Invest. Dermatol.* 67:507, 1976.

166. Seah, P. P., Fry, L., Holborow, E. J., et al. Antireticulin antibody: incidence and diagnostic significance. *Gut* 14:311, 1973.

167. Lancaster-Smith, M., Kumar, P., Clark, M. L., et al. Antireticulin antibodies in dermatitis herpetiformis and adult coaliac disease. Their relationship to a gluten-free diet and jejunal histology. *Br. J. Dermatol.* 92:37, 1975.

168. Fry, L., Seah, P. P., Riches, D. J., et al. Clearance of skin lesions in dermatitis herpetiformis after gluten withdrawal. *Lancet* 1:288, 1973.

169. Reunala, T., Blomqvist, K., and Tarpila, S. Gluten-free diet in dermatitis herpetiformis. I. Clinical response of skin lesions in 81 patients. *Br. J. Dermatol.* 97:473, 1977.

170. Marks, J., Shuster, S., and Watson, A. J. Small bowel changes in dermatitis herpetiformis. *Lancet* 2:1280, 1966.

171. Brow, J. R., Parker, F., Weinstein, W. M., et al. The small intestinal mucosa in dermatitis herpetiformis. I. Severity and distribution of the small intestinal lesion and associated malabsorption. *Gastroenterology* 60:355, 1971.

172. Weinstein, W. M. Latent celiac sprue. *Gastroenterology* 66:489, 1974.

173. Katz, S. I., Falchuk, Z. M., Dahl, M. V., et al. HL-A8: a genetic link between dermatitis herpetiformis and gluten-sensitive enteropathy. *J. Clin. Invest.* 51:2977, 1972.

174. Gebhard, R. L., Katz, S. I., Marks, J., et al. HL-A antigen type and small-intestinal disease in dermatitis herpetiformis. *Lancet* 2:760, 1973.

175. Seah, P. P., Fry, L., Kearney, J. W., et al. A comparison of histocompatibility antigens in dermatitis herpetiformis and adult coeliac disease. *Br. J. Dermatol.* 94:131, 1976.

176. Reunala, T., Salo, O. P., Tiilikainen, A., et al. Histocompatibility antigens and dermatitis herpetiformis with special reference to jejunal abnormalities and acetylator phenotype. *Br. J. Dermatol.* 94:139, 1976.

177. Solheim, B. G., Ek, J., Thune, P. O., et al. HLA antigens in dermatitis herpetiformis and coeliac disease. *Tissue Antigens* 7:57, 1976.

178. Berrens, L., Jankowski, E., and Jankowski-Berntsen, I. Complement component profiles in urticaria, dermatitis herpetiformis, and alopecia areata. *Br. J. Dermatol.* 95:145, 1976.

179. Seah, P. P., Fry, L., Mazaheri, M. R., et al. Alternate-pathway complement fixation by IgA in the skin in dermatitis herpetiformis. *Lancet* 2:175, 1973.

180. Mowbray, J. F., Hoffbrand, A. V., Hol-

borow, E. J., et al. Circulating immune complexes in dermatitis herpetiformis. *Lancet* 1:400, 1973.

181. Mohammed, I., Holborow, E. J., Fry, L., et al. Multiple immune complexes and hypocomplementaemia in dermatitis herpetiformis and coeliac disease. *Lancet* 2:487, 1976.

182. Cooney, T., Doyle, C. T., Buckley, D., et al. Dermatitis herpetiformis: a comparative assessment of skin and bowel abnormality. *J. Clin. Pathol.* 30:976, 1977.

183. Beutner, E. H., and Jordon, R. E. Demonstration of skin antibodies in sera of pemphigus vulgaris patients by indirect immunofluorescent staining. *Proc. Soc. Exp. Biol. Med.* 117:505, 1964.

184. Beutner, E. H., Lever, W. F., Witebsky, E., et al. Autoantibodies in pemphigus vulgaris: response to an intercellular substance of epidermis. *J.A.M.A.* 192:682, 1965.

185. Jordon, R. E., Beutner, E. H., Witebsky, E., et al. Basement zone antibodies in bullous pemphigoid. *J.A.M.A.* 200:751, 1967.

186. Chorzelski, T. S., Jablónska, S., Blaszczyk, M., et al. Autoantibodies in pemphigoid. *Dermatologica* 136:325, 1968.

187. van Joost, T., Cormane, R. H., and Pondman, K. W. Direct immunofluorescent study of the skin on occurrence of complement in pemphigus. *Br. J. Dermatol.* 87:466, 1972.

188. Jordon, R. E., Schroeter, A. L., Rogers, R. S., et al. Classical and alternate-pathway activation of complement in pemphigus vulgaris lesions. *J. Invest. Dermatol.* 63:256, 1974.

189. Jordon, R. E., Schroeter, A. L., Good, R. A., et al. The complement system in bullous pemphigoid. II. Immunofluorescent evidence for both classical and alternate-pathway activation. *Clin. Immunol. Immunopathol.* 3:307, 1975.

190. Jordon, R. E., Sams, W. M., Jr., Diaz, G., et al. Negative complement immunofluorescence in pemphigus. *J. Invest. Dermatol.* 57:407, 1971.

191. Jordon, R. E., Nordby, J. M., and Milstein, H. The complement system in bullous pemphigoid. III. Fixation of C1q and C4 by pemphigoid antibody. *J. Lab. Clin. Med.* 86:733, 1975.

192. Jordon, R. E., Day, N. K., Sams, W. M., Jr., et al. The complement system in bullous pemphigoid. I. Complement and component levels in sera and blister fluids. *J. Clin. Invest.* 52:1207, 1973.

193. Jordon, R. E., Day, N. K., Luckasen, J. R., et al. Complement activation in pemphigus vulgaris blister fluid. *Clin. Exp. Immunol.* 15:53, 1973.

194. Jordon, R. E., and McDuffie, F. C. Serum and blister fluid anticomplementary activity in pemphigus and bullous pemphigoid. Sucrose density gradient studies. *Proc. Soc. Exp. Biol. Med.* 151:594, 1976.

195. Tappeiner, G., Heine, K. G., Kahl, J. C., et al. C1q binding substances in pemphigus and bullous pemphigoid. Detection with a C1q binding assay. *Clin. Exp. Immunol.* 28:40, 1977.

196. Brun, C., Bryld, C., Fenger, L., et al. Glomerular lesions in adults with the Schönlein-Henoch syndrome. A light and electron microscopy study. *Acta Pathol. Microbiol. Scand. (A)* 79:569, 1971.

197. Borges, W. H. Anaphylactoid purpura. *Med. Clin. North Am.* 56:201, 1972.

198. Faille-Kuyper, E. H., Kater, L., Kooiker, C. J., et al. IgA-deposits in cutaneous blood-vessel walls and mesangium in Henoch-Schönlein syndrome. *Lancet* 1:892, 1973.

199. Ullman, S., Halberg, P., Nielsen, B., et al. Deposits of immunoglobulins and complement in the dermoepidermal junction of patients with anaphylactoid purpura. *Acta Derm. Venereol. (Stockh.)* 55:359, 1975.

200. Evans, D. J., Williams, D. G., Peters, D. K., et al. Glomerular deposition of properdin in Henoch-Schönlein syndrome and idiopathic focal nephritis. *Br. Med. J.* 3:326, 1973.

201. Sams, W. M., Jr., Claman, H. N., Kohler, P. F., et al. Human necrotizing vasculitis: immunoglobulins and complement in vessel walls of cutaneous lesions and normal skin. *J. Invest. Dermatol.* 64:441, 1975.

202. Cochrane, C. G., and Weigle, W. O. The cutaneous reaction to soluble antigen-antibody complexes: a comparison with the Arthus phenomenon. *J. Exp. Med.* 108:591, 1958.

203. Whitsed, H. M., and Penny, R. IgA-IgG cryoglobulinaemia with vasculitis. *Clin. Exp. Immunol.* 9:183, 1971.

204. Verrier-Jones, J., Cumming, R. H., Asplin, C. M., et al. Necrotizing vasculitis: a circulating immune complex producing inflammatory skin lesions. *Br. J. Dermatol.* 94:123, 1976.

205. Tuffanelli, D. L. Cutaneous immunopathology: recent observations. *J. Invest. Dermatol.* 65:143, 1975.

206. Bullock, W. E., Callerame, M. L., and Panner, B. J. Immunohistologic alteration of skin and ultrastructural changes of glomerular basement membranes in leprosy. *Am. J. Trop. Med. Hyg.* 23:81, 1974.

207. Ullman, S., Halberg, P., Nielsen, B., et al. Deposits of immunoglobulins and complement in the dermoepidermal junction of patients with anaphylactoid purpura. *Acta Derm. Venereol. (Stockh.)* 55:359, 1975.

CHAPTER 12

Renal Disease

Documentation of immune-complex material in glomerular structures probably represents one of the most sensitive assays for the presence of circulating or tissue-reactive immune complexes. Thus, slight mesangial deposition of immunoglobulins, complement components, and antigens related to *Salmonella typhosa* in typhoid fever (1) provides evidence for immune complexes as an epiphenomenon during the acute clinical illness. With rare exceptions, the same considerations apply to apparent subclinical immune-complex deposition in a host of other clinical disease states, including infectious mononucleosis (2), some parasitic infections (3), or mild viral illnesses of no apparent serious medical consequence.

The relevance of immune complexes to clinical medicine was emphasized several decades ago by the pioneering work of Germuth, Dixon, Cochrane, and others (4–6). The spectrum of human disorders where renal immune-complex deposition has now been demonstrated will comprise the major focus of this chapter. As more apparently irrelevant diseases have been investigated by renal biopsy or postmortem immunofluorescent studies, the picture has become a trifle blurred. It seems important to focus here on clinically significant renal disease and to attempt to define as precisely as possible areas of agreement and disagreement as to mechanisms of actual disease pathogenesis. A schematic representation of the entire spectrum with emphasis on significant renal disease is shown in Figure 12-1.

Poststreptococcal Glomerulonephritis

Poststreptococcal glomerulonephritis presents an interesting enigma. This disorder predictably follows infection with certain nephritogenic strains of group A hemolytic streptococci (7, 8) as evidenced by many careful epidemiologic and clinical studies; type 12 is notorious in this regard. However, studies of nephritis associated with pyogenic skin infections caused by other higher numbered streptococcal serotypes (types 49, 55, and many others) have reemphasized the complexity of the problem. With each epidemic of skin-associated nephritis in Trinidad (9, 10) or among the Red Lake Indians in northern Minnesota (11, 12), a new serotype is often defined. The recognizable features by which an isolated strain could be designated as nephritogenic are not yet apparent, making the current typing system something of a scientific anachronism, since it most often identifies nephritogenic strains in retrospect. New data have recently been presented by Villareal and co-workers (13) using acrylamide gel electrophoretic analysis, which identifies a low-molecular-weight streptococcal membrane antigen from multiple strains associated with nephritis. Studies by Treser and co-workers (14) and Markowitz and Lange (15) have also characterized cross-reacting antigens isolated from streptococcal plasma membranes and human glomeruli. Streptococcal antigenic components have been identified on glomerular membranes from patients with acute post-

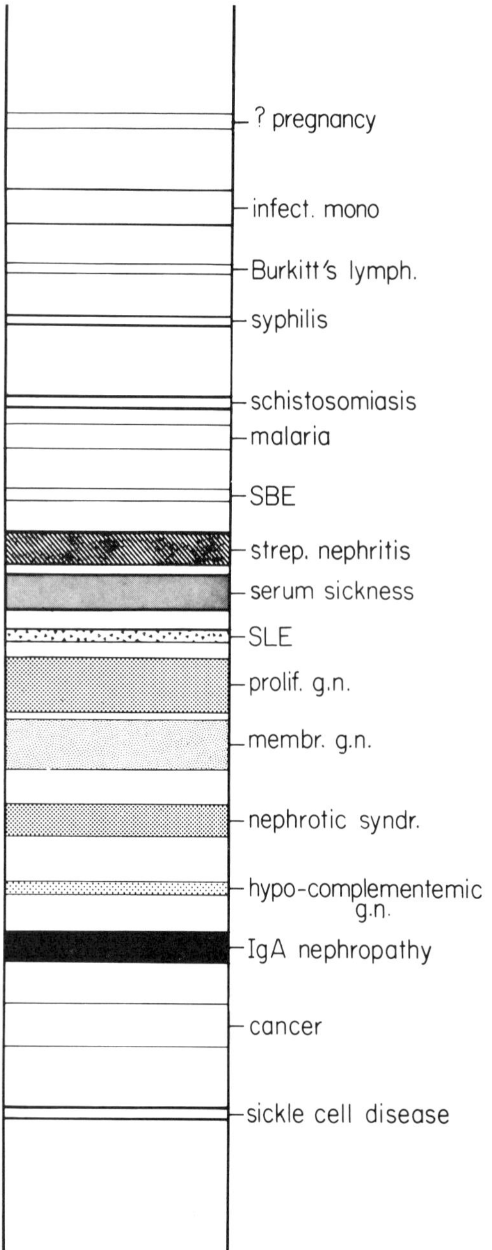

Figure 12-1 Representation of the spectrum of renal disease for which evidence exists for immune-complex involvement. Emphasis in this chapter is on the middle portion of the spectrum shown in the darker bands.

streptococcal glomerulonephritis which were initially felt to represent lipoprotein of 120,000 Daltons (16). More recently Lange and colleagues (17) have described a streptococcal antigen in glomerular tissues during the acute phases of nephritis. It was found that streptococcal antigen could be detected in sites on glomeruli early in the clinical course of nephritis which apparently had not yet been masked by antibody. These sites were located on the endothelial side of the glomerular basement membrane and in the mesangial matrix. Antigen was detected in water-soluble extracts from a variety of nephritogenic streptococci, and was analyzed by chromatography and acrylamide gel electrophoresis. Rabbit antibody to this fraction fixed to glomerular structures taken from biopsies early in the course of nephritis. Similarly, immunoglobulin from patients with a history of poststreptococcal glomerulonephritis reacted with the same antigen. Control observations indicated no reaction with glomeruli from patients with other forms of renal disease or normal kidney tissues. Unlabeled rabbit antibody to the presumed streptococcal nephritic antigen blocked staining by previous patients' sera. These reactions were recorded with streptococcal antigens obtained from various nephritogenic strains regardless of M or T type. If confirmed by other groups, these findings suggest that there may indeed be a common feature about certain streptococci making them predisposed to be associated with acute glomerulonephritis. Initial glomerular localization of such antigens to glomeruli may precede subsequent conglomeration of immunoglobulin and activated complement. These concepts now require confirmation and extension by other workers in this area.

Clinical Picture

Patients with acute poststreptococcal glomerulonephritis often present with peripheral and facial edema, mild to severe hypertension, gross hematuria, and generalized malaise. Usually diagnosis is quickly made on the basis of examination of fresh urine which shows microscopic hematuria, heavy proteinuria, and red-blood cell casts. Acute glomerulonephritis occurs most commonly during the school-age years. In most studies, ages of patients range from two to thirteen years (18–20) with a mean of six to seven years. An upper respiratory infection including mild coryza, sore throat, or otitis media is often noted prior to onset of symptoms. Skin infections particularly in cases studied in the southeastern United States (21), Red Lake epidemics (11, 12), or in Trinidad (9, 10) have frequently been recorded. Examples of streptococcal pyoderma seen in association with epidemic nephritis are shown in Figure 12-2. Serological evidence of antecedent streptococcal infection as manifested by elevation of antistreptolysin O (ASO) titers is present in approximately 80 percent of cases. If ASO, antihyaluronidase, and anti-DNase B titers are tested, an elevation is noted in virtually all subjects (21, 22). Blood pressure elevations of greater than 140/90 are noted in approximately half of children hospitalized with nephritis. Edema is present in two-thirds and in this group one-half of the subjects show ascites (23). In one prospective study of 144 children, 78 percent of those hospitalized were found to be azotemic (18) and two-thirds showed creatinine clearances more than two standard deviations below the normal mean.

Large numbers of white blood cells in urine

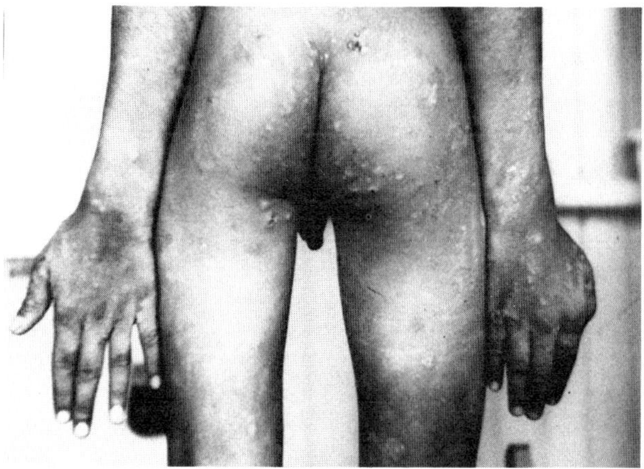

Figure 12-2 Infected scabies (culturing group A hemolytic streptococci) in a patient from Trinidad studied during epidemic nephritis. (Photograph courtesy of Elisabeth Potter, Northwestern University Medical Center, Chicago.)

samples may initially obscure the diagnosis and suggest urinary tract infection. However, in most cases the presence of red blood cell casts confirms active nephritis. A correct diagnosis is sometimes extremely difficult in elderly subjects or in patients who present with moderate to severe hypertension and anuria. Quite early during clinical studies of the disease it was recognized that acute poststreptococcal nephritis was also accompanied by marked hypocomplementemia (24). The presence of red-blood-cell casts signifying an acute glomerulitis along with depression of serum hemolytic complement represent manifestations attributed to glomerular immune-complex deposition and intense activation of the complement system. Evidence for concomitant presence of a diffuse vasculitis associated with a serum cryoprotein during acute illness has recently been presented in a patient studied by Ingelfinger and co-workers (25).

The latent interval between streptococcal infection and onset of acute glomerulonephritis generally has a mean of 10 to 14 days and appears to be somewhat shorter than the latent interval noted in acute rheumatic fever. The latent interval between streptococcal infection and onset of nephritis may be somewhat longer in cases where skin infection is the initiating event (12). It is also of interest that poststreptococcal glomerulonephritis and rheumatic fever seldom occur together or following the same streptococcal exposure. Very little direct insight is currently available concerning this point. One might postulate that thymic dependent and independent antigens could be responsible for these interval differences and clinical exclusions of rheumatic fever or nephritis respectively.

A number of studies have recorded the occurrence of glomerular immune-complex deposits at the time of acute illness and clinical onset (26–30). Paradoxically, in a disorder with a presumed identifiable streptococcal etiology, reports documenting the actual presence of streptococcal antigen within immune-complex deposits have been conflicting. Several groups (16, 17, 26, 28) have reported definite identification of streptococcal antigens in glomerular deposits by immunofluorescence and electron microscopy. Others, however, have documented moderate to heavy IgG and C deposition, but not distinct streptococcal antigens. As noted in the review of this question by Zabriskie (31), precise identification of streptococcal antigens in the anatomic sites of acute glomerulonephritis may be technically difficult because of masking by gammaglobulins and complement. Characteristic granular deposits of both immunoglobulin and streptococcal antigen in glomeruli of patients with poststreptococcal glomerulonephritis are shown in Figures 12-3 and 12-4. Demonstration of streptococcal antigens actually present within such immune deposits is dependent on obtaining biopsy material early in the course of the disease, before tissue accumulation of immunoglobulin and complement components obscure underlying antigenic material.

The nature of streptococcal antigens involved in production of acute nephritis remains a matter of controversy among several groups examining this question. Original studies by Treser and co-workers (14) claimed that the antigen was derived from group A streptococcal membrane. This result was not confirmed by Zabriskie (31), using highly specific antisera prepared against membranes of four different streptococcal strains; absorption of positive staining was accomplished only using preparations containing streptococcal cell walls. The recent report by Lange and co-workers (17) of a streptococcal antigen showing no particular M-type or T-type restriction is of considerable importance and must, as noted above, be confirmed in other laboratories before there is final agreement on this point.

An ancillary problem in pathogenesis of poststreptococcal glomerulonephritis concerns the role of fibrin deposition during the acute or subacute lesions. Studies by Kantor (32) showed that streptococcal materials such as M protein have a particular binding affinity for

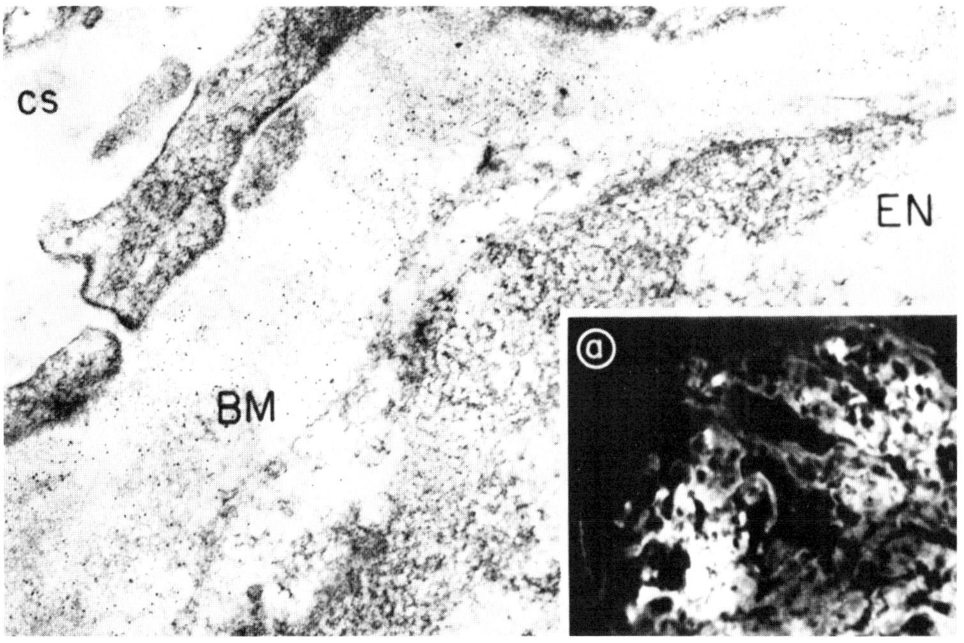

Figure 12-3 A portion of a glomerular capillary wall. Ferritin-conjugated antibody to products of the streptococcus group A, type 12, are localized in the glomerular basement membrane (BM). The small focal subepithelial deposit does not contain ferritin. EN indicates part of an endothelial nucleus; CS, the capsular space. Magnification ×39,000. Inset *a* illustrates the localization of fluorescein-conjugated antistreptococcal serum in the glomerular structures. Magnification × 200. (Reproduced with permission, G. A. Andres, L. Accinni, K. C. Hsu et al., *J. Exp. Med.* 123:399, 1976.)

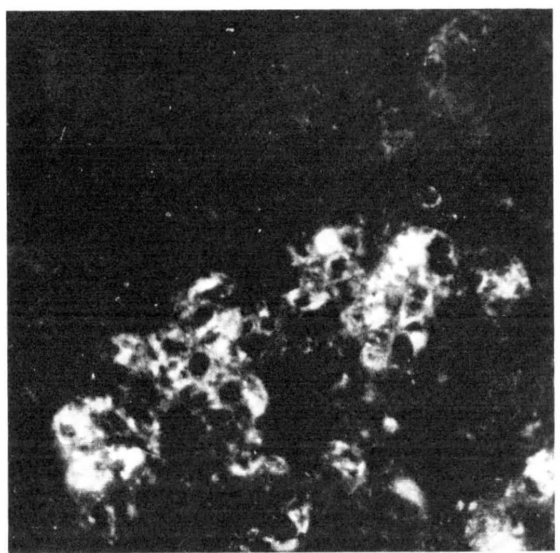

Figure 12-4 Tissue showing a portion of a glomerulus obtained from a patient 8 days after onset of acute glomerulonephritis, stained with fluroescein-conjugated rabbit antibody against a ground-cell preparation of a nephritogenic group A, type 1, β-hemolytic streptococcus. The discrete fluorescence cannot be anatomically localized with respect to the basement membrane, but appears to be present between cells or within the cytoplasm. Fluorescent microscopy $\times$ 350. (Reproduced with permission, A. F. Michael, K. N. Drummond, R. A. Good et al., *J. Clin. Invest.* 45:237, 1966.)

fibrinogen. Injection of M-protein–fibrinogen complexes in experimental animals produced glomerular localization between epithelial cells of glomerular tufts (33). It is possible that M protein may play an adjuvant role in the acute glomerular inflammatory process in this disease. This could also explain the findings by several groups of investigators of fibrinogen deposition within some of the acute lesions of the disorder (26, 27, 29).

Long-Term Sequelae

Considerable controversy exists about the long-term sequelae associated with acute post-streptococcal glomerulonephritis. Early studies by several groups suggested that long-term prognosis was considerably better in children than in adults who developed the disease (34, 35). The careful, early analysis of Jennings and Earle (36) recorded a significant proportion (13/36) of patients who progressed to chronic disease on the basis of clinical follow-up and changes on renal biopsy.

One of the most important aspects is identification of actual clinical prevalence of acute glomerulonephritis. This is illustrated in the studies of Kaplan and co-workers (12) where reintroduction of type 49 streptococci within the Red Lake Indian reservation was followed by acute glomerulonephritis in 25 individuals. In this study over 50 percent of the patients with nephritis were entirely asymptomatic and were only discovered by routine surveillance for microscopic hematuria. Corresponding laboratory studies from many of these same patients showed no marked abnormalities despite clear biopsy evidence of active nephritis. Thus, during epidemic streptococcal nephritis a substantial proportion of cases would go undetected unless there were extensive screening of the population group at risk. Similar findings have also been presented by Sagel and colleagues (37), who conducted weekly screening examinations in 248 children after group A streptococcal infections. Of these subjects 54 showed either transient CH 50 depression or mild urinary abnormalities. Renal biopsy specimens from the latter subjects frequently showed changes ranging from mild mesangial increase to endothelial proliferation characteristic of acute nephritis. The difficulties in initial identification of all patients experiencing acute poststreptococcal glomerulonephritis makes hard and fast predictions about long-term prognosis ambiguous.

Conventional morphological studies of the pathological changes occurring during acute poststreptococcal glomerulonephritis have been carefully documented by a number of workers (18–23, 35, 36, 38–41). During the acute stage glomeruli appear to be enlarged and relatively bloodless with increased lobular pattern and glomerular intracapillary cellularity increase. Mesangial proliferation is present with uniform appearance in most glomerular lobules. Polymorphonuclear leukocytes are noted infiltrating some glomerular tufts and in some cases epithelial cell proliferation, presumably related to crescent formation, is observed. In most cases the glomerular basement membranes remain thin and delicate and glomerular necrosis is absent. Electron microscopic studies of glomeruli during acute poststreptococcal nephritis again show marked increases in intracapillary cells chiefly from the mesangium. Electron-dense deposits are noted close to the glomerular basement membrane under the epithelial cells. Typical histological changes present during the acute phase of poststreptococcal glomerulonephritis are shown in Figure 12-5.

Baldwin and co-workers have reevaluated the long-term course of poststreptococcal glomerulonephritis in a number of studies (42–45). An analysis of 126 patients (89 adults and 37 children) included two to 15-year follow-up in 60 patients (42). Terminal uremia was noted within six months in 9 patients, in two years in 1 patient, and within six years in another patient. After long-term follow-up, proteinuria, hypertension, or significant reduction in filtration rate was recorded in half of the remaining patients. The histological parallels with this clinical outcome showed that as glomerular proliferation subsided during the first three years, irregular glomerular sclerosis became apparent. These changes were recorded in two-thirds of patients during follow-up years. Granular glomerular IgG deposits were noted usually during the first year, but thereafter linear deposits of IgG persisted in one-half of the subjects. Of 29 patients who showed proteinuria at two years after onset of nephritis, all but 6 had other evidence of irreversible disease.

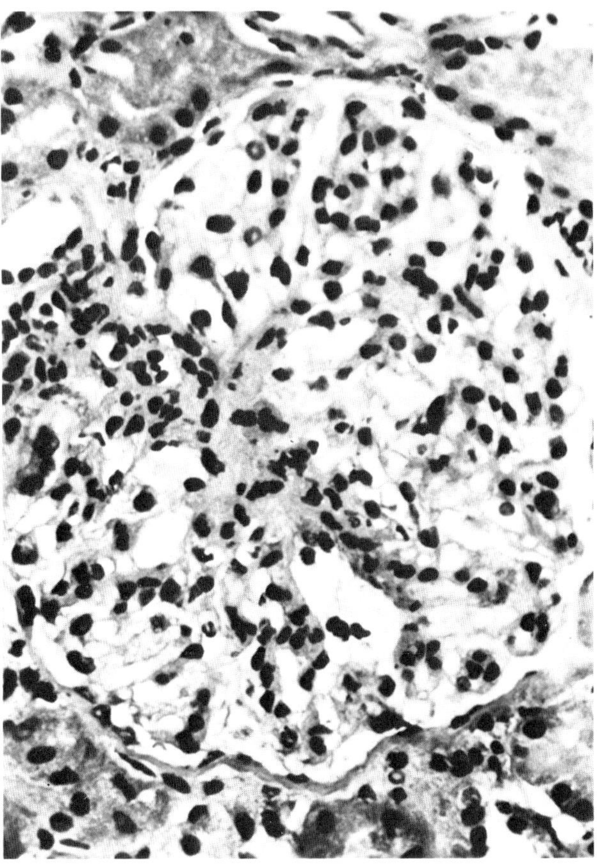

Figure 12-5 Extensive glomerular changes noted in a patient with acute glomerulonephritis. Local hypercellularity with patent capillaries is present. H&E × 250. (Reproduced with permission, P. Freedman, H. P. Meister, H. J. Lee et al., *Medicine* 49:433, 1970.)

From this study it would appear that chronic renal disease, as judged by proteinuria and hypertension alone, was present in about one-half of patients after long-term follow-up. In particular one-third of the patients, in whom proteinuria had disappeared two years or more after onset, showed the development of hypertension. A high correlation was also noted between hypertension, reduced filtration rate, and glomerular sclerosis.

The pathogenetic mechanisms involved in such disease evolution have not been clearly elucidated. If the initial renal insult in poststreptococcal glomerulonephritis is caused by deposition of antigen-antibody complexes within glomeruli, it is difficult to understand how local proliferative changes and later glomerular sclerosis can extend over so long a time course. In the sequential studies by Baldwin (42–44) granular glomerular IgG and C3 was recorded during the first year after onset, but subsequently such immune deposits were rarely seen. Later occasional linear glomerular IgG deposits were noted, but were not accompanied by persistent depression of total serum hemolytic complement. It was suggested that the subsequent chronic progression of renal disease might be related to replacement of the original exogenous immune-complex mechanism by autologous generation of antiglomerular basement membrane antibody reactivity. However, no substantial evidence has been produced to reinforce this concept. There is still a great deal to be learned about the basic mechanisms mediating healing and complete remission after acute glomerulonephritis or alternatively insidious progression to chronic renal disease.

From a historical standpoint clinical prognosis after acute poststreptococcal nephritis has changed or fluctuated considerably. Early reports analyzing outcome in the 1940s indicated that the disease evolved to complete healing in most patients and to chronic renal disease in 10 to 40 percent, with a few patients dying during the first few months of illness (38, 46–48). Many observers who have analyzed this problem have recognized that the acute nephritic episode can be followed by a prolonged transitional state, which may be characterized by few salient clinical abnormalities but which generates significant chronic renal disease as a final product in a certain proportion of individuals. Long-term follow-up of pediatric patients with well-defined clinical acute glomerulonephritis suggested that the recovery rate was higher than in adults: approaching 80 percent in most studies (49–54). In many of the early studies criteria for recovery were usually limited to absence of persistent clinical abnormalities and of persistent abnormal urine findings after several years of follow-up.

Studies dealing exclusively with poststreptococcal glomerulonephritis conducted in the 1950s focused largely on the outcome of well-defined epidemics (35, 55, 56). In the Red Lake study (35) minimal glomerular changes were noted in some children biopsied 10 years after onset, but evidence for clinical chronic renal disease was not found. Later, with the increasing use of renal biopsy, well-defined sets of patients with poststreptococcal glomerulonephritis were studied by a number of groups. These studies (22, 36, 57) bore a parallel to those recorded by Baldwin and colleagues (42–45) in that after follow-up periods of months to four years following onset, one-third to one-half of the patients showed absence of healing as judged by persistence of proteinuria. Few of these studies provided renal biopsy material on patients followed as long as 10 years. More recently, renal biopsy and long-term clinical follow-up on patients presumably healed after previous acute glomerulonephritis have consistently shown glomerular abnormalities in a significant proportion of individuals (19, 58). Thus, it would seem that one of the most challenging aspects related to the evolution of either healing or progression of chronic renal abnormalities in this group of patients is a clear definition of the pathological processes involved. Although the evidence for participation of immune-complex–mediated injury during the acute exudative stage of nephritis is convincing, it is not at all clear how the transition to a chronic, eventually sclerotic lesion comes about. If immunologic mechanisms are indeed involved in such pathogenetic changes, it seems possible that cell-mediated immunity plays a role in some instances. Studies reported by Zabriskie (31) are of considerable interest in this regard: attention was specifically directed toward patients with progressive glomerulonephritis, with the idea that the continuing clinical nature of the disease, the presence of both linear and occasionally granular immune deposits in the renal biopsy material, and the presence of mononuclear cells in histological sections of renal tissue all suggested an alteration in cell-mediated immune reactivity in the ongoing disease process. A group of patients with clinical, pathological, and immunofluorescent evidence of progressive glomerulonephritis were studied for altered cellular reactivity to various well-defined streptococcal antigens. Representative results from these studies are shown in Table 12-1, where lymphocyte-macrophage migration inhibition tests were carried out. Evidence for cell-mediated immune reactivity to streptococcal membrane and cell-wall antigens was obtained only when particulate rather than soluble streptococcal antigens were used. These general changes were also supported by results using lymphocyte transformation and the same general panel of streptococcal antigens (59). Similar studies by Rocklin and co-workers (60) in patients with progressive glomerulonephritis suggested positive cell-mediated immune reactions using renal glomerular material as antigens. Cellular reactivity to both glomerular antigens and streptococcal-derived substances could in such instances actually reflect known cross-reactivities between the two separate materials. Unfortunately, extensive cross-stimulation or inhibition of such cell-mediated immune reactions with glomerular and streptococcal antigens in the same patients has not as yet been adequately studied. A recent report by Bhat and colleagues (61) has actually noted decreased lymphocytic transformation in 12 subjects, with evidence of persistent disease 4 to 18 years after an initial bout of poststreptococcal nephritis using membrane antigens from two known nephritogenic strains, types 12 and 57. It was thought that the depression of lymphocyte reactivity in these patients was probably not a direct result of general immune depression, since concurrent lymphocyte reactivity to nonspecific mitogens such as phytohemagglutinin was not significantly reduced. These results stand in contrast to those previously recorded by Zabriskie and co-workers on a more broadly defined general group of progressive glomerulonephritis (31, 59). There are many examples, however, of a dissociation between lymphocyte reactivity and lymphokine production (62, 63). It is clear that a uniform picture has not emerged from these and other studies (64, 65) attempting to relate changes in cell-mediated immunity to persistence or progression of chronic renal changes in poststreptococcal glomerulonephritis.

Other Immunologic and Pathological Studies

In a number of ways the immunopathological changes of acute poststreptococcal glomeru-

Table 12-1 Cellular inhibition of leukocytes from patients with progressive glomerulonephritis.

Disease states	No. of patients	Type 12 membranes	Type 12 cell walls	Type 5 membranes
		Degree of inhibition to streptococcal antigens (percent)		
Progressive glomerulonephritis[a]	19	34 (±2)	27 (±3)	22.2 (±2)
Nonglomerular renal disease[b]	15	8.1 (±1)	8.1 (±2)	5.1 (±1)
Normal controls	10	8.8 (±2.6)	10.9 (±2.3)	Not tested

Source: Reproduced with permission, J. B. Zabriskie, *J. Exp. Med.* 134:1803, 1971.

[a] Cases with clinical and renal biopsy evidence of glomerular diseases.

[b] Patients with pyelonephritis, polycystic disease, lipoid nephrosis.

lonephritis represent a clinical situation analogous to the acute serum sickness model of glomerulonephritis induced in rabbits by intravenous injection of foreign proteins. In the latter model, circulating complexes localize in renal glomerular microcapillary beds and the vasculature of many other organs (66). Early workers including Schick (67), Von Pirquet (68), Volhard (69), and Klinge (70) suggested that antigen-antibody reactions and clinical manifestations such as fluid retention and hypertension were the result of a universal capillary inflammation resulting from hypersensitivity. This impression has been substantiated by occasional reports of acute arteritis in spleen or kidney tissues of such patients (30, 71). A patient recently studied by Ossi and co-workers (72) showed extensive granular deposits of C3, properdin, and IgG in the walls of splenic venous sinuses, arterioles, and in renal glomeruli. These observations support the concept of poststreptococcal glomerulonephritis as a generalized vasculitic disorder.

Ultrastructural studies of glomerular lesions in acute nephritis have documented characteristic electron-dense humps or immune deposits on the epithelial side of the basement membrane (40–42, 73). The deposits in acute post-streptococcal nephritis resemble those seen with membranous glomerulonephritis. However, the deposits associated with post-streptococcal disease usually disappear within a few weeks after disease onset. This sequential change has recently been carefully documented by Törnroth (73) in a series of elegant ultrastructural studies. Dense subepithelial deposits seven days after disease recognition are shown in Figure 12-6 from this study. Later multiple intramembranous rather lucent deposits were noted that slowly resolved or persisted with apparent gradual clinical resolution. Observations using immunofluorescence showed that IgG or C3 were generally present as long as ultrastructural alterations persisted. Eventual complete resolution of immune deposits was attributed to gradual catabolic activity of epithelial and residual mesangial cells along with absence of continuing endogenous supply of new immune-complex material.

A number of key areas necessary for eventual complete understanding of the pathogenesis of acute poststreptococcal glomerulonephritis are still not clear. The first relates to essential ingredients of nephritogenic stains of group A streptococci. The relation to impetigo or streptococcal pyoderma is particularly intriguing in this regard. Rheumatic fever as a sequel to streptococcal infection classically follows pharyngeal infection, whereas pharyngeal or skin infection may precede poststreptococcal nephritis. Local modulating factors related to these various portals of entry may play an important part in clinical evolution of this particular type of poststreptococcal complication. In this regard more attention must be directed to the actual antigens involved in these phenomena presumably mediated at least in part by immune complexes. The possible role of potent streptococcal extracellular products, such as streptolysin S, in modifying tissue fixation—either of streptococcal antigens or antigen-antibody complexes— must also be examined. It is possible that the inability of certain streptococcal materials to degrade, as has been demonstrated for components of cell walls (74–76), may relate to long-term persistence or aggravation of initial normal immune-complex phenomena. No evidence has yet been presented for prolonged persistence of such streptococcal antigens in poststreptococcal nephritis itself, although the data in the animal experimental models of myocarditis or arthritis are extremely convincing. Immune-complex–mediated mechanisms may indeed represent only the tip of the iceberg. Other still poorly defined phenomena may be of equal or potentially greater importance, particularly in the transition from acute immune-complex–mediated glomerulitis to eventual proliferative changes and sclerosis followed by chronic renal insufficiency.

Antigens Identified in Human Immune-Complex Nephritis

The demonstration of immunoglobulin and complement deposits in many human glomerular disorders points to immune-complex etiology. In marked contrast to most of the well-defined animal models of immune-complex disease, identification of antigens responsible for formation of such immune deposits in

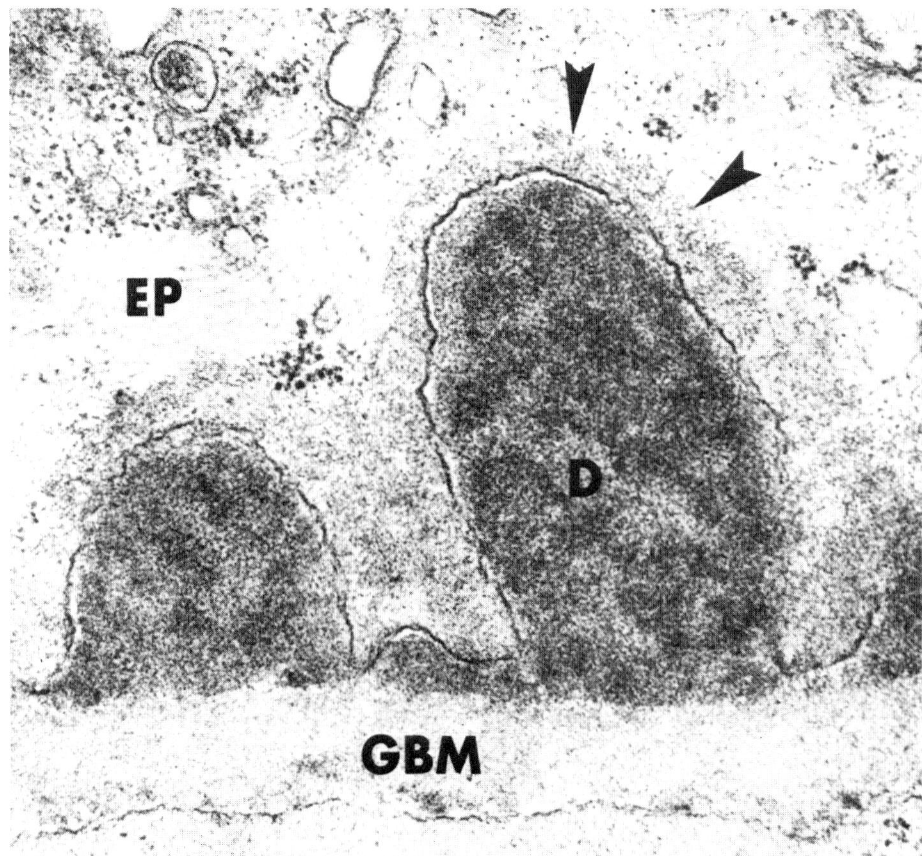

Figure 12-6   Subepithelial electron-dense deposits (D) surrounded by a zone of condensed epithelial cytoplasm (*arrows*). Capillary basement membrane (GBM) is normal. EP = epithelial cell. Magnification × 24,000.(Reproduced with permission, T. Törnroth, *Lab. Invest.* 35:461, 1976.)

human disease has proven more difficult. It seems worthwhile, therefore, to review antigens clearly documented to date in various forms of human immune-complex glomerular injury. Chronic glomerulonephritis itself represents one of the most common causes of uremia requiring dialysis and transplantation. Since immune mechanisms are thought to be directly involved in its inception and perhaps progression to eventual renal failure, it is useful to review current data identifying distinct endogenous or exogenous antigens involved. Definite identification of antigens implicated in such pathogenesis is now possible in only a minority of instances.

Endogenous Antigens

Deoxyribonucleic Acid

Antigens responsible for human immune-complex glomerulonephritis can be classified as endogenous or exogenous. The first demonstration of immune-complex glomerulopathy caused presumably by an endogenous antigen was the identification of DNA–anti-DNA complexes associated with the nephritis of systemic lupus erythematosus (SLE) (77–79). As noted in Chapter 7, complexes containing immunoglobulins, complement, and DNA are noted in renal glomeruli and occasionally by us along tubular basement membranes (TBMs). Subsequent extensive conventional morphological studies have indicated that deposition of

DNA–anti-DNA complexes may be associated with a wide spectrum of structural changes ranging from minimal glomerular alterations to diffuse proliferative or membranoproliferative changes and renal failure. Circulating immune complexes are present during active disease, and activation of the complement system signifies intrinsic participation of complement deposition and catabolism during the active process (80). Direct studies of glomerular eluates have shown high concentrations of DNA, other nuclear antigens, anti-DNA, and antinuclear antibodies compared with concurrent presence in serum (77, 78). Whether DNA–anti-DNA complexes alone or in concert with a number of other endogenous antigen-antibody systems are solely responsible for glomerular injury in SLE still remains to be determined.

Several aspects of the nephropathy of SLE remain elusive. Although it is abundantly clear that DNA–anti-DNA complexes represent a well-defined phlogistic entity in the glomerular immune-complex injury of SLE, the actual mechanism of deposition is not completely understood. Several studies have demonstrated high levels of circulating immune complexes during the clinical course of SLE nephritis (81, 82). There is also evidence for an increase in avidity of such complexes when studied in comparative analyses with DNA–anti-DNA complexes concurrently present in serum (83). There may, however, be unique mitigating factors in DNA causing it to show intrinsic physicochemical adherence to glomerular basement membrane collagen (84, 85). Izui and co-workers (86) found no evidence of direct correlation between actual detectable circulating immune complexes and DNA–anti-DNA immune complex deposition in glomeruli of active SLE patients. Thus, local important modulating factors may influence the deposition and eventual resolution of DNA–anti-DNA complexes more directly than either their concentration in plasma or their molecular composition. The high levels of immune complexes detected in the serum of various patients with active SLE in the past (81, 82, 87) may possibly bear no relation to actual materials deposited in the SLE renal lesion. It

seems likely that many complexes detected in the circulation of SLE patients represent one or more reactions encompassing the wide spectrum of autoantibodies present in individual lupus patients. Thus, direct correlation between levels of circulating immune complexes and tissue lesions in various disorders using the very sensitive radioimmunoassay techniques currently available may not be feasible. Elution studies matched with precise identification of the antigens involved and a study of the physical properties of the antigens are of great importance. Recent studies by Emlen and Mannik (88) are pertinent to this problem: clearance of exogenous single-stranded DNA (ssDNA) in mice showed rapid removal from circulation by hepatic Kupffer cells, with kinetics closely approximating a Michaelis-Menten model. The clearance mechanism, however, was saturable and with increasing amounts, persistence of circulating ssDNA was noted. High-molecular-weight DNA was rapidly cleaved to fragments of 20,000 to 30,000 Daltons by endonucleases presumably on the surface of hepatocytes or Kupffer cells.

Renal Tubular Antigen

The pathogenesis of membranous nephropathy is enigmatic and will be discussed in detail in a subsequent section; however, Naruse and co-workers (89, 90) have indicated the finding of renal tubular antigen in the form of autologous immune complexes in a series of patients with membranous glomerulonephritis. If confirmed by other groups, this mechanism of glomerular injury in membranous nephritis would provide a fascinating explanation for the origin of antigens participating in immune-complex injury in this disorder. Similar mechanisms of generation of an autoimmune response to autologous renal tubular antigen have been demonstrated using immunofluorescence and electron microscopic studies in patients with sickle cell disease immune-complex nephropathy (91, 92), in rare cases of tubulointerstitial disease associated with Fanconi's syndrome (93), or other discrete renal tubular functional abnormalities. The precipitating event that renders materials within renal tubules antigenic is unclear.

Thyroglobulin

Several reports have also documented the occurrence of thyroglobulin in glomeruli from patients with various inflammatory thyroid conditions and apparent immune-complex glomerulonephritis resulting from deposition of thyroglobulin-antithyroglobulin immune aggregates (94, 95). Thyroglobulin, a high-molecular-weight protein of about 19S, presumably is released after prolonged inflammatory reactions within the gland, with continuous or intermittent release of thyroid antigens. Complexes have also been attributed to antigen-antibody reactions in α-1 antitrypsin deficiency (96). The presence of cirrhosis or chronic active liver disease in this instance raises serious questions concerning the basic process, as chronic hepatic insufficiency itself has been connected to occasional immune-complex–mediated phenomena.

Tumors

The whole question of endogenous antigens and immune-complex glomerulonephritis associated with various tumors also represents a biological phenomenon of uncertain importance. As noted in Chapter 8, there are numerous examples of apparent immune-complex glomerulitis associated with a wide spectrum of human tumors (97–101). For the most part, endogenous tumor antigens represent materials derived from the inside of cells rather than more readily accessible antigens localized to or associated with cell membranes. This curious phenomenon may be partially understandable if one recognizes that intracellular, relatively buried, autologous antigens such as native DNA or thyroglobulin may produce subsequent immune-complex reactions on the basis of being relatively sequestered and therefore recognized as different when presented to the host in slightly altered or denatured form.

Exogenous Antigens

Analysis of identifiable exogenous antigens is useful considering the large residual fraction of immune-complex–mediated chronic renal disease represented by membranous, mem-

branoproliferative, or mixed histological types of chronic glomerulonephritis of unknown etiology but associated with immunofluorescent evidence of immune-complex deposition manifested by granular or discrete immunoglobulin and/or complement deposition. A partial catalogue of various clinical states is presented with appropriate references in Table 12-2. Currently, a conservative estimate of identification of distinct antigen in human immune-complex–mediated glomerulonephritis would be no more than 30 percent. An overview of the clinical picture and histological findings in many of the disease states shown in Table 12-2 indicates histological association ranging from minimal changes to proliferative, membranoproliferative, or membranous nephropathy. Whether all glomerular diseases associated with this wide spectrum of histological change are directly linked to an immune-complex etiology is as yet unclear. Several major morphological and clinical groups will be addressed in the following sections and both direct and indirect evidence supporting immune-complex participation will be considered.

Membranous or Membranoproliferative Glomerulonephritis

Membranous glomerulonephritis was first defined as an immunologic and clinical entity in 1965 by West and co-workers (133) and Gotoff and co-workers (134). Subsequent studies have provided continuing morphological definition for this important chronic renal disorder (135–139). Two major subtypes account for the majority of patients seen with this disease: the first subtype is characterized by subendothelial deposits, mesangial cell interposition, and glomerular basement membrane splitting. This variety has been called pure membranoproliferative glomerulonephritis (MPGN). With predominantly subendothelial immune deposits, MPGN accounts for 50 to 80 percent of reported cases. The second type, now referred to as dense-deposit disease (DDD), shows dense longitudinal intramembranous deposits. Two additional subtypes have also been described. One, designated by Burk-

Table 12-2 Exogenous antigens in immune-complex glomerulonephritis of differing types.

Antigens	References
Viral antigens	
Coxsackie B	Burch et al. (102); Burch and Colcolough (103)
Hepatitis B	Combes et al. (104); Myers et al. (105); Kohler et al. (106); Knieser et al. (107); Brzosko et al. (108)
Subacute sclerosing panencephalitis	Dayan and Stokes (109)
Oncorna-like virus	Sutherland and Mardiney (110)
Epstein-Barr viral antigen	Sonnabend et al. (111, 112)
Bacterial antigens	
Streptococcal (group A)	Treser et al. (14, 16); Lange et al. (17); Andres et al. (30)
Staphylococcal	Kaufman and McIntosh (113); Dobrin et al. (114)
Corynebacterium species	Bolton et al. (115)
Streptococcus viridans	Perez et al. (116); Keslin et al. (117)
Pneumonococcal	Hyman et al. (118)
Treponemal	Tourville et al. (119); Gamble and Reardan (120); Braunstein et al. (121)
S. typhosa	Sitprija et al. (1)
Parasitic antigens	
P. malariae	Ward and Kibukamusoke (122)
P. falciparum	Hendrickse et al. (123); Bhamarapravati et al. (124)
Schistosomiasis	Falcão and Gould (125); Silva et al. (126)
Toxoplasma	Shahin et al. (127); Ginsberg et al. (128)
Trypanosomiasis	Nagle et al. (129); de Brito, et al. (130)
Fungal antigens	
Candidiasis	Roberts and Rabson (131); Chesney et al. (132)

holder as type III (139), shows structural changes in common with both MPGN and membranous nephropathy; an intermediate form noted by Strife and colleagues (140) shows subendothelial deposits, basement membrane duplication, subepithelial deposits, and deposits within the glomerular basement membrane. At present it is not at all clear whether such extensive morphological subclassification is warranted or whether all such forms of nephritis—sharing in common the uniform accompanying clinical feature of persistent hypocomplementemia—actually represent variations of the same underlying disease process. The most significant aspect of these disorders is that all generally show reduced serum levels of the third complement component (C3). Eventual renal failure appears to be the

end result of most varieties of this pathological process (135, 137, 138, 140–144). Steroid therapy rarely produces convincing evidence of long-term clinical involvement and only rare instances of spontaneous amelioration have been recorded (138, 145, 146).

The hypocomplementemia present in the group of patients originally described with MPGN (133, 134) has been the subject of extended debate and discussion. Serum from these patients frequently contains nephritic factor, so named for the ability of such sera to activate the complement pathway through C3. For this reason MPGN has often been designated as a distinct entity called hypocomplementemic nephritis. Careful study of this fascinating syndrome has provided considerable longitudinal insight into many of the mechanisms that appear to be involved in the immunopathogenesis of chronic renal disease.

Clinical and Pathological Picture

Patients with hypocomplementemic nephritis or MPGN present either with asymptomatic proteinuria and hematuria, mild nephrotic syndrome, or gross hematuria and an apparent acute nephritis. Age at onset varies from four to thirty years. Hypertension is frequently present and in 85 percent of patients no selective proteinuria is noted. As indicated above, the disease frequently leads to progressive renal insufficiency.

Despite the subdivisions of the disease, several common pathological findings are usually present. These include enlargement of glomerular tufts with lobulation, mesangial cell hyperplasia, and increased mesangial matrix. There is often an apparent splitting of glomerular basement membrane (GBM) with interposition of mesangial fibrils and cytoplasm and nonargyrophilic deposits between endothelium and thickened GBM. A typical example of membranous nephritis is shown in Figure 12-7. Both endothelial and basement membrane deposits are present. Immunopathological studies show characteristic peripheral lobular deposition of C3 and properdin in glomerular capillaries. In at least two-thirds of patients, IgG and/or IgM are seen in glomeruli and C1q and C4 are also often present.

Sera of patients with hypocomplementemic nephritis generally show reduction of total hemolytic complement activity (CH 50) together with reduction of C3. Levels of C1, C2, and C4 can be normal or decreased. A heat-labile factor is present in these sera, causing inactivation of C3t of guinea pig serum (147). Early studies of the complement-activating properties of sera from patients with MPGN indicated increased in vivo breakdown of C3 with presence of a serum factor (C3NeF) termed nephritic factor, which cleaves C3 to $\beta_1 A$ and $\alpha_2 D$ globulins (147–150).

In view of the glomerular immunoglobulin and complement deposition and the dense deposits as seen by ultrastructural studies, the disease has been thought to be related to immune-complex etiology. Presently, a number of cases have noted C3, C1q, C4, or other complement immunofluorescent deposits in the absence of concurrent immunoglobulin. This discrepancy has been resolved in part by careful serial studies in some patients showing glomerular IgG early in the course of the disease, but none demonstrable subsequently notwithstanding persistence of C3 (151, 152). Such findings may relate to relative differences in clearance rates of various immune reactants.

Much interest in this disease has focused on the so-called serum nephritic factor, or C3NeF, since it is theoretically capable of prolonging or accelerating the nephritic process. Early studies by several groups (150, 152) demonstrated persistence of the hypocomplementemia after nephrectomy prior to renal transplantation. These findings together with studies of in vivo survival of labeled C3 (152) suggest a significant extrarenal site for complement activation and catabolism. Nephritic serum was not shown to be active on C3 contained within the euglobulin fraction of normal human sera unless the pseudoglobulin fraction was also present to supply an essential cofactor to the reaction (149); this cofactor was later identified as factor B. Early studies of C3NeF indicated that it was a gamma globulin of 150,000 Daltons. Recently there has been some disagreement about whether C3NeF is an immunoglobulin or a distinct globulin with slow gamma electrophoretic mobility but different from usual immunoglobulin molecules (146–154). However, current evidence supports the idea that C3NeF is indeed an immunoglobulin (154).

Studies with purified C3NeF showed that C3 activation did not occur if factors B, D, or properdin had been selectively depleted and it appeared that a major part of C3NeF action on C3 occurred through the alternative complement pathway (155, 156). Four plasma proteins of this pathway have now been isolated and characterized: C3; B (also termed C3 proactivator or C3PA); D, the C3PA convertase; and properdin with a molecular weight of 223,000 Daltons. Sequential steps of alternate pathway activation and feedback control are shown diagrammatically in Figure 12-8.

When these findings were applied in the past to patients with MPGN or hypocomplemente-

Figure 12-7 Typical histological changes associated with membranous glomerulonephritis, showing marked thickening of glomerular loops, splitting of basement membranes, and interposition of mesangial fibrils and cytoplasm. Magnification × 650. (Photomicrograph courtesy of David J. Evans, Royal Postgraduate Medical School, London.)

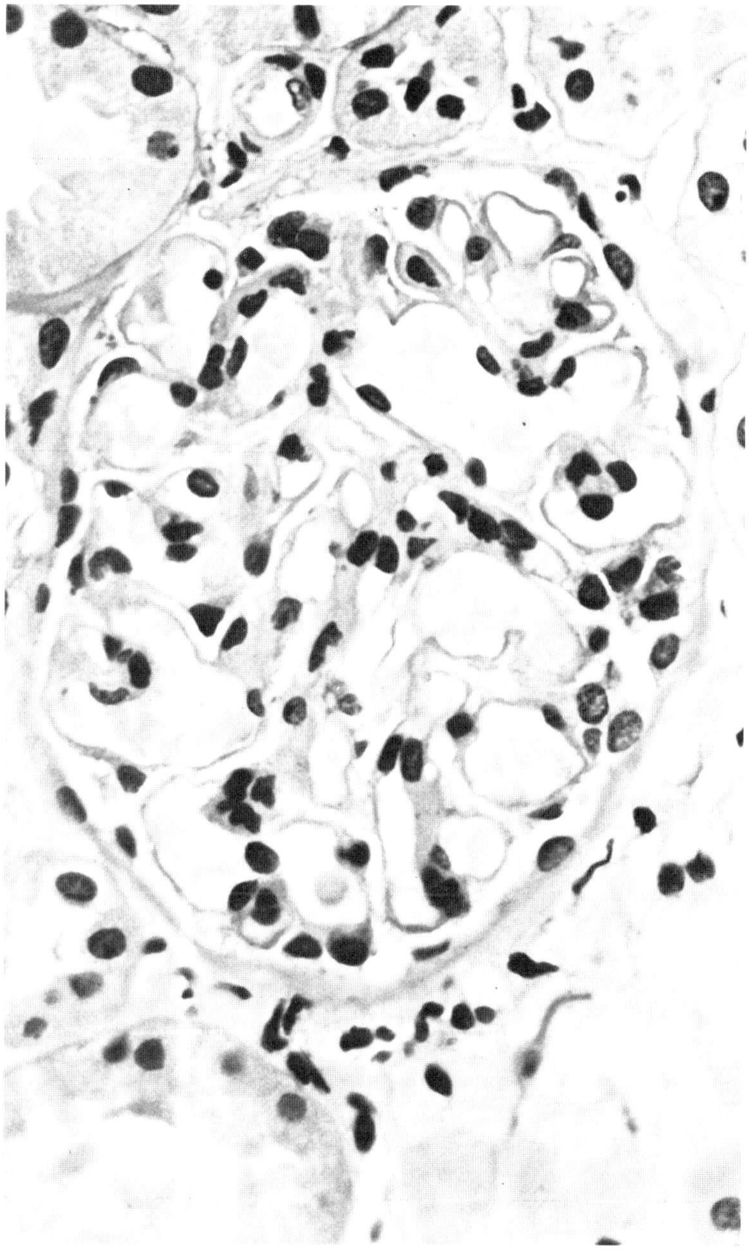

mic nephritis, confusion resulted, since immune deposits containing various complement components without apparent concurrent immunoglobulin have frequently been recorded in individual cases. It is important to point out that the findings in so-called dense-deposit disease (136, 137, 157, 158) and the other more common general picture of MPGN associated with subendothelial deposits are different. In

DDD, immunofluorescence usually shows C3 alone without early complement components C1, C2, or C4 and without immunoglobulins. In the subendothelial variety, IgG, IgM, and early complement components C1q and C4 in association with C3 are often present. Likewise in dense-deposit disease immunofluorescence for properdin is usually negative, but in subendothelial-deposit disease properdin is usually

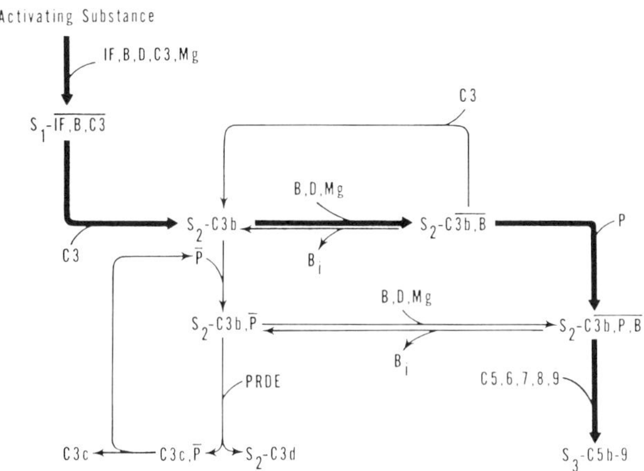

Figure 12-8 Schematic representation of the molecular dynamics of the properdin pathway. S_1 represents the site of initiation at which the properdin receptor forming enzyme is generated. S_2 denotes the site of attachment of C3b doublets, which serve as properdin receptors. S_2 is also the site of formation of the properdin activating principle that acts as the $\overline{P}$–C5 convertase. S_3 represents the site of binding of the C5b–9 membrane attack complex. The properdin receptor destroying enzyme (PRDE) acts on several different sites. (Reproduced with permission, R. G. Medicus, R. D. Schreiber, O. Götze et al., *Proc. Natl. Acad. Sci. USA* 73:612, 1976.)

detected in close association with C3 and immunoglobulin. In neither of these histological variants is factor B of the alternate complement pathway detected by immunofluorescence. Parallel clinical studies found hypocomplementemic sera in the majority of subjects with DDD. Serum complement profile shows normal C1, C4, and C2 with marked reduction in C3 and C5. Direct measurement of alternate complement components properdin, factor D, and factor B are normal and C3NeF is present. Alternatively, hypocomplementemia may be variable in subendothelial-deposit disease. Reduced concentrations of C1, C4, and C2 may be present; C5 is low. In this instance C3NeF is less frequently detectable (159). The variability of actual complement component profiles and the differences noted in immunofluorescent findings among large series of these patients indicate that a clear or uniform definition of all the events occurring during the immunologic progression of this disorder has been difficult.

From data accumulated to date, the precise mechanisms underlying hypocomplementemia and C3 activation in this interesting disease are probably not directly related only to complement consumption in the renal parenchyma. This thesis is supported by persistent hypocomplementemia following nephrectomy and numerous clinical observations that no correlation could be made between degree of disease activity and serum complement measurements. From the work of Daha and co-workers (154), the precise mechanism of C3NeF now appears to be in binding to C3 convertases (C3b$\overline{\text{B}}$ and C3B$\overline{\text{b}}$) to stabilize these labile enzymes, with prolongation of their active half-lives by a factor of ten. The nephritic-factor–stabilized enzymes are, therefore, resistant to the normal regulatory controlling mechanisms of C3b inactivator and β1H (160). Precisely how nephritic factor acts in potentiating the nephritic process is still a matter of some debate. Recent work in several laboratories indicates that C3NeF is indeed an immunoglobulin occurring quite often as a component of relatively restricted electrophoretic mobility in many sera (161). Whether this component in sera of afflicted individuals allows fixation or ready attachment of immune complexes to glomerular structures is not yet clear. Nevertheless, this particular question is of considerable practical importance, since recurrence of MPGN has been increasingly recognized after renal transplantation (162). Peters and colleagues (163) have suggested that rather than acting in a direct way to augment glomerular immune-complex deposition, C3 activation induced by C3NeF predisposes to numerous subclinical infections eventually resulting in immune-complex glomerulonephritis. It is also possible that continuing C3 activation might facilitate glomerular localization of complexes by releasing endogenous vasoactive amines, as has been previously noted during the course of experimental immune-complex nephritis (164, 165). In support of such a hypothesis are the increasingly frequent reports of isolated complement component deficiencies in association with nephritis, lupus-like states, or in many instances of clear-cut SLE (166–170). These associations between complement component deficiencies and a wide variety of presumed immune-complex disorders suggests by analogy that MPGN and hypocomplementemic nephritis may be acting by similar but as yet incompletely defined basic mechanisms.

Hypocomplementemia and Partial Lipodystrophy

Partial lipodystrophy (PLD) is apparently an acquired disease, characterized by relatively rapid symmetrical loss of subcutaneous fat from face, arms, and trunk. At times the areas involved are restricted primarily to the face, where loss of buccal fat pads produces a characteristic facial appearance. Typical physical findings associated with PLD are shown in Figure 12-9. Generally the onset of this curious disorder is during childhood and is noted following an infection. In 1958 PLD was first noted to be related to renal disease by Gellis and co-workers (171). It was found that 14 of the 77 patients previously recorded in the literature showed evidence of renal disease. Subsequently, PLD was determined to be specifically associated with mesangiocapillary nephritis, usually of the dense-deposit type. These findings are especially pertinent since the patients with PLD show the same abnormalities

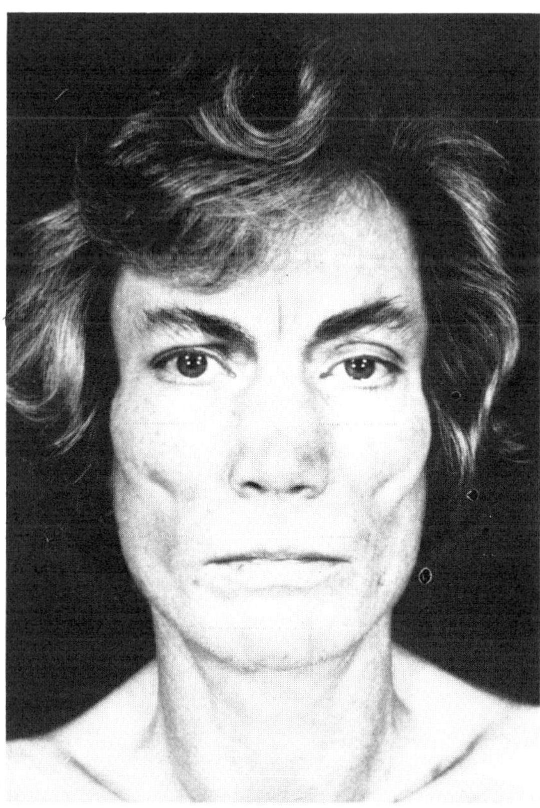
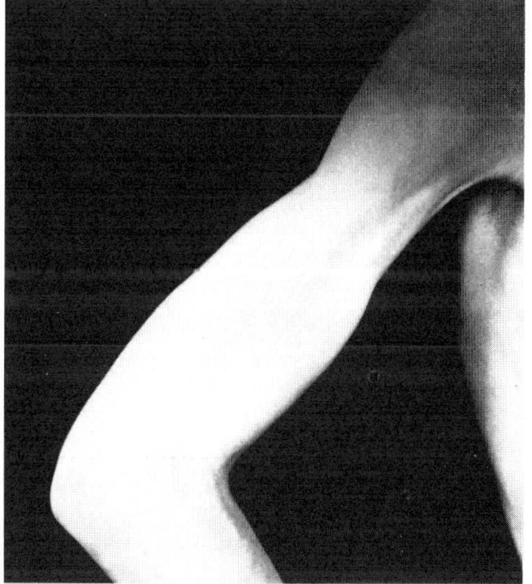

Figure 12-9 Characteristic facies in patient with partial lipodystrophy (*left*) and localized loss of subcutaneous fat in upper arm (*right*). (Photographs courtesy of Barry Bresnihan and G. R. V. Hughes, Hammersmith Hospital, London.)

of the complement system as do the children with MPGN and hypocomplementemia. PLD subjects show low C3, C3 breakdown products in fresh plasma, C3NeF, hypercatabolism of C3, reduced C3 synthesis, and normal C5 metabolism (172, 173). Renal abnormalities do not always parallel the serum complement deviations or presence of C3NeF in these patients (173, 174). Though clinically undetectable, MPGN has been noted at renal biopsy in a patient with PLD (175). Other complement abnormalities have also been described in association with PLD: Frank and co-workers (176) noted PLD in association with hereditary angioedema and C1 inhibitor deficiency; a patient with localized lipodystrophy was noted by Sissons and co-workers (173) to have low C1, C4, and C2.

The direct relation between PLD and other diseases provides a fascinating spectrum of associations. Diabetes occurs in approximately 20 percent of PLD patients. Changes in lipid metabolism, hypertriglyceridemia, elevated free fatty acids and increase in pre-beta lipoproteinemia may result from a depletion of total fat cell stores in the body as a whole (177). Other associations include hepatomegaly, liver dysfunction, fatty infiltration, cirrhosis, hyperpigmentation, and acanthosis nigricans. In addition, PLD has now been reported in association with systemic lupus, Sjögren's syndrome (178, 179), inflammatory bowel disease (180), and autoimmune thyroid disease (181). These broad associations with a number of disease entities suggest that PLD is related somehow to a basic missetting of the immune system, possibly in favor of autoimmune or self-aggressive reactions in a number of systems. The remarkable association between presence of C3NeF, PDL, and glomerulonephritis must remain the focus of considerable study. Moreover, the parallels between PDL and hypocomplementemic nephritis or MPGN suggest a final or shared common pathway in pathogenesis.

The clinical observations related to onset of PDL are intriguing in this respect. Little is understood about the genesis of the peculiar distribution of atrophy occurring in PDL. In some reports (182, 183) both partial and total lipodystrophy have followed measles. The ana-

tomic distribution of measles rash in some cases closely parallels subsequent areas affected by subcutaneous fat cell loss. Whether or not these changes represent direct or more distant sequelae of measles virus persistence in such individuals requires considerably more study. It seems unlikely that chronic activation of the complement system by C3NeF is alone capable of producing ongoing and often progressive chronic glomerulonephritis. Experimental data in animals have shown that such prolonged activation does not induce chronic sustained renal injury (184). Furthermore, a recent report involving studies of identical twins, only one of whom actually developed PLD and MPGN with C3NeF (185), indicates that genetics alone cannot account for expression of the disorder. No data are available, moreover, on whether the C3NeF antedates the development of PLD. Some of these interrelationships are shown diagrammatically in Figure 12-10. One might look on the nephritic factor as analogous to an autoantibody to a neoantigen on activated com-

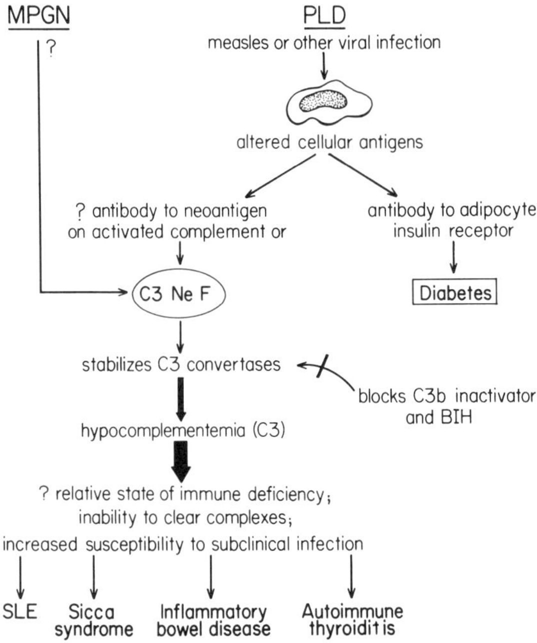

Figure 12-10 Possible interrelated mechanisms in membranoproliferative glomerulonephritis (MPGN) and partial lipodystrophy (PLD).

plement. This antibody is then capable of inducing a prolonged functional hypocomplementemic state. Changes in the handling of circulating immune complexes by the normal glomerular clearing mechanisms may increase individual susceptibility to autoimmune disorders such as SLE, Sjögren's syndrome, or inflammatory bowel disease. The final test of such a hypothesis will require experiments in which purified C3NeF is infused into primates and handling of immune complexes studied in vivo.

Physical Considerations

Although membranous glomerulonephritis is related to immune complexes, the conventional morphological and ultrastructural differences from other renal diseases in which an immune-complex etiology has been conclusively demonstrated, such as SLE or poststreptococcal glomerulonephritis, present some difficulty in interpretation. This has recently been discussed by Evans (186) in an analysis of what might be expected depending on the relative sizes of antigens involved in glomerular immune-complex phenomena. Previous work (187) indicated that the earliest lesions observed in membranous or membranoproliferative glomerulonephritis were deposition of electron-dense materials under the foot processes of epithelial cells. These deposits appeared to lie outside the basement membrane. Later during evolution of these lesions, spikes of basement membrane material were recognized between deposits, which were subsequently completely surrounded by basement membrane. During evolution the deposits may show dissolution and dispersal or progression to a process ending in glomerular sclerosis and hyalinization. This sequential change is shown in Figure 12-11. Differential concentration effects of antigen, antibody, and complexes within various glomerular structures might theoretically account for final localization of immune complexes within certain sites and in particular for the intramembranous dense deposits often seen in membranous disease. Thus, experiments by Graham and Karnovsky (188) have shown that low-molecular-weight marker proteins such as horseradish peroxi-

dase (40,000 Daltons) can enter the glomerular basement membrane and mesangium without apparent restriction or concentration gradient from the endothelial side through the GBM. Alternatively an intermediate-sized molecule such as myeloperoxidase (160,000 to 180,000 Daltons) showed heavy concentration in the regions under the epithelial cells' foot processes, with much less in the more proximal membrane and glomerular lumen. Higher-molecular-weight proteins (catalase: 250,000 Daltons; ferritin: 400,000 Daltons) have also been studied (189, 190) and although both enter the GBM, their concentrations are reduced. Accumulation of these two high-molecular-weight materials occurs mainly in the mesangium rather than in the GBM. It might, therefore, be assumed that low-molecular-weight antigens (30,000 to 60,000 Daltons), free antigen, antibody, and circulating complexes containing such low-molecular-weight antigens could diffuse into the GBM and eventually produce dense deposits. With high-molecular-weight antigens, equivalence between antigens and

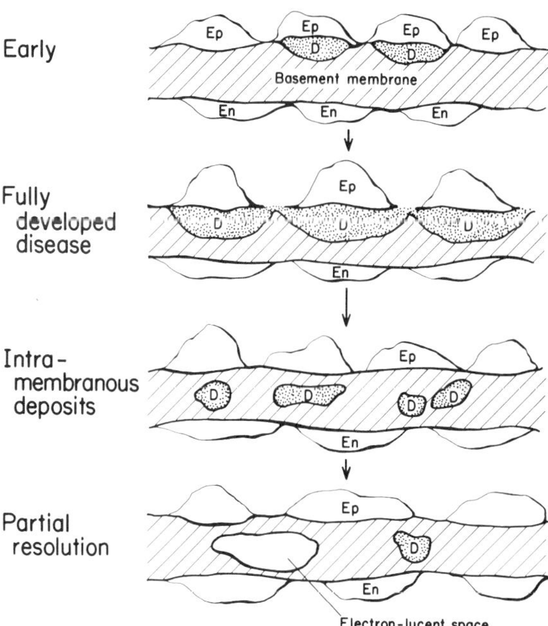

Figure 12-11 Possible mechanisms involved in the development of dense deposits (D) during evolution of membranous or membranoproliferative nephritis.

antibodies might be reached in the midportion or subepithelial areas of the GBM, also leading to immune precipitates and dense deposits. Since immune complexes are entrapped within GBM structures, leukocytic infiltration and chemotaxis may not be an important phenomenon. Immune precipitates would be in equilibrium with soluble reacting components and with time might be subject to gradual resolution. Since GBM appears to be made by epithelial cells (191), replacement from above might also favor the observed gradual inward migration of dense deposits or resolution in some cases. At the present time this hypothesis cannot be directly tested as no definitive antigens have been identified. However, if the hypothesis is correct, it would implicate either low-molecular-weight or medium-sized antigens in such reactions.

Correlations with Detectable Circulating Immune Complexes

A report by Ooi and colleagues (192) has analyzed detectable circulating immune complexes using the sensitive C1q radioimmunoassay in patients with membranoproliferative and other glomerulopathies. Patients with both subendothelial and mesangial immune deposits and those with intramembranous dense deposits were studied. Of interest were studies of 4 patients with dense-deposit disease (DDD) who underwent renal transplantation. Two patients had evidence of recurrence of DDD within the transplanted kidney. Half of the 20 MPGN patients showed elevations of immune complexes by C1q binding assay. Analysis of immune complexes present in these sera showed materials sedimenting in the 13.8 to 19.5S region, indicating the relatively high molecular weight of the complexes detected by these assay methods. A comparison of similar analyses done on SLE sera and sera from a few patients with presumed poststreptococcal acute glomerulonephritis is shown in Figure 12-12 from this study. In all cases of MPGN studied, IgG and C3 were noted both in circulating complexes and by immunofluorescence of renal tissue. However, there was no correlation between composition of immune complexes with respect to presence of IgA or IgM and positive immunofluorescence on biopsy. A

general correlation appeared when presence of detectable circulating complexes was compared to clinical status in patients with MPGN. It is clear from the hypotheses raised by Evans (186) that an attempt must now be made to examine the immune complexes circulating in these patients for the physicochemical properties of the presumed antigens present. Comparative studies of complement levels and C1q binding activities in the patients studied by Ooi and co-workers (192) indicated that detectable immune complexes were present in some patients without abnormalities in serum complement levels and, conversely, that complement might be low in the absence of detectable circulating complexes. Diminished synthesis of C3 or relative biological activity of C3NeF might influence such a comparison. Direct correlations between renal immunohistology and the presence of circulating immune complexes may finally provide the most meaningful data in practical clinical analysis.

Recurrence of MPGN after Transplantation and Response to Treatment

Even in transplanted patients where recurrent disease is not suspected clinically, renal biopsy material may show characteristic electron-dense deposits within the GBM (193, 194). Several groups have noted that regardless of electron-dense deposits in both GBM and TBM structures, there appeared to be no clinical evidence of recurrent glomerulonephritis in these patients as soon as 7 months following transplantation (193, 194) or evidence that recurrent disease of MPGN type was responsible for allograft failure. The lesion of intramembranous dense deposits can be quite widespread in the absence of clinical signs of recurrent MPGN and appearance of the electron-dense deposits may precede eventual appearance of epithelial and mesangial cell alterations within the renal parenchyma (195).

Membranous Nephropathy

The general pathological entity of membranous nephritis encompasses more patients than those with MPGN or hypocomplementemic nephritis and also includes patients with membranous glomerular lesions secondary to SLE, diabetes, specific chemical reactions such

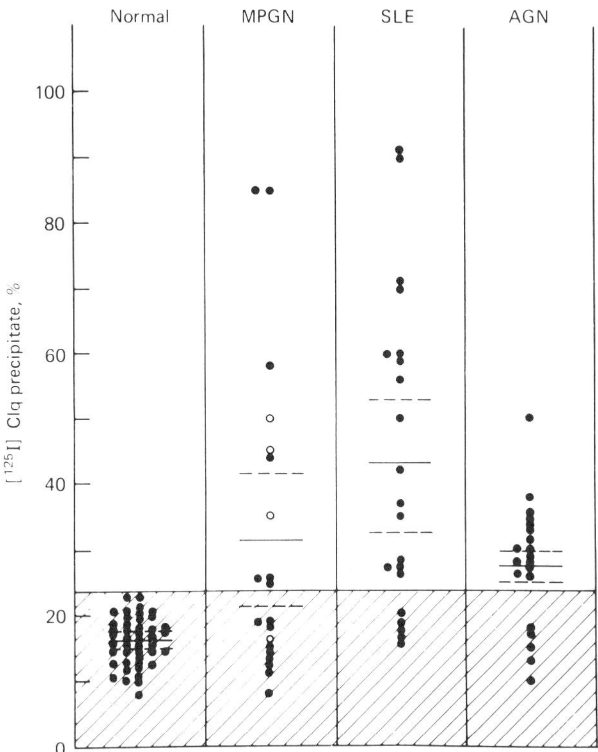

Figure 12-12 C1q binding assay of sera from normal subjects and patients with membranoproliferative glomerulonephritis (MPGN), systemic lupus erythematosus (SLE), and acute poststreptococcal glomerulonephritis (AGN). (Reproduced with permission, Y. M. Ooi, E. H. Vallota, and C. D. West, *Kidney Int.* 11:275, 1977.)

as gold or penicillamine, or certain chronic infections (syphilis, quartan malaria, or infective endocarditis). There is a wide range of opinion regarding whether specific immunosuppressive therapy has any beneficial effect on the clinical course of patients with membranous disease. Most series have indicated that patients with membranous nephropathy derive little benefit from either corticosteroid (196–200) or immunosuppressive treatment (201, 202). Occasional reports have shown what was thought to be a favorable therapeutic response with or without comparison to a control group (203–205). Any disease in which remission or relapses may occur without any treatment, and which follows a chronic course, is difficult to evaluate. A recent retrospective study of 167 cases of membranous nephropathy (206) provided 91 adults and 12 children in whom follow-up was available for a mean of 6.5 years. It appeared that clinical cure and improvement were greater in the treated than in the non-

treated groups. Moreover, prognosis was better in patients who responded to therapy. Fifty-four subjects received corticosteroids and 15 patients received corticosteroids and immunosuppressants. Control patients, selected prospectively to match those being treated, were not included in this study. The practical clinical problem posed by the large group of individuals with membranous nephropathy is an important one. What is needed now is insight into the pathological process itself—particularly local or distant factors that may govern or modulate eventual resolution or progressive sclerosis and obliteration of glomerular units.

Glomerulonephritis Mediated by Antibody to GBM

Immune-complex–mediated glomerulonephritis is found in a small proportion of patients who show presence in sera or glomerular eluates of antibody reacting directly with antigens present within the glomerular basement membrane itself. This type of nephritis is apparently not mediated so much by circulating immune complexes as by direct fixation of autologous antibody to glomerular antigens. Originally recognized largely in association with Goodpasture's syndrome, it is now clear that a small proportion of patients with a wide variety of clinical presentations may in fact show immunopathological evidence of this basic underlying mechanism. Very little is understood as yet concerning the events inducing the synthesis of antibody to GBM components, but the striking immunofluorescent findings in such patients emphasize the generalized immune reaction (presumably against self- or cross-reacting antigens) that characterizes these phenomena.

Antigenic Structure of GBM

Glomeruli obtained from animal sources or human cadavers can readily be prepared after passage of minced tissues through calibrated sieves. The glomeruli are then disrupted by sonication and several techniques used to solubilize constituents for study. Cleaving enzymes, such as collagenase or pronase, or heating GBM preparations at 110° C for three hours have been employed by various workers (207–210). Glomerular basement membrane is composed of glycoproteins containing 10 percent carbohydrates. These sugar moieties consist of two oligosaccharide chains: a disaccharide with equal amounts of glucose and galactose and a heterogeneous polysaccharide with galactose, mannose, fucose, sialic acid, and osamines. Glomerular basement membrane shows close structural similarity to collagens in that both contain hydroxyproline and hydroxylysine; GBM differs in that it also contains cystine and 3-hydroxyproline. Studies of GBM antigenicity reveal several distinct groups of antigens: pepsin digestion shows two groups of antigens (211): one is solubilized by trypsin and capable of neutralization of 75 percent of nephrotoxic antibodies and the other is an insoluble fraction reacting with the remainder of nephrotoxic antibody. In similar fashion trichloroacetic acid treatment separates several GBM antigens (212). Soluble GBM antigens isolated from urine by McPhaul and Dixon (213) are capable of producing glomerulonephritis after injection with adjuvant. These materials were between 100,000 and 200,000 Daltons.

Glomerular basement membrane appears to share antigenic reactivities with many diverse organs and with some bacteria such as the streptococcus. The most highly vascularized tissues such as lung, placenta, heart, gut, liver, and muscle are most useful in producing nephrotoxic antisera (214). Cross-reactions of GBM with collagen are present, but to a much lesser degree than with other extrarenal basement membranes.

Goodpasture's Syndrome

In 1919 Goodpasture described the association of rapidly progressive glomerulonephritis and a hemorrhagic pulmonary disorder (215). Since that time numerous cases have been recorded and several reviews of well-studied cases have been published (216–219). The clinical picture of the disease is well delineated: most patients are young men. No clear hereditary pattern has been shown, although cases occurring together in families have occsionally been noted (217, 218). Onset of the pulmonary disorder usually occurs first but may actually follow the onset of glomerulonephritis. Severe hemoptysis, often recurrent, may be the primary cause of death. Chest x-rays often show bilateral diffuse infiltrates with prominent hilar, basilar, and apical extensions. Radiological abnormalities on chest x-rays frequently clear rapidly after cessation of hemoptysis. The glomerulonephritis associated with this disease often leads to rapid progressive renal failure. Proteinuria, hematuria, and numerous red blood cell casts are present, but hypertension is not a prominent feature of the acute illness. Renal biopsy shows necrotic focal or diffuse glomerulonephritis with early changes of fibrinoid necrosis. Later endocapillary proliferation and crescent formation occur with progression to diffuse lesions. Electron microscopic examination shows thickening of GBMs by intramembranous deposits (217) (Figure 12-13). The lungs show edema and extensive intraalveolar hemorrhage with macrophages

Figure 12-13 Dense intramembranous deposits (*arrows*) seen in association with anti-GBM antibody. Magnification × 6,800. (Reproduced with permission, J. J. McPhaul, Jr., and J. D. Mullins, *J. Clin. Invest.* 57:351, 1976.)

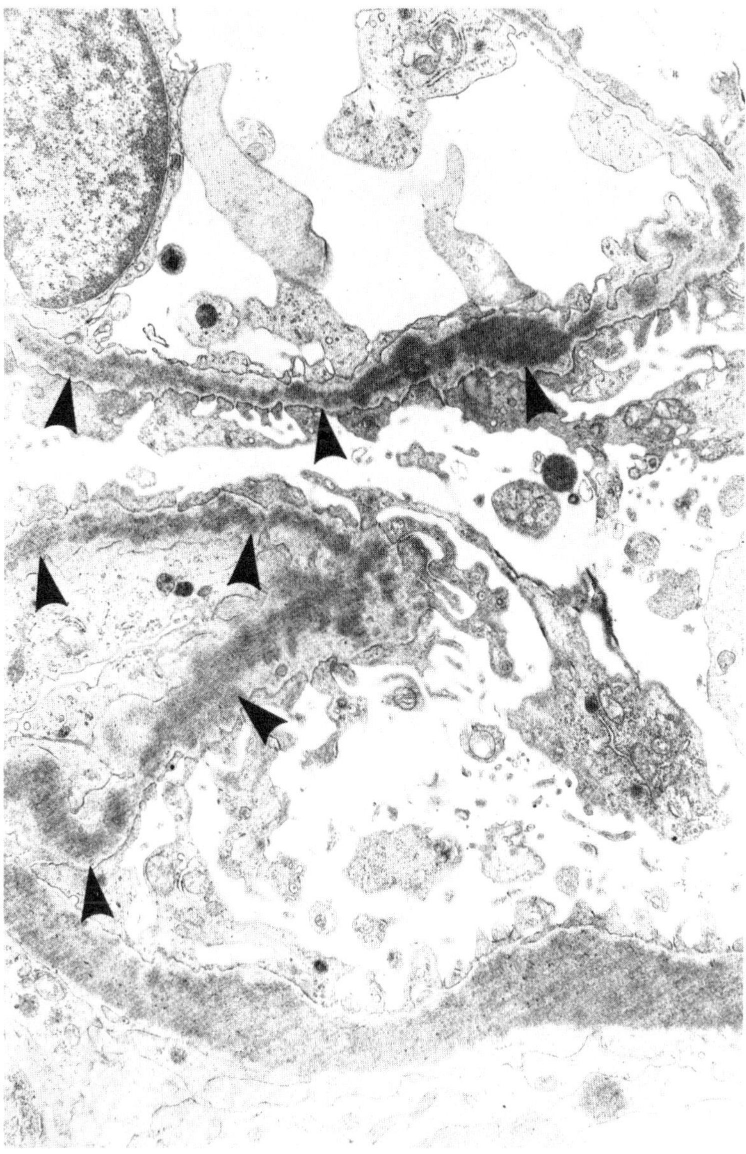

filled with hemosiderin. In more advanced or subacute lesions there are often extensive or patchy areas of alveolar fibrosis. Electron microscopic examination of these areas may show deposits along alveolar basement membranes quite similar to those seen in GBMs (217).

The most characteristic laboratory finding is the presence of antibody to GBM, usually demonstrated by immunofluorescence. A typical reaction is shown in Figure 12-14, showing characteristic linear IgG GBM staining. Concurrent linear or occasionally more granular deposition of C3 is also seen in many cases. The distinct linear quality of GBM staining in this disorder makes it clearly different from the usual lumpy-bumpy or granular irregular deposits generally associated with other immune-complex–mediated forms of nephritis, such as lupus or poststreptococcal nephritis (217–221). Immunoglobulins representing all of the four H-chain subgroups (IgG1, IgG2, IgG3, and IgG4) are present, although subgroup distribution may be variable in any individual case (222, 223). Molecules containing

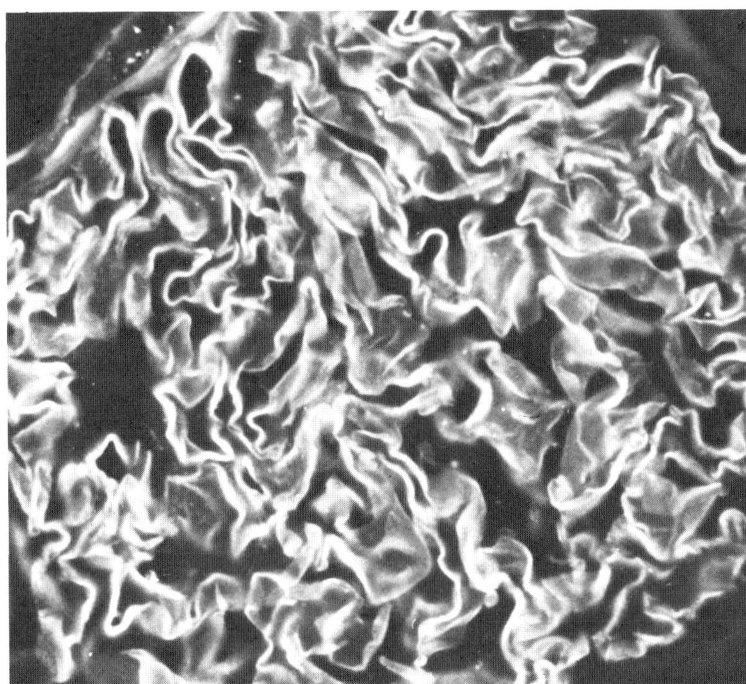

Figure 12-14 Photomicrograph illustrating typical linear fixation of IgG along glomerular basement membrane of native diseased kidney of patient with Goodpasture's syndrome, visualized by indirect immunofluorescence. Magnification × 350. (Reproduced with permission. J. J. McPhaul, Jr., and F. J. Dixon, *J. Clin. Invest.* 49:308, 1970.)

kappa or lambda light chains are present in approximately equal proportions, with a few exceptions (217, 223). In some patients it is possible to demonstrate anti-GBM serum antibodies present in excess by incubation of serum with sections of normal kidney (224). Eluates often show more relative concentration of antibody activity than is present in serum (225), and in some instances anti-GBM antibody activity may be present in eluates from kidney although undetectable in serum studied concurrently.

An analysis of fixation or cross-specificity to other tissues was performed using radiolabeled human glomerular eluates containing anti-GBM antibody infused into squirrel monkeys. A summary of these data taken from the work of McPhaul and Dixon (225) is shown in Table 12-3. Predominant tissue fixation was to kidney, with lesser degrees of reactivity in lungs, heart, spleen, or liver. Despite evidence for active in vivo fixation to lung in these primate passive transfer experiments, it could be shown that eluates did indeed fix to alveolar septae of lung if studied in greater relative protein concentration in vitro. In keeping with these latter findings are several reports showing linear deposits in lung alveolar membranes in patients with Goodpasture's syndrome (226, 227). Antigenic cross-reactivity between GBM of kidney and lung has been recognized for some time (228, 229). More recent studies of the cross-specificities of anti-GBM antibodies with pulmonary alveolar antigens have been reported by Koffler and co-workers (226). From a clinical and therapeutic standpoint, it is important to delineate this relationship; approximately 20 percent of patients with Goodpasture's syndrome have shown antecedent upper-respiratory infections prior to development of hemoptysis and nephritis (216). Direct microscopic examination of pulmonary tissues in many patients has not, however, provided much support for the concept that active infection itself is capable of inducing the symptom complex. Anti-GBM antibody was directly eluted from the lung of a patient with Goodpasture's syndrome (226). Some interesting quantitative data with respect to relative reactivities were noted. The minimum gamma-globulin concentration with anti-GBM antibody activity demonstrable by immunofluorescence in serum was 6.70 mg; for lung eluate, 0.09 mg; for kidney eluate, 0.03 mg. Thus, the lung and

Table 12-3   Organ fixation of radiolabeled human eluates containing antiglomerular basement membrane antibodies injected into squirrel monkeys.

Eluate	Percentage of fixation to—				
	Kidney	Lungs	Heart	Spleen	Liver
Control	17	6	2	4	71
Goodpasture					
B	78	2	2	3	15
F	85	1	0	2	12
O lung	71	1	0	4	23
O kidney	89	1	1	4	6
S absorbed	44	3	2	2	50
S unabsorbed	51	3	1	3	42
Non-Goodpasture					
DE	90	7	2	1	0
C	92	5	3	0	0
Du	53	5	2	2	36
Du 3 day transfer	66	2	1	3	28
Du 8 day transfer	55	3	1	2	40

Source: Reproduced with permission, J. J. McPhaul, Jr., and F. J. Dixon, *J. Clin. Invest.* 49:308, 1970.

kidney eluates contained 75 to 200 times as much anti-GBM antibody activity as the sera. Furthermore, it was shown that complete inhibition of both lung and glomerular eluate immunofluorescence could be achieved using sonicated GBM. These experiments indicate that anti-GBM antibodies themselves may participate in the damage to pulmonary alveolar membranes. In this regard, autoimmune glomerulonephritis can be induced in sheep immunized with human lung (230). The apparent close immunologic relationship of kidney and lung that is presumed from these studies of Goodpasture's syndrome suggests that selective sensitization to certain basement membrane antigens present in GBM and alveolar walls must certainly occur during natural induction of the disease. Precisely how this occurs is not at all clear. From his clinical descriptions of the disease occurring at a time of epidemic influenzal infection, Goodpasture presumed that antecedent respiratory infection somehow triggered the disease process. It seems possible that the anti-GBM and the antialveolar antibodies associated with this disorder may both represent cross-reacting antibodies to some primary viral or infectious agent. Cross-reactions reported between glomerular antigens and streptococcal antigens (15) would be in line with this concept. Alternatively, there is also strong clinical evidence to favor the idea that initial immunization may occur in the lung itself. Thus an infectious agent primarily in the lung might be capable of altering pulmonary basement membranes in such a way as to favor primary immune responsiveness to GBM.

Natural Course of the Disease

From the patients recorded soon after Goodpasture's description and in the several decades that followed, it appeared initially that the disease usually showed rapid progression and a high mortality. Viewed in retrospect today, subsequent to well over a hundred reported cases, the prognosis—although still unfavorable in many patients—may not be as ominous as was formerly believed. In some patients regardless of interval dialysis support, renal failure progresses rapidly and is accompanied by persistent hemoptysis, superimposed nosocomial infection, and rapid demise. In other patients the outlook may be considerably more favorable, and relative stabilization or apparent improvement have been recorded (217, 218). As a generality, the results with corticosteroid or combined immunosuppressive treatment have not been uniformly favorable. However, nephrectomy followed by renal transplantation may be the treatment of choice in some patients. This was initially reported by Maddock and colleagues (231) in a patient who showed what was considered to be a dramatic cessation of pulmonary hemorrhage following nephrectomy. It was postulated that removal of the source of one primary antigen—the kidneys and therefore all intrinsic autologous GBM—might be instrumental in lowering subsequent ongoing immune response to such antigens thereby modulating the severity of the disease. Since these initial observations a number of groups have reported their experience with nephrectomy and transplantation in this disorder (232–234). In general, bilateral nephrectomy can be judged to be life-saving in some patients but in 13 subjects reviewed by Wilson and Dixon (219), 6 subjects continued to experience pulmonary symptoms after nephrectomy. Five of 13 nonnephrectomized or unilaterally nephrectomized patients included in this latter study eventually died of pulmonary failure. In many patients circulating anti-GBM antibody persisted for an average of 6 to 8 months after nephrectomy. Transplantation appeared to be more often successful when delayed until circulating anti-GBM antibodies had disappeared or showed substantial decline. This analysis also presented data indicating evidence of recurrent glomerulonephritis developing in 19 of 34 transplanted patients, resulting in graft failure in at least 7 patients. Severe recurrences of anti-GBM–mediated renal disease appeared to be most often related to brief anephric periods and persistent elevations of anti-GBM antibody.

In view of these impressions, it is difficult to formulate a working plan of action for the individual patient afflicted with ongoing active Goodpasture's syndrome. It seems obvious that nephrectomy itself may act as a two-edged sword, since abrupt removal of a large mass of tissue containing the primary source of putative antigen could from a theoretical standpoint backfire by releasing considerable free circulating anti-GBM antibody of moderate affinity, which would then be free to circulate and attack cross-reactive pulmonary basement membranes or other vulnerable structures. With advancing disease, the mass of GBM in the severely damaged kidney could be acting as a sink or sponge sopping up high-affinity, potentially dangerous antibody. The results documented in nephrectomized and transplanted patients to date might support such a mechanism being operative in some, but the fact that a favorable result has been obtained in about half of the transplanted and nephrectomized patients so treated to date emphasizes the complexity of the problem. Clinical results in such patients probably represent amount and avidity of residual circulating anti-GBM antibody left after therapeutic nephrectomy and the number and immunologic state of residual GBM-antigen activated B cells in such individuals.

A new approach to this whole problem has been implemented with the use of extensive plasmapheresis, with or without combined immunosuppression. Several recent reports documenting favorable outcomes using plasmapheresis have now appeared (235, 236). In one (236), no return of renal function was noted after such treatment; extensive changes on renal biopsy had already become established, but life-threatening pulmonary hemorrhage in one patient was rapidly controlled. Of interest was the fact that plasmapheresis was accompanied by volume replacement using plasma protein fraction, fresh-frozen group-compatible plasma, or purified protein fraction. Whether the latter materials were somehow indirectly or directly involved in improvement of clinical status cannot at present be determined. It is possible that reconstitution with plasma containing potentially active complement components effective in dissolving immune precipitates may have serendipitously contributed to a beneficial effect as well. These theoretical aspects of plasmapheresis or plasma exchange were discussed in detail in Chapter 5. Regardless of these possibilities, the encouraging results obtained to date using intensive plasmapheresis in patients with active Goodpasture's syndrome suggest that this may represent the treatment of choice.

Anti-GBM Antibodies in Other Renal Disorders

Several surveys have been made of large numbers of serial renal biopsies for the incidence and clinical correlations with anti-GBM antibodies. In the study of 409 consecutive biopsies by McPhaul and Mullins (237), 43—or 11 percent of the entire group—showed anti-GBM antibody staining as defined by diffuse and linear localization of host Ig. Of note was the fact that two badly scarred renal samples in this study showed anti-GBM antibody in eluates while being negative by direct immunofluorescent study. On routine histological examination half of the patients studied showed minor and nonspecific glomerular abnormalities or mild focal glomerulonephritis. More severe involvement was seen with focal necrotizing changes (17 percent), rapidly progressive (7 percent) and chronic sclerosing glomerulonephritis (27 percent). The clinical course associated with presence of anti-GBM antibody in this large series was extremely variable. Some patients showed only indolent microhematuria, while others developed progressive renal failure or nephrotic syndrome. The presence of circulating anti-GBM antibodies confirmed by hemagglutination or radioimmunoassay was noted in a considerable proportion of patients. The variety of clinical and histological pictures observed in this series indicates that rather than being confined only to the distinct and often rapidly progressive picture of Goodpasture's syndrome, the occurrence of anti-GBM antibody may indeed represent a phenomenon of rather broad distribution within the entire spectrum of renal disease. Similar diversity of the clinical picture in non-Goodpasture's glomerulonephritis associated with presence of anti-GBM antibody has been noted by other workers (219, 238). The relative rarity of clear-cut Goodpasture's syndrome and the apparent overlap of linear anti-GBM staining

in other heterogeneous renal diseases is a phenomenon of considerable importance. It is appropriate to note that in several large French surveys systematic study of 1,200 cases showed no linear deposits (239, 240), and in one published American series of 340 biopsies, Goodpasture's or linear GBM staining was noted in only two cases (241).

When linear anti-GBM staining is seen in association with other renal diseases beside the glomerulonephritis of Goodpasture's syndrome, the spectrum of reactivities against pulmonary or other vascular membrane antigens appears to be considerably more restricted than with Goodpasture's syndrome itself. In patients with rapidly progressive glomerulonephritis and linear GBM staining the precise role of such antibody is not entirely clear. In some cases a similar syndrome can be transferred to monkeys with eluates from affected kidneys (242). In the patient studied by Lerner and co-workers (242), anti-GBM antibodies had not been detected in the serum but became evident 5 days after bilateral nephrectomy. When a transplant was subsequently done, the serum antibodies again became undetectable and linear immunofluorescent findings were noted in the transplant within 75 minutes following the arterial anastomosis. In other similar patients, such a dramatic rise and fall in anti-GBM antibodies has not generally been observed.

In summary, the role of antibody to GBM represents an immune-complex–mediated phenomenon of considerable theoretical importance. Because of its characteristic and rather distinctive appearance on direct examination of biopsy or pathological material, much interest has been focused on attempts to understand its real significance among the spectrum of patients in which it is found. It seems entirely possible that other directly reacting antitissue antibodies may be of similar importance in the modulation or direct pathogenesis of many other human disorders. Perhaps the lessons that have thus far been learned regarding the basic mechanisms involved in rare diseases such as Goodpasture's syndrome may now be applied to other diseases where antibodies reacting directly with various tissue components have been described.

IgA Nephropathy

In 1968 Berger first described a nephropathy associated with glomerular mesangial deposition of IgA with less prominent concomitant IgG and C3 deposition in a group of patients who showed no general evidence of systemic disease (243, 244). Most of the patients originally described showed normal renal function with either gross or microscopic hematuria and some degree of proteinuria that was frequently exacerbated by upper-respiratory infections. Histological examination often revealed a focal glomerulonephritis. This disorder is included under the discussion of immune-complex renal disease, even though much of the basic insight into pathogenesis or etiology is still largely unknown. As yet there is no clear identification of what antigen-antibody complex systems are involved, if indeed any are. In many ways IgA nephropathy or Berger's syndrome remains somewhat of an enigma: first, because IgA antibodies classically are not felt to be potent activators of the complement system and second, because no underlying antigen or mechanism of direct pathogenesis has yet been elucidated. The disorder might be considered one characterized by many of the features of an immune-complex nephropathy. Since the initial description, many other workers have studied patients more or less fitting the original definition. McEnery and co-workers (245) found IgA, IgG, and C3 localization without IgM in the glomeruli of a group of 9 subjects similar to those first studied by Berger. Other groups, however, have noted IgA as the predominant immunoglobulin in glomerular deposits along with IgM, IgG, and C3 (246). Accurate figures of the prevalence of this clinical entity are difficult to arrive at. However, the percentage of routine clinical material in most series fitting the general clinical characteristics and immunofluorescent profile of Berger's disease ranges between 2 and 5 percent.

Clinical and Pathological Picture

A majority of the patients with IgA nephropathy are male. The most common presenting complaint is related to persistent or intermittent recurrent hematuria. A history of repeated episodes of hematuria is obtained often associated either with antecedent febrile illness or a distinct upper-respiratory infection. In some patients streptococci have been isolated on throat culture, but in general elevated AS0 titers and other serological parameters of intense antistreptococcal immune response are not present. Urine examination usually shows hematuria with occasional documentation of red blood cell casts. Slight to moderate proteinuria is often present, occasionally at levels as high as 2 gm per 24 hours (247). In some instances the clinical picture is indistinguishable from the ordinary profile of nephrotic syndrome, and moderate diminution of creatinine clearance has also been noted. Total hemolytic serum complement tends to be normal, although specific immunochemical or functional measurement of C3 may show a moderate depression. Hypertension or severe peripheral edema is not encountered in most patients. The clinical course is marked by episodic recurrences of hematuria. In some patients the disorder appears to terminate spontaneously; in most patients repeated acute episodes occur but are rarely followed by progressive renal functional deterioration and failure. A review of the clinical profile in patients with IgA nephropathy by Zimmerman and Burkholder (248) indicated that approximately 10 percent of patients have shown decreased renal function.

Very little is yet understood concerning the precise immunopathological events occurring in patients with Berger's syndrome. The pathology associated with the disorder in general appears to be relatively mild. Glomeruli may show focal segmental capillary hypercellularity along with some degree of sclerosis or mesangial thickening caused by an actual increase in numbers of mesangial cells. Serum complement is not reduced and IgA is present in the form of diffuse, rather nodular deposits as seen by immunofluorescence (Figure 12-15).

Both IgG and C3 deposits are also often noted. In the patients studied by Zimmerman and Burkholder (248), properdin deposits were noted in 5 of 6 cases; C4 only infrequently. Similar predominance of properdin in 14 of 15 samples with absence of detectable C1q and C4 was also noted by McCoy and colleagues (247). When the nature of the IgA deposits has been examined, only rarely has secretory IgA been demonstrated in glomerular localization along with antigens present in serum IgA. Participation of secretory IgA in the glomerular dysfunction associated with IgA nephropathy has been seriously questioned by Dobrin and coworkers (249), who failed to find significant glomerular localization of secretory IgA in any of 24 patients with glomerular deposits of alpha chain. By contrast significant amounts of secretory component without concomitant alpha chain in tubular epithelial cells and casts in tissues from 51 patients with morphological evidence of significant renal damage secondary to a variety of causes were noted. Thus, no general support for the *primary* role of secretory IgA in the pathogenesis of IgA nephropathy has been presented.

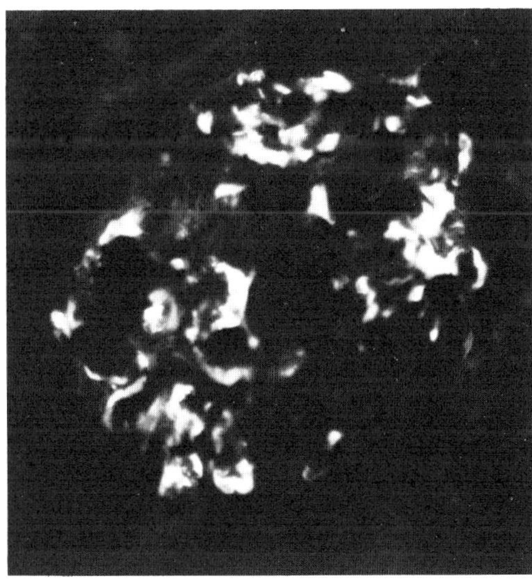

Figure 12-15 Typical IgA deposits in Berger's disease. Magnification × 350. (Photograph courtesy of A. F. Michael, University of Minnesota, Minneapolis.)

The presence of alpha chain and IgA deposits is still poorly understood with respect to IgA nephropathy. The frequent clinical association of exacerbations of hematuria with upper-respiratory infection suggests that IgA may be participating in immune complexes that subsequently lodge in the glomeruli and result in the immunofluorescent findings of IgA nephropathy. The IgA may possibly be present in such deposits as a secondary event —as, for instance, an IgA rheumatoid factor with specificity for IgG-C3 activated complexes. No data are yet available using renal tissue eluates or other serological techniques ruling out the latter possibility.

Complement fixing does not occur via the classical pathway with IgA, but it has been shown to activate complement through the alternate pathway mechanism. Thus aggregates of IgA are shown to function in this way in vitro (250). Studies by Michael and co-workers (251) have demonstrated that various aggregated proteins show preferential localization in mesangium rather than glomeruli. The well-known tendency for IgA to occur in polymeric or self-associating molecular profile may be related to the pathogenesis of Berger's syndrome. In most of the carefully studied cases, other immunoglobulins, particularly IgG and to a minor extent IgM, have also been detected by immunofluorescence. The presence of C3 and properdin without parallel extensive evidence for other complement components participating in the conventional sequence certainly implies that alternate complement pathway activation constitutes the major amplification system present in vivo. In this regard the relationship of IgG deposition in such cases is also unclear. In patient material originally described by Berger and colleagues (243, 244), IgG and IgA deposition was generally noted in parallel within individual patients. The combination of these two immunoglobulin reactants in the right proportions might be a particularly effective activator of the lesions themselves, predisposing to alternate pathway activation. That IgG is not essential for pathogenesis is apparent by the finding of patients who show IgA deposits alone, without parallel or concomitant IgG or IgM. Nevertheless, it is probably of importance that IgA deposits in association with C3 and properdin constitute the major underlying immune reactivity associated with Berger's syndrome.

The rarity of subsequent progression to serious functional renal impairment and chronic renal failure appears to reflect the absence of conventional pathway augmentation. Basic mechanisms involved in this sequence of events may, when completely unraveled, produce information of considerable practical therapeutic usefulness. Thus, it might be possible to redirect an ongoing immune process into similar channels in which direct complement pathway activation is bypassed and only alternate pathway activity utilized. Depending on the local tissue substrates or other modulating factors, this might ultimately result in a milder form of disease in conditions generally associated with progression to chronic renal failure. One of the key features in the whole sequence of postulated events thought to occur during IgA nephropathy is the exact identity of the antigens involved. Since the clinical features of the patients are often so similar, it would appear that sensitization to some putative antigen occurs resulting in production of complexes containing predominantly IgA. Immunoglobulin class specificity of immune responses is still not clearly understood. Certain bacterial polysaccharides such as the lipopolysaccharides of Gram-negative bacteria seem to be potent antigenic stimuli for IgM production, particularly when presented as particulate antigens. The antigenic stimulus in IgA nephropathy is especially inclined toward production of an IgA immune response. Other more subtle differences between the types of IgA complexes and the subclasses of IgA molecules involved also need further study in this disease. Two major IgA subclasses have been described that show differing H-chain specific antigens (252). No data are yet available on the relative proportions of IgA-1 or IgA-2 molecules in the IgA glomerular deposits in this disease.

Perhaps pertinent to IgA nephropathy is the well-known tendency for IgA molecules to bind to other plasma proteins through various nonimmunologic associative forces. Conceivably, something bound to the IgA in glomerular deposits but not IgA nor even an immunoglobulin may somehow be involved in glomerular dysfunction. There are now numerous documented examples of this nonimmune IgA binding phenomenon. Examples include binding to albumin and α-1 antitrypsin in several reports (253, 254). Perhaps more insight regarding the basic pathogenesis of IgA nephropathy will be gained when a number of these patients are studied sequentially for levels of detectable circulating immune complexes. Two of the most widely used methods to detect complexes, the Raji-cell and C1q-binding radioimmunoassays, may not be useful because they function through complement activation. Other methods programmed specifically to detect complexes composed of IgA molecules such as those recently devised by Levinsky and Soothill (255) might be employed in an effort to settle this question. It is also possible that the IgA-containing materials noted in glomerular structures of patients with IgA nephropathy may represent mesangial and glomerular localization of antigens that initially lodge in these anatomic areas and later pull out immunoglobulin A and subsequent reactants from circulating plasma.

Nephrotic Syndrome

The nephrotic syndrome itself represents a clinical symptom complex associated with edema, hypoalbuminemia, moderate to massive proteinuria, and frequently hypercholesterolemia. An example of facial edema associated with the nephrotic syndrome is shown in Figure 12-16. A number of diseases have been described in conjunction with this disorder ranging from gold or penicillamine-induced nephropathy to renal vein thrombosis, secondary syphilis, or shunt nephritis.

The nephrotic syndrome may present without impressive morphological or ultrastructural change, particularly in association with so-called minimal change lesions in childhood. Many of the latter patients can be classified as steroid responsive, and treatment with combined corticosteroids and other potent immunosuppressive drugs such as cyclophospha-

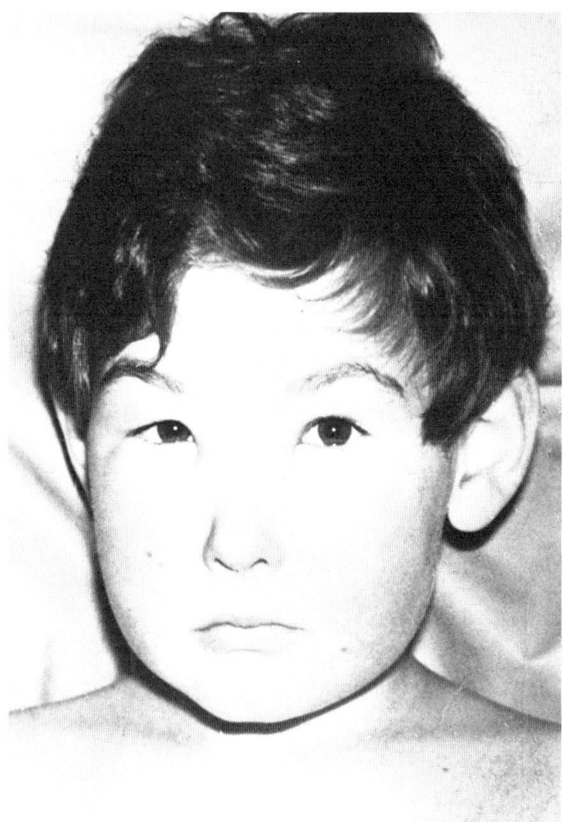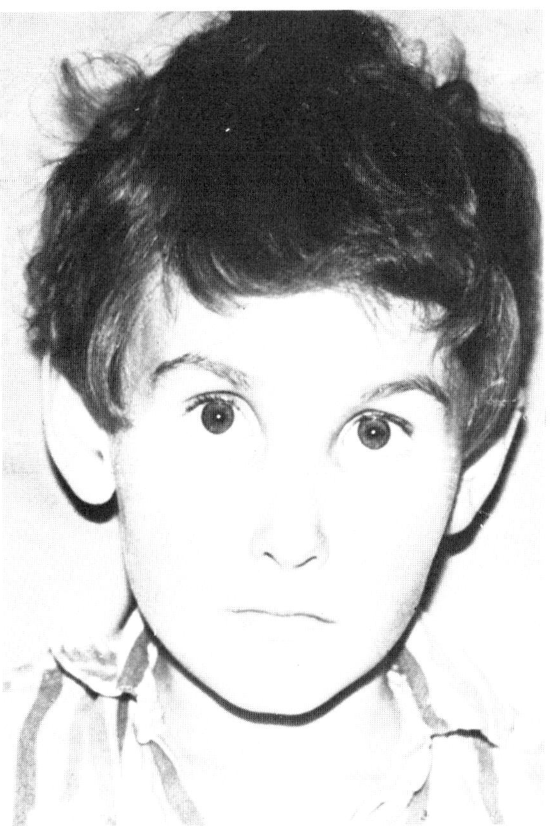

Figure 12-16 Facial edema associated with nephrotic syndrome before (*left*) and after (*right*) successful diuresis. (Photographs courtesy of J. S. Cameron, Guys Hospital, London.)

mide or chlorambucil may induce a distinct remission (256, 257). These patients have long perplexed clinicians and those who favor an immunologic etiology as the basic cause of the disorder. Other disease entities associated with a nephrotic picture such as malarial nephropathy or the full-blown nephritis of SLE show a variety of morphological changes characteristic of what the renal pathologist classifies as membranous nephritis or proliferative glomerular injury. The structural changes of minimal-change nephrotic syndrome are slight and in general there is no consistent evidence for in vivo fixation of immune-complex materials such as immunoglobulin or complement when renal tissues are examined using immunofluorescent techniques.

Nevertheless, several observations favor a possible role for altered immunologic mechanisms in the pathogenesis of the disorder.

First, as noted above, one may point to the impressive effects in some patients of corticosteroid and/or immunosuppression in inducing remission. Several isolated observations suggest association with atopy (258) and occasional patients with hay fever show a relapse or exacerbation after exposure to grass pollens (259). Immunoconglutinin, an antibody to C3, rises during the early period of relapse (260) and serum samples from some patients show inhibition of rosette formation of complement-coated erythrocytes suggesting in vivo activation of complement and the presence of circulaing immune complexes in some patients (261). Evidence for the participation of cell-mediated immunity in minimal-change nephrotic syndrome patients has been noted via a direct lymphocytotoxicity test against cultured epithelial cells derived from human kidney (262). Kidney-cell cytotoxicity was observed with T cells from patients with minimal-change nephrotic syndrome. Moreover, plasma from patients with the latter disorder was shown to inhibit mitogen-induced lymphocyte transformation and response of lymphocytes to allogeneic stimulus in mixed leukocyte cultures (263).

In 1975 a study by Giangiacomo and co-workers (264) suggested that alterations in serum immunoglobulin levels in patients with minimal-change nephrotic syndrome might reflect subtle deficiencies in T-cell control of immunoglobulin production. Thus serum IgG and IgA were reduced whereas IgM was elevated when compared to normal controls or to children with nephrotic syndrome associated with chronic glomerulonephritis. Urinary loss of IgG could not account for lowered serum IgG in idiopathic nephrotic syndrome, since low serum IgG often was observed to persist in nonproteinuric patients in long-term remission. It was suggested that elevation in IgM together with depression of IgA and IgG might reflect a deficiency in T-cell function necessary to provide the normal switch from IgM to IgG production during the course of an immune response. A parallel was drawn between the immunoglobulin profile in minimal-change idiopathic nephrotic syndrome and individuals showing the x-linked immunodeficiency syndrome with elevated IgM (265) in that the latter showed a male predominance with onset at a similar age and a familial pattern of occurrence (266). No direct experimental support for a defect in IgM to IgG switch mechanisms or T-cell deficiency in helper function was presented in the Giangiacomo study. Other workers subsequently have confirmed the findings of lowered serum IgG and IgA in minimal-change nephrotic syndrome but not uniform marked IgM elevations (267, 268). Any hypothesis that postulates a basic derangement in T-cell control should be strengthened by substantial data from patients showing that such does actually exist.

The question of an immune-complex–mediated change occurring in the course of steroid responsive minimal-change nephrotic syndrome has recently been directly addressed by Levinsky and co-workers (269), who re-corded raised levels in 17 of 18 children studied in relapse. Seven of 9 children studied sequentially showed elevated levels of complexes in early remission that later became normal. Complexes detected in these nephrotic children were apparently *not* capable of binding C1q. The patients showed a broad molecular size of complexes ranging from 2.0 to 2.5 $\times$ 10^6 Daltons and smaller complexes of 3 to 5 $\times$ 10^5 Daltons. Presumably the complexes detected during this survey were IgG, since a rabbit IgM antibody to human IgG was utilized in an inhibition of agglutination assay. It was postulated that absence of direct C1q binding might suggest predominance of noncomplement-fixing IgG subclasses such as IgG-2 or IgG-4 in these materials. Comparative assays of serum sample gel-filtration patterns from SLE patients also containing immune complexes indicated a different spectrum with 1.0 to 1.5 $\times$ 10^6 Daltons and 2.5 to 4 $\times$ 10^6 Daltons. Complexes were thought to be related clinically to renal and extrarenal SLE manifestations, respectively.

The exact relation of these observations to the pathogenesis of the proteinuria in minimal-change nephrotic syndrome is undetermined. Many immunofluorescent studies have failed to document direct renal or glomerular immune deposits in this condition (270). The occurrence of detectable elevations of immune complexes in this disorder poses a difficult question in interpretation: are the increases in such materials an epiphenomenon in no way directly related to the glomerular protein leak or are they somehow causally related? Studies by Valdez and co-workers (271) demonstrated that immune-complex glomerulonephritis may occasionally occur in the absence of demonstrable immune deposits during variations of the serum sickness renal-injury model. It is possible that minimal-change nephrotic syndrome could be mediated by such a mechanism. This explanation at present appears unlikely. Studies have demonstrated elaboration of a soluble vascular permeability factor from lymphocytes of patients with nephrotic syndrome (272). If immune complexes are in some way involved with the massive proteinuria seen in this disorder, such a mechanism triggering potent lymphocyte-derived factors seems much more likely. The growing sophistication and sensitivity of current methods for measurement of circulating complexes has far surpassed our basic understanding of the disease process. Final judgment on their relative importance must be withheld until basic mechanisms of renal injury or dysfunction in this disease are understood.

Potentiation of Immune-Complex–Mediated Renal Injury

Assuming that many primary or secondary renal lesions derive from glomerular immune-complex injury, a number of modulating factors can influence the rate or extent of the underlying process. The most important factor is the amplification system provided by the conventional and alternate complement pathways. A second, recently explored factor concerns the participation of anti-γ-globulins in conjunction with autologous immune complexes. The question of whether anti-γ-globulins amplify the inflammatory or destructive processes occurring in renal mesangium or at the glomerular basement membrane has not been completely settled as yet.

A series of observations supports the possibility that in certain patients this may contribute significantly to ongoing renal injury. The first of these observations was presented by McCormick and co-workers (273), who showed that administration of rheumatoid arthritis serum containing high levels of 19 S IgM rheumatoid factor markedly potentiated the immediate phase of nephrotoxic nephritis in experimental animals. It seemed possible, therefore, that sera containing such anti-γ-globulins were capable of augmenting immune injury in glomeruli already damaged or fixed to heterologous antibody to glomerular basement membranes or other autologous renal antigens. This concept has been extended by Rossen and co-workers (274), who studied renal biopsies and sera from 41 consecutive patients for evidence of anti-γ-globulin activities. The patients were classified into three groups on the basis of their renal functional and histological findings. One group was composed of 12 patients with

normal renal function and minimal evidence of histological changes in glomeruli; a second group comprised 18 patients with normal renal function, but distinctly abnormal biopsies or proteinuria; and a third group of 11 patients showed both decreased renal function and abnormal renal histology. Positive tests for serum rheumatoid factor were noted in none of the first group, but were present in 22 and 45 percent of the second and third groups respectively. A second assay for anti-immunoglobulins was used in which the amounts of ^{125}I-labeled patient globulin were tested for binding to immunoadsorbents coated with Cohn fraction II in competition with an equal quantity of labeled globulin from pooled normal plasma. This assay revealed increased binding in the first and second groups but definite binding in 8 of 9 patients from the third group with decreased renal function and abnormal histology. Severity of disease as judged by glomerular damage and diminished function correlated with presence of both serum and tissue-fixed anti-γ-globulin activity. Of interest was the finding of relatively high titers of antiglobulins (1 : 640 to 1 : 10,240) in several patients with diminished renal function and abnormal morphological changes. In many of the patients studied, immune deposits of IgG and IgM were present on routine immunofluorescence. Examples of the glomerular binding of fluorescein-labeled aggregated IgG recorded in this study are shown in Figure 12-17. No correlation was noted between quantitative levels of serum C3 and anti-γ-globulin activity in the various groups studied. It seemed possible that something in glomeruli other than anti-γ-globulins such as C1q might be responsible for direct tissue binding of fluorescein-labeled IgG aggregates. In one case heating the tissue sections, which theoretically would have inactivated C1q, did not block labeled IgG aggregate binding, whereas blockage was noted by preincubating the sections with unconjugated anti-IgM suggesting that glomerular binding was occurring secondary to IgM rheumatoid factors already present within the glomerular immune deposits.

Other workers have attempted to study glomerular eluates for anti-γ-globulin activity

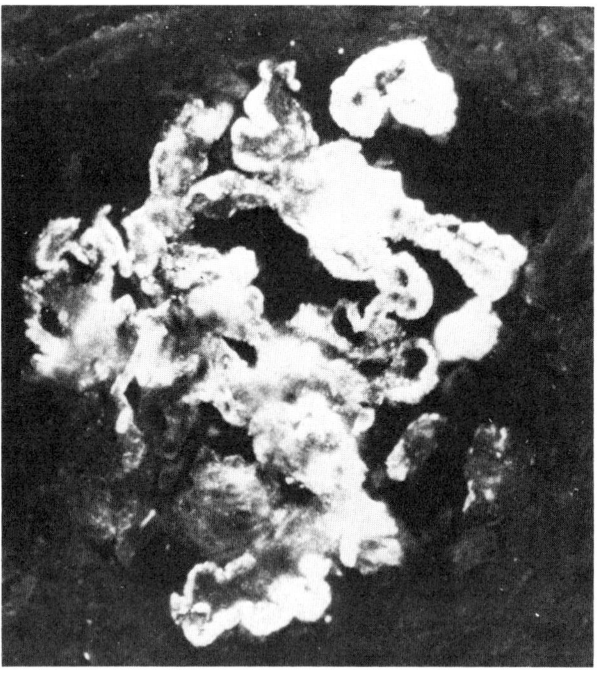

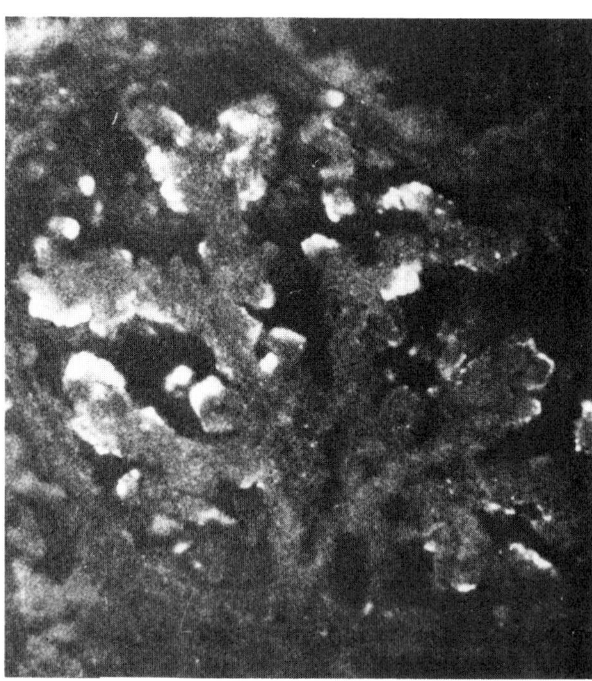

Figure 12-17 Examples of immunofluorescence in glomeruli that bound fluorescein-labeled aggregated IgG. Both photographs, magnification × 264.

(Reproduced with permission, R. D. Rossen, M. A. Reisberg, J. T. Sharp et al., *J. Clin. Invest.* 56:427, 1975.)

with less in the way of positive evidence for their presence in such materials (275, 276) particularly in patients with SLE. Examination of glomerular eluates may be difficult to interpret with certainty, as methods used to prepare eluates could conceivably also dissociate IgG antigen capable of inhibition of anti-γ-globulin reactivity after eluates are subsequently returned to neutrality.

No experimental evidence has been derived in previous studies that anti-γ-globulins themselves are directly nephrotoxic (273). The striking absence of immune-complex–mediated renal disease in patients with rheumatoid arthritis showing high levels of rheumatoid factors supports this contention. It has actually been proposed that presence of circulating anti-γ-globulins might protect the glomerulus by increasing the physical size of circulating complexes allowing for more efficient reticuloendothelial system clearance in the liver and spleen before glomerular deposition could occur (277).

Several mechanisms might be postulated to explain the possible interactions of anti-γ-globulins and immune complexes in various forms of renal injury. First, the presence in serum of antibodies showing reactivity for antigenic determinants somehow uncovered or exposed on immunoglobulin molecules participating in immune-complex formation might influence glomerular localization if they facilitated activation of the complement system. In some experimental systems rheumatoid factors and complement may actually compete for the same or adjacent fixation sites on the Fc portions of immunoglobulin molecules. It can be shown that anti-γ-globulins actually block Fc-receptor–mediated functions that also are facilitated by complement activation. Phagocytosis is an example of this type of phenomenon (278). Alternatively, several elegant studies have indicated that naturally occurring rheumatoid factors are themselves capable of inducing complement activation (279, 280). Part of the difficulty in assigning degrees of importance to these various phenomena relates to the heterogeneity of anti-γ-globulin factors.

Measurement of serum rheumatoid factor activity using the latex fixation test in patients with renal disease is not sufficiently sensitive to assign a clear priority to its pathogenetic role in a patient with circulating immune complexes and glomerular immune-complex injury. The actual class and binding specificities of the anti-γ-globulin factors are undoubtedly of great importance. If they are IgM anti-γ-globulins and show particular reactivity for conformational sites on either native or complexed autologous IgG, they may indeed accelerate glomerular deposition of circulating immune-complex materials. If, however, they are IgA anti-γ-globulins, reaction with autologous complexes may lead to a more benign disposal mechanism without significant direct conventional complement pathway activation. Also, if anti-γ-globulins of IgG-3 subclass are present, their specificity may be for production of self-associating 11 to 16S complexes rather than for larger immune aggregates. These aspects of the problem are most important and have yet to be thoroughly examined. It is also possible that certain idiotypic features of anti-γ-globulins occurring in association with immune-complex renal disease are of more practical importance than immunoglobulin subclass or other genetically determined anti-γ-globulin specificities.

Thus the anti-γ-globulins occurring in tissue deposits of a wide spectrum of patients with immune-complex renal injury must be examined in light of true autospecificity. Clearly anti-γ-globulins occur with surprising frequency in subacute bacterial endocarditis, syphilis, malarial nephrotic syndrome, schistosomiasis, trypanosomiasis, SLE, or in association with idiopathic membranous nephritis. The spectrum of these anti-γ-globulin reactivities may actually be more narrowly focused for primary specificities inherent in determinants encountered in autologous immune complexes than is generally appreciated. If such were the case, the specificity might show highest energies of binding for tissue-fixed complexes rather than for circulating materials of the same composition. The greatest chance of uncovering such unique specificities of anti-γ-globulins lies in disease states in which the putative antigens have been well characterized, such as in SLE (nDNA–anti-nDNA) or schistosomiasis in which parasitic antigens have been chemically characterized and defined (281). A certain fraction of anti-γ-globulins may conceivably show unique reactivity for deposited autologous complexes. If this is the case, it would be easy to visualize such complexes acting as an insoluble fixed-tissue immunoadsorbent extracting anti-idiotypic anti-γ-globulins from the circulating plasma and adding them to the same sites as the original immune deposits. The specificity of anti-γ-globulins present in immune deposits associated with immune-complex renal diseases needs further detailed examination. This will await application of newer techniques of elution and reactivity of eluates from a variety of diseased glomeruli. Our own efforts in this regard have recently convinced us that anti-idiotypic anti-γ-globulins with unique binding energies for autologous immune precipitates may play a significant role in the augmentation and acceleration of renal lesions in a number of heterogeneous clinical conditions. These various possibilities are shown diagrammatically in Figure 12-18.

Further studies on the immunologic profile of anti-γ-globulin binding to glomerular tissues in a variety of patients with renal disease are presented by Rossen and co-workers (282) in patients with glomerulonephritis, and following renal transplantation. Localization of fluorescein-labeled heat-aggregated IgG was used as the primary assay in these studies. Heavy localization of presumed tissue-fixed rheumatoid factor was noted particularly in association with substantial IgM, C3, and C4 immune deposits. Binding to tissues by aggregates depended on integrity of the Fc portion of IgG and no binding was noted using F(ab)$'_2$ fragments studied in parallel. The likelihood that tissue-fixed C1q was involved in binding was ruled out by enzymatic and chemical treatments designed to inactivate C1q activity. In this study glomerular binding of fluorescent IgG aggregates did not correlate with amounts of circulating immune complexes detected in concurrent serum samples using the sensitive C1q-binding method. When renal tissues from patients who had undergone renal transplant

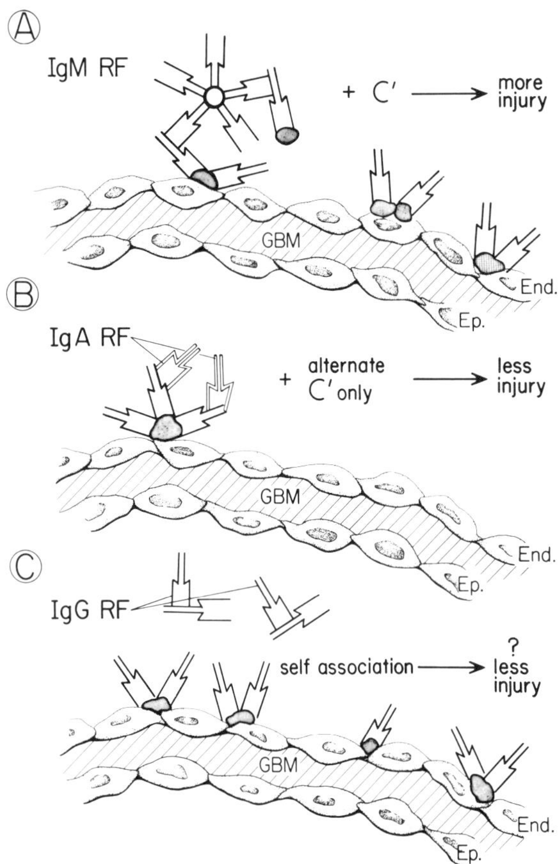

Figure 12-18 Various ways in which different classes of rheumatoid factors may function in conjunction with immune-complex renal injury on glomerular basement membranes.

were studied, aggregate binding was recorded in 18 of 21 kidney allografts. However, factors responsible for this binding were heat labile and thus could have represented C1q.

The fact that the glomerular localization of fluorescein-labeled aggregates in this study did not show a correlation with measurable circulating immune complexes raises some interesting questions regarding the relative roles of each in the pathogenesis of the actual glomerular pathology. It would appear likely that the immune deposits present in the glomeruli represent complexes and their reactants most likely to be extracted from circulation and that the anti-γ-globulin activity associated with immune deposits in severely damaged kidneys shows a unique or idiotypic specificity for com-

plexes in these sites. Anti-γ-globulin activity was detected in serum samples from only 3 of 16 patients whose kidneys contained material indicating tissue-fixed anti-γ-globulin activity. Studies of anti-γ-globulin activity in tissue eluates were hampered by insolubility of immunoglobulin recovered in the eluates. These studies emphasize gaps in our current understanding of the relationship between tissue saturation and adherence of immune complexes and such reactants as anti-γ-globulins, and the importance of circulating immune complexes as detected by sensitive assays. However, both the C1q-binding test and the Raji-cell radioimmunoassay measure complexes capable of activating the complement system. Therefore, the presence of complexes in glomeruli associated with tissue-fixed anti-γ-globulins might represent a subpopulation of immune reactants capable of reactivity not only with intrinsic receptors within diseased renal tissues but also with those bound in the area by reaction with antiglobulins in preference to direct complement pathway activation.

Detection of Soluble Complexes in Renal Disease

In many forms of renal disease there is evidence that derangement of immune mechanisms and especially glomerular localization of immune-complex material plays a basic role in the primary pathogenesis of a number of distinct lesions. In some problem areas such as that related to the idiopathic or minimal-change nephrotic syndrome, the relative importance of immune-complex–mediated phenomena still eludes us. However, in most morphological types of glomerulonephritis ranging from rapidly progressive or membranous nephritis to diffuse or focal proliferative glomerular injury immune deposits have repeatedly been demonstrated both by immunofluorescent procedures and by ultrastructural examination.

A number of attempts have been made to apply the newer sensitive assay techniques for circulating complexes to a broad spectrum of patients with renal disease. In one early study by Rossen and colleagues (283), C1q binding was measured at the time of renal biopsy in 104 consecutive patients in whom immunofluorescent findings appeared to document immune-complex disease, supported by the presence of granular immunoglobulin and/or complement deposits. Surprisingly, sera from only 21 percent of these patients showed elevated C1q binding in comparison to those of normal healthy controls. Elevation in C1q binding did, however, appear to follow clinical and histological severity, being highest in those with the most marked histological and functional derangements. Patients showing the highest levels of C1q binding for circulating immune complexes often showed immunofluorescent patterns characterized by heavy C3 and C4 deposition. In addition, a rough correlation was noted between elevated C1q binding and immunofluorescent deposits showing both glomerular IgG and IgM. No general elevation of C1q binding was noted in patients showing predominant IgA glomerular immunofluorescence.

A much higher incidence (67 percent) of detectable immune complexes was recorded by Theofilopoulos and colleagues (284), who studied 42 patients with immune-complex nephritis using the Raji-cell method. One problem inherent in such comparisons is that the data obtained by renal biopsy probably represent a kaleidoscopic or long-range view of immune-complex injury in the particular disease process examined, while a single determination of the level of soluble complexes in a heterogeneous group of patients may not accurately reflect the long-term load of immune complexes that the kidney in the individual patient has had to bear.

Subsequent studies have frequently reflected these methodological and temporal problems. However, the presence of detectable complexes seems to correlate with the degree and type of glomerular injury. A study by Woodroffe and colleagues (285) utilized three parallel assays for circulating complexes to minimize profiles of positivity depending on the test system used. The Raji-cell radioimmunoassay, the radiolabeled C1q-binding assay, and the microcomplement fixation test were each performed in parallel. Immune complexes were present in 87 percent of patients with SLE, 65 percent with glomerulonephritis associated with other systemic diseases, and 39 percent with primary glomerulonephritis. Elevations in detectable complexes appeared more frequently in patients with acute glomerulonephritis processes than in subjects with chronic disease and complexes correlated to an extent with lowered serum C3, C4, and properdin factor B levels. Comparative assessment of the profiles for immune-complex reactivity using the three tests in parallel from this study is shown in Table 12-4. From these results and our own experience, no single immune-complex assay is uniformly applicable to any such heterogeneous group of renal disease sera tested. However, a significant number of individuals with various forms

Table 12-4 Prospective study of glomerulonephritis (GN) sera for circulating immune complexes[a].

	Percent positive by—			
Patients	IRCA	IC1q BA	MCT	Any test
SLE ($n = 23$)	74	35	27	87
Other systemic GN ($n = 17$)	29	41	18	65
Primary GN ($n = 36$)	14	17	14	39
Control ($n = 31$)	3	3	6	10

Source: Reproduced with permission, A. J. Woodroffe, W. A. Border, A. N. Theofilopoulos et al., *Kidney Int.* 12:268, 1977.

[a] Abbreviations used are IRCA, Raji-cell radioimmune assay; IC1qBA, radiolabeled C1q-binding assay; MCT, microcomplement consumption test; SLE, systemic lupus erythematosus; n, number of patients studied.

of immune-complex nephropathy clearly show detectable circulating complexes particularly when studied during the acute phases of their illness. The specific factors influencing tissue deposition and consequent glomerular injury still require further definition. In particular, the influence of specific localizing capacities of certain antigens and especially final identification of the antigens involved appear to be of more practical importance in designing effective long-term programs of management, immunosuppression, or therapy. It is possible that the most nephrotoxic complexes associated with various clinical disorders rarely are detected by the current assays for soluble complexes, for they may achieve only a few passes through the circulation before glomerular entrapment.

Recurrent Glomerulonephritis in Human Renal Homografts

The recurrence of glomerulonephritis in a proportion of renal transplants is one of the most salient features emphasizing the importance of understanding underlying disease mechanisms in human immune-complex glomerular injury. That such a process occurs and sometimes compromises the long-term survival of the allograft has become increasingly apparent to the clinician, nephrologist, or surgeon charged with the ongoing care of such patients. In view of the tremendous expenditure of money and human effort involved in the case of chronic dialysis patients and individuals subsequently receiving renal allografts, it is of critical logistic importance to examine what is known concerning mechanisms involved in glomerulonephritis recurring de novo in a newly transplanted kidney.

While this general problem has received part of the attention it deserves, very little of it has come from surgical transplantation teams, whose main focus has been features immediately surrounding the transplantation event itself. Glassock and co-workers (286, 287) noted recurrence of glomerulonephritis in 11 of 17 twin renal isograft recipients. Additional reports indicated an immune-complex type of recurrent glomerulonephritis in 3 of 71 cases

studied by Porter and co-workers (288, 289). Dixon and co-workers (290) described 13 cases with anti-GBM–mediated nephritis and 26 allografts showing immune-complex nephritis in the transplanted kidney; the prevalence of recurrent nephritis may indeed be higher than was appreciated at the time of this study. A report by Seibel and colleagues (291) focused attention on the process previously present in the recipient's own kidneys prior to transplantation. Studies of 4 patients with glomerulonephritis were conducted. Observations included wedge biopsies of the donor kidney to rule out transfer of subclinically damaged renal tissue prior to the actual transplantation procedure. Ultrastructural examination of renal transplants showed electron-dense deposits in thickened basement membranes along with subepithelial humps in all 4 cases. Examples of these changes are shown in Figure 12-19. Immunofluorescent examination showed IgG and complement deposits in all instances with IgM deposition in 2 cases. Of especial interest was the finding of subepithelial humps, IgG, and complement deposits in patients studied only one hour after completion of the transplant procedure. In general, the ultrastructural and immunofluorescent changes noted approximated those seen in the host or recipient kidneys prior to transplantation. Subsequent short-term follow-up of this small group of individuals indicated preservation of renal function with continuation of immunosuppressive therapy.

Similar studies with particular emphasis on changes in serum complement component profiles were recorded by McLean and co-workers (292). Sixteen patients with membranoproliferative glomerulonephritis were studied after renal transplantation. In 12 patients where transplant histology could be studied, 7 showed recurrent membranoproliferative glomerulonephritis. In 4 patients hypocomplementemia was present, characterized by decreases in total hemolytic assay. Immunofluorescence showed more intense C3 and properdin deposition in the patients with documented hypocomplementemia. Electron microscopy showed intramembranous deposits thought to be typical of dense-deposit disease

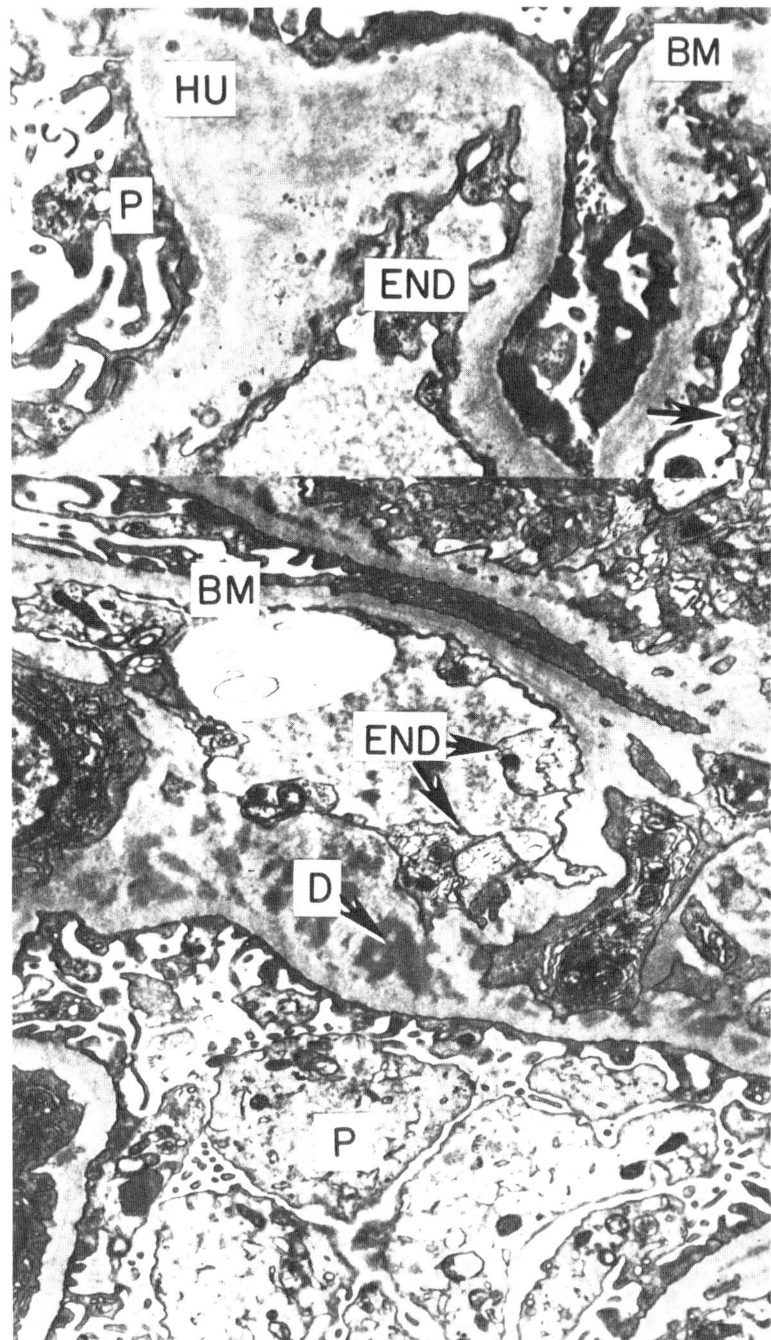

Figure 12-19 *Upper pattern:* electron micrographs of kidney removed at nephrectomy showing subepithelial hump (HU). Pedicels of the podocytes (P) exhibit some fusion and delineation. There is moderate endothelial spreading (*arrow*) and a decrease in the number of pores. BM = basement membrane; N = nucleus. Magnification × 7,570. *Lower pattern:* patient 12 weeks posttransplant. Deposits (D) of irregular shape and density are illustrated within basement membrane (BM). Endothelial (END) hypertrophy is also present. Magnification × 8,660. (Reproduced with permission, H. R. Seibel, R. J. Weymouth, S. S. Craig et al., *Virchow's Arch.* [*Pathol. Anat.*] 371:5, 1976.)

in 1 subject with persistent marked hypocomplementemia. Of note was the high death rate in patients with persistent and unremitting hypocomplementemia. In many instances the characteristic complement profile suggesting predominant alternate complement pathway activation was noted before and after renal transplantation and was not altered by the transplant nor immunosuppressive treatment. These findings suggest that the transplant procedure itself is not an effective long-term treatment if the basic underlying pathological process is capable of leapfrogging into the normal allografted donor organ.

The overall frequency of recurrence or superimposition of glomerulonephritis in allografted kidneys is not well documented. Such an occurrence may result from three separate potential mechanisms: (1) persistence of an active nephritogenic mechanism present in the host; (2) immunologic factors elicited in the host by way of the special allogenic features involved in tissue incompatibility; and (3) a new mechanism not derived from alloantibodies. No clear evidence to support the latter two mechanisms in a substantial number of patients has been presented. However, certain forms of immunologically distinct chronic renal disease appear to have an unusual tendency to reappear after allografts. Among these are IgA-glomerulopathy (293), glomerular disease manifested by anti-GBM antibody (290), and focal sclerosing glomerulonephritis (294). From data available at present, it would appear that the basic underlying immune-complex–mediated nephropathy or at least chronic renal disease involving a derangement of normal immunologic balance survives the immunosuppressive regimen involved with ordinary renal transplantation and is quite capable of reestablishing itself in the new, albeit immunosuppressed, environment. This fact appears to be the single most direct and compelling argument for the importance of extending insight into the pathogenesis of all immune-complex renal diseases. When achieved, renal transplantation will itself become an anachronism as vestigial a procedure as cupping or bleeding in the Middle Ages.

Glomerulonephritis and IR Gene Control

In a general category of disorders, many of which appear to be fundamentally related to immune-complex deposition in renal glomeruli, one might not expect to find a priori a single gene or even a few immune-response genes implicated in modifying susceptibility to immune-complex deposition. The diverse number of separate disease entities ranging from SLE to Henoch-Schönlein purpura, membranoproliferative nephritis, or IgA nephropathy represent a broad range of clinically distinct renal disorders sharing only glomerular immune-complex deposition as a common feature. Currently there is a great deal of interest in identifying HLA associations with immunopathology, particularly in terms of the antigen-specific IR gene hypothesis originally proposed by Benacerraf and McDevitt (295). From the spectrum of primary disorders associated with glomerular immune-complex pathology, it must be assumed that a variety of separate and distinct antigens per se is involved and therefore the influence of IR genes on clinical expression of disease must of necessity be similarly diverse. On the contrary, since IR gene control of the immune response may function at a number of separate and distinct levels, it is also possible that a common gene might somehow be involved at some level in regulating either antigen processing, qualitative aspects of humoral antibody response, or most important of all the physical characteristics and actual anatomic density of putative receptors for immune complexes in vulnerable structures, such as the glomeruli. For these reasons large numbers of patients with various forms of immune-complex glomerulonephritis have been examined. In most instances results do not provide clear evidence for any uniform pattern or predilection toward the formation or deposition of immune complexes with glomerular localization. However, interesting preliminary reports indicate that certain subsets of patients may indeed show an order of IR gene control that can be perhaps eventually related to the major histocompatibility system.

A report by Thomson and co-workers (258) has directly addressed these problems, with the rationale that since atopic symptoms appear to be more common in children with steroid-responsive nephrotic syndrome, some link to IR genes might be defined by HLA typing. Analysis of clinical evidence for allergy in this group showed that atopic diathesis such as hay fever, positive prick tests with grass pollen allergens, and a higher mean serum concentration of IgE antibody to timothy grass pollen were more common in nephrotic children with HLA–B12 than in those without the latter HLA type. In addition an increase in haplotype HLA–A1 and HLA–B8 was noted particularly among nonatopic nephrotic patients. Of steroid-responsive nephrotic children, 38 percent had a history of asthma, eczema, or hay fever in contrast to 18 percent of age-matched controls, giving a relative risk factor of 2.8. Further analysis of these data indicated that in children who showed both HLA–B12 and a history of atopy, the risk of developing steroid-responsive nephrotic syndrome was 13 times greater than in those with neither attribute. Associations such as these could result from a linkage of HLA–B12 and atopy, or a linkage with steroid-responsive nephrotic syndrome; however, current available data do not support a relationship between HLA–B12 and atopic populations. As noted by the authors of this report, a strict interpretation in terms of the antigen-specific IR gene concept (295) might imply a common antigen to which all patients with nephrotic syndrome might be sensitized. This also may be the case in some steroid-sensitive nephrotic syndrome children; however, it is unlikely, since relapses in most subjects are not confined to the hay fever or grass pollen season. Alternative explanations of these interesting data must therefore include postulating IR gene control at a different level such as target organ susceptibility, liability to more widespread antigen dissemination, antigen-nonspecific differences in overall immune responsiveness, or differences in the function of modulating factors such as the complement or lymphokine systems.

Clinical relevance of the possible association between atopy and nephrotic syndrome in children is emphasized by the occasional reports of atopic patients with seasonal nephrotic syndrome (296, 297) and the clinical impression of some investigators that relapses often occur after an ordinary or even mild upper-respiratory infection. Thomson and associates (258) have suggested that allergy itself may arise as a consequence of defective antigen processing and elimination—a subtle form of immunodeficiency previously proposed by Soothill (298). Thus nephrotic syndrome in some children might not be caused directly by the mechanism envisioned for hay fever (IgE and mast cells) but perhaps by lymphokines directly released after excessive stimulation of T cells or other lymphoid elements.

The HLA system in glomerulonephritis has been studied by several groups (299–302). Their reports support an apparent increase in HLA–A2 among patients with glomerulonephritis (299–301), but a recent study by Nyulassey and co-workers (303) found no deviations from normal in 105 patients. Of interest, however, in this last report was the finding of a significant association between HLA–Bw35 and Henoch-Schönlein nephritis ($p > .0005$). Relative risk associated with HLA–Bw35 in this study was calculated to be 4.91. Since Henoch-Schönlein's nephritis is associated with an immune-complex form of glomerular injury, it might represent IR gene control focused on a particular set of individual antigens. Several other disease associations with Bw35 have been reported, including subacute thyroiditis (303) and Hodgkin's disease (304). Currently no uniform data implicate a single group of antigens associated with these diverse conditions.

Recent interest has centered on the possible close linkage between HLA antigens coded for by the D locus and IR genes in humans. This typing system employs differentiation of HLA–DR antigens using B cells from individual patients. A report by Friend and co-workers (305) indicates possible association of membranoproliferative glomerulonephritis with a B-cell alloantigen. One typing serum appeared to react with a B-cell antigen present in 77 percent of such patients tested. Exact serological definition of this system has not yet been completed and must be confirmed by other groups before a designated HLA-DRw specificity is agreed upon. The primary defect in this form of nephritis appears somehow to relate to presence of C3 nephritic factor and chronic alternative complement pathway activation. The HLA-DR system is felt by most researchers to be analogous to human Ia antigens. These antigens in the mouse have shown strong apparent relationships to immune-response genes. Further exploration of possible relationships between HLA-DR typing and various well-defined forms of human immune-complex glomerulonephritis will be forthcoming.

Practical application of well-defined HLA typing systems toward the understanding of a number of chronic human renal diseases has been disappointing to date. Even when well-defined population groups are categorized as actually bearing IR genes that might predipose them to eventual development of various forms of immune-complex glomerular injury, the practical problems of management and treatment of the disease itself will remain unsolved until preprogrammed genetic expression can be modified to modulate or completely shut off mechanisms producing glomerular injury. When insight is finally gained into how the presence of various cell surface markers coded for by independent genetic mechanisms can be used to predict disease susceptibility or perhaps even prognosis, the practicing physician will still be left with the care of the patient. It seems imperative to look far beyond eventual understanding of the precise mechanisms regulating built-in genetic regulation of the immune response. More attention must be directed to modification of the disease process itself. We now know the precise biochemical defects that determine abnormal hemoglobin structure, such as those genetic deletions or misplacements involved in the production of sickle or thalassemic hemoglobins. While these genetic mechanisms have been defined for over two decades, no decisive approach has been successful in actually modifying or curing unfortunate patients with these abnormalities.

Interstitial Nephritis and Antitubular Basement-Membrane Antibodies

In the studies of immune-complex–mediated renal injury great emphasis has been placed on events occurring in the glomerulus and its capillary and mesangial networks. This is understandable since the glomeruli represent the single most important filtering apparatus for fluid and solute exchange within the kidney proper, and progressive glomerular sclerosis or obliterative scarring incident to immune-complex deposition are critical processes in eventual functional deterioration and renal failure. However, the interstitial areas of the kidney and in particular the renal tubules and their basement membranes also often may be involved in immune-complex injury. This area of renal immunopathology is less well understood and the antigen-antibody systems less clearly defined than those studied with respect to glomerular injury. Tubular structures and their collecting systems actually comprise the vast bulk of the kidney and although often less prominent than the lesions involving glomeruli, tubular interstitial immune-complex deposits are surprisingly frequent in a wide variety of heterogeneous renal disorders. Tubulointerstitial disease is an important and sometimes neglected area involving vital fluid, solute, and electrolyte exchange essential for normal body function. This section will attempt to review some of the evidence implicating interstitial immune-complex–mediated phenomena in a variety of disease processes.

Mechanisms Documented in Immune Interstitial Disease

Several types of immunopathology have been described in the production of tubular injury or tubulointerstitial immune-complex disease. Linear deposition of IgG on the tubular basement membrane has been reported in association with patients showing clear evidence for anti-GBM antibody–mediated renal disease (230, 236, 237). Subsequent inflammation is presumed to be secondary to direct fixation of antibody to TBM structures that show cross-reactions with GBM. Fixation of antibody to tissue then presumably is capable of inducing a chemotactic response and local infiltration of polymorphonuclear and other inflammatory cells eventually resulting in various degrees of tissue injury and destruction. Similar linear deposition of IgG directly on basement membranes has also been now described in methicillin interstitial nephritis (306), rapidly progressive glomerulonephritis (307), and in renal homograft recipients (308–310).

An interesting patient studied in some detail by Bergstein and Litman (311) showed interstitial nephritis of unknown primary cause in association with anti-TBM antibody demonstrated by immunofluorescence of kidney biopsy material. Linear staining of these structures with anti-IgG and anti-C3 was noted. Serum from this patient showed staining of similar structures in sections of normal human kidney. Staining could be eliminated by prior absorption of patient serum with purified TBM, although *not* with purified GBM material. The findings in this patient are of particular interest, since they represent evidence for autoantibody apparently specific for antigens concentrated in tubular basement membranes not sharing a variety of cross-reacting determinants with antigens in glomerular basement membranes. These findings are therefore considerably different from the apparent cross-reactions between renal GBM antibodies and tubular and other basement membranes described in patients with Goodpasture's syndrome or other conditions associated with such antibodies. Routine microscopic examination of renal biopsy tissues in this patient showed extensive interstitial cellular infiltrates and general disorganization of renal architecture. Also of interest were the clinical findings of glucosuria, phosphaturia, and amino aciduria suggesting a variety of tubular transport functional defects associated with the anti-tubular-basement-membrane antibody and interstitial inflammatory cell infiltration. No evidence for glomerular immune-complex deposits was presented in this subject. The mechanism of production of TBM antibody in these patients was not defined. It is conceivable that induction of the antibody occurred after interstitial and tubular damage

with release of endogenous membrane antigens.

A survey of the general events possibly involved in the generation of tubular and interstitial renal immune-complex disease was presented by McCluskey and Klassen (312) who emphasized that conspicuous tubular cell damage and interstitial inflammatory response or eventual fibrosis were common in several forms of glomerulonephritis in which glomerular lesions were thought to depend on immunologic mechanisms. No hard evidence could be mustered to support the idea that these tubular changes were somehow secondary to primary glomerular damage. Moreover, cases where marked tubular or interstitial lesions were present were often summarily diagnosed by pathologists as chronic pyelonephritis, even though a clear history of chronic or recurrent urinary tract infection was lacking. Therefore a fair proportion of such cases might indeed be the result of immune-complex or cell-mediated lesions. In direct support of this contention are data accumulated in several excellent experimental animal models of tubular immune-complex–mediated renal injury. Rabbits given repeated allografts or immunized with homologous renal tissue in complete Freund's adjuvant develop lesions associated with immune-complex deposition involving TBMs (313, 314). In one study after immunization with renal tissue antigens largely free of GBM, rabbits showed irregular interstitial fibrosis accompanied usually by sparse mononuclear cell infiltration (314). Initially glomeruli appeared normal; however, several months later experimental animals showed mild proliferative glomerulonephritis accompanied by severe tubular damage and interstitial fibrosis. Functional tubular defects of glycosuria, generalized aminoaciduria, and elevated blood urea nitrogen were present; the morphological and functional changes were accompanied by granular deposits of IgG and C3 along tubular basement membranes. Transfer of serum from affected rabbits to normals was associated with similar lesions in the normal recipients. The granular and localized nature of the IgG and C3 deposits in the experimental animals suggest that they represented immune-complex deposits rather than the accumulation of autoantibody against local tubular basement membrane structures. This interpretation was supported by the absence of detectable serum antibody against tubular basement membranes. However, these animals did show antibodies against renal tubular cell cytoplasmic antigens suggesting that the deposits detected by immunofluorescence represented union of circulating autoantibodies with autologous tubular antigens as they diffused from tubular cells.

Similar lesions have subsequently been documented in a variety of human disease states (312). Proof that such lesions represent actual deposition of immune complexes was derived from electron microscopic examination showing granular materials deposited in or along tubular basement membranes (315). Interstitial changes were often noted on conventional histological study that included fibrosis, mononuclear cell infiltration, and tubular cell damage. Clinical diagnosis of patients showing these findings included lupus nephritis, rapidly progressive glomerulonephritis, lipoid nephrosis, and idiopathic interstitial and tubular disease associated with mild proteinuria and hematuria (312, 315). In general, such extensive lesions are not considered common but may occur in a broad spectrum of diverse renal disorders.

Cell-Mediated Renal Disease

In the eyes of most renal immunopathologists, the concept that cell-mediated immune reactions could play an important role in the genesis of some lesions has met with a fair amount of skepticism and doubt (316). However, several histological and clinical features relating to tubulointerstitial disease suggest that delayed hypersensitivity against autologous antigens may be involved at some level in pathogenesis. The experimental models of tubular basement membrane disease or interstitial nephritis mentioned above are often associated with an impressive histological infiltration with lymphocytes and mononuclear cells. The mere finding of such a cellular profile within the lesions does not prove that delayed hypersensi-

tivity is a primary mechanism; similar infiltrates may be noted in several forms of experimental immune-complex injury including autoimmune thyroiditis. Direct support for the participation of sensitized lymphocytes in such reactions was provided by the finding that lymphocytes from animals immunized with renal tubular antigens produced specific MIF and delayed-type hypersensitivity skin reactions and lymphocyte transformation in vitro (317, 318). In humans, evidence that such reactions are mediated predominantly by cell-directed mechanisms is much less substantial, and further work is needed in this area.

Sjögren's Syndrome

One of the best-studied examples of predominant interstitial renal disease is Sjögren's syndrome. In this disorder the tissue response in the kidney is most often characterized by a mild tubulointerstitial infiltrate. Renal functional abnormalities are common, and a correlation between the interstitial nephritis and changes in tubular function seems probable. Histological lesions that have been documented in many of these patients are quite impressive and are frequently accompanied by marked lymphocytic and mononuclear cell reactions. Examples of these changes taken from several carefully studied cases along with immunofluorescent findings are shown in Figures 12-20 and 12-21. Electron microscopy has revealed electron-dense deposits often in thickened proximal TBMs and irregular granular areas of IgG and C3 deposition in the same locations (319).

Obvious or latent renal functional abnormalities described in association with Sjögren's syndrome have included renal tubular acidosis, impaired renal concentrating ability, glycosuria without concomitant hyperglycemia, and abnormalities in amino acid transport (320, 321). Predominant glomerular abnormalities are distinctly uncommon, but when present have included membranous nephropathy (322) or proliferative glomerulonephritis (321–324) occasionally associated with the presence of cryoglobulins (325, 326). Originally the studies of Tu and co-workers (327)

Figure 12-20 Light microscopic appearance of renal biopsy in a patient with Sjögren's syndrome, showing intense interstitial inflammation and a relatively unaffected glomerulus. H&E × 75. (Reproduced with permission, R. L. Winer, A. H. Cohen, A. S. Sawhney et al., *Clin. Immunol. Immunopathol.* 8:494, 1977.)

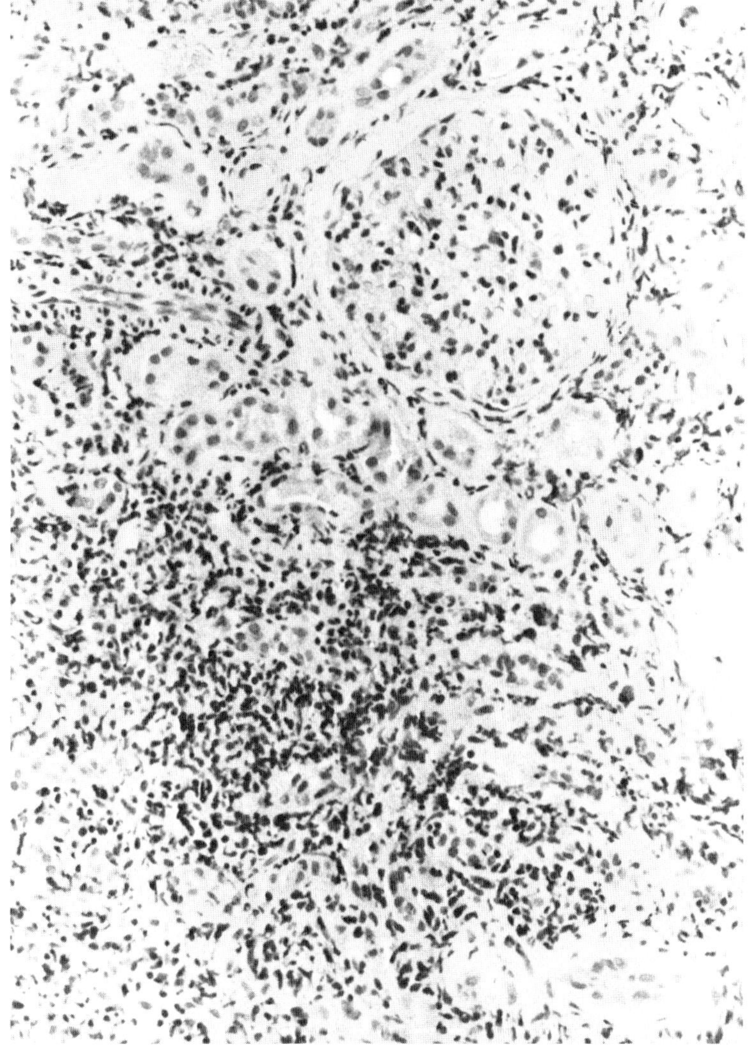

indicated that various forms of interstitial nephritis were the predominant lesion in Sjögren's syndrome. Later the finding of immunoglobulins and complement with cells comprising the interstitial infiltrates (321) supported the idea of an active immunologic process. Direct extension of this notion has now been provided by the studies of Winer and co-workers (319). The precise identity of the antigens involved in the immune complexes deposited near tubular basement membranes in Sjögren's syndrome remains a matter of some doubt (328). It is possible that autologous renal tubular antigens represent a source of the putative antigen and that some of the lymphocytes and occasional plasma cells present within interstitial infiltrates are synthesizing antibody locally reactive with such autologous tubular antigens. Talal has suggested that the lymphocytic infiltrates within such renal interstitial areas may be partially analogous to similar infiltrates within affected salivary glands in this disorder (329). Circulating antibody to salivary gland epithelial antigen is cross-reactive with renal tubular antigen (330). Such circulating antibody could conceivably combine directly with renal tubular antigens being released into interstitial areas, providing the mechanism by which immune-complex deposits are actually formed.

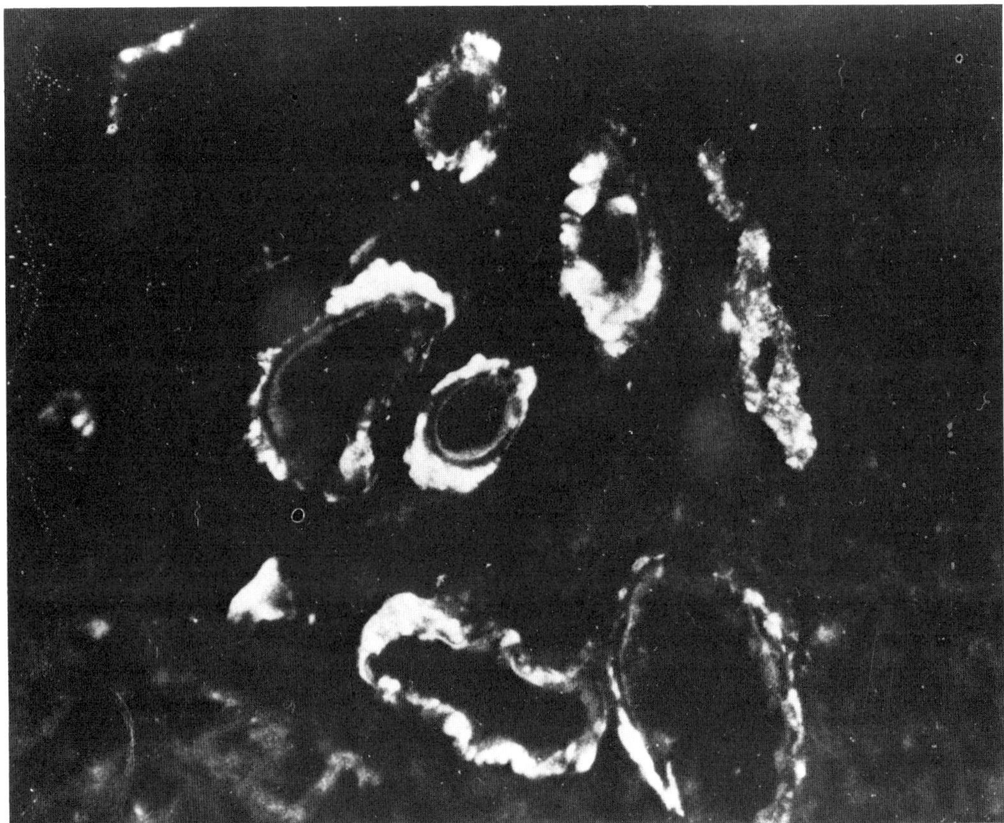

Figure 12-21 Immunofluorescent study of renal biopsy in a patient with Sjögren's syndrome, showing focal tubular basement membrane deposits of C3. The appearance and distribution of IgG were similar. Magnification × 281. (Reproduced with permission, R. L. Winer, A. H. Cohen, A. S. Sawhney et al., *Clin. Immunol. Immunopathol.* 8:494, 1977.)

Other Cell-Mediated Phenomena

The precise nature of the antigens—whether endogenous or exogenous—involved in interstitial renal immune-complex–mediated tissue injury is still a matter of some controversy. In some patients evidence implicates the participation of autologous renal tubular antigens in the disease process. Thus, a report by Shwayder and co-workers (331) noted deposition of renal tubular antigen, IgG, and C1q in glomeruli and proximal tubules of a patient with nephrosis and associated Fanconi syndrome. In this case circulating antibody to renal tubular antigen was present, but not antibody to tubular basement membrane. This case appears to differ from a patient described by Levy and co-workers (332), who showed immune-mediated Fanconi syndrome in association with antibody to TBMs, and from a similar patient studied in detail by Bergstein and Litman (311). Interstitial tubular injury may arise from direct reactions with tubular-basement membrane antigens or from immune-complex–mediated deposits containing either well-characterized tubular antigens or other antigens as in Sjögren's syndrome.

An entirely different mechanism has recently been reported by Cochrane and co-workers (333) in studies of patients with autoimmune liver disease and renal tubular acidosis (RTA). Renal tubular acidosis was present in a significant proportion of patients with primary biliary cirrhosis or chronic active hepatitis (334). The Tamm-Horsfall glycoprotein was selected for study, since this material is secreted by renal tubular cells in the same anatomic location as that involved with urinary acidification. Lymphocytes from 10 of 13 patients with chronic active hepatitis or primary biliary cirrhosis and associated RTA showed cytotoxicity for a kidney cell line known to secrete the Tamm-Horsfall protein. The cytotoxic reaction could be blocked by the protein. In addition, significant diminution in cytotoxicity was observed in the presence of aggregated IgG, suggesting participation of cells bearing Fc receptors in the killing process. It therefore seems possible that direct sensitization of circulating lymphocytes to a natural product of some renal tubular epithelial cells may serve as a basis for immunologic injury in some patients. Possibly pertinent to these findings are reports that liver-cell membranes may show cross-reactivity or antigenic similarity to Tamm-Horsfall proteins when studied in indirect immunofluorescence (335). During the process of liver-cell damage, cross-reacting antigens are possibly released that sensitize the host to materials naturally produced by renal tubular epithelial cells, and a setting is thereby induced for subsequent immunologic injury. More work on this interesting system is needed to determine whether similar or related mechanisms may be operating in other forms of poorly understood interstitial or tubular cell dysfunction.

An Approach to Treatment

Despite the fact that a great deal of information is now available on the probable mechanisms influencing the course of immune-complex–mediated glomerulonephritis, there is still much to be learned about rational and effective treatment. Most of the major practical therapeutic procedures available for various forms of immune-complex glomerulonephritis are aimed at counteracting undesirable clinical manifestations secondary to established renal injury. Relief of edema by judicious use of diuretics, control of hypertension with an increasing array of potent hypotensive agents, and treatment of superimposed infection using effective antibiotics encompass some of the most practical forms of therapy. None of these measures address the basic underlying disease. However, practical methods of therapeutic intervention such as diuretics and antihypertensives often mean the difference between survival or demise in sick patients.

Patients with certain forms of immune-complex glomerular injury do not require specific treatment other than supportive care. An example might be found in subjects recovering from acute poststreptococcal glomerulonephritis associated with mild proliferative glomerular changes. The normal built-in capacity for healing and resolution of such changes seems to suffice in effective preservation of renal function necessary for healthy survival. Similarly, patients who sustain repeated attacks of IgA-mediated nephropathy with minimal changes or normal histological examination rarely progress to uremia. Cameron (336) has estimated that one-quarter of adult patients and at least one-half of children with membranous nephropathy will show complete clinical resolution of the disease within two years. Thus in situations where long-term effects are uncertain, it is recommended that treatment be applied judiciously and reserved primarily for groups of individuals who are most likely to fare badly and least likely to show spontaneous or natural remissions.

The actual tissue injury that occurs in patients with glomerular or other renal structural immune-complex injury may be caused by several mechanisms, all of which tend to localize sufficient amounts of complexes to result in local injury. For one reason or another the patient is presented with a particular qualitative type or amount of immune complex that cannot be handled by ordinary disposal or clearing mechanisms, and immune-complex deposition with consequent tissue injury ensues. A reasonable direct approach to treatment might therefore be divided into three major categories as described by Cameron and shown in Table 12-5. First, if feasible, one might attempt direct removal of the offending antigen. Unfortunately in most instances of immune-complex glomerulonephritis, the antigen is unknown. If, however, the antigens implicit in glomerular immune-complex disease arise from infections with identifiable agents

Table 12-5   Methods of treatment in immune-complex renal disease.

Antigen removal:	Change of immune status and/or balance:	Decrease or abrogation of the following inflammatory mediators:
Specific removal by treatment or immune-absorbents	Suppression or removal of excess antibody production	Anticomplement or C′ deficiency
Antigen avoidance	Addition of excess[a] antigen	White blood cell proteases
Antibody administration[a]	Increase in cell-mediated immune control of humoral antibody	Coagulation process
Plasmapheresis	Surgical or radiological removal of lymphoid tissue	Antikinins
		Lymphokines
		Antiprostaglandins
		Antihistamine or SRS–A

[a] To avoid equivalence zone or production of soluble complexes.

such as in infective endocarditis, shunt nephritis, or even schistosomiasis, direct therapeutic benefit can often be achieved by treatment of the primary infection. The problem of antigen identification looms largest in this context in the major proportion of patients with immune-complex glomerulonephritis secondary to antigens which are virtually unknown, such as membranous or idiopathic proliferative glomerular disease. In the case of lupus nephropathy, where DNA and antibody to DNA may play an important part in the eventual immune-complex destruction of functioning renal tissue, several current approaches directed at extracorporeal immunoabsorbents using insolubilized DNA or anti-DNA may eventually prove to be of therapeutic benefit, but there is much to be learned in this regard. Likewise, plasmapheresis should be considered an alternative to specific antigen removal if there is sufficient clinical or laboratory evidence to indicate large potential pools of offending antigen circulating in plasma or freely exchangeable with the circulating plasma volume.

A second major approach relates to therapeutic intervention that would alter immune responsiveness in such a way as to reduce the formation and level of circulating or tissue-fixed complexes. The various programs aimed at immunosuppression employing antimetabolites, corticosteroids, or cytotoxic agents are used with this in mind. Immunosuppression is a powerful tool aimed at decreasing formation of humoral antibody and therefore the capacity of the organism to produce sufficient levels of circulating complexes for tissue saturation and glomerular deposition. From long clinical experience with many of these agents, it is apparent that they also reduce the normal protective immune responses and allow easy access to nosocomial infections. A second rather opposite approach has been suggested, namely stimulation of the immune response that might conceivably be modulating an uncontrolled humoral immune response via cell-mediated mechanisms, at the same time decreasing the extent or avidity of humoral antibody formation. Such a general effect has in some clinical situations been ascribed to levamisole, a drug originally used with some success in various helminthic infections. Unfortunately, the use of both cytostatic or immunosuppressive agents and partial immunostimulators has been accompanied by undesirable side effects including leukopenia, occasional thrombocytopenia, or granulocytopenia, making them a two-edged sword.

A third major approach has at times followed quite naturally upon the use of immunosuppressive or cytostatic agents, in that these same drugs may also have the ability to alter the process of immune inflammation. Thus potent agents such as corticosteroids, cyclophosphamide, chlorambucil, or azathioprine also exert profound anti-inflammatory effects in a variety of modulating systems. Such effects may be mediated by changes in local prostaglandin synthesis, blood coagulability, platelet adhesiveness, or alterations in interaction of complement components.

In summary, it would appear that the most

effective treatment of immune-complex disease of the kidney would be effective and complete elimination of the offending antigen. If this proves to be impossible since the antigens themselves are furnished by changes in autologous tissues, then the next most important and practical goal of therapy should be an effective system of shutting off the local consequences of immune-complex deposition. Because of the wide variety of disease processes involved, this latter step will be quite variable. In the case of hypocomplementemic membranous nephropathy it may eventually involve direct correction of the fundamental defect in control of complement activation. On the other hand, in the case of disease mediated by antibody to GBM, it would involve induction or reintroduction of tolerance to external cross-reacting or autologous antigens of GBM structures. Each clinical example would appear to involve a separate and carefully defined approach. From the experience already gained with over two decades of controlled trials of immunosuppression and renal transplantation it seems likely that measures now generally available to the practicing clinician cannot be applied en bloc as a panacea for the many intricate derangements unique to particular clinical disorders.

These general comments are made with a hopeful eye to the future, since it is obvious that a great deal has already been learned about many of the processes occurring in a number of immune-complex renal disorders of widely different basic etiology. The general level of interest and the momentum of knowledge already accumulated about the unique immunologic features of each type of immune-complex renal disease augur well.

References

1. Sitprija, V., Pipatanagul, V., Boonpucknavig, V., et al. Glomerulitis in typhoid fever. *Ann. Intern. Med.* 81:210, 1974.

2. Andres, G. A., Kano, K., Elwood, C., et al. Immune deposit nephritis in infectious mononucleosis. *Int. Arch. Allergy Appl. Immunol.* 52:136, 1976.

3. Lambert, P. H., and Houba, V. Immune complexes in parasitic diseases. In L. Brent and J. Holborow, eds., *Progress in Immunology II,* vol. 5, p. 57. North-Holland Publishing Co., Amsterdam, 1974.

4. Germuth, F. G., Jr. A comparative histologic and immunologic study in rabbits of induced hypersensitivity of the serum sickness type. *J. Exp. Med.* 97:257, 1953.

5. Cochrane, C. G., and Koffler, D. Immune complex disease in experimental animals and man. *Adv. Immunol.* 16:185, 1973.

6. Dixon, F. J., Feldman, J. D., and Vasquez, J. J. Experimental glomerulonephritis: the pathogenesis of a laboratory model resembling the spectrum of human glomerulonephritis. *J. Exp. Med.* 113:899, 1961.

7. Rammelkamp, C. H., Jr. Microbiologic aspects of glomerulonephritis. *J. Chron. Dis.* 5:28, 1957.

8. Wannamaker, L. W. Epidemiology of acute glomerulonephritis. In J. Metcoff, ed., *Acute Glomerulonephritis,* P. 39. Little, Brown and Co., Boston, 1967.

9. Potter, E. V., Siegel, A. C., Simon, N. M., et al. Streptococcal infections and epidemic acute glomerulonephritis in South Trinidad. *J. Pediatr.* 72:871, 1968.

10. Poon-King, T., Mohammed, I., Cox, R., et al. Recurrent epidemic nephritis in South Trinidad. *N. Engl. J. Med.* 277:728, 1967.

11. Wannamaker, L. W., and Pierce, H. C. Family outbreak of acute nephritis associated with type 49 streptococcal infection. Journal/Lancet 81:561, 1961.

12. Kaplan, E. L., Anthony, B. F., Chapman, S. S., et al. Epidemic acute glomerulonephritis associated with type 49 streptococcal pyoderma. I. Clinical and laboratory findings. *Am. J. Med.* 48:9, 1970.

13. Villarreal, H., Jr., Fischetti, V. A., Van de Rijn, I. et al. The occurrence of a protein in the extracellular products of streptococci isolated from patients with acute glomerulonephritis. *J. Exp. Med.* 149:459, 1979.

14. Treser, G., Semar, M., Ty, A., et al. Partial characterization of antigenic streptococcal plasma membrane components in acute glomerulonephritis. *J. Clin. Invest.* 49:762, 1970.

15. Markowitz, A. S., and Lange, C. F., Jr. Streptococcal related glomerulonephritis. I. Isolation, immunochemistry, and comparative chemistry of soluble fractions from type 12 nephritogenic streptococci and human glomeruli. *J. Immunol.* 92:565, 1964.

16. Treser, G., Semar, M., McVicar, M., et al. Antigenic streptococcal components in acute glomerulonephritis. *Science* 163:676, 1969.

17. Lange, K., Ahmed, U., Kleinberger, H., et al. A hitherto unknown streptococcal antigen and its probable relation to acute poststreptococcal glomerulonephritis. *Clin. Nephrol.* 5:207, 1976.

18. Lewy, J. E., Salinas-Madrigal, L., Herdson, P. B., et al. Clinicopathologic correlations in acute poststreptococcal glomerulonephritis: a correlation between renal functions, morphologic damage and clinical course of 46 children with acute poststreptococcal glomerulonephritis. *Medicine* 50:453, 1971.

19. Dodge, W. F., Spargo, B. H., Travis, L. B., et al. Poststreptococcal glomerulonephritis. A prospective study in children. *N. Engl. J. Med.* 286:273, 1972.

20. Callis, L., Vila, A., Castello, F., et al. Postinfectious glomerulonephritis of acute onset in childhood: a review of 175 cases. In J. Strauss, ed., *Pediatric Nephrology II*, p. 89., Stratton Intercontinental Medical Book Corp., New York, 1976.

21. Travis, L. B., Dodge, W. F., Beathard, G., et al. Acute glomerulonephritis in children: a review of the natural history with emphasis on prognosis. *Clin. Nephrol.* 1:169, 1973.

22. Dodge, W. F., Spargo, B. H., Bass, J. A., et al. The relationship between the clinical and pathologic features of poststreptococcal glomerulonephritis. A study of the early natural history. *Medicine* 47:227, 1968.

23. Lewy, J. E. Acute poststreptococcal glomerulonephritis. *Pediatr. Clin. North Am.* 23:751, 1976.

24. Fischel, E. E. Immune reactions in human glomerulonephritis. *J. Chronic Dis.* 5:34, 1957.

25. Ingelfinger, J. R., McCluskey, R. T., Schneeberger, E. E., et al. Necrotizing arteritis in acute poststreptococcal glomerulonephritis. *J. Pediatr.* 91:228, 1977.

26. Michael, A. F., Jr., Drummond, K. M., Good, R. A., et al. Acute poststreptococcal glomerulonephritis: immune deposit disease. *J. Clin. Invest.* 45:237, 1966.

27. Feldman, J. D., Mardiney, M. R., and Shuler, S. E. Immunology and morphology of acute poststreptococcal glomerulonephritis. *Lab. Invest.* 15:283, 1966.

28. Seegal, B. C., Andres, G. A., Hsu, K. C., et al. Studies on the pathogenesis of acute and progressive glomerulonephritis in man by immunofluorescein and immunoferritin techniques. *Fed. Proc.* 24:100, 1965.

29. McCluskey, R. T., Vassalli, P., Gallo, G., et al. An immunofluorescent study of pathogenic mechanisms in glomerular diseases. *N. Engl. J. Med.* 274:695, 1966.

30. Andres, G. A., Accinni, L., Hsu, K. C., et al. Electron microscopic studies of human glomerulonephritis with ferritin-conjugated antibody: localization of antigen-antibody complexes in glomerular structures of patients with acute glomerulonephritis. *J. Exp. Med.* 123:399, 1966.

31. Zabriskie, J. B. The role of streptococci in human glomerulonephritis. *J. Exp. Med.* 134:180s, 1971.

32. Kantor, F. S. Fibrinogen precipitation by streptococcal M protein. I. Identity of the reactants, and stoichiometry of the reaction. *J. Exp. Med.* 121:849, 1965.

33. Kantor, F. S. Fibrinogen precipitation by streptococcal M protien. II. Renal lesions induced by intravenous injection of M protein into mice and rats. *J. Exp. Med.* 121:861, 1965.

34. Lieberman, E., and Donnell, G. N. Recovery of children with acute glomerulonephritis. *Am. J. Dis. Child.* 109:398, 1965.

35. Perlman, L. V., Herdman, R. C., Kleinman, H., et al. Poststreptococcal glomerulonephritis. A ten-year follow-up of an epidemic. *J.A.M.A.* 194:63, 1965.

36. Jennings, R. B., and Earle, D. P. Poststreptococcal glomerulonephritis: histopathologic and clinical studies of the acute, subsiding acute and early chronic latent phases. *J. Clin. Invest.* 40:1525, 1961.

37. Sagel, I., Treser, G., Ty, A., et al. Occurrence and nature of glomerular lesions after group A streptococci infections in children. *Ann. Intern. Med.* 79:492, 1973.

38. Ellis, A. Natural history of Bright's disease. Clinical, histological and experimental observations. *Lancet* 1:1, 1942.

39. Grishman, E., and Churg, J. Acute glomerulonephritis: a histopathologic study by means of thin sections. *Am. J. Pathol.* 33:993, 1957.

40. Herdson, P. B., Jennings, R. B., and Earle, D. P. Glomerular fine structure in poststreptococcal acute glomerulonephritis. *Arch. Pathol.* 81:117, 1966.

41. Kimmelstiel, P., Kim, O. J., and Beres, J. Studies on renal biopsy specimens, with the aid of

the electron microscope. II. Glomerulonephritis and glomerulonephrosis. *Am. J. Clin. Pathol.* 38:280, 1962.

42. Baldwin, D. S., Gluck, M. C., Schacht, R. G., et al. The long-term course of poststreptococcal glomerulonephritis. *Ann. Intern. Med.* 80:342, 1974.

43. Baldwin, D. S., and Schacht, R. C. Late sequelae of poststreptococcal glomerulonephritis. *Annu. Rev. Med.* 27:49, 1976.

44. Schacht, R. G., Gluck, M. C., Gallo, G. R., et al. Progression to uremia after remission of acute poststreptococcal glomerulonephritis. *N. Engl. J. Med.* 295:977, 1976.

45. Baldwin, D. S. Poststreptococcal glomerulonephritis. A progressive disease? *Am. J. Med.* 62:1, 1977.

46. Longcope, W. T. Some observations on the course and outcome of hemorrhagic nephritis. *Trans. Am. Clin. Climatol. Assoc.* 53:153, 1937.

47. Murphy, F. D., and Peters, B. J. Treatment of acute nephritis: the immediate results and the outcome ten years later in eighty-nine cases. *J.A.M.A.* 118:183, 1942.

48. Ramberg, R. The prognosis for acute nephritis. *Acta Med. Scand.* 127:396, 1947.

49. Hill, L. W. Studies in the nephritis of children. Clinical considerations of classification, etiology, prognosis and treatment. *Am. J. Dis. Child.* 17:270, 1919.

50. James, R. F. The prognosis of nephritis in childhood. *J.A.M.A.* 76:505, 1921.

51. Guild, H. G. The prognosis of acute glomerular nephritis in childhood. *Bull. Johns Hopkins Hosp.* 48:193, 1931.

52. Gachet, F. S. Course and prognosis of hemorrhagic nephritis in children. *Am. J. Dis. Child.* 61:1175, 1941.

53. Davis, J. H., and Faber, H. K. The prognosis in acute glomerulonephritis in children. *J. Pediatr.* 27:453, 1945.

54. Frisk, A., and Klackenberg, G. A study of the onset and prognosis of nephritis in children. *Acta Paediatr. Scand.* 33:349, 1946.

55. Kleinman, H. Epidemic acute glomerulonephritis at Red Lake. *Minn. Med.* 37:479, 1954.

56. Stetson, C. A. Rammelkamp, C. H., Jr., Krause, R. M., et al. Epidemic acute nephritis: studies on etiology, natural history and prevention. *Medicine (Baltimore)* 34:431, 1955.

57. McCluskey, R. T., and Baldwin, D. S. Natural history of acute glomerulonephritis in the adult. *Medicine (Baltimore)* 40:203, 1961.

58. Treser, G., Ehrenreich, T., Ores, R., et al. Natural history of "apparently healed" acute post-streptococcal glomerulonephritis in children. *Pediatrics* 43:1005, 1969.

59. Zabriskie, J. B., Lewshenia, G., Möller. G., et al. Lymphocytic responses to streptococcal antigens in glomerulonephritic patients. *Science* 168:1105, 1970.

60. Rocklin, R. E., Lewis, E. J., and David, J. R. *In vitro* evidence for cellular hypersensitivity to glomerular-basement-membrane antigens in human glomerulonephritis. *N. Engl. J. Med.* 283:497, 1970.

61. Bhat, J. G., Gombos, E. A., and Baldwin, D. S. Depressed cellular immune response to streptococcal antigens in poststreptococcal glomerulonephritis. *Clin. Immunol. Immunopathol.* 7:230, 1977.

62. Bloom, B. R., Gaffney, J., and Jiminez, L. Dissociation of MIF production and cell proliferation. *J. Immunol.* 109:1395, 1972.

63. Rocklin, R. E. Production of migration inhibitory factor by non-dividing lymphocytes. *J. Immunol.* 110:674, 1973.

64. Dardenne, M., Zabriskie, J., and Bach, J. F. Streptococcal sensitivity in chronic glomerulonephritis. *Lancet* 1:126, 1972.

65. Krzymanski, M., Möller, E., and Bergström, J. Cell-mediated and humoral immunity to streptococcal cell wall antigenic extract in patients with glomerulonephritis and in healthy controls. *Scand. J. Immunol.* 4:295, 1975.

66. Dixon, F. J. The role of antigen-antibody complexes in disease. In *The Harvey Lecture Series 58,* p. 21. Academic Press, New York, 1963.

67. Schick, B. Die Nach Krankheiter des Scharlach. *Jb. Kinderheilk.* 65:132, 1907 (suppl.).

68. Von Pirquet, C. E. Allergy. *Arch. Intern. Med.* 7:259, 1911.

69. Volhard, F. Die doppelseitigen hämotogenen Nierenerkrankungen (Bright'sche Krankheit), in L. Mohr and R. Staenelin, eds., *Handbuch der Inneren Medizin,* vol. 3, pt. 2, p. 1149. Springer, Berlin, 1918.

70. Klinge, F. Die Eiweifsüberempfindlichkeit (Gewebsanaphylaxie) der Gelenke. Experimentelle pathologisch-anatomische Studien zur Pathogenese des Gelenkrheumatismus. *Beitr. Pathol.* 83:185, 1929.

71. Fordham, C. C., Epstein, F. H., Huffines, W. D., et al. Polyarteritis and acute post-streptococcal glomerulonephritis. *Ann. Intern. Med.* 61:89, 1964.

72. Ossi, E., Prezyna, A., Sepulveda, M., et al. Immune deposits in the spleen of a patient with acute poststreptococcal glomerulonephritis (APSGN). *Clin. Immunol. Immunopathol.* 6:306, 1976.

73. Törnroth, T. The fate of subepithelial de-

posits in acute poststreptococcal glomerulonephritis. *Lab. Invest.* 35:461, 1976.

74. Schwab, J. H., Cromartie, W. J., Ohanian, S. H., et al. Association of experimental chronic arthritis with the persistence of group A streptococcal cell walls in the articular tissue. *J. Bacteriol.* 94:1728, 1965.

75. Cromartie, W. J., and Craddock, J. G. Rheumatic-like cardiac lesions in mice. *Science* 154:285, 1966.

76. Cromartie, W. J., Craddock, J. G., Schwab, J. H., et al. Arthritis in rats after systemic injection of streptococcal cells or cell walls. *J. Exp. Med.* 146:1585, 1977.

77. Krishnan, C., and Kaplan, M. H. Immunopathologic studies of systemic lupus erythematosus. II. Antinuclear reaction of γ-globulin eluted from homogenates and isolated glomeruli of kidneys from patients with lupus nephritis. *J. Clin. Invest.* 46:569, 1967.

78. Koffler, D., Schur, P. H., and Kunkel, H. G. Immunological studies concerning the nephritis of systemic lupus erythematosus. *J. Exp. Med.* 126:607, 1967.

79. Koffler, D., Agnello, V., Thoburn, R., et al. Systemic lupus erythematosus: prototype of immune complex nephritis in man. *J. Exp. Med.* 134:169s, 1971.

80. Kohler, P. F. Clinical immune complex disease. Manifestations in systemic lupus erythematosus and hepatitis B virus infection. *Medicine (Baltimore)* 52:419, 1973.

81. Theofilopoulos, A. N., Wilson, C. B., and Dixon, F. J. The Raji cell radioimmune assay for detecting immune complexes in human sera. *J. Clin. Invest.* 57:169, 1976.

82. Zubler, R. H., Lange, G., Lambert, P. H., et al. Detection of immune complexes in unheated sera by a modified ^{125}I-C1q binding test. Effect of heating on the binding of C1q by immune complexes and application of the test to systemic lupus erythematosus. *J. Immunol.* 116:232, 1976.

83. Winfield, J. B., Faiferman, I., and Koffler, D. Avidity of anti-DNA antibodies in serum and IgG glomerular eluates from patients with systemic lupus erythematosus. Association of high avidity anti-native DNA antibody with glomerulonephritis. *J. Clin. Invest.* 59:90, 1977.

84. Izui, S., Lambert, P. H., Fournié, G. J., et al. Features of systemic lupus erythematosus in mice injected with bacterial lipopolysaccharides. Identification of circulating DNA and renal localization of DNA-anti-DNA complexes. *J. Exp. Med.* 145:1115, 1977.

85. Izui, S., Lambert, P. H., and Miescher, P. A. *In vitro* demonstration of a particular affinity of glomerular basement membrane and collagen for DNA. A possible basis for a local formation of DNA-anti-DNA complexes in systemic lupus erythematosus. *J. Exp. Med.* 144:428, 1976.

86. Izui, S., Lambert, P. H., and Miescher, P. A. Failure to detect circulating DNA-anti-DNA complexes by four radioimmunological methods in patients with systemic lupus erythematosus. *Clin. Exp. Immunol.* 30:384, 1977.

87. Nydegger, U. E., Lambert, P. H., Gerber, H., et al. Circulating immune complexes in the serum in systemic lupus erythematosus and in carriers of hepatitis B antigen. Quantitation by binding to radiolabeled C1q. *J. Clin. Invest.* 54:297, 1974.

88. Emlen, W., and Mannik, M. Kinetics and mechanisms for removal of circulating single-stranded DNA in mice. *J. Exp. Med.* 147:684, 1978.

89. Naruse, T., Kitamura, K., Miyakawa, Y., et al. Deposition of renal tubular epithelial antigen along the glomerular capillary walls of patients with membranous glomerulonephritis. *J. Immunol.* 110:1163, 1973.

90. Naruse, T., Miyakawa, Y., Kitamura, K., et al. Membranous glomerulonephritis mediated by renal tubular epithelial antigen-antibody complex. *J. Allergy Clin. Immunol.* 54:311, 1974.

91. Strauss, J., Pardo, V., Koss, M. N., et al. Nephropathy associated with sickle cell anemia: an autologous immune complex nephritis. I. Studies on the nature of the glomerular-bound antibody and antigen identification in a patient with sickle cell disease and immune deposit glomerulonephritis. *Am. J. Med.* 58:382, 1975.

92. Pardo, V., Strauss, J., Kramer, H., et al. Nephropathy associated with sickle cell anemia: an autologous immune complex nephritis. II. Clinicopathologic study of seven patients. *Am. J. Med.* 59:650, 1975.

93. Shwayder, M., Ozawa, T., Boedecker, E., et al. Nephrotic syndrome associated with Fanconi syndrome. Immunopathogenic studies of tubulo-interstitial nephritis with autologous immune-complex glomerulonephritis. *Ann. Intern. Med.* 84:433, 1976.

94. Weigle, W. O. Experimental autoimmune thyroiditis. *Pathol. Annu.* 8:329, 1973.

95. O'Regan, S., Fong, J. S. C., Kaplan, B. S., et al. Thyroid antigen-antibody nephritis. *Clin. Immunol. Immunopathol.* 6:341, 1976.

96. Moroz, S. P., Cutz, E., Balfe, J. W., et al. Membranoproliferative glomerulonephritis in childhood cirrhosis associated with alpha$_1$-anti-trypsin deficiency. *Pediatrics* 57:232, 1976.

97. Lewis, M. G., Loughridge, L. W., and Phillips, T. M. Immunological studies in nephrotic syndrome associated with extrarenal malignant disease. *Lancet* 2:134, 1971.

98. Costanza, M. E., Pinn, V., Schwartz, R. S., et al. Carcinoembryonic antigen-antibody complexes in a patient with colonic carcinoma and nephrotic syndrome. *N. Engl. J. Med.* 289:520, 1973.

99. Couser, W. G., Wagonfeld, J. B., Spargo, B. H., et al. Glomerular deposition of tumor antigen in membranous nephropathy associated with colonic carcinoma. *Am. J. Med.* 57:962, 1974.

100. Weksler, M. E. Nephrotic syndrome in malignant melanoma: demonstration of melanoma antigen-antibody complexes in the kidney. *Kidney Int.* 6:112A, 1974.

101. Ozawa, T., Pluss, R., Lacher, J., et al. Endogenous immune complex nephropathy associated with malignancy. I. Studies on the nature and immunopathogenic significance of glomerular bound antigen and antibody, isolation and characterization of tumor specific antigen and antibody and circulating immune complexes. *Q. J. Med.* 44:523, 1975.

102. Burch, G. E., Chu, K. C., Colcolough, H. L., et al. Immunofluorescent localization of coxsackievirus B antigen in the kidney observed at routine autopsy. *Am. J. Med.* 47:36, 1969.

103. Burch, G. E., and Colcolough, H. L. Progressive coxsackie viral pancarditis and nephritis. *Ann. Intern. Med.* 71:963, 1969.

104. Combes, B., Stastny, P., Shorey, J., et al. Glomerulonephritis with deposition of Australia antigen-antibody complexes in glomerular basement membrane. *Lancet* 2:234, 1971.

105. Myers, B. D., Griffel, B., Naveh, D., et al. Membranoproliferative glomerulonephritis associated with persistent viral hepatitis. *Am. J. Clin. Pathol.* 60:222, 1973.

106. Kohler, P. F., Cronin, R. E., Hammond, W. S., et al. Chronic membranous glomerulonephritis caused by hepatitis B antigen-antibody immune complexes. *Ann. Intern. Med.* 81:448, 1974.

107. Knieser, M. R., Jenis, E. H., Lowenthal, D. T., et al. Pathogenesis of renal disease associated with viral hepatitis. *Arch. Pathol.* 97:193, 1974.

108. Brzosko, W. J., Krawczyński, K., Nazarewicz, T., et al. Glomerulonephritis associated with hepatitis-B surface antigen immune complexes in children. *Lancet.* 2:477, 1974.

109. Dayan, A. D., and Stokes, M. I. Immune complexes and visceral deposits of measles antigens in subacute sclerosing panencephalitis. *Br. Med. J.* 2:374, 1972.

110. Sutherland, J. C., and Mardiney, M. R., Jr. Immune complex disease in the kidneys of lymphoma-leukemia patients: the presence of an oncornavirus-related antigen. *J. Natl. Cancer Inst.* 50:633, 1973.

111. Sonnabend, W., Kistler, G. S., Thiel, G., et al. Chronische Herdglomerulitis und chronischpersisterende Hepatitis nach Nierentransplantation: Nachweis von Hepatitis-B und Epstein-Barr-Virus-Antigen. *Schweiz. Med. Wochenschr.* 104:1205, 1974.

112. Oldstone, M. B. A., Theofilopoulos, A. N., Gunvén, P., et al. Immune complexes associated with neoplasia: presence of Epstein-Barr virus antigen-antibody complexes in Burkitt's lymphoma. *Intervirology* 4:292, 1974.

113. Kaufman, D. B., and McIntosh, R. The pathogenesis of the renal lesion in a patient with streptococcal disease, infected ventriculo-atrial shunt, cryoglobulinemia and nephritis. *Am. J. Med.* 50:262, 1971.

114. Dobrin, R. S., Day, N. K., Quie, P. G., et al. The role of complement, immunoglobulin and bacterial antigen in coagulase-negative staphylococcal shunt nephritis. *Am. J. Med.* 59:660, 1975.

115. Bolton, W. K., Sande, M. A., Normansell, D. E., et al. Ventriculojugular shunt nephritis with Corynebacterium bovis. Successful therapy with antibiotics. *Am. J. Med.* 59:417, 1975.

116. Perez, G. O., Rothfield, N., and Williams, R. C., Jr. Immune complex nephritis in bacterial endocarditis. *Arch. Intern. Med.* 136:334, 1976.

117. Keslin, M. H., Messner, R. P., and Williams, R. C., Jr. Glomerulonephritis with subacute bacterial endocarditis. Immunofluorescent studies. *Arch. Intern. Med.* 132:578, 1973.

118. Hyman, L. R., Jenis, E. H., Hill, G. S., et al. Alternate C3 pathway activation in pneumococcal glomerulonephritis. *Am. J. Med.* 58:810, 1975.

119. Tourville, D. R., Byrd, L. H., Kim, D. U., et al. Treponemal antigens in immunopathogenesis of syphilitic glomerulonephritis. *Am. J. Pathol.* 82:479, 1976.

120. Gamble, C. N., and Reardan, J. B. Immunopathogenesis of syphilitic glomerulonephritis. Elution of anti-treponemal antibody from glomerular immune complex deposits. *N. Engl. J. Med.* 292:449, 1975.

121. Braunstein, G. D., Lewis, E. J., Galvanek, E. G., et al. The nephrotic syndrome associated with secondary syphilis. An immune deposit disease. *Am. J. Med.* 48:643, 1970.

122. Ward, P. A., and Kibukamusoke, J. W. Evidence for soluble complexes in the pathogenesis of the glomerulonephritis of quartan malaria. *Lancet* 1:283, 1969.

123. Hendrickse, R. G., Glasgow, E. F., Adeniyi, A., et al. Quartan malarial nephrotic syndrome. Collaborative clinicopathological study in Nigerian children. *Lancet* 1:1143, 1972.

124. Bhamarapravati, N., Boonpucknavig, S., Boonpucknavig, V., et al. Glomerular changes in acute *Plasmodium falciparum* infection. An immunopathologic study. *Arch. Pathol.* 96:289, 1973.

125. Falcão, H. A., and Gould, D. B. Immune complex nephropathy in schistosomiasis. *Ann. Intern. Med.* 83:148, 1975.

126. Silva, L. C. D., de Brito, T., Camargo, M. E., et al. Kidney biopsy in the hepatosplenic form of infection with *Schistosoma mansoni* in man. *Bull. WHO* 42:907, 1970.

127. Shahin, B., Papadopoulou, Z. L., and Jenis, E. H. Congenital nephrotic syndrome associated with congenital toxoplasmosis. *J. Pediatr.* 85:366, 1974.

128. Ginsberg, B. E., Wasserman, J., Huldt, G., et al. Case of glomerulonephritis associated with acute toxoplasmosis. *Br. Med. J.* 3:664, 1974.

129. Nagle, R. B., Ward, P. A., Lindsley, H. B., et al. Experimental infections with African trypanosomes. VI. Glomerulonephritis involving the alternate pathway of complement activation. *Am. J. Trop. Med. Hyg.* 23:15, 1974.

130. de Brito, T., Hoshino-Shimizu, S., Amato Neto, V., et al. Glomerular involvement in human Kala-azar. A light, immunofluorescent, and electron microscopic study based on kidney biopsies. *Am. J. Trop. Med. Hyg.* 24:9, 1975.

131. Roberts, W. C., and Rabson, A. S. Focal glomerular lesions in fungal endocarditis. *Ann. Intern. Med.* 56:610, 1962.

132. Chesney, R. W., O'Regan, S., Guyda, H. J., et al. Candida endocrinopathy syndrome with membranoproliferative glomerulonephritis: demonstration of glomerular candida antigen. *Clin. Nephrol.* 5:232, 1976.

133. West, C. D., McAdams, A. J., McConville, J. M., et al. Hypocomplementemic and normocomplementemic persistent (chronic) glomerulonephritis; clinical and pathologic characteristics. *J. Pediatr.* 67:1089, 1965.

134. Gotoff, S. P., Fellers, F. X., Vawter, G. F., et al. The Beta$_{1\gamma}$ globulin in childhood nephrotic syndrome. Laboratory diagnosis of progressive glomerulonephritis. *N. Engl. J. Med.* 273:524, 1965.

135. Habib, R., Kleinknecht, C., Gubler, M. C., et al. Idiopathic membrano-proliferative glomerulonephritis in children. Report of 105 cases. *Clin. Nephrol.* 1:194, 1973.

136. Habib, R., Gubler, M. C., Loirat, C., et al. Dense deposit disease: a variant of membranoproliferative glomerulonephritis. *Kidney Int.* 7:204, 1975.

137. Antoine, B., and Faye, C. The clinical course associated with dense deposits in the kidney basement membranes. *Kidney Int.* 1:420, 1972.

138. Bohle, A., Gärtner, H. V., Fischbach, H., et al. The morphological and clinical features of membranoproliferative glomerulonephritis in adults. *Virchows Arch. (Pathol. Anat.)* 363:213, 1974.

139. Burkholder, P. M. Membranoproliferative glomerulonephritis. In *Atlas of Human Glomerular Pathology,* p. 185. Harper and Row, New York, 1974.

140. Strife, C. F., McEnery, P. T., McAdams, A. J., et al. A third ultrastructural variety of membranoproliferative glomerulonephritis. Abstract. Presented to Am. Soc. Nephrol. 8th Annual Meeting. Washington, D.C., 1975.

141. Cameron, J. S., Ogg, C. S., White, R. H. R., et al. The clinical features and prognosis of patients with normocomplementemic mesangiocapillary glomerulonephritis. *Clin. Nephrol.* 1:8, 1973.

142. Ooi, Y. M., Vallota, E. H., and West, C. D. Classical complement pathway activation in membranoproliferative glomerulonephritis. *Kidney Int.* 9:46, 1976.

143. Cameron, J. S., Glasgow, E. F., Ogg, C. S., et al. Membranoproliferative glomerulonephritis and persistent hypocomplementaemia. *Br. Med. J.* 4:7, 1970.

144. Mandalenakis, N., Mendoza, W., Pirani, C. L., et al. Lobular glomerulonephritis and membranoproliferative glomerulonephritis. A clinical and pathologic study based on renal biopsies. *Medicine (Baltimore)* 50:319, 1971.

145. McAdams, A. J., McEnery, P. T., and West, C. D. Mesangiocapillary glomerulonephritis: changes in glomerular morphology with long-term alternate-day prednisone therapy. *J. Pediatr.* 86:23, 1975.

146. Davis, A. E., Schneeberger, E. E., McCluskey, R. T., et al. Mesangial proliferative glomerulonephritis with irregular intramembranous deposits. Another variant of hypocomplementemic nephritis. *Am. J. Med.* 63:481, 1977.

147. Pickering, R. J., Gewurz, H., and Good, R. A. Complement inactivation by serum from patients with acute and hypocomplementemic chronic glomerulonephritis. *J. Lab. Clin. Med.* 72:298, 1968.

148. West, C. D., Winter, S., Forristal, J., et al. Evidence for *in vivo* breakdown of B$_{1c}$ globulin in hypocomplementemic glomerulonephritis. *J. Clin. Invest.* 46:539, 1967.

149. Spitzer, R. E., Vallota, E. H., Forristal, J.,

et al. Serum C'3 lytic system in patients with glomerulonephritis. *Science* 164:436, 1969.

150. Vallota, E. H., Forristal, J., Spitzer, R. E., et al. Continuing C3 breakdown after bilateral nephrectomy in patients with membranoproliferative glomerulonephritis. *J. Clin. Invest.* 50:552, 1971.

151. Michael, A. F., Herdman, R. C., Fish, A. J., et al. Chronic membranoproliferative glomerulonephritis with hypocomplementemia. *Transplant. Proc.* 1:925, 1969.

152. Herdman, R. C., Pickering, R. J., Michael, A. F., et al. Chronic glomerulonephritis associated with low serum complement activity. (chronic hypocomplementemic glomerulonephritis). *Medicine* 49:207, 1970.

153. Thompson, R. A. C3 inactivating factor in the serum of a patient with chronic hypocomplementaemic proliferative glomerulonephritis. *Immunology* 22:147, 1972.

154. Davis, A. E. III, Ziegler, J. B., Gelfand, E. W., et al. Heterogeneity of nephritic factor and its identification as an immunoglobulin. *Proc. Natl. Acad. Sci. (USA)* 74:3980, 1977.

155. Vallota, E. H., Götze, O., Spiegelberg, H. L., et al. A serum factor in chronic hypocomplementemic nephritis distinct from immunoglobulins and activating the alternate pathway of complement. *J. Exp. Med.* 139:1249, 1954.

156. Pillemer, L., Blum, L., Lepow, I. H., et al. The properdin system and immunity. I. Demonstration and isolation of a new serum protein, properdin, and its role in immune phenomena. *Science* 120:279, 1954.

157. Galle, P., and Berger, J. Dépôts intercapillaires. *J. Urol. Nephrol. (Paris)* 68:123, 1962.

158. Levy, M., Loirat, C., and Habib, R. Idiopathic membranoproliferative glomerulonephritis in children: correlations between light, electron, immunofluorescent microscopic appearances and serum C3 and C4 levels. *Biomedicine Express* 19:447, 1973.

159. Williams, D. G., Peters, D. K., Fallows, J., et al. Studies of serum complement in the hypocomplementaemic nephritides. *Clin. Exp. Immunol.* 18:391, 1974.

160. Weiler, J. M., Daha, M. R., Austen, K. F., et al. Control of the amplification convertase of complement by the plasma protein β1H. *Proc. Natl. Acad. Sci. USA* 73:3268, 1976.

161. Muller-Eberhard, H. Personal communication, 1978.

162. Berthoux, F. C., Carpentier, C. B., Blanc-Brunat, N., et al. Récidives des glomérulonéphrites mesangioprolifératives après transplantation rénale-Rôle des systèmes complément et properdine. In M. Fondation, ed., *International Course on Transplantation.* Simep-Editions, Lyon, 1973.

163. Peters, D. K., and Williams, D. G. Complement and mesangiocapillary glomerulonephritis: the role of complement deficiency in glomerulonephritis. In J. Crosnier and M. Maxwell, eds., *Advances in Neurology,* p. 67. Year Book Medical Publishing, Chicago, 1974.

164. Cochrane, C. G. Mechanisms involved in the deposition of immune complexes in tissues. *J. Exp. Med.* 134:75s, 1971.

165. Peters, D. K., Martin, A., Weinstein, A., et al. Complement studies in membranoproliferative glomerulonephritis. *Clin. Exp. Immunol.* 11:311, 1972.

166. Pickering, R. J., Michael, A. F., Herdman, R. C., et al. The complement system in chronic glomerulonephritis: three newly associated aberrations. *J. Pediatr.* 78:30, 1971.

167. Day, N. K., Geiger, H., McLean, R., et al. The association of respiratory infection, recurrent hematuria and focal glomerulonephritis with activation of the complement system in the cold. *J. Clin. Invest.* 52:1698, 1973.

168. Agnello, V., de Bracco, M. M. E., and Kunkel, H. G. Hereditary C2 deficiency with some manifestations of systemic lupus erythematosus. *J. Immunol.* 108:837, 1972.

169. Sussman, M., Jones, J. H., Almeida, J. D., et al. Deficiency of the second component of complement associated with anaphylactoid purpura and presence of mycoplasma in the serum. *Clin. Exp. Immunol.* 14:531, 1973.

170. Kohler, P. F. Hereditary angioedema (HAE) and "Familial" systemic lupus erythematosus (SLE) in identical twin boys. *J. Immunol.* 111:307, 1973 (abstract).

171. Gellis, S. S., Green, S., and Walker, D. Chronic renal disease in children with lipodystrophy. *Am. J. Dis. Child.* 96:605, 1958.

172. Peters, D. K., Williams, D. G., Charlesworth, J. A., et al. Mesangiocapillary nephritis, partial lipodystrophy, and hypocomplementaemia. *Lancet* 2:535, 1973.

173. Sissons, J. G. P., West, R. J., Fallows, J., et al. The complement abnormalities of lipodystrophy. *N. Engl. J. Med.* 294:461, 1976.

174. Thompson, R. A., and White, R. H. R. Partial lipodystrophy and hypocomplementaemic nephritis. *Lancet* 2:679, 1973.

175. Bennet, W. M., Bardana, E. J., Wuepper, K., et al. Partial lipodystrophy, C3 nephritic factor

and clinically inapparent mesangiocapillary glomerulonephritis. *Am. J. Med.* 62:757, 1977.

176. Frank, M. M., Gelfand, J. A., and Atkinson, J. P. Hereditary angioedema: the clinical syndrome and its management. *Ann. Intern. Med.* 84:580, 1976.

177. Boucher, B. J., Cohen, R. D., Frankel, R. J., et al. Partial and total lipodystrophy: changes in circulating sugar, free fatty acids, insulin and growth hormone following the administration of glucose and of insulin. *Clin. Endocrinol. (Oxford)* 2:111, 1973.

178. Mansour, A., Worsdall, P. A., and Roy, L. P. Complement studies in partial lipodystrophy. Presented at 6th Int. Congr. Nephrol., Florence, 1975.

179. Alarçon-Segovia, D., and Ramos-Niembro, F. Association of partial lipodystrophy and Sjögren's syndrome. *Ann. Intern. Med.* 85:474, 1976.

180. Senior, B., and Gellis, S. S. The syndromes of total lipodystrophy and of partial lipodystrophy. *Pediatrics* 33:593, 1964.

181. Rooney, P. J. Case of lipodystrophy. *Br. Med. J.* 2:464, 1970.

182. Poley, J. R., and Stickler, G. B. Progressive lipodystrophy. A clinical study of 50 patients. *Am. J. Dis. Child.* 106:356, 1963.

183. Davis, J. Generalized lipodystrophy, infectious mononucleosis, mild infantile hemiplegia. *Proc. R. Soc. Med.* 47:128, 1954.

184. Verroust, P. J., Wilson, C. B., and Dixon, F. J. Lack of nephritogenicity of systemic activation of the alternate complement pathway. *Kidney Int.* 6:157, 1974.

185. Reichel, W., Köbberling, J., Fischbach, H., et al. Membranoproliferative glomerulonephritis with partial lipodystrophy. Discordant occurrence in identical twins. *Klin. Wochenschr.* 54:75, 1976.

186. Evans, D. J. Pathogenesis of membranous glomerulonephritis. *Lancet* 1:1143, 1974.

187. Bariéty, J., Druet, P., LaGrue, G., et al. Les glomérulonéphrites parietoprolifératives: étude histopathologique en microscopic optique, électronique et en immuno-histochimie de 49 cas: corrélations anatomo-cliniques. *Pathol. Biol. (Paris)* 19:259, 1970.

188. Graham, R. C., and Karnovsky, M. J. Glomerular permeability. Ultrastructural cytochemical studies using peroxidases as protein tracers. *J. Exp. Med.* 124:1123, 1966.

189. Venkatachalam, M. A., Karnovsky, M. J., Fahimi, H. D., et al. An ultrastructural study of glomerular permeability using catalase and peroxidase as tracer proteins. *J. Exp. Med.* 132:1153, 1969.

190. Farquhar, M. G., Wissig, S. L., and Palade, G. E. Glomerular permeability. I. Ferritin transfer across the normal glomerular capillary wall. *J. Exp. Med.* 113:47, 1961.

191. Walker, F. The origin, turnover, and removal of glomerular basement-membrane. *J. Pathol.* 110:233, 1973.

192. Ooi, Y. M., Vallota, E. H., and West, C. D. Serum immune complexes in membrano-proliferative and other glomerulonephritides. *Kidney Int.* 11:275, 1977.

193. Turner, D. R., Cameron, J. S., Bewick, M., et al. Transplantation in mesangiocapillary glomerulonephritis with intramembranous dense "deposits": recurrence of disease. *Kidney Int.* 9:439, 1976.

194. Lamb, V., Tisher, C. C., McCoy, R. C., et al. Membranoproliferative glomerulonephritis with dense intramembranous alterations. A clinicopathologic study. *Lab. Invest.* 36:607, 1977.

195. Galle, P., and Mahieu, P. Electron dense alteration of kidney basement membranes: a renal lesion specific of a systemic disease. *Am. J. Med.* 58:749, 1975.

196. Pollak, V. E., Rosen, S., Pirani, C. L., et al. Natural history of lipoid nephrosis and of membranous glomerulonephritis. *Ann. Intern. Med.* 69:1171, 1968.

197. Miller, R. B., Harrington, J. T., Ramos, C. P., et al. Long-term results of steroid therapy in adults with idiopathic nephrotic syndrome. *Am. J. Med.* 46:919, 1969.

198. Forland, M., and Spargo, B. H. Clinicopathological correlations in idiopathic nephrotic syndrome with membranous nephropathy. *Nephron* 6:468, 1969.

199. Black, D. A. K., Rose, G., and Brewer, D. B. Controlled trial of prednisone in adult patients with the nephrotic syndrome. *Br. Med. J.* 3:421, 1970.

200. Row, P. G., Cameron, J. S., Turner, D. R., et al. Membranous nephropathy: long-term follow-up and association with neoplasia. *Q. J. Med.* 44:207, 1975.

201. Medical Research Council Working Party. Controlled trial of azathioprine and prednisone in chronic renal disease. *Br. Med. J.* 2:239, 1971.

202. Donadio, J. V., Jr., Holley, K. E., Anderson, C. F., et al. Controlled trial of cyclophosphamide in idiopathic membranous nephropathy. *Kidney Int.* 6:431, 1974.

203. Rastogi, S. P., Hart-Mercer, J., and Kerr, D. N. S. Idiopathic membranous glomerulonephritis in adults: remission following steroid therapy. *Q. J. Med.* 38:335, 1969.

204. Bolton, W. K., Atuk, N. O., Sturgill, B. C., et al. Therapy of the idiopathic nephrotic syndrome

(INS) with alternate day steroids. *Kidney Int.* 8:407, 1975.

205. Coggins, C. H. An interhospital study of the adult idiopathic nephrotic syndrome and its response to treatment. *Kidney Int.* 8:408, 1975.

206. Ehrenreich, T., Porush, J. G., Churg, J., et al. Treatment of idiopathic membranous nephropathy. *N. Engl. J. Med.* 295:741, 1976.

207. Spiro, R. G. Studies on the renal glomerular basement membrane. Preparation and chemical composition. *J. Biol. Chem.* 242:1915, 1967.

208. Spiro, R. G. Studies on the renal glomerular basement membrane. Nature of the carbohydrate units and their attachment to the peptide portion. *J. Biol. Chem.* 242:1923, 1967.

209. Kefalides, N. A. Chemical properties of basement membranes. *Int. Rev. Exp. Pathol.* 10:1, 1971.

210. Mahieu, P. M., and Winand, R. J. Carbohydrate and amino-acid composition of human glomerular-basement-membrane fractions purified by affinity chromatography. *Eur. J. Biochem.* 37:157, 1973.

211. Yagi, Y., Korngold, L., and Pressman, D. Purification of kidney components capable of neutralizing kidney localizing anti-rat kidney antibodies. *J. Immunol.* 77:287, 1956.

212. Yagi, Y., and Pressman, D. Multiplicity of the components of rat kidney antigen responsible for the localization of anti-rat kidney antibodies. *J. Immunol.* 81:7, 1958.

213. McPhaul, J. J., Jr., and Dixon, F. J. Basement membrane antigens in serum and urine. *Transplant. Proc.* 1:964, 1969.

214. Unanue, E. R., and Dixon, F. J. Experimental glomerulonephritis: immunological events and pathogenetic mechanisms. *Adv. Immunol.* 6:1, 1967.

215. Goodpasture, E. W. The significance of certain pulmonary lesions in relation to the etiology of influenza. *Am. J. Med. Sci.* 158:863, 1919.

216. Benoit, F. L., Rulon, D. B., Theil, G. B., et al. Goodpasture's syndrome: a clinicopathologic entity. *Am. J. Med.* 37:424, 1964.

217. Poskitt, T. R. Immunologic and electron microscopic studies in Goodpasture's syndrome. *Am. J. Med.* 49:250, 1970.

218. Proskey, A. J., Weatherbee, L., Easterling, R. E., et al. Goodpasture's syndrome: a report of five cases and review of the literature. *Am. J. Med.* 48:162, 1970.

219. Wilson, C. B., and Dixon, F. J. Anti-glomerular basement membrane antibody-induced glomerulonephritis. *Kidney Int.* 3:74, 1973.

220. Duncan, D. A., Drummond, K. N., Michael, A. F., et al. Pulmonary hemorrhage and glomerulonephritis. Report of six cases and study of the renal lesion by the fluorescent antibody technique and electron microscopy. *Ann. Intern. Med.* 62:920, 1965.

221. Sturgill, B. C., and Westervelt, F. B. Immunofluorescence studies in a case of Goodpasture's syndrome. *J.A.M.A.* 194:914, 1965.

222. McPhaul, J. J., Jr., and Dixon, F. J. Characterization of immunoglobulin G anti-glomerular basement membrane antibodies eluted from kidneys of patients with glomerulonephritis. II. IgG subtypes and *in vitro* complement fixation. *J. Immunol.* 107:678, 1971.

223. Lewis, E. J., Busch, G. J., and Schur, P. H. Gamma G globulin subgroup composition of the glomerular deposits in human renal diseases. *J. Clin. Invest.* 49:1103, 1970.

224. McPhaul, J. J., Jr., and Dixon, F. J. The presence of anti-glomerular basement membrane antibodies in peripheral blood. *J. Immunol.* 103:1168, 1969.

225. McPhaul, J. J., Jr., and Dixon, F. J. Characterization of human anti-glomerular basement membrane antibodies eluted from glomerulonephritic kidneys. *J. Clin. Invest.* 49:308, 1970.

226. Koffler, D., Sandson, J., Carr, R., et al. Immunologic studies concerning the pulmonary lesions in Goodpasture's syndrome. *Am. J. Pathol.* 54:293, 1969.

227. Markowitz, A. S., Battifora, H. A., Schwartz, F., et al. Immunological aspects of Goodpasture's syndrome. *Clin. Exp. Immunol.* 3:585, 1968.

228. Korngold, L., and Pressman, D. The *in vitro* purification of tissue localizing antibodies. *J. Immunol.* 71:1, 1953.

229. Baxter, J. H., and Goodman, H. C. Nephrotoxic serum nephritis in rats. I. Distribution and specificity of the antigen responsible for the production of nephrotoxic antibodies. *J. Exp. Med.* 104:467, 1956.

230. Steblay, R. W., and Rudofsky, U. Autoimmune glomerulonephritis induced in sheep by injections of human lung and Freund's adjuvant. *Science* 160:204, 1968.

231. Maddock, R. K., Jr., Stevens, L. E., Reemtsma, K., et al. Goodpasture's syndrome: cessation of pulmonary hemorrhage after bilateral nephrectomy. *Ann. Intern. Med.* 67:1258, 1967.

232. Shires, D. L., Pfaff, W. W., De Quesada, A., et al. Pulmonary hemorrhage and glomerulonephritis. Treatment of two cases by bilateral

nephrectomy and renal transplantation. *Arch. Surg.* 97:699, 1968.

233. Siegel, R. R. The basis of pulmonary disease resolution after nephrectomy in Goodpasture's syndrome. *Am. J. Med. Sci.* 259:201, 1970.

234. Halgrimson, C. G., Wilson, C. B., Dixon, F. J., et al. Goodpasture's syndrome. Treatment with nephrectomy and renal transplantation. *Arch. Surg.* 103:283, 1971.

235. Lockwood, C. M., Boulton-Jones, J. M., Lowenthal, R. M., et al. Recovery from Goodpasture's syndrome after immunosuppressive treatment and plasmapheresis. *Br. Med. J.* 2:252, 1975.

236. Lockwood, C. M., Rees, A. J., Pearson, T. A., et al. Immunosuppression and plasma-exchange in the treatment of Goodpasture's syndrome. *Lancet* 1:711, 1976.

237. McPhaul, J. J., Jr., and Mullins, J. D. Glomerulonephritis mediated by antibody to glomerular basement membrane. Immunological, clinical, and histopathological characteristics. *J. Clin. Invest.* 57:351, 1976.

238. Bach, J. F., Dardenne, M., Hinglais, N., et al. Role of anti-basement membrane immunity in human glomerulonephritis. *Adv. Nephrol.* 2:75, 1972.

239. Berger, J., Yaneva, H., and Hinglais, N. Immunofluorescence des glomerulonephrites. In *Actualités Nephrologiques de l'Hôpital Necker,* p. 17. Flammarion, Paris, 1971.

240. Bariéty, J., and Druet, P. Résultats de l'immunohistochemie de 589 biopsies rénales (transplantés exclus). *Ann. Med. Intern. Fenn.* 122:63, 1971.

241. McIntosh, R. M., Tinglof, B., Kaufman, D., et al. Immunohistology in renal disease. Diagnostic, prognostic, therapeutic, and etiology value and limitations. *Q. J. Med.* 40:385, 1971.

242. Lerner, R. A., Glassock, R. J., and Dixon, F. J. The role of anti-glomerular basement membrane antibody in the pathogenesis of human glomerulonephritis. *J. Exp. Med.* 126:989, 1967.

243. Berger, J., and Hinglais, N. Les dépôts intercapillaires d'IgA-IgG. *J. Urol. Nephrol. (Paris)* 74:694, 1968.

244. Berger, J. IgA glomerular deposits in renal disease. *Transplant. Proc.* 1:939, 1969.

245. McEnery, P. T., McAdams, A. J., and West, C. D. Glomerular morphology, natural history and treatment of children with IgA-IgG mesangial nephropathy. In P. Kincaid-Smith, ed., *Glomerulonephritis: Morphology, Natural History and Treatment,* p. 305. John Wiley & Sons, New York, 1973.

246. Lowance, D. C., Mullins, J. D., and McPhaul, J. J., Jr. Immunoglobulin A (IgA) associated glomerulonephritis. *Kidney Int.* 3:167, 1973.

247. McCoy, R. C., Abramowsky, C. R., and Tisher, C. C. IgA nephropathy. *Am. J. Pathol.* 76:123, 1974.

248. Zimmerman, S. W., and Burkholder, P. M. Immunoglobulin A nephropathy. *Arch. Intern. Med.* 135:1217, 1975.

249. Dobrin, R. S., Knudson, F. E., and Michael, A. F. The secretory immune system and renal disease. *Clin. Exp. Immunol.* 21:318, 1975.

250. Götze, O., and Müller-Eberhard, H. J. The C3-activator system: an alternate pathway of complement activation. *J. Exp. Med.* 132:90s, 1971.

251. Michael, A. F., Fish, A. J., and Good, R. A. Glomerular localization and transport of aggregated proteins in mice. *Lab. Invest.* 17:14, 1967.

252. Tomasi, T. B., Jr., and Bienenstock, J. Secretory immunoglobulins. *Adv. Immunol.* 9:1, 1968.

253. Mannik, M. Binding of albumin to gamma-A-myeloma proteins and Waldenström macroglobulins by disulfide bonds. *J. Immunol.* 99:899, 1967.

254. Tomasi, T. B., Jr., and Hauptman, S. P. The binding of α-1 antitrypsin to human IgA. *J. Immunol.* 112:2274, 1974.

255. Levinsky, R. J., and Soothill, J. F. A test for antigen-antibody complexes in human sera using IgM of rabbit antisera to human immunoglobulins. *Clin. Exp. Immunol.* 29:428, 1977.

256. Barratt, T. M., and Soothill, J. F. Controlled trial of cyclophosphamide in steroid-sensitive relapsing nephrotic syndrome of childhood. *Lancet* 2:479, 1970.

257. Grupe, W. E., Makker, S. P., and Ingelfinger, J. R. Chlorambucil treatment of frequently relapsing nephrotic syndrome. *N. Engl. J. Med.* 295:746, 1976.

258. Thomson, P. D., Barratt, T. M., Stokes, C. R., et al. HLA antigens and atopic features in steroid-responsive nephrotic syndrome of childhood. *Lancet* 2:765, 1976.

259. Hardwicke, J., Soothill, J. F., Squire, J. R., et al. Nephrotic syndrome with pollen hypersensitivity. *Lancet* 1:500, 1959.

260. Ngu, J. L., Barratt, T. M., and Soothill, J. F. Immunoconglutinin and complement changes in steroid sensitive relapsing nephrotic syndrome of children. *Clin. Exp. Immunol.* 6:109, 1970.

261. Smith, M. D., Barratt, T. M., Hayward, A. R., et al. The inhibition of complement-dependent lymphocyte rosette formation by the sera of children with steroid-sensitive nephrotic syndrome and other renal diseases. *Clin. Exp. Immunol.* 21:236, 1975.

262. Eyres, K., Mallick, N. P., and Taylor, G. Evidence for cell-mediated immunity to renal antigens in minimal-change nephrotic syndrome. *Lancet* 1:1158, 1976.

263. Moorthy, A. V., Zimmerman, S. W., and Burkholder, P. M. Inhibition of lymphocyte blastogenesis by plasma of patients with minimal-change nephrotic syndrome. *Lancet* 1:1160, 1976.

264. Giangiacomo, J., Cleary, T. G., Cole, B. R., et al. Serum immunoglobulins in the nephrotic syndrome. A possible cause of minimal-change nephrotic syndrome. *N. Engl. J. Med.* 293:8, 1975.

265. Cooper, M. D., Faulk, W. P., Fudenberg, H. H., et al. Meeting report of the Second International Workshop on Primary Immunodeficiency Disease in Man, held in St. Petersburg, Florida, February, 1973. *Clin. Immunol. Immunopathol.* 2:416, 1974.

266. Goldman, A. S., Ritzmann, S. E., Houston, E. W., et al. Dysgammaglobulinemic antibody deficiency syndrome. *J. Pediatr.* 70:16, 1967.

267. Sobel, A. T., Intrator, L., Lagrue, G., et al. Serum immunoglobulins in idiopathic minimal-change nephrotic syndrome. *N. Engl. J. Med.* 294:50, 1976.

268. Ingelfinger, J. R., Link, D. A., Davis, A. E., et al. Serum immunoglobulins in idiopathic minimal-change nephrotic syndrome. *N. Engl. J. Med.* 294:50, 1976.

269. Levinsky, R. J., Malleson, P. N., Barratt, T. M., et al. Circulating immune complexes in steroid-responsive nephrotic syndrome. *N. Engl. J. Med.* 298:126, 1978.

270. Mallick, N. P. The pathogenesis of minimal-change nephropathy. *Clin. Nephrol.* 7:87, 1977.

271. Valdez, A. J., Germuth, F. G., and Rodriguez, E. Fatal immune complex glomerulonephritis without deposits. *Fed. Proc.* 34:878, 1975.

272. Lagrue, G., Xheneumont, S., Branellec, A., et al. A vascular permeability factor elaborated from lymphocytes. I. Demonstration in patients with nephrotic syndrome. *Biomedicine* 23:37, 1975.

273. McCormick, J. N., Day, J., Morris, C. J., et al. The potentiating effect of rheumatoid arthritis serum in the immediate phase of nephrotoxic nephritis. *Clin. Exp. Immunol.* 4:17, 1969.

274. Rossen, R. D., Reisberg, M. A., Sharp, J. T., et al. Antiglobulins and glomerulonephritis. Classification of patients by the reactivity of their sera and renal tissue with aggregated and native human IgG. *J. Clin. Invest.* 56:427, 1975.

275. Koffler, D., Schur, P. H., and Kunkel, H. G. Immunological studies concerning the nephritis of systemic lupus erythematosus. *J. Exp. Med.* 126:607, 1967.

276. Koffler, D., Agnello, V., Carr, R. I., et al. Variable patterns of immunoglobulin and complement deposition in the kidneys of patients with systemic lupus erythematosus. *Am. J. Pathol.* 56:305, 1969.

277. Davis, J. S., IV. A hypothesis: a hypothetical common mechanism in systemic lupus erythematosus and rheumatoid arthritis. *Arthritis Rheum.* 9:631, 1966.

278. Messner, R. P., Laxdal, T., Quie, P. G., et al. Serum opsonin, bacteria, and polymorphonuclear leukocyte interactions in subacute bacterial endocarditis. Anti-γ-globulin factors and their interaction with specific opsonins. *J. Clin. Invest.* 47:1109, 1968.

279. Zvaifler, N. J., and Schur, P. Reactions of aggregated mercaptoethanol treated gamma globulin with rheumatoid factor-precipitin and complement fixation studies. *Arthritis Rheum.* 11:523, 1968.

280. Schmid, F. R., Roitt, I. M., and Rocha, M. J. Complement fixation by a two-component antibody system: immunoglobulin G and immunoglobulin M anti-globulin (rheumatoid factor). Paradoxical effect related to immunoglobulin G concentration. *J. Exp. Med.* 132:673, 1970.

281. Nash, T. E., Nasir-Ud-Din, and Jeanloz, R. W. Further purification and characterization of a circulating antigen in schistosomiasis. *J. Immunol.* 119:1627, 1977.

282. Rossen, R. D., Rickaway, R. H., Reisberg, M. A., et al. Renal localization of antiglobulins in glomerulonephritis and after renal transplantation. *Arthritis Rheum.* 20:947, 1977.

283. Rossen, R. D., Reisberg, M. A., Singer, D. B., et al. Soluble immune complexes in sera of patients with nephritis. *Kidney Int.* 10:256, 1976.

284. Theofilopoulos, A. N., Wilson, C. B., Bokisch, V. A., et al. Binding of soluble immune complexes to human lymphoblastoid cells. II. Use of Raji cells to detect circulating immune complexes in animal and human sera. *J. Exp. Med.* 140:1230, 1974.

285. Woodroffe, A. J., Border, W. A., Theofilopoulos, A. N., et al. Detection of circulating immune complexes in patients with glomerulonephritis. *Kidney Int.* 12:268, 1977.

286. Glassock, R. J., Feldman, D., Reynolds, E. S., et al. Recurrent glomerulonephritis in human renal isotransplants: a clinicopathologic study. Proc. 1st Int. Congr. Transplant. Soc., Paris, p. 230, 1967.

287. Glassock, R. J., Feldman, D., Reynolds, E. S., et al. Human renal isografts: a clinical and pathologic analysis. *Medicine* 47:411, 1968.

288. Porter, K. A., Andres, G. A., Calder, M. W., et al. Human renal transplants. II. Immunofluorescent and immunoferritin studies. *Lab. Invest.* 18:159, 1968.

289. Porter, K. A., Dossetor, J. B., Marchioro,

T. L., et al. Human renal transplants. I. Glomerular changes. *Lab. Invest.* 16:153, 1967.

290. Dixon, F. J., McPhaul, J. J., Jr., and Lerner, R. L. Recurrence of glomerulonephritis in the transplanted kidney. *Arch. Intern. Med.* 123:554, 1969.

291. Seibel, H. R., Weymouth, R. J., Craig, S. S., et al. Recurrent glomerulonephritis in human renal homografts. *Virchows Arch.* 371:5, 1976.

292. McLean, R. H., Geiger, H., Burke, B., et al. Recurrence of membranoproliferative glomerulonephritis following kidney transplantation. Serum complement component studies. *Am. J. Med.* 60:60, 1976.

293. Berger, J., Yaneva, H., Nabarra, B., et al. Recurrence of mesangial deposition of IgA after renal transplantation. *Kidney Int.* 7:232, 1975.

294. Noël, L. H., Berger, J., Descamps, B., et al. Recurrence of glomerulonephritis after renal transplantation. In Proc., 6th Int. Congr. Nephrol., p. 1026 (abstract), 1975.

295. Benacerraf, B., and McDevitt, H. O. Histocompatibility-linked immune response genes. *Science* 175:273, 1972.

296. Wittig, H. J., and Goldman, A. S. Nephrotic syndrome associated with inhaled allergens. *Lancet* 1:542, 1970.

297. Reeves, W. G., Cameron, J. S., Johansson, S. G. O., et al. Seasonal nephrotic syndrome. Description and immunological findings. *Clin. Allergy* 5:121, 1975.

298. Soothill, J. F. President's address. Some intrinsic and extrinsic factors predisposing to allergy. *Proc. R. Soc. Med.* 69:439, 1976.

299. Patel, R., Mickey, M. R., and Terasaki, P. I. Leukocyte antigens and disease. I. Association of HL-A2 and chronic glomerulonephritis. *Br. Med. J.* 2:424, 1969.

300. Mickey, M. R., Kreisler, M., and Terasaki, P. I. In P. I. Terasaki, ed., *Histocompatibility Testing, 1970,* p. 237. Munksgaard, Copenhagen, 1970.

301. Jensen, H., Ryder, L. P., Nielsen, L. S., et al. HLA antigens and glomerulonephritis. *Tissue Antigens* 6:368, 1975.

302. Nyulassy, S., Buc, M., Sasinka, M., et al. The HLA system in glomerulonephritis. *Clin. Immunol. Immunopathol.* 7:319, 1977.

303. Nyulassy, S., and Iványi, P.: HL-A systém a choroby. Prehľad súcasných poznatkov. *Cas. Lék. Cesk.* 114:287, 1975.

304. Iványi, P. The major histocompatibility antigens in various species. *Curr. Top. Microbiol. Immunol.* 53:1, 1970.

305. Friend, P. S., Noreen, H. J., Yunis, E. J., et al. B-cell alloantigen associated with chronic mesangiocapillary glomerulonephritis. *Lancet* 1:562, 1977.

306. Border, W. A., Lehman, D. H., Egan, J. D., et al. Antitubular basement-membrane antibodies in methicillin-associated interstitial nephritis. *N. Engl. J. Med.* 291:381, 1974.

307. Morel-Maroger, L., Kourilsky, O., Mignon, F., et al. Antitubular basement membrane antibodies in rapidly progressive poststreptococcal glomerulonephritis: report of a case. *Clin. Immunol. Immunopathol.* 2:185, 1974.

308. Andres, G. A., Accinni, L., Hsu, K. C., et al. Human renal transplants. III. Immunopathologic studies. *Lab. Invest,* 22:588, 1970.

309. Williams, G. M., Lee, H. M., Weymouth, R. F., et al. Studies in hyperacute and chronic renal homograft rejection in man. *Surgery* 62:204, 1967.

310. Klassen, J., Kano, K., Milgrom, F., et al. Tubular lesions produced by autoantibodies to tubular basement membrane in human renal allografts. *Int. Arch. Allergy Appl. Immunol.* 45:675, 1973.

311. Bergstein, J., and Litman, N. Interstitial nephritis with anti-tubular-basement-membrane antibody. *N. Engl. J. Med.* 292:875, 1975.

312. McCluskey, R. T., and Klassen, J. Immunologically mediated glomerular, tubular and interstitial renal disease. *N. Engl. J. Med.* 288:564, 1973.

313. Klassen, J., and Milgrom, F. Autoimmune concomitants of renal allografts. *Transplant. Proc.* 1:605, 1969.

314. Klassen, J., McCluskey, R. T., and Milgrom, F. Nonglomerular renal disease produced in rabbits by immunization with homologous kidney. *Am. J. Pathol.* 63:333, 1971.

315. Klassen, J., Andres, G. A., Brennan, J. C., et al. An immunologic renal tubular lesion in man. *Clin. Immunol. Immunopathol.* 1:69, 1972.

316. Dixon, F. J. What are sensitized cells doing in glomerulonephritis? *N. Engl. J. Med.* 283:536, 1970.

317. Grupe, W. E. An *in vitro* demonstration of cellular sensitivity in experimental autoimmune nephrosis in rats. *Proc. Soc. Exp. Biol. Med.* 127:1217, 1968.

318. Litwin, A., Adams, L. E., Levy, R., et al. Cellular immunity in experimental glomerulonephritis of rats. I. Delayed hypersensitivity and lymphocyte stimulation studies with renal tubular antigens. *Immunology* 20:755, 1971.

319. Winer, R. L., Cohen, A. H., Sawhney, A. S., et al. Sjögren's syndrome with immune-complex tubulointerstitial renal disease. *Clin. Immunol. Immunopathol.* 8:494, 1977.

320. Shearn, M. A., and Tu, W. H. Latent renal

tubular acidosis in Sjögren's syndrome. *Ann. Rheum. Dis.* 27:27, 1968.

321. Talal, N., Zisman, E., and Schur, P. H. Renal tubular acidosis, glomerulonephritis, and immunologic factors in Sjögren's syndrome. *Arthritis Rheum.* 11:774, 1968.

322. Safar, M., Bariéty, J., Lagrue, G., et al. Association d'un syndrome néphrotique et d'un syndrome de Gougerot-Sjögren. *Sem. Hop. Paris* 40:1423, 1964.

323. Perreau, P., Jouband, F., Simard, C., et al. Syndrome de Gougerot-Sjögren et glomérulonéphrite. *Sem. Hop. Paris* 48:973, 1972.

324. Bucher, U. G., and Reid, L. Sjögren's syndrome; report of a fatal case with pulmonary and renal lesions. *Br. J. Dis. Chest* 53:237, 1959.

325. Meltzer, M., and Franklin, E. C. Cryoglobulins, rheumatoid factors, and connective tissue disorders. *Arthritis Rheum.* 10:489, 1967.

326. Scully, R. E., and McNeely, B. U. Case records of the Massachusetts General Hospital. *N. Engl. J. Med.* 292:1285, 1975.

327. Tu, W. H., Shearn M. A., Lee, J. C., et al. Interstitial nephritis in Sjögren's syndrome. *Ann. Intern. Med.* 69:1163, 1968.

328. Pasternack, A., and Linder, E. Renal tubular acidosis: an immunopathological study on four patients. *Clin. Exp. Immunol.* 7:115, 1970.

329. Talal, N. Sjögren's syndrome, lymphoproliferation, and renal tubular acidosis. *Ann. Intern. Med.* 74:633, 1971.

330. Miettinen, A., and Linder, E. Membrane antigens shared by renal proximal tubules and other epithelia associated with absorption and excretion. *Clin. Exp. Immunol.* 23:568, 1976.

331. Shwayder, M., Ozawa, T., Boedecker, E., et al. Nephrotic syndrome associated with Fanconi syndrome: immunopathogenic studies of tubulointerstitial nephritis with autologous immune-complex glomerulonephritis. *Ann. Intern. Med.* 84:433, 1976.

332. Levy, M., Gagnadoux, M. F., and Habib, R. An immunologic Fanconi syndrome. Abstract. Proc. 3rd Int. Symp. Pediatr. Nephrol., Washington, D.C., p. 13, 1974.

333. Cochrane, A. M. G., Tsantoulos, D. C., Moussouros, A., et al. Lymphocyte cytotoxicity for kidney cells in renal tubular acidosis of autoimmune liver disease. *Br. Med. J.* 2:276, 1976.

334. Golding, P. L., Smith, M., and Williams, R. Multisystem involvement in chronic liver disease. Studies on the incidence and pathogenesis. *Am. J. Med.* 55:772, 1973.

335. Tsantoulos, D. C., McFarlane, I. G., Portmann, B., et al. Cell-mediated immunity to human Tamm-Horsfall glycoprotein in autoimmune liver disease with renal tubular acidosis. *Br. Med. J.* 4:491, 1974.

336. Cameron, J. S. Diseases of the urinary system. Treatment of glomerulonephritis by drugs. II. *Br. Med. J.* 1:1520, 1977.

CHAPTER 13

Experimental Models

An increasing number of naturally occurring diseases such as NZB/W F_1 hybrid systemic-lupus-like syndromes in mice, lymphocytic choriomeningitis murine infection, the natural SLE present in some canine models, and even equine infectious anemia, have provided important data on immune complexes and diseases of presumed autoimmune etiology. The following chapter will not seek to provide any sort of encyclopedic catalogue of all the animal models that have been studied, but rather will focus on basic questions pertinent to our understanding of immune-complex–mediated phenomena in human disease states. Of great interest is the possible relation of viral infection to certain features of diseases such as the nephropathy, central nervous system lesions, hemolytic anemia, or salivary gland lesions in the NZB/W hybrid model of SLE. There seem to be a number of fundamental effects of immune complexes themselves on regulatory or primary immune processes, which bear directly on our understanding of pathological processes in human disease states. A group of experimental models have been selected for discussion; these relate directly to the host of human disorders already covered in preceding chapters.

The use of antigen-antibody complexes and human or animal lymphoid cells in vitro has highlighted many specific effects of immune complexes. Several early reports (1, 2) indicated that preformed immune complexes were capable of stimulating human lymphocytes from normal unprimed donors. Studies by So-derberg and Coons (3) also demonstrated stimulation of normal rabbit lymphocytes by antigen-antibody complexes. This effect appeared to be dependent on the presence of complement in the culture media. The reaction was supported by C4-deficient serum, suggesting that the alternate complement pathway could provide the necessary amplification. Rabbit lymphocytes from peripheral blood, bone marrow, spleen, and lymph nodes showed complement-dependent lymphocyte stimulation by immune complexes, but no response was noted using rabbit thymocytes. Of particular note was the inability of aggregated IgG, often considered analogous to immune complexes, to induce lymphocyte stimulation. Other work has shown that complexes injected into unprimed experimental animals may induce a rapid enhanced specific antibody response with kinetics and immunoglobulin profile resembling a secondary immune response (4). Stimulatory effects of immune complexes were not documented in other research directed at this problem (5, 6). It seems likely that the types of complexes used—for example, whether formed in antibody excess and amounts of protein per cell stimulated—may have a significant bearing on the results of such in vitro experiments.

A complement requirement for lymphocyte activation by complexes is a provocative concept. More and more experimental evidence has linked complement components and their activated sequences directly to lymphocyte membranes (7, 8). Immune-complex activation or stimulation of lymphocytes could occur through Fc receptors on such cells or through receptors for C3, C3b, C3d (9), or C4 (10). Dukor and co-workers (11) have suggested that complement might be involved in lymphocyte triggering of interactions between T and B cells. This line of reasoning was based largely on evidence that T-independent antigens were capable of activating C via the alternative pathway. Other experimental support for such a concept was provided by reports showing direct stimulation of mouse lymphocytes by isolated C3b (12). Complement components adsorbed to immune complexes may somehow lower the threshold for lymphocyte activation by processes not yet completely understood. In the experiments described by Möller and Coutinho (13) the presence of complement was capable of reducing the required dose of polyclonal B-cell activators by a factor of ten. Thus it is possible that activated complement components bound to immune complexes may provide additional ligands fixing to lymphocyte cell-surface membranes, focusing activating stimuli in these regions.

The fact that immune complexes may be capable of inciting lymphoid cells to an active division process in vitro, and possibly also in vivo, bears directly on several naturally occurring diseases in man. Some of the most obvious ramifications of this principle are in the case of SLE or in patients with large amounts of circulating immune complexes associated with malignancy or parasitic infection. Determination of how immune-complex materials of a particular range of ratios or molecular characteristics may be capable of stimulating B cells pertains also to secondary effects of major therapeutic manipulations of large amounts of circulating antibody (plasmapheresis, for instance). A number of experimental studies suggest that amounts of antibody within the host may be one of the most important factors governing the setting of the "immunostat" that influences various types of humoral antibody formation (14). If the direct effects of preformed immune complexes are also considered, then most of the self-regulating adjustments in the immune reaction may well be accounted for. Should it be conclusively demonstrated that a certain qualitative type of humoral immune response is indeed harmful to a host afflicted with any one of a number of diseases, fundamental insight into how to shut off such a response would become very useful. Precise knowledge of the mechanics of generating humoral antibody response for both thymic-dependent and thymic-independent antigens is obviously important; this is where the action is in eventual production of antibodies and other immune reactants making up immune complexes themselves.

The problem is further illustrated by the opposite side of the coin—namely, that in certain situations antigen-antibody complexes seem capable of abrogating the immune response. Under some circumstances immune complexes, particularly when adsorbed to potential antigen-binding cells, may be involved in the phenomenon of immune suppression. Such effects have been demonstrated in hosts with progressively growing tumors (15, 16), in recipients who maintain apparently healthy allografts (17, 18), or even in various forms of immunologic tolerance (18–20). When immunosuppressive effects of immune complexes are carefully studied, it generally becomes apparent that the effect cannot be generated by antigen or antibody alone. It may in many systems be related to the presence of Fc portions of antibody reacting with appropriate Fc cell-surface structures (21).

From these and a number of other studies the profound biologic effects of immune complexes are evident. Much of the recent clinically oriented work aimed at applying sensitive methods of radioimmunoassay for quantitative estimation of circulating immune complexes may be slightly off the mark as far as elucidating the exact role of complexes as stimulators or inhibitors of various immune reactions; quantities and particular types of immune complexes trapped within key sites of immune stimulation may not correlate with complexes still circulating and detectable in the host. This problem is especially pertinent in interpretation of data showing high levels of apparent circulating complexes in the sera of patients with malignancy. The whole area needs much additional study and the development of other in vitro assays to predict the effects of tissue or cell-fixed complexes on specific immune responses.

Target Organs Other Than the Kidney

Thyroiditis

Immunization of mice with soluble heterologous thyroglobulin results in the development of an intense interstitial thyroiditis characterized by deposition of autologous immune complexes at the follicular basement membranes and within interstitial spaces (22). This lesion is felt to result from termination of unresponsiveness or tolerance to autologous thyroglobulin and induction of autoantibody production (23). The necessary role of antibody to autologous thyroglobulin has been demonstrated by so-called antigen suicide experiments, in which administration of highly labeled ^{125}I-syngeneic thyroglobulin affects only bone-marrow–derived B cells and markedly diminishes the severity of lesions, presumably by direct killing of antigen-binding cells, the precursors of humoral antibody production. A number of workers have shown that passive transfer of thyroglobulin-specific antibody will produce thyroiditis in rabbits (24), guinea pigs (25, 26) and mice (27). These results provide an interesting concept closely linked to one of the leading theories explaining autoimmune reactions. It has been postulated that T cells are generally unresponsive to or tolerant of autologous thyroglobulin, and for that matter other autologous "self"-antigens. However, B cells are fully competent, and autoantibody and subsequent thyroiditis result from direct stimulation of immunocompetent B cells, bypassing the need for antigen-specific helper T cells (28, 29).

Experimental support for such a concept has been provided by observations documenting the occurrence of potentially self-reactive B cells in normal individuals for such antigens as thyroglobulin, DNA, or polynucleotides (30–32). The finding that passive transfer of autoantibody alone does not induce autoimmune disease, coupled with the demonstration of potential autoantibody-producing cells in virtually all normals tested, emphasizes that autoimmune responsiveness is a built-in feature of all normal individuals and that there must exist some regulatory mechanism in most normal subjects which protects them from such sequelae. This basic hypothesis is shown diagrammatically in Figure 13-1. Various mechanisms may be postulated whereby a number of potential antigen-binding B cells can become activated and, bypassing the need for T-cell modulation, proliferate to such an extent that an ongoing autoimmune reaction is initiated. This mechanism is further emphasized by recent observations on the potential of

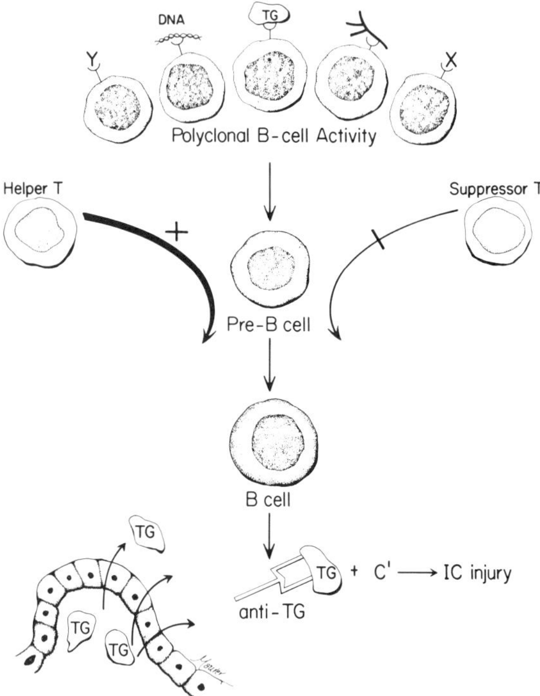

Figure 13-1 Potential antigen-binding cells are shown above. When various antigens are bound, pre-B cells differentiate to B cells capable of forming humoral antibody. In the case of antithyroglobulin antibody, reaction with thyroglobulin (TG) released from thyroid follicles may then produce immune complexes (IC), which react with the complement system and induce injury. Helper and suppressor T cells modulate this process. C' refers to complement.

the heterogeneous group of compounds called polyclonal B-cell activators in inducing autoantibody production in normal hosts (33–37).

It has also been claimed that autoreactive T cells may exist normally because neonatal lymphoid cells can react against syngeneic spleen lymphocytes (38). Autosensitization of lymphocytes can be demonstrated by culturing on syngeneic fibroblasts or reticular cells (39). A proper balance between suppressor cells and helper cells has been suggested as a key surveillance mechanism that protects the normal host against potentially injurious autoimmune reactions (40, 41). This concept is illustrated graphically in Figure 13-2, which shows the difference between possible control mechanisms in normal subjects and those with SLE. This explanation for immunologic surveillance has

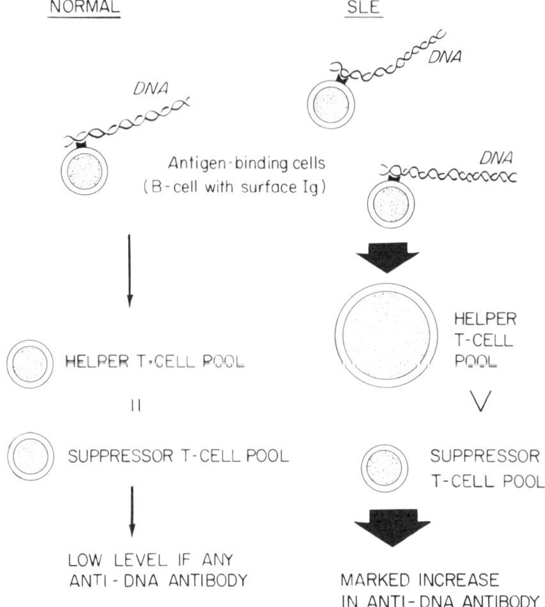

Figure 13-2 Possible differences between the balance of immune regulatory influences in patients with SLE and normal subjects. Since subjects with SLE as well as normal individuals show detectable levels of potential antigen-binding cells, a deficiency in the suppressor-cell population and functional overactivity of the helper-cell pool may combine to produce excessive anti-DNA antibody and, therefore, increments in DNA–anti-DNA immune complexes.

been exhaustively explored in a number of naturally occurring disease models, including NZB/W hybrid lupus-like syndrome (40–44) and in fact in SLE itself (45–47), where a number of observations support a decrease in functional suppressor T-cell activity. Some interesting data presented by Primi and colleagues (37) indicate that polyclonal B-cell activators and this particular mechanism inducing the formation of autoantibody may not be as susceptible to suppressor T-cell modulation as has been generally assumed. Treatment of cultured cells activated with lipopolysaccharide from *Escherichia coli* as a B-cell activator produced autoantibody to albumin regardless of elimination or presumed inactivation of mouse T cells using anti–T-cell antiserum. Such findings suggest that suppressor T cells may not in fact play a major role in the maintenance of long-standing self-tolerance. Although suppressor T cells per se may not be involved in controlling autoantibody response to potent polyclonal B-cell activators, suppressor-cell modulation may proceed from other cell types such as adherent cells or monocytes and macrophages.

Observations concerning interstitial immune-complex–mediated thyroiditis in mice (23) are of great interest, for they clearly relate the development of inflammatory and destructive lesions within the thyroid gland to the temporal appearance and quantitative amounts of serum antibody to thyroglobulin. It was postulated that upon induction of ongoing production of antithyroglobulin antibody in these animals, as the antibody became available within the interstices of thyroid glands actively secreting thyroglobulin, interstitial immune-complex deposition took place. Moreover, when immune complexes capable of complement fixation were present, rapid ingress of neutrophils and tissue damage became apparent. Interstitial immune complexes noted in this experimental model were granular or lumpy in appearance and often formed at the basal areas of thyroid follicular cells in close association with follicular basement membranes. Electron microscopic examination of the lesions showed electron-dense deposits between follicular basement membrane areas and the plasma membranes of cells. Examples of these immune deposits are shown in Figure 13-3, which indicates the granular IgG deposition of antithyroglobulin antibody during the development of this experimental model.

Immunologic and histopathological occurrences in experimental mouse thyroiditis thus appeared to resemble an Arthus reaction, in which circulating antibody to autologous antigen was capable of reacting directly with autologous antigen escaping from thyroid follicles. Interstitial immune-complex injury was associated with intense PMN cell infiltration at early stages of the lesions. The importance of this cellular phase, presumably initiated by local release of large amounts of chemotactic

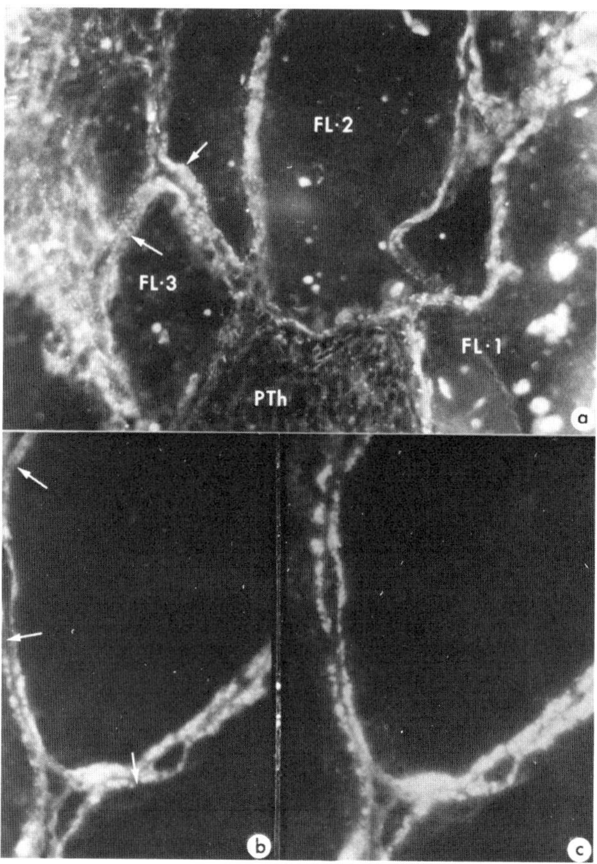

Figure 13-3   Granular immunofluorescent deposits (*arrows*) of mouse Ig in presumed immune complexes are shown in *A*. These were present in the thyroid glands of immunized mice from day 48 throughout the experimental period (up to 75 days after immunization). Heavy granular Ig deposits in a follicle disrupted by inflammatory cells are apparent adjacent to follicle 3 (FL-3). No Ig deposits are observed in the parathyroid (PTh) gland. Staining is with fluorescein-conjugated goat antimouse Fab (IgG) serum. Magnification × 750. The photomicrograph in *B* depicts the follicular basement membrane and the IgG deposits in the thyroid of an immunized mouse. Ig deposits stained with rhoda-mine-conjugated rabbit antimouse IgG are shown in intimate relation to the follicular basement membrane (*arrows*) outlined by indirect immunofluorescence using horse antirabbit renal basement membrane antiserum. Magnification × 330, KP-500 exciter filter. The thyroid follicle in Figure 13-3*B* was then photographed with a different exciter filter, which allows viewing in *C* of the rhodamine-labeled antimouse IgG antibody alone. Note the granular Ig deposits along the outline of the follicle. Magnification × 330, KP-546 exciter filter. (Reproduced with permission, J. A. Claggett, C. B. Wilson, and W. O. Weigle, *J. Exp. Med.* 140:1439, 1974.)

complement-generated factors, has been emphasized by early studies of the sequence of such reactions (48–50). Another significant feature revealed by these studies (23) was that local thyroid injury occurred without evidence of extensive extrathyroidal immune-complex injury. It is assumed that in the situation of experimental thyroiditis induced by immunization with heterologous thyroglobulin, immune complexes formed are present in zones of antigen excess where a variety of molecular ratios of soluble complexes might be expected. Experimental models in which thyroglobulin-antithyroglobulin immune deposits were noted in renal tissues have generally involved manipulation of the model in such a way as to allow thyroglobulin antigen more access to the circulation and more opportunity for formation of soluble circulating immune complexes (51, 52).

Clinical implications of these findings for human disease states are suggested by the finding of IgM, IgE, IgG, C1q, and C3 distributed in focal granular deposits and often in association with the thyroid follicular basement membrane in 70 percent of the patients with Graves' disease (53). IgG, IgA, and C3 were noted in heavy granular pattern in only 1 of 8 patients with Hashimoto's thyroiditis studied by Kalderon and co-workers (54). However, all 8 individuals showed electron-dense deposits at the junction of the follicular and basal plasma membranes. It is important to point out that the great renewal of interest in immune mechanisms is directly responsible for perpetuating the autonomous hyperactivity of the thyroid gland in Graves' disease (55). Antibodies capable of reacting with thyroid-stimulating hormone (TSH) receptors in the gland itself may be involved in direct release of excess active thyroid hormone in a situation that escapes the normal feedback control mechanisms.

The work illustrating the effects of locally deposited immune complexes in experimental thyroiditis may have much broader implications than merely the tissue injury related to thyroiditis. It has, for instance, been demonstrated that γ-globulin fractions present in the serum of patients with thyrotoxicosis are capable of directly stimulating TSH receptors as well as the cAMP pathway involved in primary thyroid hormonal release from the gland (56–58). Whether such pathways also involve participation of complement-activating mechanisms by local deposition of immune complexes is not yet clear. At the present time there are a number of clinical phenomena that may be directly related to antibody reactions with various key cell receptors. Rather than presenting as clinical problems related to extensive tissue injury, such conditions manifest themselves in well-defined functional disturbances. The increasing number and diversity of this set of human disorders is astounding; extensions of the concept appear to be proliferating rapidly. A partial listing of such functional human disorders is given in Table 13-1.

It is not at all clear that deposition of immune complexes per se is directly involved in the pathogenesis of these conditions or whether, for instance, complement amplification by local deposition or activation of circulating complement components represents an essential feature in all of these disease states. Thus, it can be shown that antibody to TSH receptors is capable of setting off a chain of reactions resulting in autonomous release of thyroid hormone in the situation encountered in Graves' disease. Likewise, antibody as well as cell-mediated immune reactions to acetylcholine receptors seems capable of inducing the clinical disorder of myasthenia gravis (59–61). In similar vein, studies of a relatively rare group of patients with profound insulin resistance associated with acanthosis nigricans have suggested that the insulin-handling disturbance in these patients may well be caused by antibodies combining directly with cell-surface insulin receptors, impeding primary transmission of hormone-cell interactions (62–64). There is a host of other human disease states that could fall within this general category— for example, disorders mediated by antibody to cell-surface receptors vital in primary cell function. Many, indeed, probably still wait to be recognized clinically. Again, the degree to which immune-complex deposition is primarily involved has not yet really been determined, since many of the disorders studied thus far are actuated by minute amounts of antibody undetectable by conventional tech-

Table 13-1   Disease states probably related to local antigen-antibody reactions involving important cell receptor mechanisms.

Disease	Key receptor site involved	Evidence supporting immunological mechanisms
Myasthenia gravis	Acetylcholine receptor site	Cell-mediated and humoral immunity demonstrable in human patients using isolated isologous or heterologous acetylcholine receptors
Insulin-resistant diabetes and acanthosis nigricans	Insulin receptors on cells	Isolated IgG, and F(ab)$'_2$ of IgG, capable of blocking insulin binding to cell receptors
Thyrotoxicosis	TSH receptor on thyroid hormone secreting TSH-responsive cells	Isolated IgG or γ-globulin components directly stimulate TSH receptor and activate second messenger (cyclic AMP) mechanisms $\rightarrow$ autonomous thyroid hormone secretion

niques of immunofluorescence or electron microscopy.

Experimental Immune-Complex Disease of the Lung

The minute capillary network present in the lung would appear to be a potential site for immune-complex injury. There has, however, been surprisingly little experimental confirmation of this probability, and rabbits with acute or chronic serum sickness generally have not been found to show pulmonary changes (65, 66). On the contrary, acute anaphylaxis appears to be a condition associated with sudden, rather massive precipitation of circulating antigen-antibody complexes within pulmonary capillaries (67–69), but seems to bear no close relationship to chronic interstitial pneumonitis or fibrosis as it appears in man.

Studies presented by Brentjens and associates (70) have indicated that rabbits producing hyperactive antibody responses to protein antigens such as bovine serum albumin (BSA) maintained in a state of relative antigen-antibody equivalence by large multiple daily doses of BSA develop membranous and proliferative lung lesions associated with deposits of injected antigen as well as host IgG, complement, and fibrinogen. The inflammatory changes within the pulmonary parenchyma induced by such local immune-complex deposits appeared to simulate many of the morphological findings

noted in human interstitial pulmonary disease. Immune deposits were localized in the alveolar capillary walls, interstitium, and walls of terminal bronchioles. Electron microscopy of tissues from such hyperimmunized rabbits often showed subendothelial electron-dense deposits. Immunofluorescent localization of both BSA antigen and autologous anti-BSA IgG antibody are shown in Figure 13-4. Many of the rabbits receiving the hyperimmunization procedure necessary to induce such lesions also showed serum-sickness–like granular immune-complex deposits in renal glomeruli. However, the granular patterns of immune-complex deposition noted were distinctly different from those recorded in association with Goodpasture's syndrome, where a rather linear

Figure 13-4   *Above,* sections of lung stained with fluorescein-conjugated antibody to BSA. Granular deposits are seen along the alveolar capillary walls and in the interstitium. *Below,* a section of lung stained with fluorescein-conjugated antibody to rabbit IgG is shown. Granular deposits are present in the alveolar capillary walls and in the interstitium. Both photographs, magnification × 1,000. (Reproduced with permission, J. B. Brentjens, D. W. O'Connell, I. B. Pawlowski et al., *J. Exp. Med.* 140: 105, 1974.)

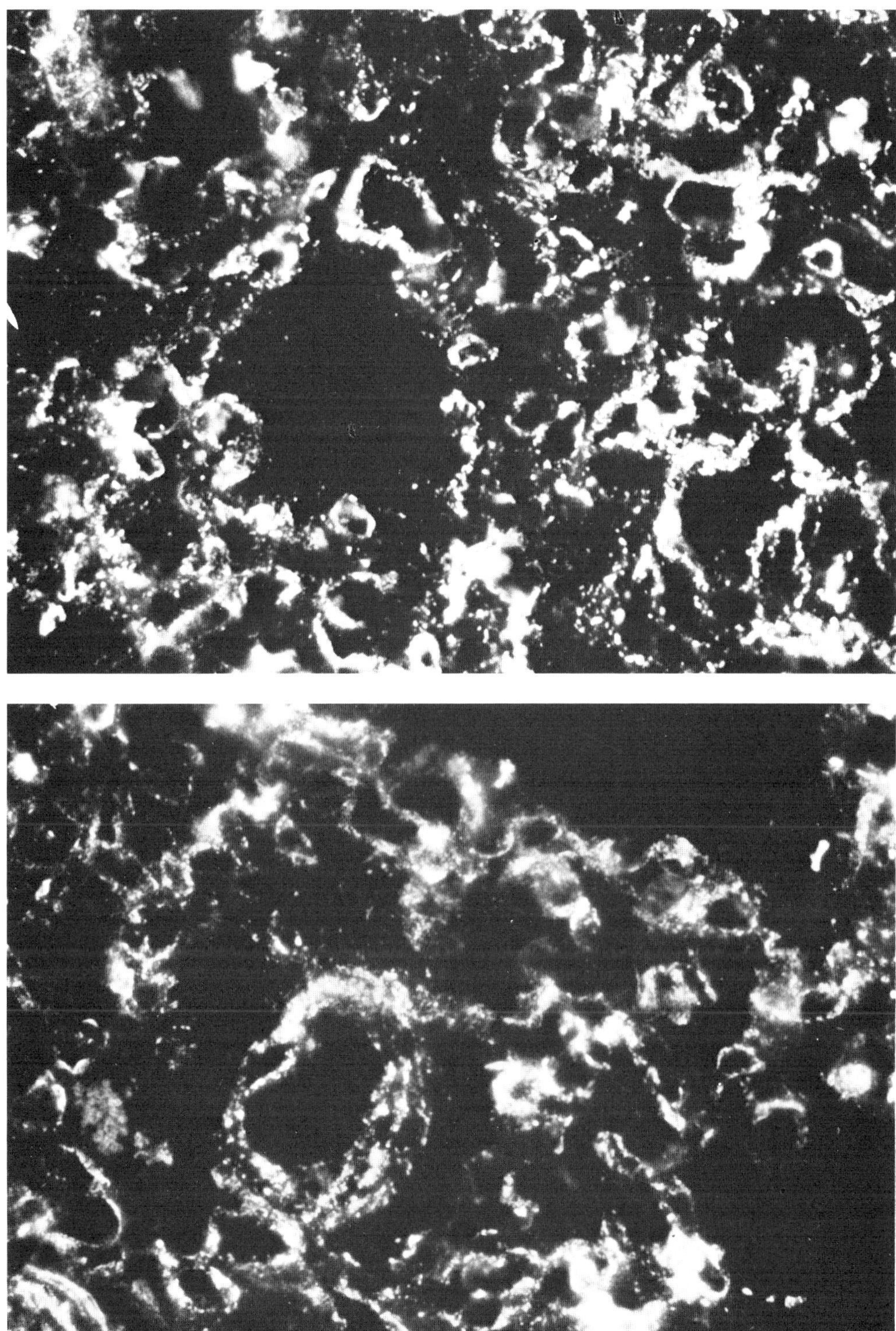

pattern of immunoglobulin deposition is often seen in pulmonary tissues.

Previous studies of the conventional model of rabbit serum sickness (65, 66) showed that the critical factor in the development of lesions was the quantity of antibody formed during the immunization procedures. This also appeared to be the case in the model for immune-complex injury to the lungs developed by the Brentjens group (70), since only animals with hyperactive immune responsiveness developed detectable pulmonary lesions.

These observations may be applicable to clinical features of human disease states associated with interstitial pneumonitis or eventual pulmonary fibrosis associated with a number of disorders. In human diseases characterized by interstitial lung changes the inflammatory process often appears to be associated with supporting pulmonary structures and the microcapillary circulation rather than the alveoli themselves. Subsequent proliferation of interstitial cells, along with interstitial edema and accumulations of polymorphonuclear leukocytes, mononuclear cells, and progressive laying down of reticulin fibrils with fibrosis, appear to be characteristic of such a process in humans (71, 72). Several human disorders included under the general rubric *hypersensitivity pneumonitis* may involve direct reaction between circulating antibody and inhaled antigen in an Arthus-type situation. Thus, sensitization to a wide variety of such inhalants (including coffee bean dust, pituitary snuff, bird droppings, or fungal contaminants of moldy hay) may relate to this latter sort of mechanism, which is commonly called *extrinsic allergic alveolitis* (73–75). Such a circumstance is quite different from that induced by circulating immune complexes. A number of clinical and histological studies suggest that circulating complexes may be participating in the genesis of pulmonary lesions in patients with SLE or mixed connective-tissue diseases associated with large amounts of so-called intermediate complexes ranging from 9 to 18S (76–79). Patients with SLE may occasionally show impairment of diffusing capacity, seemingly because of an increase in membrane resistance (79).

Also, in occasional patients with SLE, interstitial fibrosis (76, 77), proliferative alveolitis (80, 81), or wire-loop lesions in pulmonary capillaries (82, 83) have been recorded. The increasing use of routine lung biopsy in the diagnosis and evaluation of a wide range of diagnostic problems may add substantially to any list of clinical conditions affecting the lung and involved in various ways with immune-complex deposition. It appears that the baseline knowledge and deftness of interpretation in the area of pulmonary immunopathology is often relatively underdeveloped in medical centers where immunofluorescent study of kidney or skin biopsy material has become part of the standard routine. In clinical situations where direct insight into the possible tissue deposition of immunoglobulins and activated complement components in lung biopsy material might be substantially useful, the tissues are promptly dropped into formalin and undergo routine tissue fixation and conventional processing.

The ramifications of understanding of a number of interesting clinical syndromes possibly related to immune-complex deposition within lung tissues are well illustrated by the findings with respect to rheumatoid lung (84), where immunofluorescent studies have demonstrated extensive granular deposits of IgG and IgM along with complement in alveolar walls and capillaries in a large proportion of patients (Figure 13-5). Homing of immune complexes to the lung, particularly in the areas of small bronchioles, interstitium, and pulmonary arteriolar capillaries obviously raises the important problem of precisely what makes them stick there. Very little information seems to be available. There is, for instance, no clear indication of built-in C3 or IgG Fc receptors in such tissues. The pharmacodynamic control of pulmonary vascular resistance and reactivity through such mediators as the prostaglandins or serotonin is still poorly understood. It seems likely that local tissue factors play an important role in the actual tissue saturation by complexes in the pulmonary interstitium or arteriolar capillaries. Careful sequential immunofluorescent and electron microscopic studies of patients with suspected immune-complex–

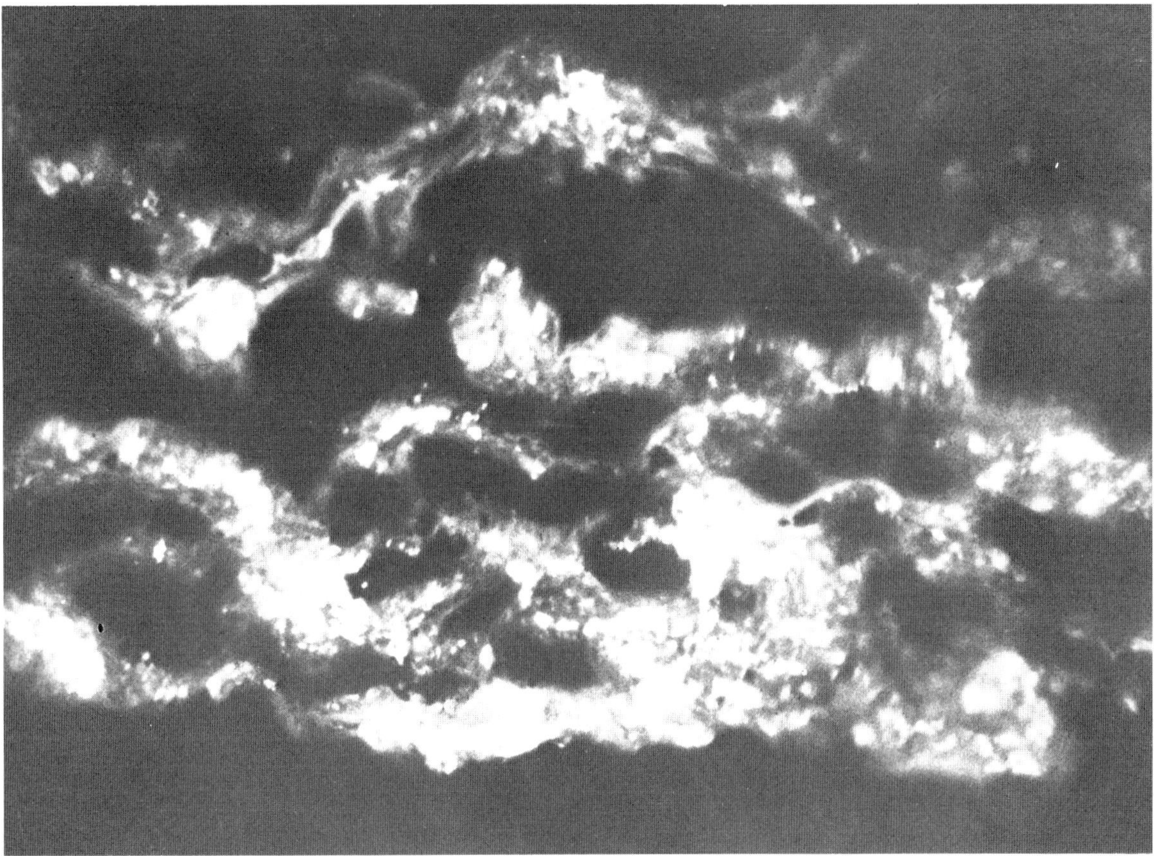

Figure 13-5 IgM deposition in alveolar capillaries in a patient with rheumatoid lung. A similar distribution of C3 was also noted in this particular instance. Magnification × 350.

mediated lesions involving the pulmonary tissues should provide further valuable insight.

Research directed at a more precise understanding of these relationships has been reported by Dreisin and co-workers (85). Circulating immune complexes were measured in a group of patients with interstitial lung disease. Levels of circulating complexes were elevated in all but 3 of 16 patients with cellular disease, but in none of 8 with diffuse fibrosis. In addition, granular deposits of IgG, usually with C3, were present in 94 percent of patients with elevations of immune complexes, but in only 11 percent of those with normal levels. Radiographic and physiological responses to corticosteroid therapy were better in patients whose assays initially showed elevated levels of complexes. A summary of the levels of circulating complexes in this group of subjects is given in Figure 13-6.

Viral Infections in Animals

Many observations relate the role of various types of circulating or tissue-fixed immune complexes to the progression of lesions or the final subversion of the host. The discussion here does not attempt to categorize or list all findings in this area, but focuses on a few areas where available information seems most relevant to the clinical problems discussed in preceding chapters. It is hoped that this selection will emphasize certain features common to many of the diseases of still unknown cause,

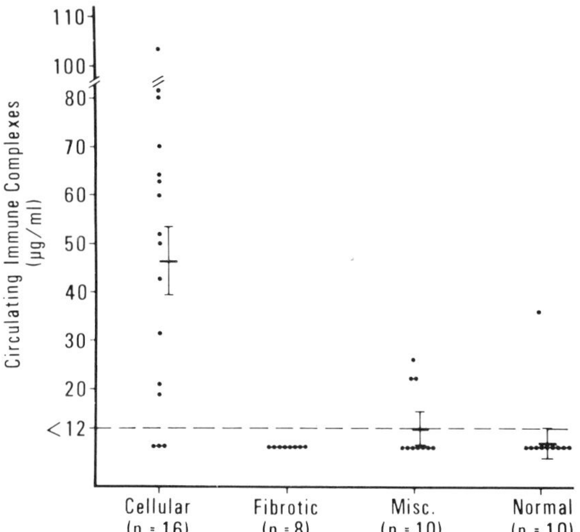

Figure 13-6 Circulating immune-complex levels, as determined by the Raji-cell method, in patients with cellular and fibrotic interstitial lung disease, patients with other lung diseases (misc.) and normal controls (means ± S.E.M. are shown as bars). (Reproduced with permission, R. B. Dreisin, M. I. Schwarz, A. N. Theofilopoulos et al., *N. Engl. J. Med.* 298:353, 1978).

where there have been repeated suggestions or experimental data implying that virus infection may be an integral part of the process.

Lymphocytic Choriomeningitis Viral Infection

Lymphocytic choriomeningitis infection (LCM) of mice produces a number of disease syndromes depending upon the strain of virus, the route of infection, and the age and particular strain of mice infected (86–90). One form of virus infection involves vertical or congenital infection, in which fetuses of infected mothers are infected by virus in utero and then exhibit chronic virus infection throughout their lives. These mice either do not respond immunologically to the viral infection or produce a chronic sustained antibody response leading to various forms of immune-complex injury including glomerulonephritis (91). The apparent unresponsiveness of some mice infected with the virus led Burnet and Fenner (92) to the concept that there existed a state of apparent immunologic tolerance to those antigens presented to the animal during fetal or neonatal development. Later the clonal selection theory developed by Burnet (93) involved a hypothesis on how this form of tolerance might be induced by deletion during ontogeny of clones of immunocytes reactive with apparent self-antigens.

Universal tolerance to viral antigens induced by fetal exposure and subsequent clonal deletion has subsequently proved *not* to be the case, since antiviral antibodies are produced in the LCM virus carrier state (91). Also, an important feature of the immune response to LCM virus infection in adult mice is the much studied phenomenon of generation of thymus-derived T cells that are capable of highly efficient lysis of LCM virus-infected target cells (94–96). T cells specifically sensitized to viral determinants appear to be responsible for recovery from primary infection in adult animals (97, 98) and also are capable of inducing acute lethal CNS damage in animals infected by the intracerebral route (99–101). On the other hand, LCM virus carriers that have acquired the infection in utero do not show cytotoxic T cells. Induction of a partially tolerant state does not, however, require in utero infection; it can also be observed in adult animals infected with a relatively high dose of virus (90).

A number of fascinating features of LCM infection provide possible analogies to much of the immunopathology of immune-complex diseases discussed at length in previous chapters of this book. Chronic infection per se usually is not associated with cytopathogenicity. Furthermore, mice persistently infected with LCM virus often demonstrate extremely high titers of virus in virtually all tissues, but show very little in the way of cellular injury (86, 88). Similarly, LCM infection of cells in tissue culture is generally not accompanied by detectable cell injury despite the active process of viral replication (102–104). Adult mice inoculated with LCM virus develop an acute fatal disease only if after inoculation with the virus they make an anti-LCM response. Thus the immune response to the infection itself produces the lesions and symptomatology of the disorder. In such cases it can also be demonstrated that various immunosuppressive regimes prevent acute disease manifestations

(105–108). In many ways this appears to be analogous to the situation in SLE, where the immune response to something is capable of inducing widespread tissue damage in a number of vulnerable areas.

The LCM carrier state develops in mice that are inoculated shortly after birth or infected transplacentally in utero. Such animals make an anti-LCM antibody response throughout their lives (109, 110) and show high titers of infectious virus in their tissues. Mouse strains carrying the largest amount of LCM virus and making the greatest anti-LCM antibody response develop the earliest and most severe manifestations of immune-complex injury.

LCM carrier mice of several strains develop a characteristic disease composed of chronic glomerulonephritis, focal hepatic necrosis, and generalized proliferation of lymphoid tissues. Renal lesions in these animals are illustrated in Figure 13-7. The nature of γ-globulin immune-complex deposits in the kidneys of these mice (Figure 13-8) was studied by testing eluates directly in microcomplement fixation. The results showed that the relative amounts of specific anti-LCM antibody found in the glomerular deposits increased with aging and chronicity of the LCM infection. Approximately half of the gamma globulin obtained in the glomerular elution procedure could be ac-

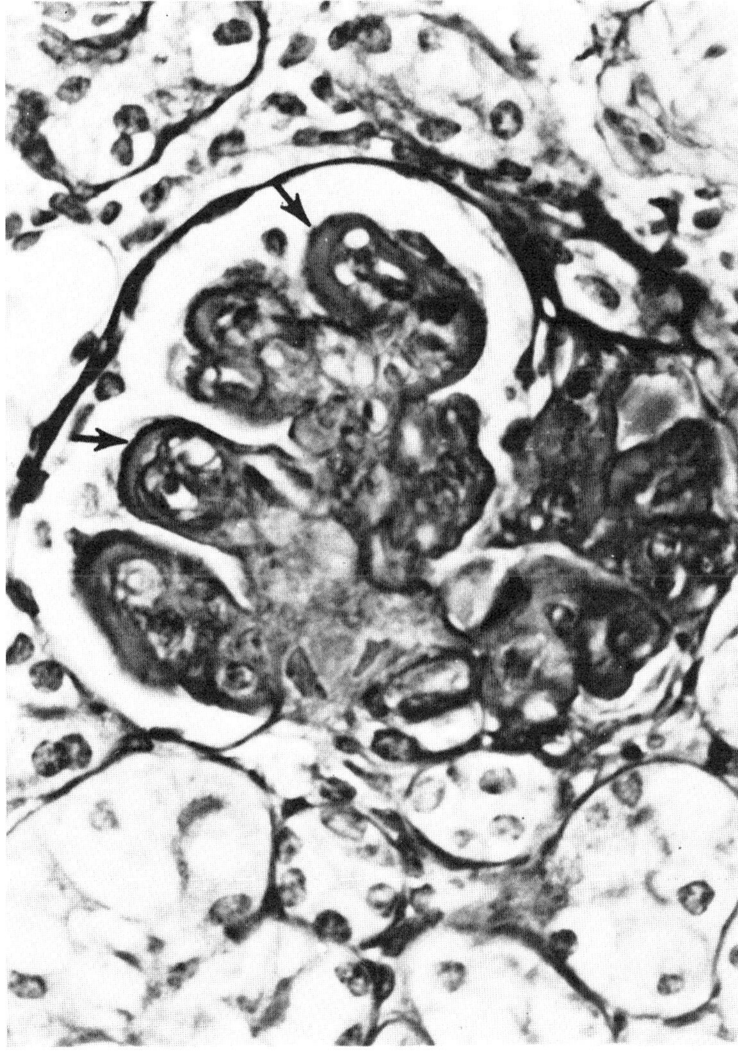

Figure 13-7 Glomerular lesions (*arrows*) in an LCM-infected mouse showing thickening of basement membranes. Magnification × 380. (Photograph courtesy of M. B. A. Oldstone, Scripps Research Foundation, La Jolla, California.)

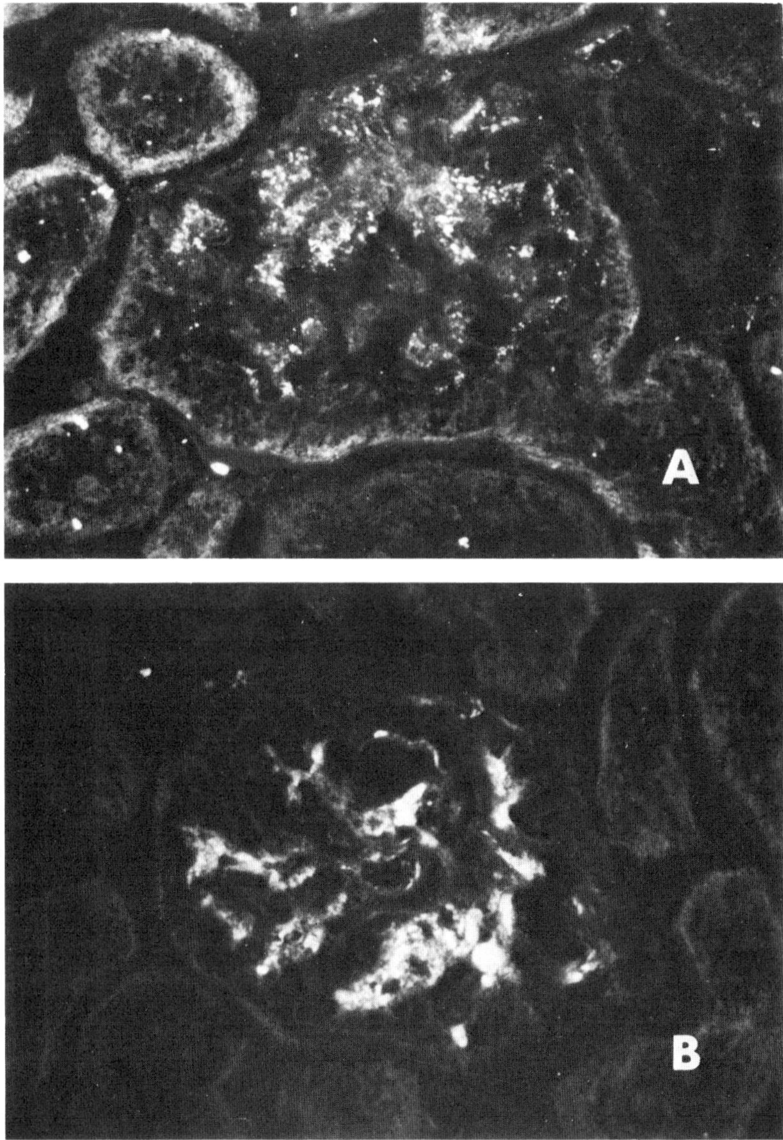

Figure 13-8 Fluorescent photomicrograph of a renal glomerulus from a mouse persistently infected with LCM virus. *A*, distribution of LCM viral antigen; *B*, staining for mouse IgG. Magnification × 200. (Photograph courtesy of M. B. A. Oldstone, Scripps Research Foundation, La Jolla, California.)

counted for as specific anti-LCM antibody. Assay of infected mouse sera for immune complexes employed treatment by antimouse γ-globulin and antimouse albumin antisera and subsequent reassay of the sera for infectivity. Infectious virus was often present bound to γ-globulins, and treatment with antimouse γ-globulin markedly diminished serum infectivity. Electron microscopic visualization of im-

mune deposits in the glomeruli of chronically infected LCM mice is shown in Figure 13-9.

There continues to be a controversy about whether or not animals with the LCM carrier state are indeed tolerant in the classic sense. Volkert and associates (111, 112), as well as workers in several other laboratories (113, 114), have maintained that essentially no anti-LCM specific antibody is manufactured during

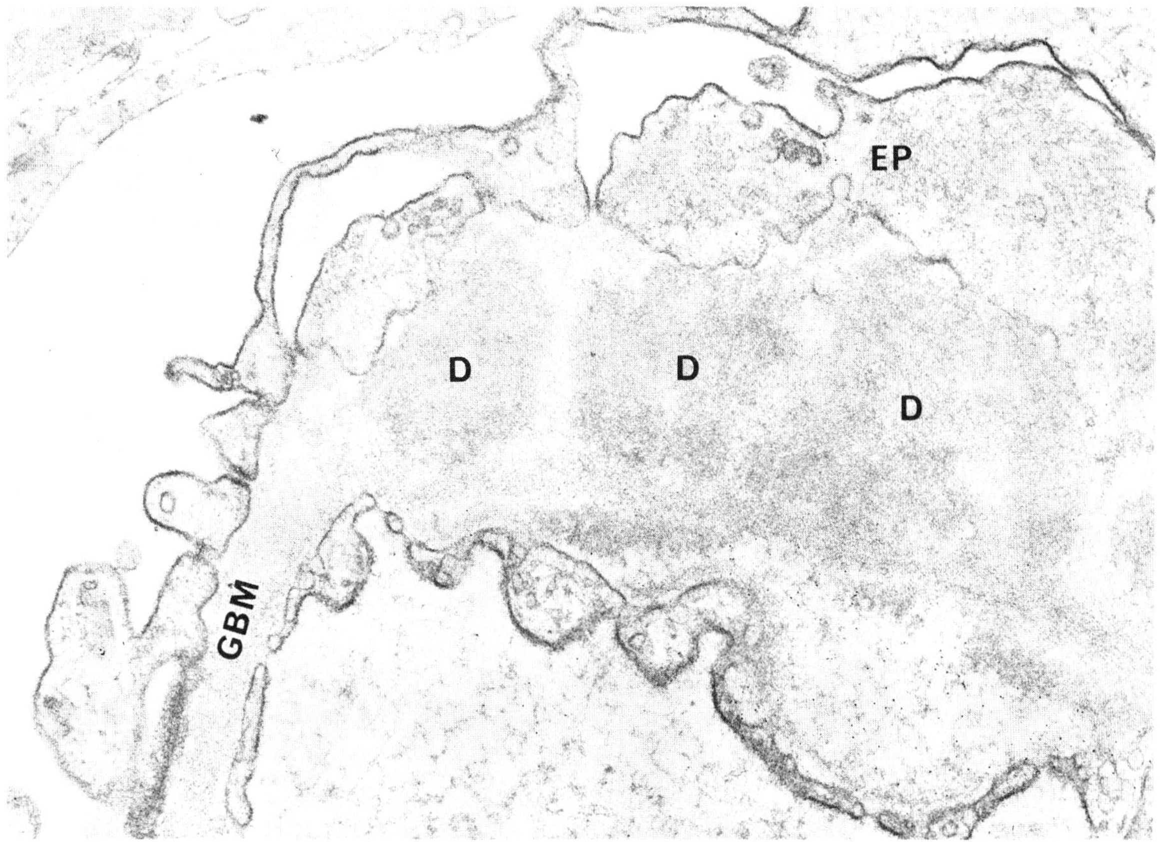

Figure 13-9 Electron photomicrograph of a glomerulus taken from an 8-month old mouse persistently infected with LCM virus. Note lumpy deposition of electron-dense material (D) along the outer aspect of the glomerular basement membrane (GBM). EP = epithelial cell. Magnification × 17,000. (Photograph courtesy of M. B. A. Oldstone, Scripps Research Foundation, La Jolla, California.)

the course of chronic LCM carrier state or infection. Thus, it was reported that LCM immune T cells did not stimulate B cells in LCM carrier mice to produce anti-LCM antibody. These findings concerning failure of adoptive immunization to stimulate specific antibody production provide evidence in favor of the original concept of true and not split immunologic tolerance in the chronic disease or LCM carrier states.

Direct evidence supporting the theory that serum from chronically infected LCM mice contains anti-LCM reactive antibody has also been presented by Welsh and colleagues (115), who demonstrated that guinea pig complement added to serum from persistently infected LCM mice lowered infectivity of this material. This in turn suggests that the LCM serum contained antigen-antibody complexes capable of direct elimination by a heterologous complement source. The importance of several immune mechanisms working in concert in the pathogenesis of LCM infection was illustrated by the experiments of Oldstone and Dixon (116), which showed that parabiosis of immune mice to isologous LCM carriers or transfer of immune lymphoid cells to isologous LCM carriers intensified chronic disease lesions in the carriers of several LCM murine strains. Also, the passive transfer of isologous or heterologous anti-LCM antibody to persistently infected carrier mice caused prompt appearance of acute necrotizing inflammatory lesions. Viral antigen could be identified by immunofluorescence in the cytoplasm or on the surface of many infected cells such as hepatic parenchymal cells, choroid cells of the brain, and within the endothelial cells of blood vessels. In lesions mediated by parabiotic or intravenous transfer of anti-LCM antibody, direct combination of antibody with viral antigen in the vessels or perivascular spaces induced PMN cell infiltration as a result of complement activation proceeding to acute necrotizing vasculitis (Figure 13-10). This interpretation was supported by observations in which carrier mice were decomplemented at time of transfer

of immune antibody, whereupon PMN accumulation and tissue necrosis did not occur. After initiation of necrotizing lesions (accomplished by transfer of immune serum in this animal model) mononuclear cells replaced PMNs within lesions which then resembled those generally associated with the development of delayed hypersensitivity reactions. The extent to which direct transfer of anti-LCM antibody participated in the development of these lesions was difficult to ascertain.

The experimental model of latent LCM infection and the participation of immune-com-

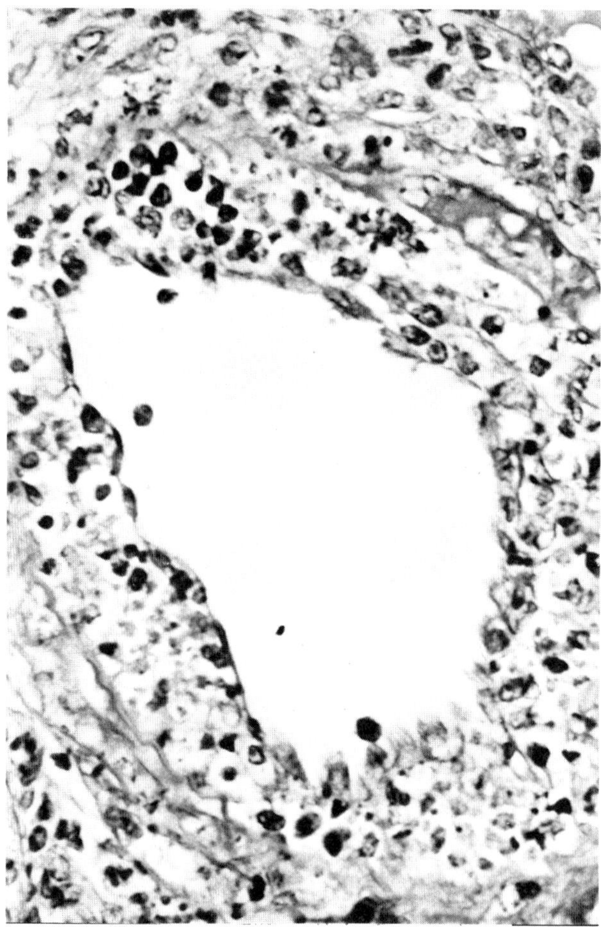

Figure 13-10 Arteritis in a mouse with chronic LCM infection in which the vascular lesions are the result of virus-antibody immune-complex deposits. Note the tearing of the intima and inflammation of the vessel wall. Parallel immunofluorescence studies showed positive staining for host IgG, C3, and viral antigen. Magnification × 281. (Photograph courtesy of M. B. A. Oldstone, Scripps Research Foundation, La Jolla, California.)

plex–mediated phenomena in such chronically infected animals has recently been reviewed by Oldstone (117). Chronic LCM infection has been useful in that it has provided a model in which to study the relationship of lifelong or chronic persistent viral infection to generation of several manifestations of immune-complex disease. One of the major advantages of this animal model is the relative ease of isolation of the virus and apparent viral-specific antigens on the surface of infected cells. The cytotoxic T-cell response engendered by LCM viral infection has also provided a fruitful arena for the study of specific effector functions related to cell-mediated immunity and the relative necessity for effector cell and infected target cells to share cell-surface recognition structures related to the mouse histocompatibility or H-2 system. A series of studies have conclusively demonstrated that the cell-mediated immune response induced in various strains of mice infected with LCM virus involves recognition by immune or immunologically committed T cells of viral-specific antigen as well as a self-marker coded for by the major histocompatibility gene complex (118–120).

Several features of the generation of cytotoxic T-effector cells during the induction of murine lymphocytic choriomeningitis infection are noteworthy. The studies of Pfizenmaier and colleagues (121) have shown that mice injected with LCM virus generate specifically sensitized T lymphocytes, which can kill and release ^{51}Cr from labeled virus-infected cells. Previous work had indicated that cytotoxic effector lymphocytes were restricted to cells infected with virus and compatible with the effector cells within definite regions of the mouse major histocompatibility locus. The Pfizenmaier studies indicated that four to six days after infection with LCM virus, the lymphocytes generated were specifically cytotoxic to syngeneic target cells irrespective of whether they contained viral antigen. However, as primary viral infection proceeded, the specificity for killing only of virally infected cells narrowed, and normal noninfected syngeneic cells were no longer preferred targets. These findings suggest that early events in LCM in-

fection are capable of inducing an autoimmune reaction in which the H-2 restricted cell-surface determinants serve as the antigenic signal for effector lymphocyte killing.

Similar evidence for microheterogeneity among effector killer cells was presented later by Dunlop and associates (122). The concepts involved in H-2 restriction and recognition of virally coded antigens on target cells are shown in Figure 13-11. A corollary of these observations, extensively studied with respect to LCM viral infections (122–124), might be that viral antigens somehow resembling or simulating histocompatibility surface markers adventitiously escape immune surveillance and killing. Alternately, close association between HLA structures and viral antigens on cell surfaces might ensure escape from surveillance and direct cytotoxic killing by immune killer cells. If such a situation were present in human disorders such as SLE, it could explain persistence of putative agents within tissues and survival of the host long enough to develop the peripheral and often fatal consequences of a prolonged but ineffective humoral immune response—namely glomerular, central nervous system, and other microcapillary end-organ damage from immune-complex disease. A potential mechanism is shown in Figure 13-11.

The concept that cells involved in viral immune reactions are most effective when effector cells and target cells share histocompatibility determinants is an important one that must be considered in all models involving attempts to demonstrate T-cell–mediated killing or other cellular interactions against model target tissues. How much H-2 or HLA restriction is required in various cell-to-cell communicative reactions in systems where a known or demonstrable virus is not apparent represents an area of intense activity in a number of laboratories. The question is particularly important in experimental models involving cultured cells from individual patients being killed by effector cells from other patients with the same disorder. A number of claims for disease-specific or nonspecific reactions need to be reexamined with this particular principle firmly in mind. Among the most obvious are reported experiments that involve killing of cultured cells

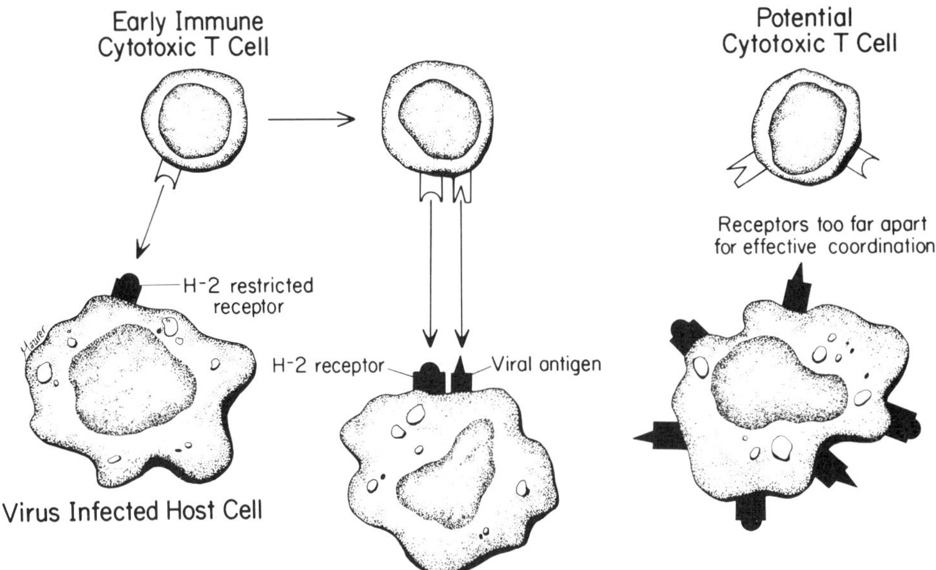

Figure 13-11 Cytotoxicity, particularly T-cell killing of virally infected cells, may involve a fit between histocompatibility antigens (H-2) and virally induced cell-surface antigens.

from rheumatoid arthritis synovia by lymphoid cells of other patients afflicted with the same disease (125–127). Without close attention to possible HLA restriction, the results of much of this work are difficult to put into any kind of meaningful perspective. Similar experiments, even using autologous cells of patients before and after remission in acute leukemia (128–130), are difficult to fathom. The requirements for cells capable of cooperating through mutual HLA or similar recognition structures in the case of acute leukemia patients before and after remission have been stressed (130).

The effects of virus infection on the immune system represent a fascinating model for possible application to a number of human diseases currently considered disorders of unknown etiology. In the case of LCM virus infections of mice, it can be shown that primary immunizing infections result in transient and sometimes lasting alterations in immune function at levels of antigen processing or recognition reflected in both humoral and cellular immunity. The study of Jacobs and Cole (131), for instance, showed depression of in vitro lymphocyte activation. Addition of normal peritoneal exudate macrophages corrected this

proliferative defect; it appeared that the acute effects of LCM virus infection had profoundly affected the essential interaction of macrophage or monocyte populations. Since this cell population is well endowed with active Fc and complement receptors, it seems possible that either transient or long-lasting changes in these cells could influence the handling of immune complexes in such a way as to allow them eventually to produce microvascular injury.

The New Zealand Mouse

For a number of years it has been apparent that New Zealand black mice, and in particular the NZB/W F_1 hybrid, show evidence for a naturally occurring animal model simulating various features of human autoimmune disorders such as SLE or Sjögren's syndrome. First recognized to be associated with spontaneous hemolytic anemia, progressive immune complex nephropathy, and antinuclear antibody, the disease seen in the NZB/W mouse bears a remarkable similarity to human SLE. The fundamental immunologic derangement in NZB mice or in NZB/W hybrid progeny has now been interpreted and applied in constructive attempts to understand the basic SLE problem. Always interwoven into the basic plot has been the suspicion—at times the implicit assumption—that viral infection per se caused the NZB syndrome and therefore somehow by analogy the same would eventually surface with regard to SLE. There are a number of lines of evidence that can be mustered to support such an argument, but the interconnecting events or mechanisms, if such be the case, are not clear. Nevertheless, the NZB/W mouse model provides abundant opportunity to examine a naturally occurring disorder in which immune-complex–mediated glomerulonephritis as well as hemolytic anemia and apparent humoral hyperresponsiveness appear to be fundamental factors in the development of clinical disease.

The most basic immunologic abnormality that has emerged from studies of New Zealand mice relates to development of numerous autoantibodies, immune-complex disease, and an age-related loss of suppressor as well as helper T-cell function (132–134). Whether the disorder relates principally to viral or genetic features or to a unique interaction of both has also not yet been clarified. Animals born to NZB/W matings appear clinically normal, but within 2 to 3 months begin to show signs of hemolytic anemia, positive Coombs' tests, antinuclear as well as anti-DNA antibodies, positive lupus cell tests, evidence of circulating immune complexes, immune-complex deposits in glomeruli and other capillary foci such as the choroid plexus, and later progressive clinical deterioration with renal insufficiency, anemia, inanition, and death within 10 to 12 months. During development of the disease NZB/W mice also show evidence of antilymphocyte antibodies with T-cell or thymocyte specificity, DNA–anti-DNA as well as IgG and complement deposits at the dermal-epidermal junction, round-cell infiltrates of salivary glands similar in many respects to the histological features of Sjögren's syndrome, and evidence of progressive defects in fundamental immune regulatory mechanisms allowing unbridled expression of humoral hyperresponsiveness and impaired thymic function. Intermingled in this clinical disorder are a number of features suggesting that C-type RNA viruses are somehow involved in many aspects of the disease. A tabular comparison of the remarkable parallels between clinical NZB/W mouse disease and human SLE is presented in Table 13-2. In only a few areas is there a significant divergence in the clinical course. One of these is the eventual development of lymphoid malignancy in 10 to 15 percent of NZB/W mice, whereas such an outcome is not customarily

Table 13-2 Comparison of NZB/W mouse disease and human systemic lupus erythematosus

	NZB/W mice	Human SLE
Hemolytic anemia	+++[a]	+
Antinuclear antibody	+++	+++
Anti-DNA antibody	+++	+++
Anti-RNA antibody	+++	+++
Anti-Sm antibody	++	+++
Immune-complex glomerulonephritis	+++	+++
Choroid-plexus immune deposits	++	++
Ig and C at dermal-epidermal junction	++	+++
Association with eventual lymphoid malignancy	++	0
Loss of suppressor-cell function	+++	++
Loss of effective helper-cell function	++	+
Anti-lymphocyte antibody (anti–T cell)	+++	++

[a] 0 to +++ refers to degree of expression in disease state.

seen with SLE patients. The immunologic process is very similar in both disorders. However, this striking analogy does not prove that the primary genesis of the disease syndrome is the same in the two conditions. It seems worthwhile to examine several of the specific manifestations and clinical findings in NZB/W mice with particular reference to information now available supporting the identity and mechanisms of action of circulating or fixed autologous immune complexes.

Hemolytic Anemia

The precise relationship between development of autoimmune hemolytic anemia in New Zealand mice and genetic influences, which could presumably be regarded as "autoimmunity genes," has not yet been delineated; the pattern of inheritance appears to be rather complex (135, 136). Early in the genetic analysis of the disease Howie and Helyer (137) pointed out that (NZB × NZC) F_1 mice showed predominant hemolytic anemia, whereas the characteristic lesion in (NZB × NZW) F_1 hybrids was nephritis. This gave rise to the concept that expression of various forms of autoimmunity among a number of NZB crosses was modified and to a large extent governed by the genetic contribution of the normal strain. The study reported by Braverman (138) was particularly enlightening; it appeared that the NZB possessed a gene dominant for production of autoantibody against erythrocytes, whereas the NZW possessed a separate, modifying gene which in the presence of the complementary NZB gene allowed for development of antinuclear antibody. Subsequent studies by Ghaffir and Playfair (139) showed that autoantibodies against erythrocytes appeared much earlier in NZB mice than in (NZB × Balb/c) F_1 hybrids and that this difference in temporal expression of autoantibody might be caused by gene dosage effects, whereby a single copy of a particular gene would produce late appearance of antierythrocyte antibody but multiple copies could correlate with a much earlier expression of the abnormality.

Immunochemical specificity of the antierythrocyte antibody produced by New Zealand mice is directed at antigen normally exposed on the red-cell surface and termed autoantigen X by Linder and Edgington (140). Studies of B lymphocytes secreting antierythrocyte antibody have indicated that a heterogeneous group of clones of cells are capable of producing the antibody and have also provided evidence that a basic defect in immune regulation is concerned with induction and perpetuation of this response (141, 142). The loss of ordinary immune regulation, permitting the emergence of clones of cells making antierythrocyte antibody, has been analyzed in ingenious ways. Transfers of spleen cells from aged Coombs-positive NZB mice to young Coombs-negative NZB, C3H, or C57B1 mice resulted in appearance of Coombs positivity only in NZB recipients (143), thereby suggesting a primary deficit in NZB animals that involves homeostatic surveillance of the immune system. Denman and associates (144) transferred spleen and bone marrow cells from aged NZB mice to normal Balb/c mice and noted weak but infrequent Coombs positivity. On the other hand, treatment of recipient mice with anti–T-cell antiserum enhanced the magnitude and frequency of Coombs-positive reactions (145). Similar experiments transferring fetal liver and bone marrow from NZB mice to lethally irradiated DBA/2 recipients produced positive Coombs' tests in 33 percent of the recipients 100 days following transfer (146, 147). Such results also implied a defect in the primordial NZB hematopoietic stem cell, which allows it to produce autoantibody if present in the right environment. More recent studies by DeHeer and Edgington (148) of critical factors allowing unbridled development of such self-reactive antibody-forming cells suggest that the formation of antierythrocyte antibody is not governed by macrophage interactions, humoral factors, or T cells but appears to be a defect somehow permitting phenotypic expression of self-reactive B lymphocytes. These observations are in many ways suggestive of the type of B-cell–driven response seen in the case of autoantibody formation associated with the polyclonal B-cell activators (33–37).

The lack of proper immunoregulatory drive has been repeatedly raised by a number of investigators in relation to the manifestations of NZB disease. It has been suggested that part of the basic disturbance in immune regulation results from a lack of effective suppressor cell function. Gershwin and Steinberg (149) have shown that autoimmune hemolytic anemia can be reversed by treatment of mice destined to develop the disease, using syngeneic young thymocytes that presumably supply sufficient quantities of active suppressor cells to modulate the response. Whether or not the immune defect relates to a functional deficiency of suppressor T cells, or more to an uncompromising autonomous driving of self-directed B-cell clones, has not yet been settled. In the case of the autoimmune hemolytic anemia of New Zealand mice, immune complexes are formed directly on the surface of circulating red blood cells and presumably create hemolysis and a shortened red-cell survival through activation of complement and normal Fc receptor reticuloendothelial system clearance mechanisms. The experiments of Linder and Edgington (140) have provided evidence that erythrocyte antigens reacting with autoantibody under such circumstances do not appear to be phenotypically new surface-membrane structures but rather naturally occurring cell-membrane antigens. Thus the spontaneously developing

acute hemolytic anemia present in the NZB mouse model is a specific example of a profound physiological disturbance generated by apparent self-directed autoantibody reacting with and facilitating destruction of autologous erythrocytes.

Immune-Complex Glomerulonephritis

One of the most striking features of disease in the NZB × NZW hybrid animals is the predictable development of immune-complex glomerulonephritis. Although this phenomenon bears a striking parallel to the clinical situation in human SLE, it appears to be governed by a rather uniform time course and pattern which have made it an irresistible animal model for study of analogous phenomena in human SLE. Beginning at about two months and steadily increasing during the remainder of the animals' lives, there is a rapid increment in proportions of animals showing antinuclear and anti-DNA antibody, glomerular immunofluorescent deposits of IgG, IgM, and C3, and proteinuria associated with progressive renal insufficiency, inanition, and finally death. Immune-complex glomerulonephritis is the major manifestation in the NZB/W hybrid. A cumulative plot is shown in Figure 13-12 taken from the review by Howie and Helyer (137). The renal pathol-

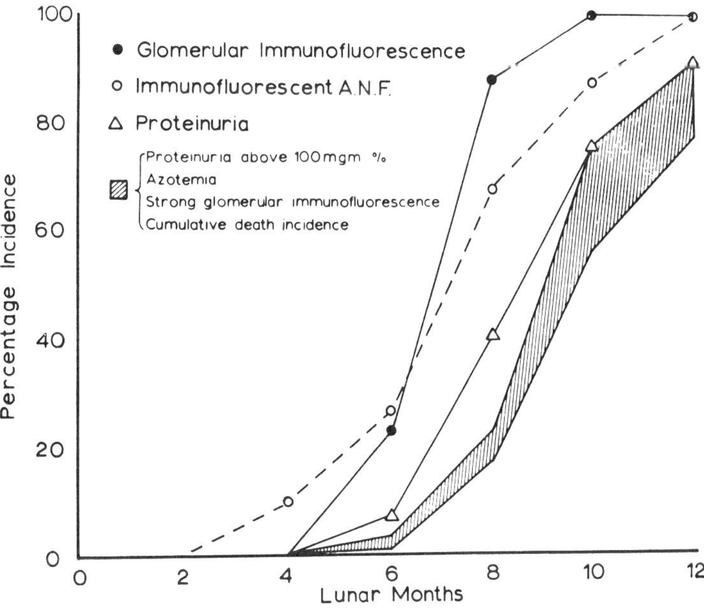

Figure 13-12 Incidence of glomerular immunofluorescence, ANF, and proteinuria in NZB/W mice, by age. (Reproduced with permission, J. B. Howie and B. J. Helyer, *Adv. Immunol.* 9:215, 1968.)

ogy frequently resembles the wire-loop lesions of membranous or proliferative glomerulo-nephritis seen in patients with systemic lupus erythematosus. Representative examples of these lesions are shown in Figure 13-13 from the classic study by Mellors (150). Immuno-fluorescent studies along with electron micro-scopic examination of the developing renal lesions provided early and clear documentation of the immune-complex nature of this process (Figures 13-14 and 13-15). Since the disorder was first recognized as an excellent parallel model for the study of human SLE, it has been the focus of examination by an ever increasing number of workers. One of the most intrigu-

ing and as yet unresolved problems related to immune-complex nephritis in the NZB/W white mice is the importance of viral infection in actually inducing the lesions.

From early studies of this model it was clear that a progressive rise in antibodies with vari-ous forms of antinuclear reactivity occurred in conjunction with the development of the ne-phritis. Positive lupus cell tests were observed in a small proportion of animals, but other more sensitive serologic and immunofluores-cent tests showed that a majority of animals eventually developed antinuclear as well as anti-DNA antibodies, closely simulating the heterogeneity and multiplicity of responses

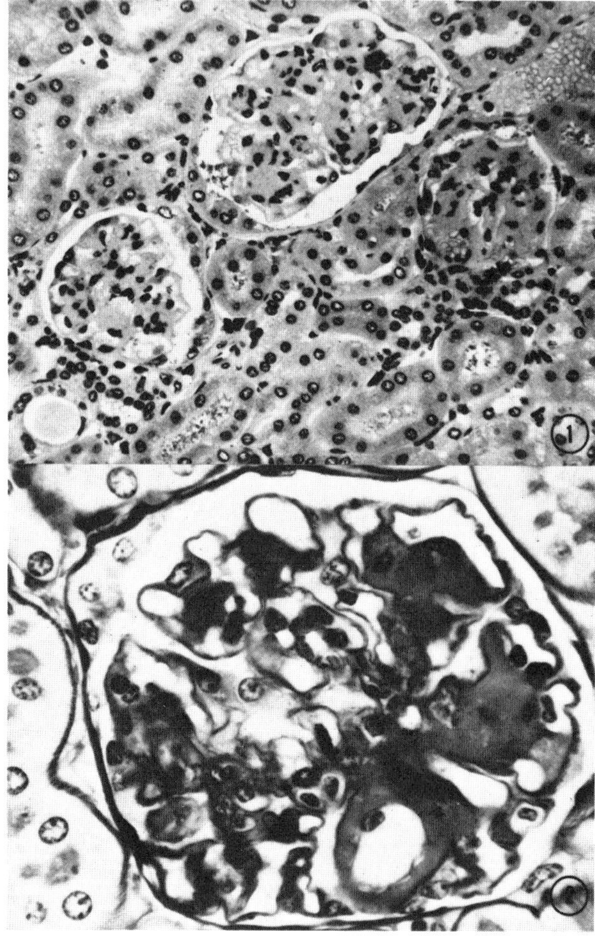

Figure 13-13 Focal membranous glomerular le-sions resembling the wire-loop lesions of lupus ne-phritis. Periodic acid–Schiff reaction. Magnification × 684. (Reproduced with permission, R. C. Mellors, *J. Exp. Med.* 122:25, 1965.)

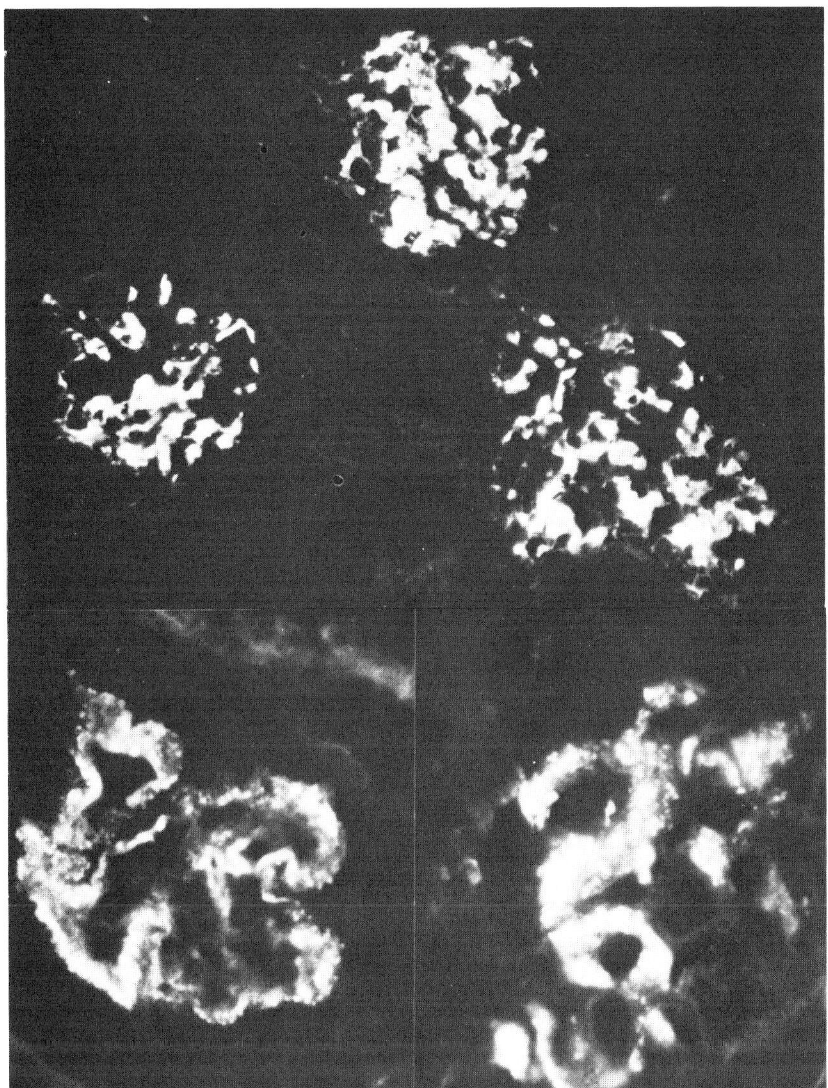

Figure 13-14 *Above,* localization of mouse immunoglobulins in three glomerular tufts in glomerulonephritis of NZB/B1 mice. Fluorescent rabbit antibodies to mouse immunoglobulins are evident (by immunofluorescence). Magnification × 318. *Left below,* membranous localization of mouse immunoglobulins in the capillary walls of a lobule of a glomerular tuft (by immunofluorescence). Magnification × 850. *Right below,* focal localization of mouse immunoglobulins in the intercapillary (mesangial) region of a glomerular tuft. Magnification × 1,300. (Reproduced with permission, R. C. Mellors, *J. Exp. Med.* 122:25, 1965.)

seen in association with human SLE (137, 151, 152). Antinuclear antibodies have been considered to be of primary importance in the pathogenesis of the immune-complex glomerulonephritis in the NZB/W model, based on sequential analysis of their occurrence in

serum and identification directly within the glomerular immune deposits. The studies by Lambert and Dixon (153) were particularly convincing in this regard: serum taken from NZB/W animals contained DNA-like antigen during the disease; eluates of gamma globulins

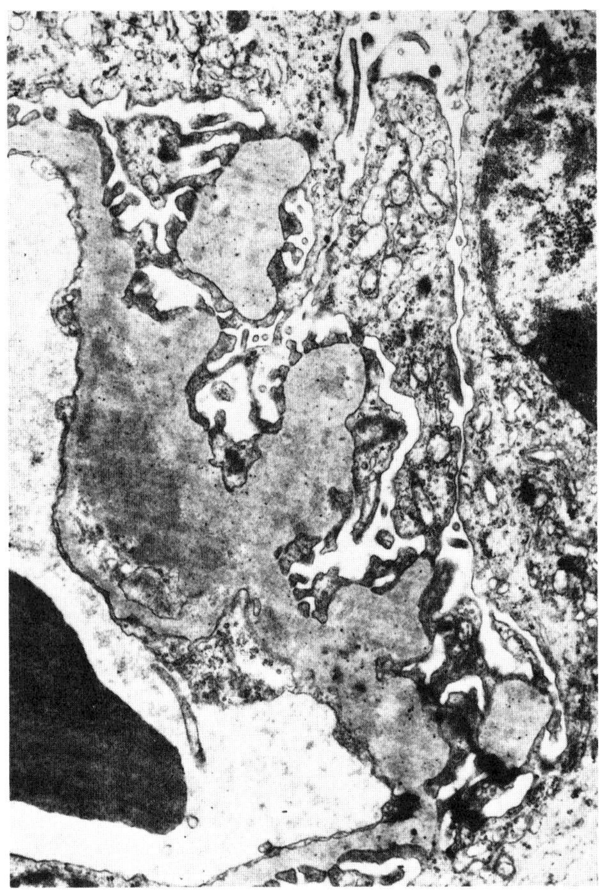

Figure 13-15 A glomerular membranous lesion with homogeneous swelling of the capillary basement membrane (along the diagonal from *upper left to lower right*) with obliteration of laminae rarae and accumulations in the subendothelial (*toward the left*) and subepithelial (*toward the right*) spaces. The foot processes of the epithelial cell (*toward the right*) and the urinary spaces appear relatively normal. Electron micrograph, magnification × 11,400. (Reproduced with permission, R. C. Mellors, *J. Exp. Med.* 122:25, 1965.)

from diseased kidneys capable of complement fixation with heat-denatured DNA as antigen produced impressive antinuclear staining when tested by immunofluorescence on normal tissue substrates; the NZB/W nephritis could be accelerated during the course of its natural development by immunization of animals with DNA but not by unrelated antigens such as bovine serum albumin (BSA). Data from this study are shown in Table 13-3. It thus appeared that DNA–anti-DNA complexes were extremely important in the production of immune lesions within the glomeruli during natural development of the disease. Again it must be pointed out how striking an analogy this bears to the situation in human SLE, where the central role of DNA–anti-DNA complexes has also been firmly established by elution and specificity studies using tissues from affected patients (154–156).

One of the most important unanswered questions appears to be what process initiates the formation of anti-DNA antibodies and the precise relation this may have to concurrent viral infection—particularly relative to C-type RNA viruses. The most revealing results have to date been derived from immunopathological and genetic studies, again with several

Table 13-3 Acceleration of NZB/W nephritis after injection of DNA.

Experimental animal	Strain	Injection	Proteinuria over 7 mg/24 hr [a]	Glomerular lesions [b]		
				Histology	γG deposits	Fibrin deposits
Mice with no serum	Swiss-Webster	DNA[c]	0/11	0/11	0/11	0/11
anti-DNA antibodies	NZB/W	DNA[c]	0.9	2/9	2/9	2/9
Mice with serum	NZB/W	BSA[d]	0.8	0/8	1/8	0/8
anti-DNA antibodies	NZB/W	DNA[c]	7/9	7/9	9/9	8/9
	AJAX	DNA[e]	0/10	0/10	—	—

Source: Reproduced with permission, P. H. Lambert and F. J. Dixon, *J. Exp. Med.* 127:507, 1968.

[a] Observed 1 day after last injection.

[b] Observed 2 days after last injection.

[c] 7 daily injections of 130 μg heat-denatured calf thymus DNA.

[d] 7 daily injections of 130 μg BSA.

[e] 7 daily injections of 130 μg, followed by intraperitoneal injections of 200 μg five times a week for an additional 4 weeks.

mouse models. Early studies appeared to implicate the murine leukemia virus (MuLV) in the pathogenesis of NZB/W disease (157–161). MuLV-related antigens appear early in the life of the NZB mice, and antibodies to these endogenous viral antigens occur later, accompanied by immune-complex glomerulonephritis. Immunoelectron microscopy showed that anti-MuLV antibodies showed reactions with viral envelope antigens (162, 163). Furthermore, studies by Mellors and colleagues (158, 159) demonstrated that MuLV-related antigens were present in eluates of nephritic kidneys and the MuLV antigens localized within glomerular lesions by immunofluorescence methods. Extensions of this approach have utilized highly defined antisera to various structural components of MuLV representing glycoproteins of the viral envelope (164).

Immunofluorescent reactions identifying the gp 69/71 MuLV glycoprotein in frozen sections of affected mouse glomeruli are shown in Figure 13-16. In addition, the gp 69/71 antigen was identified in glomerular eluates from diseased kidneys. The serum and tissues of NZB, NZW, and their F_1 hybrids contained high concentrations of this viral envelope glycoprotein, which suggests that immune complexes in affected mice were derived from endogenous MuLV infection. One of the problems with an assumption that MuLV is indeed the cause of

murine lupus is that it should therefore be possible to mimic the disease by infecting susceptible but otherwise normal mouse strains. Studies presented by Croker and co-workers (165) have indicated that an SLE-like syndrome can be induced in immunologically normal mice by injection of neonates with a murine leukemia virus isolated from NZB lymphoblasts. This SLE syndrome was characterized by antinuclear antibodies and immune-complex glomerulonephritis. Both antinuclear antibody titers and incidence of glomerulonephritis were higher in females than in males, but no Coombs positivity or hemolytic anemia was observed.

These studies are still difficult to interpret, for the MuLV agents or other oncornaviruses are ubiquitous in many strains of mice and the changes seen in murine SLE of the NZB/W type cannot be ascribed only to MuLV. Cannat and Varet (166) have noted induction of antinuclear antibody but not glomerulonephritis by the Friend-Moloney-Raucher group of MuLV in several mouse strains. Moreover, immune-complex glomerulonephritis has been reported in association with leukemia induced by the FMR group of viruses (167, 168). The glomerulonephritis that develops spontaneously in aging mice of several different strains appears to be related to immune complexes and ubiquitous MuLV antigens (169–181). It

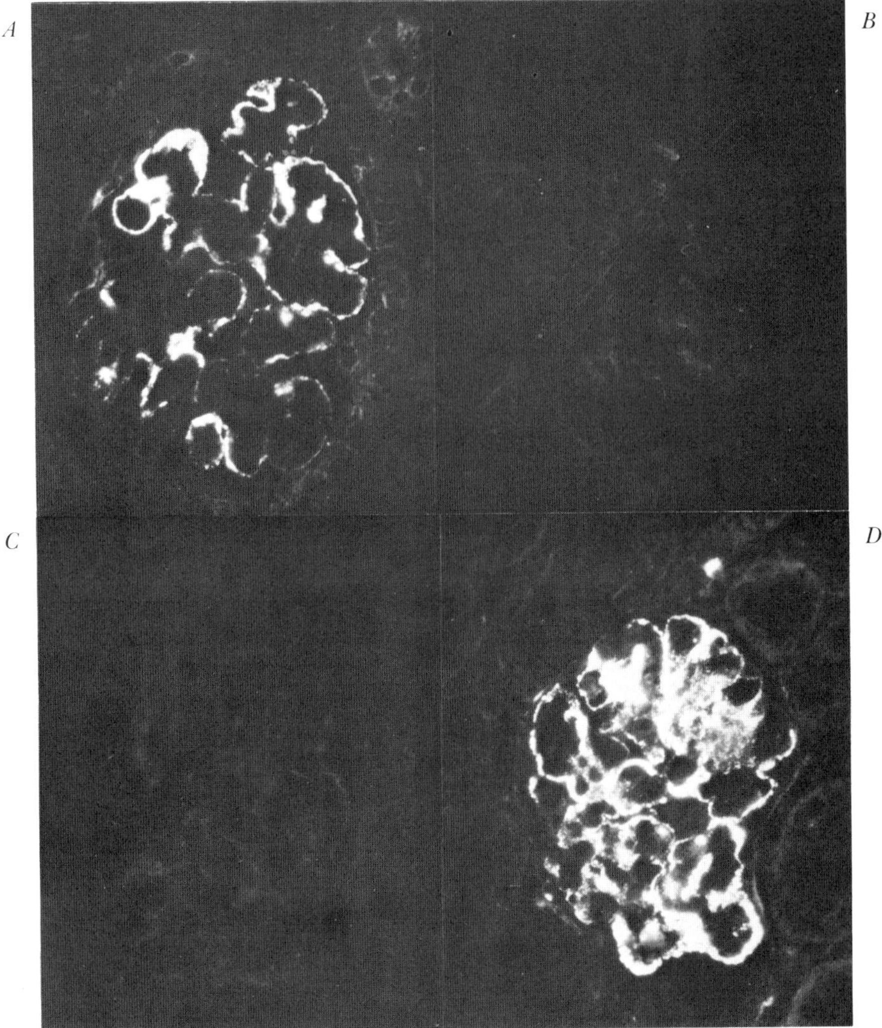

Figure 13-16 Immunofluorescent photomicrographs of frozen sections of perfused kidneys of mice, B/WF$_1$, 11 months. Specificity of immunofluorescence reaction by anti-gp69/71: *A*, absorbed with sonicated C57BL/6J thymus; *B*, absorbed with intact Rauscher MuLV suspension; *C*, absorbed with sonicated E'G2 cells; *D*, bound immunoglobulins in the wall of the peripheral capillary loops and mesangium in a section of the same kidney. Note the specific absorption of the fluorescence reaction (*B* and *C*), and the similar distribution of gp69/71 and bound immunoglobulins (*A* and *D*). Magnification × 500. (Reproduced with permission, T. Yoshiki, R. C. Mellors, M. Strand et al., *J. Exp. Med.* 140:1011, 1974.)

seems clear, however, that in the immune-complex glomerular disease of NZB/W mice, antinuclear as well as anti-Gross viral antigens are important in inducing injury. An attempt to quantitate the relative contribution of each was made by Dixon and colleagues (172); they found evidence for both types of immune complexes in eluates of glomeruli from diseased animals. Still vitally needed is an understanding of the basic derangements in the immune response that allow animals to manufacture marked elevations of antibody to such potential antigens. Whether unregulated immune hyperresponsiveness is responsible or some other primary immune defect remains to be determined.

A recent contribution to our understanding of the relationship between endogenous viral infection and the expression of autoimmune immune-complex injury in NZB mice is that of Datta and colleagues (173, 174). The basic problem involved in studying the relationship between C-type RNA viruses and NZB/W mouse disease is that the viruses most closely implicated in the etiology of the disease are xenotropic—that is, they can only be demonstrated conclusively by transfer to tissues or tissue cultures of a different species. Using genetic and backcross analyses, the Datta group showed that the phenotypic expression of such infectious viruses was determined by at least two genes, Nzv-1 and Nzv-2, which behaved independently of the development of autoantibodies and glomerulonephritis (173). Expression of the viral envelope glycoprotein gp70 was analyzed in relation to expression of infectious xenotropic virus, autoantibody formation, and the development of both immune-complex nephritis and lymphomas (174). Since gp70 appears to be the major glycoprotein component of C-type RNA viruses, it serves as a useful marker for their presence. However, it can be found in the tissues and serum of virtually all mice tested (172, 175, 176). Structural studies of serum gp70 indicate that it is the same in all mouse strains and resembles the gp70 of the NZB xenotropic virus (176). The presence of gp70 appears to be independent of the expression of complete viral particles. In the serum of NZB mice there is 1,000-fold greater concentration of this marker glycoprotein than of the viral core protein. Metabolic studies of gp70 production have also indicated that its levels reflect its rate of synthesis. Therefore, in NZB mice high levels in sera reflect a very high rate of synthesis as well as abundant expression of the C-type RNA xenotropic virus itself.

The Datta analyses (174) indicate that serum levels of gp70 are controlled by a complex system of genes that are probably recessive in contrast to the dominant Nzv-1 and Nzv-2 genes. Regardless of their viral (Nzv) phenotype, in studies of virus-negative progeny of NZB ×

SWR mice, nephritis developed which did not appear to contain detectable viral antigens (including gp70) as determined by immunofluorescence techniques (173). Deposition of gp70 antigen within nephritic immune deposits might therefore be occurring as a secondary rather than a primary event. It is conceivable that the fundamental defect in NZB mice relates more directly to primordial defects in gene regulation, which allow both marked increment of gp70 protein expression and unregulated B-cell–driven synthesis of numerous autoantibodies including anti-DNA, other antinuclear factors, and antilymphocyte antibodies.

Type C Viruses and Human SLE

Type C oncornaviruses in general belong to the retrovirus family, which possesses an RNA genome and an RNA-dependent DNA polymerase (177). Retroviruses either are transmitted horizontally or are vertically integrated within the host genome. Some retroviruses appear to be factors in leukemia or various solid tumors, others are associated with neurologic or immunologic disease but may appear to be unrelated to any clinical disorder (177). Although from one standpoint these agents can be considered as equivalent to host genes, they can also be thought of as independent infectious agents. There are a number of recently isolated mammalian retroviruses, which differ from other C type viruses and are not yet classified (178).

Experimental work on the possible role of C-type viruses in SLE still presents the intriguing possibility that they are somehow related to the human disease. Lewis and associates (179), using indirect immunofluorescence and serum antibody from another patient with SLE, found an antigen possibly related to C-type viral infection on rare peripheral blood lymphocytes from patients with SLE. The serum antibody used could be partially absorbed with a type C virus from a mouse tumor that had developed after inoculation of material from a dog with SLE. Antisera to this mouse virus also recognized antigens present on a small proportion of SLE lymphocytes, but the antigen has not been further defined.

Strand and August (180), using competitive radioimmunoassay, also provided evidence for C-type related glycoproteins in tissues from 3 SLE patients. The molecular size of one competing tissue protein in this report was similar to that of core type C viral protein, but competitors from different tissues behaved like antigens from different viruses. These findings contrast to other negative studies by several groups using normal, neoplastic, or other SLE tissues (181–183).

Immunofluorescence studies by Mellors and Mellors (184) detected C-type viral antigen in immune glomerular deposits of 3 patients with SLE. In this carefully done research appropriate absorption of specific anti–C-type viral antisera blocked positive immunofluorescence. Subsequent attempts to extend these remarkable observations have not indicated similar specificity in a much larger batch of renal biopsy material. Panem and co-workers (185) claimed C-type viral antigens in all of 11 SLE patients' kidneys examined by immunofluorescence. However, the specificity of the reagents used in the study are dubious. In particular, no absorption of antisera was reported using uninfected cells from the same source as those used to cultivate the virus.

Although much of the work just described provides enticing evidence that C-type viral infection may somehow be involved in human SLE, a complete picture has not emerged. Some of the gaps in our understanding have been reviewed by Phillips (186). C-virus–like particles were identified in both normal and SLE placentas (187), but no C-related antigens were found in crude extracts of 14 tissues (some of which contained virus-like particles) using sensitive radioimmunoassay procedures. During these studies a 70,000 M.W. C-type related antigen was found on both SLE and normal subjects' lymphocytes, via lactoperoxidase labeling and anti-baboon or anti-RD114 virus antisera (188). Furthermore, attempts by Phillips and co-workers to isolate type C viruses directly from patients with SLE have thus far been negative (189, 190). The relationship of type C virus infection and SLE is still ambiguous. Enough bits and pieces of evidence have emerged, however, to make further concentrated effort in this area worthwhile and perhaps eventually decisive.

Features of NZB/W Mouse Disease That Suggest a Regulatory Defect

The rapid development of humoral autoantibody in NZB/W mice can be shown to be related to a defect in T-cell–B-cell control mechanisms. There is now extensive evidence to support the concept of defective T-cell reactivity, regarding both tolerance induction and immune surveillance or suppressor T-cell activity (134). There also appears to be clear evidence for an age-dependent loss of both helper and suppressor T-cell function. Whether this results from defects in T cells themselves or from intermediary messenger molecules such as lymphokines acting to synergize intercellular communication is not yet known.

There are some indications that thymic humoral factors may be deficient in NZB/W mice (191, 192). A number of studies indicate premature thymic epithelial cell involution with prominent degeneration and vacuolization of cells, which are critical for maintenance of normal thymic function (193–195). Studies by Gershwin and associates (196) of the morphologic and functional characteristics of thymic epithelial cells have indicated marked age-dependent changes in such material cultured in vitro. After several weeks in culture the majority of epithelial-like cells showed increase in size, contained a number of vacuoles, and appeared to undergo degenerative changes. The source of the substances widely regarded as being thymic hormones is felt to be the thymic epithelial cells (197). Despite the demonstrated influence of thymic humoral factors on the immune system, research reported to date has failed to show much in the way of dramatic improvement or change in the natural course of disease in NZB or NZB/W mice treated with thymic extracts (198, 199).

With respect to alterations in thymic activity in NZB/W and human SLE, it is interesting that naturally occurring antilymphocyte antibodies present in both disorders may well play some role in modulating immune function. In NZB mice the antilymphocyte antibody appears to show some specificity for thymus cells and increases in titer with age of the animals. Its presence has also been demonstrated to affect the traffic patterns of lymphocytes by incubation of sera positive for the antibody and subsequent assay for lymphocyte homing or tissue distribution (200, 201). The fact that the NZB/W disease state actually induces an autoantibody to its own T cells may reflect the penultimate in autoimmune dysfunction and complete loss of control for basic homeostatic mechanisms usually operative in the normal immune system.

The model still appears to provide an excellent ground for attempts to manipulate or impede progression of the disease state as a whole. It is obvious that any effective therapeutic program must address itself to ablating the unbridled self-destructive hyperresponsiveness of the humoral immune system and the capacity to generate immune complexes. Whether this will eventually involve restoration of immune balance through appropriate suppressor T-cell control or through programs designed specifically to shut off self-reactive B cells remains to be seen.

Recently, primarily through experiments in mice, there have been a number of advances in identification of various subsets of lymphocytes that may be involved in fundamental lymphocyte interaction. Instead of merely referring to T-cell subsets as helper, killer, or suppressor on the basis of in vitro functional analysis, it has become possible to identify lymphocyte subpopulations on the basis of cell-surface markers defined by alloantisera obtained by immunization of one strain of mice with lymphocyte antigens from another. Cantor and co-workers have thus defined an antigenic marker system on mouse lymphocytes using such antisera which is called the Ly system (202–204). Mouse lymphocytes that express the Thy1+, Ly1+, Ly23− surface phenotype appear to be programmed for helper function. In contrast, T cells that are Ly23+ cells are destined to act as suppressor cells. A third major T-cell subclass—expressing the surface phenotype Ly123+—can react to antigen and differentiate to produce cytotoxic effector cells, perhaps suggesting that this particular T-cell subclass contains potential antigen-binding

or antigen-reactive cells, but has not yet been committed to become helper or suppressor. Moreover, it has recently been learned that stimulation of Ly1+,2− T cells results in T-helper cells but that such Ly1+ helper cells also induce a subset of nonimmune uncommitted T cells to exert a potent feedback inhibition of the immune response. The surface phenotype of these "feedback inhibitor cells" is Ly123+ Qa1+ (205). This sequence of events is shown diagrammatically in Figure 13-17.

The importance of these findings is illustrated when the phenotypes of such cells are analyzed in the New Zealand mouse. Cantor and colleagues (206) have found that during the first year of life NZB mice show high concentrations and absolute numbers of Ly1+,2,3− cells, but substantially reduced numbers of Ly1,2,3+ "feedback inhibitor" cells. We now have an opportunity to investigate the precise steps at which immunologic control appears to break down. It is not yet clear whether the naturally occurring antilymphocyte antibody present in NZB mice shows particular specificity or predilection for the Ly, 123+ feedback inhibitor cell or whether, alternatively, this built-in control mechanism merely reflects ungoverned antigenic stimula-

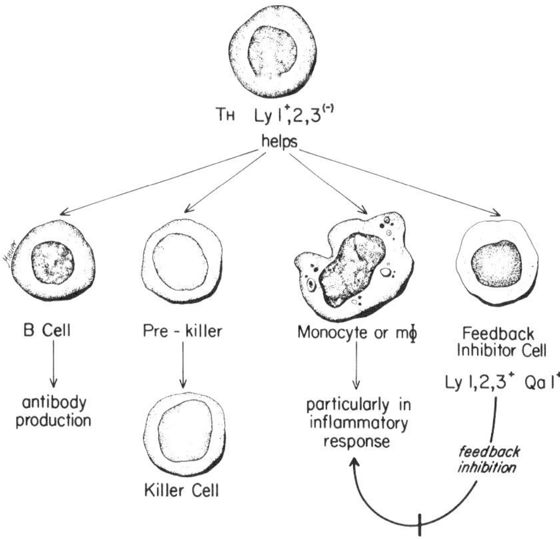

Figure 13-17 Interrelationships among the cell types involved in immune inflammation. Φ refers to macrophages.

tion at some other level. No similar reagents are yet available to help sort out the process going on in patients with loss of feedback inhibition to the immune response. There is some indication that T-helper and T-suppressor cells in humans may be defined by T-cell subsets bearing receptors for Fc of IgM and Fc of IgG respectively (207). But highly discriminating reagents such as are available in the mouse Ly system must await further laboratory development.

Canine Systemic Lupus

Occurrence in dogs of a disorder resembling human systemic lupus erythematosus was first described in 1965 by Lewis and associates (208). This disease was associated with autoimmune hemolytic anemia, idiopathic thrombocytopenic purpura, and nephritis; one dog actually showed a malar eruption. Positive LE cell tests, antithyroid antibody, and occasional presence of rheumatoid factor were also described in these animals. Wire-loop lesions and changes of chronic membranous nephritis were noted, but not splenic periarterial onion-skin lesions. Subsequent laboratory study of these dogs provided evidence for antinuclear antibodies, complement fixation with DNA-histone complexes, and positive antiglobulin tests. Initial analysis did not demonstrate a distinct predilection for any one breed of dogs to acquire the disease; for this reason a colony of SLE dogs was established, and attempts were made to breed them in order to analyze both genetic and environmental factors that might influence the expression of the disease itself. A subsequent analysis of this breeding colony (eventually 480 animals) was presented by Lewis and Schwartz (209.) This study indicated a relatively high frequency of perinatal death —however, there was no distinct evidence of SLE by histological analysis. Thymic abnormalities, mainly consisting of lymphoid follicles, were frequently recorded among the dogs of this colony. In addition, a high frequency of serologic abnormalities including positive LE cell tests and antinuclear antibodies was present. Backcross as well as outbreeding experiments aimed at demonstrating possible genetic

control of some of these abnormalities failed to reveal clear evidence of a single gene associated with either serological abnormalities or disease expression, and the possibility of vertical transmission by an infectious agent, though not documented directly, was considered (208).

Interesting extensions of this work by the same group (210) utilized cell-free filtrates prepared from spleens of dogs with presumed SLE. When injected into newborn dogs, these cell-free filtrates induced development of antinuclear antibody and positive LE cell tests. In some instances mice injected with the same materials produced antinative DNA antibodies. Some murine recipients developed malignant lymphomas; murine leukemia viruses were identified in these tumors by serological, virological, and electron microscopic techniques. An example of the lymphomas induced in mice injected with canine SLE cell-free filtrates is shown in Figure 13-18. Puppies inoculated with the SLE-filtrate–induced mouse lymphomas developed positive tests for antinuclear antibody and positive LE cell tests within four months. These results were interpreted to mean that dogs with SLE harbored a virus which when passed to other dogs in cell-free filtrates was somehow capable of inducing formation of antinuclear antibody and LE cell production. When canine SLE filtrates were given to mice, endogenous murine leukemia viruses were activated, and in some animals this was associated with development of lymphoma. No definite isolation of primary virus material from canine SLE filtrates occurred, but the results of these experiments indicating transmission across species of possible agents capable of inducing serological abnormalities, as well as positive SLE tests, again suggests that similar transmission of agents from household pets to man may play an important role in SLE.

Aleutian Disease in Mink

Aleutian mink disease is a fascinating naturally occurring model of immune-complex disease in which a viral agent has been recovered after prolonged searching and with long foreknowledge that an infectious agent must indeed be

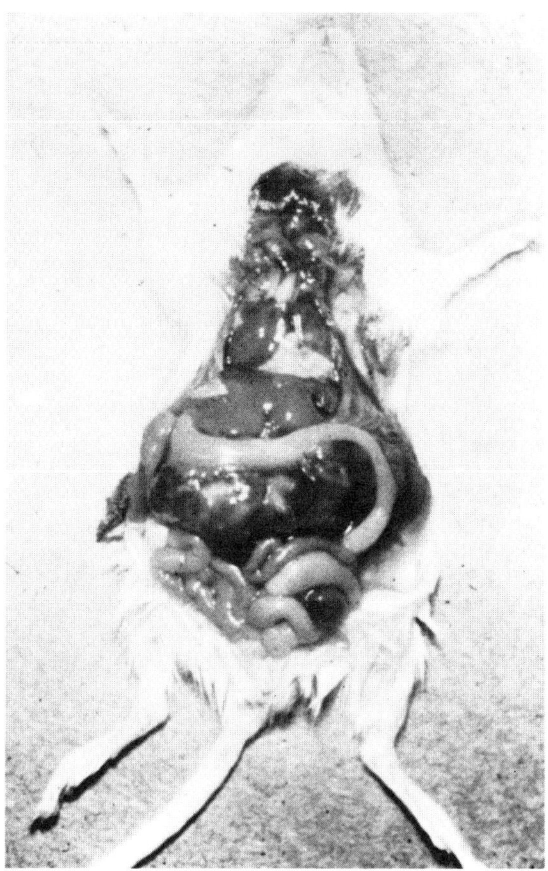

Figure 13-18 SLE dog-induced murine lymphoma. Splenomegaly, hepatomegaly, generalized lymphadenopathy, and an enlarged thymus characterize the gross features of the tumor. (Reproduced with permission, R. M. Lewis, J. André-Schwartz, G. S. Harris et al., *J. Clin. Invest.* 52:1893, 1973.)

present. In 1941 a spontaneous mutation occurred in a population of ranch mink, which was accompanied by a distinctive change in coat color. The color was felt to represent phenotypic expression of a homozygous recessive gene, and the mink affected were said to possess the "Aleutian trait." The major gene types were AA, aa, and aA—with the aa mink representing animals homozygous for the trait expressed.

These Aleutian mink developed an illness characterized by widespread arteritis, chronic active hepatitis, and glomerular injury, along with abundant interstitial nephritis (211, 212). The predominance of plasma cells within the

lesions initially raised the question of a primary plasma cell disorder (213), but experimental transmission of the disease clearly established that an agent present in blood, urine, feces, saliva, or extracts of virtually all infected tissues contained the transmissible material (214, 215). One of the most striking features of the clinical picture was the extreme hypergammaglobulinemia in the chronic or terminal stages. Transmission of the disease was more readily achieved to aa mink than to Aa or AA phenotypes. One of the characteristics of the disease was the development of immune-complex glomerular deposits, with a granular pattern of IgG and complement notable in immunofluorescence studies (216, 217). In addition, weak staining for viral antigen was often present in tissues only early in the disease process (217). Electron microscopic examination of glomerular lesions showed lumpy deposits of electron-dense materials corresponding to the immune deposits noted by immunofluorescence (216). Moreover, elution of diseased kidneys yielded IgG that bound to particulate antigen in cells of diseased mink (218).

Antibodies to the virus, and in particular the remarkable degree of IgG elevation in this naturally occurring animal model, are of interest. In our own experience it is not unusual for γ-globulin levels to reach 4 to 5 gm%. In some animals the electrophoretic mobility of gamma globulins becomes restricted, and oligoclonal or occasionally monoclonal bands are seen. Presence of large amounts of antibody to virus or antigens associated with virus infection does very little to alter the infectiousness of the serum or gamma globulin–containing fractions; such serum fractions can be shown to produce infections when injected into test animals (219). This particular viral infection appears to be somewhat unusual in that infectious virus coexists unimpeded in serum with large amounts of apparent virus-specific antibody. The situation is shown in Figure 13-19.

The fact that infectious complexes of virus and antibody molecules do exist in serum was first demonstrated by Porter and Larsen (220), who showed that infectivity of serum could be precipitated or removed by treatment with antibody to mink γ-globulin. In the case of Aleu-

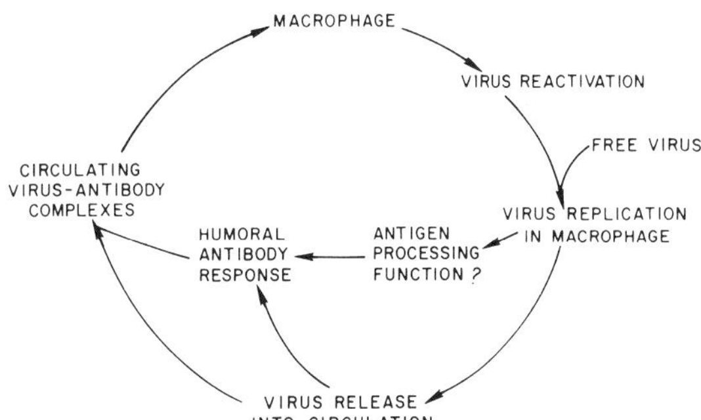

Figure 13-19 The hypothetical mechanism leading to viral persistence in Aleutian disease viral (ADV) infection of mink. The macrophages are thought to phagocytize ADV-antibody complexes, reactivate the virus, and thus allow the virus to replicate in the phagocyte cell. This mechanism would negate any effect of antiviral antibody in terminating infection and might promote viral persistence. (Reproduced with permission, D. D. Porter, A. E. Larsen, and H. G. Porter, *J. Exp. Med.* 130:575, 1969.)

tian mink disease the investigator has the distinct advantage that an excellent assay for the presence of virus exists in merely inoculating test materials into aa or Aa strains; if the agent is present, characteristic Aleutian disease will eventually develop. Moreover, shortly after virus inoculation Aleutian disease viral antigen can be demonstrated in local lymphoid tissue.

Animals with Aleutian disease show presence of both DNA and anti-DNA, as monitored by complement fixation and Ouchterlony analysis (221). The viral agent appears to be remarkably resistant to heating or chemical treatments that usually inactivate viruses. Recent immunochemical and electron microscopic analysis of Aleutian disease virus antigens by Notani and colleagues (222) revealed icosahedral virus particles as well as ring-like structures in one antigenic preparation. Similar findings have been described by Cho and Ingram (223). Subunit component analysis of one of the 80S antigens described by Notani indicated molecular weights of 30,000, 25,000, and 15,000, which he and his associates felt were typical of a picornavirus polypeptide configuration. A summary of knowledge concerning the purification and structure of the

Aleutian disease virus was presented by Cho (224), who considers the virus to be most typical of the parcovirus group. An electron microscopic view of viral antigen-antibody complexes is shown in Figure 13-20.

The earlier difficulties encountered in attempts to characterize this virus are an object lesson to those interested in possible identification of other diseases of unknown etiology. Much useful information may be gained as more insight is available about the assembly and expression of this infectious virus in its natural tissue habitat. At the moment Aleutian disease has a great deal more direct information to offer the clinical investigator than the NZB/W mouse, since an agent has now been identified that produces sustained chronic infection when inoculated into appropriate strains of mink, and that is associated with immune-complex end-organ damage while at the same time demonstrating lifelong persistence of the infectious agent.

Other Viral Agents and Glomerulonephritis

Since viruses have been implicated in a number of experimental models of glomerular and microcapillary bed injury—including lymphocytic choriomeningitis NZB/W mice, Aleutian disease, and LDH virus, as well as coxsackie B4 infection (225), equine infectious anemia (226), and leukemia (227)—it seems likely that a considerable portion of chronic glomerulonephritis in humans may be caused by immune-complex injury caused by viral illnesses that have not yet been clinically identified. A report by Wright and co-workers (228) described experimental production of immune-complex glomerulonephritis by administration of soluble complexes prepared from adenovirus-antiviral antibodies. Viral antigen, C3, and IgG antibody were readily apparent in glomerular structures, but only 17 percent of inoculated mice developed proliferative glomerulonephritis. It is apparent that viral antigens of diverse types can be associated with glomerular immune-complex injury. Local factors such as the ability of the mesangium to clear autolo-

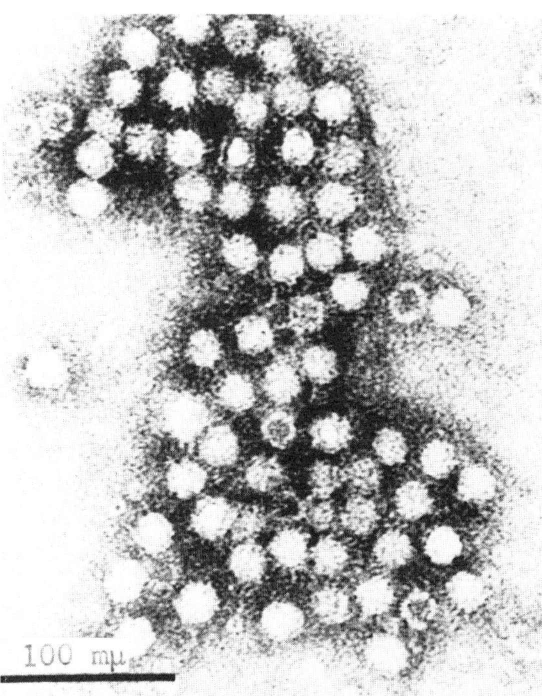

Figure 13-20 Aleutian mink disease virus-antibody complexes, negative stained with 2-percent phosphotungstic acid, pH 7.0. (Reproduced with permission, H. J. Cho and D. G. Ingram, *J. Immunol. Methods* 4:217, 1974.)

gous complexes or the type of lattice engendered within complexes themselves undoubtedly are major determinants in this process.

A number of reports document the occurrence of spontaneous glomerulonephritis in an ever increasing number of animal models including mice, cats, dogs, sheep, goats, hogs, steers, and horses (226, 227, 229–233). In all these instances demonstration of host gamma globulin and complement along the glomerular basement membrane as well as ultrastructural evidence for electron-dense deposits in the same areas or within the mesangium indicate an immune-complex etiology. In some of these naturally occurring models such as hog cholera (233) or equine infectious anemia (226), the antigens have been identified. A spontaneously occurring immune-complex nephritis has also been described in monkeys (234). All of these models bear a close resem-

blance to the clinical picture seen in human disease and may eventually afford an opportunity for more insight into mechanisms governing this sort of pathological process.

Experimental Models of Renal Injury

One area responsible for the development of a large body of useful knowledge in the field of immune-complex–mediated tissue injury relates to the development of animal models as possible analogues for acute or chronic glomerulonephritis in man. Experimental (Masugi) nephritis has been produced by administration of heterologous antikidney serum made in another species. The sequence of events involves fascinating interactions between the host immune system and heterologous antibody, which deposits in renal tissues and appears to start a self-perpetuating series of inflammatory reactions. After preliminary work established the sequential development of lesions mediated first by heterologous antibody and later by interaction with autologous host complement and host antibody, a great deal of interest focused on precise identification of renal tissue antigens—glomerular basement membrane, tubular basement membrane, and other antigens within renal tubular tissues. This orientation clarified the basic immunochemical and physical arrangement of specific tubular, glomerular, and membrane antigens. Heymann's experimental nephritis, produced by immunization with whole kidney homogenates prepared from either isologous or heterologous sources, was developed and extensively studied. More precise knowledge of the chemical composition of glomerular basement membrane (GBM) and its possible relation to diseases associated with anti-GBM antibody emerged.

Finally in the fifties and early sixties, with application of the rapidly emerging technique of immunofluorescence, it became apparent that a number of autologous and presumably immune reactants were identifiable within glomeruli of various patients with the clinical or pathological picture of acute or chronic glomerulonephritis. In many instances these immune deposits were recognized within capillaries in microvascular sites such as glomeruli, which were somehow particularly vulnerable to injury. Against this background the experimental models of acute and chronic serum sickness and much of what is now known concerning basic phenomena of autologous immune-complex renal injury emerged. Some of this experimental work and its clinical application has been described in previous chapters. Additional aspects presented here will focus on more recent developments, or in some cases on extensions and refinements of perception involved in the three major models of experimental renal injury: serum sickness, immunization by renal antigens, and Masugi nephritis. Despite persisting gaps in our basic understanding, there is probably no area of modern clinical immunology where so much useful insight has been generated by careful study of experimental models.

The Serum Sickness Model

A number of studies between 1957 and 1960 indicated that intravenously administered soluble antigen-antibody complexes were capable of inducing a number of potent peripheral effects in various experimental animals. Studies by Germuth and McKinnon (235) emphasized the importance of such materials in the induction of anaphylactic shock when administered to normal unsensitized guinea pigs. Moreover, reports by Benacerraf and co-workers indicated an impressive acute glomerulonephritis in rats or mice after intravenous application of soluble antigen-antibody complexes (236, 237). Immunofluorescence techniques earlier had been sharpened to allow precise localization of reactants in tissues (238), and McLean and co-workers (239) had demonstrated that it was possible to induce glomerulonephritis in rabbits by small intravenous injections of horse serum.

In 1961 Dixon and associates (240) first described a model for the production of acute and chronic glomerulonephritis in the rabbit by repeated daily injections of foreign protein antigens. This model involved administration of repeated amounts of bovine serum albumin (BSA), human serum albumin (HSA), bovine

gamma globulin (BGG), or human gamma globulin (HGG), with variation in dosage of antigen to match the quantities of antibody being produced by the experimental animal to keep the relative amounts of each near the equivalence point (or in slight antigen excess) in the circulation. In order to neutralize all of the antibody formed by the most responsive rabbits, daily injections on the order of 100 to 200 mg of antigen were required, and in some situations fatal anaphylaxis eliminated such responders from the experimental protocol. After the procedures had been initiated, onset of acute glomerulonephritis was frequently noted within 1 or 2 weeks.

Functional and morphological changes induced by the four different antigens were quite similar. When injections were continued for periods longer than several weeks, a morphological picture closely resembling chronic glomerulonephritis included proliferation of glomerular capillary endothelium as well as moderate accumulation of polymorphonuclear leukocytes within glomeruli. These changes were very similar to those seen during acute glomerulonephritis in humans. Moreover, immunofluorescence studies showed granular antigen scattered throughout glomeruli without any obvious anatomic localization. Electron-dense materials were also identified on the luminal side of the capillary basement membranes. When injections of antigens were discontinued, most of these pathological changes gradually resolved.

In the rabbits developing chronic glomerulonephritis, the most consistent finding was that most of these animals (43 of 45) were in the equivalence zone when proteinuria developed. After each injection of antigen, free antigen-antibody complexes persisted in the circulation for several hours and then were replaced by an excess of antibody prior to the next daily injection. For each of the four foreign protein antigens administered, the incidence of chronic glomerulonephritis appeared to be *independent* of the amounts of antigen given. This finding is significant in view of the parallel situations that may exist in the case of chronic human glomerular injury with regard to various viral infections, infective endocarditis, or clinical situations such as schistosomiasis, trypanosomiasis or malaria.

In the initial Dixon studies none of the 37 rabbits failing to make detectable antibody developed kidney lesions in spite of continued injections over many months. It was also observed that the bovine antigens (BSA and BGG) were more effective in producing chronic glomerulonephritis than those of human origin (HSA and HGG). Twenty-nine percent of rabbits receiving BSA and 42 percent of those receiving BGG developed chronic glomerulonephritis, while only 9 and 16 percent respectively of the animals receiving HSA or HGG showed nephritis. Attempts to manipulate the immune response by administering x-ray or endotoxin with the first injection did not appear to alter the incidence of subsequent glomerulonephritis.

Morphological changes in rabbits developing subacute and chronic glomerulonephritis were remarkably similar to those seen in human lesions. The earliest finding was a diffuse amorphous thickening of the glomerular capillary basement membrane. Some of the alterations in chronic lesions resembled similar findings in human membranous nephropathy. The most common changes, however, were associated with lobulation of glomerular capillaries, inflammation, proliferation of glomerular epithelial and endothelial cells, and eventual scarring and obliteration of glomeruli. Thickened basement membrane structures showed strong immunofluorescent staining for specific antigen, host gamma globulin, and specific antibody. These granular immune deposits appeared to be independent of the kind of antigen injected and were related primarily to the degree of thickening of basement membranes; in no case were they present without concurrent basement membrane thickening. Glomerular capillaries in some animals showed both polymorphonuclear and mononuclear leukocytes containing granular antigen, presumably in complex form. The only extraglomerular antigen deposits observed in these chronic rabbits were fine deposits within walls of splenic arterioles.

When injections of antigen were discontinued in chronic nephritis rabbits, many showed what appeared to be irreversible renal damage. There was some corresponding reduction in the inflammatory reaction within glomeruli after injections had ceased, but membrane thickening and proliferative changes did not diminish within 5 to 6 months in any of these animals. Immunofluorescent monitoring of renal lesions, however, showed gradual disappearance of granular stainable antigens from previous glomerular distribution. These findings were confirmed in sequential electron microscopic observation.

Studies of acute and subsequent chronic glomerular injury using the serum sickness model have made it possible to extend many of the concepts covered in previous chapters. The acute serum sickness model of Cochrane and associates (241, 242) emphasized the importance of both complement and circulating polymorphonuclear leukocytes initiating microvascular foci of inflammation. Moreover, it appeared that the larger complexes of 19 S or above were more prone than smaller ones to deposit in vessels or glomeruli and induce tissue injury. The experimental model of "one-shot" serum sickness or its counterpart, chronic glomerulonephritis, by hyperimmunization with various materials in a number of experimental animals has become a standard technique for the investigation of immune-complex injury.

These classic studies emphasized a relationship between the size or quantitative amounts of antibody response in experimental animals and the occurrence of acute glomerulonephritis. Two-thirds of the experimental rabbits with early proteinuria were among the very best antibody responders, and the majority of animals developing acute glomerulonephritis made a large antibody response. At the time, these observations seemed to match the expectation that those rabbits with the largest quantitative antibody response would show the largest concentrations of circulating complexes, albeit for the shortest intervals of time. The experimental findings are paralleled by clinical data. For instance, those children who develop acute nephritis following streptococcal infection usually are individuals making large antibody responses to various streptococcal antigens (243, 244), much as in the serum sickness model.

Several theoretical difficulties still exist when we attempt to transcribe the events documented in Dixon's model of chronic glomerulonephritis (240) into the actual situation observed in the spectrum of human chronic glomerulonephritis. The foremost is obviously the source and nature of the antigens involved. This is a point that was obvious 18 years ago when the model was first developed, and it is still not completely resolved today. In the rabbit model exogenous antigen is repeatedly introduced during the development of the lesions, but in many human disease states accompanied by chronic immune deposition and apparent immune-complex glomerulonephritis, the precise antigens involved—whether exogenous or endogenous—have not yet been clearly defined. Also, the quantitative amounts of antigen involved in the glomerular immune-complex injury of chronic serum sickness are probably larger on a mg/kg of body weight basis than in many human conditions such as malaria, schistosomiasis, syphilis, infective endocarditis, or SLE. The most important aspect of the chronic serum sickness model for chronic glomerulonephritis was the demonstration that immune-complex injury could be produced by exogenous antigens such as BSA or BGG, which bore no antigenic similarity to and had no derivation from renal material. This finding alone shifted emphasis in the study of chronic or acute renal injury away from immune mechanisms involving autologous kidney antigens to the potential pathogenetic significance of immune complexes themselves. The acute and chronic serum sickness model produced a number of important observations: the acute form of the disease was associated with a hyperactive antibody response, whereas the subacute and chronic forms were accompanied by relatively poor antibody response. Complexes of antigen and antibody were shown to localize in the kidney without any apparent immunologic specificity, presumably as a result of anatomic or other physiological responses. Antigen-antibody complexes not specifically oriented against kidney appeared to be able to produce changes

quite similar to those associated with antikidney antiserum. Complexes themselves were capable of directly mediating tissue injury after localizing within the kidney.

Experimental models of acute and chronic serum sickness have been studied by a number of different groups as in vivo models of immune-complex–mediated reactions. Systemic involvement of several highly vascularized organs outside the kidney is also of general interest and closely resembles some of the vasculitis lesions associated with SLE. In this regard, one of the most common manifestations of SLE is polyserositis (245).

Recently Albini and co-workers (246) studied the induction of serum sickness in rabbits using BSA and prolonged intravenous administration as established in the original Dixon model (240), attempting to keep the ratio of antigen to antibody near equivalence in the circulation. Particular attention was directed at serous membranes of pleura, peritoneum, and pericardial surfaces. Serous effusions were specifically examined for the presence of complexes by the Raji-cell technique. In addition, changes in local vascular permeability were performed using fluorescein-conjugated dextrans of molecular weights 20,000, 70,000, and 150,000.

In the course of these studies serous effusions developed in 18 of 19 rabbits with acute serum sickness and in 28 of 39 animals with chronic disease. The serous membranes of serum sickness animals showed an increase in polymorphonuclear leukocytes (PMNs). Some vessels were obliterated by aggregates of PMNs, platelets, or fibrin. Electron microscopy revealed arteriolar or venular obstruction by neutrophils, basophils, and platelets. The capillary endothelium was swollen and had lost its contact with the basement membrane. Leukocytes and platelets showed extensive degranulation, and a large number of free granules were observed within the lumina of vessel walls or the perivascular tissues. In addition, electron-dense deposits were identified by electron microscopy between endothelium and basement membranes, particularly in the acute serum sickness model. Granular immunofluorescence localization of host IgG, C3, and

BSA antigen was frequently present within the peritoneal, pleural, and pericardial microvasculature. Examples of these findings are shown in Figure 13-21.

The deposits were noted most commonly at the entrance of anastomosing branches of glomerulus-like structures in the omentum and at vascular bifurcations in all of the serosal surfaces (Figure 13-22). Immune deposits were identified in vessels of pleura, pericardium, and peritoneum in 75 percent of rabbits with chronic serum sickness and serous exudates. Raji-cell tests for immune complexes in the rabbits with serous effusions were strongly positive. Of particular interest was the finding that development of serous effusions during BSA serum sickness was accompanied by increased vascular permeability which allowed 150,000-Dalton dextrans access to the effusions. The visceral and parietal serosal surfaces constitute semipermeable membranes probably involved in the normal process of filtration.

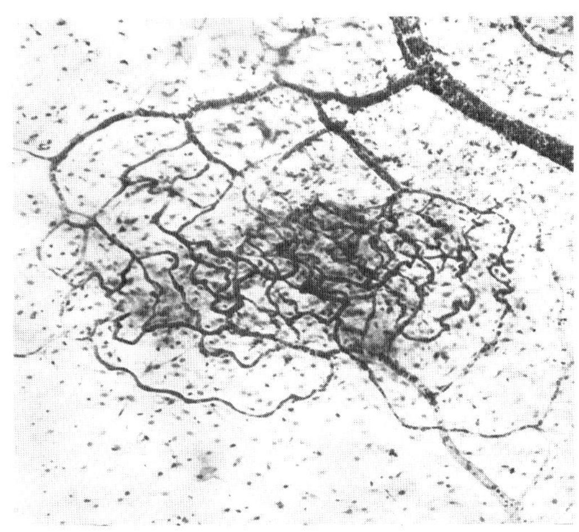

Figure 13-22 A rabbit with chronic serum sickness, showing an enlarged" glomerulus-like" structure in the peritoneum. Numerous cells are present in the loose connective tissue between the vascular anastomoses. H&E × 150. (Reproduced with permission, B. Albine, E. Ossi, and G. Andres, *Lab. Invest.* 37:64, 1977.)

Serosal fluid maintains a chemical and osmotic equilibrium with plasma and diffuses back out of the potential spaces into interstitial tissues and thence into lymphatics. Since inflammatory cells appeared to localize preferentially in vessels specifically involved in this filtration process, it seems possible that these particular sites within serosal surfaces represent a preferential target for immune-complex–mediated injury. Furthermore, the accumulation of neutrophils and platelets in vessels near serosal surfaces suggests that local release of potent vasoactive amines (247) may play a role in the accumulation of serous effusions during this process.

These observations are directly relevant to the polyserositis seen in many connective-tissue diseases such as SLE, rheumatoid arthritis, and mixed connective-tissue disorders. Active SLE may be associated with ascites (248), and in such patients granular deposits of IgG and C3 may be seen in peritoneal tissues obtained at laparotomy or autopsy. Pleural or pericardial fluids obtained from patients with active SLE may show a diminution in levels of early complement components (249–251), presumably reflecting the accumulation of complexes

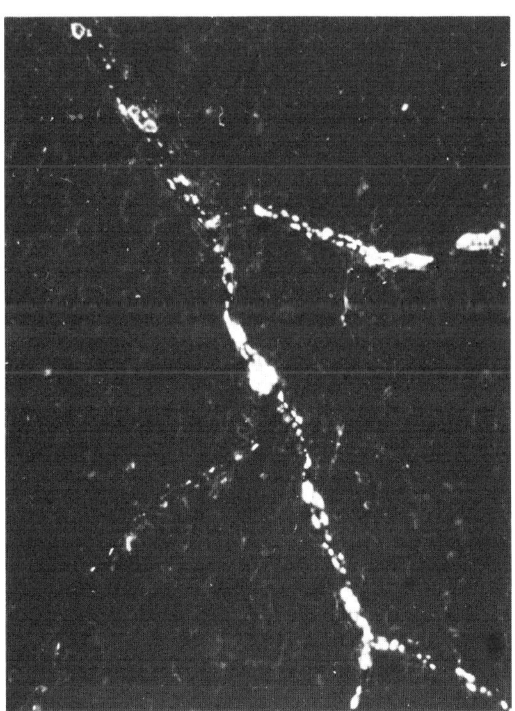

Figure 13-21 Granular deposits of IgG in the vessel walls in the pericardium of a rabbit. Magnification × 200. (Reproduced with permission, B. Albini, E. Ossi, and G. Andres, *Lab. Invest.* 37:64, 1977.)

in these materials. The Albini experiments (246) document several mechanisms involved in the serositis accompanying acute or chronic deposition of complexes near visceral surfaces. It seems likely that similar studies concentrating on the mechanics and sequence of immune-complex injury in other extrarenal sites during the induction of immune-complex deposition in the general serum sickness model will provide further insight into important local phenomena in other tissues.

Following establishment of the acute or chronic BSA serum sickness model, observers noted that the chronic lesions that developed in experimental animals could be classified as crescentic (240, 252, 254), membranous (240, 253), or mesangiopathic (254). The variety of morphological changes presumably ensuing from the single basic process of immune-complex deposition reflected similar, rather·disparate histological changes seen in the whole gamut of chronic human glomerular disease. These differences have been reexamined by Germuth and colleagues (255). Animals were immunized with two different regimes. One group received 12.5 mg of BSA per day throughout the immunization period, and the second group was given increasing doses of BSA in an attempt to parallel the immune response. In the first group of animals, marked differences were noted in the incidence of membranous lesions; 50 percent showed membranous changes, versus only 15 percent in the group given doses of BSA paralleling the immune response. Moreover, crescentic changes were noted in none of the animals receiving the fixed 12.5 mg per day dose, whereas 27 percent showed crescentic nephritis in the variable dosage regime. Mesangiopathic changes were noted in 31 percent of the latter group, in contrast to only 11 percent of the fixed-dosage animals. It was concluded that occurrence of membranous glomerulonephritis was favored by presence in the circulation of small concentrations of soluble complexes, whereas crescentic changes were more likely to occur with high concentrations of such immune-complex material. This study documents the influence of different quantitative amounts of complexes flooding glomerular structures either intermit-

tently or at a slow, steady state and determining the type of pathological changes that eventually ensue. Direct proof is needed, in which temporal fluctuations in the relative amounts of circulating complexes are measured by one or several of the current radioimmunoassays in conjunction with similar histological studies.

Glomerular Clearing Mechanisms

One of the critical features in the way the host handles immune complexes relates to the specific function of built-in clearing mechanisms. This feature becomes particularly important in studies of experimental models such as one-shot or multiple-dose serum sickness nephritis in rabbits or other experimental animals. In the kidney itself it appears that the mesangium functions as an extension of the conventional reticuloendothelial system, since it has the capacity to take up a wide variety of macromolecular materials (256–260). The localization and handling of materials of a size range corresponding to a broad spectrum of immune complexes reveals a substantial capacity within functioning mesangium to trap and eventually clear macromolecular materials entering the glomerulus. Moreover, evidence obtained largely from electron microscopic observations using various identifiable tracer molecules indicates that small proteins appear to be rapidly and completely filtered into the urinary space, while larger molecules may be held up at the epithelial slit pore or within the GBM itself (260). Very large molecules may proceed as far as the lamina rara interna, but most are excluded by the GBM from the subendothelial space entering the area of the glomerular mesangium (257, 261). After localization within the mesangial spaces, they are removed by mechanisms that are only poorly understood. Complement may not be required for mesangial or RES uptake of circulating IgG aggregates, since it has been demonstrated that antigen-antibody complexes may be eliminated from the circulating blood volume at a normal rate in complement-depleted animals (262). However, the removal of complexes from the circulation in vivo (262) and also the uptake of aggregated IgG by peritoneal macrophages in vitro (263) may be partially dependent on their abilities to activate the complement system. With respect to human disease states, corticosteroids appear to alter transit of macromolecules across vascular walls in experimental immune-complex disease (264).

One sidelight of the theoretical and pathological problems involved in disorders such as experimental serum sickness relates to the mechanism of glomerular hypercellularity induced during the development of immune-complex–mediated injury. The general term *proliferative glomerulonephritis* has often been applied to conditions where there appears to be an excess of cells within the glomerulus (265, 266). Larger numbers of mononuclear cells within the glomerulus could be derived from endothelial, mesangial, or infiltrating cells originating from outside of the kidney. This problem has recently been examined by Bradfield and Cattell (267), using the one-shot active immune-complex nephritis model in rabbits. It was found that most of the extra cells were mononuclear, with a few polymorphonuclear leukocytes. Glomerular mitoses were more common in hypercellular glomeruli, providing evidence of local proliferation. In addition, kidney biopsies taken an hour after administration of tritiated thymidine contained locally labeled cells. By electron microscopy both mesangial and endothelial cells were identified in mitosis; however, the origin of the majority of mononuclear cells in hypercellular glomeruli could not be identified. Glomerular infiltration by some cells of extraglomerular origin including macrophages, lymphocytes, and plasma cells was also noted.

A second experimental model was employed by this same group (268), using intravenous administration of Habu snake venom to induce focal glomerulonephritis in the rat (this particular venom causes mesangiolysis in rabbits and subsequent mesangial cell hypercellularity). Again by means of radiolabeling techniques, it was shown that the glomerular hypercellularity induced was caused by local proliferation of mesangial cells and that there was no evidence for origin of increased mononuclear cells in mesangium from bone marrow.

It would appear that the adaptive capacity of the mesangium may well determine how the kidney reacts to various types of immune-complex injury. In many of the clinical disorders we have discussed, immunofluorescent identification of immune-complex deposits has shown them to be largely mesangial, whereas in other diseases immune-complex deposition appears to be more peripheral and localized close to the GBMs. Unique features associated with various disorders must be clarified before we understand the precise mechanisms of mesangial processing and the factors that govern observed differences in immune-complex localization. One of the most important factors may well be unique differences in the localizing affinities of particular antigens involved in the complexes themselves. This has been emphasized by the work of Izui and colleagues (269), where a special affinity between DNA and GBM collagen was demonstrated. Such factors may well be as important in the glomerular localization of immune complexes as the capacity for the mesangium to process or keep up with clearing of loads of circulating material entering afferent glomerular arterioles.

Mesangial function per se in the development of various lesions associated with immune-complex disease is extremely important. The experiments of Michael and co-workers (260) utilized injection of ferritin-conjugated IgG aggregates into mice, and although mesangial localization was noted, there was no apparent glomerular injury. As noted above, Germuth and co-workers (264) demonstrated that immune complexes in the BSA serum sickness model could be deflected into the mesangium during cortisone administration but did not appear to produce tissue injury there. More recently, experiments by Mauer and associates (270) have shown that antigen-antibody reactions occurring in the mesangium can induce histological lesions similar to those seen in certain types of human glomerulonephritis associated with mesangial deposits. Kidneys with mesangial deposits of antigen were transplanted to recipients with circulating antibodies to the mesangial antigen. An acute inflammatory reaction was seen, which was followed by mesangial cell proliferation, mesangial matrix increase, and focal glomerular necrosis with PMN cell exudation.

Another study by Stilmant and colleagues (271) utilized immunization of mice with cadmium-free ferritin. After 5 to 8 weeks of immunization mice developed proteinuria and a proliferative glomerular lesion with considerable mesangial hypercellularity. Iron stains for the iron-binding ferritin protein showed prominent mesangial iron, and IgG as well as C3 were observed to be mainly localized within mesangial areas. Electron microscopy showed ferritin-containing immune complexes in what appeared to be an expanded mesangial matrix. Many of these changes resembled the histology associated with human membranoproliferative glomerulonephritis.

In the case of mesangial localization of immune complexes the rabbit chronic serum sickness model has demonstrated that animals with intermediate levels of antibody responsiveness form circulating complexes of approximately 1 $\times$ 10^6 Daltons in slight antibody excess, and that often such complexes localize within mesangial structures (254, 272). Complexes with similar properties may be formed in the case of IgM antibodies reacting with antigen or, in the case of IgG antibodies, reacting with relatively large antigens. Germuth and Rodriguez (272) observed mesangial hyperplasia and increased cellularity in association with mesangial immune-complex deposition, but clinical nephritis and proteinuria were present only when deposits extended to contiguous capillary loop structures. Although it is generally held that altered permeability of GBM in immune-complex glomerulonephritis is produced by glomerular deposition of complexes on GBMs, there is very little clear perception of precisely how such complexes pass from the circulation and are localized in these areas. The studies of the Stilmant group have been useful, since complexes were observed passing across the basement membrane and being arrested at the site of epithelial slit pores to form subepithelial electron-dense deposits. Continuation of such a process might be capable of accumulating masses of immune deposits sufficient to produce the subepithelial "humps" noted in a number of presumed immune-complex lesions. Further careful definition of the processes by which macromolecules such as complexes are handled within the glomerulus is necessary.

Autologous Immune-Complex Nephropathy

A model of experimental immune-complex nephritis originally developed by Heymann and associates (273) has been extensively studied by a number of groups. This particular animal model bears a striking resemblance to membranous glomerulonephritis in man, both in its immunofluorescent and ultrastructural features. The basic pathogenesis of lesions appears to involve induction of autoantibodies against renal antigens, which are normally present in the brush border of renal tubular cells (274–276). The tubular antigen has been characterized as a well-defined lipoprotein. It is thought to enter the circulation in small amounts and complex with host autoantibody to form immune aggregates, which then deposit in glomeruli (274). Complexes are subsequently detected as typical granular deposits of immunoglobulin and complement along the epithelial side of the GBM. The experimental animal model is often accompanied by heavy proteinuria similar to its possible human counterpart, membranous glomerulonephritis. If a comparable mechanism is involved in the generation of human membranous glomerulonephritis, it is still not clear what process induces the initial autoimmunization to tubular brush border antigens.

During the induction of autologous immune-complex Heymann's nephritis, definite changes occur in the permeability of the GBM. These have been studied by Schneeberger and associates (277), using enzymatic tracer molecules of known molecular weights as well as electron-opaque 500,000 M.W. ferritin. Previous studies had established considerable insight into the ultrastructural basis for protein filtration within the normal glomerulus. Most utilized tracer molecules of known molecular weight, which could be visualized directly in the electron microscope. Farquhar and co-workers (278) showed that the lamina densa of the GBM behaved as a filtration barrier for rather large protein molecules such as ferritin. Later work indicated that a second filtration barrier occurred at the region of the slit pore complex (279). Thus the glomerulus may be thought of as containing two serial filters: (1) the GBM, which acts as a coarse filter restricting large proteins; and (2) the slit pore complex, which acts as a fine filter restricting smaller proteins. Subsequent experiments have indicated that the slit diaphragm, which spans the space between epithelial foot processes, is actually a highly ordered isoporous structure (280). The actual central filament and adjacent cross bridges form rectangular pores measuring 50×150Å. The slit diaphragm of the glomerulus apparently represents the fine filtering mechanism for proteins and other macromolecules.

In the tracer studies reported by the Schneeberger group (277), direct evidence for increased glomerular permeability in the course of autologous immune-complex nephropathy was supported by the finding of permeability to larger proteins, ferritin, and catalase. By electron microscopic monitoring it was determined that increased permeability was present only in those regions of the glomerulus where immune deposits were also identified. Leukocytes or other extraneous cells did not appear to be involved in the increase in glomerular permeability. Direct apposition of immune-complex materials up to and including slit pore diaphragm structures provided evidence that such deposits altered functioning of this fine filter system as well, perhaps allowing passage of much larger proteins than those that were normally excluded. This distribution of early epimembranous complex deposits is now known to correspond to the localization of polyanionic glomerular sialoprotein on epithelial cells and in regions of filtration slits beneath slit pore diaphragms (281–283). Moreover, a number of recent ultrastructural and physiological studies have suggested that the negatively charged sialoproteins may be related to the permeability of circulating macromolecules (284–287).

This specific problem has recently been directly addressed in Heymann's autologous immune-complex–mediated nephritis through use of an ingenious experimental manipulation (288). Rats were rendered proteinuric by injection or unilateral renal perfusion with the aminonucleoside of puromycin before they developed immune-complex deposition following immunization with proximal tubular antigen to induce autologous immune-complex nephropathy. Control animals immunized with renal tubular antigens alone developed the usual diffuse granular deposits of IgG and tubular antigen on the subepithelial surface of the GBM. In sharp contrast, it was found that rats already nephrotic from the aminonucleoside developed few or no GBM deposits and that a significant increase in mesangial localization of IgG and tubular antigen occurred. This dramatic alteration in immune-complex localization was documented both in rats with aminonucleoside nephrosis and in unilaterally nephrotic kidneys that appeared to exclude any generalized effect of the aminonucleoside administration on the underlying basic immune process of Heymann's autoimmune nephritis. Absence of glomerular basement membrane localization of immune deposits correlated closely with reduced staining for the polyanionic glomerular sialoprotein in nephrotic kidneys. Thus, aminonucleoside-perfused kidneys studied several weeks after resolution of proteinuria demonstrated return of normal sialoprotein and subsequent development of subepithelial immune-complex deposits.

These studies emphasize that basic properties of the glomerulus itself appear to determine localization of immune-complex deposition. It seems unlikely that changes of built-in receptors for immune complexes such as the C3b receptor described by Gelfand and others (289, 290) play a role in this sequence of events, since such receptors have not been demonstrated in the rat and subepithelial deposits are noted experimentally before localization of complement. The most likely interpretation of the data presented by Couser and co-workers (288) is that aminonucleoside alternations in the electrophysical properties of the capillary wall reduce the affinity of complexes for the GBM, and shunting inward to the mesangial system occurs. There is a large body of evidence favoring a relationship between reduction of glomerular polyanion and onset of proteinuria and aminonucleoside nephrosis (283). Histochemical and ultrastructural studies also have indicated that the major sites of negative charge are located on the subepithelial site of the glomerulus (281–283). Furthermore, studies by Rennke and associates (291) have shown that neutral and anionic ferritin molecules do not penetrate normal GBM, but that negatively charged ferritin molecules of the same size reach the subepithelial surface and accumulate as aggregates in filtration slits very similar to the early deposits in Heymann's nephritis. Other highly charged macromolecules such as heparin-protamine polyelectrolyte complexes seem to localize in the subepithelial space and near slit pores (292, 293).

These experimental results suggest that the charge of glomerular capillary walls may be an important determinant in some instances of subepithelial complex localization. Subepithelial deposits have been demonstrated in a broad variety of human diseases associated with a number of different immune complexes including SLE (294), hepatitis B antigen (295), tumor antigens (296), and membranous nephritis (297). The elegant studies of glomerular permeability cited above have been extended by Schneeberger and Grupe (298), again using Heymann's autologous immune-complex model. Changes in the slit diaphragm and glomerular epithelium areas of rats with autologous nephritis were examined by electron microscopy after fixation with tannic acid –glutaraldehyde. Displacement of epithelial foot processes by immune-complex deposits and associated slit diaphragms toward the urinary space were present. After onset of proteinuria associated with autologous immune-complex deposition, the epithelial foot processes were observed to spread, so that there was a net decrease in epithelial-cell surface area and a diminution in length of the interepithelial slits. The redundant slit diaphragm area became pleated in the remaining interepithelial spaces. No primary ultrastructural defect within the slit diaphragm was observed

that would account for the severe proteinuria. Instead, areas of detached epithelial cells and an occasional slit pore lacking a slit diaphragm were felt to represent probable sites for protein loss into the urinary spaces. Although the exact process by which glomerular protein loss occurs in this disease model is not yet fully understood, many factors that bear directly on the problem have been elucidated.

Masugi Nephritis

The experimental production of nephritis using heterologous antiserum to kidney was first extensively developed by Masugi in 1934 (299). Administration of antikidney antibody produced in another species was followed by fixation of antibody to renal structures (including glomeruli and portions of renal tubules) and subsequent fixation of host gamma globulin and complement in similar distribution later in the development of lesions in association with proteinuria. Masugi nephritis can be induced in rats by a single intravenous injection of rabbit antirat kidney serum. In such animals the proteinuria then occurs in two phases. The early or heterologous phase, which includes the first 24 hours, is associated with binding of heterologous rabbit antibody to the GBM; the late or delayed autologous phase of proteinuria, beginning after several days, is associated with induction of autologous rat antibody fixed to the rat glomerular capillaries. The pattern of fixation of heterologous antibody to rat glomeruli usually shows linear deposition of IgG along GBM very much like that associated with Goodpasture's syndrome in the human. During the heterologous phase glomerular IgG binding occurs as the result of fixation of the hetero-antirat kidney antibody within glomeruli, whereas in the second reactive phase the IgG fixed to the glomerulus is eventually derived from the host (300–302).

One of the most interesting features of the disease is its persistence, often with progression of the autologous nephritis phase long after the original injection of antikidney antiserum. Some of the first studies on the initial behavior of the heterologous antikidney antibody were presented by Sarre and Wirtz (303), who demonstrated that duration of the original antikidney antibody within the circulation was very short in spite of the subsequent development of chronic nephritis. Later radio-labeling experiments by Pressman (304) established interaction of the heterologous antibody with renal and nonrenal tissues and provided direct evidence for its persistence in renal tissues. In rabbits the heterologous phase of Masugi nephritis depends on the amount of antikidney antibody actually fixing to tissues. Much of the early experimental work in this species employed duck antibody to rabbit kidney. This model has raised some interesting basic questions about the role of complement activation in the progress of the disease, since avian antibodies are relatively deficient in their ability to activate the complement sequence.

Pathologic studies of the glomerulus show impressive immunofluorescence and ultrastructural evidence of fixation of nephrotoxic heterologous antibody to glomeruli. An example of such lesions may be seen in Figure 13-23. The initial lesion appears to be on the luminal side of the basement membrane where irregular electron-dense deposits are seen to accumulate. These early changes are slightly different from those associated with other forms of immune-complex renal disease, where deposits often are noted on the epithelial side of the glomerular capillary. Subsequent subacute and chronic changes that occur in the experimental animals show some variation depending on the species used. Rabbits, dogs, and sheep appear to develop proliferative glomerular injury.

There is still some uncertainty about the role of complement in the final immunologic glomerular damage after injection of the nephrotoxic serum. Much of the earlier work done with nephrotoxic antibodies used rabbit, sheep, or duck nephrotoxic serum. Quite early in the course of experimental work it was noted that in kidneys perfused in vitro with rabbit nephrotoxic antibody, a drop was noted in the complement activity of the renal perfusate, whereas if duck nephrotoxic serum was utilized, no such diminution in complement activity occurred (305). Quantitative complement-fixation tests showed little actual fixation of guinea pig complement by duck nephro-

toxic serum and rat kidney antigens (306). On the other hand, rabbit nephrotoxic antibodies and kidney antigens can be readily shown to fix complement.

There does not appear to be a distinct correlation between the complement-fixing ability of such sera and their nephrotoxic effects in vivo (307, 308). Direct proof that in vivo complement fixation may occur in some forms of nephrotoxic nephritis has been obtained by in vitro fixation of complement in which frozen sections of kidney from an animal previously injected with nephrotoxic serum were exposed to fresh heterologous serum, and subsequently to fluorescent antiserum to complement proteins of the heterologous species (309). A second approach has generally employed staining of sections of nephritic kidneys with fluorescent antisera to complement proteins (310, 311). Experimental results in a number of laboratories have shown that rats injected with rabbit nephrotoxic serum or rabbits injected with sheep antibody show immediate in vivo localization of complement along glomerular capillary walls in a pattern identical to that exhibited by the gamma-globulin distribution of the nephrotoxic antibody. However, no in vivo fixation of complement was seen when nephrotoxic duck antisera were given to rats (306). When rats were decomplemented by various methods, subsequent injection of rabbit nephrotoxic antibody failed to induce proteinuria (310), which was noted during the second or autologous phase of the disease. Rats made immunologically tolerant to rabbit γ-globulin, and decomplemented prior to injection of moderate doses of nephrotoxic rabbit antibody, never developed proteinuria (310).

Subsequent work using this interesting model showed that complement mediated some of the acute immunologic injury in nephrotoxic nephritis by inducing chemotaxis of PMN leukocytes into the glomeruli (311). The number of PMNs infiltrating glomeruli was proportional to the amount of nephrotoxic antibody injected and presumably to the amount of locally activated complement. It appeared that the acute transitory phase characterized by glomerular accumulation of

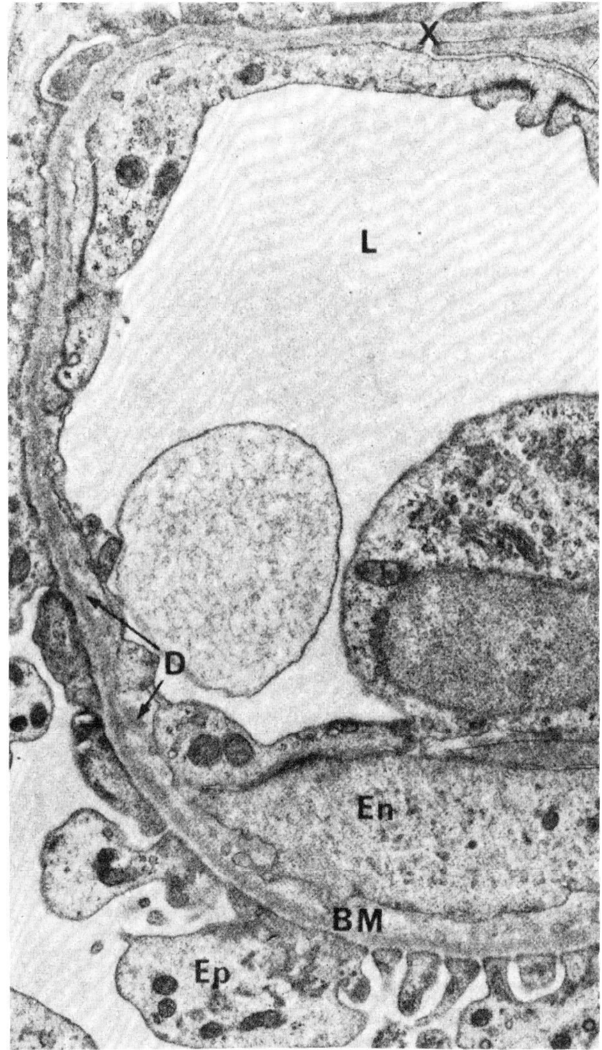

Figure 13-23 Electron micrograph of the glomerular capillary of a rat with nephrotoxic nephritis sacrificed 3 days after injection of rabbit NTAb. The basement membrane is thickened and shows an irregular deposit (D) along its luminal side. An area of normal-appearing basement membrane is shown at X. The endothelial cytoplasm is swollen, the epithelial foot processes are broad. BM = basement membrane; En = endothelial cell; Ep = epithelial cell; L = lumen. Magnification × 6,000. (Reproduced with permission, E. R. Unanue and F. J. Dixon, *Adv. Immunol.* 6:1, 1967.)

PMNs was essential for glomerular injury; extreme depletion of PMNs before injection of nephrotoxic serum prevented the onset of proteinuria despite the glomerular fixation of complement and nephrotoxic antibody. Large doses of nephrotoxic antibody in rats depleted of PMNs induced proteinuria, though in much lesser amounts than when normal levels of PMNs were present. The additional observations that duck nephrotoxic nephritis can be induced in rats without detectable participation of either PMNs or complement indicates that other mediators may be capable of causing glomerular injury in this system. The exact way in which such avian antibodies are capable of inducing glomerular damage, apparently without active PMN infiltration or complement activation, is still under study.

During the two phases of this experimental disease, proteinuria is felt to be related to increased permeability of the glomerular basement membrane. Studies by Gang and colleagues (312, 313) have focused on the chemical, morphological, and functional changes in GBM during the evolution of nephrotoxic nephritis. These investigations showed that degree of proteinuria was quantitatively related to loss of lipid phosphorus from GBM as well as to degree of thickening of the membrane in association with the deposit of first heterologous and second autologous host antibody. The proteinuria itself was first related to loss of lipid phosphorus in the membrane and later accentuated by influx of inflammatory cells (313). Glomerular basement membrane injury can be correlated with excretion of antigens related to GBM in the urine. Gross changes in the ultrastructure of the GBM have not been demonstrated during this process; however, use of lanthanum hydroxide tracers (a small colloidal particle <20 Å) showed considerable segments of the membrane (600 to 1,000 Å in length) in which the entire width appeared to be filled with these small colloidal particles (314). This type of ultrastructural change was correlated in its timing to onset of urinary excretion of GBM-like protein and the beginning of frank proteinuria.

In summary, three useful models for understanding immune-complex renal disease have been discussed: (1) serum sickness; (2) the autologous immune nephritis induced by immunization with whole kidney or purified brush border antigens; and (3) the Masugi nephrotoxic serum model. Each of these systems has produced a vast amount of detailed information that is outside the scope of this volume. It is hoped, however, that new models or adaptations of experimental protocols already in existence may provide increasing insight into the diverse number of human conditions that involve antigen-antibody reactions and therefore, eventually, immune complexes.

New Models of Possible Relevance

Inflammatory Bowel Disease

The precise association between the presence of immune complexes and actual tissue lesions in a number of clinical conditions has not yet been completely defined. It is well established, for instance, that circulating immune complexes are detectable in sera from patients with inflammatory bowel disease, including both regional enteritis and ulcerative colitis (315–318). The presence of complexes detectable by various tests also appears to bear some clinical relation to occurrence of extraintestinal manifestations such as iritis, arthritis, or erythema nodosum (315). It is not clear whether the presence of circulating complexes in these conditions is somehow a primary event or whether they arise from the extensive denudation of the mucosal surfaces associated with severe bowel involvement.

Recently Hodgson and colleagues (319) have developed an interesting animal model that may shed light on this question. An experimental colitis in rabbits was observed after intravenous injection of preformed immune complexes made from human serum albumin and anti-HSA. Injections were given to unsensitized rabbits. Prior irritation of tissue was initiated by rectal instillation of dilute formalin solutions. The formalin irritant alone produced transient changes that reverted to normal within 24 hours, but in rabbits given intravenous immune complexes formed in antigen excess, a severe colitis developed. Histological features of these lesions, shown in Figure 13-24, included mucosal ulceration, mixed inflammatory cell infiltrations of lamina propria, and crypt abscess formation. Many of the histological changes noted were felt to be compatible with immune-complex–mediated phenomena, including perivascular edema and infiltration by polymorphonuclear cells. Administration of complexes without prior irritation of the colon, however, produced no detectable lesions.

Several other previously studied models of experimental colitis in animals may have been partially dependent on immune-complex phenomena. Goldgraber and Kirsner (320) were able to induce severe local inflammatory changes associated with necrosis by mucosal injections of egg albumin into rabbits previously sensitized to the same antigen. A second model developed by Kraft and co-workers (321) involved prior sensitization of rabbits to egg albumin antigen and mild colonic inflammation,

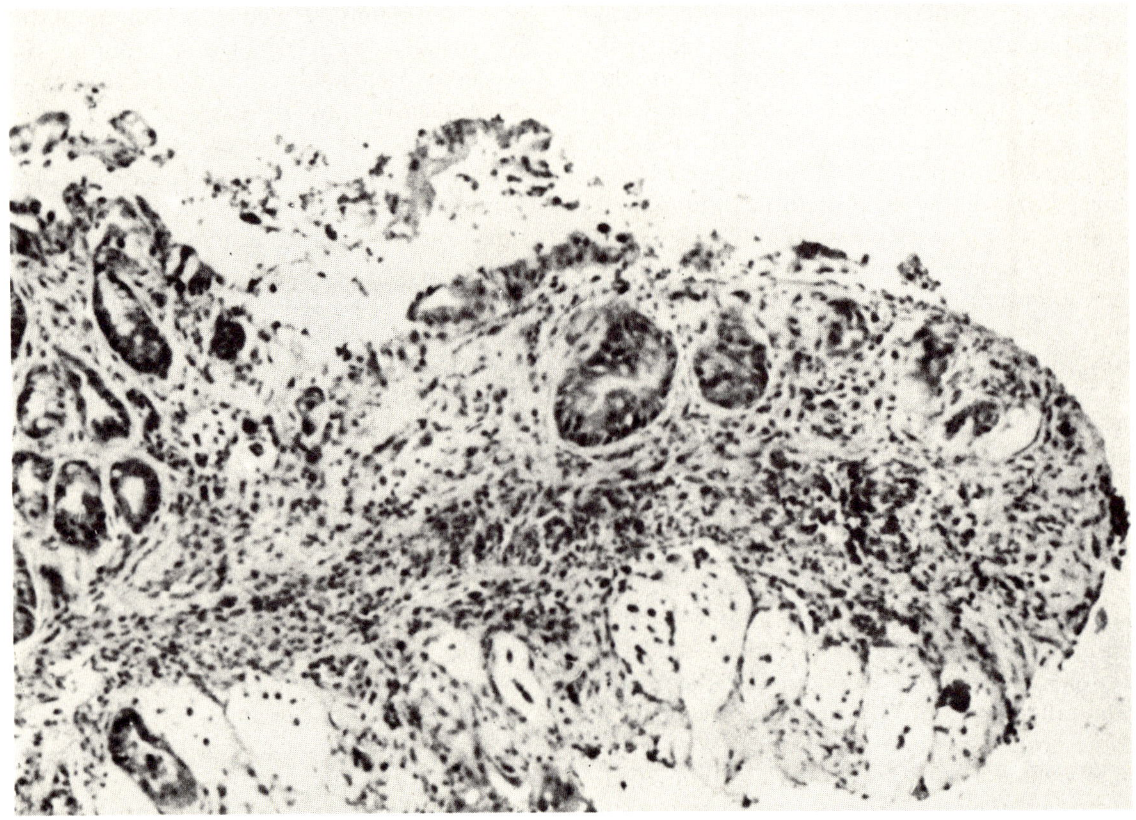

Figure 13-24   Rabbit rectal biopsy 22 hours after injection of antigen-antibody complexes. There is mucosal ulceration, loss of goblet cells from the glands, and inflammation throughout the lamina propria. H&E × 176. (Reproduced with permission, H. J. F. Hodgson, B. J. Potter, J. Skinner et al., *Gut* 19:225, 1978.)

again with dilute formalin solutions. Intravenous injections of egg albumin led to subsequent mucosal edema and ulceration, along with perivascular round-cell infiltration and a mixed cellular inflammatory response. Specific antigen was observed within the affected areas. It seems unlikely that human inflammatory bowel disease or ulcerative colitis is caused only by activation of immune complexes. A number of alternative possibilities including both cell-mediated and cross-reactive antibody mechanisms have been implicated at various times in direct pathogenesis (322, 323). Of late there has been increased attention to the possibility that an infectious agent may be involved (324). All of these animal models require some sort of prior or concomitant irritative process in the gut before immune-complex localization can augment or potentiate the process.

Chronic Liver Disease and Disturbances of Portal-Systemic Circulation

A number of observations support the possible relevance of circulating immune complexes in various types of chronic liver disease. In the case of hepatitis B viral infection, viral antigens are directly demonstrable (325, 326). Studies by Thomas and associates (327) document the prevalence of circulating complexes in sera from both hepatitis A and hepatitis B patients. In chronic active hepatitis and in alcoholic liver disease there appeared to be a significant correlation between C1q binding and the severity of hepatitis. Of particular interest were the findings of elevation of circulating complexes in patients with primary biliary cirrhosis. Inasmuch as the primary pathology occurs in the liver itself, the finding of a broad spectrum of immune complexes of varying size and undoubtedly differing constitution raises the important possibility that one of the central clearing mechanisms—namely the large bed of fixed macrophages, Kupffer cells, and splenic monocytes—is deranged secondary to the primary hepatic pathology.

An interesting series of experiments relating directly to this problem has been reported by van Marck and colleagues (328). Portosystemic collateral circulation was implemented in mice infected with *Schistosoma mansoni* by partial ligation of the portal vein. This experimental intervention was used to compare immune glomerular deposits to unoperated infected, sham-operated, and normal mice. Extensive mesangial immune deposits of IgM, IgA, IgG, and C3 were detected via immunofluorescence techniques, more frequently in operated than in unoperated infected mice. Schistosomal antigen within immune deposits appeared more frequently in infected animals who had undergone partial portal-vein obstruction. An interesting sidelight was the high percentage of glomerular immune-complex deposits (71 percent) found in uninfected mice that had undergone portal-vein ligation. These results suggest an influence on the prevalence of glomerular deposits of portal draining venules proceeding from the gastrointestinal tract.

In this model, after partial portal-vein occlusion, functioning collaterals linking the portomesenteric and caval system increased, as documented by much higher schistosomal egg counts in the lungs of operated and infected animals. Since clearance of immune complexes appears to occur predominantly in hepatic Kupffer cells (329), it might be expected that in a chronic disorder such as schistosomiasis, antigens released within the portal venous radicles might in the presence of portal obstruction bypass the Kupffer cell system and be free to participate in glomerular immune-complex deposition. The presence of a remarkable increase in glomerular immune-complex deposits in uninfected operated animals with subsequent portal bed obstruction came as a distinct surprise, and might be interpreted to indicate that many intestinal antigens beside those associated with schistosomal infection can be shunted into the systemic circulation and induce glomerular immune-complex injury. This experimental approach obviously should now be correlated with direct measurement of levels of detectable complexes in experimental animals before and after portal-vein occlusion. It also raises some fundamental questions about the high prevalence of detectable circulating complexes in any heterogeneous group of patients with liver disease (327), since the levels of complexes may merely reflect portal-systemic shunting. Common clinical conditions in which circulating complexes have now been detected also include prominent liver involvement either by well-defined microfoci of granulomata (as in sarcoidosis or lepromatous leprosy) or massive reticuloendothelial system activation, such as must be the case in infective endocarditis or malaria. The observation of circulating complexes in many of these states may merely reflect saturation of the usual handling and processing depots within such primary organs as the liver and spleen. This view emphasizes the real need for a useful, workable assay of immune-complex handling such as labeled C1q turnover or similar methods now being explored in a number of laboratories.

Direct Therapeutic Attempts to Influence Immune-Complex Deposition

Any rational consideration of this important area might lead to the immediate conclusion that the most effective way to stop immune-complex deposition is of course to remove the antigen completely from the host. Such a solution is indeed possible when the infecting organism is eliminated with antibiotics in situations like infective endocarditis or shunt nephritis. Unfortunately, in many clinical conditions either the antigen is unknown or it has been identified as being related somehow to autologous tissues. Antigen-specific plasmaphersis or immunoadsorbent columns might also provide a direct approach to ridding the host of offending antigens when these have been well characterized and appear to be the agents responsible for ongoing immune-complex injury.

Modifications of the Coagulation System

From time to time a certain degree of enthusiasm seems to arise for various forms of anticoagulation in the modification of what is presumed, on the basis of immune mediated mechanisms, to be ongoing renal injury. There are very few hard data to suggest that various forms of anticoagulation employed in experimental models of glomerulonephritis significantly affect the outcome of pathological lesions. Border and associates (330) studied chronic serum sickness induced in rabbits by daily injections of BSA as well as antiglomerular basement membrane nephritis induced by intravenous injection of known amounts of heterologous anti-GBM antibody. Heparin administration was begun 2 to 6 weeks after the start of BSA injections or before the administration of heterologous anti-GBM antibody. In this carefully designed study no significant differences were observed in proteinuria, severity of glomerular lesions, or immunofluorescent patterns of immunoglobulin or fibrinogen-related antigens in anticoagulated and control animals. Heparin in the maximum permissible doses did alter the progression of several forms of experimental immune-complex nephritis.

Humphrey and Jaques (331) were the first to observe in 1955 that antigen-antibody complexes unrelated to platelet antigens were associated with platelet aggregation and release of factors such as histamine and serotonin. It has subsequently become clear that many factors released from platelets, including platelet permeability factors and an assortment of vasoactive amines, can theoretically facilitate immune-complex deposition and subsequent microvascular inflammation. Later, in 1968, Kniker and Cochrane (332) showed that in BSA serum sickness nephritis, prior platelet depletion using specific platelet antisera or inhibition of platelets by potent inhibitors of platelet vasoactive amines markedly reduced vascular inflammation and immune-complex deposition. There is also some evidence that platelet localization may in fact be correlated with differences in renal pathology (333). Such features of platelet localization could contribute through a number of mechanisms to chronic, slowly progressive glomerular scarring in many conditions. Studies by Clark and co-workers (334) have demonstrated signifi-

cant decreases in intracellular platelet serotonin concentrations in patients with active SLE and biopsy-proven glomerulonephritis.

A number of attempts to detect fibrin or fibrinogen-related materials within renal biopsy or autopsy material have suggested that the coagulation process may be a primary mediator in immunologic renal disease. However, convincing evidence for a primary role of the coagulation process per se in mediation of tissue damage appears to be lacking. Direct turnover studies of platelets, fibrinogen, and plasminogen indicate that the major homeostatic abnormality in a variety of renal diseases is platelet consumption (335).

Studies by Bolton and co-workers (336) indicated that administration of cyproheptadine, an agent with antihistamine and antiserotonin properties, delayed onset and degree of proteinuria in autologous Heymann's type nephritis in rats. A typical result recorded in this study is shown in Figure 13-25. Although the use of this potent antagonist of serotonin and histamine appeared to alter the course of immune-complex deposition, it did not abolish or completely reverse the natural features of the disorder. In view of the therapeutic failures using other regimes like combinations of immunosuppressive agents (337, 338), it appears worthwhile to seek further for drugs capable of modulating the peripheral effects of immune-complex phenomena such as antiserotonins, antihistamines and antiplatelet permeability factors.

Other Experimental Manipulations

A number of references have been made in earlier sections to the fact that in both SLE and its natural animal model, the NZB/W mouse, a basic imbalance appears to exist between control and feedback modulation of humoral and cellular immunity. Beside numerous combinations of immunosuppressive regimes (which will not be discussed here), several imaginative approaches have recently been proposed. Krakauer and colleagues (339) treated mice prospectively with soluble lymphocyte supernates (termed SIRS) produced by activation of normal mouse lymphocytes by plant mitogens such as concanavalin A. These experiments

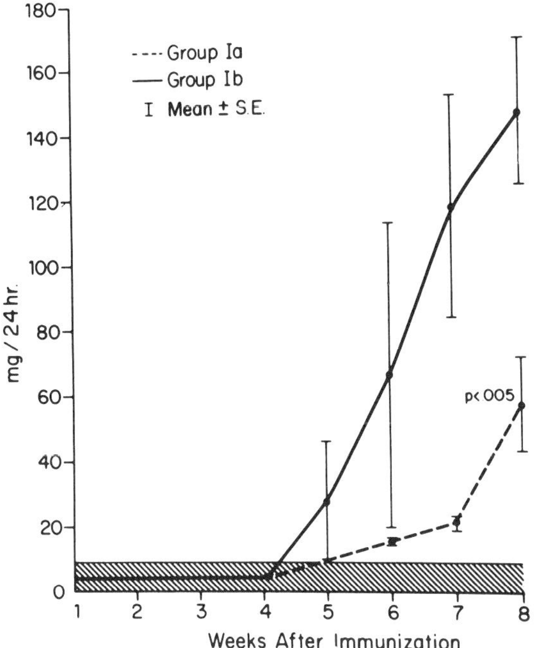

Figure 13-25 Proteinuria in experimental immune-complex glomerulonephritis. The amount of proteinuria excreted by animals who became proteinuric at each weekly interval is noted to be significantly less in animals treated with antihistamine, antiserotonin agent (group Ia) than in the controls (group Ib). (Reproduced with permission, W. K. Bolton, B. A. Spargo, and E. J. Lewis, *J. Lab. Clin. Med.* 83:695, 1974.)

were devised with the idea that lymphocyte-derived factors—particularly those obtained from T cells—might be broadly deficient in the disease and that restoration of normal T-cell–B-cell modulation might be achieved by administration of a heterogeneous spectrum of such factors in a sort of "lymphokine soup" to NZB or NZB/W mice before the sixth to eighth week of life, when the inexorable progression of the disease begins. Initial results with this regime have been dramatic, with virtual abolition of many of the peripheral immune-complex–mediated phenomena during the natural course of the disease. An example of results from this study is shown in Table 13-4. Much more precise analysis of the events involved in this fascinating model are needed before any final evaluation of the prospect for similar treatment of human disease is possible.

Another ingenious approach that has produced some striking changes in the natural course of NZB/W mouse lupus has been directed at rendering animals tolerant to DNA before the temporal onset of the disease itself (340, 341). This work has indicated that induction of tolerance to at least one of the antigens involved in the progressive immune-complex glomerulonephritis in NZB/W mice can markedly alter the incidence of subsequent natural occurrence of the nephritis. Again, whether application to the human state is feasible or practical remains to be seen. In this particular model advantage was taken of the massive body of evidence implicating DNA–anti-DNA complexes as one of the fundamental processes in glomerular immune-complex injury. Animals were rendered tolerant using nucleic acids or other nuclear antigens fixed to isologous carrier proteins derived from the same species. Immediate application of similar approaches to other human conditions must await precise identification of the antigens involved. This point has been repeatedly emphasized in other parts of this book; relevance, for instance, to the problem of "blocking" immune complexes in various types of cancer or parasitic infection is obvious.

A number of experimental models have been devised to investigate the effects of immune complexes on both immune cells and cell interactions in vitro as well as experimental animals in vivo. Although a great deal of primary insight into basic mechanisms has emerged, a number of vague areas still require clarification and amplification. In particular, more precise insight into the mechanisms governing local immune-complex disposal and degradation of immune complexes lodged in various microcirculatory beds needs to be developed. It is not yet clear whether ancillary factors, such as lymphokines or vasoactive amines released by activated immune cells, alter the local disposal mechanisms for immune complexes. It is possible that receptors for materials intrinsic to immune complexes (Fc receptors or C3b receptors) may be modulated by extracellular products of various bacteria—or even by materials released locally by inflammatory cells in sites of tissue injury.

Table 13-4 Effects of treatment with soluble lymphocyte supernates (SIRS) on renal pathology (graded 0 to 4+) encountered in individual NZB/W mice at different time points after initiation of SIRS treatment at 4 weeks of age.

	Renal pathology in mice of age (weeks)—				
Preparation	10	16	22	28	34
BALB/c SIRS	+ [a]	+	0	+ +	+
	+	0	0	0	0
	0		+	0	0
Young (4-week) NZB/W SIRS	+	+	+	+	0
	+	+	0	+	+
	+	+	+	+	+
Control preparation[b]	+ +	+ +	+ +	+ + +	+ + + +
	+ +	+ +	+ +	+ + +	+ + +
	+	+ +	+ + +	+ + +	+ + +
Untreated	+	+ +	+ +	+ + + +	+ + + +
	+ +	+	+ + +	+ + +	+ + +
	+	+ +	+ +	+ + +	+ + + +

Source: Reproduced with permission, R. S. Krakauer, W. Strober, D. L. Rippeon, et al., *Science* 196:56, 1977.

[a] 0 to + + + + refers to grading of severity of renal pathology.

[b] Supernatant fluid obtained from BALB/c spleen cells exposed to concanavalin A for several minutes.

References

1. Möller, G. Induction of DNA synthesis in normal human lymphocyte cultures by antigen-antibody complexes. *Clin. Exp. Immunol.* 4:65, 1969.

2. Bloch-Shtacher, N., Hirschhorn, K., and Uhr, J. W. The response of lymphocytes from non-immunized humans to antigen-antibody complexes. *Clin. Exp. Immunol.* 3:889, 1968.

3. Soderberg, L. S. F., and Coons, A. H. Complement-dependent stimulation of normal lymphocytes by immune complexes. *J. Immunol.* 120:806, 1978.

4. Terres, G., Morrison, S. L., Habicht, G. S., et al. Appearance of an early "primed state" in mice following the concomitant injections of antigen and specific antiserum. *J. Immunol.* 108:1473, 1972.

5. Ryan, J. L., Arbeit, R. D., Dickler, H. B., et al. Inhibition of lymphocyte mitogenesis by immobilized antigen-antibody complexes. *J. Exp. Med.* 142:814, 1975.

6. Wahl, S. M., Iverson, G. M., and Oppenheim, J. J. Induction of guinea pig B-cell lymphokine synthesis by mitogenic and nonmitogenic signals to Fc, Ig, and C3 receptors. *J. Exp. Med.* 140:1631, 1974.

7. Sundsmo, J. S., Kolb, W. P., and Müller-Eberhard, H. J. Leukocyte complement: neoantigens of the membrane attack complex on the surface of human leukocytes prepared from defibrinated blood. *J. Immunol.* 120:850, 1978.

8. Sundsmo, J. S., Curd, J. G., Kolb, W. P., et al. Leukocyte complement: assembly of the membrane attack complex by human peripheral blood leukocytes in the presence and absence of serum. *J. Immunol.* 120:855, 1978.

9. Theofilopoulos, A. N., Dixon, F. J., and Bokisch, V. A. Binding of soluble immune complexes to human lymphoblastoid cells. I. Characterization of receptors for IgG, Fc and complement and description of the binding mechanism. *J. Exp. Med.* 140:877, 1974.

10. Ross, G. D., and Polley, M. J. Specificity of human lymphocyte complement receptors. *J. Exp. Med.* 141:1163, 1975.

11. Dukor, P., Schumann, G., Gisler, R. H., et al. Complement-dependent B-cell activation by cobra venom factor and other mitogens? *J. Exp. Med.* 139:337, 1974.

12. Hartmann, K. U., and Bokisch, V. A. Stimulation of murine B lymphocytes by isolated C3b. *J. Exp. Med.* 142:600, 1975.

13. Möller, G., and Coutinho, A. Role of C′3

and Fc receptors in B-lymphocyte activation. *J. Exp. Med.* 141:647, 1975.

14. Weigle, W. O. Cyclical production of antibody as a regulatory mechanism in the immune response. *Adv. Immunol.* 21:87, 1975.

15. Baldwin, R. W., Price, M. R., and Robins, R. A. Blocking of lymphocyte-mediated cytotoxicity for rat hepatoma cells by tumor-specific antigen-antibody complexes. *Nature* 238:185, 1972.

16. Sjögren, H. O., Hellström, I., Bansal, S. C., et al. Suggestive evidence that the 'blocking antibodies' of tumor-bearing individuals may be antigen-antibody complexes. *Proc. Natl. Acad. Sci. USA* 68:1372, 1971.

17. Stuart, F. P., Saitoh, T., and Fitch, F. W. Rejection of renal allografts: specific immunologic suppression. *Science* 160:1463, 1968.

18. Voisin, G. A., Kinsky, R. G., and Duc, H. T. Immune status of mice tolerant of living cells. II. Continuous presence and nature of facilitation-enhancing antibodies in tolerant animals. *J. Exp. Med.* 135:1185, 1972.

19. Wright, P. W., Hargreaves, R. E., Bansal, S. C., et al. Allograft tolerance: presumptive evidence that serum factors from tolerant animals that block lymphocyte-mediated immunity *in vitro* are soluble antigen-antibody complexes. *Proc. Natl. Acad. Sci. USA* 70:2539, 1973.

20. Halliday, W. J., and Walters, B. A. The mechanism of tolerance in contact hypersensitivity to dinitrochlorobenzene in guinea-pigs. *Clin. Exp. Immunol.* 16:203, 1974.

21. Sinclair, N. R., Lees, R. K., Abrahams, S., et al. Regulation of the immune response. X. Antigen-antibody complex inactivation of cells involved in adoptive transfer. *J. Immunol.* 113:1493, 1974.

22. Clagett, J. A., Wilson, C. B., and Weigle, W. O. Interstitial immune complex thyroiditis in mice: the role of autoantibody to thyroglobulin. *J. Exp. Med.* 140:1439, 1974.

23. Clagett, J. A., and Weigle, W. O. Roles of T and B lymphocytes in the termination of unresponsiveness to autologous thyroglobulin in mice. *J. Exp. Med.* 139:643, 1974.

24. Nakamura, R. M., and Weigle, W. O. Transfer of experimental autoimmune thyroiditis by serum from thyroidectomized donors. *J. Exp. Med.* 130:263, 1969.

25. Käresen, R., and Godal, T. Induction of thyroiditis in guinea-pigs by intravenous injection of rabbit anti-guinea-pig thyroglobulin serum. I. Light microscopic study. *Immunology* 17:847, 1969.

26. Käresen, R., and Godal, T. Induction of thyroiditis in guinea-pigs by intravenous injection of rabbit anti-guinea-pig thyroglobulin serum. II. Studies with fluorescent antibody technique. *Immunology* 17:863, 1969.

27. Vladutiu, A. O., and Rose, N. R. Transfer of experimental autoimmune thyroiditis of the mouse by serum. *J. Immunol.* 106:1139, 1971.

28. Clinton, B. A., and Weigle, W. O. Cellular events during the induction of experimental thyroiditis in the rabbit. *J. Exp. Med.* 136:1605, 1972.

29. Weigle, W. O. Recent observations and concepts in immunological unresponsiveness and autoimmunity. *Clin. Exp. Immunol.* 9:437, 1971.

30. Bankhurst, A. D., Torrigiani, G., and Allison, A. C. Lymphocytes binding human thyroglobulin in healthy people and its relevance to tolerance for autoantigens. *Lancet* 1:226, 1973.

31. Bankhurst, A. D., and Williams, R. C., Jr. Identification of DNA-binding lymphocytes in patients with systemic lupus erythematosus. *J. Clin. Invest.* 56:1378, 1975.

32. Sawada, S., Pillarisetty, R. J., Michalski, J. P., et al. Lymphocytes binding polyriboadenylic acid and synthesizing antibodies to nucleic acids in autoimmune and normal mice. *J. Immunol.* 119:355, 1977.

33. Biberfeld, G., and Gronowicz, E. *Mycoplasma pneumoniae* is a polyclonal B-cell activator. *Nature* 261:238, 1976.

34. Hammarström, L., Smith, E., Primi, D., et al. Induction of auto-antibodies to red blood cells by polyclonal B-cell activators. *Nature* 263:60, 1976.

35. Primi, D., Hammarström, L., Smith, C. L., et al. Characterization of self-reactive B-cells by polyclonal B-cell activators. *J. Exp. Med.* 145:21, 1977.

36. Primi, D., Smith, C. I. E., Hammarström, L., et al. Evidence for the existence of self-reactive human B lymphocytes. *Clin. Exp. Immunol.* 29:316, 1977.

37. Primi, D., Smith, C. I. E., and Hammarström, L. Role of suppressor T cells in autoimmune responses induced by polyclonal B cell activators. *Scand. J. Immunol.* 7:121, 1978.

38. Howe, M. L., Goldstein, A. L., and Battisto, J. R. Isogeneic lymphocyte interaction: recognition of self-antigens by cells of the neonatal thymus. *Proc. Natl. Acad. Sci. USA* 67:613, 1970.

39. Gronowicz, E., and Coutinho, A. Functional analysis of B cell's heterogeneity. *Transplant. Rev.* 24:3, 1975.

40. Allison, A. C. Interactions of T and B lymphocytes in self-tolerance and autoimmunity. In D. H. Katz and B. Benacerraf, eds., *Immunological Tolerance,* p. 25. Academic Press, New York, 1974.

41. Allison, A. C. Unresponsiveness to self-antigens. *Lancet* 2:1401, 1971.

42. Talal, N., and Steinberg, A. D. The pathogenesis of autoimmunity in New Zealand black mice. *Curr. Top. Microbiol. Immunol.* 64:79, 1974.

43. Bach, J. F., Dardenne, M., and Salomon, J. C. Studies on thymus products. IV. Absence of serum 'thymic activity' in adult NZB and (NZB × NZW) F$_1$ mice. *Clin. Exp. Immunol.* 14:247, 1973.

44. Gerber, N. L., Hardin, J. A., and Chused, T. M. Loss with age in NZB-W mice of thymic suppressor cells in the graft-vs-host reaction. *J. Immunol.* 113:1618, 1974.

45. Abdou, N. I., Sagawa, A., Pascual, E., et al. Suppressor T-cell abnormality in idiopathic systemic lupus erythematosus. *Clin. Immunol. Immunopathol.* 6:192, 1976.

46. Bresnihan, B., and Jasin, H. E. Suppressor function of peripheral blood mononuclear cells in normal individuals and in patients with systemic lupus erythematosus. *J. Clin. Invest.* 59:106, 1977.

47. Horowitz, S., Borcherding, W., Moorthy, A. V., et al. Induction of suppressor T cells in systemic lupus erythematosus by thymosin and cultured thymic epithelium. *Science* 197:999, 1977.

48. Cochrane, C. G. Immunologic tissue injury mediated by neutrophilic leukocytes. *Adv. Immunol.* 9:97, 1968.

49. Henson, P. M. Pathologic mechanisms in neutrophil-mediated injury. *Am. J. Pathol.* 68:593, 1972.

50. Ward, P. A. Leukotactic factors in health and disease. *Am. J. Pathol.* 64:521, 1971.

51. Weigle, W. O., and Nakamura, R. M. Perpetuation of autoimmune thyroiditis and production of secondary renal lesions following periodic injections of aqueous preparations of altered thyroglobulin. *Clin. Exp. Immunol.* 4:645, 1969.

52. Koffler, D., Sandson, J., and Kunkel, H. G. Elution studies on tissues from patients with Goodpasture's syndrome and other forms of subacute glomerulonephritis. *J. Clin. Invest.* 47:55a (abstract), 1968.

53. Werner, S. C., Wegelius, O., Fierer, J. A., et al. Immunoglobulins (E,M,G) and complement in connective tissues of the thyroid in Grave's disease. *N. Engl. J. Med.* 287:421, 1972.

54. Kalderon, A. E., Bogaars, H. A., and Diamond, I. Ultrastructural alterations of the follicular basement membrane in Hashimoto's thyroiditis. Report of eight cases with basement deposits. *Am. J. Med.* 55:485, 1973.

55. Kahn, C. R., Megyesi, K., Bar, R. S., et al. Receptors for peptide hormones. New insights into the pathophysiology of disease states in man. *Ann. Intern. Med.* 86:205, 1977.

56. Smith, B. R., and Hall, R. Thyroid-stimulating immunoglobulins in Grave's disease. *Lancet* 2:427, 1974.

57. Yamashita, K., and Field, J. B. Effects of long-acting thyroid stimulator on thyrotropin stimulation of adenyl cyclase activity in thyroid plasma membranes. *J. Clin. Invest.* 51:463, 1972.

58. Adams, D. D., Fastier, F. N., Howie, J. B., et al. Stimulation of the human thyroid by infusions of plasma containing LATS protector. *J. Clin. Endocrin. Metab.* 39:826, 1974.

59. Patrick, J., and Lindstrom, J. M. Autoimmune response to acetylcholine receptor. *Science* 180:871, 1973.

60. Lindstrom, J. M., and Patrick, J. Purification of the acetylcholine receptor by affinity chromatography. In M. V. L. Bennett, ed., *Synaptic Transmission and Neuronal Interaction,* p. 191. Raven Press, New York, 1974.

61. Almon, R. R., Andrew, C. G., and Appel, S. H. Serum globulin in myasthenia gravis: inhibition of α-bungarotoxin binding to acetylcholine receptors. *Science* 186:55, 1974.

62. Bruce, D. H., Bernard, W., and Blackard, W. G. Spontaneous disappearance of insulin-resistant diabetes mellitus in a patient with a collagen disease. A case report with review of the literature for conditions associated with insulin resistance. *Am. J. Med.* 48:268, 1970.

63. Flier, J. S., Kahn, C. R., Roth, J., et al. Antibodies that impair insulin receptor binding in an unusual diabetic syndrome with severe insulin resistance. *Science* 190:63, 1975.

64. Kahn, C. R., Flier, J. S., Bar, R. S., et al. The syndromes of insulin resistance and acanthosis nigricans. Insulin-receptor disorders in man. *N. Engl. J. Med.* 294:739, 1976.

65. Dixon, F. J., Feldman, J. D., and Vazquez, J. J. Experimental glomerulonephritis. The pathogenesis of a laboratory model resembling the spectrum of human glomerulonephritis. *J. Exp. Med.* 113:899, 1961.

66. Dixon, F. J. The role of antigen-antibody complexes in disease. In *The Harvey Lectures,* ser. 58, p. 21. Academic Press, New York, 1963.

67. Gregory, J. E., and Rich, A. R. The experimental production of anaphylactic pulmonary lesions with the basic characteristics of rheumatic pneumonitis. *Bull. Johns Hopkins Hosp.* 78:1, 1946.

68. McKinnon, G. E., Andrews, E. C., Jr., Heptinstall, R. H., et al. An immunohistologic study on the occurrence of intravascular antigen-antibody

precipitation and its role in anaphylaxis in the rabbit. *Bull. Johns Hopkins Hosp.* 101:258, 1957.

69. Weigle, W. O., Cochrane, C. G., and Dixon, F. J. Anaphylactogenic properties of soluble antigen-antibody complexes in the guinea pig and rabbit. *J. Immunol.* 85:469, 1960.

70. Brentjens, J. R., O'Connell, D. W., Pawlowski, I. B., et al. Experimental immune complex disease of the lung. The pathogenesis of a laboratory model resembling certain human interstitial lung diseases. *J. Exp. Med.* 140:105, 1974.

71. Liebow, A. A. New concepts and entities in pulmonary disease. In A. A. Liebow and D. E. Smith, eds., *The Lung,* p. 332. Williams & Wilkins Co., Baltimore, 1968.

72. Spencer, H. Chronic interstitial pneumonia. In A. A. Liebow and D. E. Smith, eds., *The Lung,* p. 134. Williams & Wilkins Co., Baltimore, 1968.

73. Turner-Warwick, M., and Pepys, J. Some aspects of immunopathology and lung disease. *Br. J. Dis. Chest* 61:113, 1967.

74. Vazquez, J. J. Immunopathologic aspects of lung disease. *Arch. Intern. Med.* 126:471, 1970.

75. McCombs, R. P. Diseases due to immunologic reactions in the lungs. *N. Engl. J. Med.* 286:1186, 1972.

76. Sperryn, P. N., and Mace, B. E. Systemic lupus erythematosus with fibrosing alveolitis. *Proc. R. Soc. Med.* 64:58, 1971.

77. Eisenberg, H., Dubois, E. L., Sherwin, R. P., et al. Diffuse interstitial lung disease in systemic lupus erythematosus. *Ann. Intern. Med.* 79:37, 1973.

78. Tomasi, T. B., Jr., Fudenberg, H. H., and Finby, N. Possible relationship of rheumatoid factors and pulmonary disease. *Am. J. Med.* 33:243, 1962.

79. Huang, C-T., Hennigar, G. R., and Lyons, H. A. Pulmonary dysfunction in systemic lupus erythematosus. *N. Engl. J. Med.* 272:288, 1965.

80. Földes, I., and Beregi, E. Immunomorphological methods in the diagnosis of lung diseases. *Scand. J. Respir. Dis.* 80:73, 1972 (suppl.).

81. Nozawa, Y. Histopathological findings of the lung in collagen diseases—especially on their differential diagnosis. *Acta Pathol. Jap.* 22:843, 1972.

82. Kapanci, Y., and Chamay, A. Lésions en anse de fil de fer des capillaires pulmonaires dans le lupue érythemateux disseminé (L.E.D.). *Virchows Arch. (Pathol. Anat.)* 342:236, 1967.

83. Kuhn, C. Systemic lupus erythematosus in a patient with ultrastructural lesions of the pulmonary capillaries previously reported in the "Review" as due to idiopathic pulmonary hemosiderosis. *Am. Rev. Respir. Dis.* 106:931, 1972.

84. DeHoratius, R. J., Abruzzo, J. L., and Williams, R. C., Jr. Immunofluorescent and immunologic studies of rheumatoid lung. *Arch. Intern. Med.* 129:441, 1972.

85. Dreisin, R. B., Schwarz, M. I., Theofilopoulos, A. N., et al. Circulating immune complexes in the idiopathic interstitial pneumonias. *N. Engl. J. Med.* 298:353, 1978.

86. Traub, E. A filterable virus recovered from white mice. *Science* 81:298, 1935.

87. Rowe, W. P. Studies on pathogenesis and immunity in lymphocytic choriomeningitis infection of the mouse. In Research Report NM 005 048.14.01, Naval Medical Research Institute, Bethesda, Md. p. 167, 1954.

88. Volkert, M., and Larsen, J. H. Immunological tolerance to viruses. *Prog. Med. Virol.* 7:160, 1965.

89. Lehmann-Grube, F. Lymphocytic choriomeningitis virus. *Virol. Monogr.* 10:1971.

90. Hotchin, J. Persistent and slow virus infections. *Monogr. Virol.* 3:1971.

91. Oldstone, M. B. A., and Dixon, F. J. Lymphocytic choriomeningitis: production of antibody by "tolerant" infected mice. *Science* 158:1193, 1967.

92. Burnet, F. M., and Fenner, F. Immunological behavior of young animals, p. 71, and Theoretical aspects of antibody production, p. 78. In *The production of antibodies,* Monographs of the Walter and Eliza Hall Institute. MacMillan and Co. of Australia, Melbourne and London, 1949.

93. Burnet, F. M. The clonal selection theory of antibody production. In *The Clonal Selection Theory of Acquired Immunity,* p. 49. Vanderbilt and Cambridge University Presses, Nashville, Tenn., 1959.

94. Marker, O., and Volkert, M. *In vitro* measurement of the time course of cellular immunity to LCM virus in mice. In F. Lehmann-Grube, ed., *Lymphocytic Choriomeningitis Virus and Other Arenaviruses,* p. 207. Springer-Verlag, New York, 1973.

95. Cole, G. A., Prendergast, R. A., and Henney, C. S. *In vitro* correlates of LCM virus-induced immune response. In F. Lehmann-Grube, ed., *Lymphocytic Choriomeningitis Virus and Other Arenaviruses,* p. 61. Springer-Verlag, New York, 1973.

96. Doherty, P. C., Zinkernagel, R. M., and Ramshaw, I. A. Specificity and development of cytotoxic thymus-derived lymphocytes in lymphocytic choriomeningitis. *J. Immunol.* 112:1548, 1974.

97. Mims, C. A., and Blanden, R. V. Antiviral action of immune lymphocytes in mice infected with lymphocytic choriomeningitis virus. *Infect. Immun.* 6:695, 1972.

98. Zinkernagel, R. M., and Welsh, R. M. H-2 compatibility requirement for virus-specific T cell-

mediated effector functions *in vivo*. I. Specificity of
T cells conferring antiviral protection against lymphocytic choriomeningitis virus is associated with H-2K and H-2D. *J. Immunol.* 117:1495, 1976.

99. Gilden, D. H., Cole, G. A., Monjan, A. A., et al. Immunopathogenesis of acute central nervous system disease produced by lymphocytic choriomeningitis virus. I. Cyclophosphamide-mediated induction by the virus-carrier state in adult mice. *J. Exp. Med.* 135:860, 1972.

100. Cole, G. A., Nathanson, N., and Prendergast, R. A. Requirement for θ-bearing cells in lymphocytic choriomeningitis virus-induced central nervous system disease. *Nature* 238:335, 1972.

101. Doherty, P. C., and Zinkernagel, R. M. T-cell-mediated immunopathology in viral infections. *Transplant. Rev.* 19:89, 1974.

102. Oldstone, M. B. A., and Dixon, F. J. Direct immunofluorescent tissue culture assay for lymphocytic choriomeningitis virus. *J. Immunol.* 100:1135, 1968.

103. Wilsnack, R. E., and Rowe, W. P. Immunofluorescent studies of the histopathogenesis of lymphocytic choriomeningitis virus infection. *J. Exp. Med.* 120:829, 1964.

104. Pedersen, I. R., and Volkert, M. Multiplication of lymphocytic choriomeningitis virus in suspension cultures of Earle's strain L cells. *Acta Pathol. Microbiol. Scand.* 67:523, 1966.

105. Rowe, W. P. Protective effect of pre-irradiation on lymphocytic choriomeningitis infection in mice. *Proc. Soc. Exp. Biol. Med.* 92:194, 1956.

106. Haas, V. H., and Stewart, S. E. Sparing effect of A-methopterin and guanazolo in mice infected with virus of lymphocytic choriomeningitis. *Virology* 2:511, 1956.

107. Hotchin, J., and Weigand, H. The effects of pretreatment with x-rays on the pathogenesis of lymphocytic choriomeningitis in mice. I. Host survival, virus multiplication, and leukocytosis. *J. Immunol.* 87:675, 1961.

108. East, J., Parrott, D. M. V., and Seamer, J. The ability of mice thymectomized at birth to survive infection with lymphocytic choriomeningitis virus. *Virology* 22:160, 1964.

109. Oldstone, M. B. A., and Dixon, F. J. Pathogenesis of chronic disease associated with persistent lymphocytic choriomeningitis viral infection. I. Relationship of antibody production to disease in neonatally infected mice. *J. Exp. Med.* 129:483, 1969.

110. Hotchin, J. E., and Cinits, M. Lymphocytic choriomeningitis infection of mice as a model for the study of latent virus infection. *Can. J. Microbiol.* 4:149, 1958.

111. Volkert, M. Studies on immunological tolerance to LCM virus. II. Treatment of virus carrier mice by adoptive immunization. *Acta Pathol. Microbiol. Scand.* 57:465, 1963.

112. Volkert, M., Bro-Jørgensen, K., Marker, O., et al. The activity of T and B lymphocytes in immunity and tolerance to the lymphocytic choriomeningitis virus in mice. *Immunology* 29:455, 1975.

113. Hoffsten, P. E., Villalobos, R., Hill, C., et al. T-cell deficiency in immune complex glomerulonephritis. *Kidney Int.* 11:318, 1977.

114. Cihak, J., and Lehmann-Grube, F. Examination of LCM virus specific immunologic tolerance in mice. *Z. Immunitaetsforsch.* 152:79, 1976.

115. Welsh, R. M., Jr., Lampert, P. W., Burner, P. A., et al. Antibody-complement interactions with purified lymphocytic choriomeningitis virus. *Virology* 73:59, 1976.

116. Oldstone, M. B. A., and Dixon, F. J. Pathogenesis of chronic disease associated with persistent lymphocytic choriomeningitis viral infection. II. Relationship of the anti-lymphocytic choriomeningitis immune response to tissue injury in chronic lymphocytic choriomeningitis disease. *J. Exp. Med.* 131:1, 1970.

117. Oldstone, M. B. A., Welsh, R. M., and Joseph, B. S. Pathogenic mechanisms of tissue injury in persistent viral infections. *Ann. N.Y. Acad. Sci.* 256:65, 1975.

118. Katz, D. H., and Benacerraf, B. The function and interrelationships of T-cell receptors, Ir genes and other histocompatibility gene products. *Transplant. Rev.* 22:175, 1975.

119. Doherty, P. C., Blanden, R. V., and Zinkernagel, R. M. Specificity of virus-immune effector T cells for H-2K or H-2D compatible interactions: implications for H-antigen diversity. *Transplant. Rev.* 29:89, 1976.

120. Zinkernagel, R. M., and Doherty, P. C. Major transplantation antigens, viruses, and specificity of surveillance T cells. *Contemp. Top. Immunobiol.* 7:179, 1977.

121. Pfizenmaier, K., Trostmann, H., Rollinghoff, M., et al. Temporary presence of self-reactive cytotoxic T lymphocytes during murine lymphocytic choriomeningitis. *Nature* 258:238, 1975.

122. Dunlop, M. B. C., Doherty, P. C., Zinkernagel, R. M., et al. Secondary cytotoxic cell response to lymphocytic choriomeningitis virus. II. Nature and specificity of effector cells. *Immunology* 31:181, 1976.

123. Zinkernagel, R. M., Dunlop, M. B., Blanden, R. V., et al. H-2 compatibility requirement for virus-specific T-cell-mediated cytolysis. Evaluation

of the role of H-21 region and non-H-2 genes in regulating immune response. *J. Exp. Med.* 144:519, 1976.

124. Zinkernagel, R. M. H-2 restriction of virus-specific T-cell-mediated effector functions *in vivo.* II. Adoptive transfer of delayed-type hypersensitivity to murine lymphocytic choriomeningitis virus is restricted by the K and D region of H-2. *J. Exp. Med.* 144:776, 1976.

125. Griffiths, M. M., Smith, C. B., Ward, J. R., et al. Cytotoxic activity of rheumatoid and normal lymphocytes against allogeneic and autologous synovial cells *in vitro. J. Clin. Invest.* 58:613, 1976.

126. Person, D. A., Sharp, J. T., and Lidsky, M. D. The cytotoxicity of leukocytes and lymphocytes from patients with rheumatoid arthritis for synovial cells. *J. Clin. Invest.* 58:690, 1976.

127. Sukernick, R., Hanin, A., and Mosolov, A. The reaction of blood lymphocytes from patients with rheumatoid arthritis against human connective tissue cells *in vitro. Clin. Exp. Immunol.* 3:171, 1968.

128. Zarling, J. M., Raich, P. C., McKeough, M., et al. Generation of cytotoxic lymphocytes *in vitro* against autologous human leukaemia cells. *Nature* 262:691, 1976.

129. Powles, R. L., Russell, J., Lister, T. A., et al. Immunotherapy for acute myelogenous leukaemia: a controlled clinical study 2½ years after entry of the last patient. *Br. J. Cancer* 35:265, 1977.

130. Lee, S. K., and Oliver, R. T. D. Autologous leukemia-specific T-cell-mediated lymphocytotoxicity in patients with acute myelogenous leukemia. *J. Exp. Med.* 147:912, 1978.

131. Jacobs, R. P., and Cole, G. A. Lymphocytic choriomeningitis virus-induced immunosuppression: a virus-induced macrophage defect. *J. Immunol.* 117:1004, 1976.

132. Bielschowsky, M., Helyer, B. J., and Howie, J. B. Spontaneous anaemia in mice of the NZB/BL strain. *Proc. Univ. Otago Med. Sch.* 37:9, 1959.

133. Lambert, P. H., and Dixon, F. J. Pathogenesis of the glomerulonephritis of NZB/NZW mice. *J. Exp. Med.* 127:507, 1968.

134. Talal, N., and Steinberg, A. D. The pathogenesis of autoimmunity in New Zealand black mice. *Curr. Top. Microbiol. Immunol.* 64:79, 1974.

135. Bielschowsky, M., and Bielschowsky, F. Observations on NZB/BL mice; differential fertility in reciprocal crosses and the transmission of the autoimmune haemolytic anaemia to NZB/BL × NZC/BL hybrids. *Aust. J. Exp. Biol. Med. Sci.* 42:561, 1964.

136. Burnet, F. M. and Holmes, M. C. Genetic investigations of autoimmune disease in mice. *Nature* 207:368, 1965.

137. Howie, J. B., and Helyer, B. J. The immunology and pathology of NZB mice. *Adv. Immunol.* 9:215, 1968.

138. Braverman, I. M. Study of autoimmune disease in New Zealand mice. I. Genetic features and natural history of NZB, NZY, and NZW strains and NZB/NZW hybrids. *J. Invest. Dermatol.* 50:483, 1968.

139. Ghaffar, A., and Playfair, J. H. L. The genetic basis of autoimmunity in NZB mice studied by progeny-testing. *Clin. Exp. Immunol.* 8:479, 1971.

140. Linder, E., and Edgington, T. S. Antigenic specificity of anti-erythrocyte autoantibody responses by NZB mice: identification and partial characterization of two erythrocyte surface auto-antigens. *J. Immunol.* 108:1615, 1972.

141. DeHeer, D. H., and Edgington, T. S. Cellular events associated with the immunogenesis of anti-erythrocyte autoantibody responses of NZB mice. *Transplant. Rev.* 31:116, 1976.

142. DeHeer, D. H., and Edgington, T. S. Clonal heterogeneity of the anti-erythrocyte autoantibody responses of NZB mice. *J. Immunol.* 113:1184, 1974.

143. Holmes, M. C., Gorrie, J., and Burnet, F. M. Transmission by splenic cells of an autoimmune disease occurring spontaneously in mice. *Lancet* 2:638, 1961.

144. Denman, A. M., Russell, A. S., and Denman, E. J. Adoptive transfer of the diseases of New Zealand black mice to normal mouse strains. *Clin. Exp. Immunol.* 5:567, 1969.

145. Denman, A. M., and Frenkel, E. P. Mode of action of anti-lymphocyte globulin. I. The distribution of rabbit anti-lymphocyte globulin injected into rats and mice. *Immunology* 14:107, 1968.

146. Morton, J. I., and Siegel, B. V. Early autoantibody formation in lethally irradiated or drug-treated H-2 compatible recipients of pre-autoimmune NZB bone marrow or fetal liver cells. *Transplantation* 17:624, 1974.

147. Morton, J. I., and Siegel, B. V. Transplantation of autoimmune potential. I. Development of antinuclear antibodies in H-2 histocompatible recipients of bone marrow from New Zealand black mice. *Proc. Natl. Acad. Sci. USA* 71:2162, 1974.

148. DeHeer, D. H., and Edgington, T. S. Evidence for a B lymphocyte defect underlying the anti-X anti-erythrocyte autoantibody response of NZB mice. *J. Immunol.* 118:1858, 1977.

149. Gershwin, M. E., and Steinberg, A. D. Suppression of autoimmune hemolytic anemia in New Zealand (NZB) black mice by syngeneic young

thymocytes. *Clin. Immunol. Immunopathol.* 4:38, 1975.

150. Mellors, R. C. Autoimmune disease in NZB/BL mice. I. Pathology and pathogenesis of a model system of spontaneous glomerulonephritis. *J. Exp. Med.* 122:25, 1965.

151. Mellors, R. C. Autoimmune and immunoproliferative diseases of NZB/BL mice and hybrids. *Int. Rev. Exp. Pathol.* 5:217, 1966.

152. East, J. Immunopathology and neoplasms in New Zealand black (NZB) and SJL/J mice. *Prog. Exp. Tumor Res.* 13:84, 1970.

153. Lambert, P. H., and Dixon, F. J. Pathogenesis of the glomerulonephritis of NZB/W mice. *J. Exp. Med.* 127:507, 1968.

154. Krishnan, C., and Kaplan, M. H. Immunopathologic studies of systemic lupus erythematosus. II. Antinuclear reaction of γ-globulin eluted from homogenates and isolated glomeruli of kidneys from patients with lupus nephritis. *J. Clin. Invest.* 46:569, 1967.

155. Koffler, D., Schur, P. H., and Kunkel, H. G. Immunological studies concerning the nephritis of systemic lupus erythematosus. *J. Exp. Med.* 126:607, 1967.

156. Tan, E. M., Schur, P. H., Carr, R. I., et al. Deoxyribonucleic acid (DNA) and antibodies to DNA in the serum of patients with systemic lupus erythematosus. *J. Clin. Invest.* 45:1732, 1966.

157. Mellors, R. C., and Huang, C. Y. Immunopathology of NZB/BL mice. VI. Virus separable from spleen and pathogenic for Swiss mice. *J. Exp. Med.* 126:53, 1967.

158. Mellors, R. C., Aoki, T., and Huebner, R. J. Further implications of murine leukemia-like virus in the disorders of NZB mice. *J. Exp. Med.* 129:1045, 1969.

159. Mellors, R. C., Shirai, T., Aoki, T., et al. Wild-type gross leukemia virus and the pathogenesis of the glomerulonephritis of New Zealand mice. *J. Exp. Med.* 133:113, 1971.

160. Mellors, R. C., and Huang, C. Y. Immunopathology of NZB/BL mice. V. Viruslike (filterable) agent separable from lymphoma cells and identifiable by electron microscopy. *J. Exp. Med.* 124:1031, 1966.

161. Mellors, R. C. Autoimmune disease and neoplasia of NZB mice—implications of murine leukemia-like virus. *Perspect. Virol.* 6:239, 1968.

162. Aoki, T., Boyse, E. A., Old, L. J., et al. G (Gross) and H-2 cell-surface antigens: location on Gross leukemia cells by electron microscopy with visually labeled antibody. *Proc. Natl. Acad. Sci. USA* 65:569, 1970.

163. Aoki, T., and Takahashi, T. Viral and cellular surface antigens of murine leukemias and myelomas. Serological analysis by immunoelectron microscopy. *J. Exp. Med.* 135:443, 1972.

164. Yoshiki, T., Mellors, R. C., Strand, M., et al. The viral envelope glycoprotein of murine leukemia virus and the pathogenesis of immune complex glomerulonephritis of New Zealand mice. *J. Exp. Med.* 140:1011, 1974.

165. Croker, B. P., Jr., Del Villano, B. C., Jensen, F. C., et al. Immunopathogenicity and oncogenicity of murine leukemia viruses. I. Induction of immunologic disease and lymphoma in (BALB/c × NZB) F_1 mice by Scripps leukemia virus. *J. Exp. Med.* 140:1028, 1974.

166. Cannat, A., and Varet, B. Induction of antinuclear antibodies in mice inoculated with Rauscher leukemogenic virus: possible role of genetic factors in "non-New Zealand" strains. *Immunol. Commun.* 2:527, 1973.

167. Richer, L., Tanaka, T., Sykes, J. A., et al. Further studies on the biological relationship of murine leukemia viruses and on kidney lesions of mice with leukemia induced by these viruses. *Natl. Cancer Inst. Monogr.* 22:459, 1966.

168. Branca, A., de Petris, S., Allison, A. C., et al. Immune complex diseases. I. Pathological changes in the kidneys of BALB/c mice neonatally infected with Moloney leukaemogenic and murine sarcoma viruses. *Clin. Exp. Immunol.* 9:853, 1971.

169. Linder, E., Pasternack, A., and Edgington, T. S. Pathology and immunology of age-associated disease of mice and evidence for an autologous immune complex pathogenesis of the associated renal disease. *Clin. Immunol. Immunopathol.* 1:104, 1972.

170. Oldstone, M. B. A., Tishon, A., Tonietti, G., et al. Immune complex disease associated with spontaneous murine leukemia: incidence and pathogenesis of glomerulonephritis. *Clin. Immunol. Immunopathol.* 1:6, 1972.

171. Porter, D. D., Porter, H. G., and Cox, N. A. Immune complex glomerulonephritis in one-year-old C57BL/6 mice induced by endogenous murine leukemia virus and erythrocyte antigens. *J. Immunol.* 111:1626, 1973.

172. Dixon, F. J., Oldstone, M. B. A., and Tonietti, G. Pathogenesis of immune complex glomerulonephritis of New Zealand mice. *J. Exp. Med.* 134:65s, 1971.

173. Datta, S. K., Manny, N., Andrzejewski, C., et al. Genetic studies of autoimmunity and retrovirus expression in crosses of New Zealand black mice. I. Xenotropic virus. *J. Exp. Med.* 147:854, 1978.

174. Datta, S. K., McConahey, P. J., Manny, N.,

et al. Genetic studies of autoimmunity and retrovirus expression in crosses of New Zealand black mice. II. The viral envelope glycoprotein gp70. *J. Exp. Med.* 147:872, 1978.

175. Strand, M., and August, J. T. Oncornavirus envelope glycoprotein in serum of mice. *Virology* 75:130, 1976.

176. Elder, J. H., Jensen, F. C., Bryant, M. L., et al. Polymorphism of the major envelope glycoprotein (gp70) of murine C-type viruses: virion associated and differentiation antigens encoded by a multi-gene family. *Nature* 267:23, 1977.

177. Dalton, A. J., Melnick, J. L., Bauer, H., et al. The case for a family of reverse transcriptase viruses: Retraviridae. *Intervirology* 4:201, 1974.

178. Callahan, R., Sherr, C. J., and Todaro, G. J. A new class of murine retroviruses: immunological and biochemical comparison of novel isolates from *Mus cervicolor* and *Mus caroli*. *Virology* 80:401, 1977.

179. Lewis, R. M., Tannenberg, W., Smith, C., et al. C-type viruses in systemic lupus erythematosus. *Nature* 252:78, 1974.

180. Strand, M., and August, J. T. Type-C RNA virus gene expression in human tissue. *J. Virol.* 14:1584, 1974.

181. Todaro, G. J., Sherr, C. J., and Benveniste, R. E. Baboons and their close relatives are unusual among primates in their ability to release non-defective endogenous type C viruses. *Virology* 72:278, 1976.

182. Stephenson, J. R., and Aaronson, S. A. Endogenous C-type viral expression in primates. *Nature* 266:469, 1977.

183. August, J. T., and Strand, M. Type-C oncornaviruses and autoimmunity. *Arthritis Rheum.* 20:64s, 1977 (suppl.).

184. Mellors, R. C., and Mellors, J. W. Antigen related to mammalian type-C RNA viral p30 proteins is located in renal glomeruli in human systemic lupus erythematosus. *Proc. Natl. Acad. Sci. USA* 73:233, 1976.

185. Panem, S., Ordoñez, N. G., Kirstein, W. H., et al. C-type virus expression in systemic lupus erythematosus. *N. Engl. J. Med.* 295:470, 1976.

186. Phillips, P. E. Viruses and systemic lupus erythematosus. *Bull. Rheum. Dis.* 28:954, 1977–78.

187. Imamura, M., Phillips, P. E., and Mellors, R. C. The occurrence and frequency of type-C virus-like particles in placentas from patients with systemic lupus erythematosus and from normal subjects. *Am. J. Pathol.* 83:383, 1976.

188. Markenson, J. A., Phillips, P. E., Brinkman, J. P., et al. Type C virus-related antigens on the surface of lymphocytes from normals and patients with SLE. *Arthritis Rheum.* 19:809 (abstract), 1976.

189. Phillips, P. E., Hargrave, R., Stewart, E., et al. Type C oncorna-virus isolation studies in systemic lupus erythematosus. I. Attempted detection by isopycnic sedimentation of ^{3}H-uridine-labelled virions. *Ann. Rheum. Dis.* 35:422, 1975.

190. Phillips, P. E., and Hargrave-Granda, R. Type C oncornavirus isolation studies in systemic lupus erythematosus. II. Attempted detection by viral RNA-dependent DNA polymerase assay. *Ann. Rheum. Dis.* 37:225, 1978.

191. Dauphinee, M. J., Palmer, D. W., and Talal, N. Evidence for an abnormal microenvironment in the thymus of New Zealand black mice. *J. Immunol.* 115:1054, 1975.

192. Bach, J. F., Dardenne, M., and Salomon, J. C. Studies on thymus products. IV. Absence of serum 'thymic activity' in adult NZB and (NZB × NZW) F_1 mice. *Clin. Exp. Immunol.* 14:247, 1973.

193. de Vries, M. J., and Hijmans, W. A deficient development of the thymic epithelium and autoimmune disease in NZB mice. *J. Pathol. Bacteriol.* 81:487, 1966.

194. Sato, V. L., Waksal, S. D., and Herzenberg, L. A. Identification and separation of pre T-cells from nu/nu mice: differentiation by preculture with thymic reticuloepithelial cells. *Immunology* 24:173, 1976.

195. Waksal, S. D., Cohen, I. R., Waksal, H. W., et al. Induction of T-cells differentiation *in vitro* by thymus epithelial cells. *Ann. N.Y. Acad. Sci.* 249:492, 1975.

196. Gershwin, M. E., Ikeda, R. M., Kruse, W. L., et al. Age-dependent loss in New Zealand mice of morphological and functional characteristics of thymic epithelial cells. *J. Immunol.* 120:971, 1978.

197. Dardenne, M., Papiernik, M., Bach, J. F., et al. Studies on thymus products. III. Epithelial origin of the serum thymic factor. *Immunology* 27:299, 1974.

198. Gershwin, M. E., Steinberg, A. D., Ahmed, A., et al. Study of thymic factors. II. Failure of thymosin to alter the natural history of NZB and NZB/NZW mice. *Arthritis Rheum.* 19:862, 1976.

199. Talal, N., Dauphinee, M., Pillarisetty, R., et al. Effect of thymosin on thymocyte proliferation and autoimmunity in NZB mice. *Ann. N.Y. Acad. Sci.* 249:438, 1975.

200. Shirai, T., and Mellors, R. C. Natural thymo-cytotoxic autoantibody and reactive antigen in New Zealand black and other mice. *Proc. Natl. Acad. Sci. USA* 68:1412, 1971.

201. Shirai, T., and Mellors, R. C. Natural cyto-

toxic autoantibody against thymocytes in NZB mice. *Clin. Exp. Immunol.* 12:133, 1972.

202. Shen, F. W., Boyse, E. A., and Cantor, H. Preparation and use of Ly antisera. *Immunogenetics* 2:591, 1975.

203. Cantor, H., and Boyse, E. A. Functional subclasses of T lymphocytes bearing different Ly antigens. I. The generation of functionally distinct T-cell subclasses is a differentiative process independent of antigen. *J. Exp. Med.* 141:1376, 1975.

204. Cantor, H., Shen, F. W., and Boyse, E. A. Separation of helper T cells from suppressor T cells expressing different Ly components. II. Activation by antigen: after immunization, antigen-specific suppressor and helper activities are mediated by distinct T-cell subclasses. *J. Exp. Med.* 143:1391, 1976.

205. Eardley, D. D., Hugenberger, J., McVay-Boudreau, L., et al. Immunoregulatory circuits among T-cell sets. I. T-helper cells induce other T-cell sets to exert feedback inhibition. *J. Exp. Med.* 147:1106, 1978.

206. Cantor, H., McVay-Boudreau, L., Hugenberger, J., et al. Immunoregulatory circuits among T-cell sets. II. Physiologic role of feedback inhibition *in vivo*: absence in NZB mice. *J. Exp. Med.* 147:1116, 1978.

207. Moretta, L., Webb, S. R., Grossi, C. E., et al. Functional analysis of two human T-cell subpopulations: help and suppression of B-cell responses by T-cells bearing receptors for IgM or IgG. *J. Exp. Med.* 146:184, 1977.

208. Lewis, R. M., Schwartz, R., and Henry, W. B., Jr. Canine systemic lupus erythematosus. *Blood* 25:143, 1965.

209. Lewis, R. M., and Schwartz, R. S. Canine systemic lupus erythematosus. Genetic analysis of an established breeding colony. *J. Exp. Med.* 134:417, 1971.

210. Lewis, R. M., André-Schwartz, J., Harris, G. S., et al. Canine systemic lupus erythematosus. Transmission of serologic abnormalities by cell-free filtrates. *J. Clin. Invest.* 52:1893, 1973.

211. Hartsough, G. R., and Gorham, J. R. Aleutian disease in mink. *Natl. Fur News* 28:10, 1956.

212. Helmboldt, C. F., and Jungherr, E. L. The pathology of Aleutian disease in mink. *Am. J. Vet. Res.* 19:212, 1958.

213. Obel, A. L. Studies on a disease in mink with systemic proliferation of the plasma cells. *Am. J. Vet. Res.* 20:384, 1959.

214. Karstad, L., and Pridham, T. J. Aleutian disease in mink. I. Evidence of its viral etiology. *Can. J. Comp. Med.* 26:97, 1962.

215. Henson, J. B., Gorham, J. R., and Leader, R. W. Hypergammaglobulinaemia in mink initiated by a cell-free filtrate. *Nature* 197:206, 1963.

216. Henson, J. B., Gorham, J. R., Tanaka, Y., et al. The sequential development of ultrastructural lesions in the glomeruli of mink with experimental Aleutian disease. *Lab. Invest.* 19:153, 1968.

217. Porter, D. D., Larsen, A. E., and Porter, H. G. The pathogenesis of Aleutian disease of mink. I. *In vivo* viral replication and the host antibody response to viral antigen. *J. Exp. Med.* 130:575, 1969.

218. Porter, D. D., Porter, H. G., and Deerhake, B. B. Immunofluorescence assay for antigen and antibody in lactic dehydrogenase virus infection of mice. *J. Immunol.* 102:431, 1969.

219. Henson, J. B., Williams, R. C., Jr., and Gorham, J. R. Isolation of serum fractions capable of producing Aleutian disease in mink. *J. Immunol.* 97:344, 1966.

220. Porter, D. D., and Larsen, A. E. Aleutian disease of mink: infectious virus-antibody complexes in the serum. *Proc. Soc. Exp. Biol. Med.* 126:680, 1967.

221. Barnett, E. V., Williams, R. C., Jr., Kenyon, A. J., et al. 'Nuclear' antigens and anti-nuclear antibodies in mink sera. *Immunology* 16:241, 1969.

222. Notani, G. W., Hahn, E. C., Sarkar, N. H., et al. Characterization of Aleutian disease antigens. *Nature* 261:56, 1976.

223. Cho, H. J., and Ingram, D. G. Isolation, purification and structure of Aleutian disease virus by immunological techniques. *Nature (New Biol.)* 243:174, 1973.

224. Cho, H. J. Purification and structure of Aleutian disease virus. *Front. Biol.* 44:159, 1976.

225. Sun, S. C., Burch, G. E., Sohal, R. S., et al. Coxsackie B_4 viral nephritis in mice and its autoimmune-like phenomena. *Proc. Soc. Exp. Biol. Med.* 126:882, 1967.

226. Banks, K. L., Henson, J. B., and McGuire, T. C. Immunologically mediated glomerulitis of horses. I. Pathogenesis in persistent infection by equine infectious anaemia virus. *Lab. Invest.* 26:701, 1972.

227. Mellors, R. C., Shirai, T., Aoki, T., et al. Wild-type Gross leukemia virus and the pathogenesis of the glomerulonephritis of New Zealand mice. *J. Exp. Med.* 133:113, 1971.

228. Wright, N. G., Morrison, W. I., Thompson, H., et al. Experimental adenovirus immune complex glomerulonephritis. *Br. J. Exp. Pathol.* 54:628, 1973.

229. Osborne, C. A., and Vernier, R. L. Glomerulonephritis in the dog and cat: a comparative review. *J. Am. Animal Hosp. Assoc.* 9:101, 1973.

230. Kurtz, J. M., Russell, S. W., Lee, J. C., et al. Naturally occurring canine glomerulonephritis. *Am. J. Pathol.* 67:471, 1972.

231. Lerner, R. A., and Dixon, F. J. Spontaneous glomerulonephritis in sheep. *Lab. Invest.* 15:1279, 1966.

232. Lerner, R. A., Dixon, F. J., and Lee, S. Spontaneous glomerulonephritis in sheep. II. Studies on natural history, occurrence in other species, and pathogenesis. *Am. J. Pathol.* 53:501, 1968.

233. Cheville, N. F., Mengeling, W. L., and Zinober, M. R. Ultrastructural and immunofluorescent studies of glomerulonephritis in chronic hog cholera. *Lab. Invest.* 22:458, 1970.

234. Poskitt, T. R., Fortwengler, H. P., Jr., Bobrow, J. C., et al. Naturally occurring immune-complex glomerulonephritis in monkeys (*Macaca* irus). I. Light, immunofluorescence and electron microscopic studies. *J. Pathol.* 76:145, 1974.

235. Germuth, F. G., Jr., and McKinnon, G. E. Studies on the biological properties of antigen-antibody complexes. I. Anaphylactic shock induced by soluble antigen-antibody complexes in unsensitized normal guinea pigs. *Bull. Johns Hopkins Hosp.* 101:13, 1957.

236. Benacerraf, B., Potter, J. L., McCluskey, R. T., et al. The pathologic effects of intravenously administered soluble antigen-antibody complexes. II. Acute glomerulonephritis in rats. *J. Exp. Med.* 111:195, 1960.

237. Miller, F., Benacerraf, B., McCluskey, R. T., et al. Production of acute glomerulonephritis in mice with soluble antigen-antibody complexes prepared from homologous antibody. *Proc. Soc. Exp. Biol. Med.* 104:706, 1960.

238. Coons, A. H., and Kaplan, M. H. Localization of antigen in tissue cells. II. Improvements in a method for the detection of antigen by means of fluorescent antibody. *J. Exp. Med.* 91:1, 1950.

239. McLean, C. R., Fitzgerald, J. D. L., Younghusband, O. Z., et al. Diffuse glomerulonephritis induced in rabbits by small intravenous injections of horse serum. *Arch. Pathol.* 51:1, 1951.

240. Dixon, F. J., Feldman, J. D., and Vazquez, J. J. Experimental glomerulonephritis. The pathogenesis of a laboratory model resembling the spectrum of human glomerulonephritis. *J. Exp. Med.* 113:899, 1961.

241. Kniker, W. T., and Cochrane, C. G. The localization of circulating immune complexes in experimental serum sickness: the role of vasoactive amines and hydrodynamic forces. *J. Exp. Med.* 127:119, 1968.

242. Cochrane, C. G., and Koffler, D. Immune complex disease in experimental animals and man. *Adv. Immunol.* 16:185, 1973.

243. Rammelkamp, C. H., Jr. Microbiologic aspects of glomerulonephritis. *J. Chron. Dis.* 5:28, 1957.

244. Fischel, E. E. Immune reactions in human glomerulonephritis. *J. Chron. Dis.* 5:34, 1957.

245. Dubois, E. L., and Tuffanelli, D. L. Clinical manifestations of systemic lupus erythematosus. Computer analysis of 520 cases. *J.A.M.A.* 190:104, 1964.

246. Albini, B., Ossi, E., and Andres, G. The pathogenesis of pericardial, pleural, and peritoneal effusions in rabbits with serum sickness. *Lab. Invest.* 37:64, 1977.

247. Benveniste, J., Henson, P. M., and Cochrane, C. G. Leukocyte-dependent histamine release from rabbit platelets. The role of IgE, basophils, and a platelet-activating factor. *J. Exp. Med.* 136:1356, 1972.

248. Bitran, J., McShane, D., and Ellman, M. H. Ascites as the major manifestation of systemic lupus erythematosus. *Arthritis Rheum.* 19:782, 1976.

249. Glovsky, M. M., Louie, J. S., Pitts, W. H., Jr., et al. Reduction of pleural fluid complement activity in patients with systemic lupus erythematosus and rheumatoid arthritis. *Clin. Immunol. Immunopathol.* 6:31, 1976.

250. Hunder, G. G., Mullen, B. J., and McDuffie, F. C. Complement in pericardial fluid of lupus erythematosus: studies in two patients. *Ann. Intern. Med.* 80:453, 1974.

251. Hunder, G. G., McDuffie, F. C., and Hepper, N. G. G. Pleural fluid complement in systemic lupus erythematosus and rheumatoid arthritis. *Ann. Intern. Med.* 76:357, 1972.

252. Briggs, J. D., Kwaan, H. C., and Potter, E. V. The role of fibrinogen in renal disease. III. Fibrinolytic and anticoagulant treatment of nephrotoxic serum nephritis in mice. *J. Lab. Clin. Med.* 74:715, 1969.

253. Germuth, F. G., Jr., Senterfit, L. B., and Pollack, A. D. Immune complex disease. I. Experimental acute and chronic glomerulonephritis. *Johns Hopkins Med. J.* 120:225, 1967.

254. Germuth, F. G., Jr., Senterfit, L. B., and Dreesman, G. R. Immune complex disease. V. The nature of the circulating complexes associated with glomerular alterations in the chronic BSA-rabbit system. *Johns Hopkins Med. J.* 130:344, 1972.

255. Germuth, F. G., Jr., Taylor, J. J., Siddiqui, S. Y., et al. Immune complex disease. VI. Some determinants of the varieties of glomerular lesions in

the chronic bovine serum albumin-rabbit system. *Lab. Invest.* 37:162, 1977.

256. Latta, H., and Maunsbach, N. B. Relations of the centrolobular region of the glomerulus to the juxta-glomerular apparatus. *J. Ultrastruct. Res.* 6:562, 1962.

257. Farquhar, M. G., and Palade, G. E. Functional evidence for the existence of a third cell type in the renal glomerulus. *J. Cell. Biol.* 13:55, 1962.

258. Benacerraf, B., McCluskey, R. T., and Patras, D. Localization of colloidal substances in vascular endothelium: a mechanism of tissue damage. I. Factors causing the pathologic deposition of colloidal carbon. *Am. J. Pathol.* 35:75, 1959.

259. Menefee, M. G., Mueller, C. B., Bell, A. L., et al. Transport of globin by the renal glomerulus. *J. Exp. Med.* 120:1129, 1964.

260. Michael, A. F., Fish, A. J., and Good, R. A. Glomerular localization and transport of aggregated proteins in mice. *Lab. Invest.* 17:14, 1967.

261. Karnovsky, M. J., and Ainsworth, S. K. The structural basis of glomerular filtration. In J. Hamberger, J. Crosnier, and M. H. Maxwell, eds., *Advances in Nephrology,* vol. 2, p. 35. Year Book Medical Publishers, Chicago, 1972.

262. Mannik, M., Arend, W. P., Hall, A. P., et al. Studies on antigen-antibody complexes. I. Elimination of soluble complexes from rabbit circulation. *J. Exp. Med.* 133:713, 1971.

263. Hess, M. W., and Lüscher, E. F. Macrophage receptors for IgG aggregates. *Exp. Cell. Res.* 59:193, 1970.

264. Germuth, F. G., Jr., Valdes, A. J., Senterfit, L. B., et al. A unique influence of cortisone on the transit of specific macromolecules across vascular walls in immune complex disease. *Johns Hopkins Med. J.* 122:137, 1968.

265. Langhans, T. Über die Veranderungen der Glomeruli bei der Nephritis nebst einigen Bemerkungen über die Entstehung der Fibrincylinder. *Virchows Arch. (Pathol. Anat.)* 76:85, 1879.

266. Volhard, F., and Fahr, K. T. B. Nephritis —diffuse glomerulonephritis. In *Die Brightische Nierenkrankheit,* p. 29. Springer-Verlag, Berlin, 1914.

267. Bradfield, J. W. B., and Cattell, V. The mesangial cell in glomerulonephritis. I. Mechanisms of hypercellularity in experimental immune complex glomerulonephritis. *Lab. Invest.* 36:481, 1977.

268. Bradfield, J. W. B., Cattell, V., and Smith, J. The mesangial cell in glomerulonephritis. II. Mesangial proliferation caused by Habu snake venom in the rat. *Lab. Invest.* 36:487, 1977.

269. Izui, S., Lambert, P. H., and Miescher, P. A. *In vitro* demonstration of a particular affinity of glomerular basement membrane and collagen for DNA. A possible basis for a local formation of DNA-anti-DNA complexes in systemic lupus erythematosus. *J. Exp. Med.* 144:428, 1976.

270. Mauer, S. M., Sutherland, D. E. R., Howard, R. J., et al. The glomerular mesangium. III. Acute immune mesangial injury: a new model of glomerulonephritis. *J. Exp. Med.* 137:553, 1973.

271. Stilmant, M. M., Couser, W. G., and Cotran, R. S. Experimental glomerulonephritis in the mouse associated with mesangial deposition of autologous ferritin immune complexes. *Lab. Invest.* 32:746, 1975.

272. Germuth, F. G., Jr., and Rodriguez, E. Experimental animal diseases. In *Immunopathology of the Renal Glomerulus,* pp. 23, 24, 33. Little, Brown and Co., Boston, 1973.

273. Heymann, W., Hackel, D. B., Harwood, S., et al. Production of nephrotic syndrome in rats by Freund's adjuvants and rat kidney suspensions. *Proc. Soc. Exp. Biol. Med.* 100:660, 1959.

274. Glassock, R. J., Edgington, T. S., Watson, J. I., et al. Autologous immune complex nephritis induced with renal tubular antigen. II. The pathogenetic mechanism. *J. Exp. Med.* 127:573, 1968.

275. Grupe, W. E., and Kaplan, M. H. Demonstration of an antibody to proximal tubular antigen in the pathogenesis of experimental autoimmune nephrosis in rats. *J. Lab. Clin. Med.* 74:400, 1969.

276. Sugisaki, T., Klassen, J., Andres, G. A., et al. Passive transfer of Heymann nephritis with serum. *Kidney Int.* 3:66, 1973.

277. Schneeberger, E. E., Leber, P. D., Karnovsky, M. J., et al. Altered functional properties of the renal glomerulus in autologous immune complex nephritis: an ultrastructural tracer study. *J. Exp. Med.* 139:1283, 1974.

278. Farquhar, M. G., Wissig, S. L., and Palade, G. E. Glomerular permeability. I. Ferritin transfer across the normal glomerular capillary wall. *J. Exp. Med.* 113:47, 1961.

279. Karnovsky, M. J., and Ainsworth, S. K. The structural basis of glomerular filtration. In *Advances in Nephrology from the Necker Hospital,* vol. 2, p. 35. Year Book Medical Publishers, Chicago, 1972.

280. Schneeberger, E. E. Glomerular permeability to protein molecules—its possible structural basis. *Nephron* 13:7, 1974.

281. Jones, D. B. Mucosubstances of the glomerulus. *Lab. Invest.* 21:119, 1969.

282. Mohos, S. C., and Skoza, L. Glomerular sialoprotein. *Science* 164:1519, 1969.

283. Michael, A. F., Blau, E., and Vernier, R. L. Glomerular polyanion: alteration in amino-nucleoside nephrosis. *Lab. Invest.* 23:649, 1970.

284. Chang, R. L. S., Deen, W. M., Robertson,

C. R., et al. Permselectivity of the glomerular capillary wall. III. Restricted transport of polyanions. *Kidney Int.* 8:212, 1975.

285. Blau, E. B., and Haas, J. E. Glomerular sialic acid and proteinuria in human renal disease. *Lab. Invest.* 28:477, 1973.

286. Bennett, C. M., Glassock, R. J., Chang, R. L. S., et al. Permselectivity of the glomerular capillary wall: studies of experimental glomerulonephritis in the rat using dextran sulfate. *J. Clin. Invest.* 57:1287, 1976.

287. Bohrer, M., Baylis, C., Robertson, C. R., et al. Mechanisms of the puromycin-induced defects in the transglomerular passage of water and macromolecules. *J. Clin. Invest.* 60:152, 1977.

288. Couser, W. G., Jermanovich, N. B., Belok, S., et al. Effect of amino-nucleoside nephrosis on immune complex localization in autologous immune complex nephropathy in rats. *J. Clin. Invest.* 61:561, 1978.

289. Gelfand, M. C., Shin, M. L., Nagle, R. B., et al. The glomerular complement receptor in immunologically mediated renal glomerular injury. *N. Engl. J. Med.* 295:10, 1976.

290. Burkholder, P. M., Oberley, T. D., Barber, T. A., et al. Immune adherence in renal glomeruli. Complement receptor sites on glomerular capillary epithelial cells. *Am. J. Pathol.* 86:635, 1977.

291. Rennke, H. G., Cotran, R. S., and Venkatachalam, M. A. Role of molecular charge in glomerular permeability: tracer studies with cationized ferritins. *J. Cell. Biol.* 67:638, 1975.

292. Seiler, M. W., Venkatachalam, M. A., and Cotran, R. S. Glomerular epithelium: structural alterations induced by polycations. *Science* 189:390, 1975.

293. Seiler, M. W., Rennke, H. G., Venkatachalam, M. A., et al. Pathogenesis of polycation-induced alterations ("fusion") of glomerular epithelium. *Lab. Invest.* 36:48, 1977.

294. Koffler, D., Schur, P. H., and Kunkel, H. G. Immunological studies concerning the nephritis of systemic lupus erythematosus. *J. Exp. Med.* 126:607, 1967.

295. Combes, B., Stastny, P., Shorey, J., et al. Glomerulonephritis with deposition of Australia antigen-antibody complexes in glomerular basement membrane. *Lancet* 2:234, 1971.

296. Couser, W. G., Wagonfeld, J. B., Spargo, B. H., et al. Glomerular deposition of tumor antigen in membranous nephropathy associated with colonic carcinoma. *Am. J. Med.* 57:962, 1974.

297. Naruse, T., Kitamura, K., Miyakawa, Y., et al. Deposition of renal tubular epithelial antigen along the glomerular capillary walls of patients with membranous glomerulonephritis. *J. Immunol.* 110:1163, 1973.

298. Schneeberger, E. E., and Grupe, W. E. The ultrastructure of the glomerular slit diaphragm in autologous immune complex nephritis. *Lab. Invest.* 34:298, 1976.

299. Masugi, M. Über die experimentelle Glomerulonephritis durch das spezifische Antinierenserum. Ein Beitrag zur Pathogenese der diffusen Glomerulonephritis. *Beitr. Pathol.* 92:429, 1934.

300. McCluskey, R. T. Immunologic mechanisms in renal disease. In R. H. Heptinstall, ed., *Pathology of the Kidney,* vol. 1, p. 273. Little, Brown and Co., Boston 1974.

301. Unanue, E. R., and Dixon, F. J. Experimental glomerulonephritis: immunological events and pathogenetic mechanisms. *Adv. Immunol.* 6:1, 1967.

302. Shigematsu, H., and Kobayashi, Y. The development and fate of the immune deposits in the glomerulus during the secondary phase of rat Masugi nephritis. *Virchows Arch. (Zellpathol.)* 8:83, 1971.

303. Sarre, H., and Wirtz, H. Geschwindigkeit und Ort der Antigen-Antikörper-Reaktion bei der experimentellen Nephritis. *Dtsch. Arch. Klin. Med.* 189:1, 1942.

304. Pressman, D. Current status of the tissue localization of I^{131}-labeled antitissue antibodies. *Ann. N. Y. Acad. Sci.* 70:72, 1957.

305. Lange, K., and Wenk, E. J. Investigations into the site of complement loss in experimental glomerulonephritis. *Am. J. Med. Sci.* 228:454, 1954.

306. Unanue, E. R., and Dixon, F. J. Experimental glomerulonephritis. IV. Participation of complement in nephrotoxic nephritis. *J. Exp. Med.* 119:965, 1964.

307. Steblay, R. W., and Lepper, M. H. Some immunologic properties of human and dog glomerular basement membranes. I. Isolation of human glomerular basement membrane; similar or identical complement-fixing antigens in human and dog glomerular basement membrane preparations. *J. Immunol.* 87:627, 1961.

308. Vogt, A. Symposium der Gesellschaft für Nephrologie. In F. Reubi and H. G. Pauli, eds., *Das Nephrotische Syndrom. II,* p. 198. Thieme, Stuttgart, 1963.

309. Klein, P., and Burkholder, P. Ein Verfahren zur fluoreszenzoptischen Darstellung der Komplementbindung und seine Anwendung zur histoimmunologischen Untersuchung der experimentellen Nierenanaphylaxie. *Dtsch. Med. Wochenschr.* 84:2001, 1959.

310. Hammer, D. K., and Dixon, F. J. Experimental glomerulonephritis. II. Immunologic events

in the pathogenesis of nephrotoxic serum nephritis in the rat. *J. Exp. Med.* 117:1019, 1963.

311. Cochrane, C. G., Unanue, E. R., and Dixon, F. J. A role of polymorphonuclear leukocytes and complement in nephrotoxic nephritis. *J. Exp. Med.* 122:99, 1965.

312. Gang, N. F., and Kalant, N. Nephrotoxic serum nephritis. I. Chemical, morphologic, and functional changes in the glomerular basement membrane during the evolution of nephritis. *Lab. Invest.* 22:531, 1970.

313. Gang, N. F., Mautner, W., and Kalant, N. Nephrotoxic serum nephritis. II. Chemical, morphologic, and functional correlates of glomerular basement membrane at the onset of proteinuria. *Lab. Invest.* 23:150, 1970.

314. Gang, N. F., Trachtenberg, E., Allerhand, J., et al. Nephrotoxic serum nephritis. III. Correlation of proteinuria, excretion of the glomerular basement membrane-like protein, and changes in the ultrastructure of the glomerular basement membrane as visualized with lanthanum. *Lab. Invest.* 23:436, 1970.

315. Doe, W. F., Booth, C. C., and Brown, D. L. Evidence for complement-binding immune complexes in adult coeliac disease, Crohn's disease, and ulcerative colitis. *Lancet* 1:402, 1973.

316. Jewell, D. P., and MacLennan, I. C. M. Circulating immune complexes in inflammatory bowel disease. *Clin. Exp. Immunol.* 14:219, 1973.

317. Nielsen, H., Binder, V., Daugharty, H., et al. Circulating immune complexes in ulcerative colitis. I. Correlation to disease activity. *Clin. Exp. Immunol.* 31:72, 1978.

318. Hodgson, H. J. F., Potter, B. J., and Jewell, D. P. Immune complexes in ulcerative colitis and Crohn's disease. *Clin. Exp. Immunol.* 29:187, 1977.

319. Hodgson, H. J. F., Potter, B. J., Skinner, J., et al. Immune-complex mediated colitis in rabbits. An experimental model. *Gut* 19:225, 1978.

320. Goldgraber, M. B., and Kirsner, J. B. The Arthus phenomenon in the colon of rabbits. A serial histological study. *Arch. Pathol.* 67:556, 1959.

321. Kraft, S. C., Fitch, F. W., and Kirsner, J. B. Histologic and immuno-histochemical features of the Auer "colitis" in rabbits. *Am. J. Pathol.* 43:913, 1963.

322. Perlmann, P., and Broberger, O. *In vitro* studies of ulcerative colitis. II. Cytotoxic action of white blood cells from patients on human fetal colon cells. *J. Exp. Med.* 117:717, 1963.

323. Bull, D. M., and Iznaczak, T. F. Eterobacterial common antigen-induced lymphocyte reactivity in inflammatory bowel disease. *Gastroenterology* 64:43, 1973.

324. Cave, D. R., Mitchell, D. N., and Brooke, B. N. Evidence of an agent transmissible from ulcerative colitis tissue. *Lancet* 1:1311, 1976.

325. Wands, J. R., Alpert, E., and Isselbacher, K. J. Arthritis associated with chronic active hepatitis: complement activation and characterization of circulating immune complexes. *Gastroenterology* 69:1286, 1975.

326. Wands, J. R., Mann, E., Alpert, E., et al. The pathogenesis of arthritis associated with acute hepatitis-B surface antigen-positive hepatitis: complement activation and characterization of circulating immune complexes. *J. Clin. Invest.* 55:930, 1975.

327. Thomas, H. C., DeVilliers, D., Potter, B., et al. Immune complexes in acute and chronic liver disease. *Clin. Exp. Immunol.* 31:150, 1978.

328. van Marck, E. A. E., Deelder, A. M., and Gigase, P. L. J. Effect of partial portal vein ligation on immune glomerular deposits in *Schistosoma mansoni* infected mice. *Br. J. Exp. Pathol.* 58:412, 1977.

329. Bjørneboe, M., and Prytz, H. The mononuclear phagocytic functions of the liver. In A. Ferguson and R. N. M. MacSween, eds., *Immunological Aspects of the Liver and Gastrointestinal Tract,* p. 251. MTP Press, Lancaster, Engl., 1976.

330. Border, W. A., Wilson, C. B., and Dixon, F. J. Failure of heparin to affect two types of experimental glomerulonephritis in rabbits. *Kidney Int.* 8:140, 1975.

331. Humphrey, J. H., and Jaques, R. J. The release of histamine and 5-hydroxytryptamine (serotonin) from platelets by antigen-antibody reactions (*in vitro*). *J. Physiol. (Lond.)* 128:9, 1955.

332. Kniker, W. T., and Cochrane, C. G. The localization of circulating immune complexes in experimental serum sickness: the role of vaso-active amines and hydrodynamic forces. *J. Exp. Med.* 127:119, 1968.

333. Clark, W. F., Lewis, M. L., Cameron, J. S., et al. Intrarenal platelet consumption in the diffuse proliferative nephritis of systemic lupus erythematosus. *Clin. Sci. Mol. Med.* 49:247, 1975.

334. Clark, W. F., Friesen, M., Linton, A. L., et al. The platelet as a mediator of tissue damage in immune complex glomerulonephritis. *Clin. Nephrol.* 6:287, 1976.

335. George, C. R. P., Slichter, S. J., Quadracci, L. J., et al. A kinetic evaluation of hemostasis in renal disease. *N. Engl. J. Med.* 291:1111, 1974.

336. Bolton, W. K., Spargo, B. A., and Lewis, E. J. Chronic autologous immune complex glomerulopathy: effect of cyproheptadine. *J. Lab. Clin. Med.* 83:695, 1974.

337. Heymann, W., Hunter, J. L. P., and

Hackel, D. B. Experimental autoimmune nephrosis in rats: III. *J. Immunol.* 88:135, 1962.

338. Lim, V. S., and Spargo, B. Immunosuppressive treatment of autologous immune complex nephritis in rats. *J. Lab. Clin. Med.* 81:661, 1973.

339. Krakauer, R. S., Strober, W., Rippeon, D. L., et al. Prevention of autoimmunity in experimental lupus erythematosus by soluble immune response suppressor. *Science* 196:56, 1977.

340. Borel, Y., Lewis, R. M., and Stollar, B. D. Prevention of murine lupus nephritis by carrier-dependent induction of immunologic tolerance to denatured DNA. *Science* 182:76, 1973.

341. Stollar, B. D., and Borel, Y. Carrier-induced tolerance to nucleic acid antigens. *J. Immunol.* 115:1095, 1975.

CHAPTER 14

Epilogue

It is clear from the abundant clinical and experimental evidence presented in this book that immune complexes play an important part in the normal mediation of most immune responses. Indeed, their generation may represent one of the fundamental modulating influences in homeostasis or feedback inhibition within the immune system. In view of the now very convincing array of data produced by Binz and Wigzell (1–4), it is apparent that immune responses specific for idiotypes or unique combining regions of both antibodies and specifically immune cells are capable of discrete, individualized control within virtually all immune reactions. This view was also predicted earlier by the "network theory" proposed by Jerne (5). Aside from the importance of immune complexes in control and modulation of immune responses generally, the clinician is faced with a number of problems in which the generation of an immune response has produced manifestations of disease. In some instances these overt clinical phenomena produce only minor irritations or disruption of normal function; in others the result may be life threatening or disastrous.

It is obvious from much of the material already covered here that considerably more precise knowledge of the whole process of immune-complex formation, disposal, and amplification during tissue deposition is necessary before completely rational or effective therapy can become available. We have already learned a tremendous amount about the immunochemical and physical aspects of immune complexes and their capacity to create microvascular injury or inflammation, largely through experimental models such as serum sickness or careful analysis of the reactants and events involved in such diseases as lupus nephritis. Yet there remain a vast number of gray areas and poorly understood phenomena. One of the most important is identification of the primary mechanisms called upon to handle complexes and dispose of them where necessary. Certainly the reticuloendothelial system and the circulating macrophage-monocyte pool are directly involved; however, there are a growing number of identifications of other intrinsic tissue receptors, which may also be important for adherence to or disposal of circulating immune complexes. Table 14-1 lists some of these potential receptors, many of which have been only partially characterized. Whether such putative immune-complex receptors have survived the evolutionary process through protection of the host remains to be seen, but their diversity in anatomical distribution and sites within the body present some fascinating theoretical questions. Thus the Fc receptors present in the placenta (16, 17) may have a completely different function from those now demonstrable within the choroid plexus (15). Likewise, the C3b receptors on the epithelial surface of the renal glomerulus (16) may subserve a number of functions that are different from those involved in impeding certain types of complexes piling up in these areas during renal immune-complex deposition. The diversity of cell types demonstrated to bear Fc receptors is also impressive, ranging from the polymorph, monocyte, and macrophage to the

Table 14-1 Potential receptors for immune complexes and their distribution in blood and human tissues.

Receptor (and reference)	Function
C3:	
Glomerulus (epithelial surface) (6)	Density inversely correlated with immune-complex deposits.
Macrophage or monocyte (7)	May be involved in phagocytosis or cell-to-cell interaction.
Lymphocyte (8)	Used in some studies as a marker for B cells.
Langerhans' cells (9)	Significance not yet clear.
Fc:	
Polymorphonuclear cells (10)	Active in phagocytosis.
Lymphocytes (11)	IgG Fc receptor cells felt to be a B-cell subpopulation and/or associated with so-called L cells (12, 13). Four different T-cell subsets show IgG (Tγ), IgM (Tμ), IgA (Tα), and IgE (Tϵ) Fc receptors.
Macrophages/monocytes (17, 11)	Clearly involved in phagocytosis and reticuloendothelial function.
Platelets (14)	Physiological function not yet clear.
Choroid plexus (15)	May be important in preservation of blood-brain barrier.
Placenta (16, 17)	Protects fetus against endogenous immune-complex injury. (?)
Certain human tumor cells (18)	May produce survival value for tumor.
Langerhans' cells (9, 19)	Important in initiating immune reactions in skin. (?)
Mast cells (20)	Bind IgE antibodies; initiate allergic responses.
Renal interstitium (25)	May determine sites of tubulointerstitial immune deposits.

lymphocyte and even the platelet. The very fact that such a wide variety of circulating cells show receptors for portions of immunoglobulin molecules exposed during formation of immune complexes suggests that complexes play a potential role in the functioning of all these cell types.

In the case of derangements of body function, the problem becomes even more intriguing. It can be shown that certain tumor cells are heavily endowed with Fc receptors (18) and that viral infection itself may cause cells to express Fc receptors, which appear to be undetectable in uninfected cells (21, 22). A number of studies have been launched with the aim of understanding the physical and chemical makeup of these important receptor structures. Chemical characterization begins to indicate that Fc structures are probably represented by complex glycoproteins of 40,000 to 60,000 Daltons (23, 24). Furthermore, a microheterogeneity in their combining specificities has begun to emerge (24). It seems likely that Fc receptors and their specificities on the placenta may be quite different from those present on B or T lymphocytes. There is also the possibility that individual phenotypic expression of Fc receptors in many of the anatomic sites alluded to above may be genetically controlled. At present there is no direct evidence to support such a hypothesis. However, among all patients who develop streptococcal pharyngitis with nephritogenic group A organisms, there may be a few whose vulnerable target cells on the epithelial surfaces of renal glomeruli have 100 or perhaps 1,000 times as many potential C3b receptors as other individuals similarly infected, but who do not subsequently get clinically apparent acute glomerulonephritis. The same might be said for gonococcal sepsis, nephrosis with schistosomiasis, hypersensitivity pneumonitis, and a number of other disorders. Methods are needed to predict phenotypes, if such actually exist, which may be inordinately susceptible to the damaging peripheral effects of circulating complexes during times of maximal potential risk or clinical exposure.

It seems apparent from the extended discussions of preceding chapters that certain organs or anatomic foci are involved over and over with presumed immune-complex injury. This distribution of lesions or clinical involvement suggests that local factors such as intrinsic receptors for complexes, or other basic influences such as the character of the antigens involved, may predispose anatomic sites in the glomerulus, renal tubular basement membranes, dermal-epidermal junction, choroid plexus, synovium, serous surfaces, pulmonary peribronchiolar areas, or interstitial spaces between thyroid follicles to tissue deposition and injury. One might draw up lists of possible sites of primary localization of immune complexes merely on the basis of accumulated clinical observations of where lesions or disturbances frequently occur, even though receptors have been defined in only a few of these sites. Such a format is shown in Table 14-2. Despite the fact that there is not yet substantial supporting evidence for some of these examples, studies of possible induction or exposure of receptors might well prove illuminating.

One of the most poorly defined areas relative to the role of immune complexes in clinical medicine is precise identification of the antigens involved. A number of examples of hepatitis B viral antigens within circulating complexes associated with the renal, cutaneous, or vasculitis lesions in this disorder have been demonstrated (26, 27); surprisingly, the same is not true for acute leukemia or for a vast number of other conditions where claims for presence of circulating complexes have been

Table 14-2   Known or possible sites for some sort of immune-complex receptor, based on frequency of involvement during various clinical conditions associated with high levels of detectable circulating complexes.

Site of localization	Clinical examples	Supporting evidence (and reference)
Glomerulus	SLE, schistosomiasis with nephrosis, acute glomerulonephritis, malarial nephropathy	C3b receptor definitely present (6)
Renal tubular basement membranes or interstitium	Interstitial immune deposits with SLE, Sjögren's syndrome	Fc receptor definitely present (25)
Dermal-epidermal junction	SLE, granuloma annulare, herpes gestationis, dermatitis herpetiformis	None
Choroid plexus	Immune deposits in experimental sickness and SLE	Fc receptor definitely present (15)
Synovium	Acute rheumatic fever, serum sickness, SLE, disseminated gonococcal infection, sarcoidosis	None
Serous surfaces: pleura, peritoneum, pericardium	Diffuse serositis in SLE, connective-tissue diseases, serum sickness	None

published. Unless a systematic search for and identification of such putative antigens is made, one cannot be entirely sure that the complexes being detected in various disease states by the highly sensitive radioimmunoassay techniques contain any extrinsic *antigens* at all; they may in fact be composed of antibody called forth by the primary disease state and self-reacting anti-idiotypic antibody directed at combining sites of the original disease-associated antibody.

Such a situation is depicted in Figure 14-1, which shows antibody reacting with anti-idiotype contrasted to the more conventional anti-antibody associated with IgG rheumatoid factors. It is probable from a brief inspection of the model in this figure that complexes containing primary antibody to primary antigen and anti-idiotypic antibody to primary antibody would show much of the sedimentation behavior (11 to 19S) associated with complexes that have been detected with neoplastic states, acute rheumatic fever, disseminated gonococcal sepsis, hepatitis B infection, or many of the parasitic diseases. Also idiotype–anti-idiotype complexes would perforce show two free Fc portions, capable presumably of activation of complement pathways and C1q binding as well as C3 activation, and consequently reactive with Raji cells or solid-phase conglutinin in respective assays. It is not clear what proportion of immune complexes currently being measured in many laboratories may be related to immune complexes of idiotypes, and therefore not related to primary disease antigens at all. It is important for the appropriate laboratories to look very hard at this possibility and to verify what extrinsic antigens are present in a variety of disease states. Mere demonstration of antigen in immune deposits does not address itself to the question.

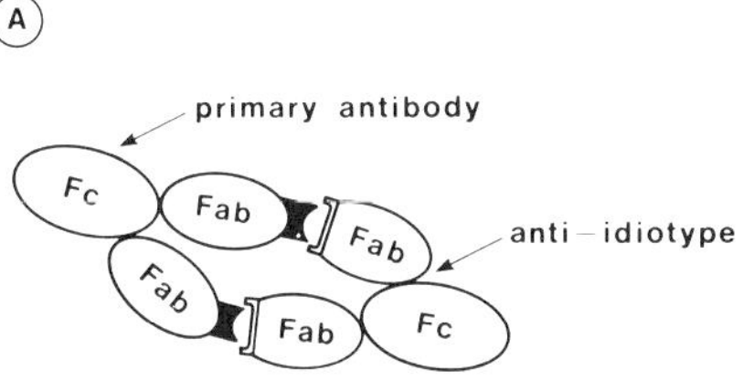

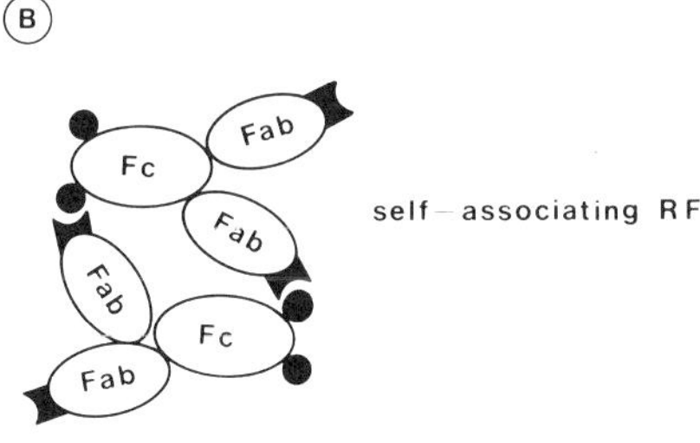

Figure 14-1 *A*, diagrammatic representation of how primary antibody called forth by a particular disease process (anti-DNA, antiparasitic antigen, antitumor, and the like) reacts with anti-idiotype. The anti-idiotype specificity is directed at the antibody combining site of the first or primary antibody. Such complexes, because of their asymmetric shape, may sediment as 11 to 18S instead of as the more compact structures shown in *B*, which depicts self-associating 7S IgG rheumatoid factors (RF).

The survey presented in this volume is intended to provide an up-to-date assessment of the state of the art. Further refinements in technique or careful clinical and immunologic study will clarify our thinking in many areas. The overall subject is an intriguing one, for it represents one of the most relevant applications of immunology to clinical medicine. It is our hope that this rather cursory look will serve to stimulate some further measure of interest on the part of the average clinician as well as the basic or clinical investigator.

References

1. Binz, H., and Wigzell, H. Shared idiotypic determinants on B and T lymphocytes reactive against the same antigenic determinants. II. Determination of frequency and characteristics of idiotypic T and B lymphocytes in normal rats using direct visualization. *J. Exp. Med.* 142:1218, 1975.

2. Binz, H., and Wigzell, H. Specific transplantation tolerance induced by autoimmunization against the individual's own, naturally occurring idiotypic, antigen-binding receptors. *J. Exp. Med.* 144:1438, 1976.

3. Binz, H., and Wigzell, H. Shared idiotypic determinants on B and T lymphocytes reactive against the same antigenic determinants. I. Demon-

stration of similar or identical idiotypes on IgG molecules and T-cell receptors with specificity for the same alloantigens. *J. Exp. Med.* 142:197, 1975.

4. Binz, H., and Wigzell, H. Antigen-binding, idiotypic T-lymphocyte receptors. *Contemp. Top. Immunobiol.* 7:113, 1977.

5. Jerne, N. K. Towards a network theory of the immune system. *Ann. Immunol. (Paris)* 125c:373, 1974.

6. Gelfand, M. C., Frank, M. M., and Green, I. A receptor for the third component of complement in the human renal glomerulus. *J. Exp. Med.* 142:1029, 1975.

7. Huber, H., Polley, M. J., Linscott, W. D., et al. Human monocytes: distinct receptor sites for the third component of complement and for immunoglobulin G. *Science* 162:1281, 1968.

8. Ross, G. D., and Polley, M. J. Assay for the two different types of lymphocyte complement receptors. In J. B. Natvig, P. Perlmann, and H. Wigzell, eds., "Lymphocytes, Isolation, Fractionation, and Characterization." *Scand. J. Immunol.* 5:99, 1976 (suppl.).

9. Stingl, G., Wolff-Schreiner, E. C., Pichler, W. J., et al. Epidermal Langerhans cells bear Fc and C3 receptors. *Nature* 268:245, 1977.

10. MacLennan, I. C. M., Connell, G. E., and Gotch, F. M. Effector activating determinants on IgG. II. Differentiation of the combining sites for C1q from those for cytotoxic K cells and neutrophils by plasmin digestion of rabbit IgG. *Immunology* 26:303, 1974.

11. Dickler, H. B. Lymphocyte receptors for immunoglobulin. *Adv. Immunol.* 24:167, 1976.

12. Horwitz, D. A., and Lobo, P. I. Characterization of two populations of human lymphocytes bearing easily detectable surface immunoglobulin. *J. Clin. Invest.* 56:1464, 1975.

13. Lobo, P. I., and Horwitz, D. A. An appraisal of Fc receptors on human peripheral blood B and L lymphocytes. *J. Immunol.* 117:939, 1976.

14. Palosuo, T., and Leikola, J. Platelet aggregation by isolated and aggregated human IgG. *Clin. Exp. Immunol.* 20:371, 1975.

15. Braathen, L. R., Førre, O., Husby, G., et al. Evidence for Fc IgG receptors and complement fac-

tor C3b receptors in human choroid plexus. *Clin. Immunol. Immunopathol.* 14:284, 1979.

16. Jenkinson, E. J., Billington, W. D., and Elson, J. Detection of receptors for immunoglobulin on human placenta by EA rosette formation. *Clin. Exp. Immunol.* 23:456, 1976.

17. Elson, J., Jenkinson, E. J., and Billington, W. D. Fc receptors on mouse placenta and yolk sac cells. *Nature* 255:412, 1975.

18. Tönder, O., Morse, P. A., Jr., and Humphrey, L. J. Similarities of Fc receptors in human malignant tissue and normal lymphoid tissue. *J. Immunol.* 113:1162, 1974.

19. Shelley, W. B., and Juhlin, L. Langerhans cells form a reticuloepithelial trap for external contact antigens. *Nature* 261:46, 1976.

20. Ishizaka, K., and Ishizaka, T. IgE and reaginic hypersensitivity. *Ann. N.Y. Acad. Sci.* 190:443, 1971.

21. Costa, J. C., and Rabson, A. S. Role of Fc receptors in herpes simplex virus infection. *Lancet* 1:77, 1975.

22. Costa, J., Rabson, A. S., Yee, C., et al. Immunoglobulin binding to herpes virus-induced Fc receptors inhibits virus growth. *Nature* 269:251, 1977.

23. Rask, L., Klareskog, L., Östberg, L., et al. Isolation and properties of a murine spleen cell Fc receptor. *Nature* 257:231, 1975.

24. Cooper, S. M., Sambray, Y., and Friou, G. J. Isolation of separate Fc receptors for IgG complexes to antigen and native IgG from a murine leukaemia. *Nature* 270:253, 1977.

25. Gelfand, M. C., Frank, M. M., Green, I., et al. Binding sites for immune complexes containing IgG in the renal interstitium. *Clin. Immunol. Immunopathol.* 13:19, 1979.

26. Theofilopoulos, A. N., Wilson, C. B., and Dixon, F. J. The Raji cell radioimmune assay for detecting immune complexes in human sera. *J. Clin. Invest.* 57:169, 1976.

27. Wands, J. R., Mann, E., Alpert, E., et al. The pathogenesis of arthritis associated with acute hepatitis-B surface antigen-positive hepatitis: complement activation and characterization of circulating immune complexes. *J. Clin. Invest.* 55:930, 1975.

Index